Pathology
of the Liver

Commissioning Editor: Geoffrey Nuttall
Project Editor: Lowri Daniels
Copy Editor: Ruth Swan
Design Direction: Sarah Cape
Production: Mark Sanderson
Sales Promotion Executive: Douglas McNaughton

THIRD EDITION

Pathology of the Liver

Edited by

Roderick N. M. MacSween
BSc MD FRCP(Edin) FRCP(Glasg) FRCPath FIBiol FRSE
Professor of Pathology, University of Glasgow; Honorary Consultant Pathologist,
University Department of Pathology, Western Infirmary, Glasgow, UK

Peter P. Anthony MB BS FRCPath
Professor of Clinical Histopathology, University of Exeter;
Consultant Pathologist, Royal Devon and Exeter Healthcare NHS Trust, Exeter, UK

Peter J. Scheuer MD BSc(Med) FRCPath
Emeritus Professor of Histopathology, Royal Free Hospital School of Medicine,
University of London, London, UK

Alastair D. Burt BSc MD MRCPath MIBiol
Senior Lecturer in Pathology, School of Pathological Sciences, University of
Newcastle upon Tyne; Honorary Consultant Histopathologist, Royal Victoria
Infirmary Trust and Freeman Hospital Trust, Newcastle upon Tyne, UK

Bernard C. Portmann MD FRCPath
Consultant Histopathologist and Honorary Senior Lecturer,Institute of Liver
Studies, King's College School of Medicine and Dentistry, London, UK

Foreword to the Third Edition by **Kunio Okuda** MD PhD
Professor Emeritus, The First Department of Medicine, Chiba University, Japan

Foreword to the First Edition by **The late Hans Popper** MD PhD
Formerly Gustave L. Levy Distinguished Service Professor, Mount Sinai School of
Medicine of the City University of New York, New York, USA

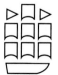

CHURCHILL LIVINGSTONE
EDINBURGH LONDON MADRID MELBOURNE NEW YORK AND TOKYO 1994

CHURCHILL LIVINGSTONE
Medical Division of Longman Group Limited

Distributed in the United States of America by Churchill Livingstone
Inc., 650 Avenue of the Americas, New York, N.Y. 10011, and by associated companies, branches and representatives throughout the world.

First edition 1979
Second edition 1987
Third edition 1994

ISBN 0-443-04454-6

British Library Cataloguing in Publication Data
A catalogue record for this book is available from the British Library.

Library of Congress Cataloging in Publication Data
A catalog record for this book is available from the Library of Congress.

Printed in Hong Kong
SP/01

The
publisher's
policy is to use
paper manufactured
from sustainable forests

Contents

Contributors

Peter P. Anthony MB BS FRCPath
Professor of Clinical Histopathology, University of
Exeter; Consultant Pathologist, Royal Devon and Exeter
Healthcare NHS Trust, Exeter, UK

P. Bannasch Dr med
Professor of Pathology, Division of Cell Pathology,
German Cancer Research Centre, Heidelberg, Germany

K. P. Batts MD
Consultant, Department of Pathology and Laboratory
Medicine, Mayo Clinic; Assistant Professor of Pathology,
Mayo Medical School, Rochester, Minnesota, USA

Leonardo Bianchi MD
Professor of Pathology, Department of Pathology,
University of Basel, Basel, Switzerland

A. D. Burt BSc MD MRCPath MIBiol
Senior Lecturer in Pathology, School of Pathological
Sciences, University of Newcastle upon Tyne; Honorary
Consultant Histopathologist, Royal Victoria Infirmary
Trust and Freeman Hospital Trust, Newcastle upon
Tyne, UK

V. J. Desmet MD PhD
Professor of Histology and Pathology, Catholic University
Leuven; Head, Department of Pathology II, University
Hospital St Raphael, Leuven, Belgium

Fred Gudat MD
Professor, Institute for Pathology, University of Basel,
Basel, Switzerland

Pauline de la M. Hall MB BS FRCPA
Senior Consultant in Pathology, Department of
Histopathology, Flinders Medical Centre; Associate
Professor of Pathology, Flinders University of South
Australia, Adelaide, South Australia, Australia

June W. Halliday AM BSc(Hons) PhD
Chairperson, Liver Unit, Queensland Institute of Medical
Research, Brisbane, Queensland, Australia

Kamal G. Ishak MD PhD
Chairman, Department of Hepatic and Gastrointestinal
Pathology, Armed Forces Institute of Pathology,
Washington DC; Clinical Professor of Pathology,
Uniformed Services University for the Health Sciences,
Bethesda, Maryland; Professorial Lecturer, Mount Sinai
School of Medicine, New York, USA

O. F. W. James FRCP
Head of Liver Group and Professor of Medicine
(Geriatrics), School of Clinical Medical Sciences,
University of Newcastle upon Tyne, Newcastle upon
Tyne, UK

John F. R. Kerr PhD FRCP FRCPath FRCPA
Professor of Pathology, University of Queensland,
Brisbane, Queensland, Australia

Sebastian Lucas FRCP FRCPath
Senior Lecturer, Department of Histopathology,
University College London Medical School, London, UK

Jurgen Ludwig MD
Professor of Pathology, Division of Anatomic Pathology,
Mayo Clinic and Mayo Foundation, Rochester,
Minnesota, USA

Roderick N. M. MacSween BSc MD FRCP(Edin)
FRCP(Glasg) FRCPath FIBiol FRSE
Professor of Pathology, University of Glasgow; Honorary
Consultant Pathologist, University Department of
Pathology, Western Infirmary, Glasgow, UK

G. H. Millward-Sadler BSc MB ChB FRCPath MHSM
Consultant Pathologist, General Hospital, Southampton;
Senior Lecturer, Southampton University Hospitals;
Medical Director, Southampton University Hospitals
Trust, Southampton, UK

Lawrie W. Powell AC MD PhD FRCP(Lond) FRACP
Director, Queensland Institute of Medical Research, The
Bancroft Centre, Brisbane, Queensland, Australia

Bernard C. Portmann MD FRCPath
Consultant Histopathologist and Honorary Senior
Lecturer, Institute of Liver Studies, King's College
School of Medicine and Dentistry, London, UK

Fenton Schaffner MS(Pathol) MD
George Baehr Professor of Medicine Emeritus, Mount
Sinai School of Medicine of the City University of New
York, New York, USA

R. J. Scothorne BSc MD FRCS(Glasg) FRSE
Emeritus Professor of Anatomy, University of Glasgow,
Glasgow, UK

Jeffrey Searle BSc MB BS MD FRCPA
Clinical Professor of Pathology, University of
Queensland; Director, Division of Anatomical Pathology,
Royal Brisbane Hospital, Queensland, Australia

Harvey L. Sharp MD
Chief, Paediatric Gastroenterology and Nutrition;
Professor of Paediatrics, University of Minnesota School
of Medicine, Minneapolis, Minnesota, USA

P. J. Scheuer MD BSc(Med) FRCPath
Emeritus Professor of Histopathology, Department of
Histopathology, Royal Free Hospital School of Medicine,
University of London, London, UK

Swan N. Thung MD
Professor of Pathology, Mount Sinai Medical Center,
New York, USA

Ian R. Wanless MD CM FRCP(C)
Associate Professor of Pathology, University of Toronto,
Toronto; Director, Canadian Liver Pathology Reference
Centre, Toronto, Ontario, Canada

David Weedon MD FRCPA
Clinical Professor of Pathology, University of
Queensland, Brisbane; Senior Visiting Pathologist, Royal
Brisbane Hospital, Brisbane, Queensland, Australia

Hyman J. Zimmerman MD
Professor of Medicine Emeritus, George Washington
University; Distinguished Scientist Emeritus, Armed
Forces Institute of Pathology, Washington DC, USA

Foreword to the Third Edition

In the 15 years that have elapsed since the late Hans Popper wrote the foreword for the first edition of this book in 1979, there has been remarkable progress in the biological sciences pertaining to hepatology, particularly molecular biology. The five major, if not all, the viruses that cause human liver disease have now been identified and characterized, which is one of the foremost achievements of the 20th century. The prevention of some of the viral hepatitides has now become a reality, and it is reasonable to predict that the incidence of viral hepatitis, the most common cause of liver disease in many countries, will decline rapidly and that this will be followed by a corresponding decrease in the incidence of primary liver cancer. Increasing numbers of hepatologists have switched their interests from conventional hepatology to the study of hepatitis viruses, and now pay less attention to the specific morphological and functional features. However, hepatology remains hepatology! There are still numerous liver diseases that are unrelated to viruses, such as alcoholic and metabolic liver diseases. Also, there is strong evidence that hepatitis viruses are not the only aetiological factors for primary liver cancer. The immunology and physiology of the liver have assumed a particular importance in the management of patients who have undergone liver transplantation, another new development that has occurred during this short period of 15 years. The diagnosis of graft rejection, however, is not possible without histopathology. Imaging technology is yet another area of progress that began with the advent of real-time ultrasonography utilizing electronically activated transducers, followed by computerized tomography (CT) and magnetic resonance imaging (MRI). All these modalities are based on sectional anatomy of the body for interpretation, reviving an interest in gross liver pathology which had nearly been forgotten. The amount of information gained by such means is enormous, and the detected gross abnormalities are clearly a result of pathomorphological changes. In other words, advanced imaging calls for a more detailed and precise knowledge of morphology. The ultrasound scanning machine is even equated, by some, with the stethoscope. With Doppler ultrasound flowmetry and MR angiography, portal venous haemodynamics can now be grossly evaluated and quantified without an invasive procedure. Thus, hepatology has acquired increasingly finer physiological and morphological nuances.

None of these new developments will ever reduce the role of histopathology in the diagnosis and management of liver disease. Rather, they will go on demanding further morphological explanations. During these 15 years, progress made in the field of liver pathology has been just as remarkable as in others. Different subsets of lymphocytes can be identified using specific antibodies against surface antigenic epitopes, and even those cells in the liver sensitized to particular antigens, including virus-induced epitopes, can now be recognized under the microscope. With the development of novel histochemical and immunohistochemical techniques, the functions of individual cell types that constitute the liver can also be much better understood. Morphology and biochemistry have advanced in parallel, the former more often helping the latter to further progress. Fat droplets in the cytoplasm, and collagen fibers in the proximity of the perisinusoidal (Ito) cells, now explain the biochemical activities of this cell, such as storage of vitamin A and collagen synthesis. Similarly, morphology and immunology are mutually interdependent, and one can visualize cytotoxic T-cells actually killing an hepatocyte. The roles of various cytokines cannot be understood without morphological evidence. Programmed cell death or apoptosis of the hepatocyte can be clearly distinguished from necrosis; the former is associated with the expression of particular genes. Liver damage, including acute massive necrosis, therefore needs reassessment in terms of these pathogenetically different types of cell death.

Molecular biology has progressed at a rapid pace and the three billion base pairs in the entire human genome are expected to be deciphered earlier than the set goal of 2006. Claims have already been made that all of the component genes will be identified within a few years. This is due to remarkable technical advances in molecular and genetic biology, and utilization of the polymerase chain reaction which has become a routine in many laboratories. Along with such advances there has been progress in our understanding of hepatocarcinogenesis, and it will not be long until the multiple molecular events that are required for malignant transformation of the hepatocyte are elucidated. In practical terms, tissue analysis for particular gene expressions will provide information on how close the hepatocytes are to malignant transformation in the diseased liver. The limitations of the conventional haematoxylin and eosin stain in the differential diagnosis of normal, premalignant and early malignant cells will soon be overcome by the demonstration of messenger (m)RNA in the cells for particular oncogenes and by identifying the products of tumour suppressor genes. Such differential diagnosis is a particular necessity because small nodular lesions seen by ultrasonography can now be destroyed by ultrasound-guided injection of ethanol as a therapeutic procedure. The potential of these nodules to develop into malignant lesions should be phenotypically, hence functionally, demonstrable. Indeed, it seems that, as our knowledge of cellular function in relation to liver disease advances, the demand for a better insight into functional morphology and pathomorphology increases and these do not remain as static characterizations. These are always changing in a progressive way, and increasingly assume dynamic features. Humans are never really convinced until they can see the event in question – as a Japanese adage puts it 'Hearing a hundred times does not exceed seeing just once!' In this respect, man is perhaps more dependent on vision that any other living species. Clearly, as a means

whereby information can be gained, visual recognition exceeds all other types of perception, and histopathology is one example of this. One liver tissue section, when properly studied, will provide more information than will a legion of liver function tests. Pathological morphology has long been the core of disease science, and will remain so. In fact, few people are aware that it has led the way for progress in immunology and biochemistry, and there have been many instances in which a false direction in medical research was corrected by the study of morphology. Accordingly, regardless of the area of interest, one has to have a sufficient knowledge of liver pathology in order to be a qualified hepatologist who is fully able to understand liver disease and make an accurate diagnosis. The definition of many liver diseases is still based on pathomorphology even though the hitherto unknown aetiological factors may now be identified.

All of the chapters in this book have been written by the foremost world authorities and are richly illustrated with high quality photographs and photomicrographs. Particular emphasis is placed, as stated in the editors' preface, on close clinico-pathological cooperation, making the book useful not only for histopathologists, but also for clinically-orientated hepatologists: this is one of the remarkable features of the text. There are several published monographs on liver histopathology, but they are directed mainly to diagnosis. This book is quite different and unique in its approach, in that it describes each disease with full references just as does a comprehensive textbook of hepatology; gross, microscopic and electron microscopic figures are included for a fuller understanding of various diseases whilst at the same time assisting the reader to achieve diagnostic capability and skill.

Chiba, Japan, 1994   Kunio Okuda

Foreword to the First Edition

At a time when the world literature devoted to the liver and its diseases abounds with monographs and textbooks, some of them superb, the question arises as to the need for and the purpose of this book. Indeed, the subject matter seems to have been covered from every point of view imaginable. One almost fears a 'paper pollution'. The justification for this new volume lies first of all in both the excellence and experience of the contributors, who have devoted decades to the study of the morphology of the abnormal liver Moreover, the role of pathology in the study of liver diseases is changing and enlarging. Two factors enter into this development: one, the specific role of pathology, a classic discipline in medicine, and the other, the specific function of hepatology, as a recently emerging discipline.

Pathology is the study of the mechanism of diseases with emphasis by most pathologists on the morphological features. Many believe that pathology is suffering from an identity crisis. Most observations possible with conventional morphologic tools seem to have been made during two or more centuries of study. 'These observations were based on human material obtained at autopsy or surgery and on various experimental models. For two reasons, however, this widespread assumption is less true for the liver than for many other organs. One is the fact that the cadaver liver cells reflect but poorly the status of the organ because premortal events change the appearance of the liver cells. Anoxia during the agonal period causes major distortions and the abundance of digestive enzymes in the liver play havoc with the structure. Liver biopsy, widely used for only 35 years, produced a new pathology of the organ. The second reason is the use of new techniques such as electron microscopy with all its applications. The observations have been made more meaningful by the simultaneous development of tissue fractionation, permitting cytochemical analysis of a relatively homogeneous organ. No wonder that the emerging molecular pathology of

mammalian tissue was greatly based on investigations of the liver and that organelle pathology was almost entirely initiated by studies on this organ. This led to a renaissance of pathology with the liver as standard model.

Thus, morphologic study by conventional and fine structural techniques of material from both human biopsy and animal models of human diseases, correlated with observations by biochemical and biophysical techniques, created a new concept of structure and function of the liver. Functional tests of the liver are notoriously less informative than in other organ systems because few widely used tests measure specific functions of the liver and because most indicate only an altered activity rather than a specific impairment of a given function. Moreover, many hepatic functions are altered in non-hepatic diseases either because hepatic blood flow is impaired or the liver reacts non-specifically to primary changes in other organ systems. Thus, in many aspects, liver biopsy appears to be a more reliable parameter than liver function tests and, except for simple screening, is widely used to establish the presence of liver disease and to establish its nature and often its aetiology. Biopsy thus serves prognosis and dictates management. This diagnostic superiority of liver biopsy in many aspects of clinical practice depends, however, on knowledge and experience in the histologic interpretation of liver biopsy specimens. Moreover, the conventional light microscopic interpretation was sharpened by fine structural investigations, including histochemistry, which permitted better appreciation of light microscopic features. Electron microscopy by itself has less diagnostic applications in liver disease than in other organs, particularly the kidney, but it has contributed to the understanding of pathogenetic mechanisms. Finally some immunopathologic techniques provide additional diagnostic parameters, particularly as these techniques become simplified and standardised and even applied to routine paraffin sections.

These developments   encouraged the acquisition of

skills in biopsy interpretation and the information presented in this book thus assumes importance for the practising clinician. It should enable him either to make his own interpretation or at least to better understand the language of the report. It should, however, be emphasized that developments in the visualization of the biliary tract by various recently introduced cholangiographic techniques are reducing the diagnostic importance of biopsy and of other laboratory methods in establishing the presence and site of mechanical biliary obstruction.

In addition to serving the management of the individual patient, the morphological investigation, again greatly based on biopsy, has become a key feature in the classification of liver diseases as illustrated in chronic hepatitis and in primary malignant and, especially, benign hepatic tumours. Classification is the basis of prognosis and communication between clinicians, pathologists and biologists is the main requirement. Moreover, classification is essential in the epidemiology of diseases, particularly if this nomenclature is to be applied world-wide. Since geographic pathology of cirrhosis and hepatic cancer may provide clues to the aetiology, an internationally accepted nomenclature is a prerequisite to potential success. This also entails the thorny problem of the evaluation of the significance of hepatic lesions in experimental animals, particularly neoplastic ones which have a bearing on environmental medicine. The interpretation of these lesions influences the actions of regulatory agencies in the increasing numbers of environmental and industrial problems calling for decisions of major influence on economic aspects and even the lifestyle of the population. Elimination of the prevailing confusion in nomenclature and evaluation will assist in reaching reasonable decisions. In all these aspects, communication, meaning agreement on a name, takes precedence over its correctness or the identification of the pathological process. In this sense, presentation of some pathologic facts in this book is a progress report rather than a final dogma, despite the century-old study of pathology.

Hepatology is a new discipline emerging in the greater part of the world only after the Second World War. It seems to have developed from the convergence of several trends in different parts of the world. In Anglo-Saxon and Germanic countries the biology of the liver has been studied with increasing intensity almost since the onset and blooming of scientific medicine after the Renaissance.

The large, homogeneous organ was a useful tool for physiologic and biochemical studies. Many general biochemical principles are based on the study of the liver and its organelles. The identification of mammalian organelles and their function was usually unravelled by investigation of the liver. These biologic studies, however, had but limited impact on the clinical work in liver disease. In the Latin countries, by contrast, concern with the clinical dysfunction of the liver was widespread and hepatology has been a respected discipline for a long time, in spite of the exaggerations so well reflected in Moliere's plays. The third contributing trend was widespread public health problems in the developing, frequently tropical countries, where liver cirrhosis, cancer and parasitic disease have been important public hazards reducing the life expectancy of a significant segment of the population. The improvement in global scientific interchange after the Second World War resulted in a unified hepatology as a new international discipline, attempting mutually beneficial and other exciting correlations between basic science and clinical medicine, with pathology contributing its share.

Several factors added to this blossoming of hepatology. One was the increasing awareness of the social impact of liver diseases at a time when the sociological and behavioural considerations challenged the primacy of biological observations in the health sciences. Increasing recognition of the role of poverty, malnutrition and alcoholism raised interest in diseases of the liver. Since the liver renders many environmental factors biologically active, its function determines environmental diseases in other organs in addition to those in the liver itself. Finally, the new radiologic and radionuclide diagnostic techniques, the former largely developed in Japan, facilitate the diagnosis of liver diseases.

Specialization entails restriction of knowledge to a circumscribed field to improve acquisition of new data by study in depth. An added justification for this restriction, however, is the application of this initially restricted information to other organ systems. The central location of the liver favours such a development which makes diseases of other organs better understood. Hope is expressed that this volume which reflects the merging of an old discipline with a new one may serve medicine as a whole.

New York, 1979   Hans Popper

Preface

In the seven years which have elapsed since the publication of the second edition, there have been continuing advances in hepatopathology and all chapters in this edition have had to be extensively revised. We believe that this volume represents the state of the art at the time of going to press, but in addition we are well aware that the rate of advance is rapid and that there have already been conceptual changes in some areas since the chapters were completed. This is particularly true with respect to acute and chronic hepatitis. However, the reader can be assured that the morphological accounts which are given are entirely appropriate although changing views, on grading and staging of chronic hepatitis in particular, will in the near future lead to a revised nomenclature. The third edition, therefore, remains 'a progress report rather than a final dogma', to reiterate the late Hans Popper's comments in his foreword to the first edition.

Hans Popper died in 1988 and the three original editors remain thankful for the enthusiastic support and encouragement which he gave us in our endeavours. His foreword to the first edition is published again, because it set the guidelines which we have since tried to follow. Kunio Okuda has done the honour of writing a foreword on this occasion and we are pleased with the emphatic way in which he stresses the continuingly-important role of the histopathologist in the understanding and the diagnosis of liver disease.

The clinico-pathological correlation which characterized the earlier editions has been maintained. The account of nutritional liver disease has been assimilated into chapter 17. We have included a section on experimental liver tumours in chapter 16, because this is a topic in which there have been considerable advances at the molecular level which are applicable to our understanding of human liver cancer, a tumour which, on a world-wide basis, remains of great importance. The increasing use of hepatic and bone marrow transplantation as therapeutic modalities is reflected in the introduction of a new chapter which deals with the pathological lesions which can develop in the liver allograft and in the native liver in graft versus host disease. We are deeply grateful to all our contributors who have collaborated wholeheartedly with us as editors, and once again our editing has given us much pleasure and the editorial pens have been used lightly.

The major change in this edition has been the introduction of colour illustrations, which was undertaken after very careful consideration. We were persuaded by the publisher that this would represent a considerable advance in presentation and that, in addition, the quality of the visual presentation would be such as to considerably enhance the text. There were those among the editors who were sufficiently conservative to feel that black-and-white illustrations were best appreciated by most histopathologists; our views have been changed by the quality of reproduction which the printers have achieved.

The editors are now five in number and the original three have consequently had their duties lightened. There has been a great sense of harmony in the 'editorial office' and, with future editions in mind, transfer of editorial responsibilities will be straightforward. The survival of *Pathology of the Liver* is assured.

Glasgow	Roddy MacSween
Exeter	Peter Anthony
London	Peter Scheuer
Newcastle	Alastair Burt
London	Bernard Portmann
1994	

Acknowledgements

Acknowledgement of illustrations from previous publications, of modifications to illustrations and diagrams, and acknowledgement of original photographic material or microscopic material is appropriately made in each chapter and in the figure legends.

We would like to thank all those who have helped with the preparation of manuscripts and figures. Secretarial assistance was provided in Exeter by Mrs Jo Wright, in London by Mrs Elisabeth Portmann and in Newcastle by Mrs Liz Tweedy and Mrs Jill Denny. Preparation of the final edited manuscript was undertaken in the University Department of Pathology, Western Infirmary, Glasgow; we are deeply grateful to Mrs Maureen Ralston who, in addition to preparing manuscripts and providing disks for each chapter, also helped with the final indexing and with much of the correspondence. Finally, it is again a pleasure to thank Churchill Livingstone, and in particular Geoffrey Nuttall and Lowri Daniels, for their advice at all times and for dealing with the few unforeseen problems which arose.

1

Developmental anatomy and normal structure

R. N. M. MacSween   R. J. Scothorne

During the period of over 300 years in which liver morphology has been studied, numerous concepts of its structural organization have emerged. These concepts have had to consider the liver as both an 'endocrine' and an exocrine gland. Its 'endocrine' functions are provided for by the intimate relationship between interconnected sheets of hepatocytes and specialized vessels, the hepatic sinusoids, which carry varying mixtures of venous and hepatic arterial blood. Its exocrine functions are revealed by the presence, within the sheets of hepatocytes, of networks of intercellular spaces — the bile canaliculi — which drain their contents into the biliary tree, whose epithelial lining is continuous at its peripheral 'twigs' with the hepatic parenchyma, and at the end of its main stem with the duodenal epithelium.

The three major concepts of the basic structural organization of the liver have been the hexagonal lobule (now 'classic lobule') described by Kiernan in 1833,[1] the portal lobule described by Mall in 1906[2] and the liver acinus defined by Rappaport and his colleagues in 1954.[3] On the basis of microscopy of the circulation in the living liver, Bloch (1970)[4] defined the dynamic functional unit as a single sinusoid with its perisinusoidal space and surrounding cylinder of hepatocytes. Each of these concepts is manmade and represents a particular way of looking at an organ of great structural complexity and with a multitude of functions. No one concept is more 'correct' than the others. The portal lobule is now largely of historical interest and will not be discussed further. In the first edition of this text in 1979 we stated that the concept of the liver acinus was proving to be of greatest value to the pathologist in the interpretation of disordered structure and function. This assertion has been amply confirmed since then and the acinus has generally come to be accepted as the structural, microvascular and functional unit. However, studies on hepatic angioarchitecture[5] and the zonal distribution of some hepatic enzymes[6] have suggested a need for some re-evaluation of the acinar concept. The

1

morphological descriptions which appear in this edition are based on the acinar concept but, insofar as the 'classic lobule' is still referred to in some hepatology texts and terms such as lobular hepatitis (e.g. in Ch. 9) continue to be used, we shall return to it later in this chapter.

Our concept of the organization of the liver is perhaps best appreciated by study of the development of the liver, before consideration of its definitive structure.

DEVELOPMENT OF THE LIVER

GENERAL FEATURES

In human embryos, the liver first appears at the end of the third week of development. Its parenchyma is of endodermal origin and arises from the liver bud or hepatic diverticulum, which develops as a hollow midline outgrowth from the ventral wall of the future duodenum. The connective tissue framework of the liver is of mesenchymal origin, and develops from two sources: (i) the septum transversum, a transvesre sheet of cells which incompletely separates the pericardial and peritoneal cavities; and (ii) cells derived from the mesenchymal lining of the associated coelomic cavity, which actively invade the septum transversum (Figs 1.1a and 1.2a).

During the fourth week, bud-like clusters of epithelial cells extend forwards and outwards from the hepatic diverticulum into the mesenchymal stroma, in which has appeared a hepatic sinusoidal plexus, fed by a vitelline venous plexus draining blood from the wall of the yolk sac. As the epithelial buds grow into the septum transversum, they break up into thick anastomosing epithelial sheets

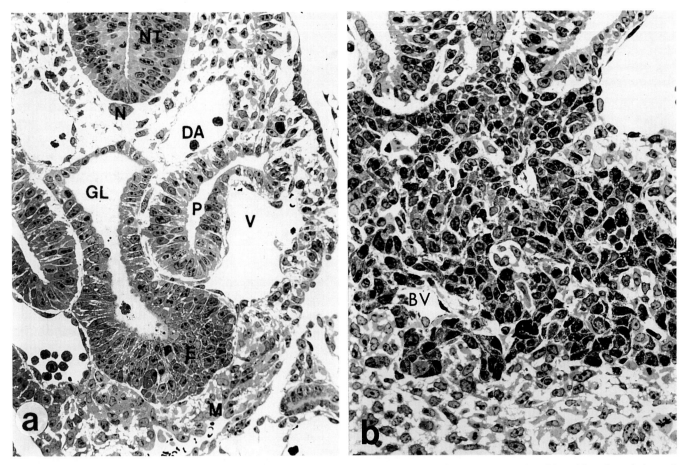

Fig. 1.1 This illustrates stages in the early development of the liver in mouse embryos of 14 somites (a), and 26 somites (b); and in a sheep embryo of 10 mm crown rump length (c) and (d). (a) The hepatic bud appears as a thick-walled hollow diverticulum of the foregut, extending ventrally into the loose mesenchyme of the septum transversum and flanked on each side by a vitelline vein. NT = Neural tube; N = notochord; DA = dorsal aorta; GL = gut lumen; P = pericardio-peritoneal canal; V = vitelline vein; E = endodermal component of the developing liver (hepatic bud); M = mesenchyme of the septum transversum. Semi-thin resin section. Toluidine blue. (b) The hepatic bud is broken up into thick anastomosing plates between which are blood vessels (BV), the primitive sinusoids. From the deep surface of the thickened mesenchymal epithelium, which lines the coelom, cells are budded off to contribute to the mesenchymal bed of the liver. Semi-thin resin section: Toluidine blue. (c) & (d) The continuity of the hepatic plates with the hepatic duct in the ventral mesentery (lesser omentum) is shown. (c) H & E. (d) H & E.

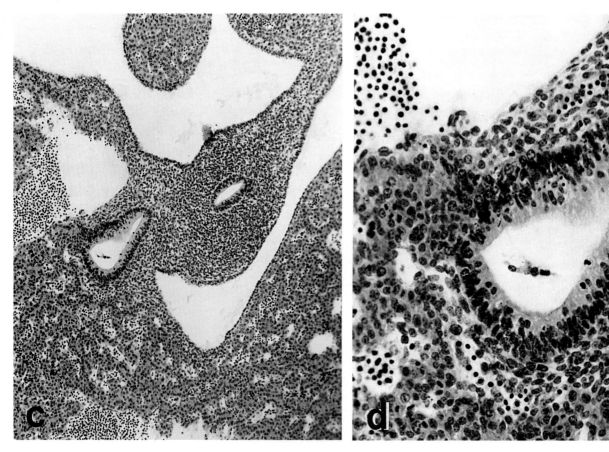

Fig. 1.1 *Contd*

which meet and enmesh vessels of the hepatic sinusoidal plexus, forming the primitive hepatic sinusoids (Figs 1.1b, 1.2b). The intimate relation between hepatocytes and sinusoidal capillaries, so characteristic of the adult organ, is therefore already anticipated in the 4-week-old embryo (Fig. 1.2c). The caudal part of the hepatic diverticulum does not contribute to the invading sheets of primitive hepatocytes but forms instead the epithelial primordium of the cystic duct and gallbladder.

Once established, the liver grows rapidly and soon extends beyond the confines of the septum transversum in whichever direction it can. It bulges dorsally on each side of the midline, into the peritoneal cavity, as right and left lobes, which are initially symmetrical. It also grows ventrally and caudally into the mesenchyme of the anterior abdominal wall, extending down to the umbilical ring. Associated with these changes, the stomach and duodenum, which were initially in broad contact with the septum transversum, draw away from it, thus producing a mid-sagittal sheet of mesoderm, the ventral mesogastrium or future lesser omentum. As the duodenum withdraws from the septum transversum, the stalk of the original hepatic diverticulum is also drawn out to form, within the lesser omentum, the epithelial elements of the extrahepatic bile ducts (Fig. 1.1c & d). The liver becomes partly

freed from its originally broad contact with the septum transversum by extensions of the peritoneal cavity, so that, in the adult, direct contact with the diaphragm persists only as the bare area of the liver. This is bounded by the attachments of peritoneal reflexions, which form the coronary and falciform ligaments.

VASCULAR ARRANGEMENTS

The fetal liver consists of anastomosing sheets of liver cells, each sheet being several cells in thickness and forming a 'muralium multiplex',[7] a condition which still pertains, in part at least, in the neonatal liver. By five months after birth, the sheets are, in general, two cells thick ('muralium duplex'). The pattern typical of the adult ('muralium simplex') is not established until about five years of age.

Initially, the hepatic sinusoidal plexus receives blood from symmetrically arranged vitelline veins and is drained into the sinus venosus by similarly symmetrical right and left hepato-cardiac channels[8] (Fig. 1.2b). As the developing liver grows, the laterally placed right and left umbilical veins, which run in the body wall and carry oxygenated blood from the placenta to the sinus venosus, also come to supply blood to the hepatic sinusoidal plexus

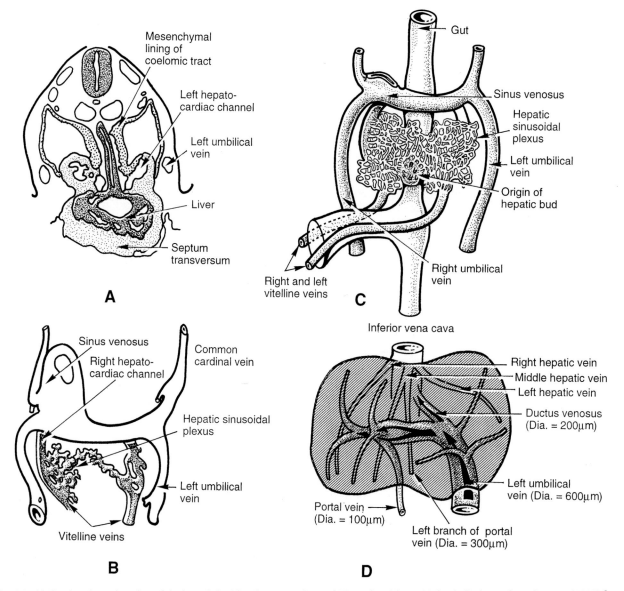

Fig. 1.2 (a) Section through region of the hepatic bud in a human embryo of 25 somites (about 26 days). Redrawn from Streeter (1942).[8] (b) Vascular channels associated with the developing liver, in a human embryo of 30 somites. Redrawn from Streeter (1942).[8] (c) Vascular channels in the human liver at a slightly later stage, showing the further extensive development of the hepatic sinusoidal plexus. Based on Streeter (1945).[9] (d) Scheme of the portal hepatic circulation, in a human embryo of 17 mm (about 7 weeks). Redrawn from Lassau & Bastian (1983)[10].

(Fig. 1.2c). Once this connection is made (in embryos of 5 mm, 5th week) the circulatory pattern within the liver changes rapidly. The left umbilical vein becomes the principal source of blood entering the liver, partly because it comes to carry all the blood returning from the placenta when the right umbilical vein withers and disappears, and partly because the volume of blood returning from the gut in the vitelline veins is small. The definitive vascular pattern of the fetal liver, already established in embryos of the seventh week (about 17 mm long), is shown in Figure 1.2d. The originally paired vitelline veins have given way to a single portal vein which, on entering the liver, divides into right and left branches. Blood in the left umbilical vein has a choice of three routes through the

liver: (i) through branches which enter the sinusoidal plexus of the left half of the liver; (ii) through the sinusoidal plexus of the right half of the liver, by retrograde flow through its connection with the left branch of the portal vein; and (iii) through the ductus venosus directly into the inferior vena cava. The ductus venosus is a new venous channel which has developed through the enlargement of pre-existing sinusoidal channels, probably in response to the obliquely directed stream of placental blood. In the fetus, therefore, the umbilical vein is seen as the major contributor to the hepatic circulation, as indeed it must be since the placenta is the role source of nutrients. Although the flow routes indicated in the embryonic liver in Figure 1.2d are merely inferred from the relative dimensions of the vessels involved, they have been clearly demonstrated by cine-radiography in the late fetal sheep.[9a] At birth, a sphincteric mechanism closes the ductus venosus at its proximal end, blood flow ceases in the umbilical vein, and the left side of the liver receives blood which now flows from right to left through the left branch of the portal vein. The closed segment of the umbilical vein between the umbilicus and the liver regresses to form the ligamentum teres; the ductus venosus undergoes fibrosis and becomes the ligamentum venosum.

HEPATOCYTES AND SINUSOIDAL CELLS

The primitive hepatocytes are derived exclusively from the endodermal outgrowths of the hepatic diverticulum. Synthesis of α-fetoprotein begins at the earliest stage of liver differentiation, some 25–30 days after conception, and continues until birth. Intestinal epithelium and yolk-sac cells also secrete α-fetoprotein. Glycogen granules are present in fetal hepatocytes at 8 weeks; glycogenesis commences at 12–14 weeks, the maximal glycogen reserve is achieved at birth, but the rapid onset of glycogenolysis depletes the storage to approximately 10% within 2–3 days post-partum.[11] Fat accumulation occurs in parallel with glycogenesis.[11] Haemosiderin deposits appear early in development, become more marked as hepatic haemopoiesis decreases and are then predominantly present in periportal hepatocytes; these are also the storage sites for copper. The specialized sinusoidal cells, Kupffer cells and perisinusoidal cells, appear at 10–12 weeks.

Bile acid synthesis begins at about 5–9 weeks and bile secretion at about 12 weeks.[12] Canalicular transport and hepatic excretory function, however, is still immature at birth (and for 4–6 weeks post-partum — Ch. 11) and, therefore, bile excretion across the placenta is important in the fetus.

THE DUCT SYSTEM

This is best understood if the liver is regarded as an exocrine gland. The hepatic bud gives rise not only to the epithelial parenchyma — the future hepatocytes — but also to the epithelial lining of the branching duct system, from its main stem, the common bile duct, to its terminal twigs, the smallest ductules, the canals of Hering.

The bile canaliculi are first seen in human embryos of the 6th week, long before bile production begins at 12 weeks. They develop from membrane foldings between junctional complexes, and appear as intercellular spaces within sheets of presumptive hepatocytes, therefore corresponding to the lumens of the secretory elements of any exocrine gland. They have no wall of their own, but simply lie between presumptive hepatocytes. At this early stage the canaliculi resemble those of the adult, except that, in a 'muralium multiplex', each canaliculus is surrounded by several cells, perhaps as many as seven in one sectional profile.

The epithelial lining of the extrahepatic bile ducts develops from the drawn-out stalk of the original hepatic outgrowth. It is continuous at its caudal end with the duodenal epithelium and at the cephalic end with the primitive hepatic sheets. Both hepatic ducts and part of the cystic duct develop from the cephalic end of the diverticulum, while the caudal segment develops into the gallbladder, part of the cystic duct and the common hepatic duct.

The intrahepatic ducts, which link the bile canaliculi and the extrahepatic ducts, develop from the limiting plate of primitive hepatocytes which surround the branches of the portal vein. This has been known since the 1920s[13] but has been confirmed more recently using immunohistochemical methods and monoclonal antibodies to cytokeratins and cell surface markers.[14–20] Cytokeratins are the intermediate filaments of epithelial cells, and 19 different types have been identified.[21] Normal adult hepatocytes express cytokeratins 8 and 18 whereas intrahepatic bile ducts, in addition, express cytokeratins 7 and 19. During the first 7–8 weeks of embryonic development no intrahepatic bile ducts are evident and the epithelial cells express cytokeratins 8, 18 and 19. At about 9–10 weeks (27–30 mm embryos) primitive hepatocytes surrounding large portal vein branches near the liver hilum express these cytokeratins more intensely and form a layer of cells (Fig. 1.3a) which ensheaths the mesenchyme of the primitive portal tracts to form the so-called ductal plate.[13] This is followed by a second but discontinuous layer of epithelial cells which show a similar phenotypic change and so a segmentally double-layered plate is formed. The liver cells which do not form ductal plates lose cytokeratin 19 expression. From 12 weeks onwards a lumen develops in segments of the ductal plates forming double-layered cylindrical or tubular structures (Fig. 1.3b). Further remodelling of the plate occurs; invading connective tissue separates it from the liver parenchyma and the tubular structures become incorporated into the mesenchyme surrounding the portal vein branches. An anastomosing network of bile ducts is formed, excess ductal epithelium undergoes resorption and bile ducts appear within the definitive portal tracts. Weak immunoreactivity for cytokeratin 7 is present in large bile ducts from about 20 weeks gestation.

The entire process of duct development progresses centrifugally from the porta hepatis and also from the larger to the smaller portal tracts. However, this process may not be complete at 40 weeks gestation and full expression of cytokeratin 7 is not found until about 1 month post-partum. Thus, the intrahepatic bile duct system is still immature at birth.[14] Failure of remodelling and resorption produces the 'ductal plate malformation'[22] and may also be significant in the production of various

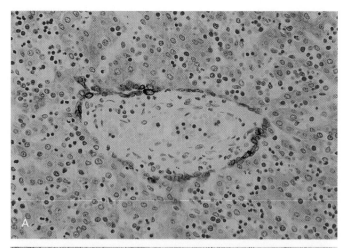

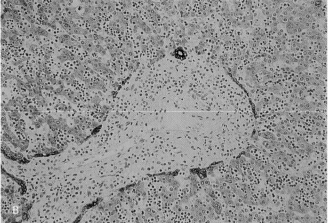

Fig. 1.3 Development of the ductal plate and of intrahepatic bile ducts. (a) Increased expression of cytokeratins in primitive hepatocytes at the interface with the mesenchyme of the primitive portal tracts; human fetus of 12 weeks gestation. (b) Later stage showing a discontinuous double-layered plate of epithelial cells at the mesenchymal interface; note the formation of tubular structures (upper right) within this plate. Human fetus of 14 weeks gestation. Immunoperoxidase staining; antibody (5D3) to low molecular weight cytokeratins. By courtesy of Dr A D Burt

congenital malformations of the intrahepatic biliary tree. Furthermore, injury to or destruction of the ductal plate in utero may be a factor in the development of intrahepatic biliary atresia[20] (see Ch. 3).

It is not known what factors determine whether immature hepatocytes differentiate in one direction, to hepatocytes, or in the other, to ductal epithelium. However, differentiation to ductal epithelium is associated, as first noted by Bloom[13] in 1925, with contact of primitive hepatic epithelium with young connective tissue developing in the portal tracts. There is now experimental evidence to indicate that the association is indeed one of cause and effect: in ectopic grafts of embryonic mouse liver, immature hepatocytes which are in contact with vascular endothelium tend to differentiate into mature hepatocytes, while those in contact with connective tissue cells differentiate into ductal epithelium.[23]

Despite their common ancestry, hepatocytes and ductal

epithelium have been considered as distinct cell types and the epithelium of the terminal twigs of the biliary tree — the canals of Hering[24] — includes typical hepatocytes and typical ductal cells, but no forms intermediate between the two. However, a change in differentiation from hepatocytes to bile-duct cells — ductular metaplasia — occurs in liver injury of various aetiologies and, in particular, contributes to the pattern of ductular proliferation seen in cholestatic liver disease (see Chs 11 and 12). Immunohistochemical investigations have shown that the metaplasia is characterized by a phenotypic change, in which hepatocytes express cytokeratins 7 and 19 which, in the normal liver, are restricted to bile-duct cells.[25-28] Whereas, previously, it was considered that duct cell proliferation contributed only duct cells and not hepatocytes, there is currently considerable interest in the possibility of metaplasia or transdifferentiation between duct cells and hepatocytes. This topic of bipotential progenitor cells or stem cells is further discussed in the section on hepatic regeneration.

HAEMOPOIESIS

Hepatic haemopoiesis is a feature of the embryonic and fetal liver of mammals including man. It begins at about six weeks (10 mm), when foci of haemopoietic cells appear extravascularly among the sheets of hepatocytes. By the twelfth week, the liver is the main site of haemopoiesis, having superseded the yolk sac; activity subsides in the fifth month, when the bone marrow becomes haemopoietic, and has normally ceased within a few weeks after birth. It is largely erythropoietic, but the stem cells may also give rise to granulocytes, megakaryocytes and monocytes. When the liver is in the haemopoietic phase it produces a stimulator which can be detected in vitro by its switching of quiescent mouse marrow stem cells into cycle. In mouse liver, declining production of stimulator in late gestation and after birth correlates with a decrease in haemopoietic stem cell numbers in the liver.[29] The source of the stem cells is now well established experimentally in the mouse; they develop *de novo* in the blood islands of the yolk sac, proliferate and migrate to colonize the fetal liver, and other lymphoid and myeloid organs.[30] Although hepatic haemopoiesis is normally erythropoietic, grafts of fetal mouse hepatic tissue to adult syngeneic hosts show granulopoiesis. The type of haemopoiesis occurring in fetal liver seems to depend, therefore, upon factors extrinsic to the liver.[31]

GROWTH OF THE LIVER

In its growth, the liver would seem to favour the traditional view of its structure: it grows by division and growth of constituent 'classic lobules'. Studies in the pig have shown that the average diameter of 'lobules' is 0.33 mm in early fetal life, 0.5 mm at birth, and about 1 mm in the adult. Growth involves increase in number and size of hepatocytes, counterbalanced in part by a reduction in diameter of sinusoids. New 'lobules' arise by division of existing ones. The process may be understood by reference to Figure 1.4. The hepatic venule, originally single, has divided, apparently sending out a side branch. This is not, in fact, a new outgrowth, but represents the enlargement of pre-existing sinusoids, as a 'preferred channel' under the moulding influence of increased blood flow.

Causal factors in hepatic development

Development of the mammalian liver involves contributions from three different sources: endodermal epithelium from the foregut, mesenchyme from the septum transversum, and mesenchymal epithelium from the coelomic lining. Is the topographical association between these three elements fortuitous, or are causative interactions between them responsible for liver development? Although the answers to these questions are uncertain for mammals, there is clear experimental evidence from the

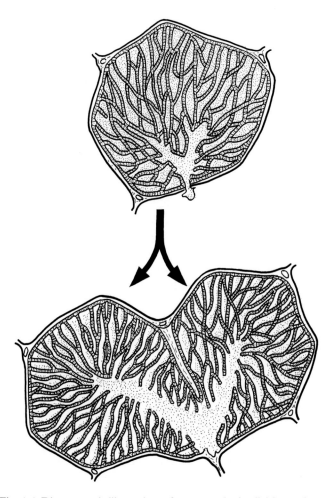

Fig. 1.4 Diagrammatic illustrations of two stages in the division and growth of a 'classic lobule.'

chick embryo that liver development is dependent on a chain of inductive interactions in which the mesodermal component takes the initial and major role.[32] At early somite stages, endoderm at the anterior intestinal portal (i.e. at the site at which the hepatic bud will later appear) becomes determined, or committed to hepatic development, through the inductive action of adjacent cardio-hepatic mesoderm. When the hepatic bud appears, as the first overt sign of liver development, at 20–22 somites, its growth and differentiation are dependent upon further inductive influence of the hepatic mesenchyme into which it grows. If the bud is separated from hepatic mesenchyme and explanted, it fails to differentiate. Isolated buds explanted in combination with hepatic or related mesenchymes, e.g. mesenteric or peritoneal, form liver; other types of mesenchyme, e.g. somitic or mesonephric, are ineffective as inducing agents.

Unlike the hepatic endoderm, which from early somite stages is localized to the midline at the anterior intestinal portal, the prospective hepatic mesenchyme is found not only in the same region, but also in wider areas extending backwards on either side of the midline. If explanted, these lateral areas of hepatic mesenchyme do not give rise to liver parenchyma since they lack the contribution of determined hepatic endoderm. If allowed to develop in situ, but experimentally isolated from contact with hepatic endoderm, the lateral hepatic mesenchyme forms masses similar in position to the right and left lobes but lacking hepatocytes. Within these masses there develop sinusoids, communicating with the vitelline veins. Sinusoidal development, often attributed to 'breaking up' of the vitelline vessels by invading hepatic endoderm, seems therefore to be autonomous in the chick. A similar conclusion was reached by Severn[33] in a descriptive study of human liver development. However, the development of a fenestrated endothelium lacking endothelial cell gaps and devoid of basement membrane is determined by the presence of hepatocytes.[34] Quite apart from their intrinsic interest, these observations may turn out to be of significance to the pathologist in understanding the interactions of epithelial parenchyma and the extracellular matrix in liver disease.

Hepatic regeneration

The liver has hitherto been regarded as an example of a conditional renewal system.[35] These are systems that ordinarily undergo little or no renewal but in which, under certain circumstances, the rate of cell production may be greatly increased. There may be an adaptive hyperplasia due to an increased functional demand or a regenerative response because of loss of functional tissue. There is now speculation, however, that the liver does have a self-renewal system for replacing ageing hepatocytes which undergo apoptosis; thus, it may be a stem cell and lineage system,[36,37] an arrangement which fits in with the concept of a 'streaming liver', as first proposed by Zajicek and his colleagues in 1985[38] and which also affords a theoretical explanation for the functional hepatocyte heterogeneity described below. The liver, however, is also capable of renewal whenever there is any pathological or experimentally-induced injury which causes a reduction in its functional hepatic cell mass. It is to this phenomenon that the term regeneration has been applied, a phenomenon which has stimulated considerable research and with an enormous literature, of which there have been a number of recent reviews.[35,39–43]

Stem cells

Stem cells may be defined as undifferentiated cells capable of proliferation, self-maintenance, and the production of a large number of differentiated functional progeny, regenerating the tissue after injury; there is flexibility in the exercise of these options. Distinction is made between actual and potential (or facultative) stem cells — the latter possess these capabilities but express them only in certain circumstances.[44] The need for a stem cell population in the liver has been argued against on the basis that mature hepatocytes are multipotential cells and able to proliferate. In addition it has, up till now, been impossible to identify a progenitor compartment in mammalian livers. In experimental carcinogenesis, mostly in rodents (see Ch. 16), proliferation of diploid so-called oval cells has been described and there is evidence that these cells may be equivalent to primitive bile-duct cells of the ductal plate, that they are located in the canals of Hering and can express α-fetoprotein, that they can proliferate in other forms of severe liver injury, and that they can give rise to hepatocytes in vivo and undergo transformation in culture with the production of a continuous cell line having features of hepatocellular carcinoma.[45] These oval cells have peculiar phenotypic features distinct from both normal and proliferating biliary epithelial cells and from mature hepatocytes.[45–47] Their precise nature, origin and fate, however, remain controversial, with debate as to whether they are derived from a postulated stem cell or are themselves facultative stem cells.[47,48] The possibility that periductular cells may also act as stem cells has not been excluded.[36]

Whether an equivalent of the oval cell exists in the human is equally controversial. However, immunophenotypic and ultrastructural studies have supported the existence of bipotential progenitor epithelial cells in human liver.[49–53] The topic has recently been briefly reviewed.[54] De Vos & Desmet,[53] in their ultrastructural study of the ductular reaction, identified a novel, small epithelial cell which they considered might be a candidate progenitor cell. These progenitor cells may normally exist in a periportal stem cell compartment in which there is a heterogeneous cell population among which are cells with neuroendocrine features[55,56]. Some of these express parathyroid hormone-related peptide,[57] an incomplete mitogen, which requires epidermal growth factor (EGF) and transforming growth factor β (TGFβ) to stimulate cell division. Thus, as Roskams and her colleagues have speculated, there are likely to be interactions between different cells in the periportal region, with complex growth factor loops, both autocrine and paracrine, which have an important role in proliferation and differentiation of progenitor cells following liver injury.[57]

The streaming liver

Studies on cell kinetics in the rat by Zajicek and his colleagues[38,58–60] suggest that there is a continuous, though extremely slow, production of hepatocytes in the periportal zones and that they move from their site of origin as part of a cell stream, comprising the parenchyma/ stromal complex (accompanied by sinusoidal cells, and probably also by its nerve supply). This cell stream advances, at a rate estimated at about 2 μm/day, towards the perivenular zone where its constituents are assumed to undergo apoptosis, although the evidence for this is at present somewhat circumstantial. The life expectancy of the hepatocyte in rats was estimated at about 200 days. This concept implies a progenitor zone in the periportal area and, in addition, implies both a chronological and a biological age for the streaming cells, the biological age equating with differentiation and being accompanied by an increased content of DNA. The functional heterogeneity of hepatocytes in the acinus is discussed below as is the composition of the extracellular matrix, which shows a gradient with different composition in zone 1 as compared with zones 2 and 3 of the acinus. Such matrix gradients may be similar to those identified in the intestine and haemopoietic tissue, and may have an important role in regulating hepatocyte and sinusoidal cell function. Reid and colleagues[37,61] have embraced the concepts of a stem cell compartment, the streaming liver, functional heterogeneity in the acinus and extracellular matrix gradients to produce a hypothetical model of liver lineage (Fig. 1.5)

Liver regeneration after experimental partial hepatectomy and toxic liver injury

If more than 10% of the liver is removed experimentally, the deficit is made good by cellular proliferation and hypertrophy in the remainder. This response is remarkable for several reasons: it occurs predictably and reproducibly in an organ in which mitotic activity is normally minimal in the adult; new hepatocytes arise by proliferation of existing ones, despite the fact that these are cells with a wide range of specialized functions; a similar response follows a second and succeeding partial hepatectomies;

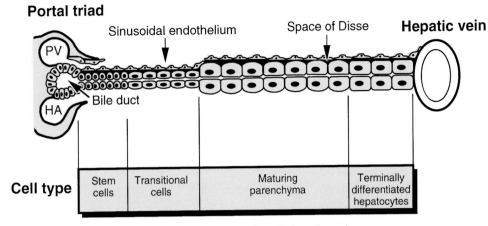

Fig. 1.5 Model illustrating a stem cell and lineage system in the liver with some details of the extracellular matrix gradient. Within the stem cell compartment in the periportal area cells capable of differentiating into biliary epithelium or hepatocytes are produced. The hepatocytes differentiate as they stream in a periportal (zone 1) to perivenular (zone 3) direction, and this is accompanied by an increase in cell size — < 20 μm in diameter for transitional cells and 30–40 μm for mature cells. The extracellular matrix comprises heparan sulphate (HS), heparin (H), chondroitin sulphate (CS) and dermatan sulphate (DS) proteoglycans (PG). Modified after Reid et al[61].

and the proliferative response subsides when the original mass of the organ is restored. Two further points should be stressed: (i) the regeneration is not morphogenetic and it does not restore the lobe or lobes removed, but involves rather the enlargement of the part which remains; and (ii) the response results not only from partial hepatectomy, but from any change, experimental or pathological, which reduces the total functioning mass of the liver.

Following experimental partial hepatectomy, there is a proliferative response which becomes synchronous and generalized throughout the liver remnant but, initially at least, occurs principally in the periportal zones (zone 1 of the acinus). The hepatocytes undergo transition from G_0 to G_1; this lasts for 12–14 hours, at which point DNA synthesis (S phase) begins, peaking at 22–24 hours. Mitotic activity follows 6–8 hours later. The non-parenchymal elements are also involved, but only after a further lag of about 24 hours. The growth spurt diminishes and finally ceases at about 7 days when the original liver weight is restored. As already mentioned, the growth potential is retained and the liver remnant can be induced to undergo further episodes of regeneration.

Whereas the precise trigger for the regenerative response is not known, there is recognition of a number of proto-oncogenes and growth factors which are both stimulatory and suppressor and which regulate the process.[62,63] Most of the growth factors involved are mitogenic for other cell types but, in the hepatectomy model, they act only on the liver. Some of the factors also act as mor-

phogens and, thus, probably have a role in the ordered nature of the growth process.

The regenerative response is associated with the expression of three proto-oncogenes, *c-fos*, *c-jun* and *c-myc* (so-called immediate early genes); the expression of these returns to normal within 3 hours.[64] The proteins encoded by these genes act as transactivators of other genes which are then involved in the progression of the hepatocytes through the cell cycle. The growth factors which are thought to mediate these patterns of proto-oncogene expression include hepatocyte growth factor (HGF) and transforming growth factors (TGF) α and β_1, the former acting as an autocrine stimulator of hepatocytes, the latter as an autocrine stimulator of non-parenchymal cells (see Ch. 10) but as a paracrine repressor of hepatocyte proliferation. Epidermal growth factor (EGF), which shares considerable sequence homology with TGFα and acts through the same receptor, may also stimulate hepatocyte regeneration, as may acidic fibroblast growth factor (aFGF).

Hepatocyte growth factor, which was cloned in 1989, is the most potent mitogen for hepatocytes and can stimulate proliferation at concentrations within its normal (physiological) serum range.[65] Following hepatectomy or liver injury serum HGF levels rapidly rise and within 12 hours there is enhanced HGF mRNA expression by perisinusoidal cells.[66] In patients with liver disease, serum HGF levels have been shown to correlate with the severity of liver injury.[67] Exogenously administered HGF augments the proliferative response of hepatocytes following hepatectomy, and can stimulate DNA synthesis in hepatocytes in normal liver.[68] HGF acts through the tyrosine kinase growth factor receptor *c-met*, a proto-oncogene product that is expressed by hepatocytes. The temporal expression of TGFα mRNA shows a pattern similar to HGF during liver regeneration, and there is experimental evidence for interaction between these two factors.[69] The precise nature of these interactions and the mechanisms involved in controlling the regenerative response are currently under intense investigation. The abrogation or suppression of the regenerative response is also of vital importance. In addition to its probable role in enhancing the synthesis of extracellular matrix protein, $TGF\beta_1$ appears to have a key role in switching off or preventing uncontrolled hepatocyte growth.[70]

MACROANATOMY OF THE LIVER

This account assumes a knowledge of the macroscopic morphology of the liver, such as could be obtained from a standard undergraduate text, and draws attention only to features of particular interest to the pathologist.

The liver lies almost completely under the protection of the rib cage, projecting below it, and coming into contact with the anterior abdominal wall only below the right costal margin and the xiphisternum. It is moulded to the undersurface of the diaphragm, the muscular part of which separates it on each side from the corresponding lung and pleural sac. It is separated by the central tendon of the diaphragm from the pericardium and the heart. The posterior surface of the liver is the least accessible and its relationships are of some clinical importance. It includes the following, form right to left:

1. The 'bare area' which is surrounded by the reflections of peritoneum which form the superior and inferior layers of the coronary ligaments. It lies in direct contact with the diaphragm, except where the inferior vena cava, the right adrenal and the upper part of the right kidney intervene.

2. The caudate lobe, which lies between the inferior vena cava on the right and, on the left, the fissure of the ligamentum venosum and the attachment of the lesser omentum. The caudate lobe projects into the right side of the superior recess of the lesser sac; behind it lies the right crus of the diaphragm, between the inferior vena cava and the aorta.

3. A small area on the left, covered by peritoneum and related to the abdominal oesophagus.

The traditional division into right and left, caudate and quadrate lobes is of purely topographical significance. A more useful and important subdivision is made on the basis of the branching pattern of the hepatic artery, portal vein and hepatic ducts. As these are followed into the liver

from the porta hepatis, each branches in corresponding fashion, accompanied by a branching tree of connective tissue, continuous with the external (Glisson's) capsule of the liver. On this basis, the liver is divided into right and left 'physiological' lobes of about equal size. The plane of separation between these two 'hemi-livers' corresponds, on the visceral surface of the liver, to a line extending from the left side of the sulcus for the inferior vena cava superiorly, to the middle of the fossa for the gallbladder inferiorly.

On a similar basis each lobe has been further subdivided into portal (or porto-biliary-arterial) segments, in studies pioneered by Hjortso (1951)[71] and extended by Couinaud (1957)[72] and many others. Within each hemi-liver, the primary branches of the portal vein divide to supply two main portal segments, each of which is further divided horizontally into superior and inferior segments. According to this scheme there are, therefore, eight segments, or nine if the caudate lobe is separately designated. In the absence of a fully agreed anatomical nomenclature, the following terms are sufficiently descriptive of the segments: *right lobe* — antero-superior and antero-inferior, postero-superior and medio-inferior; *left lobe* — medio-superior and medio-inferior, latero-superior and latero-inferior. The *caudate lobe* stands at the watershed between right and left vascular and ductal territories; its right portion in particular may be served by right or left vessels and duct, although its left part is almost invariably supplied by the transverse portion of the left branch of the portal vein.

These nine hepatic segments are separate in the sense that each has its own vascular pedicle (arterial, portal venous and lymphatic) and biliary drainage. There are said to be no intrahepatic anastomoses between the right and left hepatic arteries, a view which is generally supported by injection studies of cadaveric livers. However, Mays & Mays[73] have shown, by selective in vivo hepatic arteriography after ligation of the right or the left hepatic artery in humans, that there exist intrahepatic translobar collateral arteries capable of perfusing the entire occluded arterial system. They found no intermediate filling of sinusoids or of portal venules. However, the virtual vascular independence of each segment has been shown by studies in the living, using computed tomography, magnetic resonance imaging, and ultrasonography together with intravenous contrast injections which allow ready recognition of the liver's major vascular structures.[74,75]

Recognition of this compartmental pattern is of considerable pathological significance: regional degeneration of a lobe or segment may follow disturbance of its blood supply by a particular portal vein branch. While this recognition might be thought to facilitate surgical segmental resection, its usefulness is at present somewhat limited by the absence of defining connective tissue septa between segments and by the topography of the hepatic veins, which run in an intersegmental position and in planes which cross those followed by the portal triad.[76] Moreover, the pattern of segments shows individual variation.

Gupta and his colleagues[77] analysed variations in the segmental pattern of the liver. In nearly one-half of 85 livers examined, the pattern and sizes of segments were similar; in the remainder there were many variants, involving principally increase or decrease in size of one or more segments at the expense of neighbouring segments. There are said to be no anastomoses between the blood vessels or hepatic ducts of adjacent segments. Anomalous origin of the arterial supply of the liver is very common. In an analysis of more than 2300 cases, Nelson et al[78] reported a left hepatic artery as arising from the left gastric artery in 14%, a right hepatic from the superior mesenteric artery in 14%, and a common hepatic from the superior mesenteric artery in 3%. Extrahepatic anastomoses have been described between hepatic arteries and a number of other arteries, mostly arising as branches of the common hepatic artery (e.g. right gastric and gastroduodenal arteries). Anastomoses also exist with branches of the superior and inferior phrenic arteries, of the internal thoracic artery and with intercostal arteries. Although normally unimportant, they may constitute the major arterial supply after ligation of the hepatic artery.[79]

Two points should be noted: (1) if, say, the 'physiological' right lobe is supplied by an artery other than the right hepatic, the intrahepatic pattern of branching is usually normal; (2) a branch of abnormal origin supplying a particular part of the liver is the sole supply of that part — it is aberrant rather than accessory. Similar anomalies not uncommonly affect the duct system. For example, an aberrant segmental duct may leave the liver independently and drain into the extrahepatic duct system, or even directly into the gallbladder.

While the branches of the hepatic artery and portal vein and the tributaries of the hepatic ducts run together and serve segments of liver, the hepatic veins run independently and are intersegmental. Like the portal vein, they lack valves. The three major hepatic veins, the right, intermediate and left (the intermediate and left often forming a common trunk) enter the upper end of the retro-hepatic segment of the inferior vena cava: the terminal portions of each are frequently at least partially exposed above the posterior surface of the liver, where they are vulnerable to trauma. In addition to these major hepatic veins, several (about 5 per liver) accessory hepatic veins open into the lower part of the hepatic segment of the inferior vena cava.[80] Since the caudate lobe regularly drains directly into the inferior vena cava, it may escape injury from venous outflow block (Ch. 14).

Obstruction of portal venous flow may be compensated for by enlargement of portal-systemic venous anastomoses which occur at several sites: lower oesophagus, anal canal, at the umbilicus, at the bare area of the liver and where parts of the gut, e.g. colon and duodenum, are in direct contact with the posterior abdominal wall. These anastomoses become functionally significant when portal hypertension develops. The effects of increased portal venous pressure are compounded by the absence of valves in the portal system.

MICROANATOMY OF THE LIVER

THE HEPATIC MICROCIRCULATION

Details of the hepatic microcirculation are given now, because it is on an understanding of this that the concept of the hepatic acinus is based.

Portal circulation

Within the liver, the portal vein divides into successive generations of distributing or conducting veins, so-called because they do not directly feed the sinusoidal circulation. According to their position in the hierarchy of branching, they may be classified as interlobar, segmental and interlobular. The smallest conducting veins are interlobular veins, about 400 μm in diameter. Further branching of these produces the portal vein branches which distribute their blood into the sinusoids. These succeeding branches are: (i) the pre-terminal portal venules, the axial vessels of the complex acini which, microscopically, are found in portal tracts of triangular cross section; (ii) the terminal portal venules, which taper to about 20–30 μm in diameter, are surrounded by scanty connective tissue in portal tracts of circular rather than triangular cross section, and supply the simple acini. From the pre-terminal and terminal portal venules there arise very short side branches, i.e. the inlet venules, which have an endothelial lining with a basement membrane and scanty adventitial fibrous connective tissue, but no smooth muscle, in their walls. They pass through the periportal limiting plate to open into the sinusoids. Some early branching of the smallest conducting veins may produce more than one portal vein within some portal canals, and these supply only those sinusoids which abut upon the canal.

Arterial circulation

The hepatic artery branches accompany the portal veins and two or more branches may be present within each portal area. The terminal distribution of the arteries is by three routes: into a periportal plexus, into a peribiliary plexus, and into terminal hepatic arterioles.

A periportal plexus is characteristically distributed around portal vein branches within the portal canal. It drains into hepatic sinusoids. Occasional arterio-portal anastomoses between periportal arterioles and terminal portal venules were reported in human liver;[81,82] however, Yamamoto et al[83] denied the existence of any arterio-portal anastomoses in human liver, although finding them frequently in rat liver.

A peribiliary plexus supplies all the intrahepatic bile ducts. Around the larger ducts, the peribiliary plexus is two-layered, with a rich inner, subepithelial layer of fine capillaries and an outer, periductular, venous network which receives blood from the inner layer. Small bile ducts have only a single layer of fine capillaries. Ultrastructural studies have shown that the capillaries are lined by fenestrated endothelium which contains pinocytic vesicles.[84] The peribiliary plexus drains principally into hepatic sinusoids. This vascular route from an hepatic artery supply through the peribiliary plexus into hepatic sinusoids has been called a 'peribiliary portal system'.[85] The peribiliary plexus develops in parallel with the development of the intrahepatic bile ducts, spreading from the hepatic hilum to the peripheral area of the liver and becoming fully developed with the full maturation of the biliary system.[86] It has been proposed that the peribiliary plexus is involved in reabsorption of bile constituents including bile acids (cholehepatic circulation) and in the uptake of vasoactive substances secreted by entero-chromaffin cells in the biliary epithelium[87,88]. Rappaport[89] suggested that, by providing for countercurrent exchange of ions between blood and bile, the peribiliary plexus was involved in both secretion and resorption of bile constituents; the ultrastructural features are consistent with active transport between the capillaries and biliary epithelial cells, and this activity may be altered to meet increased functional demands in bile-duct obstruction.[84]

Terminal hepatic arterioles have an internal elastic lamina and a layer of smooth muscle cells, and open into periportal sinusoids. Reports of hepatic arterioles which penetrate deeply into the parenchyma before entering sinusoids near to the hepatic veins have not been confirmed, either by SEM studies of resin casts of the vascular tree[81,83] or in studies of the hepatic circulation in vivo.[90]

Venous drainage

Having perfused the parenchyma via the sinusoids, the blood enters the terminal hepatic venules (the central veins of the 'classic lobules'). Several collecting venules may drain the blood from individual abutting acini into the terminal venules. Scanning electron microscopy has clearly demonstrated in the walls of veins the fenestrations through which the sinusoids open.[91] The terminal vein branches unite to form intercalated veins which in turn form larger hepatic vein branches whose macroanatomy has already been described.

FUNCTIONAL HISTOLOGY OF THE MICROCIRCULATION

This account is based immediately on the work of McCuskey which has been reviewed by him,[90-93] but derives ultimately from the pioneering studies of Knisely et al[94] using quartz rod transillumination of living liver. Arterio-portal relationships are summarized in Fig. 1.6 which shows a terminal portal venule from which a series of sinusoids originates, and an accompanying terminal hepatic arteriole (internal diameter approximately 10 μm). There are various kinds of connection between arteriole and sinusoid, all of them being found in the periportal areas, and all of internal diameter no greater than the diameter of an erythrocyte. Approximately two-thirds of the blood supply comes from the portal venules whose inlets are controlled by sphincters — afferent or inlet sphincters — composed of sinusoidal lining cells. Flow of arterial blood to the sinusoids is intermittent, and determined by independently contractile smooth muscle sphincters in the walls of hepatic arterioles and their arteriolo-sinusoidal branches. Blood flowing into a group of sinusoids could therefore be arterial, venous or mixed, depending upon sphincteric and contractile activity. Flow of blood through the sinusoids is probably controlled in the sinusoid itself, and here the endothelial cell is known to be responsive to a variety of vasoactive substances. The perisinusoidal cells may also have a role in regulation, and McCuskey[92,93] has been a proponent of the view that Kupffer cells, which are capable of contracting and swelling, may also affect the patency of the sinusoidal lumen.

There is heterogeneity in the blood flow through the sinusoids. In the periportal zones the sinusoids form an

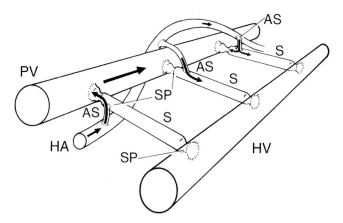

Fig. 1.6 Scheme to show relationships of hepatic arteriole (HA), portal venule (PV), sinusoids (S) and hepatic venule (HV). Arterio-sinusoidal branches (AS) may open in various ways into the sinusoids and blood flowing to a group of sinusoids could therefore be arterial, venous or mixed. Blood flow through the sinusoids is determined by the activity of 'sphincters' (SP) in the arteriolar wall and of sphincteric mechanisms at the inlet and outlet of the sinusoids. Based on McCuskey[90].

interconnecting polygonal network. Downstream, however, they become organized as parallel vessels which open into the terminal hepatic venule; short intersinusoidal sinusoids connect adjacent parallel sinusoids. Blood entering the hepatic venules passes through efferent or outlet sphincters which, like the inlet sphincters, are composed of sinusoidal lining cells. Blood may sometimes be stored in sinusoids with closed outlet sphincters, and released as an 'autotransfusion' when the sphincters open. The precise neural and humoral mechanisms which may operate are unknown. Many of the in vivo observations were made on mice and rabbits. If similar mechanisms exist in human liver for regional variation in sinusoidal blood flow at microscopic level, it is evident that statements about relative contributions of hepatic arterial and portal venous flow to overall hepatic blood flow must be treated with caution. Moreover, it must be remembered that the portal venous system is a low pressure one, and that the major factor in the control of blood flow through it is arteriolar resistance in the gastrointestinal and splenic circulations.

It should be said that there are those who dissent from these views on the hepatic microcirculation, derived from transillumination of livers in anaesthetized, immobilized animals. Greenway & Lautt[95,96] have reviewed the evidence and point out that studies using microspheres show a uniform distribution of portal venous blood throughout the liver; substances reaching the liver via the hepatic artery or portal vein are equally well extracted; elevation in venous pressure, reduction of portal venous flow and stimulation of hepatic nerves do not result in flow redistribution within the liver. While the portal vein does supply the larger amount of the blood supply to liver, the liver is not capable of directly controlling this flow and, thus, the only control of flow within the liver is via the hepatic artery. It has been postulated that the hepatic arterial flow is not regulated by liver metabolic demands but changes inversely in response to altered portal blood flow, a response which is controlled by a unique intrinsic mechanism in which adenosine plays a key role.[95,97,98]

THE HEPATIC ACINUS

Kiernan's concept of the polyhedral or classic lobule has already been mentioned.[1] It is traditionally represented as hexagonal in outline with, at its centre, a central vein, a terminal tributary of the hepatic vein. The boundaries of such a lobule are well defined in only a few species (e.g. pig) by interlobular septa of connective tissue. In most other species, including man, connective tissue is sparse, except in the portal canals which lie between the 'corners' of adjacent lobules. It is evident from Figure 1.7 that the blood from the terminal afferent vessels perfuses through sinusoids which pass into segments only of adjacent hexagonal lobules. It seemed improbable, therefore, that

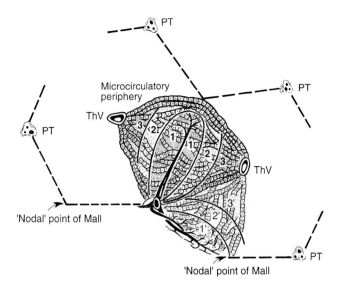

Fig. 1.7 Diagrammatic representation of the simple acinus and the zonal arrangement of hepatocytes. Two neighbouring classic lobules are outlined by the discontinuous lines, and the acinus occupies adjacent sectors of these. Although only one channel is shown as forming the central core of the acinus, the acinus is arranged round the terminal branches of the portal vein, hepatic artery and bile ductule. Zones 1, 2 and 3 represent areas which receive blood progressively poorer in nutrients and oxygen; zone 3 thus represents the microcirculatory periphery, and the most peripheral portions of zone 3 from adjacent acini form the perivenular area. The nodal points of Mall represent vascular watershed areas where the terminal afferent vessels from neighbouring acini meet. PT = portal tract; ThV = terminal hepatic vein (central vein of 'classic lobule'); 1,2,3 = microcirculatory zones; 1^1, 2^1, 3^1 = microcirculatory zones of neighbouring acinus; – – – – – – = outline of 'classic lobule'. Based on Rappaport[99] and published with permission.

such a hexagonal mass of parenchyma could subserve the role of a functional unit.

Rappaport and his colleagues,[3] on the basis of elegant studies of the hepatic microcirculation, defined a unit or acinus related to the terminal branches of the afferent microcirculation. This concept was extended in subsequent papers and reviews[89,99–101] in which it was suggested that the hepatic parenchyma is divisible into structural units of first order, second order and third order, as illustrated diagrammatically in Figure 1.8. The division into acini was initially based on the terminal portal circulation as illustrated in Figure 1.7, but it must be borne in mind that the arterial blood supply and the biliary drainage system follow a similar distribution pattern.

The *simple acinus* is defined as a small parenchymal mass, irregular in size and shape, arranged around a small round portal tract containing a terminal portal vein and its accompanying hepatic arteriole and bile duct; the acinus lies between two (or more) terminal hepatic venules into which it drains; it has no investing capsule; in a two-dimensional view it occupies part only of two adjacent classic lobules (Fig. 1.9) and in a three-dimensional view it

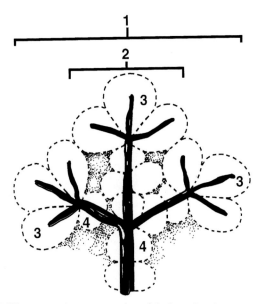

Fig. 1.8 Diagrammatic representation of the hepatic acinar structure: this shows an acinar agglomerate — 1, three complex acini — 2, and a number of simple acini — 3. The acinar agglomerate is supplied by a portal vein (and hepatic artery) branch which subdivides into three preterminal branches supplying each complex acinus; these branches in turn subdivide into terminal branches supplying the simple acini. The acinuli — 4, are arranged as a sleeve around the preterminal and the main supplying vessels. Modified with permission from Rappaport et al[103].

appears as a berry-like structure at the end of the terminal vascular/biliary stalk. The simple acini abut against one another and, as shown in Figure 1.7, the sites where the terminal arterioles and venules from neighbouring acini give out into their final capillaries constitute watershed areas and correspond to the 'nodal' points of Mall.[102] The approximate dimensions of the simple acinus are 1480 μm in length, 1070 μm in width and 800 μm in thickness.[103]

The *complex acinus* comprises at least three simple acini and a sleeve of parenchyma around the preterminal portal vein branches and their accompanying arterial and biliary elements (Fig. 1.10). The sleeve of parenchyma around the preterminal vessels comprises small clumps — *acinuli* — which are supplied by venular and arteriolar branches from the preterminal vessels.

The *acinar agglomerate* is composed of three or four complex acini and the acini forming the sleeve of parenchyma around the large triangular or oval-shaped portal tract supplying the agglomerate. The supplying portal vein is between 300 and 1200 μm in diameter (average 600 μm). The unity of the agglomerate is again determined by the fact that the vascular supply and the biliary drainage are common to the whole agglomerate as well as to its acinar subdivisions.

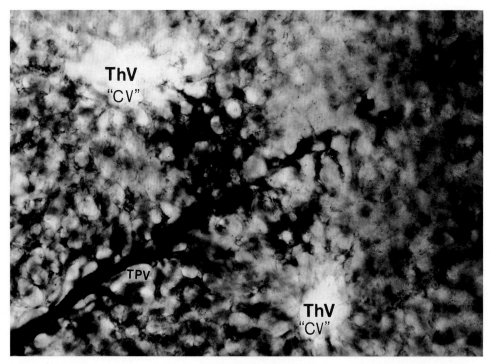

Fig. 1.9 Human liver, simple acinus. The terminal portal vein (TPV) branch of the structural unit is injected with India ink, and runs perpendicular to the two terminal hepatic vessels (ThV) or central veins ("CV") with which it interdigitates. Comparison with Figure 1.7 indicates how the acinus occupies sectors of two adjacent classic lobules and extends between the two hepatic venule branches. Thick cleared section. Illustration supplied by Professor A M Rappaport, Toronto, and published with permission.

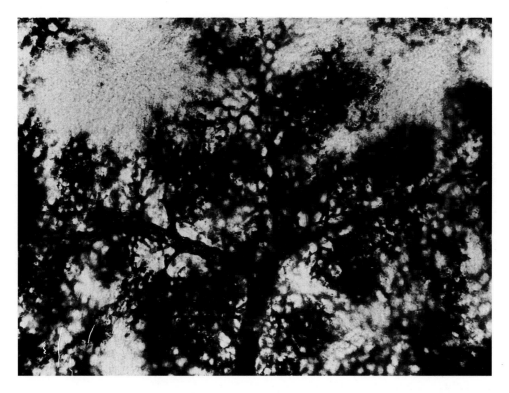

Fig. 1.10 Human liver, complex acinus. The sinusoids injected with India ink are supplied by three terminal portal vein branches arising from a single large preterminal vessel. Thick cleared section. Illustration supplied by Professor A M Rappaport, Toronto, and published with permission.

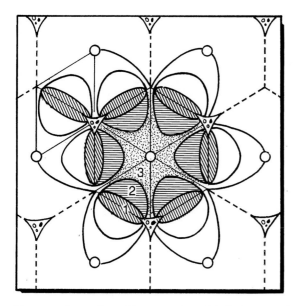 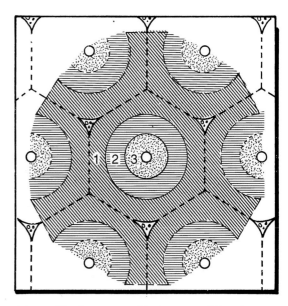

Fig. 1.11 Comparison of Rappaport's model of acinar zonation and the modifications proposed by Lamers and his colleagues. In Rappaport's model on the left (compare with Fig. 1.7) there is continuity between acinar zones 3 producing a stellate configuration of zones 3 around the (terminal) hepatic venules (○); acinar zones 1 are discrete. In Lamers et al's modification (right) acinar zones 3 are discrete, producing a circular configuration around the hepatic venules; there is continuity between acinar zones 1, however, producing a reticular configuration around the terminal portal tracts (▽). Modified after Lamers et al[6].

Within the simple acinus there is further subdivision into zones 1, 2 and 3 (Fig. 1.7) and we shall shortly discuss the evidence of functional heterogeneity based on this zonation. In Figure 1.7 there is apparent continuity between zone 3 of adjacent simple acini. Although subdivision of the complex acini into circulatory zones is difficult to demonstrate in the normal liver, ischaemic and viral injury extending through adjacent zones 3 — pericomplex acinar — provides indirect morphological evidence of continuity between these zones. However, Lamers and his colleagues,[6] in a re-evaluation of the concept of the liver acinus based on three-dimensional assessment of hepatic enzyme zonation, suggested that the perivenular zone was circular and discrete rather than stellate, whereas the periportal zone was reticular and contiguous between adjacent acini rather than discrete. This is illustrated in Figure 1.11, and this 'metabolic acinus' is therefore of a different configuration from the 'micro-circulatory acinus' of Rappaport.

The hepatic muralium. Within the acini the hepatocytes appear, in single sections, to form irregularly arranged cords (see Fig. 1.13a). The tri-dimensional reconstructions of Elias[104,105] showed that the hepatocytes are in fact arranged in the form of plates or laminae, one cell in thickness, and these elegant studies have been fully confirmed by scanning electron microscopy (SEM).[91,106,107] These hepatic laminae branch and anastomose with one another to form a complicated system of walls, the hepatic muralium, a maze-like arrangement of partitions between which the sinusoids interweave and interconnect in a continuous labyrinth.

Immediately deep to the external capsule of the liver is a single continuous sheet of hepatocytes, forming the external limiting plate. Elias[108] described this as extending inwards at the porta hepatis, to follow the branching of the portal vein and hepatic artery, and forming an internal periportal limiting plate. This bounds the portal tracts and forms an interface between the connective tissue of the tract and the hepatic parenchyma. In similar fashion, the external limiting plate extends into the liver as an investment around the hepatic veins and their tributaries, forming around these an internal perivenular limiting plate. Both the periportal and perivenular limiting plates are discontinuous where perforating vascular and biliary radicles pass through them.

Matsumoto and Kawakami's primary lobule

Detailed studies of the hepatic angio-architecture by Matsumoto & Kawakami[5] led them to suggest that each 'classic lobule' consisted of six to eight primary lobules, as illustrated in Figure 1.12. Each primary lobule is cone-shaped, with a convex surface at the periphery of the 'classic lobule', and its apex at, and draining into, a hepatic venule. Terminal portal venules, together with the

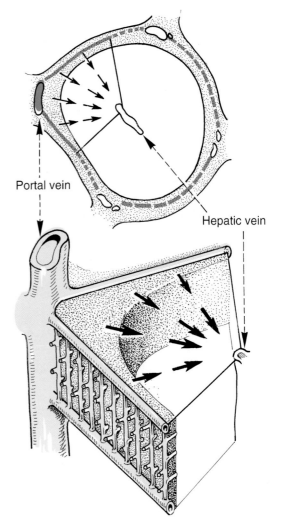

Fig. 1.12 Matsumo and Kawakami's primary lobule concept. An outline of the 'classic lobule' is shown above; this is thought to comprise several cone-shaped primary lobules, one of which is outlined, and arrows indicate the direction of blood flow. A three-dimensional reconstruction of a primary lobule is shown below; septal branches (which correspond to the terminal portal vein branches at the centre of Rappaport's acinus) extend from the portal veins and break up into a network of sinusoids which supply the lobule; the periseptal zone (corresponding to acinar zone 1) is shaded ▦ and the remainder of the lobule is cone-shaped (corresponding to acinar zones 2 and 3); arrows indicate the direction of blood flow. Modified after Matsumoto & Kawakami[5].

sinusoids which arise from them, form a 'vascular septum' between adjacent units. The objection to this functional unit is that it does not derive its blood supply from a single distributing portal vein; however, it does fit in better with those species like the pig which have fibrous septa enclosing 'classic lobules'.

Thus, there is continuing debate about the definitive functional unit in the liver. In the earlier edition of this text we indicated our support for Rappaport's acinus in preference to the lobule (the acinar and lobular terminology are compared in Table 1.1). The acinus, in our opinion, still best fits the concept of a functional unit, defined as the smallest amount of tissue in an organ which

Table 1.1 Comparison of lobular and acinar terminologies

Lobular	Acinar
Central; centrilobular; centrizonal	Perivenular; acinar zone 3
Mid-zonal	Acinar zone 2
Peripheral; periportal	Periportal; acinar zone 1
Multilobular	Multiacinar
Panlobular	Panacinar
Central/central (necrosis or bridging)	Peri-acinar (complex) (necrosis or bridging)
Central/portal (necrosis or bridging)	Peri-acinar (simple), peripheral acinar, zone 3 (necrosis or bridging)
Portal/portal (necrosis or bridging)	Portal-portal (necrosis or bridging)

subserves that organ's functions and whose supply is normally and exclusively provided by terminal or 'end' vessels.

Functional heterogeneity in the liver acinus

Inherent in the concept of microvascular zonality within the acinus is the possibility that there may also be functional heterogeneity of the hepatocytes within each zone. This, however, is not an entirely new concept and Jones (1853)[109] expressed the view that, while all hepatocytes were potentially alike, it did not follow that they all did the same thing at the same time, nor that each did the same thing all the time. The foregoing account of the microcirculation indicates that hepatocytes in zone 1 are the first to be supplied by blood rich in oxygen and nutrients, whereas zone 3 cells are at the microcirculatory periphery (Fig. 1.7) and this, in part at least, affords an explanation for their greater susceptibility to ischaemic injury.

There is now substantial evidence favouring such zonal heterogeneity, and this concept has recently been reviewed.[110,111] The heterogeneity may variously comprise: (i) morphological differences e.g., at the light microscopic level, variation in the fraction of parenchymal volume occupied by sinusoids and variation in the arrangement of the sinusoidal network (see earlier), or, ultrastructurally, differences in canalicular diameter and in the size and distribution of mitochondria, and smooth endoplasmic reticulum; (ii) metabolic differences with variation in the distribution pattern of many enzymes reflected in turn by differences, e.g. in drug metabolism, which may determine the site at which liver-cell injury is morphologically seen; and (iii) zonal variation in bile formation (see Ch. 11) with differences in the proportion of the bile salt-dependent and bile salt-independent secretion.

The concept of metabolic zonation was demonstrated in respect of carbohydrate metabolism, periportal hepatocytes being glucose-forming cells and perivenous hepatocytes glucose-utilizing cells. The uptake of bile is normally a function of periportal hepatocytes and they were predominantly responsible for the secretion of the bile salt-

dependent fractions of bile. However, increasing the bile salt load demonstrated that all the acinar hepatocytes were capable of taking up bile salts. These types of 'hepatocytic' metabolic heterogeneity were due to the availability of rate limiting factors in the sinusoidal blood and were also determined by the direction of blood perfusion.

However, other more complex types of hepatocytic heterogeneity also exist. Thus, glutamine synthetase and ornithine aminotransferase, important enzymes in nitrogen detoxification, are preferentially expressed in, and indeed strictly limited to, a narrow rim of hepatocytes surrounding terminal hepatic venules, and cytochrome P-450 induction by phenobarbitol is selectively confined to perivenous hepatocytes. Detailed investigations of these examples of hepatocyte heterogeneity have suggested that there may be zonal modulation of gene expression and that, in the case of glutamine synthetase and ornithine aminotransferase expression, this is dependent on cell–cell interaction — perivenous hepatocytes interacting with the endothelial cells of hepatic veins.[112,113]

Thus, functional heterogeneity within the acinus may be due, in part, to substrate delivery from the sinusoidal blood and in part to differential modulation of gene expression. If the concept of the 'streaming liver' (see above) is shown to be correct then this implies that hepatocytes, as they move from a periportal to a perivenous position, show different patterns of gene expression. Consequently, there is not simply zonal heterogeneity so much as hepatocytic or functional heterogeneity. The precise mechanisms by which the functional heterogeneity is regulated are likely to be very complex and are not yet fully understood, and it is not clear whether it is controlled at the transcriptional or post-transcriptional level.

Transcriptional regulation of hepatocyte gene expression

There has been considerable progress in understanding the factors that regulate transcription of the genes that control the many and varied functions of the hepatocyte, such as the synthesis of albumin and α_1-antitrypsin. These transcription factors are nuclear proteins that bind to short, specific, DNA sequences, termed promoters and enhancers, located upstream and/or downstream of a given gene. Any gene will have perhaps ten such sites to which individual transcription factors can bind, and only when a full complement of factors is present is a gene effectively transcribed.

Examination of the DNA regulatory elements in a number of hepatocyte-specific genes has revealed that many carry similar sequences, though for each gene the combination and arrangement of these sites is different. In some cases the presence of a particular sequence can be used to group genes into families. For example, the acute phase response genes, C-reactive protein, haptoglobin and haemopexin all employ similar regulatory sequences.[114]

A number of sequence-specific DNA binding proteins that are important in the regulation of hepatocyte gene expression have been identified; most bind as dimers and many belong to families of similar proteins with which they can form heterodimers. The best characterized of these groups of proteins are the CCAAT enhancer binding proteins (C/EBP family), hepatocyte nuclear factors (HNF) 1α and β, HNF-3 and HNF-4. Although all are expressed in the liver, none is liver specific. Thus, the maintenance of fully differentiated hepatocyte function appears to be dependent on a complex interplay of a large number of DNA binding proteins and their specific binding elements.[115,116]

Transcription factors and the DNA sequences to which they bind are crucial in maintaining normal gene expression. As yet there is only one known example of a role for these factors in the pathogenesis of liver disease. Patients with haemophilia B Leyden, who suffer from low levels of factor IX in childhood, have a point mutation in the DNA binding site for HNF-4, thus greatly reducing the ability of HNF-4 to activate the factor IX promoter. It seems likely, however, that a role for these factors in the pathogenesis of other liver diseases will soon become apparent.

THE HEPATOCYTE

The hepatocyte is a polyhedral epithelial cell approximately 30–40 μm in diameter and, in common with other epithelial cells, it is highly polarized, with transport directed from its sinusoidal surface to the canalicular surface (Fig. 1.13). Within its plasma membrane, three specialized regions, or domains, are recognized: *basolateral* (or sinusoidal), which faces the sinusoid and the perisinusoidal space; *canalicular*, bounding that part of the intercellular space which constitutes the bile canaliculus; and *lateral*, facing the rest of the intercellular space.[88,117–119] This polarity is largely maintained by the tight junctions formed between adjacent hepatocytes in the lateral domain, which create a barrier between the two domains and also between the plasma in the intercellular space and the bile in the canaliculus. In addition to tight junctions there are also gap junctions and desmosomes in the lateral domain, and it is across this domain that intercellular communication takes place. Stereological studies in the rat have shown that the basolateral, canalicular and lateral domains comprise approximately 70%, 15% and 15% respectively of the total cell surface area.[120] Various techniques (reviewed by Meier in 1988[119]) have been used to characterize these domains, mainly in rat liver. Separation and isolation of basolateral and canalicular fractions have recently been achieved for human liver[121] and there may be differences in certain membrane marker enzymes as compared with the rat.

The *basolateral surface* is covered with abundant microvilli (Fig. 1.13b), each measuring 0.5 μm long and not evident, even as a brush or striated border, by optical microscopy. Microvilli may protrude through the fenestrae of the endothelial cells and into the sinusoidal lumen. The surface specialization is related here, as elsewhere, to absorptive and/or secretory activity; it obviously increases the surface area, but by a factor (approximately × 6) smaller than one might expect. Between the bases of the microvilli SEM shows small surface indentations or pits.[91] Some of these represent secretory vacuoles discharging into the plasma by a process of exocytosis, and others are coated pits involved in selective receptor-mediated endocytosis. The perisinusoidal space of Disse is a tissue space between the hepatocytes and the endothelial sinusoidal lining cells. Within the space of Disse extracellular matrix proteins are present in low density and they may also have a role in maintaining the polarity of the hepatocyte. However, the hepatocyte has no basement membrane and the exchange of material between the blood and hepatocytes is a function, solely, of its plasma membrane.

Canalicular surface. The bile canaliculus has no wall proper to itself. It is an intercellular space (Fig. 1.14a), formed by the apposition of the edges of gutter-like hemicanals on the adjacent surfaces of neighbouring hepatocytes (Fig. 1.14b). Its diameter varies from 0.5–1.0 μm in the perivenular area and from 1–2.5 μm in acinar zone 1. The surface is unevenly covered by microvilli (Fig. 1.14a) which are more abundant along a 'marginal ridge' at each edge of the hemi-canaliculus. In experimental biliary obstruction the canaliculi become dilated and the microvilli disappear, except along the marginal ridges. Microfilaments are particularly concentrated around the canaliculi, forming a distinct, organelle-free pericanalicular sheath, and they also extend into the microvilli. The presence of contractile elements in the pericanalicular zone can be demonstrated by indirect immunofluorescence (Fig. 1.14c) using a smooth-muscle antibody-containing serum.[122] The microfilaments are contractile, influence the calibre of the canaliculi, are functionally important in bile flow, regulate the permeability of the tight junctions and help to maintain the structural integrity of the canalicular domain[88,123,124] (see Ch. 11). The presence of ATP can be demonstrated histochemically (Fig. 1.14d), beautifully outlining the canalicular network. Accumulations of lipofuscin or haemosiderin (Fig. 1.14e) may also outline the canalicular pole of the hepatocyte.

The canalicular surface is isolated from the rest of the intercellular surface by junctional complexes, which include tight junctions, gap junctions and desmosomes (Fig. 1.14a). Tight junctions are belt-like zones of intimate contact between the plasma membranes of adjacent hepatocytes. In freeze-fracture replicas (see Fig. 11.21), the junction usually consists of no more than 3–5 parallel strands on the P-face of the membrane. The strand

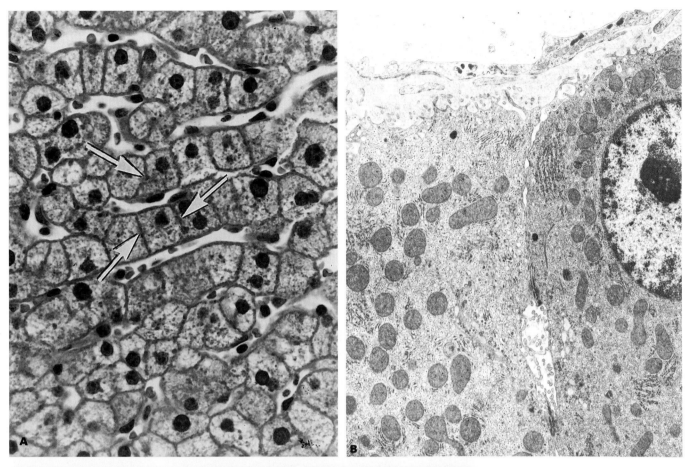

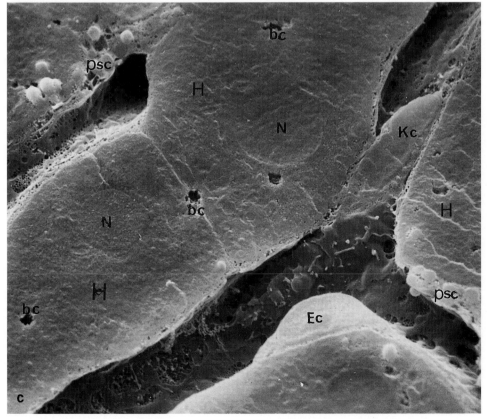

Fig. 1.13 Light microscopy. Liver-cell plates cut longitudinally show (i) a centrally placed nucleus and occasional binucleate cells, (ii) the sinusoidal surface against which Kupffer cell nuclei are abutting, (iii) the canalicular pole (arrows), (iv) the intercellular surface. (b) Transmission electron micrograph (TEM). Electron micrograph of parts of two hepatocytes, illustrating their three surfaces: sinusoidal, canalicular and intercellular. Note the microvilli on the sinusoidal surface projecting into the space of Disse. Baboon liver, × 8775 (c) Scanning electron micrograph (SEM) showing several cell types. Hepatocytes (H) contain a nucleus (N), and at the junction between cells the bile canaliculus (bc) and the intercellular surface are clearly defined. The sinusoidal surface is seen and in the sinusoidal area a Kupffer cell (Kc), endothelial cell (Ec) and two perisinusoidal cells (psc) are present. This SEM and most of the others shown in this chapter were kindly provided by Prof E Wisse, Brussels. They are all preparations of rat liver.

nearest to the canaliculus is uninterrupted and anasto-moses with those more laterally placed. The tight junc-tions constitute a permeability barrier to macromolecules between the bile canaliculus and the rest of the intercel-lular space. 'Tightness' is, however, a relative term; there seems to be a positive correlation between degrees of tight-ness and the number of strands forming the junction. On this basis the canalicular tight junctions are comparable with those elsewhere in the body (e.g. in the rete testis and vasa efferentia) which are regarded as only 'moderately tight'. Detailed descriptions of structure and function of tight and other junctions are found in chapter 11.

The *lateral surface* is the least complex of the three; it extends from the bile canaliculus to the margin of the sinusoidal surface and is specialized for cell attachment and cell–cell communication. It is not entirely plane: microvilli may extend on to it from the sinusoidal surface and protrude into narrow extensions of the space of Disse; there are occasional folds (plicae) and round-mouthed openings, which may represent pinocytic vesicles.[91] There are also seen, by SEM, knob-like protrusions and corre-sponding indentations which, fitted into one another, would form the 'press-stud' or 'snap-fastener' type of intercellular attachment long familiar in transmission electron microscopy (TEM).

There are also specialized areas called gap (or, better, communicating) junctions. These are seen by TEM as patches of close approximation of the two membranes and,

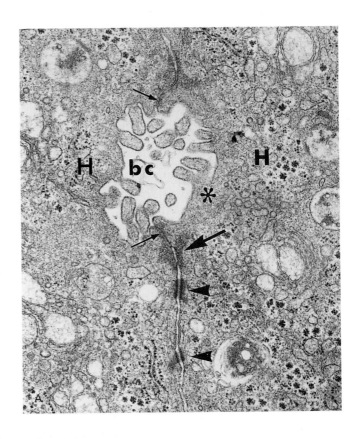

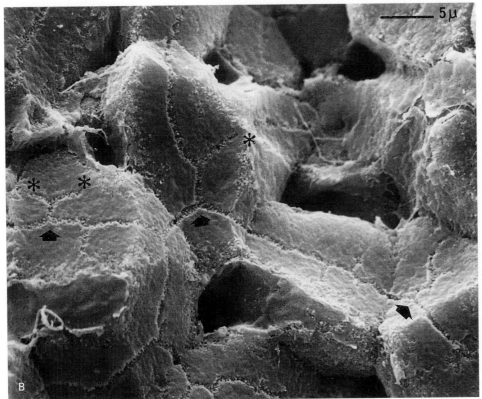

Fig. 1.14 (a) TEM. Bile canaliculus (bc). Note microvilli projecting into the lumen and the organelle-free pericanalicular cytoplasm (*). Tight junctions (broad arrow) intermediate junctions (thin arrows) and desmosomes (arrow heads) are present between the two adjacent hepatocytes (H). Human liver. Print kindly provided by Professor P Bioulac-Sage. (b) SEM. On the surface of a number of neighbouring hepatocytes, an interconnected network of bile hemi-canaliculi can be observed. The canaliculi show bifurcations (arrows) together with blunt ends (asterisks). (c) Bile canaliculi in rabbit liver: immunofluorescence preparation in which the section was reacted with a human serum containing smooth-muscle antibody: the pericanalicular microfilaments have produced strong positive immunofluorescence. (d) Pattern of bile canaliculi shown by histochemical demonstration of ATPase in pericanalicular cytoplasm. (e) Hepatocytes in iron overload; note how the pericanalicular accumulation of haemosiderin outlines the canalicular network. Perls' reaction.

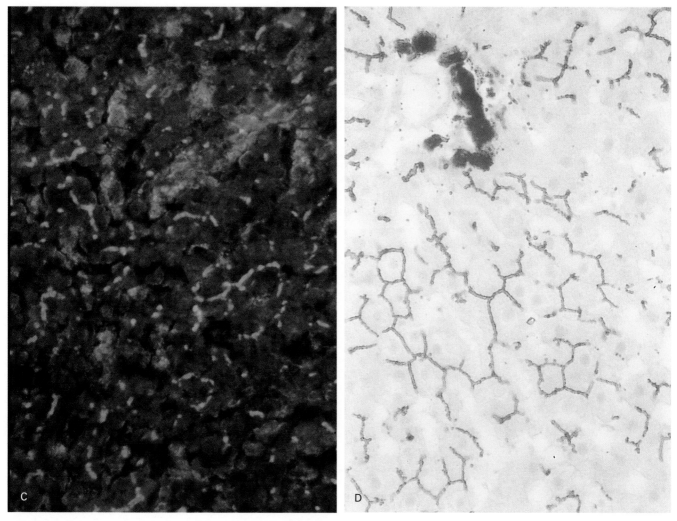

Fig. 1.14 *Contd.*

in freeze-fracture preparations, as irregularly shaped aggregates of particles on the P-face. The gap between the two membranes is 2–4 nm wide and is bridged by the intramembrane particles (of protein or lipid) which project like 'bobbins' from the external surface of each of the two membranes. Since each 'bobbin' is perforated by a central pore and apposed 'bobbins' are in contact, communications are established which provide for the transfer of ions or metabolites, or both, between hepatocytes. Such communications have been shown to play a role in the regulation of hepatocyte functions, e.g. hepatic carbohydrate metabolism by sympathetic nerve fibres.[125]

Hepatocytes in the limiting plates have a surface which abuts on the adjacent fibrous tissue, and which is irregularly covered with microvilli and may be moulded round connective tissue fibres, producing irregular indentations. The space of Mall, between the hepatocyte in the periportal area and the fibrous tissue, corresponds to the perisinusoidal space of Disse.

The domains of the hepatocyte plasma membrane are not simply topographical entities. They are specialized to subserve different functions: the isolation and study of canalicular and basolateral membrane fractions in various species, including man, have shown that there are many differences including differences in protein and lipid composition, fluidity, and the presence of various enzymes, receptors and transport systems.[118,121,126] The hepatocytes can decrease or increase the concentration of specific proteins in each domain. In addition, recycling of the plasma membrane occurs such that following receptor-mediated endocytosis or 'internalization' the receptor can be recycled back to the cell surface. The precise mechanisms by which the hepatocyte regulates and maintains the heterogeneity of its surface domains are still not clear, nor do we know how alterations in liver-cell plasma membranes contribute to, or result in, specific liver diseases.

Nucleus

This shows the characteristics one would expect in the nucleus of a cell actively engaged in protein synthesis: it is large, occupying 5–10% of the volume of the cell, and

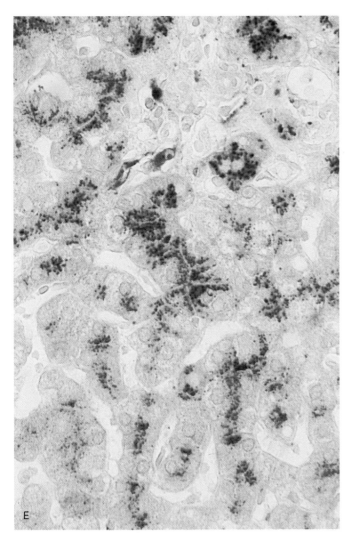

E

Fig. 1.14 *Contd.*

spherical, with one or more prominent nucleoli and scattered chromatin. There is considerable variation in both number and size of nuclei. About 25% of the cells are binucleate: the two nuclei are similar in size and staining properties and they divide simultaneously. At birth, all but a few hepatocytes are mononuclear. Hepatocyte nuclei fall into various size classes, with volumes in the ratio 1:2:4:8. This variation reflects polyploidy, the DNA content increasing correspondingly.[127] At birth, in man, nearly all hepatocytes are diploid (and mononucleate). From the eighth year, when more than 90% of hepatocytes are diploid, the number of tetraploid nuclei (i.e. those with twice the normal DNA content) increases, to reach about 15% in children of 15 years.[128] Tetraploid cells are thought to arise by mitosis of cells with two diploid nuclei. The DNA content of each nucleus doubles, but the chromosomes are then arranged on a single mitotic spindle, so that division produces two daughter cells, each with a single tetraploid nucleus. The significance of polyploidy in hepatocytes is unknown. Since cell size is proportional to cell ploidy,[129] polyploidy does not provide an increased amount of genetic material per unit volume of cytoplasm.

Mitotic division provides for embryonic and early post-natal growth, but the adult liver has a very low mitotic index, with estimates ranging from one mitosis per 10–20 000 cells, to 2.2 mitoses per 1000 cells. The liver has hitherto been classified as a conditional renewal system,[35] and the individual hepatocyte is correspondingly long-lived: cell life may be up to 300 days or even measured in years in laboratory rodents.[130] However, these figures may need downward revision if the liver is shown to be a stem cell and lineage system (p. 8).

Endoplasmic reticulum

This topic has recently been reviewed by De Pierre and his colleagues.[131]

Optical microscopy of liver from a well-fed animal shows granular clumps of basophilic material (the 'ergastoplasm') which, like similar material in other cells, was identified on electron microscopy with rough endoplasmic reticulum (RER). This consists of a network of parallel, flattened sacs or cisternae on whose cytoplasmic surfaces are attached polyribosomes (Fig. 1.15a,b). Clusters of RER are scattered randomly throughout the cytoplasm and constitute approximately 60% of the endoplasmic reticulum. The remaining 40% constitutes the smooth endoplasmic reticulum (SER), which also forms anastomosing networks of tubules and vesicles of varying diameter and which are continuous with the cisternae of the RER; they lack a ribosomal coating, hence the designation smooth or agranular (Fig. 1.16). The outer nuclear membrane also has attached ribosomes, and continuity between the outer nuclear membrane and the outer membrane of the RER has been demonstrated. The SER is often found in the region of the Golgi apparatus and communicates with it; there is frequently a close topographical relationship of the SER with glycogen (Fig. 1.16). Following cell disruption and differential centrifugation the RER is a principal constituent of the so-called microsomal fraction. Studies of isolated rat microsomes suggest that the membrane of the ER comprises about 10% protein and 30% lipid, of which 85% is phospholipid. The ER occupies 15% of the total cell volume and its surface area — approximately 60 000 μm^2 per hepatocyte — is more than 35 times the area of the plasma membrane. There is also zonality in the distribution of the ER; the surface area of SER in zone 3 of the acinus is twice that in zone 1.

A variety of electron microscopic and biochemical techniques has shown the synthesis of protein at the polyribosomes, and its entry into the cisternae of the RER through which it passes via the SER to the Golgi ap-

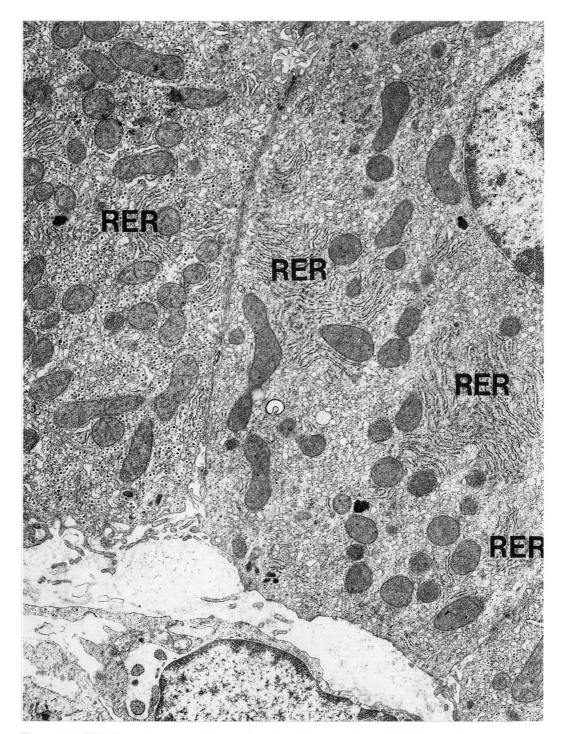

Fig. 1.15 (a) TEM illustrating scattered clumps of rough endoplasmic reticulum (RER) in two adjacent hepatocytes. Baboon liver, × 6150. (The TEMs of baboon liver were prepared by H. Johnston)

paratus. It travels from here to be 'packaged for export' in Golgi-derived secretory vesicles.

The cell functions which are associated with the ER include: (i) protein synthesis, both secretory proteins and some of the protein constituents of the cell and organelle membranes; (ii) the metabolism of fatty acids, phospho-lipids and triglycerides; (iii) the production and metabolism of cholesterol and, possibly, the production of bile acids; (iv) xenobiotic metabolism; (v) ascorbic acid synthesis; and (vi) haem degradation.

Not all protein synthesis in the hepatocyte involves the ER however; some, including structural proteins of the

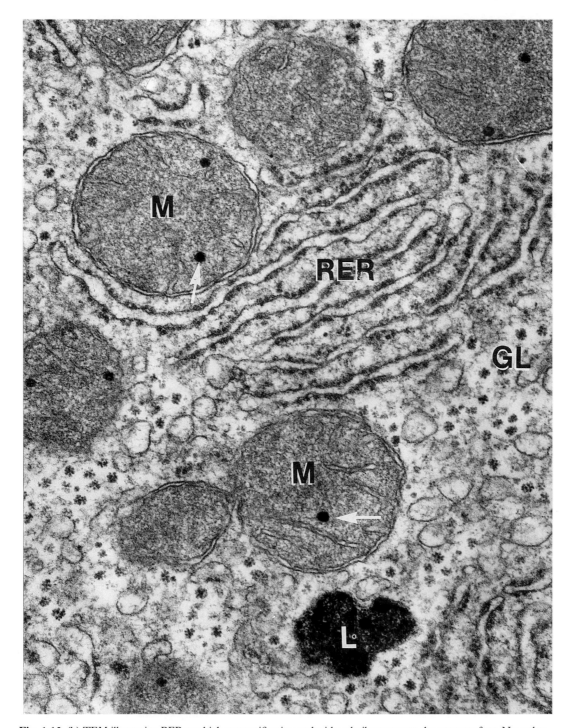

Fig. 1.15 (b) TEM illustrating RER at a higher magnification and with polyribosomes on the outer surface. Note also mitochondria (M) in which matrix granules (arrows) are conspicuous, a lysosome (L), and glycogen rosettes (GL). Baboon liver, × 35 000

cell itself, are formed by free ribosomes, a process which is particularly active during development and regeneration when the number of these organelles can fluctuate considerably. The cytochrome P-450 system is localized in the ER and this is the system whereby the liver cell functions in the metabolism and detoxification of xenobiotics. This enzyme system can be reversibly induced by certain xeno-

biotics, e.g. phenobarbitol (see Ch. 15), and this is accompanied by the synthesis and hypertrophy of ER; the mechanisms involved in new membrane production are not clear.

Glucose-6-phosphatase is localized on the ER but the role, if any, of the ER in glycogen metabolism is not clear. The SER proliferates during synthesis of glycogen and

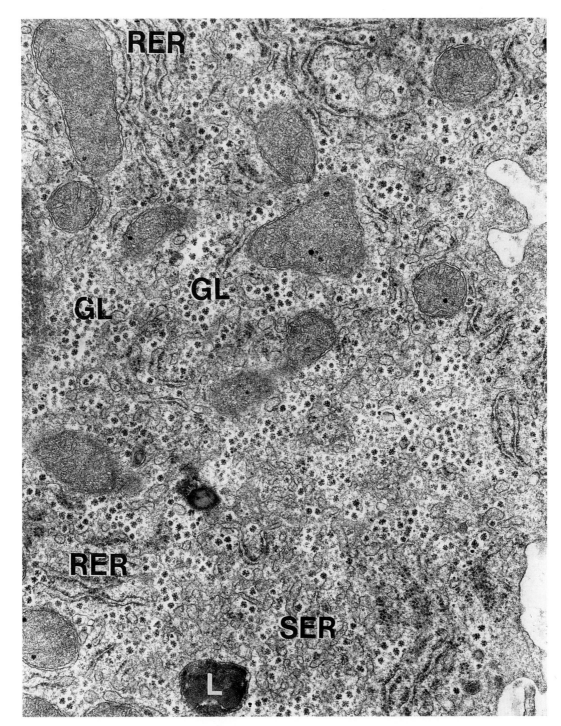

Fig. 1.16 TEM illustrating networks of smooth endoplasmic reticulum (SER) contrasting with RER. Note also glycogen rosettes (GL) and a lysosome (L). Baboon liver, × 16 650.

during its degradation in fasting animals.[132] However, SER is absent during the period of rapid glycogenolysis which occurs in mammalian livers just after birth.[133]

Golgi complex

Each hepatocyte contains as many as 50 Golgi zones (which may not be separate but rather form a tri-dimen-sional continuity) situated most commonly near to the bile canaliculus or beside the nucleus.[131] Each complex appears as a stack of four to six curved, flattened parallel sacs, often with dilated bulbous ends containing electron-dense material. The convex or cis surface is directed towards the ER and small vesicles in the cis-Golgi transfer synthesized proteins from the ER. The concave or trans surface is the origin of the secretory vesicles. Vesicles break off from the ends of the sacs and carry the contained secretory proteins, including lipoproteins, for discharge at the sinusoidal surface. Numerous small primary lysosomes are also present in the vicinity of the Golgi complex. The complex and its associated cytoplasm constitutes approximately 2–4% of the cell volume. In addition to its role in the secretion of lipoproteins the Golgi complex is important in the glycosylation of secretory proteins and in the synthesis and recycling of membrane glycoprotein receptors.[131]

The close and frequent juxtaposition of Golgi zones and the bile canaliculus has long suggested a role for the Golgi in bile secretion. When hepatocytes are disaggregated by enzyme perfusion, the bile canaliculi disappear and the peripheral location of the Golgi complexes is lost; however, after 24 hours in vitro monolayer culture, new bile canaliculi are formed and the Golgi–biliary polarity is restored.[134] In recent years bile acids have been demonstrated within Golgi vesicles[135] and there is now good evidence that the Golgi complex is functionally important in bile secretion.[88]

Lysosomes

The existence of lysosomes was first predicted by De Duve on the basis of biochemical studies on liver homogenates,[136] and it was he who subsequently identified them with the 'peribiliary dense bodies' found in electron micrographs of liver, and who established them as a new species of cell organelle. Their functions in health and disease have been reviewed,[137,138] and thus are of particular importance to pathologists because of their involvement in a number of storage diseases (see Ch. 4).

Lysosomes present a variety of appearances in electron micrographs of liver (Figs 1.15 and 1.16), but basically they are vesicles, bounded by a single membrane, containing acid hydrolases — e.g. acid phosphatase, aryl sulphatase, esterase and β-glucuronidase. Their form is so variable that unequivocal identification depends on histochemical demonstration of one of the contained enzymes, most conveniently acid phosphatase.

Lysosomes of this type are essentially storage granules for enzymes, sequestered by membranes from contact with the cytoplasm; the enzymes are elaborated by the usual mechanism of protein synthesis — RER–SER–Golgi complex. Lysosomes number about 15–20 per hepatocyte in the rat and, although they are found particularly in the neighbourhood of the bile canaliculus, there is at present no evidence of their direct involvement in the production or excretion of bile.

Their pleomorphism reflects a variety of functions:

1. Although the liver cell is long-lived, there is evidence for turnover of its cytoplasm and organelles: e.g. the half-life of hepatocyte mitochondria is estimated at approximately ten days and that of the RER at much less. Cytoplasmic constituents may become incorporated within, and digested by, the primary lysosome, forming with it an autophagic vacuole, one variety of secondary lysosome. Autophagic vacuoles, therefore, show fragments of organelles or of cell inclusions in various stages of digestion. The phenomenon is seen most strikingly in the liver of starving animals when parts of hepatocyte cytoplasm are sacrificed to meet the metabolic needs of the organism. Very rapid glycogenolysis, as in the immediate postnatal period in mammals, is associated with the appearance of 'glycogenosomes' — lysosomes which have incorporated glycogen particles, and, presumably, break them down. Autophagic vacuoles are also conspicuous during periods of rapid growth and differentiation in liver, both in development and in regeneration.

2. Lysosomes also incorporate lipofuscin pigment, which may accumulate, undigested, over long periods, forming so-called residual bodies, and material of exogenous origin, including iron, stored as ferritin, which accumulates in large quantities in iron overload states (see Ch. 5).

3. Coated vesicles and multivesicular bodies result from receptor-mediated endocytosis.[140] Following aggregation of ligand–receptor complexes in clathrin-coated pits on the basolateral cell surface these vesicles are internalized to form endosomes or endocytic vesicles. Ligands which are internalized by hepatocytes in this way include insulin, low-density lipoproteins, transferrin, IgA and asialoglycoproteins. Fusion of endosomes occurs to form multivesicular bodies. Some of these vesicles are responsible for transcytosis or intracellular transport from the basolateral domain to the canalicular domain; others fuse with primary lysosomes and their contents undergo partial degradation before being exocytosed at the canalicular or basolateral domain; still others undergo complete degradation and become increasingly electron dense with the formation of dense bodies.[88,138,139] Microtubules (p. 28) appear to have an important role in sorting the pathways along which endocytic vesicles move within the hepatocyte.[141]

Peroxisomes (microbodies)

These are ovoid, single, membrane-bound granules 0.2–1.0 μm in diameter, first described as microbodies by Rouiller & Bernhard in 1956.[141] Each hepatocyte may contain 300–600 peroxisomes and they comprise 1.5–2% of cell volume. There is morphological heterogeneity between species; in the rat, peroxisomes contain a paracrystalline striated core or nucleoid in which urate oxidase is concentrated; human peroxisomes lack a core.[142] Peroxisomes contain oxidases which use molecular oxygen to oxidize a number of substrates with the production of hydrogen peroxide (hence the name of the organelle) which, in turn, is hydrolysed by peroxisomal catalase. Approximately 20% of the oxygen consumption of the liver is used in peroxisomal activity. The energy produced by this oxidation is dissipated as heat. Alcohol may be metabolized in the liver by peroxisomal catalase (see Ch. 10). Drugs, such as clofibrate, which lower blood lipids cause a proliferation of peroxisomes, an increase that has been causally linked to their hypolipidaemic action.[143] Alterations in hepatocyte perixosomes have been reported in bacterial infections, viral hepatitis, Wilson's disease, alcoholic liver diseases and cirrhosis.[145,145a] Since the last edition of this text a number of metabolic disorders have been described in which there is either an absence of peroxisomes or a deficiency of peroxisomal enzymes.[145,146] The liver involvement in these is discussed in chapter 4.

Mitochondria

These are large organelles (1.5 μm in diameter and up to 4 μm long), approximately 1000 per cell, constituting about 20% of the cytoplasmic volume of hepatocytes.[149] They show the features commonly regarded as characteristic of mitochondria in general: an outer membrane, separated by a gap from an inner membrane, from which highly convoluted cristal folds project into the interior of the organelles, to be surrounded by matrix (Figs 1.15b and 1.17). The cristae considerably increase the area of the inner membrane and, in liver cells, it constitutes about a third of the total membrane of the cell. Stains such as Janus green used to demonstrate mitochondria in living cells by light microscopy do so by virtue of their oxidation by the mitochondria. Fluorescent dyes can also be used to study mitochondria in living cells; these dyes are lipid-soluble cations and accumulate in mitochondria because of the large, interior, negative membrane potential.[148] The matrix contains electron-dense granules (Fig. 1.15b), which may represent concentration of Ca^{2+}, a small circular DNA and ribosomes. Crystalloid structures may also be present but are a non-specific feature and are not related to any disease. The DNA codes for some of the mitochondrion's own proteins which are synthesized on the ribosomes within the organelles. The larger proportion of the organelles' protein, however, is encoded by nuclear DNA and then 'imported'. Mitochondria are self-replicating, with a half-life of about 10 days. Mutations in the mitochondrial genome account for various mitochondrial myopathies,[149] but no liver-associated disease has yet been attributed to such a lesion. Mitochondria may fuse and are remarkably mobile organelles which move about in the cytoplasm, closely associated with microtubules.

In three important papers, Candipan & Sjostrand[150–152] have shown that the methods almost universally used to prepare liver for electron microscopic study may produce appearances in the mitochondria which, though widely

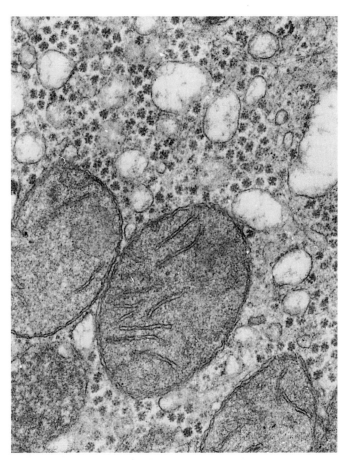

Fig. 1.17 TEM to show mitochondria, illustrating the matrix and cristae comprising outer and inner membranes separated by an intermembrane gap. Human liver, × 39 000.

accepted as real, are probably artefactual. In particular, their findings suggest: (i) that the inner and outer membranes are closely apposed and that there is no space within the crista; (ii) that the cristal membrane is not simply an infolding of the inner membrane but differs structurally from it; (iii) that there is no evidence that the cristae undergo 'conformational changes' in different metabolic states; (iv) that the two size classes of mitochondria often referred to as 'condensed' and 'orthodox' are preparative artefacts. These findings, and the knowledge that mitochondria move and change their shape in living cells, make difficult the interpretation of changes in mitochondrial morphology thought to be related to disease processes.

The structural compartmentation of mitochondria provides for topographical localization of various enzyme systems, the details of which form almost a science in themselves. It need only be said here that the outer membrane is relatively unimportant as a locus for enzymes; it keeps the inner membrane together and contains porin, a transport protein which forms channels which are permeable to molecules less than 2 kD.[147] The inner membrane and cristal lamellae support the respiratory chain enzymes concerned with oxidative phosphorylation which generates ATP. The matrix contains most of the components of the citric acid cycle and the enzymes involved in beta oxidation of fatty acids and in the urea cycle. Mitochondria are randomly distributed within individual hepatocytes but are smaller and more numerous in acinar zone 3 than in acinar zone 1 cells, and occupy only 13% of cell volume in the periportal cells.[153] These differences may, as already discussed, be of functional significance.

The cytoskeleton

The major components of the cytoskeleton of most eukaryotic cells, including the hepatocytes, comprise 6 nm microfilaments, 8–10 nm intermediate filaments and 20 nm microtubules. These are structurally, chemically and functionally distinct and are dynamic structures capable of rapid modulation and adaptation in response to functional demands. In addition, there are a number of accessory proteins which modulate these components, and which link them to one another, to cell organelles and to the cell membrane; these are part of a microtrabecular lattice or cytomatrix. These structures interact to regulate internal organization, cell shape, movement, secretion and division.[117,154–156] They can be visualized on TEM and SEM, but more recently the use of polyclonal and monoclonal antibodies in immunohistochemical methods has allowed their investigation by light microscopy.

Microfilaments are double-stranded molecules of polymerized fibrous (F) actin; the monomeric form of the protein is globular (G) actin and these two forms exist in equilibrium in the cell. The microfilaments are present in bundles and form a three-dimensional intracellular meshwork. There is extensive intracellular binding and cross-linking with other intracellular proteins such as myosin, lamin, and spectrin. The filaments are mainly located at the cell periphery; they attach to the plasma membrane and extend into microvilli. They are particularly concentrated in the pericanalicular ectoplasm and attach to the junctional complexes which limit the canaliculus. The functional roles for microfilaments involve cell membrane motility, endo- and exocytosis, secretion and vesicle transfer. Their major role in bile secretion is discussed in chapter 12.

Microtubules are a family of unbranched rigid tubules of variable length which are structurally similar in all cells. They are polymers composed of two subunits of tubulin, α and β. Polymerization and growth take place from organizing centres including centrioles. Microtubules are part of the mitotic apparatus. They are also present in cell cilia. Like the microfilaments, they attach to and cross-link a number of proteins. In addition to their role in cell division, microtubules contribute to the maintenance of cell shape, cell movement, intracellular move-ment and transfer, protein secretion and canalicular membrane activity (see Ch. 11). The precise mechanisms by which they exert these functions have recently been reviewed.[157]

Intermediate filaments are a family of self-assembling protein fibres. They are structurally similar in all cells, comprising a central 'backbone' of assembled rods. In addition the individual polypeptides in intermediate filaments are arranged in an α-helical coiled-coil arrangement which confers tensile strength. Unlike the microtubules and microfilaments, intermediate filaments are heterogeneous in subunit composition and antigenicity, and are grouped into five immunologically distinct types whose distribution is cell specific:[158] cytokeratin, desmin, vimentin, glial fibrillary acidic protein and neurofilaments. Cytokeratins are the intermediate filaments of epithelial cells and are present in hepatocytes and, in greater amounts, in bile-duct epithelium. The are thought to act as an intracellular scaffold and are most numerous where there is cellular mechanical stress. In the liver cells, they are located just inside the plasma membrane and are particularly condensed in the pericanalicular sheath. They are linked to desmosomes on the lateral plasma membrane of hepatocytes. They attach to other components of the cytoskeleton, and to organelles such as the RER and vesicles. They function as 'the mechanical integrators of cellular space'.[154]

The cytokeratins can be further divided on the basis of their molecular weight into 19 subtypes.[21] Most epithelial cells contain at least two, one of which is acidic and the other basic. In hepatocytes, cytokeratins 8 and 18 are present, while bile-duct epithelium also contains cytokeratins 7 and 19, a phenotypic difference which, as discussed earlier, becomes established during embryogenesis. Intermediate filaments are present in Mallory bodies. In alcoholic liver disease and other types of liver injury Mallory bodies are thought to form as a result of microtubule depolymerization (Fig. 1.18) with a consequent collapse of the intermediate filament network.

The microtrabecular lattice or *cytomatrix* comprises an extremely fine filamentous network in the cell cytoplasm which, as first suggested by Frey-Wyssling in 1948,[159] confers a 'molecular framework' on it. This microtrabecular lattice divides the cytoplasm into two continuous phases, one protein-rich and the other water-rich.[160] The other cytoskeletal components interact with the microtrabecular lattice which, like them, is readily modulated and altered to ensure normal cell function.

Glycogen

A principal function of liver is the synthesis of glycogen (from glucose, or from lactic and pyruvic acids or glycerol), its storage and its breakdown and release as glucose into the circulation. It is depleted in fasting

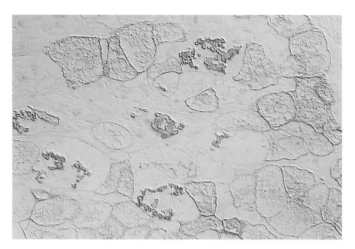

Fig. 1.18 Liver biopsy from a patient with alcoholic liver disease: immunoperoxidase staining of cytokeratin with antibody CAM 5.2. The cytokeratin microfilaments form a regular network within most of the liver cells but, in some, the network pattern is lost and the microfilaments are aggregated to form coarse, discrete Mallory bodies. By courtesy of Dr A D Burt.

animals, disappearing last from the cells in acinar zone 3; on refeeding, it appears first in periportal cells and in well-fed animals becomes uniformly distributed throughout the acinus. In electron micrographs, glycogen appears as dense granules of two types, β particles 15–30 nm in diameter, and α particles, aggregates of the smaller particles arranged in rosettes (Fig. 1.16). Intranuclear glycogen usually appears as β particles.

The zonal pattern of distribution of glycogen has been beautifully demonstrated by using density gradients to separate 'light' and 'heavy' hepatocytes from suspensions of dissociated cells.[161] Glycogen concentrations are similar in the two types, but in the perivenular ('light') cells, the glycogen granules are dispersed between the SER tubules, whereas in the heavy cells they are packed in large aggregates. It is not clear how far these and other differential characteristics of hepatocytes are a function of their topographical location and how far they depend on intrinsic genetic differences.

THE HEPATIC SINUSOID AND THE SINUSOIDAL CELLS

Sinusoids (Fig. 1.19a) have an average diameter of about 10 μm, but they may distend to about 30 μm. Periportal sinusoids are more tortuous than the perivenular ones.[162] Four distinct types of sinusoidal cell can be identified, each with its own characteristic morphology, topography and population dynamics:[163] the lining of the sinusoids is formed by endothelial cells; the perisinusoidal cells are found in the space of Disse which lies between the sinusoidal endothelial cells and the hepatocytes; the Kupffer cells and liver-associated lymphocytes lie on the luminal aspect of the endothelium.

Sinusoidal endothelial cells

These form an attenuated cytoplasmic sheet (about 50–80 nm in maximum thickness) perforated by numerous holes (fenestrae) and, unlike endothelial cells elsewhere, they apparently do not form junctions with adjacent endothelial cells. The fenestrae are so abundant that, in SEM, the greater part of the cell has a net-like appearance, forming a tenuous barrier, reinforced here and there where adjacent endothelial cells overlap one another (Fig. 1.19b). The fenestrae measure 0.1–0.2 μm in diameter and are grouped in clusters forming so-called sieve plates. The diameter of the fenestrae is greater in the perivenular zone but there is also a marked increase in their number. Thus, endothelial cell porosity is higher in the perivenular zone (acinar zone 3) than in the periportal zone (acinar zone 1).[164] The smaller fenestrae are intracellular and appear in cultured endothelial cells. The larger are usually intercellular, and some workers consider that they may be artefacts due to fixation.[162] There is evidence that fenestrae are labile structures whose diameters may change in response to endogenous mediators (e.g. serotonin)[164] and exogenous agents such as alcohol.[165] The fenestrae lack diaphragms and since, in most species, a basement membrane is absent on the deep surface of the sinusoidal endothelium, there is continuity between the sinusoidal lumen and the perisinusoidal space of Disse.

This unique structure allows the endothelial cells to filter the sinusoidal blood. Solutes pass freely through the fenestrae from the lumen into the space of Disse and come into contact with the hepatocytes. Large particles such as newly generated chylomicrons, however, are excluded. Wisse and co-workers[166] have postulated that transport of materials through the fenestrae may be facilitated by the pressure effect of blood cells in the sinusoidal lumen— flexible erythrocytes pressing plasma and small particles into the space of Disse ('forced sieving') and rigid leucocytes squeezing fluid out ('endothelial massage' — see Fig. 1.26).

Sinusoidal endothelial cells show a number of phenotypic differences compared with vascular endothelium. They do not bind the lectin *Ulex europaeus* and, in most species, do not express factor VIII-related antigen (von Willebrand factor),[163] although the cells assume these properties in chronic liver disease.[167,168] Furthermore, they do not normally contain other molecules characteristically found in vascular endothelium, such as GMP-140 and CD34, but do express Fcγ IgG receptors (CD16 and CDw32), CD4, CD14 and aminopeptidase N.[163,169] They also exhibit membrane immunoreactivity for ICAM-1.[169] The natural ligand for this adhesion molecule, LFA-1, is present on Kupffer cells; this receptor may therefore be involved in adhesion of Kupffer cells to the endothelial lining.[169] Up-regulation

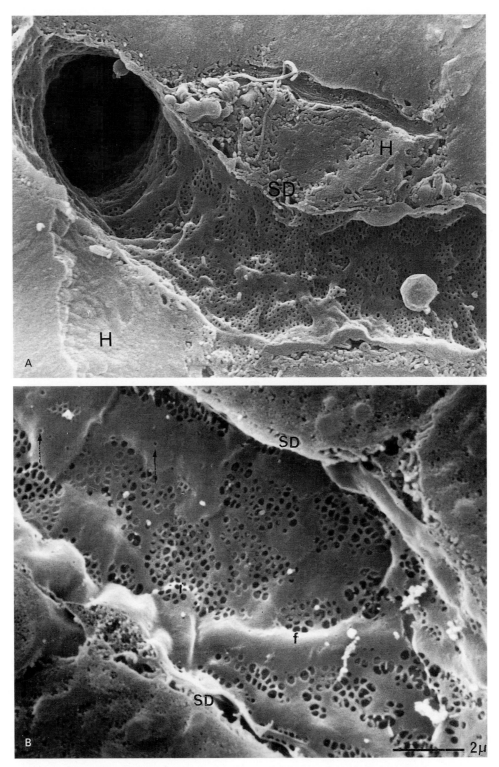

Fig. 1.19 (a) SEM. Normal hepatic sinusoid in rat liver. Note the regular distribution of fenestrae in the sieve plates which are separated by intervening cytoplasmic processes. H = hepatocyte; SD = space of Disse. (b) SEM. Endothelial fenestrations (f) of about 0.1 μm are grouped together in sieve plates. Processes of endothelial cells show small holes, most probably representing the pinching off of micropinocytotic vesicles (arrows). SD = Space of Disse.

of ICAM-1 expression in sinusoidal endothelial cells may be important in 'trapping' LFA-1 positive lymphocytes in inflammatory liver diseases.[170] There is also sinusoidal endothelial cell heterogeneity within the acinus: the increased porosity in acinar zone 3 has already been mentioned but, in addition, heterogeneous lectin binding and expression of various receptors have also been demonstrated.[169,171]

Another unusual feature of sinusoidal endothelial cells is their high endocytotic activity.[166] This process appears to be directed towards uptake and lysosomal degradation of compounds rather than providing an alternative route for their transport from the sinusoidal lumen to the space of Disse. The intracellular handling of denatured proteins such as formaldehyde-treated albumin has been well documented in isolated sinusoidal endothelial cells.[172] The protein binds to so-called scavenger receptors on the cell membrane and is rapidly internalized with the formation of vesicles. These are transferred to smooth, membrane-lined endosomes which become transformed into dense-body type lysosomes when they receive hydrolytic enzymes from transfer tubules, probably derived from the Golgi complex. Other receptors, now identified on these cells, may mediate endocytosis of a large number of endogenous compounds, some of which are effete molecules and are cleared from the circulation and others which are modified and undergo transcytosis to hepatocytes.[173] The sinusoidal endothelial cells also have synthetic activity and produce prostaglandins, endothelin and possibly cytokines such as interleukin-1 and interleukin-6.[173]

The space of Disse and the perisinusoidal cells

The space of Disse lies primarily between the sinusoidal wall and the outer sinusoidal surface of the hepatocyte, from which abundant microvilli project into the space and may be of importance in keeping the space open. This space is not normally discernible in biopsy material but in autopsy liver the hepatocytes shrink from the sinusoids and the space is then characteristically evident. Studies with SEM show extensions of the space outwards between adjacent hepatic cells and this considerably expands the perisinusoidal compartment.[174] It forms, therefore, an extensive and almost unique extravascular space. As noted earlier, the sinusoidal endothelium is not only discontinuous and extensively fenestrated, but in many species (including man) lacks a basement membrane. It is thus freely permeable to blood plasma, which enters the space and comes into direct contact with the hepatocytes. This extravascular plasma constitutes the immediate medium of exchange between blood and hepatocytes, whose surface area of contact is increased by the abundant microvilli. The plasma is then presumed to flow towards the centre of the hepatic acini; some, however, is taken up by lymphatic spaces in the periportal zone and some may re-enter the sinusoidal blood. The movement of plasma in the space of Disse may, in part, be due to the 'endothelial massage' effect of leucocytes (p. 39). The nature of the anatomical link between the periportal ends of the space of Disse and the lymphatics is discussed later.

The space of Disse contains striated collagen fibres composed of type III and type I collagen;[175] this constitutes the 'reticulin' framework of the liver. Several other extracellular matrix components, however, can be demonstrated by immunohistochemistry. In spite of the absence of an identifiable basement membrane at this site, basement membrane components — collagen type IV, laminin and heparan sulphate proteoglycan — are present. The composition of the perisinusoidal matrix is thought to be crucial for maintaining the function of hepatocytes. The importance of altered cell–matrix interactions in chronic liver disease has recently been reviewed[176] and is discussed in chapter 10.

Within the space of Disse are stellate cells whose long cytoplasmic processes surround the sinusoids (Fig. 1.20a–c). The perikarya of the cells are usually found within recesses between hepatocytes. They have been referred to under a variety of terms — Ito cells, hepatic lipocytes, fat-storing cells, stellate cells and parasinusoidal cells[177–179] — but, throughout this text, we call them perisinusoidal cells. They contain many small lipid droplets (Fig. 1.20c) which are rich in vitamin A; this can be demonstrated by fluorescence microscopy when excitation light of 328 nm wavelength is used and by gold chloride impregnation. Rough endoplasmic reticulum and Golgi apparatus are well developed in these cells (Fig. 1.20c). They are considered to have two major functions: storage of vitamin A and production of extracellular matrix proteins.[177,179–181]

In most species they represent the major site of storage for vitamin A. Dietary retinyl esters reach the liver in chylomicron remnants. These pass from the sinusoidal lumen through the endothelial fenestrae and are taken up by hepatocytes. Most of the endocytosed retinol is rapidly transferred to the perisinusoidal cells for storage by, an as yet poorly defined, transport mechanism.[180] The cells contain a high concentration of cellular retinoid-binding protein and cellular retinol-acid binding protein.

There is now overwhelming evidence that perisinusoidal cells are the major source of extracellular matrix proteins in normal and fibrotic liver[176,179–181]. They proliferate in response to acute and chronic liver injury and undergo phenotypic changes to so-called transitional cells and myofibroblasts; this is associated with enhanced matrix protein synthesis and is mediated by cytokines released by activated Kupffer cells, platelets and, possibly, compounds released by damaged sinusoidal endothelium and hepatocytes.[176]

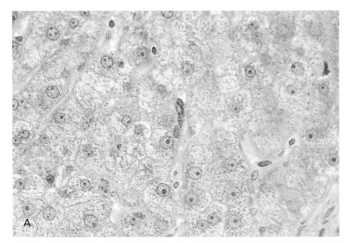

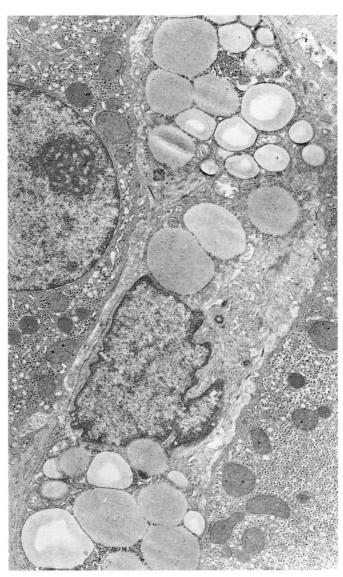

Fig. 1.20 Perisinusoidal cells. (a) These may ocasionally be seen on optical microscopy; the fat globules are phloxinophilic in this section stained by Masson's trichrome and the perisinusoidal location of the cell is readily appreciated. (b) Rat liver: immunoperoxidase stain for desmin; the perisinusoidal cells show extensive prolongation of their cytoplasm within the space of Disse. (c) TEM showing a perisinusoidal cell, lying within Disse's space. Note numerous non-membrane-bound fat globules and the profiles of rough endoplasmic reticulum. Human liver × 7375.

The morphological similarities between perisinusoidal cells and pericytes of other tissues, their ultrastructural appearance, and the demonstration of the muscle-associated protein desmin in their cytoplasm (Fig. 1.20b) have all raised the possibility that they may be contractile.[182] In vitro evidence of cytokine-mediated contractility has been reported.[183] However, the role of perisinusoidal cells in controlling intrasinusoidal blood flow remains speculative.

The Kupffer cells

Kupffer cells are hepatic macrophages and are present in the lumen of hepatic sinusoids (Fig. 1.21a,b). They belong to the mononuclear phagocytic system but manifest phenotypic differences which distinguish them from other macrophages. They are of considerable importance

in host defence mechanisms and in addition have an important role in the pathogenesis of various liver diseases.[184] On SEM, Kupffer cells have an irregular stellate shape[185] and within the sinusoidal lumen the cell body rests on the endothelial lining (Fig. 1.21c). They are more numerous in the periportal sinusoids[186] and there is some evidence that, like hepatocytes, Kupffer cells also manifest functional heterogeneity in the liver acinus.[186,187] They never form junctional complexes with endothelial cells, but they may be found in gaps between adjacent endothelial cells and their protoplasmic processes may extend through larger endothelial fenestrae into the perisinusoidal space (Fig. 1.21a). The luminal surface shows many of the structural features associated with macrophages: small microvilli and microplicae and sinuous invaginations of the plasma membrane. These features together give to the surface the appearance of a micro-labyrinth (Fig. 1.21c).

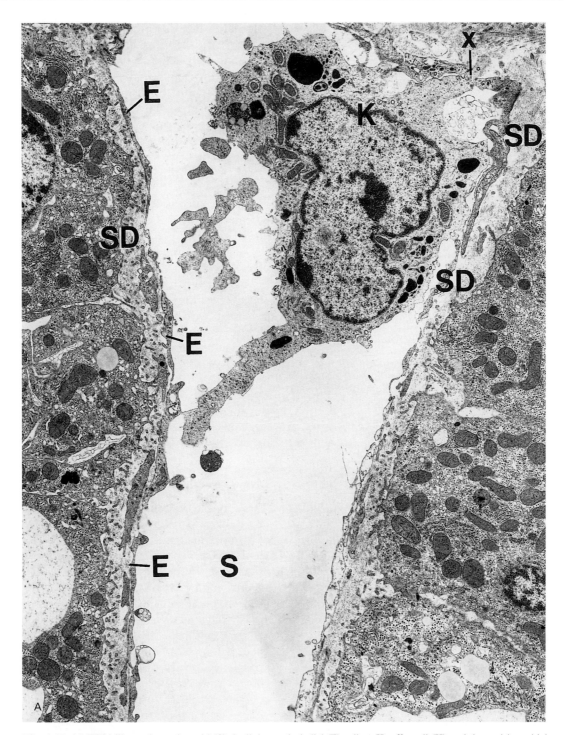

Fig. 1.21 (a) TEM illustrating a sinusoid (S), its lining endothelial (E) cells. a Kupffer cell (K) and the perisinusoidal spaces of Disse (SD). At 'x' a Kupffer cell cytoplasmic process extends into the perisinusoidal space through an endothelial fenestra. Baboon liver, × 2500. (b) TEM of rat liver Kupffer cell; note the irregular cell surface; numerous lysosomes are present in the cytoplasm. L = sinusoidal lumen; SD = space of Disse. × 9600. Courtesy of Prof E Wisse. (c) SEM. Part of Kupffer cell lying in a sinusoid and showing characteristic microvilli projecting at the cell surface (arrows). Small rims of fenestrated endothelium can be observed at both sides of the Kupffer cell-f. A small bundle of collagen fibres-c is situated in the space of Disse (SD) on the right.

Kupffer cells have been considered to be fixed tissue macrophages, but they appear capable of actively migrating along the sinusoids, both with and against the blood flow, and can migrate into areas of liver injury and into regional lymph nodes.[188] They selectively phagocytose vital dyes, particulate material and effete erythrocytes. They contain lysosomes and phagosomes, and the cisternae of their endoplasmic reticulum are rich in peroxi-

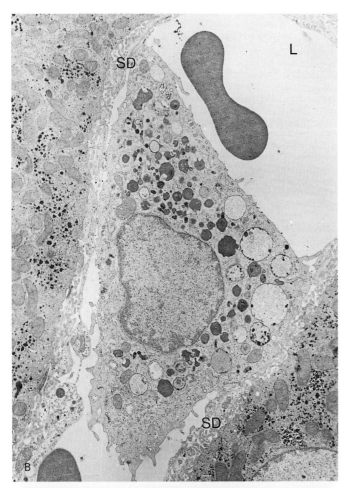

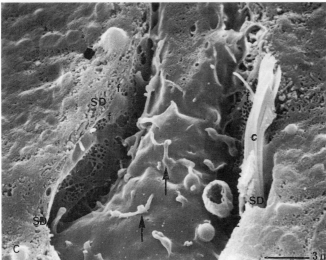

Fig. 1.21 *Contd.*

dase. Their primary function is the ingestion and degradation of particulate and soluble material in portal blood. The efficiency of this clearance function is shown by the fact that removal of particulate material is limited only by the magnitude of hepatic blood flow and that removal of particles may approach single-pass efficiency. Kupffer

cells play a major role in clearance of endotoxin from the blood.[186] This leads to the release of a variety of mediators including interleukins 1 and 6, tumour necrosis factor α (TNFα), interferons and eicosanoids which participate in the host response to infection and are responsible for some of the clinical manifestations of endotoxaemia. Several cytokines released by activated Kupffer cells are also thought to have local effects, modulating microvascular responses[93] and the functions of hepatocytes and perisinusoidal cells[189] (see Chs 2 and 10). Although Kupffer cells can express class II histocompatibility antigens[190] and can function in vitro as antigen-presenting cells, they appear to be considerably less efficient at this than macrophages at other sites.[191] Their principal roles in the immune response therefore, appear to be antigen sequestration by phagocytosis and clearance of immune complexes.[192]

There is firm evidence from bone marrow transplant and liver transplant studies that Kupffer cells are derived, at least in part, from circulating monocytes.[193] However, Kupffer cells are capable of replication and their local proliferation accounts for a substantial part of the expansion of this cell population in response to liver injury.[194,195] Furthermore, Kupffer cells appear in the fetal liver of the mouse before there are circulating monocytes and there is evidence that they are derived from primitive macrophages which first appear in the yolk sac.[196] These data suggest that Kupffer cells may have a dual origin.[196]

Liver-associated lymphocytes (pit cells)

Wisse et al[197] described so-called pit cells in the sinusoids of rat liver. These were characterized by the presence of cytoplasmic granules. Similar cells have now been identified in the livers of various species including humans.[198,199] Immunophenotyping of these cells, both in rodents and in humans, has shown that they are a heterogeneous population and it seems more appropriate to speak of liver-associated lymphocytes rather than a single cell type (i.e. pit cell).[197–199] The ultrastructural appearances are similar to those of large granular lymphocytes in peripheral blood. They are generally found in loose contact with Kupffer cells or endothelial cells. The cells contain characteristic electron-dense granules, rod-cored vesicles and parallel tubular arrays; these organelles are often polarized within the cytoplasm (Fig. 1.22). In the rat these cells express markers of natural killer lymphocytes, and isolated liver-associated lymphocytes have been shown to exhibit natural killer activity in vitro.[200] Liver-associated lymphocytes are thought to be recruited from the peripheral blood. They manifest characteristic phenotypic differences, however, and these are acquired by processes of differentiation in the liver, probably in response to cytokines which are secreted by other sinusoidal cells.[201] In addition to natural killer activity they also exhibit lymphokine-activated killer activity.[200] The liver-

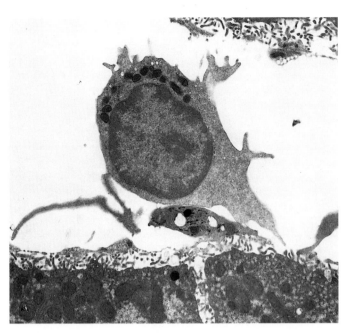

Fig. 1.22 Liver-associated lymphocyte lying within a sinusoid; the granular organelles within the cytoplasm are polarized, × 6425. By courtesy of Dr A D Burt.

associated lymphocytes are thought to play an important role in immunological defences in the liver, against metastasizing tumour cells and viral infections.

THE BILIARY SYSTEM

As already described, the bile canaliculi form a complicated polygonal network with many anastomotic interconnections. They drain into periportal cholangioles or terminal ductules which have a basement membrane and which are lined by three to six cells which may be ductal cells or hepatocytes (Fig. 1.23). This represents the commencement of the biliary tree and these early ductules are also known as the canals of Hering, some of which may show dilatation where several canaliculi converge to form them. The ductules extend through the limiting plate and unite, within the smallest portal tracts, to form the interlobular bile ducts, the smallest branches of which are 15–20 μm in diameter. They are lined by a single layer of flattened cuboidal epithelium, have a basement membrane and are in turn ensheathed in the fibrous tissue of the portal tracts (Fig. 1.24). The interlobular ducts anastomose freely, increase in size and form larger septal or trabecular ducts which are more than 100 μm in diameter and which are lined by a simple tall columnar epithelium with basally situated nuclei. The portal tract fibrous tissue shows some condensation round these ducts, but there is no well-marked concentric orientation.

These larger ducts further anastomose to form the large hilar intrahepatic bile ducts, 1–1.5 mm in diameter, which give rise to the main hepatic ducts. Studies by Terada and

his colleagues[202,203] have demonstrated the presence of glandular elements around the larger intrahepatic bile ducts. These glands are of two types: (i) intramural mucous glands which communicate directly with the bile-duct lumen, and (ii) extramural mixed seromucinous glands which form branching tubulo-alveolar lobules and secretory ducts that drain into the bile-duct lumen (Fig. 1.25). These peribiliary glands are found in relation to the common hepatic ducts, the hilar ducts and a proportion of the larger septal ducts. Scanning electron microscopy showed that hilar ducts may also have irregular side branches and pouches in which bile may be stored and probably modified.[204] The precise functions of these peribiliary glands are still uncertain. They share some antigenic determinants with pancreatic exocrine acini, secrete a number of enzymes, and must be of importance in normal biliary function.[204a,204b]

Since the last edition of this text there has been a considerable increase in our knowledge of the structure and function of bile ductular cells,[19,87,88,205,206] studies which have confirmed the view of Rous & McMaster[207] in 1921 that bile ducts have an important role in modifying canalicular bile, a role to which the intrahepatic peribiliary glands may also contribute. Ultrastructurally, the biliary epithelial cell has a prominent Golgi complex, numerous cytoplasmic vesicles and short luminal microvilli. Studies in the rat suggest that 10–15% of basal bile flow is produced by ductal epithelium[208] and it has been estimated that the corresponding contribution in humans is 40%.[88] This function is thought to be under the influence of secretin, which is released from the duodenum following vagal stimulation and the presence of acid in the duodenum, and which stimulates the secretion of bicarbonate-rich bile.[205] In addition there is evidence that bile acids are reabsorbed via biliary epithelium, and recirculated by a cholehepatic shunt pathway via the peribiliary plexus, and that this promotes bile-acid-dependent bile flow in the ducts.[209,210] Reabsorption of urate and glucose occurs across the bile-duct epithelium; the cells also secrete IgA, and IgM (but not IgG) has been shown immunohistochemically on human biliary epithelial cells.[87,211] The intrahepatic peribiliary glands secrete seromucinous fluid,[204] IgA and secretory piece,[211] and contain hormones.[212] The epithelia of large intrahepatic bile ducts and their accompanying peribiliary glands contain pancreatic α-amylase and trypsin.[213] Normally the biliary epithelial cells express class I MHC antigens but not class II; cytokine-induced expression of class II antigen is seen in graft-versus-host disease, allograft rejection, primary biliary cirrhosis and primary sclerosing cholangitis (see Chs. 12 and 18) and this may be important in the pathogenesis of the bile-duct injury in these diseases. Bile-duct epithelium also expresses γ-glutamyl-transpeptidase (γGT), carcinoembryonic antigen (CEA) and epithelial membrane antigen (EMA), representing

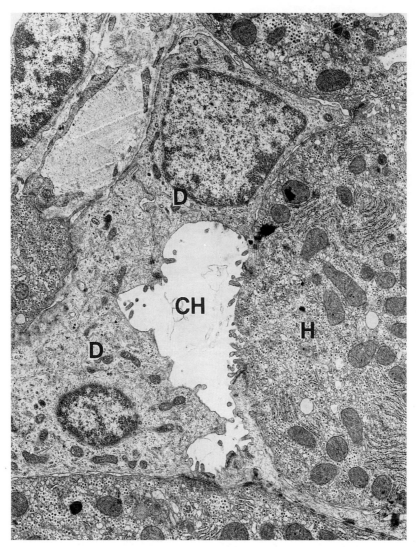

Fig. 1.23 TEM of a section through a canal of Hering (CH) whose wall shows two ductal cells (D) and a hepatocyte (H). Baboon liver. × 5265.

other phenotypic differences when compared with hepatocytes, but the precise significance of this is, as yet, uncertain.[87]

OTHER CONSTITUENT TISSUES

The extracellular matrix

The liver normally has only a small amount of connective tissue in relation to its size. Whereas in the human body collagen constitutes about 30% of the total protein, the corresponding figure for the liver is 5–10%. Underlying the visceral peritoneum or serosa there is a layer of dense connective tissue admixed with elastic fibres which varies in thickness from 40–70 μm. This constitutes Glisson's capsule, irregular prolongations of which extend into the superficial parenchyma, producing some architectural distortion which must not be misinterpreted when wedge biopsies are examined. Condensation of Glisson's capsule

occurs at the porta hepatis, and the fibrous tissue then extends into the liver, supporting and accompanying the portal vein, hepatic artery and bile-duct branches and constituting the portal tracts. Some extension of the capsular tissue also accompanies the large hepatic vein branches, but there is no fibrous sheath surrounding the terminal hepatic venules which are in direct contact with perivenular hepatocytes. Within the acini the extracellular matrix is confined to the space of Disse and this so-called reticulin network or framework is usually visualized by silver impregnation staining methods (Fig. 1.26). The extracellular matrix in the liver, in common with that in other organs, serves to provide cohesiveness between cells, induces cell polarization, allows intercellular communication and affects gene expression and cellular differentiation. A brief outline of the extracellular matrix in the normal liver is given in the ensuing paragraphs and is based on detailed reviews which have recently been published.[176,214–216]

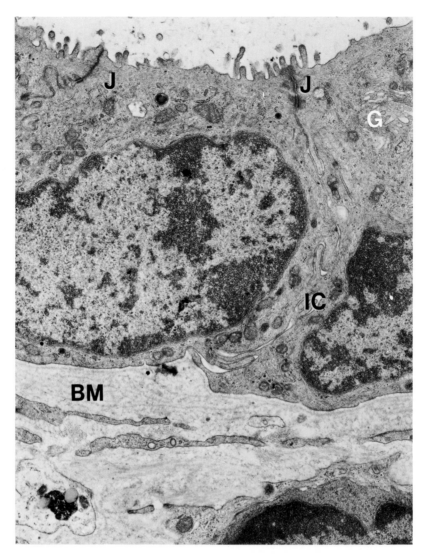

Fig. 1.24 TEM of simple cuboidal epithelium of a bile duct. Note the contorted intercellular space (IC), open basally and closed apically by a junctional complex (J). A Golgi complex (G) is seen in one of the cells and a basement membrane (BM) is present. Baboon liver, × 10 530.

Hepatic fibrosis and cirrhosis are serious consequences of many types of liver injury and the mechanisms involved in this are discussed in detail in chapter 10. The components of the extracellular matrix are collagens, glycoproteins and proteoglycans.

Collagens are composed of three identical or similar polypeptide chains folded into a triple helix to give the molecule stability. Thirteen types of collagen have been described and of these types I, III, IV, V and VI are found in the liver; types I and III comprise more than 95% of the collagen in normal liver with IV, V and VI contributing approximately 1%, 2–5% and 0.1% respectively.[217]

The matrix glycoproteins are highly cross-linked and insoluble. They are multivalent and have well-defined domains that interact with cell surface receptors and other components of the extracellular matrix. Some are involved in cell adhesion and, thus, may be present in serum and other body fluids. Laminin is the major glycoprotein in basement membrane and interacts there with type IV collagen; small amounts are normally present in the space of Disse but increased amounts are present in so-called capillarization of the sinusoids. Fibronectin exists in two isoforms, one of which, plasma fibronectin, is produced by hepatocytes. Fibronectin is also produced by perisinusoidal cells and endothelial cells. It mediates cell adhesion to collagen. Other glycoproteins present in the liver are vitronectin which is co-distributed with fibronectin, undulin which is closely associated with collagen types I and III, nidogen (entactin) which forms a complex with laminin, and elastin which is found in the walls of blood vessels and in portal tracts.

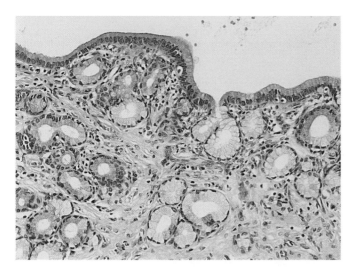

Fig. 1.25 Large intrahepatic bile duct near the hilum. Note the surrounding mucous and seromucinous peribiliary glands; one mucous gland opens into the duct lumen. H & E.

The proteoglycans are macromolecules consisting of a central protein core to which glycosaminoglycans and oligosaccharide side chains are attached. The proteoglycans have been classified according to the type of glycosaminoglycan present. They contain specific functional domains which interact with cell surface receptor molecules. In the liver, heparan sulphate is the most abundant and is present in portal tracts, in basement membrane and on the surface of hepatocytes.

The regulation of extracellular matrix production is discussed in chapter 10. The perisinusoidal cells are mainly responsible for the production of both collagen and the non-collagenous proteins; hepatocytes may produce some collagen and some proteoglycans: the role of Kupffer cells and sinusoidal endothelial cells is mediated through the production of cytokines which modulate the synthetic activity of perisinusoidal cells, but they may also produce small amounts of proteoglycans. Reference has already been made to the importance of extracellular matrix inter-action with hepatocytes and non-parenchymal cells in maintaining normal liver function (p. 1.8). There is a gradient in the extracellular matrix in the space of Disse (Fig. 1.5), with variation in its amount and composition with increasing distance from the portal tracts.[61,218] Thus, for example, laminin, collagen type IV and heparan sulphate predominate in the periportal zone whereas in the perivenular zones fibronectin, collagen type III, and dermatan sulphate are more abundant.[61] The extracellular matrix in the normal liver is considered to be of major importance in regulating and modulating hepatocyte function in the acinus,[61,219] contributes to the mainte-nance of hepatocyte polarity[22] and has some regulatory effect on the functional role of non-parenchymal cells.[221] The extracellular matrix is a dynamic structure which also undergoes degradation.[218,222] This is a function of various

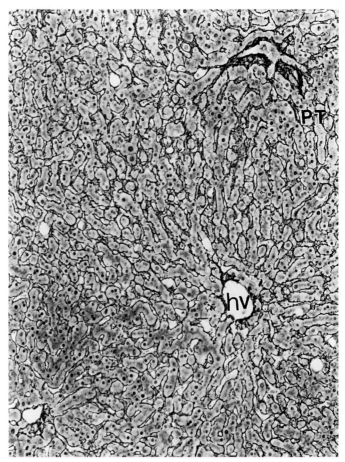

Fig. 1.26 Low power view to show normal portal tract/hepatic vein relationships. PT = portal tract; hV = hepatic vein. Gordon and Sweets' reticulin

metalloproteinases which include type-specific collage-nases.

Lymphatics

The liver is the largest single source of lymph in the body, producing 15–20% of the overall total volume[223] and 25–50% of the thoracic duct flow.[224] Hepatic lymph has an unusually high protein content (about 85–95% of that in plasma) and a high content of cells, of which about 80% are lymphocytes and the remainder macrophages. Indeed, it has been calculated that, in the sheep, more lympho-cytes migrate through the liver in the lymph than through any other non-lymphoid organ, and that about 2×10^8 macrophages leave the liver in lymph each day.[225]

The terminal twigs of the intrahepatic lymphatic tree are found as a fine, valved plexus of flattened endothelial tubes, associated with terminal branches of the hepatic artery. Traced towards the porta hepatis, the plexus en-larges and remains primarily periarterial, although in the larger portal canals it becomes associated also with portal vein branches and bile-duct tributaries, adding a fourth element to the traditional 'portal triad'. Similar but much smaller and functionally less important lymphatic plexuses are associated with the hepatic vein branches. A third plexus, found in the capsule, forms significant anastomoses with intrahepatic lymphatics. Most of the collecting lymphatics leave the liver at the porta hepatis and drain into hepatic nodes located along the hepatic artery and thence to coeliac nodes. There are other important efferent routes: via the falciform ligament and the superior epigastric vessels to the parasternal nodes; from the bare area to posterior mediastinal nodes; and from the visceral surface to the left gastric nodes. As efferent collecting lymphatics leave the liver their walls suddenly thicken, through the acquisition of a muscle layer.[226,227] The importance of the anastomoses between intrahepatic and capsular lymphatics is evident when hepatic venous pressure is increased. There follows a great increase in production of hepatic lymph, of protein content identical with that of plasma, indicating unrestricted leakage of protein into Disse's space.[228] The capsular efferent lymphatics enlarge in response to the increased lymph flow, and exudation of excess lymph from the capsular plexus forms protein-rich ascitic fluid.[229]

The function of lymphatics is to drain excess fluid and protein from the interstitial spaces of an organ. In the liver the interstitial space of Disse is the most prominent and it is assumed that hepatic lymph is mainly formed there with a small supplement from the peribiliary capillary plexus in the portal tracts. A protein-rich filtrate is produced in the space of Disse because of the free permeability of the sinusoidal endothelium and the consequent absence of a colloid osmotic block.[230] A protein-poor filtrate is formed by the less permeable peribiliary capillaries and this may dilute the protein of the sinusoidal filtrate.[224]

The route followed by interstitial fluid formed in Disse's space to its entry into the first-order lymphatic plexus has been controversial.[224,230] It is agreed that lymphatic capillaries are absent within the acini and that there are no direct channels, with a continuous lining, between Disse's space and the primary lymphatics. Wisse and his colleagues[231,232] have suggested that 'endothelial massaging' by blood cells may be of importance in causing fluid movement in the space of Disse (Fig. 1.27). Henriksen et al[231] suggested that, as in other tissues, the terminal lymphatics in the portal tracts had anchoring filaments between opposing endothelial cells which regulated the direction of flow from the interstitial space into the lymphatics. An electron microscopic study of the rat's liver[233] has established the following pathway, by the use of natural markers (precipitated lymph protein and chylomicrons) and artificial tracers injected intravenously (ferritin, pontamine blue and monastral blue). Fluid formed in Disse's space escaped at the periphery of the portal tract through gaps between hepatocytes of the limiting plate. These gaps contained hepatocyte microvilli, delicate 'wicks' of collagenous fibres and occasional

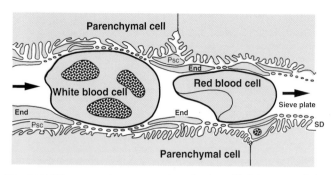

Fig. 1.27 Diagrammatic reconstruction of a sinusoid. It is proposed that blood cells deform the sinusoidal wall, effectively 'massaging' fluid through the space of Disse (SD). End = endothelial cell; Psc = perisinusoidal cell. Modified after Wisse & de Leeuw[162]

slender processes of portal tract fibroblasts, extending into the parenchyma from the periportal space of Mall. Here long flattened processes of fibroblasts formed discontinuous linings of 'spaces' which contained tracer material, occasional lymphocytes and macrophages, and collagen bundles. These 'spaces' were not true lymphatics, since they lacked an endothelial lining, but they appeared to function as prelymphatic channels, leading fluid towards the terminal twigs of the lymphatic tree.

Nerve supply and innervation

Nerve fibres reach the liver in two separate but intercommunicating plexuses around the hepatic artery and portal vein, and are distributed with their branches. They include preganglionic parasympathetic fibres derived from both vagi, and sympathetic fibres which are mostly postganglionic with cell bodies in the coeliac ganglia, and which receive their preganglionic sympathetic connections from spinal segments T7–T10. The hilar plexuses also include visceral afferent fibres and some phrenic nerve fibres, probably also afferent in character.[234] Current knowledge of the intrahepatic distribution of neural elements and of the various effector humoral mechanisms, including the role of various cytokines, eicosanoids and nitric oxide (NO), has recently been reviewed.[93,235]

It is of historical interest that von Kupffer, in his original study, proposed to examine the nerves within the liver but was unable to demonstrate any. Immunohistochemical studies of human liver, however, using antibodies to common neural proteins such as protein gene product (PGP) 9.5 and N-CAM, have shown that nerve fibres not only are present around vascular structures in portal tracts but extend into the parenchyma (Fig. 1.28), running along the sinusoids. Fluorescence histochemistry[236] and immunohistochemistry using antibodies to dopamine-β-hydroxylase and tyrosine hydroxylase[237] have shown that the majority of intrasinusoidal fibres are sympathetic; many contain neuropeptide tyrosine (NPY), a regulatory peptide commonly found in adrenergic nerves.[237]

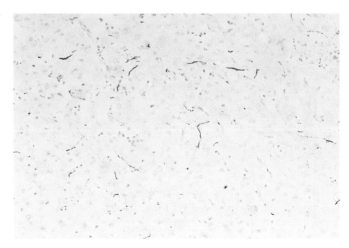

Fig. 1.28 Human liver reacted with an antibody to the neural protein gene product (PGP) 9.5; positive-staining nerve fibres are present in a perisinusoidal distribution. By courtesy of Dr A D Burt.

Unmyelinated nerve fibres can be seen in the space of Disse using TEM.[238] They are frequently surrounded by Schwann cell processes but a few bare nerve endings or varicosities are found in close apposition to hepatocytes or perisinusoidal cells. Synaptic clefts have been identified at points of contact suggesting that there is direct innervation of these cells, although true synapses are not found.

Release of neurotransmitters from the intrasinusoidal sympathetic fibres may modulate hepatocyte and perisinusoidal cell function. There is evidence that adrenergic nerves play a role in the control of hepatocyte carbohydrate and lipid metabolism, and in intrahepatic haemodynamics. Stimulation of hepatic sympathetic nerves in vivo produces hyperglycaemia. This effect is caused by enhanced glycogenolysis in hepatocytes and appears to be under α-adrenergic control.[239] The regulation of hepatic carbohydrate metabolism by sympathetic nerve fibres may be mediated by gap junctional communication.[126] Hepatic vascular resistance is increased by hepatic nerve stimulation, but it does not appear to be under sympathetic tone; this response is mediated through adrenergic receptors.[240,241] Bioulac-Sage and co-workers have speculated that adrenergic nerves may induce contraction in perisinusoidal cells, thereby regulating intrasinusoidal blood flow.[238]

An extensive cholinergic (parasympathetic) network is found in rat liver.[242] In human liver, Amenta et al[243] described parasympathetic cholinergic innervation of portal tract vessels with only limited innervation of the parenchyma. Immunohistochemical studies have also identified intrahepatic fibres containing two neuropeptides, substance P and calcitonin gene-related peptide (CGRP), which are commonly found in afferent nerves.[244,245] Such afferent fibres may be involved in chemo- and osmoreception as well as in vasomotor regulation.[234]

The ability of orthotopic allografts to function satisfactorily suggests that neural mechanisms have only a minor

regulatory role, at least under basal conditions; only limited re-innervation occurs in the transplanted human liver.[246,247] However, there is some evidence in experimental animals,[248,249] and possibly in humans,[249] that the liver's normal response to hypovolaemic shock is impaired by denervation and may result in hepatic ischaemic injury. Loss of intrasinusoidal fibres in the cirrhotic liver may contribute to impaired metabolic function.[250]

THE LIVER IN BIOPSY AND AUTOPSY SPECIMENS

Now that the constituent tissues of the liver have been described in turn, it is proposed to discuss the overall histological patterns and their physiological variations as seen in liver biopsy and autopsy material. It is of interest, however, to look at the relative contribution of each to the whole (Table 1.2). The data are of volumetric composition of rat liver; information for the human liver is less complete, but probably comparable.[251]

In the examination of liver tissue attention should be paid to the overall architecture, the portal tracts and their constituent parts, the acinar parenchyma inclusive of hepatocytes, sinusoids and sinusoidal cells, and the hepatic veins. The normal portal tract/hepatic vein relationships are as shown in Figure 1.26. Surrounding the hepatic veins the individual hepatocytes tend to have a more regular arrangement resembling cords, and correspondingly the sinusoidal network radiates out for a short distance into the perivenular area with a more regular radial pattern of the reticulin framework. Outside the perivenular zone the liver-cell plates are arranged less regularly, and correspondingly the sinusoidal network and reticulin framework do not demonstrate a distinct radial arrangement. Within the reticulin framework the liver-cell plates are two cells thick up to the age of about 5 years (Fig. 1.29a,b); thereafter the normal pattern is for these to be one cell thick (Fig. 1.29c). In the adult, the presence of twin-cell liver plates and the formation of rosettes indicates regeneration (Fig. 1.29d).

The individual hepatocyte is polygonal in shape and in haematoxylin and eosin preparations the cell margins are clearly outlined. In the liver-cell plates cut in a longitudinal plane it is possible to define the sinusoidal margin

Table 1.2 Volumetric composition of rat liver

	%
Hepatocytes	77.8
Endothelial cells	2.8
Kupffer cells	2.1
Perisinusoidal cells	1.4
Disse's space	4.9
Sinusoids	10.6
Bile canaliculi	0.4
Extra-hepatocytic space (total)	22.2

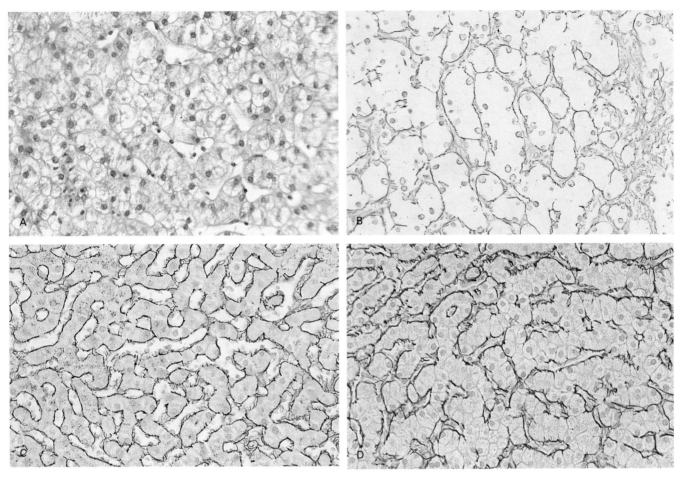

Fig. 1.29 (a) Liver biopsy from a child of 17 months; note the twin-cell liver plates: these are better shown on a reticulin preparation at the same magnification in (b), in which the nuclei are seen in a perisinusoidal position; (c) adult liver showing normal single-cell liver plates with centrally placed nuclei; (d) adult liver at same magnification as (c) showing a regenerative response with twin-cell liver plates; as in (b) the nuclei tend to be in a perisinusoidal position; there is also rosette formation. Gordon & Sweets' reticulin.

or pole and also the canalicular pole at the junction between adjacent cells (see Fig. 1.13). The cytoplasm is granular and eosinophilic, but within it basophilic aggregates of RER can be defined in a perinuclear distribution and at the canalicular poles, the intervening cytoplasm tending to be paler in appearance. The nucleus is centrally placed and one or more nucleoli are easily identified. In childhood there is virtually no nuclear pleomorphism. Thereafter, variation in nuclear size develops and, with increasing age, nuclear polyploidy with increased haematoxyphilia is a normal finding, the majority of nuclei being diploid but with a few tetraploid or even larger nuclei being found. This pleomorphism is more marked in acinar zone 2. The hepatocytes in the portal limiting plates are smaller than other parenchymal cells (<20 μm in diameter), show more intense nuclear staining and have a uniform, more basophilic cytoplasm. Binucleate cells may occasionally be found. Mitoses are rarely seen in biopsy material. Nuclear displacement to the sinusoidal pole with hyperchromasia is a cytological indication of regenerative activity (Fig. 1.29d).

The liver cell is rich in glycogen, but in routine haematoxylin and eosin preparations its presence is discerned only with difficulty, imparting a fine reticulated and foamy appearance to the cell cytoplasm. Staining by the PAS method readily demonstrates the glycogen (Fig. 1.30a) and it is usually uniformly distributed. The amount and distribution, however, show diurnal and diet-related variations. An irregular distribution pattern may sometimes be found in biopsies and is not of diagnostic significance (Fig. 1.30b). Glycogen accumulation in nuclei produces a vacuolated appearance, is common in childhood, and may be conspicuous in certain adult conditions (chronic cardiac failure, diabetes and Wilson's disease, for example), but is not per se of diagnostic significance.

Lipofuscin forms a further intracytoplasmic inclusion, occurring as fine, light brown, PAS-positive and acid-fast granules at the canalicular pole, predominantly of perivenular hepatocytes. Normally, lipofuscin is not abundant until the second decade, and thereafter there appears to be a progressive increase in its amount both in individual hepatocyte content and also in the extent of hepatocyte

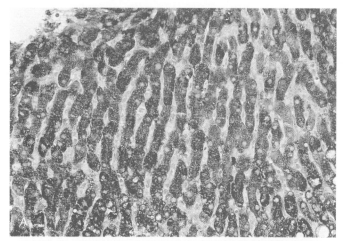

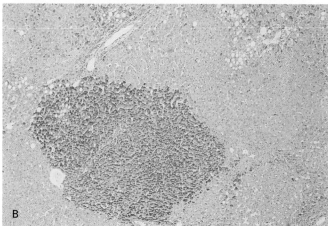

Fig. 1.30 (a) Glycogen accumulation within liver cells shown in a PAS preparation. (b) Irregular distribution of PAS-positive glycogen in a wedge biopsy of liver; there are scattered positive cells and also one large positive area showing an acinar-like configuration.

involvement. Lipofuscin is a breakdown product of lysosomal material, reflecting cell activity, and is referred to as 'wear and tear' pigment. It is not found in recently regenerated hepatocytes.

It is not unusual in otherwise apparently normal livers to note a very few, single, hyalinized, necrotic liver cells within cell plates, representing apoptosis of hepatocytes; and also occasional foci where more than one hepatocyte has been lost and is replaced by an aggregate of three or four chronic inflammatory cells. The occasional hepatocyte may also normally contain fat. Stainable iron is absent or demonstrable in only scant amounts.

The sinusoids form an apparently discontinuous system of narrow channels between the liver-cell plates, their diameter varying from 4–15 μm. Sinusoids in the perivenular area are normally of larger dimension, and with ageing and atrophy of liver-cell cords there may be apparent dilatation of these sinusoids, a normal variation however. The sinusoids are cylindrical and appear circular in transverse section, running parallel to aligned liver cells.

In the normal biopsy specimen the lining cells are not conspicuous, and are represented by their flattened elongated nuclei at the sinusoidal margin (Fig. 1.13a). Plumper cells containing PAS-positive (diastase-resistant), acid-fast granular aggregates of ceroid pigment (similar to lipofuscin) represent Kupffer cells (Fig. 1.31a). Their numbers increase with age and, in addition, the presence of aggregates of such cells is a manifestation of liver-cell injury (Fig. 1.31b). Normal blood cells are present within the sinusoids. Extramedullary haemopoiesis is normal only within the first few weeks of life. Sequestration of lymphocytic or mononuclear cells within sinusoids is abnormal, and may be an early manifestation of some myeloproliferative disorders (see Ch. 17).

The perisinusoidal space of Disse is not seen in biopsy material, but in autopsy livers the space becomes dilated, reticulin fibres can be seen traversing it, and the sinusoidal lining cells and Kupffer cells now appear to be free and separate from the adjacent hepatocytes

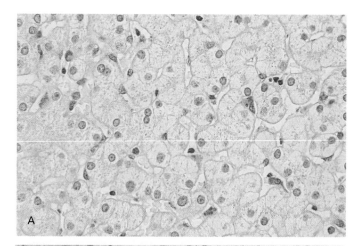

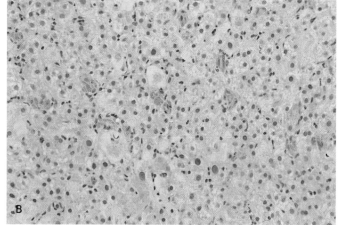

Fig. 1.31 (a) Kupffer cells in a PAS/diastase preparation: granular aggregates of ceroid pigment are present in a number of cells lying within or at the periphery of sinusoids. (b) Focal aggregates of PAS-positive ceroid-containing Kupffer cells in a liver biopsy from a patient with acute hepatitis.

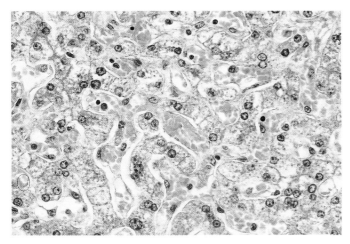

Fig. 1.32 Liver 'biopsy' performed within one hour of the patient's death: note how the sinusoidal endothelium has become separated from the liver-cell plates; the endothelial cells, Kupffer cells and the reticulin framework enclose the intraluminal blood cells and there is 'expansion' of the space of Disse. Masson's trichrome.

(Fig. 1.32). The perisinusoidal cell (Fig. 1.20) cannot be distinguished with certainty on routine stains but can be identified by staining for fat, by demonstration of vitamin A fluorescence, in resin sections and on electron microscopy.[252,253]

The large intrahepatic bile ducts (internal diameter greater than 100 μm) — septal or trabecular ducts — are lined by tall columnar epithelial cells with basally situated nuclei and clear, faintly eosinophilic cytoplasm, which contains granular PAS-positive material at their luminal pole (Fig. 1.33). The fibrous tissue of the portal tracts is arranged in a rather irregular circumferential manner round these ducts. Lymphocytes may occasionally be present within the lining epithelium. The small intrahepatic bile ducts — interlobular — are lined by low columnar or cuboidal epithelium, whose cells contain

basally situated nuclei in the larger branches; PAS-positive material is also present at the luminal pole. More than one interlobular duct may be present in a portal tract. The ducts connect with the bile canaliculi via ductules or canals of Hering. Ductules have a low columnar epithelium and are not accompanied by portal vein and hepatic artery branches; they are in part lined by ductal cells and in part by liver cells, but normally the junction of these with canaliculi and in turn, of ductules with ducts is not clearly defined and is not discernible in routine sections of normal liver.

The microanatomy of the portal vein and hepatic artery has already been described. Progressive hyalinization of the terminal hepatic artery branches is an ageing phenomenon occurring even in the absence of systemic hypertension. The type I collagen fibres of portal tracts become denser with age, and in disease processes accompanied by swelling and fibrosis in portal tracts, the outlines of the normal tracts can be distinguished because of the increased density of the collagen, its doubly refractile properties and its brownish staining reaction in untoned reticulin preparations, contrasting with a yellower staining of young, newly laid down collagen.

The portal tracts (Fig. 1.34) normally contain a few lymphocytes and macrophages but polymorphs and plasma cells are abnormal findings. Increasing numbers of lymphocytes and macrophages may appear in older persons, the density of their distribution varying between portal tracts. The relationship of such chronic inflammatory cell infiltration of portal tracts to natural 'wear and tear' or undefined hepatotoxins is uncertain. Focal aggregation only within some portal tracts should be regarded as probably not significant, whereas generalized portal tract involvement is abnormal. The differential diagnosis of such infiltrates and non-specific reactive hepatitis is further discussed in chapter 17.

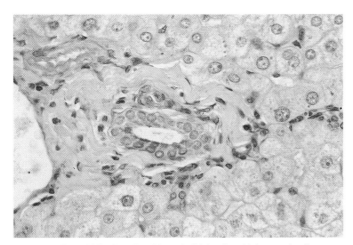

Fig. 1.33 Septal bile duct lined by cuboidal cells which contain discrete supranuclear PAS-positive granules.

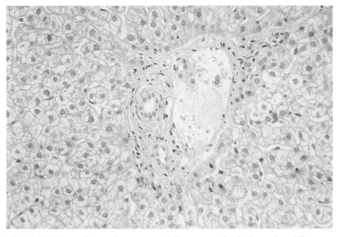

Fig. 1.34 Normal portal tract containing a portal vein branch, a bile duct and a hepatic arteriole.

REFERENCES

1. Kiernan F. The anatomy and physiology of the liver. Philosophical Transactions of the Royal Society of London, Series B 1833; 123: 711–770
2. Mall F P. A study of the structural unit of the liver. Am J Anat 1906; 5: 277–308
3. Rappaport A M, Borowy Z J, Lougheed W M, Lotto W N. Subdivision of hexagonal liver lobules into a structural and functional unit; role in hepatic physiology and pathology. Anat Rec 1954; 119: 11–34
4. Bloch E H. The termination of hepatic arterioles and the functional unit of the liver as determined by microscopy of the living organ. Ann NY Acad Sci 1970; 60: 78–87
5. Matsumoto T, Kawakami M. The unit-concept of hepatic parenchyma: A reexamination based on angioarchitectural studies. Acta Pathol Jpn 1982; 32 (suppl 2): 285–314
6. Lamers W H, Hilberts A, Furt E et al. Hepatic enzymic zonation: A reevaluation of the concept of the liver acinus. Hepatology 1989; 10: 72–76
7. Elias H, Sherrick J C. Morphology of the liver. New York: Academic Press, 1969
8. Streeter G L. Developmental horizons in human embryos. Age groups XI and XII. Contributions to Embryology of the Carnegie Institution of Washington 1942; 30: 213–244
9. Streeter G L. Developmental horizons in human embryos. Contributions to embryology of the Carnegie Institution of Washington 1945; 31: 29–36
9a. Barclay A E, Franklin F J, Pritchard M M L. The fetal circulation. Oxford: Blackwell Scientific, 1944
10. Lassau J P, Bastian D. Organogenesis of the venous structure of the human liver. A haemodynamic theory. Anatomia Clinica 1983; 5: 97–102
11. Dubois A M. The embryonic liver. In Rouiller C L, ed. The liver. New York: Academic Press, 1963; pp 1–39
12. Suchy F J, Bucuvalas J C, Novak D A. Determinants of bile formation during development: ontogeny of hepatic bile acid metabolism and transport. Semin Liver Dis 1987; 7: 77–84
13. Bloom W. The embryogenesis of human bile capillaries and ducts. Am J Anat 1925–26; 36: 451–466
14. Van Eyken P, Sciot R, Callea V, Van der Steen K, Moerman P, Desmet V J. The development of the intrahepatic bile ducts in man: a keratin-immunohistochemical study. Hepatology 1988; 8: 1586–1595
15. Van Eyken P, Sciot R, Desmet V J. Intrahepatic bile duct development in the rat: a cytokeratin-immunohistochemical study. Lab Invest 1988; 59: 52–59
16. Burt A D, Stewart J A, Aitchison M, MacSween R N M. Expression of tissue polypeptide antigen (TPA) in fetal and adult liver: changes in liver disease. J Clin Pathol 1987; 40: 719
17. Gall J A M, Bhathal P S. Morphological and immunohistochemical assessment of intrahepatic bile duct development in the rat. J Gastroenterol Hepatol 1989; 4: 241–250
18. Shah K, Gerber M A. Development of intrahepatic bile ducts in humans. Immunohistochemical study using monoclonal cytokeratin antibodies. Arch Pathol Lab Med 1989; 113: 1135
19. Desmet V J. Embryology of the liver and intrahepatic biliary tract, and an overview of malformations of the bile duct. In: MacIntyre N, Benhamou J-P, Bircher J, Rizzetto M, Rodes J, eds. Oxford textbook of clinical hepatology, vol 1. Oxford: Oxford University Press, 1991: pp 495–519
20. Desmet V J. Congenital diseases of intrahepatic bile ducts: variations on the theme "ductal plate malformation". Hepatology 1992; 16: 1069–1083
21. Moll R, Franke W W, Schiller D A, Geiger B, Krepler R. The catalog of human cytokeratins: patterns of expression in normal epithelia, tumors and cultured cells. Cell 1982; 31: 11
22. Jørgensen M J. The ductal plate malformation. Acta Path Micr Scand 1977; 257: 1–88
23. Shiojiri N. The origin of intrahepatic bile duct cells in the mouse. J Embryol Exp Morphol 1984; 79: 25–39
24. Hering E. Ueber den Bau der Wirbeltierleber. Sitzungberichte der Akademie der Wissenschaften in Wien, Mathematisch-Naturwissen Schaftiche Klasse 1866; 54: 496–515
25. Desmet V J. Modulation of biliary epithelium. In: Reutter W, Popper H, Arias I M, Heinrich P C, Keppler D, Landmann L, eds. Modulation of liver cell expression. Lancaster: MTP Press, 1987: pp 195–214
26. Van Eyken P, Sciot R, Van Damme B, De Wolf-Peeters C, Desmet V J. Keratin immunohistochemistry in normal human liver. Cytokeratin pattern of hepatocytes, bile ducts and acinar gradient. Virchows Arch (A) 1987; 412: 63–72
27. Van Eyken P, Sciot R, Desmet V J. A cytokeratin immuno-histochemical study of alcoholic liver disease: evidence that hepatocytes can express 'bile duct-type' cytokeratins. Histopathology 1988; 13: 605–617
28. Van Eyken P, Sciot R, Desmet V J. A cytokeratin immuno-histochemical study of cholestatic liver disease: evidence that hepatocytes can express 'bile duct-type' cytokeratins. Histopathology 1989; 15: 125–135
29. Dawood K A, Briscoe C V, Thomas D B, Riches A C. Regulation of haemopoietic stem cell proliferation by stimulatory factors produced by murine fetal and adult liver. J Anat 1990; 168: 209–216
30. Moore M A S, Owen J J T. Stem cell migration in the developing myeloid and lymphoid systems. Lancet 1967; ii: 658–659
31. Moore M A S, Johnson G R. Hemopoietic stem cells during embryonic development and growth. In: Cairnie A B, Lala P K, Osmond D G, eds. Stem cells of renewing cell populations. New York: Academic Press, 1976
32. Croisille Y, Le Douarin N M. Development and regeneration of the liver. In: DeHaan R L, Ursprung R L, eds. Organogenesis. New York: Holt, Rinehart & Winston, 1965
33. Severn C B. A morphological study of the development of the human liver. II. Establishment of liver parenchyma, extrahepatic ducts and associated venous channels. Am J Anat 1972; 133: 85–108
34. Modis L, Martinez-Hernandez A. Hepatocytes modulate the hepatic microvascular phenotype. Lab Invest 1991; 65: 661–669
35. Wright N, Alison M. The liver. In: The biology of epithelial cell populations, vol 2. Oxford: University Press, 1984: pp 880–956
36. Aterman K. The stem cells of the liver — a selective review. J Cancer Res Clin Oncol 1992; 118: 87–115
37. Reid L M. Stem cell biology, hormone/matrix synergies and liver differentiation Curr Opinion Cell Biol 1990; 2: 121–130
38. Zajicek G, Oren R, Weinreb M Jr. The streaming liver. Liver 1985; 5: 293–300
39. Leffert H L, Lock R S, Lad P J, Shapiro I P, Skelly H, de Hemptinne B. Hepatocyte regeneration, replication and differentiation. In: Arias I M, Jakoby W B, Popper H, Schachter D, Shafritz D A, eds. The liver, biology and pathobiology, 2nd edn. New York: Raven Press, 1988: pp 833–850
40. Fausto N, Mead J E. Biology of disease. Regulation of liver growth: protooncogenes and transforming growth factors. Lab Invest 1989; 60: 4–13
41. Michalopoulos G K. Liver regeneration: molecular mechanisms of growth control. FASEB J 1990; 4: 176–187
42. Fausto N. Molecular biology of the liver. In: Prieto J, Rodes J, Shafritz D A, eds. Hepatobiliary diseases. Berlin: Springer-Verlag, 1992: pp 73–93
43. Weinbren K. Compensatory hyperplasia/hepatic regeneration. In: McIntyre N, Benhamou J-P, Bircher J, Rizzetto M, Rodes J, eds. Oxford textbook of clinical hepatology, vol 1. Oxford: Oxford University Press, 1991: pp 102–106
44. Potten C S, Loeffler M. Stem cells: attributes, cycles, spirals, pitfalls and uncertainties. Lessons for and from the crypt. Development 1990; 110: 1001–1020
45. Fausto N, Lemire J M, Shiojiri N. Oval cells in liver carcinogenesis: cell lineages in hepatic development and the identification of facultative stem cells in normal livers. In: Sirica A E, ed. The role of cell types in hepatocarcinogenesis. Boca Raton: CRC Press, 1992: pp 89–108
46. Sirica A E, Cihla H P. Isolation and partial characterizations of oval and hyperplastic bile ductular cell-enriched populations from

the livers of carcinogen and noncarcinogen-treated rats. Cancer Res 1984; 44: 3454–3466

47. Sirica A E, Mathis G A, Sano N, Elmore L W. Isolation, culture and transplantation of intrahepatic biliary epithelial cells and oval cells. Pathobiology 1990; 58: 44–64

48. Sell S. Is there a liver stem cell? Cancer Res 1990: 50: 3811–3815

49. Gerber M A, Thung S N, Shen S, Stromeyer F W, Ishak K G. Phenotypic characterization of hepatic proliferation. Antigenic expression by proliferating eptihelial cells in fetal liver, massive hepatic necrosis, and nodular transformation of the liver. Am J Physiol 1983; 110: 70–74

50. Shah K D, Gerber M A. Development of intrahepatic bile ducts in humans. Possible role of laminin. Arch Pathol Lab Med 1990; 113: 1135–1138

51. Desmet V J, van Eyken P, Sciot R. Cytokeratins for probing cell lineage relationships in developing liver. Hepatology 1990; 12: 1249–1251

52. Zajicek G. Hepatocytes and intrahepatic bile duct epithelium originate from a common stem cell. Gastroenterology 1991; 100: 582–583

53. De Vos R, Desmet V J. Ultrastructural characteristics of novel epithelial cell types identified in human pathologic liver specimens with chronic ductular reaction. Am J Pathol 1992; 140: 1141–1450

54. Burt A D, MacSween R N M. Bile duct proliferation — its true significance. Histopathology 1993; 23: 599–602

55. Roskams T, Van den Oord J J, De Vos R, Desmet V J. Neuroendocrine features of reactive bile ductules in cholestatic liver disease. Am J Pathol 1990; 137: 1019–1025

56. Roskams T, de Vos R, van den Oord J J, Desmet V J. Cells with neuroendocrine features in regenerating human liver. APMIS 1991; 23: 32–39

57. Roskams T, Campos R V, Drucker D J, Desmet V J. Reactive human bile ductules express parathyroid hormone-related peptide. Histopathology 1993; 23: 11–19

58. Zajicek G, Ariel I, Arber N. The streaming liver. II. Hepatocyte life history. Liver 1988; 8: 80–87

59. Zajicek G, Ariel I, Arber N. The streaming liver. III. Littoral cells accompany the streaming hepatocyte. Liver 1988; 8: 213–218

60. Zajicek G. Hepatocytes and intrahepatic bile duct epithelium originate from a common stem cell. Gastroenterology 1991; 100: 582–583

61. Reid L M, Fiorino A S, Sigal S H, Brill S, Holst P A. Extracellular matrix gradients in the space of Disse: relevance to liver biology. Hepatology 1992; 15: 1198–1203

62. Fausto N, Webber E M. Control of liver growth. Crit Rev Eukaryol Gene Exper 1993; 3: 117–135

63. Bucher N L R. Liver regeneration: an overview. J Gastroenterol Hepatol 1991; 6: 615–624

64. Fausto N, Mead J E. Role of proto-oncogene and transforming growth factors in normal and neoplastic liver growth. In: Popper H, Schaffner F, eds. Progress in liver diseases, vol IX. Philadelphia: W B Saunders, 1990: pp 51–71

65. Michalopoulos G, Zarnegar R. Hepatocyte growth factor. Hepatology 1992; 15: 149–155

66. Konoshita T, Tashio K, Makamura T. Marked increase of HGF mRNA in non parenchymal cells of rats treated with hepatotoxin. Biochem Biophys Res Comm 1989; 165: 1229–1234

67. Hioki O, Watanabe A, Minemura M, Tsuchida T. Clinical significance of hepatocyte growth factor levels in liver diseases. J Med 1993; 24: 35–46

68. Fujiwara K, Nagoshi S, Ohno A et al. Stimulation of liver growth by exogenous human hepatocyte growth factor in normal and partially hepatectomised rats. Hepatology 1993; 18: 1443–1449

69. Webber E M, Fitzgerald M J, Brown P I, Bartlett M H, Fausto N. Transforming growth factor α expression during liver regeneration after partial hepatectomy and toxic injury, and potential interactions between transforming growth factor-α and hepatocyte growth factor. Hepatology 1993; 18: 1422–1431

70. Strain A J. Transforming growth factor-β: the elusive hepatic chalone. Hepatology 1991; 16: 269–270

71. Hjortso C-H. The topography of the intrahepatic duct systems. Acta Anat 1951; 11: 599–615

72. Couinaud C. Le foie; etudes anatomiques et chirurgicales. Paris: Masson et Cie, 1957

73. Mays E T II, Mays E T. Are hepatic arteries end arteries? J Anat 1983; 137: 637–644

74. Bismuth H, Aldridge M C, Kunstlinger F. Macroscopic anatomy of the liver. In: McIntyre N, Benhamou J P, Bircher J, Rizzetto M, Rodes J, eds. Oxford textbook of clinical hepatology, vol 1. Oxford: Oxford University Press, 1991: pp 3–11

75. Menu Y. Modern imaging of the liver and biliary tract. In: McIntyre N, Benhamou J P, Bircher J, Rizzetto M, Rodes J, eds. Oxford textbook of clinical hepatology, vol 1. Oxford: Oxford University Press, 1991: pp 326–343

76. Ger R. Surgical anatomy of the hepatic venous system. Clin Anat 1988; 1: 15–22

77. Gupta S C, Gupta C D, Arora A K. Subsegmentation of the human liver. J Anat 1977; 124: 413–423

78. Nelson T M, Pollack R, Jonasson O, Abcarian H. Anatomic variants of celiac, superior mesenteric and inferior mesenteric arteries and their clinical relevance. Clin Anat 1988; 1: 75–91

79. Michels N A. Newer anatomy of liver and its variant blood supply and collateral circulation. Am J Surg 1966; 112: 337–347

80. Chang R W H, Quan S-S, Yen W W C. An applied anatomic study of the ostia venae hepaticae and the retrohepatic segment of the inferior vena cava. J Anat 1989; 164: 41–48

81. Ohtani O, Murakami T, Jones A L. Microcirculation of the liver with special reference to peribiliary portal system. In: Motta P M, Didio L J A, eds. Basic and clinical hepatology. The Hague: Martinus Nijhoff: 1982

82. Mitra S K. The terminal distribution of the hepatic artery with special reference to arterio-portal anastomosis. J Anat 1966; 100: 651–663

83. Yamamoto K, Sherman I, Phillips M J, Fraser M M. Three dimensional observations of the hepatic arterial termination in rat, hamster and human liver by scanning electron microscopy of microvascular casts. Hepatology 1985; 5: 452–456

84. Kono N, Nakanuma Y. Ultrastructural and immuno-histochemical studies of the intrahepatic peribiliary capillary plexus in normal liver and extrahepatic obstruction in human beings. Hepatology 1992; 15: 411–418

85. Murukami T, Itoshima T, Shimada Y. Peribiliary portal system in the monkey liver as evidenced by the injection replica scanning electron microscopy method. Arch Histol Jpn 1974; 37: 245–260

86. Terada T, Nakanuma Y. Development of human peribiliary capillary plexus: a lectin-histochemical and immunohistochemical study. Hepatology 1993; 18: 529–536

87. Tavolini N. The intrahepatic biliary epithelium: an area of growing interest in hepatology. Semin Liver Dis 1987; 7: 280–292

88. Nathanson M H, Boyer J L. Mechanisms and regulation of bile secretion. Hepatology 1991; 14: 551–566

89. Rappaport A M. Hepatic blood flow: morphological aspects and physiological regulation. Int Rev Physiol 1980; 21: 1–63

90. McCuskey R S. A dynamic and static study of hepatic arterioles and hepatic sphincters. Am J Anat 1966; 119: 455–478

91. Grisham J W, Nopanitaya W, Compagno J. Scanning electron microscopy of the liver: a review of methods and results. In: Popper H, Schaffner F, eds. Progress in liver diseases, vol V. New York: Grune & Stratton, 1976: pp 1–23

92. McCuskey R S. Hepatic microcirculation. In: Bioulac-Sage P, Balabaud C, eds. Sinusoids in human liver: health and disease. The Kupffer Cell Foundation: Rijswijk, 1988: pp 151–164

93. McCuskey R S, Reilly F D. Hepatic microvasculature: dynamic structure and its regulation. Semin Liver Dis 1992; 13: 1–12

94. Knisely M H, Bloch E H, Warner L. Selective phagocytosis. I. Microscopic observations concerning the regulation of the blood flow through the liver. Kongelige Danske Videnskabernes Selskab Biologiske Skrifter 1948; 4: 1–93

95. Lautt W W, Greenway C V. Conceptual review of the hepatic vascular bed. Hepatology 1987; 7: 952–963

96. Greenway C V, Lautt W W. Hepatic circulation. In: Schultz S G, Wood J D, Rauner B B, eds. Handbook of physiology — the gastrointestinal system I. American Physiological Society, New York: Oxford University Press, 1989; 1: 1519–1564

97. Lautt W W, Legare D J, Ezzat W R. Quantitation of the hepatic

arterial buffer response to graded changes in portal blood flow. Gastroenterology 1990; 98: 1024–1098

98. Lautt W W. Reciprocity not proven in hepatic blood flow. Gastroenterology 1991; 100: 1483–1484

99. Rappaport A M. The microcirculatory acinar concept of normal and pathological hepatic structure. Beiträge zu Pathologie 1976; 157: 215–243

100. Rappaport A M. Hepatic blood flow: morphological aspects and physiological regulations. Int Rev Physiol 1980; 21: 1–63

101. Rappaport A M. Physioanatomic considerations. In: Schiff L, Schiff E R, eds. Diseases of the liver, 5th edn. Philadelphia: Lippincott, 1982: pp 1–57

102. Rappaport A M, General consideration of the physioanatomy of the hepatic circulation. In: Abramson D I, Dobrin P B, eds. Blood vessels and lymphatics of organ systems. New York: Academic Press, 1984: pp 469–477

103. Rappaport A M, MacPhee P J, Fisher M M, Phillips M J. The scarring of the liver acini (cirrhosis). Virchows Archiv (A) 1983; 402: 107–137

104. Elias H. A re-examination of the structure of mammalian liver. I. Parenchymal architecture. Am J Anat 1949; 84: 311–334

105. Elias H. A re-examination of the structure of mammalian liver. II. The hepatic lobule and its relation to the vascular and biliary system. Am J Anat 1949; 85: 379–456

106. Grisham J W, Nopanitaya W, Compagno J. Scanning electron microscopy of normal rat liver: the surface structure of its cells and tissue components. Am J Anat 1976; 144: 295–322

107. Motta P M, Muto M, Fujita T. The liver. An atlas of scanning electron microscopy. Tokyo: Igaku-Shoin, 1978

108. Elias H. Anatomy of the liver. In: Rouiller C, ed. The liver: morphology, biochemistry, physiology, vol 1. New York: Academic Press, 1963: p. 41

109. Jones C H. Further enquiries as to the structure, development and function of the liver. Philosophical Transactions of the Royal Society of London Series B: Biological Science 1853; 143: 1–28

110. Gumucio J J. Hepatocyte heterogeneity: the coming of age. From the description of a biological curiosity to a partial understanding of its physiological meaning and regulation. Hepatology 1989; 9: 154–160

111. Jungeman K, Katz N R. Functional specialisation of different hepatocyte populations. Physiol Rev 1989; 69: 708–764

112. Kuo F C, Damell J E. Evidence that interaction of hepatocytes with the collecting (hepatic) veins triggers position-specific transcription of the glutamine synthetase and ornithine aminotransferase genes in the mouse liver. Mol Cell Biol 1991; 11: 6050–6058

113. Gebhardt R. Cell–cell interactions: clues to hepatocyte heterogeneity and beyond. Hepatology 1992; 16: 843–845

114. Baumann H, Morella K K, Campos S P et al. Role of CAAT-enhancer binding protein isoforms in the cytokine regulation of acute-phase plasma protein genes. J Biol Chem 1992; 267: 19744–19751

115. Lai E. Regulation of hepatic gene expression and development. Semin Liver Dis 1992; 12: 246–251

116. Crabtree G R, Schibler U, Scott M P. Transcriptional regulatory mechanisms in liver midgut morphogenesis of vertebrates and invertebrates. In: McKnight S L, Yamamoto K R, eds. Transcriptional regulation, vol 2. Cold Spring Harbor Laboratory Press, 1992: pp 1063–1102

117. Philips M J, Satir P. The cytoskeleton of the hepatocyte: organisation, relationships and pathology. In: Arias I M, Jakoby W B, Popper H, Schachter D, Shafritz D A, eds. The liver: biology and pathobiology. New York: Raven Press, 1988: pp 11–27

118. Schachter D. The hepatocyte plasma membrane: organisation and differentiation. In: Arias I M, Jakoby W B, Popper H, Schachter D, Shafritz D A, eds. The liver: biology and pathobiology. New York: Raven Press, 1988: pp 131–140

119. Meier P J. Transport polarity of hepatocytes. Semin Liver Dis 1988; 8: 293–307

120. Hubbard A L, Wall D, Ma A. Isolation of rat hepatocyte plasma membranes. I. Presence of the three major domains. J Cell Biol 1983; 96: 217–229

121. Wolters H, Spiering M, Gerding A, Slooff M J H, Kuipers F, Hardonk M J, Vonk R J. Isolation and characterisation of canalicular and basolateral plasma membrane fractions from human liver. Biochim Biophys Acta 1991; 1069: 61–69

122. Armstrong E M, MacSween R N M. Demonstration of bile canaliculi by an immunofluorescent staining technique. Anat Rec 1973; 177: 311–317

123. Philips M J, Oshio C, Miyami M, Katz H, Smith C R. A study of bile canalicular contractions in isolated hepatocytes. Hepatology 1982; 2: 763–768

124. Arias I M, Che M, Gatmaitan Z, Leveille C, Nishida T, St Pierre M. The biology of the bile canaliculus. Hepatology 1993; 17: 318–329

125. Seseke F G, Gardemann A, Jungerman K. Signal propagation via gap junctions, a key step in the regulation of liver metabolism by the sympathetic hepatic nerves. FEBS Letters 1992; 301: 265–270

126. Doyle D, Byanover Y, Petill J K. Plasma membrane: biogenesis and turnover. In: Arias I M, Jakoby W B, Popper H, Schachter D, Shafritz D A, eds. The liver: biology and pathobiology. New York: Raven Press 1988: pp 141–164

127. Feldmann G. Liver ploidy. J Hepatol 1992; 16: 7–10

128. Adler C P, Ringlage W P, Bohm N, DNA content and cell number in heart and liver of children. Path Res Pract 1981; 172: 25–41

129. Epstein C J. Cell size, nuclear content and development of polyploidy in mammalian liver. Proc Natl Acad Sci USA 1967; 57: 327–334

130. MacDonald R A. 'Lifespan' of liver cells. Arch Int Med 1981; 107: 335–343

131. De Pierre J W, Andersson G, Dallner G. Endoplasmic reticulum and Golgi complex. In: Arias I M, Jakoby W B, Popper H, Schachter D, Shafritz D A, eds. The liver: biology and pathobiology. New York: Raven Press, 1988: pp 165–187

132. Cardell R R. Action of metabolic hormones on the fine structure of rat liver cells. I. Effects of fasting on the ultrastructure of hepatocytes. Am J Anat 1971; 131: 21–54

133. Philips M J, Unakar N J, Doornewaard G, Steiner J W. Glycogen depletion in the new born rat liver. J Ultrastructural Res 1967; 18: 142–165

134. Wanson J C, Drochmans P, Mosselmans R, Ronveaux M F. Adult rat hepatocytes in primary monolayer culture. J Cell Biol 1977; 74: 858–877

135. Lamri Y, Roda A, Dumont M, Feldmann G, Erlinger S. Immunoperoxidase localization of bile salts in rat liver cells. Evidence for a role of the Golgi apparatus in bile salt transport. J Clin Invest 1988; 82: 1173–1182

136. De Duve. Lysosome concept. In: de Reuck A V J, Cameron M P, eds. Ciba Foundation Symposium on Lysosomes. Boston: Little Brown, 1963: pp 1–31

137. Bainton D F. The discovery of lysosomes. J Cell Biol 1981; 91: 66s–76s

138. Novikoff A B, Novikoff P M. Lysosomes. In: Arias I M, Jakoby W B, Popper H, Schachter D, Shafritz D A, eds. The liver: biology and pathobiology, New York: Raven Press, 1988: pp 227–239

139. Forgac M. Receptor-mediated endocytosis. In: Arias I M, Jakoby W B, Popper H, Schachter D, Shafritz D A, eds. The liver: biology and pathobiology. New York: Raven Press, 1988: 207–225

140. Goltz J S, Wolkoff A W, Novikoff P M, Stockert R J, Satir P. A role for microtubule in sorting endocytic vesicles in rat hepatocytes. Proc Natl Acad Sci USA 1992; 89: 7026–7030

141. Rouiller C, Bernhard W. 'Microbodies' and the problem of mitochondrial regeneration in liver cells. J Biophys Biochem Cytol 1956; (suppl) 2: 355–358

142. Lazarow P B. Peroxisomes. In: Arias I M, Jakoby W B, Popper H, Schachter D, Shafritz D A, eds. The liver: biology and pathobiology. New York: Raven Press, 1988: pp 241–254

143. Staubli W, Schweizer W, Suter J, Weibel E R. The proliferative response of hepatic peroxisomes of neonatal rats to treatment with SW-13 437 (Nafenopin). J Cell Biol 1977; 74: 665–669

144. Sternlieb I, Quintara N. The peroxisomes of human hepatocytes. Lab Invest 1977; 36: 140–149
145. Goldfischer S L. Peroxisomal diseases. In: Arias I M, Jakoby W B, Popper H, Schachter D, Shafritz D A, eds. The liver: biology and pathobiology. New York: Raven Press, 1988: pp 255–267
145a. De Creamer D, Pauwels M, Roels F. Peroxisomes in cirrhosis of the human liver: A cytochemical ultrastructural and quantitative study Hepatology 1993; 17: 404–410
146. Roels F. Peroxisomes. A personal account. Brussels: VUB Press, 1991
147. Hinkle P C. Mitochondria. In: Arias I M, Jakoby W B, Popper H, Schachter D, Shafritz D A, eds. The liver: biology and pathobiology. New York: Raven Press, 1988: pp 269–275
148. Johnson L V, Walsh M L, Chen L B. Localisation of mitochondria in living cells with rhodamine 123. Proc Natl Acad Sci USA 1980; 77: 990–994
149. Lestienne P. Mitochondrial DNA mutations in human disease — a review. Biochemie 1992: 74: 123–130
150. Candipan R C, Sjostrand F S. Water movement from intra-cristal spaces in isolated liver mitochondria. J Ultrastructure Res 1984; 89: 249–260
151. Candipan R C, Sjostrand F S. Freeze fracture analysis of isolated liver mitochondria in different metabolic states. J Ultrastructure Res 1984; 89: 274–280
152. Candipan R C, Sjostrand F S. An analysis of the contribution of the preparatory techniques to the appearance of condensed and orthodox conformations of liver mitochondria. J Ultrastructure Res 1984; 89: 281–294
153. Loud A V. A quantitative stereological description of the ultrastructure of normal rat liver parenchymal cells. J Cell Biol 1968; 37: 27–46
154. Lazarides E. Intermediate filaments as mechanical integrators of cellular space. Nature 1980; 283: 249–256
155. Denk H, Franke W W. Cytoskeletal filaments. In: Arias I M, Popper H, Schachter D, Shafritz D A, eds. The liver: pathology and pathobiology. New York: Raven Press, 1985: pp 57–60
156. Feldmann G. The cytoskeleton of the hepatocyte. Structure and functions. J Hepatology 1989; 8: 380–386
157. Schroer T A, Sheetz M P. Functions of microtubule-based motors. Ann Rev Physiol 1991; 53: 629–652
158. Wang E, Fischman D, Liem R K H, Sun T T. Intermediate filaments. Ann NY Acad Sci 1985; 455: 32–56
159. Frey-Wyssling A. Submicroscopic morphology of protoplasm and its derivatives. New York: Elsevier, 1948
160. Porter K R. Cytomatrix. In: Arias I M, Jakoby W B, Popper H, Schachter D, Shafritz D A, eds. The liver: biology and pathobiology. New York: Raven Press, 1988: pp 29–45
161. Drochmans P, Wanson J C, Mosselmans R. Isolation and subfractionation on Ficoll gradients of adult rat hepatocytes. J Cell Biol 1975; 66: 1–22
162. Wisse E, De Leeuw A M. Structural elements determining transport and exchange processes in the liver. In: Davis S S, Illum L, McVie J G, Tomlinson E, eds. Microspheres and drug therapy. Pharmaceutical, immunological and medical aspects. Amsterdam: Elsevier, 1984: pp 1–23
163. Burt A D, Le Bail B, Balabaud C, Bioulac-Sage P. Morphologic investigation of sinusoidal cells. Semin Liver Dis 1993; 13: 21–38
164. Arias I M. The biology of hepatic endothelial fenestrae. In: Schaffner F, Popper H, eds. Progress in liver diseases, vol IX. Philadelphia: W B Saunders, 1990: pp 11–26
165. Mak K M, Lieber C S. Alterations in endothelial fenestration in liver sinusoids of baboons fed alcohol. A scanning electron microscopic study. Hepatology 1984; 4: 386–391
166. Wisse E, De Zanger R B, Charels K, Van der Smissen M, McCuskey R S. The liver sieve: considerations concerning the structure and function of endothelial fenestrae, the sinusoidal wall and the space of Disse. Hepatology 1985; 5: 683–689
167. Petrovic L M, Burroughs A, Scheuer P J. Hepatic sinusoidal endothelium: Ulex lectin binding. Histopathology 1989; 14: 233–243
168. Babbs C, Haboubi N Y, Mellor J M et al. Endothelial cell transformation in primary biliary cirrhosis: a morphological and biochemical study. Hepatology 1990; 11: 723–729

169. Scoazec J-Y, Feldmann G. In situ phenotyping study of endothelial cells of the human hepatic sinusoid: results and functional implications. Hepatology 1991; 14: 789–797
170. Volpes R, Van den Oord J J, Desmet V J. Immunohistochemical study of adhesion molecules in liver inflammation. Hepatology 1990; 12: 65–69
171. Vidal-Vanaclocha F, Rocha M, Asumendi A, Barberá-Guillem E. Isolation and enrichment of two sublobular compartment-specific endothelial cell subpopulations from liver sinusoids. Hepatology 1993; 18: 328–339
172. Eskild W, Kindberg G M, Smedsrod B, Blomhoff R, Norum K R. Intracellular transport of formaldehyde-treated serum albumin in liver endothelial cells after uptake via scavenger receptor. Biochem J 1989; 258: 511–520
173. Reider H, Meyer zum Buschenfelde K H, Ramadori G. Functional spectrum of sinusoidal endothelial liver cells. Filtration, endocytosis, synthetic capacities and intercellular communication. J Hepatol 1992; 15: 237–250
174. Motta P, Porter K. Structure of rat liver sinusoids and associated tissue spaces as revealed by scanning electron microscopy. Cell Tissue Res 1974; 148: 111–125
175. Geerts A, Schuppan D, Lazerans S, De Zanger R, Wisse E. Collagen type I and III occur together in hybrid fibrils in the space of Disse of normal rat liver. Hepatology 1990; 12: 233–241
176. Burt A D. Cellular and molecular aspects of hepatic fibrosis. J Pathol 1993; 170: 105–114
177. Wake K. Perisinusoidal stellate cells (fat storing cells, interstitial cells, lipocytes) their related structure in and around the liver sinusoids and vitamin A-storing cells in extrahepatic organs. Int Rev Cytol 1980; 66: 303–353
178. Aterman K. The parasinusoidal cells of the liver: a historical account. Histochem J 1986; 18: 279–305
179. Ramadori G. The stellate cell (Ito-cell, fat storing cell, lipocyte, perisinusoidal cell) of the liver. New insights into an intriguing cell. Virchow Archiv [B] 1991; 61: 147–158
180. Blomhoff R, Wake K. Perisinusoidal stellate cells of the liver: important roles in retinol metabolism and fibrosis. FASEB J 1991; 5: 271–277
181. Hendriks H F J, Bosma A, Brouwer A. Fat-storing cells: hyper- and hypovitaminosis A and the relationships with liver fibrosis. Semin Liver Dis 1993; 13: 72–80
182. Burt A D, Robertson J L, Heir J, MacSween R N M. Desmin containing stellate cells in rat liver; distribution in normal animals and response to experimental acute liver injury. J Pathol 1986; 150: 29–35
183. Kawadu N, Klein H, Decher K. Eicosanoid-mediated contractility of hepatic stellate cells. Biochem J 1992; 285: 367–371
184. Winwood P J, Arthur M J P. Kupffer cells: their activation and role in animal models of liver injury and human liver disease. Semin Liver Dis 1993; 13: 50–59
185. Motta P M. A scanning electron microscopic study of the rat liver sinusoid. Cell Tissue Res 1975; 164: 371–385
186. Wake K, Decker K, Kirn A, Knook D L, McCuskey R S, Bouwens L, Wisse E. Cell biology and kinetics of Kupffer cells in the liver. Int Rev Cytol 1990; 118: 173–229
187. Te Koppele J M, Thurman R G. Phagocytosis by Kupffer cells predominate in pericentral region of the liver lobule. Am J Physiol 1990; 259: G814–G821
188. MacPhee P J, Schmidt E E, Groom A C. Evidence for Kupffer cell migration along liver sinusoids, from high-resolution in vivo microscopy. Am J Physiol 1992; 263: G17–G23
189. Andus T, Bauer J, Gerok W. Effects of cytokines on the liver. Hepatology 1991; 13: 364–377
190. Barbatis C, Kelly P, Greveson J, Heryet A, McGee JO'D. Immunocytochemical analysis of HLA class II (DR) antigens in liver disease in man. J Clin Pathol 1987; 40: 879–884
191. Rogoff T M, Lipsky P E. Role of the Kupffer cells in local and systemic immune responses. Gastroenterology 1981; 80: 854–860
192. Rifai A, Mannik M. Clearance of circulatory IgA immune complexes is mediated by a specific receptor on Kupffer cells in mice. J Exp Med 1984; 160: 125–137

193. Gale R P, Sparkes R S, Golde D W. Bone marrow origin of hepatic macrophages (Kupffer cells) in humans. Science 1978; 201: 937–938

194. Bouwens L, Baekeland M, Wisse E. Cytokinetic analysis of the expanding Kupffer cell population in rat liver. Cell Tissue Kin 1986; 19: 217–226

195. Johnson S J, Hines J E, Burt A D. Macrophage and perisinusoidal cell kinetics in acute liver injury. J Pathol 1992; 166: 351–358

196. Naito M, Takahashi K, Ohno H, Nishikawa S I. Yolk sac macrophages — a possible Kupffer cell precursor in the fetal mouse liver. In: Wisse E, Knook D L, Decker K, eds. Cells of the hepatic sinusoid. Rijswijk: Kupffer Cell Foundation, 1989; 2: 419–420

197. Wisse E, van't Noordende J M, van der Meulen J, Daems W Th. The pit cell: description of a new cell type occurring in rat liver and peripheral blood. Cell Tiss Res 1976; 173: 423–435

198. Winnock M, Lafon M-E, Boulard A et al. Characterisation of liver-associated natural killer cells in patients with liver tumours. Hepatology 1991; 13: 676–682

199. Winnock M, Barcina M G, Lukomska B, Bioulac-Sage P, Balabaud C. Liver-associated lymphocytes: role in tumor defense. Semin Liver Dis 1993; 13: 81–92

200. Bowwens L, Remels L, Baekeband M et al. Large granular lymphocytes or "pit cells" from rat liver: isolation, ultrastructural characterisation and natural killer activity. Eur J Immunol 1987; 17: 37–42

201. Vanderkerken K, Bouwens L, De Neve W et al. Origin and differentiation of hepatic natural killer cells (pit cells). Hepatology 1993; 18: 919–925

202. Terada T, Nakanuma Y, Ohta G. Glandular elements around the intrahepatic bile ducts in man: their morphology and distribution in normal livers. Liver 1987; 7: 1–8

203. Ishida F, Terada T, Nakanuma Y. Histologic and scanning electron microscopic observations of intrahepatic peribiliary glands in normal human livers. Lab Invest 1989; 60: 260–265

204. Yamamoto K, Fisher M M, Phillips M J. Hilar biliary plexus in human liver. Lab Invest 1985; 52: 103–106

204a. Nakanuma Y, Katayanagi K, Terada T, Saito K. Intrahepatic peribiliary glands of humans. I. Anatomy, development and presumed functions. J Gastroenterol Hepatol 1994; 9: 75–79

204b. Nakanuma Y, Sasaki M, Terada T, Harada K. Intrahepatic peribiliary glands of humans. II. Pathological spectrum. J Gastroenterol Hepatol 1994; 9: 80–86

205. Reichen J. Physiology of bile formation and of the mobility of the biliary tree. In: McIntyre N, Benhamou J-P, Bircher J, Rizzetto M, Rodes J, eds. Oxford textbook of clinical hepatology. Oxford: Oxford University Press, 1991: pp 87–94

206. Sirica A E. Biology of biliary epithelial cells. In: Bruyer J L, Ockner R E, eds. Progress in liver diseases, vol X. Philadelphia: Saunders, 1992: pp 63–87

207. Rous P, McMaster P D. Physiological causes for the varied character of stasis bile. J Exp Med 1921; 24: 75–95

208. Alpini G, Lenzi R, Zhai W-R et al. Bile secretory function of intrahepatic biliary epithelium in the rat. Am J Physiol 1989; 257: G124–G133

209. Yoon Y B, Hogey L R, Hofmann A F et al. Effect of side chain shortening on the physiological properties of bile acids: hepatic transport and effect on biliary reaction of 23 urodeoxycholate in rodents. Gastroenterology 1986; 90: 837–852

210. Lamri Y, Erlinger S, Dumont M, Roda A, Feldmann G. Immunoperoxidase localisation of urodeoxycholic acid in rat biliary epithelial cells. Evidence for a cholehepatic circulation. Liver 1992; 12: 351–354

211. Sugiura H, Nakanuma Y. Secretory components and immunoglobulins in the intrahepatic biliary tree and peribiliary glands in normal livers and hepatolithiasis. Gastroenterol Jpn 1989; 24: 308–314

212. Kurumaya H, Nakanuma Y, Ohta G. Endocrine cells in the intrahepatic biliary tree in normal livers and hepatolithiasis. Arch Pathol Lab Med 1989; 113: 143–147

213. Terada T, Nakanuma Y. Immunohistochemical demonstration of pancreatic α-amylase and trypsin in intrahepatic bile ducts and peribiliary glands. Hepatology 1991; 14: 1129–1135

214. Rojkind M. Extracellular matrix. In: Arias I M, Jakoby W B, Popper H, Schachter D, Shafritz D A, eds. The liver: biology and pathobiology. New York: Raven Press, 1988: pp 707–716

215. Schuppan D. Structure of the extracellular matrix in normal and fibrotic liver: collagens and glycoproteins. Semin Liver Dis 1990; 10: 1–10

216. Friedman S L. Cellular sources of collagen and regulation of collagen production in liver. Semin Liver Dis 1990; 10: 20–29

217. Pares A, Caballera J. Metabolism of collagen and other extracellular proteins. In: McIntyre N, Benhamou J-P, Bircher J, Rizzetto M, Rodes J, eds. Oxford textbook of clinical hepatology, vol 1. Oxford: Oxford University Press, 1991: pp 199–211

218. Martinez-Hernandez A, Amenta P S. Morphology, localization and origin of the hepatic extracellular matrix. In: Zern M, Reid L, eds. Extracellular matrix: chemistry, biology, pathology. New York: Marcell Dekker, 1993

219. Bircher N, Robinson G, Farmer S. Effects of extracellular matrix on hepatocyte growth and gene expression: implications for hepatic regulation and the repair of liver injury. Semin Liver Dis 1990; 10: 11–19

220. Murat A I, Sattler C A, Sattler G L, Pitot H C. Reestablishment of cell polarity of rat hepatocytes in primary culture. Hepatology 1993; 18: 198–205

221. McGuire R F, Bissell D M, Boyle J, Roll F J. Role of extracellular matrix in regulating fenestrations of sinusoidal endothelial cells isolated from normal rat liver. Hepatology 1992; 15: 989–997

222. Arthur M J P. Matrix degradation in the liver. Semin Liver Dis 1990; 10: 47–55

223. Witte M H, Witte C L. Lymphatic system in the liver. In: Abramson D I, Dobrin P B, eds. Blood vessels and lymphatics in organ systems. New York: Academic Press, 1984

224. Barrowman J A. Hepatic lymph and lymphatics. In: McIntyre N, Benhamou J-P, Bircher J, Rizzetto M, Rodes J, eds. Oxford textbook of clinical hepatology, vol 1. Oxford: Oxford University Press, 1991: pp 37–40

225. Smith J B, McIntosh G H, Morris B. The traffic of cells through tissues: a study of peripheral lymph in sheep. J Anat 1970; 107: 87–100

226. Comparini L, Bastianini A. Graphic reconstructions in the morphological study of the hepatic lymph vessels. Angiologica 1965; 2: 81–95

227. Comparini L. Lymph vessels of the liver in man. Angiologica 1969; 6: 262–274

228. Granger D N, Miller T, Allen R, Parker R E, Parker J C, Taylor A E. Permselectivity of cat blood-lymph barrier to endogenous macromolecules. Gastroenterology 1979; 77: 103–109

229. Witte M H. Ascitic, thy lymph runneth over. Gastroenterology 1979; 76: 1066–1068

230. Henriksen J H, Horn T, Christoffersen P. The blood-lymph barrier in the liver. A review based on morphological and functional concepts of normal and cirrhotic liver. Liver 1984; 4: 221–232

231. Wisse E, de Zanger R B, Jacobs R. Lobular gradients in endothelial fenestrae and sinusoidal diameter favour centro-lobular exchange processes: a scanning EM study. In: Knook D C, Wisse E, eds. Sinusoidal liver cells. Amsterdam: Elsevier, 1982: pp 61–67

232. Wisse E, de Zarger R B, Jacobs R, McCuskey R S. Scanning electron microscope observations on the structure of portal veins, sinusoids and central veins in rat liver. Scanning Electron Microscopy 1983; 3: 1441–1452

233. Al-Jomard A, Reid O, Scothorne R J. An EM study of the route of drainage of interstitial fluid from the space of Disse into portal tract lymphatics. Proceed XIIth Int Anatomical Congress, 1985; p. 9 (abstract)

234. Friedman J M. Hepatic nerve function. In: Arias I M, Popper H, Jakoby W B, Schachter D, Shafritz D A, eds. The liver, biology and pathobiology. New York: Raven Press, 1988: pp 949–959

235. Maher J J, Friedman S L. Parenchymal and nonparenchymal cell interactions in the liver. Semin Liver Dis 1993; 13: 13–20

236. Moghimzadeh E, Nobin A, Rosengren E. Fluorescence microscopical and chemical characterization of the adrenergic innervation in mammalian liver tissue. Cell Tiss Res 1983; 230: 605–613

237. Burt A D, Tiniakos D, MacSween R N M et al. Localization of adrenergic and neuropeptide tyrosine-containing nerves in the mammalian liver. Hepatology 1989; 9: 839–845

238. Bioulac-Sage P, Lafon M E, Saric J, Balabaud C. Nerves and perisinusoidal cells in human liver. J Hepatol 1990; 10: 105–112

239. Hartmann H, Beckh K, Jungermann K. Direct control of glycogen metabolism in the perfused rat liver by the sympathetic innervation. Eur J Biochem 1982; 123: 521–526

240. Lautt W W. Hepatic nerves: a review of their function and effects. Can J Physiol Pharmacol 1980; 58: 105–123

241. Lautt W W. Afferent and efferent neural roles in liver function. Prog Neurobiol 1983; 1: 323–348

242. Skaaring P, Bierring F. On the intrinsic innervation of normal rat liver. Histochemical and scanning electron microscopic studies. Cell Tiss Res 1976; 171: 141–155

243. Amenta F, Cavallotti C, Ferrante F et al. Cholinergic nerves in the human liver. Histochem J 1981; 13: 419–424

244. Goehler L E, Sternini C, Brecha N C. Calcitonin gene-related peptide immunoreactivity in the biliary pathway and liver of the guinea-pig: distribution and colocalization with substance P. Cell Tiss Res 1988; 253: 145–150

245. Feher E, Fodor E, Feher J. Ultrastructural localization of somatostatin- and substance P-immunoreactive nerve fibers in the feline liver. Gastroenterology 1992; 102: 287–294

246. Dhillon A P, Sankey E A, Wang J H et al. Immunohistochemical studies on the innervation of human transplanted liver. J Pathol 1992; 167: 211–216

247. Boon A P, Hubscher S G, Lee J L, Hines J E, Burt A D. Hepatic reinnervation following orthotopic liver transplantation in man. J Pathol 1992; 167: 217–222

248. Ozier Y, Braillon A, Gaudia C, Roulat D, Hadengue A, Lebrec D. Hepatic denervation alters haemodynamic response to haemorrhage in conscious rats. Hepatology 1989; 10: 473–476

249. Henderson J M, Mackay G J, Lumsden A B, Alta H M, Brouillard R, Kutner M H. The effect of liver denervation on hepatic haemodynamics during hypovolaemic shock in swine. Hepatology 1992; 15: 130–133

250. Lee J A, Ahmed Q, Hines J E, Burt A D. Disappearance of hepatic parenchymal nerves in human liver cirrhosis. Gut 1992; 33: 87–91

251. Blouin A, Bolender R P, Weibel E R. Distribution of organelles and membranes between hepatocytes and non-hepatocytes in rat liver parenchyma. J Cell Biol 1977; 72: 441–455

252. Bronfenmajer S, Schaffner F, Popper H. Fat-storing cells (lipocytes) in human liver. Arch Pathol 1966; 82: 447–453

253. Hopwood D, Nyfors A. Effect of methotrexate therapy in psoriatics on the Ito cells in liver biopsies, assessed by point-counting. J Clin Pathol 1976; 29: 698–703

2

Pathophysiology of the liver

A. D. Burt   O. F. W. James

The liver plays many pivotal roles in intermediary metabolism and in the clearance of toxins. These are facilitated by its unique anatomical relationships, in particular by the presence of a dual blood supply. Many of the conditions described in subsequent chapters lead to profound disturbances in liver function and to alterations in the hepatic circulation. In this chapter we briefly consider the physiological basis of the major metabolic processes in normal liver. The clinical manifestations of liver disease are then discussed in relation to their pathophysiology. Finally, methods available for the assessment of liver function will be described; an understanding of biochemical tests and imaging techniques that are commonly used in clinical hepatology is essential for those involved in liver biopsy interpretation. Several textbooks of hepatology are recommended for a more comprehensive review of liver pathophysiology.[1-5]

PHYSIOLOGY OF HEPATIC FUNCTION

HEPATIC CIRCULATION

The high level of metabolic activity in the liver is reflected in the magnitude of its blood supply. Total hepatic blood flow in normal adults under resting conditions is between 1500 and 1900 ml/min,[6] which amounts to approximately 25% of cardiac output. Clearance studies have shown values to be higher in males than females and to fall with advancing age.[6] Hepatic blood flow increases after feeding[7] and decreases during sleep[8] and exercise.[9] The liver receives blood from two sources: the hepatic artery normally contributes approximately one-third and the remainder is supplied by the portal vein.[10] Arterial and portal venous blood becomes admixed within the sinusoids. The proportions contributed by the hepatic artery and portal vein vary considerably under different conditions.[11] In cirrhosis, for example, the amount derived from the arterial supply is greatly increased, due largely to portal-systemic shunting.

Hepatic artery

The hepatic artery is a branch of the coeliac axis. At the porta hepatis it lies in front of the portal vein and medial to the common bile duct. It divides into right and left branches and each branch supplies one of the two 'functional' halves of the liver. Each 'functional' half comprises two sectors which can be further subdivided into segments (p. 10).[12] Additional branches of the hepatic artery include the right gastric and gastroduodenal arteries. Variations in the anatomy and distribution of the hepatic artery are common and aberrant branches are frequently observed in imaging studies; they are rarely of clinical importance. Within the liver, branches of the hepatic artery lie in the portal tracts and drain into the sinusoids of acinar zone 1; arterio-portal anastomoses have been demonstrated in several species[13] but are not present in the human liver.

Portal vein

The portal vein is formed by the confluence of the superior mesenteric and splenic veins (Fig. 2.1). It is approximately 6–8 cm in length and has a mean diameter of 12 mm.[14] The superior mesenteric vein receives blood from the small intestine, colon and head of pancreas. The splenic vein is formed from several tributaries originating at the splenic hilum and also receives blood from the pancreas and from the left gastroepiploic and inferior mesenteric veins. At the porta hepatis, the portal vein divides into two branches before entering the liver. Portal vein radicles accompany hepatic artery branches and have an identical intrahepatic distribution. Portal venous blood has a considerably higher oxygen content than that of systemic veins and it contributes over 60% of the total oxygen supply to the liver under normal circumstances.

Regulation of hepatic blood flow

The pressure in the hepatic artery is equivalent to that of the systemic blood pressure while that in the portal system is between 6 and 10 mmHg; these pressures are equilibrated within the sinusoids where it is estimated to be approximately 3 mmHg above that in the inferior vena cava. Alterations to total hepatic blood flow are largely determined by changes in the hepatic artery. As in other tissues, a relatively constant arterial flow is maintained by autoregulation. Thus, over the physiological range, vascular resistance rises or falls in parallel with the arterial pressure; this effect may be mediated by adenosine.[15] However, unlike most other organs, hepatic arterial flow rates are not significantly altered by changes in hepatic oxygen demand. The liver normally extracts less than 40% of oxygen supplied and, in situations where demand is increased, this is met by enhanced extraction.[16] Reduction in portal venous flow leads to an increase in hepatic arterial flow. The mechanisms responsible for this pressure-flow relationship are uncertain but may also involve adenosine.[17] There is no autoregulation in the portal venous system and changes in flow within the portal vein are largely determined by factors affecting intestinal blood supply.

Under normal circumstances, the liver contains an amount of blood disproportionate to its weight and may serve as a reservoir. Experimental studies have shown that in massive haemorrhage the liver can expel up to 50% of hepatic blood volume as part of a compensatory mechanism and that this is mediated by sympathetic nerves.[18]

Hepatic lymph

Lymphatic channels are found in portal tracts, around some hepatic vein branches and in Glisson's capsule,[19] but not within hepatic acini. The relationship between these networks and the generation of hepatic lymph is discussed in chapter 1. As in other tissues, lymph flow is involved in the maintenance of fluid homeostasis. In contrast to other organs, however, accumulated interstitial fluid in the liver can be removed not only via the lymphatic circulation but also into the peritoneal cavity through the capsule. Hepatic lymph is estimated to account for up to 50% of total thoracic duct flow, a rate equivalent to approximately 0.75 ml/min.

BILIRUBIN METABOLISM

The liver is responsible for the disposal of bile pigments. Bilirubin is formed from the breakdown of the porphyrin moiety of haem-containing compounds such as haemoglobin, myoglobin, cytochromes and catalase.[20] Daily bilirubin production in normal adults amounts to approxi-

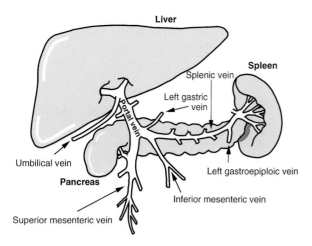

Fig. 2.1 Anatomy of the portal venous system.

mately 300 mg. Kinetic studies using radiolabelled haem precursors such as ε-aminolaevulinic acid have demonstrated that over 80% of this is derived from catabolism of haemoglobin from senescent erythrocytes.[21] The major peak of labelled bile pigments is observed between 90 and 150 days, which is equivalent to the normal red blood cell life span. 'Early-labelled bilirubin', excreted within a few days, is derived from hepatic haem compounds (in particular cytochromes P-450) and from prematurely destroyed erythrocyte precursors; the latter fraction increases in conditions of ineffective erythropoiesis.[21]

Synthesis of unconjugated bilirubin involves two distinct enzyme systems and occurs mainly in cells of the mononuclear phagocyte system.[22] Haem oxygenase cleaves the porphyrin ring of haem; this is an oxygen- and NADPH-dependent reaction and leads to generation of biliverdin. The enzyme has a remarkable stereoselectivity for the α-meso bridge of haem. As a result, although other isomers are formed, the predominant fraction of bile pigments in man are of IXα type. In the second system, biliverdin is converted to bilirubin by the cytosolic enzyme biliverdin reductase.[22] Unconjugated IXα bilirubin is lipid-soluble and in the fully protonated diacid form has a biplanar ridge-tile configuration. The molecular structure of bilirubin determines its ionization, solubility, binding to serum proteins and subsequent handling by the hepatocyte.[23,24]

Bilirubin formed in the mononuclear phagocyte system (and approximately 40% of that derived from hepatic haem) is released into the blood stream where it is attached to a high affinity binding site on albumin. This interaction can be altered by some drugs such as sulphonamides. Under normal circumstances, circulating free bilirubin is present in only trace amounts. Bilirubin is efficiently removed from plasma by hepatocytes. Although this was originally thought to be mediated through a specific albumin receptor, it appears to involve other carrier proteins present at the sinusoidal domain or basolateral membrane of hepatocytes. At least three putative carriers have been described for the uptake of non-bile acid organic anions — bilitranslocase, bilirubin-BSP binding protein and organic anion binding protein.[24,25] The relative roles of these systems in the uptake of bilirubin are yet to be elucidated. There is evidence that some bilirubin may be transported into hepatocytes by simple physico-chemical partitioning in the absence of specific carriers. The process is seen as a series of potentially reversible steps — dissociation from albumin, influx through hepatocyte membranes, intracytoplasmic transport and conjugation — each of which contributes to determine the rate of uptake.[26] Within the hepatocyte, bilirubin is bound to ligandin and Z (or fatty acid binding) protein, both of which prevent reflux back into the plasma. The lipid-soluble unconjugated bilirubin is converted to a water-soluble compound by conjugation with UDP-xylose, UDP-glucose and UDP-glucuronic acid. Glucuronidation is the most important form of bilirubin conjugation in humans and is catalysed by microsomal UDP glucuronosyl transferases.[20] These are classified into two subfamilies; only those in subfamily 1 are involved in bilirubin metabolism. This enzyme family catalyses glucuronidation not only of bilirubin but of other endogenous and exogenous compounds such as thyroid hormones, catecholamines and morphine. The four enzymes identified thus far in subfamily 1 are encoded by a single gene, distinct mRNA species being the result of alternative splicing.[27] Deficiency of bilirubin UDP glucuronosyl transferase activity is a feature of the inherited conjugated hyperbilirubinaemias, Crigler–Najjar and Gilbert's syndromes. Knowledge of the molecular biology of the controlling gene has led to a greater understanding of the clinical expression of these disorders.

Monoglucuronide and diglucuronide forms of conjugated bilirubin are generated, the latter being the predominant type secreted in human bile. The mechanisms responsible for transport from the smooth endoplasmic reticulum, where conjugation takes place, to the canalicular membrane of the hepatocyte remain elusive but may be regarded as carrier mediated since the system appears saturable and susceptible to competitive inhibitors. The relative roles of cytosolic flow, binding to proteins such as ligandin, and Golgi-derived vesicular transport, remain to be determined. Excretion of conjugated bilirubin into the canaliculus involves are ATP-dependent multispecific organic anion transporter.[28] Within the biliary system, conjugated bilirubin is incorporated into mixed micelles. It is not absorbed from the small intestine, but in the colon bacterial β-glucuronidases hydrolyses conjugated bilirubin with the formation of urobilinogens. These are lipid-soluble and absorption occurs to only a very limited extent in the colon. Any urobilinogen and small amounts of unconjugated bilirubin which are absorbed are re-excreted by the kidneys and liver. Thus, enterohepatic circulation of bile pigments is of minor physiological significance. When liver function is impaired, however, or in haemolysis, the relative amount re-excreted by the kidneys increases leading to urobilinogenuria.[29]

BILE ACID METABOLISM

The principal functions of bile acids are:

(i) maintenance of cholesterol homeostasis,
(ii) stimulation of bile flow in the biliary system, and
(iii) emulsification/absorption of dietary lipid in the intestine.

Bile acids are highly conserved in nature although the chemical composition of the major bile acids in lower vertebrates differs from the 24 carbon atom structure seen in man.[30] The liver plays a pivotal role in bile acid metabolism in that the hepatocyte is the only cell with the ability to enzymatically convert cholesterol to bile acids.[31] Cholesterol for this process is derived from two sources: (i) chylomicron remnants containing dietary cholesterol and (ii) de novo synthesis from acetyl-CoA by liver cells. The biosynthetic pathways for the generation of bile acids have been reviewed in detail.[32,33] Structurally, the bile acid molecule has two distinct components: a steroid nucleus and an aliphatic side-chain; this basic skeleton is termed cholane. The two principal cholanoic acids formed from cholesterol in the human liver (the so-called *primary bile acids*) are cholic acid and chenodeoxycholic acid. Synthesis from cholesterol is a multi-step process, the key elements of which are: (i) modifications to the steroid nucleus, including reduction of a carbon double bond and epimerization of the 3-hydroxyl group, and (ii) subsequent oxidation of the aliphatic side chain with loss of the terminal three carbon atoms (Fig. 2.2). The rate-limiting step in the conversion of cholesterol to 7α-hydroxycholesterol involves the microsomal enzyme 7α-hydroxylase.[34] The activity of this cytochrome P-450-dependent mono-oxygenase is regulated by the level of bile acids returning to the liver in the enterohepatic circulation and is a classic example of a negative feedback system.[31] Bile acids with side-chains of variable length are found under certain circumstances. C20 forms are present in the meconium of newborn infants[35] and larger molecules have been described in children with inherited deficiencies of bile acid synthesis.[36] Bile acids with modifications to the steroid nucleus (e.g. trihydroxy- and tetrahydroxy- forms), which differ from those in the common primary bile acids, can be detected at low levels in normal adults and are more abundant in conditions associated with cholestasis.

More than 99% of bile acids are conjugated before being secreted by the hepatocytes. This is important not only for their interaction with other components of bile (e.g. phospholipids, cholesterol) but also in preventing precipitation of the protonated form in the acidic environment of the upper small intestine. The most common conjugates are N-aminoacyl forms containing either taurine or glycine; this results from the action of two enzymes — bile acid CoA synthetase and an N-acyltransferase. Other methods of bile acid conjugation (e.g. glucuronidation, sulphation) occur to a limited extent in normal individuals but to a much greater degree in cholestasis. The conjugated bile acids are secreted into the canaliculi against a large concentration gradient. This is partly mediated by electrical forces due to the high potential across the canaliculus (–30 mV),[37] and partly by a specific 100 kD carrier protein.[38] Bile acids secreted into the canaliculi exert a large osmotic effect; this is one of the mechanisms responsible for the induction of bile flow (bile acid-dependent flow).[38] An additional effect is induction of secretion by hepatocytes of vesicles containing phospholipids and cholesterol. The bile acids solubilize these vesicles with the formation of mixed micelles. These pass through the biliary system and enter the duodenum, although during fasting, when the sphincter of Oddi is contracted, bile acids are stored in the gallbladder. Within the small intestine bile acids help to solubilize monoglycerides and fatty acids which have been formed from the digestion of dietary triglyceride; this enhances absorption of lipids and fat-soluble vitamins. Some of the bile acids are deconjugated in the jejunum and ileum and these can be reabsorbed by passive diffusion.

Conjugated bile acids are efficiently taken up by ileal enterocytes. This involves an active transport system located at the basolateral domain of these cells.[39] Reabsorbed bile acids are transported back to the liver in the portal venous blood. Uptake by hepatocytes is an efficient process involving transport systems distinct from those involved in bilirubin uptake.[40] Transport of bile acids through the hepatocyte involves a number of cytosolic proteins which include sulphotransferase and glutathione S-transferase.[41] Deconjugated bile acids are reconjugated and secreted once more into the canaliculus. This enterohepatic circulation leads to efficient conservation of bile acids. Cycling between the liver and intestine is estimated

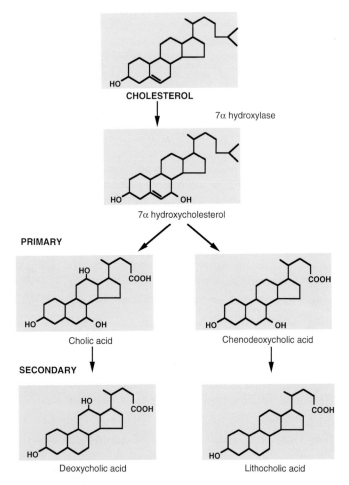

Fig. 2.2 Pathways of bile acid biosynthesis.

to occur up to 15 times a day. Primary bile acids which are not reabsorbed in the ileum undergo biotransformation by bacterial enzymes in the colon. Loss of the 7-hydroxyl group is catalysed by anaerobes, leading to the formation of deoxycholic and lithocholic acid from cholic acid and chenodeoxycholic acid respectively — the so-called *secondary bile acids* (Fig. 2.2); these are the four main constituents of the bile acid pool. Other changes which may occur include oxidation of hydroxyl groups with subsequent reduction and epimerization. By this mechanism, cholic acid is transformed to the 7β-hydroxyl form and chenodeoxycholic acid becomes ursodeoxycholic acid. This form of biotransformation also occurs in the liver but is trivial in normal man.

Less than a quarter of the secondary bile acids generated are reabsorbed from the colon, enter the portal venous system and are removed by the hepatocytes, thus forming an additional component to the enterohepatic circulation. Absorption of deoxycholic acid occurs more readily than that of lithocholic acid; the latter undergoes only limited enterohepatic cycling. Under normal circumstances, very little bile acid enters the systemic circulation and urinary excretion is therefore negligible. Daily faecal bile acid excretion (principally in the form of lithocholic and deoxycholic acid) amounts to approximately 500 mg and is balanced by biosynthesis from cholesterol. In liver disease, measurement of serum bile acid levels has been proposed as a liver function test but experience has shown that such measurements carry no advantage over other measures of hepatic dysfunction.

LIPID METABOLISM

Several forms of lipid are normally present in plasma — cholesterol and cholesterol esters, triglycerides and phospholipids. These are water insoluble and are present as lipoproteins which are classified on the basis of their ultracentrifugal properties into very low density lipoprotein (VLDL), low density lipoprotein (LDL) and high density lipoprotein (HDL); chylomicrons form a further class of lipoprotein. Lipoproteins are spherical particles with a hydrophobic core, covered by a single layer of amphipathic molecules — phospholipid, cholesterol and one or more apoproteins. The apoproteins are polypeptide chains originally classified into three major forms but it is now recognized that a large number of distinct molecules exist. VLDL, LDL and HDL differ in their apoprotein composition. A novel lipoprotein fraction Lp(a), whose function has yet to be established and whose concentration varies widely between individuals, has recently been described.[42] High levels of Lp(a) are associated with increased risk of coronary heart disease. The liver plays a central role in lipoprotein metabolism and cholesterol homeostasis and is frequently involved in diseases affecting lipid metabolism (see Ch. 4).

Cholesterol metabolism

Cholesterol is a component of all cell membranes, where it exists as free sterol. In plasma and in some organs such as the liver, cholesterol esters are also found in which a long chain fatty acid is attached to the 3β-hydroxyl group. Cholesterol can be synthesized by most cell types but in the liver synthesis occurs predominantly within hepatocytes. The amount synthesized daily in the liver of normal individuals is approximately double that obtained from dietary sources. Over 1.2 g of cholesterol is lost in the faeces daily in the form of free sterol or as bile acids. Cholesterol synthesis involves a complex pathway. Mevalonate is initially formed from acetyl-CoA via 3-hydroxy-3-methylglutaryl CoA (HMG CoA) and subsequently phosphorylated and decarboxylated to form isopentenyl pyrophosphate. Condensation of several molecules of this leads to generation of squalene. The subsequent conversion to cholesterol is a multi-step process with lanosterol as an intermediate. The rate-limiting step is production of mevalonate from HMG CoA, a reaction which is catalysed by HMG CoA reductase.[43] The activity of this enzyme is controlled by cholesterol — another example of negative feedback inhibition. Cholesterol synthesized in the hepatocyte can be further metabolized by acyl-CoA cholesterol-acyl transferase (ACAT) to cholesterol ester which is packaged into lipoproteins and secreted into the blood stream. Alternatively, it can be excreted via the biliary system either as neutral lipid or following conversion to bile acids.

Fatty acid metabolism

Hepatocytes are capable of endogenous fatty acid synthesis. This pathway involves two cytosolic enzymes — acetyl-CoA carboxylase and fatty acid synthase. The former catalyses the formation of palmitoyl-CoA from malonyl-CoA and acetyl-CoA.[44] Liver cells can also take up exogenous non-esterified fatty acids from the blood. They are principally derived from adipose tissue following triglyceride hydrolysis by a hormone-sensitive lipase. Smaller amounts also come from absorption of dietary non-esterified fatty acids and from circulating triglyceride-rich lipoproteins by the action of lipoprotein lipase. For fatty acids to be metabolized by the hepatocyte they must first be 'activated' to acyl-CoA esters. These can then be utilized in the formation of triglyceride, phospholipid or cholesterol esters, or alternatively can be oxidized in mitochondria to yield acetyl-CoA.[45] The latter process is dependent on a specific transporter system involving carnitine acyl transferase which enables fatty acyl-CoA to gain access to the mitochondrial matrix. A small amount of fatty acid metabolism also occurs in peroxisomes.[46] This process does not have any requirement for specific transporters, but complete oxidation to acetyl-CoA does not occur.

Triglyceride and phospholipid metabolism

Esterification of fatty acyl-CoA with glycerol 3-phosphate produces triglyceride. Microsomal and cytosolic phosphatidate phosphohydrolase catalyses the formation of diacylglycerol from phosphatidate and this is an important control enzyme in triglyceride synthesis.[47] Diacylglycerol acyl transferase catalyses the final step in the pathway; this is the only step unique to triglyceride synthesis (the others are shared with phospholipid synthesis). The triglyceride thus formed is either utilized for the generation of lipoproteins for export or metabolized within the hepatocyte (Fig. 2.3). This occurs through the action of hepatic lipases located in lysosomes and, to a lesser extent, in the endoplasmic reticulum. Phospholipid synthesis requires activation of its constituent bases (e.g. choline and ethanolamine) before reaction with diacylglycerol.

Lipoprotein metabolism

The role of the liver in lipoprotein metabolism is complex.[48] The main features are: (i) secretion of HDL and VLDL; (ii) removal of chylomicron remnants and LDL; and (iii) secretion of lecithin-cholesterol acyl transferase (LCAT) into the blood.

High density lipoprotein is secreted as a nascent particle containing the apoproteins ApoAI and ApoAII[49] which are synthesized by the hepatocyte. The particle plays an important role in 'reverse' cholesterol transport and thus in cholesterol turnover. Further metabolism of HDL in the plasma requires LCAT which forms cholesterol ester from cholesterol and phosphatidylcholine and involves the interaction of several apoproteins.[50] VLDL is a triglyceride-rich lipoprotein containing ApoB100, ApoC and ApoE. These particles are assembled within the endoplasmic reticulum and Golgi apparatus of the hepatocyte before being secreted.

Chylomicron remnants and LDL are removed from the circulation following interaction of their surface apoproteins with specific hepatic receptors. Uptake and degradation of LDL by the hepatocyte alters hepatic cholesterol

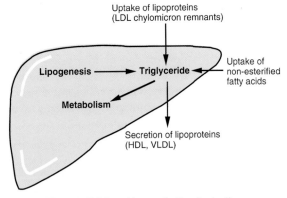

Fig. 2.3 Triglyceride metabolism in the liver.

metabolism by inhibiting HMG CoA reductase activity and by stimulating ACAT activity.

AMINO ACID, PROTEIN AND AMMONIA METABOLISM

Amino acids

The liver is of prime importance in amino acid metabolism. Amino acids are removed from the plasma by hepatocytes and are used for protein synthesis or as a source of energy through gluconeogenesis. Under normal circumstances plasma amino acids are derived from intestinal absorption but skeletal muscle becomes the major source when there is dietary protein deprivation.[51] The 'essential' amino acids must be present in the diet as these cannot be synthesized de novo. The liver is the principal site for the synthesis and modification of non-essential amino acids and for the re-amination of most essential amino acids. It may also release amino acids for utilization by peripheral tissues.[52] Furthermore, it plays a major role in the breakdown of amino acids with the production of urea.[53]

While twenty different amino acids are utilized for protein synthesis in man, more than this number are found in proteins since some (e.g. proline) undergo post-translational modifications. The metabolism of the individual amino acids varies considerably. Some (e.g. glycine) can be converted to glucose while others (e.g. leucine) are transaminated or de-aminated to keto-acids. The branched chain essential amino acids leucine, valine and isoleucine are unlike other amino acids in that they are taken up to only a limited extent by the liver, and most are extracted and metabolized by skeletal muscle.[54]

The daily turnover of amino acids is high in normal individuals (250–300 g/day in a 70 kg man). A large proportion of those released following protein degradation are re-utilized for synthesis. However, over 30 g per day is irreversibly catabolized and lost to the amino acid/protein pool, and this must be balanced by dietary intake. In many liver diseases protein catabolism is considerably increased. Nitrogen released from the complete catabolism of amino acids can be removed by a variety of routes but the principal pathway is urea synthesis and excretion. With the exception of the branched chain amino acids, all essential amino acids are degraded in the liver. Non-essential amino acids can be oxidized in liver and skeletal muscle.

Urea, ammonia and nitrogen balance

Catabolism of amino acids yields ammonia. This can be used for the synthesis of other nitrogenous compounds but it is highly toxic and the liver is largely responsible for its removal. Other endogenous sources of ammonia in-

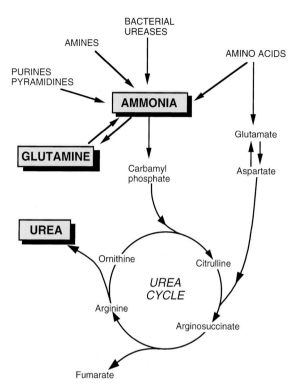

Fig. 2.4 Pathways of ammonia metabolism.

clude purines and pyramidines from nucleic acids and amines such as noradrenaline; up to 25% comes via the portal system from the intestine where it is generated by bacterial ureases. The major pathways of ammonia metabolism are outlined in Figure 2.4.[55] Over 90% of surplus nitrogen is disposed of by conversion of ammonia to urea which is then excreted by the kidneys. The urea cycle occurs almost exclusively in liver. Two of the key enzymes — carbamyl synthetase I and ornithine transcarbamylase — are found in only trace amounts in other tissues. They are expressed most abundantly by periportal (zone 1) hepatocytes.[56] Urea synthesis is regulated by intrahepatic levels of N-acetylglutamate and is also under hormonal control which involves glucagon and glucocorticoids.[57] The other major pathway for ammonia removal is through the production of glutamine. In contrast to urea cycle enzymes, glutamine synthetase is found only in perivenular (zone 3) liver cells.[58]

Protein metabolism and the liver

Hepatic protein synthesis accounts for approximately 15% of total body protein production. A small fraction of this relates to synthesis of structural proteins and cytoplasmic enzymes but the bulk of it is accounted for by secretory products — the plasma proteins.[59] These are generated on the polyribosomes of the rough endoplasmic reticulum of hepatocytes and are released into the circulation at the sinusoidal domain of the cells. The multiple steps involved

in gene transcription, RNA processing and translation have now been elucidated.[60-62] Some data on transcriptional regulation have come from studies of liver-specific proteins such as albumin. With many genes, there are regulatory sequences upstream from the transcriptional start point, which control the rate of transcription.[60] In the case of albumin, this comprises two sequences common to other genes (promoters) — the TATA- and CAAT-boxes — and two liver-specific control sequences (enhancers).[63] The regulatory function of promoters is mediated by specific proteins — the so-called transcription factors. The effects of enhancer sequences may also be influenced by specific proteins but the mechanisms are less clearly understood. Newly synthesized protein is transported from the ribosomes into the lumen of the endoplasmic reticulum, a process which involves binding of a signal sequence on the molecule to a signal recognition particle.[64] Once inside the endoplasmic reticulum, the signal sequence is cleaved and the protein undergoes further post-translational modifications as it is transported along the secretory pathway via the cis- and trans-Golgi apparatus. These include formation of disulphide bonds and glycosylation. Some blood coagulation proteins synthesized in the liver (factors II, VII, IX, X) contain an N-terminal γ-carboxyglutamic acid residue which is essential for their normal function. This modification involves a vitamin K-dependent carboxylase. Abnormal secretory proteins resulting from gene mutations (e.g. Z-type α_1-antitrypsin) may show impaired transport along the secretory pathway resulting in an endoplasmic reticulum storage disorder (p. 143). Proteins are finally transported from the trans-Golgi to the cell surface in secretory vesicles[65] by the action of microtubules. The mechanisms responsible for directing secretory proteins to the sinusoidal domain of the cell are thought to involve 'sorting carrier proteins' within the Golgi apparatus.[66]

Various factors influence the level of protein synthesis in the liver. Nutritional status is important. In starvation, the rate of synthesis drops due to decreased availability of amino acids, decreased RNA stability and disaggregation of ribosomes.[67] Several hormones are known to alter hepatic protein synthetic rates. Insulin, for example, increases synthesis (possibly via transcription factors), whereas glucagon has an inhibitory effect. The synthesis and secretion of some proteins (e.g. C-reactive protein, serum amyloid A, C3) by hepatocytes is increased in the face of tissue injury and inflammation — the so-called *acute phase response*. Synthesis of serum amyloid A may be increased several hundred-fold. Under such circumstances, however, the rate of synthesis of other proteins such as albumin may decrease. These are referred to as negative acute phase proteins. The acute phase response is mediated principally by cytokines released by lymphocytes and macrophages. Interleukin-1 and tumour necrosis factor α are known to play a role but interleukin-6 is thought to be the most important mediator. These molecules have effects at both transcriptional and post-transcriptional levels.[68] Interleukin-6 induces the interaction of DNA-binding proteins with promoter elements of several acute phase genes. It may also enhance the secretion rate of some proteins including α_2-macroglobulin.

The major proteins secreted by the hepatocyte are listed in Table 2.1. Albumin is the most abundant with a normal plasma concentration of 40–50 g/l. It has two principal functions: the regulation of plasma oncotic pressure and as a major transport protein.[69] Transferrin is the carrier protein for iron in plasma; the role of this molecule in iron transport and storage has been reviewed extensively[70,71] and the subject is discussed in chapter 5. Caeruloplasmin is an α_2-glycoprotein which acts as a specific copper-binding protein. The liver is the sole site of synthesis of all components of the coagulation cascade, apart from factor VIII which can be synthesized at other sites. In addition, it produces many of the proteins involved in fibrinolysis, although plasminogen activators are mainly synthesized at extrahepatic sites. The complement system is important in host defence against microorganisms and in inflammation.[72] It can be activated via the classical or alternative pathways and a number of inhibitory control proteins are known to exist. The whole system involves more than 20 proteins, most of which are synthesized by hepatocytes, but other cells, in particular macrophages, have the capacity to produce complement proteins.[73] α_1-Antitrypsin is the most abundant of the protease inhibitors (Pi) produced in the liver, with a concentration of 2–4 g/l. It is an inhibitor of serine proteases and is mainly involved in inhibiting the activity of neutrophil elastase. There is considerable polymorphism of the α_1-antitrypsin gene; some phenotypes, most notably PiZZ, are associated with reduced serum levels and may be accompanied by pan-acinar emphysema and cirrhosis. Kupffer cells also produce α_1-antitrypsin and several other plasma proteins such as C3[74] but, in quantitative terms, their contribution is small.

In addition to being a major protein producer, the liver also plays a role in their degradation. Endogenous cytoplasmic proteins are degraded by lysosomal proteases, and the amino acids generated are re-utilized for protein synthesis or energy. Circulating glycoproteins are also degraded by hepatocytes, Kupffer cells and sinusoidal endothelial cells following uptake by receptor-mediated endocytosis. A number of elegant studies have characterized the nature and distribution of the asialoglycoprotein receptor present at the sinusoidal domain of hepatocytes and have elucidated the pathways which lead to lysosomal degradation of glycoproteins following their internalization into the cell.[75,76]

CARBOHYDRATE METABOLISM

The liver plays an important role in the maintenance of plasma carbohydrate levels.[77,78] After a meal, glucose and fructose are removed by hepatocytes from the portal venous blood. This has two beneficial effects: it provides a readily accessible energy store and it prevents wide fluctuations in plasma osmolality. The efficiency of first pass uptake of glucose by the liver is disputed; values obtained using different methods range between 25 and 60%.[79] Hepatic uptake is determined by the levels of glucose in sinusoidal blood and by the action of insulin. The ratio of glucagon to insulin may be more important and other hormones such as glucocorticoids are also involved. Within the hepatocyte, glucose is converted to glucose-6-phosphate which is then used for synthesis of glycogen or glycerol and fatty acids and hence VLDL. The liver is the predominant site for the metabolism of fructose — principally to lactate and glycogen — and of galactose to either glucose or glycogen.

During fasting, the liver becomes an essential source of energy for other tissues. Glucose is generated by two routes in the hepatocyte: glycogenolysis and gluconeogenesis. During overnight fasting the former is the more important but its contribution falls rapidly after 24 hours.[79] Gluconeogenesis in the liver utilizes lactate, pyruvate, amino acids and glycerol. Quantitatively, lactate is the most important precursor. Glycogenolysis and gluconeo-

Table 2.1 Plasma proteins synthesized in the liver

Albumin

Transport proteins
　　Lipoproteins
　　Transferrin
　　Transcortin
　　α_1 Acid glycoprotein
　　Caeruloplasmin
　　Thyroid hormone-binding proteins
　　Retinol-binding proteins
　　Vitamin D-binding proteins

Coagulation and fibrinolysis proteins
　　Fibrinogen
　　Factor II, V, VII–XIII
　　Prekallikrein
　　Kininogen
　　Prothrombin
　　Protein C
　　Plasminogen

Complement
　　C1q,r,s
　　C2–C9
　　Factor B
　　Factor D

Protease inhibitors
　　α_1-Antitrypsin
　　α_1-Antichymotrypsin
　　α_2-Macroglobulin
　　Antithrombin III
　　α_2-Antiplasmin
　　C1 inhibitor

Miscellaneous acute phase proteins
　　C-reactive protein
　　Serum amyloid A

genesis are controlled by factors similar to those regulating glucose uptake and glycogen synthesis. Thus, autoregulation by the glucose level and by insulin, glucagon and other hormones, all exert effects through complex interactions. Sympathetic nerves may also play a role.[80] There is evidence for reciprocal heterogeneity within the hepatic acinus in the activity of enzymes involved in glycogen synthesis and gluconeogenesis.[81]

XENOBIOTIC METABOLISM

Most drugs and related xenobiotics are lipophilic and this property enables such compounds to gain access to their cellular targets. The major pathways for excretion of xenobiotics are via the bile or urine and they must first be rendered hydrophilic for this to occur. This biotransformation is considered to have two distinct phases.[82] Phase I reactions convert the compound to a more polar metabolite by oxidation, reduction or hydrolysis. For some xenobiotics this is sufficient for effective excretion. Many compounds, however, require to be conjugated with an endogenous molecule such as glucuronic acid — a phase II reaction. Although both forms of biotransformation occur at a variety of extrahepatic sites (e.g. skin, intestine, kidneys, lungs), the liver is the principal site of metabolism for most drugs and related xenobiotics. Many of the enzymes involved have broad substrate specificities and have evolved for the metabolism of endogenous compounds such as steroids. However, they can also utilize xenobiotics as alternative substrates. Drug metabolism often leads to generation of an inactive compound but reactive and highly toxic intermediates may be formed. This phenomenon explains the hepatotoxicity of many therapeutic agents[83] and the final product can be more toxic than the parent compound — so-called metabolic activation. The major enzyme systems involved in hepatic metabolism of xenobiotics are outlined in Table 2.2.

One of the most important systems for the oxidation of endogenous substrates and a wide range of drugs and carcinogens involves cytochrome P-450. Although this was originally thought to be a single haem-containing enzyme with a broad substrate specificity,[84] it is now recognized that there is a group of closely related isoenzymes encoded by separate genes.[85,86] The cytochromes P-450 are classified according to their molecular structure[87] and over 70 distinct types have been identified which can be grouped into families and subfamilies. They have different but overlapping substrate specificities and their activity can be selectively enhanced by a variety of foreign compounds. Cytochromes P-450 are located within the smooth endoplasmic reticulum of hepatocytes in the so-called microsomal compartment. There is zonal heterogeneity in the expression of most isoenzymes within the acinus. The ethanol-inducible form, P-450 2E1, for example, is found most abundantly in hepatocytes of acinar zone 3. This phenomenon of zonal heterogeneity is recognized with other drug-metabolizing enzymes (Fig. 2.5). Some cytochromes P-450 are expressed by extrahepatic tissues such as gastric mucosa and renal tubular epithelium. Polymorphisms for cytochrome P-450 genes have been identified and some of these may explain differences within a population in the propensity to develop adverse drug reactions. Recently, aberrant splicing of cytochrome P-450 2D6 RNA has been demonstrated in individuals who are poor metabolizers of the drug debrisoquine.[88]

Enhancement of cytochrome P-450-dependent metabolism can be seen following exposure to a large number of agents including alcohol, tobacco smoke and drugs such as barbiturates and phenytoin.[89] This phenomenon of induction is mediated by increased expression of the genes, although the precise control mechanisms are unclear. With many drugs that are oxidized by cytochromes P-450, induction will lead to increased degradation and thus, decreased pharmacological activity. With others

Table 2.2 Hepatic enzyme systems involved in xenobiotic metabolism

Phase I reactions
 Cytochrome P-450-dependent mono-oxygenase system
 Microsomal flavin-containing mono-oxygenase
 Prostaglandin endoperoxide synthetase
 Esterases
 Epoxide hydrolase
 Dehydrogenases

Phase II reactions
 UDP-glucuronosyltransferases
 UDP-glycosyltransferase
 Glutathione S-transferases
 Methyltransferases
 Acetyltransferases
 Sulphotransferases

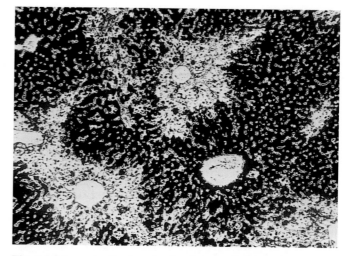

Fig. 2.5 Immunolocalization of carboxylesterase in human liver. The predominant signal is seen in hepatocytes of acinar zone 3. Rabbit polyclonal anti-carboxylesterase; indirect peroxidase. Specimen photographed using confocal scanning laser microscopy. Courtesy of Dr D J Harrison.

however, (e.g. paracetamol), induction leads to more rapid generation of reactive metabolites and may therefore exacerbate drug-induced hepatotoxicity. In the case of P-450 2E1, induction may be an important step in nitrosamine-induced carcinogenesis. Other drugs can selectively decrease cytochrome P-450 activity by competitive inhibition.

Whereas phase I oxidative metabolism may in some instances lead to more rather than less reactive metabolites, the conjugates produced by phase II metabolism are usually unreactive. A large number of commonly used drugs such as morphine and chlorpromazine are conjugated by glucuration before excretion. This is catalysed by UDP glucuronosyl transferases which belong to the same supergene family as those involved in bilirubin metabolism. Other endogenous compounds which are substrates for these enzymes include serotonin, steroids, some bile acids and catecholamines.[90] The glutathione S-transferases are another family of proteins involved in phase II reactions but they also act as intracellular binding proteins.[91] Unlike cytochromes P-450 and UDP glucuronosyl transferases, they are largely cytosolic enzymes. Several isoforms have been identified and these can be classified into three types — alpha, mu and pi — depending on their isoelectric point.[92] Glutathione S-transferases are expressed in all tissues; in the adult liver, hepatocytes express the alpha isoform but not the pi form. By contrast, bile-duct epithelium contains pi and alpha forms (Fig. 2.6).[93] Alterations to this pattern of expression occur in alcoholic liver disease, cholestasis and in hepatocellular carcinoma.[94] Recent evidence has suggested that the pi isoform may play a role in the multidrug-resistance (MDR) phenomenon observed in some human tumours, where treatment with one anticancer drug confers resistance to further treatment by that agent and other chemo-

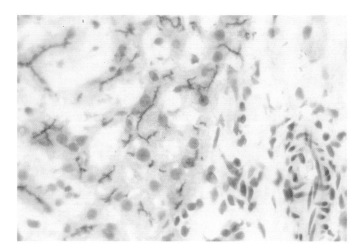

Fig. 2.7 Immunolocalization of p-glycoprotein in human liver. The protein is present at the canalicular domain of hepatocytes. Indirect immunoperoxidase. Courtesy of Dr D Tiniakos.

therapeutic agents. Hepatocytes contain another protein involved in this process, p-glycoprotein.[95] This 170 kD product of the MDR1 gene is found at the canalicular domain of hepatocytes (Fig. 2.7). It may act as a transcanalicular transporter for organic cations in the normal liver.

PORTAL HYPERTENSION

A large number of conditions lead to increased resistance and a rise in pressure in the portal venous system. This may occur from obstruction to blood flow in the portal vein itself, within the liver sinusoids or in the hepatic veins. Portal hypertension exists when pressure exceeds 10 mmHg. A collateral circulation develops which diverts blood from the portal system into the systemic veins. Pre-existing anastomotic channels open up where portal vein tributaries lie in close proximity to veins draining into the superior and inferior vena cavae.[96] These occur at five main sites:[97] in the submucosa of the oesophagus and stomach, in the submucosa at the anorectal junction, in the anterior abdominal wall, between the left renal and the splenic veins, and in the falciform ligament. When portal hypertension is due to extrahepatic obstruction as in portal vein thrombosis, additional anastomoses develop at the porta hepatis, in the suspensory ligament of the liver and in the diaphragm and omentum. These can be considered as an attempt by the portal venous flow to reach the liver by bypassing the obstruction.

Pathology

Anastomotic channels at the lower end of oesophagus are clinically the most significant and bleeding from varices at this site remains a major cause of morbidity and mortality. Vianna and co-workers used a combination of radiology,

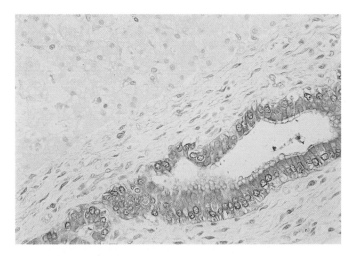

Fig. 2.6 Distribution of pi glutathione S-transferase in normal human liver. Staining is restricted to biliary epithelium. Polyclonal pi GST antibody. Indirect immunoperoxidase.

corrosion casting, histology and morphometry to study the detailed anatomy of the intrinsic and extrinsic venous systems of the gastric cardia and oesophagus in normal subjects[96] and in patients with portal hypertension.[98] The intrinsic veins, i.e. those within the wall of the stomach or oesophagus, are found in four well-defined areas (from below upwards): gastric, palisade, perforating and truncal zones. The gastric zone extends from the proximal cardia to the level of the gastro-oesophageal junction. Unlike the rest of the stomach, in which veins exist in an irregular network, the veins just below the gastro-oesophageal junction become arranged longitudinally; they are in direct continuity with the palisade zone which extends 2–3 cm cranially from the junction. At this level the veins are almost exclusively present in the lamina propria and it is this area which acts as the main watershed between the portal and systemic circulations. In the perforating zone, there is communication between the intrinsic veins and larger channels surrounding the oesophagus which form the extrinsic system. The perforating 'treble clef' veins receive blood from the longitudinal veins of the palisade zone below and the descending submucosal venous trunks of the longer oesophageal truncal zone above. The truncal zone is the most proximal and extends to approximately 15 cm above the gastro-oesophageal junction. In portal hypertension, intrinsic veins within any of these zones may become dilated and tortuous, forming varices. Extrinsic veins are also dilated in up to 60% of cases and in a minority they may be present in the absence of intrinsic varices, the so-called para-oesophageal varices. Histologically, the varicose veins show proliferation of the medial smooth muscle cells and increased elastic tissue. Thrombi may be present within the lumen, particularly after recent sclerotherapy. Ectasia of the venous channels in the palisade zone may lead to rupture and gastrointestinal haemorrhage. Turbulent flow in the perforating zone together with thinning of the muscularis mucosa may also be responsible.[99,100] Rupture of oesophageal varices occurs only when portal pressure exceeds 12 mmHg. Sometimes it is the extrinsic oesophageal veins which dilate to form para-oesophageal varices and, in a small proportion of individuals, these can exist in the absence of gastro-oesophageal varices.[98]

Although gastric varices are mainly confined to the cardia, subtle intramucosal vascular abnormalities have been described throughout the stomach in patients with portal hypertension. Histologically, ectatic capillaries and venules are seen in the lamina propria which communicate with deeper vessels. Microthrombi may be present and there may be increased numbers of vertically orientated smooth muscle fibres in the mucosa[101] (Fig. 2.8). This is referred to as *portal or congestive gastropathy*.[102] Gross lesions in the antrum have been described in which the striking endoscopic appearances led to the term 'watermelon stomach';[103] longitudinal rugal folds which contain

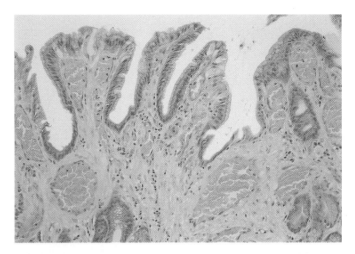

Fig. 2.8 Portal gastropathy in a gastrectomy specimen from a patient with primary biliary cirrhosis. Smooth muscle fibres course upwards in the lamina propria. H & E.

dilated vessels converge on the pylorus. The gastric manifestations of portal hypertension may arise more frequently in patients whose oesophageal varices have been obliterated by sclerotherapy. The development of collaterals between the superior haemorrhoidal (portal) vein and the middle and inferior haemorrhoidal (systemic) veins results in anorectal varices which may lead to rectal bleeding. Colonic varices are also found occasionally (*portal colopathy*). The remnant of the umbilical vein may open up and serve as an anastomosis between the main left portal vein and the epigastric veins of the anterior abdominal wall. These dilated collaterals are seen radiating from the umbilicus ('caput medusae'). The splenic and portal veins are tortuous and dilated and there may be subendothelial haemorrhages, mural thrombi and even atheromatous plaques.

At autopsy, the changes of portal hypertension may be difficult to ascertain. Oesophageal varices tend to collapse but a number of methods such as injection with barium/gelatin or mucosal stripping and clearing with benzene[104] can be used to demonstrate their presence (Fig. 2.9). The spleen is usually enlarged, and has a firm, congested cut surface and a thickened capsule. There may be scattered, hard nodules throughout the splenic pulp — the so-called Gamna–Gandy bodies. Microscopically, these are composed of fibro-elastic tissue with abundant iron and calcium deposits. They represent the residuum of previous haemorrhage into splenic follicles (Fig. 2.10).

Aetiology

The major causes of portal hypertension are listed in Table 2.3. They can be classified anatomically into *prehepatic, intrahepatic or post-hepatic*. Haemodynamic studies, including assessment of sinusoidal pressures, allow a

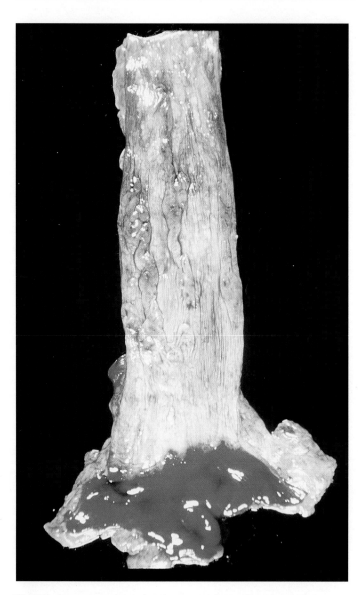

Fig. 2.9 Autopsy specimen showing ruptured oesophageal varices. Courtesy of Dr A J Malcolm.

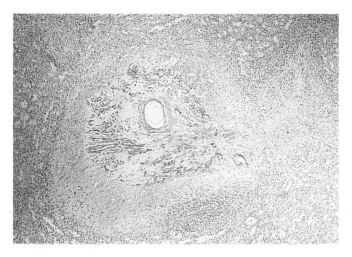

Fig. 2.10 Gamna–Gandy body in spleen. H & E.

Table 2.3 Major causes of portal hypertension

Prehepatic
  Portal vein thrombosis
  Tropical splenomegaly
  Splenic vein thrombosis

Intrahepatic
  Cirrhosis
  Non-cirrhotic and pre-cirrhotic conditions:
    Nodular regenerative hyperplasia
    Schistosomiasis
    Alcoholic hepatitis
    Drug-induced hepatitis
    Hypervitaminosis A
    Sarcoidosis
    Ductal plate malformations—congenital hepatic fibrosis
    Idiopathic portal hypertension

Post-hepatic
  Veno-occlusive disease
  Budd–Chiari syndrome
  Congestive cardiac failure, constrictive pericarditis

further subclassification into pre-sinusoidal, intrasinusoidal and post-sinusoidal.[105] There is some degree of overlap, and some post-sinusoidal conditions also have a sinusoidal component. In alcoholic hepatitis, for example, ballooning degeneration and pericellular fibrosis lead to sinusoidal-type portal hypertension but there may also be obliteration of hepatic vein branches producing a post-sinusoidal component. Although intrahepatic portal hypertension is usually due to chronic liver disease, it may be seen in severe acute hepatitis[106] and in acute fatty liver of pregnancy.[107] Rare causes of portal hypertension include hereditary haemorrhagic telangiectasia,[108] systemic mastocytosis,[109] and metastatic carcinoma in the liver.[110] The most frequent cause of prehepatic portal hypertension is portal vein thrombosis although rarely the site of obstruction may occur more proximally in the splenic and/or mesenteric veins. In adults, thrombosis in the portal system is almost always associated with intra-abdominal sepsis or tumour, or with blood disorders associated with a hypercoagulable state such as myeloproliferative diseases. Venous outflow obstruction may also occur as a result of an underlying thrombogenic condition although intrinsic lesions of the hepatic veins and external compression or tumour invasion of the hepatic vein are probably more common.

Pathogenesis

The level of portal pressure is determined by flow rate and vascular resistance. The fundamental abnormality in almost all forms of portal hypertension is increased resistance. In cirrhosis, increased intrahepatic vascular resistance results from a combination of factors which include: reduced sinusoidal calibre due to hepatocyte enlargement or nodular regeneration, impaired sinusoidal wall elasticity, compression of hepatic venules by nodules, peri-venular fibrosis and possibly veno-occlusive changes. Some or all of these phenomena may also contribute to the development of portal hypertension in pre-cirrhotic disorders such as alcoholic hepatitis.

Within the cirrhotic liver some portal venous blood is shunted through collateral vessels in fibrous septa thus bypassing the sinusoids. Hepatocytes in regenerating nodules may therefore lose their portal venous blood supply and become dependent on the hepatic artery for oxygen and nutrients.[111] In addition to purely structural factors, it is now thought likely that increased resistance occurs, in part, because of an abnormal pressor response in the portal vasculature to vasoactive compounds such as catecholamines,[112] serotonin[113] and endothelin.[114] Although impediment to flow is important, increased portal venous inflow may also play a role (the 'forward hypothesis'). Portal pressure is initially lowered by the opening up of collaterals, and portal hypertension is subsequently maintained by increasing the portal blood flow.[115] This results from the development of a hyperdynamic splanchnic circulation due to increased cardiac output, vasodilatation and a decreased responsiveness to vasoconstrictors. This may be mediated by nitric oxide.[116]

Portal hypertension has a number of important effects. It contributes to the development of ascites and hepatic encephalopathy and, possibly by diminishing the supply of hepatotrophic factors to the liver, it may interfere with liver regeneration. The most serious complication, however, is rupture of oesophageal varices with gastrointestinal haemorrhage, and most therapeutic attempts are geared towards their prevention or control. Acute bleeding varices are generally managed by balloon tamponade and vasoconstrictor therapy using either vasopressin (or an analogue)[117] or somatostatin[118] (or a synthetic analogue). Sclerotherapy is also used in most centres, either at the time of the initial endoscopy for diagnosis or after haemorrhage has been controlled.[119] A number of approaches have been used for prophylaxis against bleeding, either to prevent a first bleed in patients with known portal hypertension or to prevent rebleeding.[120] Those who fail to respond to therapeutic measures or sclerotherapy may require surgical intervention, either in the form of devascularization or the creation of a porto-caval shunt. Many shunt procedures are complicated by the development or exacerbation of encephalopathy and can interfere with subsequent transplant surgery. A novel shunt procedure has recently been developed using an angiographic approach. In this, a channel between a large branch of the intrahepatic portal vein and a large tributary of the hepatic vein is produced and maintained by insertion of an expandable stent between the vessels (the TIPPS procedure).[121] Early results are promising but long-term development of encephalopathy, stent occlusion and redevelopment of portal hypertension have yet to be evaluated.

JAUNDICE

Jaundice is the term used to describe the yellow discolouration of skin which occurs when the level of plasma bilirubin is increased.[122] Bile pigments bind avidly to tissues with a high elastin content; jaundice is thus often first detectable in the sclerae, when plasma levels rise above 35 μmol/l. In prolonged cholestasis, the skin may be greenish due to the deposition of other bile pigments, in particular biliverdin.

A large number of disorders may interfere with the metabolism of bilirubin. There may be an increased load of unconjugated bilirubin as seen in haemolytic conditions, or there may be an abnormality of conjugated or unconjugated bilirubin uptake and transport in hepatocytes. Defective conjugation is a further mechanism. This may either be due to acquired liver injury or result from an inherited enzyme deficiency (Gilbert's or Crigler–Najjar syndromes).[123] Impaired excretion of conjugated bilirubin into the canaliculus is a feature of the Dubin–Johnson syndrome and of some cases of drug-induced jaundice.[124] Finally, any obstruction to the intra- or extra-hepatic biliary tract, such as gallstones, cholangiocarcinoma, benign stricture and carcinoma of the head of the pancreas, will interfere with conjugated bilirubin excretion. The various causes of jaundice are frequently classified into prehepatic, hepatic and cholestatic; there is, however, considerable overlap between the latter two forms. In alcoholic hepatitis, for example, there is defective transcanalicular transport but conjugation may also be deficient. In some situations, such as jaundice in the postoperative period, the pathogenesis is multifactorial.[125] Prehepatic jaundice is characterized by elevated plasma levels of unconjugated bilirubin, while hepatic jaundice is associated with a mixed hyperbilirubinaemia, and cholestatic jaundice with a predominantly conjugated hyperbilirubinaemia. Bile pigment in the intestine is reduced or absent in the presence of obstruction and the faeces are pale. As conjugated bilirubin is water-soluble, increased amounts are excreted by the kidney and the urine becomes dark. At the same time, urinary urobilinogen levels are low. Bilirubin is absent from the urine in prehepatic jaundice. Other biochemical abnormalities are associated with each of the three types. Raised serum alkaline phosphatase, for example, is an important feature of cholestatic jaundice.

On the basis of clinical history, physical examination, urinalysis, simple haematological and biochemical tests (including measurement of the proportion of conjugated and unconjugated bilirubin in the serum), it is generally possible to establish the type of jaundice in an individual patient. In addition to the above investigations an acceptable routine screen for common causes of hepatic jaundice would include viral serology, serum ferritin and autoantibodies. A number of algorithms have been formulated for

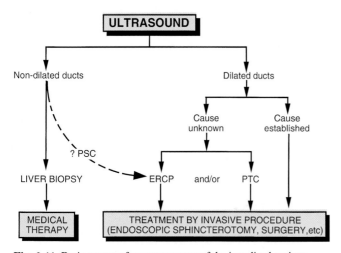

Fig. 2.11 Basic strategy for management of the jaundiced patient. PSC = primary sclerosing cholangitis; ERCP = endoscopic retrograde cholangiopancreatography; PTC = percutaneous transhepatic cholangiography.

the differential diagnosis of jaundice.[126,127] Some of these have been validated in clinical studies[128] and have led to the suggested use of expert systems in hepatology, but computer-aided diagnostics lack specificity at present.[129] When it is established that a patient has cholestatic jaundice the following important questions must be addressed: is it due to intra- or extra-hepatic disease, and if the latter, what is the level of the obstruction? Ultrasonography is the first line of investigation (Fig. 2.11). It is a non-invasive procedure which distinguishes between extrahepatic biliary obstruction and other causes of cholestasis by the demonstration of dilated bile ducts; it has an accuracy of over 90%.[130] Further imaging methods include endoscopic retrograde cholangiopancreatography (ERCP) or percutaneous transhepatic cholangiography (PTC). Isotope scans and intravenous cholangiography are of limited value. PTC is most successful when there is marked intrahepatic bile-duct dilatation and it can be combined with the insertion of stents for the palliative relief of malignant strictures. Sphincterotomy and gallstone removal or the insertion of low stents can be carried out at the time of ERCP.

Retention of conjugated bilirubin in hepatic and cholestatic jaundice is in itself of little consequence and it is the associated metabolic effects of hepatic failure or cholestasis which are of greater clinical relevance. By contrast a high level of unconjugated bilirubin is neurotoxic, particularly in the neonatal period when it leads to irreversible damage to the basal ganglia (*kernicterus*).[131] Unconjugated bilirubin is virtually absent in normal bile but its concentration may increase in conditions of unconjugated hyperbilirubinaemia and result in the precipitation of calcium bilirubinate salts and the development of pigment gallstones.[132]

CHOLESTASIS

Any impairment of bile secretion, from the level of canalicular membrane of hepatocytes to the ampulla of Vater, is termed *cholestasis*. The mechanisms responsible for normal canalicular bile flow are reviewed elsewhere in this book (p. 427), as is the contribution of bile ductular cells to modification of bile content (p. 35). In cholestasis, impaired bile flow leads to retention in the blood of substances that are normally excreted in the bile. These are bile acids, conjugated bilirubin and cholesterol.

Serum bile acids can be measured by enzymatic bioluminescence assays which are capable of detecting them in the picomolar range. Raised serum levels for total bile acids are specific for liver disease but are not confined to cholestatic disorders. Indeed, it has been suggested that measurement of serum levels of conjugated cholic acid is a sensitive and specific screening test for all forms of hepatic disease,[133] but this has not been widely adopted. Individual bile acids can be distinguished by radio-immunoassay or gas-liquid chromatography and mass spectrometry[134] but these techniques are not used routinely in clinical practice. There is an increase in the amount of trihydroxy bile acids such as hyocholic acid in cholestasis[135] and a substantial rise in conjugated forms — particularly of sulphates — which are excreted by the kidneys. The synthesis of bile acids and cholesterol by hepatocytes is decreased but plasma levels of the former remain elevated several-fold above the normal. Bile acids have been implicated in the pruritus of cholestasis but the pathogenesis of this troublesome complication is far from clear. There is no direct relationship with plasma or cutaneous bile acid concentrations,[136] and other mechanisms, involving endogenous opioids[137,138] or mast cell-derived mediators,[139] may play a role.

Secretion of cholesterol and phospholipid vesicles into canalicular bile is impaired in cholestasis; instead, these vesicles are exocytosed into the blood stream. They can bind to lipoproteins, leading to the generation of so-called lipoprotein X.[140] Total serum cholesterol is elevated, and when cholestasis persists for several months, this may be associated with the development of cutaneous xanthomas. These typically occur around the eyes (xanthelasmas), on the neck and in palmar creases. The hyperlipidaemia of cholestasis, however, does not increase the risk of patients for atheromatous disease.[141]

Lack of intestinal primary bile acids in cholestasis leads to impaired emulsification of dietary fat. In prolonged severe cholestasis this produces steatorrhoea and, in turn, leads to inadequate uptake of vitamins A, D, K and E and calcium. Vitamin D deficiency with secondary hyperparathyroidism is thought to contribute to the osteoporosis which occurs in chronic cholestatic disorders such as primary biliary cirrhosis[142] and primary sclerosing cholangitis.[143] The pathogenesis of this so-called *hepatic osteodystrophy*, however, is complex and treatment with high dose vitamin D has little effect on bone density. Osteomalacia also occurs in chronic liver disease but it is not confined to cholestatic conditions.[144] Osteoporosis is the dominant form of metabolic bone disease in cholestasis, and osteomalacia is a late feature. The liver is the site of 25-hydroxylation of vitamin D_2 and vitamin D_3 and of synthesis of vitamin D-binding protein. These functions appear to be preserved even in advanced liver disease[145] and other factors, including reduced exposure to sunlight in the chronically sick patient and low dietary intake, may be more important.

HEPATIC FAILURE

A generalized impairment of hepatic metabolic function can complicate most forms of liver disease. It may present acutely, as in massive hepatic necrosis due to toxins or viral hepatitis, or have an insidious onset as in chronic liver diseases. In cirrhosis, the clinical features may develop rapidly when decompensation is precipitated by haemorrhage or sepsis. *Fulminant hepatic failure* is defined as 'a potentially reversible condition resulting from severe liver injury with onset of coma within 8 weeks of appearance of the first symptoms and in the absence of pre-existing liver disease'. The term *subfulminant hepatic failure* is now applied to those patients with a slower onset of cerebral dysfunction (8 weeks to 6 months).[146,147] An alternative terminology has been proposed to recognize three forms — *hyperacute, acute and subacute*; this classification also relies upon the interval between the onset of jaundice and encephalopathy.[148] The term 'acute liver failure' is probably suitable to include all of the above.[147] There are a number of features which are common to all forms of hepatic failure. Some complications however, (e.g. cerebral oedema, hypoglycaemia) are peculiar to acute liver failure[148] while others such as endocrine changes and cutaneous spider naevi are limited to chronic liver disease.

While there are many heterogeneous causes of acute liver failure its common features suggest a similar pathogenesis. Endotoxaemia and associated elevations in circulating tumour necrosis factor α may play a role. It has also been suggested that there are decreased levels of the protein which binds and sequesters actin released during hepatic necrosis — G_c protein — leading to precipitation of actin filaments in the peripheral microcirculation.[147]

HEPATIC ENCEPHALOPATHY

Neuropsychiatric disorders are common in acute and chronic liver diseases. They vary from mild personality changes and sleep disorders to profound coma. These are collectively referred to as *hepatic encephalopathy*.[149,150] Similar features have occasionally been observed after surgically created portal-systemic shunts in the absence of parenchymal liver disease,[151] and the term *portal-systemic encephalopathy* has been applied.[152] Other features of hepatic insufficiency however are also present in most patients. In acute hepatic failure, the onset is rapid; coma with decerebrate rigidity may develop within 24 hours. Subtle personality changes and mild intellectual impairment are seen in the prodromal stages of encephalopathy in chronic liver disease. In cirrhosis, episodes of clinically apparent encephalopathy occur at intervals, with exacerbations being precipitated by factors such as gastrointestinal haemorrhage, sepsis, electrolyte disturbance, constipation or the administration of sedatives. The severity of encephalopathy in a patient can be graded on the basis of clinical examination, the most commonly used system recognizing four stages.[153] Psychometric tests such as the Reitan number connection test can be used for a more quantitative assessment and these are particularly suited for the detection of early changes.[154] A number of abnormalities have been described on electroencephalography (EEG). There is a bilateral slowing of the normal alpha rhythm with the appearance of delta waves (1.5–3 Hz) and in the later stages, triphasic waves appear.[155] Visual and auditory-evoked potentials have also been used for the detection of early encephalopathy.[156] In more severe encephalopathy (stage 3–4) the Glasgow coma scale is of value.

The neuropathological changes seen in most cases of hepatic encephalopathy are subtle. The most frequent finding is the presence of so-called Alzheimer type II astrocytes in the corpus striatum, in layers 5 and 6 of the cerebral cortex and in the cerebellar dentate nucleus. These cells have an enlarged, pale nucleus with a prominent nucleolus. Much less common are Alzheimer type I cells which have large hyperchromatic multilobated nuclei. Neither form is specific for hepatic encephalopathy.[157] These changes are probably reversible, but when encephalopathy is chronic, progressive loss of astrocytes and cortical neurons occurs.

Cerebral oedema occurs in over 75% of patients with fulminant hepatic failure but is rarely seen in those with chronic liver diseases.[158] A consequence of this cerebral oedema is decreased intracerebral blood flow, sometimes leading to ischaemia.[159] Evidence from animal models of fulminant hepatic failure suggests that this may result from increased permeability of the blood-brain barrier, but direct injury to neuroglial cells has also been implicated.[160] The oedema may be severe enough to produce raised intracranial pressure and lead to brain stem coning. This is one of the commonest modes of death in fulminant hepatic failure.[149] Additional neuropathological features, including mamillary body changes of Wernicke's encephalopathy, central pontine myelinolysis and Marchiafava–Bignami disease, may be present in the brains of alcoholic patients who die with encephalopathy.[161]

The pathogenesis of hepatic encephalopathy has been the subject of considerable debate.[150,152] Some indication of the likely mechanisms involved is derived from simple clinical observations. The reversible nature of the cerebral dysfunction of early encephalopathy suggests that it is a metabolic abnormality rather than direct toxic injury, and changes previously regarded as irreversible have been found to resolve completely following transplantation.[162] The global nature of the neurophysiological changes also points to a metabolic mechanism for pathogenesis.[155] Hepatic encephalopathy only occurs when portal venous blood enters the systemic circulation without being processed by the liver. In cases of massive necrosis, the 'shunt' is due to a combination of ineffective liver-cell metabolism and inadequate perfusion, whereas in cirrhosis the portal blood bypasses hepatocytes through extrahepatic and intrahepatic anastomoses although diminished liver-cell function also plays a part. This suggests that the agent(s) involved is at least partly gut-derived and is normally eliminated or metabolized by the liver. Encephalopathy is exacerbated by any substantial intestinal protein load due to haemorrhage or a high-protein diet, which suggests that the agent is related to protein or one of its breakdown products. Furthermore, as intestinal decontamination with oral antibiotics ameliorates encephalopathy, it is likely that intestinal bacteria play a role, either by producing or modifying the compound. The substance must be capable of crossing the blood-brain barrier and altering neuronal function by either impairing cerebral energy metabolism or interfering with neurotransmission. Cerebral oxygen and glucose consumption are reduced in hepatic encephalopathy but this occurs late and probably reflects a decreased demand.[163] Most recent interest has focused on altered inhibitory and excitatory neurotransmission and a number of hypotheses have been formulated incriminating different agents.[150] Many of the studies used to test these hypotheses have utilized animal models of fulminant hepatic failure such as thioacetamide- or galactosamine-induced hepatic necrosis[164] but there are no satisfactory experimental models of chronic hepatic encephalopathy. A large proportion of studies in humans have relied upon the biochemical measurement of substances in peripheral blood. A few have examined fresh cerebral tissue at autopsy and some clinical intervention studies have provided additional data. In vivo magnetic resonance spectroscopy has recently been used in studies of patients with cirrhosis and encephalopathy.[165,166]

The ammonia hypothesis. Ammonia was the first compound to be implicated as a mediator of encephalopathy.[167,168] Arterial blood ammonia levels are frequently elevated in hepatic encephalopathy and there is a relationship between blood levels and the degree of cerebral dysfunction.[169] Ammonia is freely permeable to the brain in the presence of an intact blood-brain barrier. It may alter cerebral blood flow and glucose metabolism

and interfere with the uptake of some amino acids.[170–172] However, its potential effect on brain glutamate levels is probably of greater importance. The brain is devoid of an effective urea cycle and almost all ammonia taken up by the cerebral cortex is incorporated into glutamine with the consequent depletion of glutamate. This is the most important excitatory neurotransmitter of the central nervous system and a disturbance in glutamatergic transmission could account for many of the features of encephalopathy.[150] Glutamate in the normal brain is present in several distinct compartments, including a labile pool for glutamatergic transmission. In the rat thioacetamide model, total cerebral glutamate is reduced but it is not clear which compartments are affected.[164] Autopsy studies in humans have also shown decreased concentrations in patients with encephalopathy.[172] A study of portacaval-shunted rats showed an increased binding of radiolabelled glutamate in the cerebral cortex consistent with a decrease of synaptic glutamate and/or up-regulation of post-synaptic receptors.[173] Recent studies using synaptosomes have shown that ammonia itself may have a direct effect on both inhibitory and excitatory neurotransmission.[174]

Synergistic hypothesis. Although ammonia appears to be a good candidate as a mediator of encephalopathy, there are some drawbacks to the ammonia hypothesis. Arterial levels are normal in up to 10% of patients with encephalopathy, and neuropsychiatric signs are sometimes absent in others with grossly elevated levels.[169] This may be explained by enhanced uptake and/or more rapid turnover in the encephalopathic brain[175] but it has been postulated that other factors may act synergistically with ammonia. Candidates include mercaptans, derived from methionine metabolism, and short chain fatty acids.[176] Although there is some experimental evidence to support such synergism, methodological difficulties for measuring mercaptans have hampered studies in humans.[177] Serotonin — a neurotransmitter whose activity may be altered in encephalopathy — may also have a synergistic interaction with ammonia.[178]

False neurotransmitter hypothesis. Alterations in intracerebral concentrations of the neurotransmitters nor-adrenaline and dopamine have also been implicated in hepatic encephalopathy[179] but findings in experimental models have been inconsistent.[180] An alternative suggestion has been that there may be increased levels of false dopaminergic neurotransmitters such as octopamine in encephalopathy.[181,182] It was postulated that these may be derived either from the gut or by de novo synthesis in the brain. This idea has not been substantiated by experimental data.[183]

GABA hypothesis. Gamma amino butyric acid (GABA) is an inhibitory neurotransmitter in the brain. It has been postulated that increased GABA-ergic tone may be involved in hepatic encephalopathy.[184] According to this hypothesis, GABA is generated by colonic bacteria.

Impaired clearance by the failing liver leads to elevated serum levels and, in the presence of an impaired blood-brain barrier, GABA is taken up by the brain. Experimental studies have yielded conflicting data on plasma and brain concentrations of GABA and on the status of post-synaptic GABA receptors.[150] This hypothesis has recently been modified to include modulation of GABA-ergic transmission by benzodiazepine agonists.[185] The $GABA_A$ receptor has three components: the binding site for GABA itself, a benzodiazepine receptor and a chloride ionophore which also contains receptors for barbiturates. Encephalopathy can be exacerbated by the administration of benzodiazepines and may be dramatically reversed by the benzodiazepine antagonist flumazenil,[186] although only in some patients. It was therefore suggested that endogenous benzodiazepine agonists, produced by colonic bacteria or present in the diet, may be involved in enhancing GABA-ergic tone in hepatic encephalopathy.[185] The presence of such substances has been described in the CSF and brain extracts from animal models and in cirrhotic patients with encephalopathy but they are, as yet, poorly characterized.[187]

Unified hypothesis. None of the above hypotheses is universally accepted. They are not mutually exclusive and each may explain some of the manifestations of encephalopathy. Attempts have been made to draw together the individual hypotheses into a unified concept which also incorporates additional disturbances such as hormonal changes; this has been reviewed elsewhere.[188]

ASCITES

Accumulation of serous fluid within the peritoneal cavity is commonly seen in patients with end-stage liver disease.[189] It may also occur in pre-cirrhotic patients with acute hepatic failure due to massive hepatic necrosis, and in conditions associated with sinusoidal portal hypertension such as alcoholic hepatitis. Gross ascites results in marked abdominal distension and eversion of the umbilicus; herniae and striae may also be present. The development of ascites in a cirrhotic patient is an ominous sign — up to 50% of patients die within a year.[190] Ascites can be partially controlled by a low sodium diet and the judicious use of diuretics but therapeutic paracentesis may also be required. In refractory cases, additional measures may be necessary, such as the insertion of a peritoneovenous (Le Veen) shunt which conserves total body protein.

The mechanisms of ascites formation in liver disease are complex. Portal hypertension plays an important role. Increased intrasinusoidal pressure appears to be crucial and ascites rarely develops in prehepatic portal hypertension. In animals with experimental hepatic outflow obstruction it has been demonstrated that raised pressure increases the flow of sinusoidal plasma into the space of Disse. The liver has a low compliance due to its capsule and interstitial pressure therefore increases. The net result of these changes is a dramatic increase in the amount of hepatic lymph flow into the thoracic duct and through the surface of the liver.[191] This phenomenon explains the development of ascites in the Budd–Chiari syndrome and in veno-occlusive disease. In cirrhosis, however, other factors must be involved. The ascitic fluid in cirrhosis usually has a significantly lower protein content — having the characteristics of a transudate with protein less than 2.5 g/dl — than that in outflow obstruction in which the ascites has a protein content above 3 g/dl. Furthermore, in the cirrhotic liver increased intrasinusoidal pressure does not lead to such dramatic changes in plasma volume within the space of Disse (and hence in the lymphatics) because of the phenomenon of capillarization (p. 413).

Sodium retention, a common feature in cirrhosis, appears to be important for the development of ascites.[192] This occurs principally through increased renal tubular reabsorption through activation of the renin–angiotensin–aldosterone[193] and sympathetic nervous systems.[194] Paradoxically, however, there is also increased activity of several endogenous natriuretic compounds[192] namely atrial natriuretic peptide, brain natriuretic peptide and natriuretic hormone (digoxin-like factor[195]). The relationship between these systems, portal hypertension, hypoalbuminaemia and peripheral circulatory disturbances is complex.

According to the classic *underfill theory*,[196] the initial event is disruption of the Starling equilibrium within the hepatic and splanchnic circulation due to increased hydrostatic pressure and low oncotic pressure. The resultant shift of fluid from the vascular to the extravascular compartment leads to contraction of the effective circulating plasma volume. This, in turn, activates the endogenous antinatriuretic systems leading to 'homeostatic' retention of sodium and water by the kidney. By contrast, in the *overfill hypothesis*[197] the primary event is considered to be inappropriate sodium retention by the kidney mediated via a hepatorenal reflex involving intrahepatic sensory receptors. Sodium and water retention in turn lead to expansion of the plasma volume and 'overflow' ascites formation. While there is evidence from experimental models to support each of these hypotheses, neither explains satisfactorily all observations made in patients with cirrhosis and ascites.

Schrier et al[198] proposed an alternative theory — the *peripheral arteriolar vasodilatation hypothesis* (Fig. 2.12) — which is more consistent with the circulatory changes that occur and it also explains the paradoxical increase in both natriuretic and antinatriuretic activities. According to this hypothesis, portal hypertension is the initial event. The associated splanchnic and peripheral vasodilatation produces arterial hypotension which, through stimulation of high pressure baroreceptors, leads to activation of the

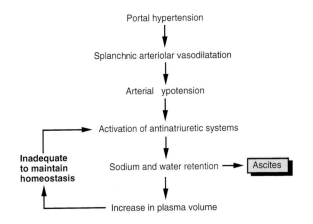

Portal hypertension

↓

Splanchnic arteriolar vasodilatation

↓

Arterial ypotension

↓

Activation of antinatriuretic systems

↓

Inadequate to maintain homeostasis → Sodium and water retention → Ascites

↓

Increase in plasma volume

Fig. 2.12 Outline of the peripheral arteriolar vasodilatation hypothesis.

renin–angiotensin–aldosterone and sympathetic nervous systems and hence sodium retention. As ascites develops, sodium and water retained by the kidneys (together with an increased cardiac output) becomes insufficient to compensate for arterial hypotension because of increasing splanchnic vasodilatation and because it is shifted into the extravascular compartment (i.e. ascites). The result is persistent activation of the antinatriuretic systems. The increased venous return which follows peripheral arteriolar vasodilatation stimulates the release of endogenous natriuretic substances but, as these do not fully counteract the effects of the antinatriuretic systems, sodium retention continues.

An important complication of ascites is *spontaneous bacterial peritonitis* which can be diagnosed by the presence of a high neutrophil count in the peritoneal fluid ($> 250 \times 10^6$ cells/l). Organisms cannot be detected in all cases but the most common are Gram-negative bacilli.[199] Spontaneous bacterial peritonitis has a high mortality rate.[200]

FUNCTIONAL RENAL FAILURE

Renal failure is common in hepatic failure. It can be due to co-existent primary kidney disease or acute tubular necrosis secondary to gastrointestinal haemorrhage or sepsis. Patients with alcoholic cirrhosis in particular may develop glomerulonephritis which is characterized by mesangial IgA deposits but this rarely leads to renal failure.[201] However, in most patients with end-stage liver disease and renal failure the kidneys show no histological abnormalities, and uraemia is thought to result from alterations in renal blood flow. This rapidly progressive functional renal failure is termed the *hepatorenal syndrome*.[202] Kidneys removed from patients dying with the syndrome assume normal function in transplanted recipients.[203] The hepatorenal syndrome may be potentially reversible in the

early stages but in some patients there is progression to acute tubular necrosis.[204]

The syndrome is characterized by a reduction in-glomerular filtration rate due to diminished renal arterial flow. Pre-glomerular vascular resistance is increased, with a resultant shift of blood from the cortex to the medulla. It is widely accepted that this is due to vasoconstriction of the renal interlobular arteries and arterioles.[205] Several mechanisms have been proposed to explain these vascular changes. Almost all patients with the hepatorenal syndrome also have ascites; Schrier et al[198] have proposed that both conditions could be explained by their peripheral arterial vasodilatation hypothesis (Fig. 2.12). Circulating vasoconstrictors have also been implicated. Several groups have shown a relationship between endotoxaemia and the development of the hepatorenal syndrome.[206] This led to the suggestion that endotoxins may stimulate the generation of vasoactive eicosanoids in the systemic and/or intrarenal circulation. Moore et al[207] demonstrated increased production of the cystinyl-leukotriene LTE_4 in patients with the hepatorenal syndrome compared with those with cirrhosis and ascites but no renal failure. There may also be decreased production of the vasodilator prostaglandin E_2.[208] Lang and co-workers[209] demonstrated a hepatorenal reflex initiated by the infusion of glutamine into the portal venous system of rats, which led to diminished renal blood flow. This raises the possibility that the liver itself may be the source of an agent with vasoconstrictor activity. Less common than the hepatorenal syndrome is a moderate and more prolonged form of functional renal failure which may develop in patients with 'stable' cirrhosis who nonetheless have ascites which is resistant to conventional diuretic treatment.

HYPERDYNAMIC CIRCULATION

Marked peripheral vasodilatation is found in all forms of hepatic failure and is manifest by a bounding pulse and flushed extremities. Cardiac output is increased[210] but arterial pressure is low; the relationship of this to the development of ascites and the hepatorenal syndrome is discussed above. Systemic vascular resistance is reduced and the arteriovenous oxygen difference is diminished. These changes are attributed to the development of multiple small arteriovenous anastomoses under the influence of a vasodilator substance. The nature of this mediator is uncertain and it may or may not be identical to the substance responsible for the hyperdynamic portal circulation. Several candidates have been suggested including GABA,[211] gut-derived neuropeptides and prostaglandins.[212] Vallance & Moncada[213] suggested that there may be excess synthesis of nitric oxide in hepatic failure because of endotoxaemia and that this may account for most of the vasodilatation.

HEPATOPULMONARY SYNDROME

A common finding in hepatic failure is reduced arterial oxygen saturation which may be accompanied by cyanosis and finger clubbing in some patients with longstanding cirrhosis. This may be the result of intrapulmonary arteriovenous shunting.[214] Marked dilatation of pulmonary arteries has been described in angiographic studies and functional studies have revealed ventilation–perfusion mismatch.[214] The mechanisms responsible are unclear but the changes are potentially reversible following transplantation.[215] Occasionally, primary pulmonary hypertension may also develop in patients with portal hypertension.[216]

CHANGES IN AMINO ACID, PROTEIN AND AMMONIA METABOLISM

Aminoaciduria is a frequent finding and the ratio of branched chain amino acids to aromatic amino acids is reduced in the plasma.[217] This is a consequence of both an increase in the aromatic acids phenylalanine and tyrosine, and a decrease in branched chain amino acids. Production of secretory proteins by hepatocytes is diminished although the mechanisms responsible are yet to be determined.[218] Of greatest clinical relevance are reduced plasma levels of albumin and coagulation factors. In the case of albumin, this is not entirely due to decreased hepatic production but partly to a shift in its distribution between vascular and extravascular compartments.[219] Plasma levels of C3 are often reduced in decompensated liver disease and may contribute to the predisposition to bacterial infections.[220]

Blood ammonia levels rise because of failure of the liver to remove that which is present in the sinusoidal blood; portal-systemic shunting contributes. There may be increased production of ammonia in the intestine because of an overgrowth of urease-containing bacteria[221] or gastrointestinal haemorrhage. Urea synthesis in the liver is decreased in hepatic failure and plasma levels may fall.[222] Diminished activity of the rate-limiting enzymes of the urea cycle has been demonstrated in livers from patients with decompensated cirrhosis.[223]

COAGULATION DISORDERS

Bleeding is a common complication of hepatic failure. Life-threatening haemorrhage occurs in up to 50% of patients with acute hepatic failure; spontaneous bleeding or bruising and cutaneous purpura indicate decompensation of hepatic function in those with chronic liver disease. As the liver synthesizes factors involved in coagulation, anti-coagulation and fibrinolysis (Table 2.1), the changes which occur are complex.[224]

Impaired synthesis of coagulation factors by hepatocytes is one of the most important factors. Plasma levels of the major components are reduced when there is significant liver-cell loss. Factors V and VII have the shortest half-lives and fall most rapidly. Assessment of factor V concentration is a useful index of the severity of acute liver failure — a value at presentation of less than 10% of normal indicates a poor prognosis.[225] The prothrombin time, however, remains the most useful test for the detection of coagulopathy in patients with liver disease. In cholestatic disorders, impaired absorption of the fat-soluble vitamin K contributes to diminished production of factors II, VII, IX and X. Even in the absence of vitamin K deficiency, however, there may be defective carboxylation of these proteins in liver disease, which results in the production of non-functional molecules.[226] Abnormal forms of fibrinogen showing defective polymerization are also found in hepatic failure.[227] Des-γ-carboxyprothrombin is found in patients with hepatocellular carcinoma and may be a useful serum marker for the disease.[228]

Production of the endogenous anticoagulants protein C, protein S and antithrombin III is impaired in hepatic failure.[229] Furthermore, clearance of activated clotting factors by the liver is decreased. This may contribute to the development of disseminated intravascular coagulation which occurs predominantly in patients with acute liver failure. Other factors involved include the release of tissue thromboplastin from the injured liver and endotoxaemia. Disseminated intravascular coagulation is less frequently found in cirrhosis[230] where it is usually of low grade. Accelerated fibrinolysis is seen in liver failure and occurs because of decreased synthesis of the plasmin inhibitors, antiplasmin, C1-inhibitor and α_2-macroglobulin, and impaired clearance by the liver of tissue plasminogen activator.[231] Enhanced fibrinolysis contributes to the increased risk of bleeding in both acute and chronic hepatic failure.

Platelet abnormalities also contribute to impaired coagulation in liver disease. In cirrhosis, thrombocytopenia occurs predominantly as a result of hypersplenism, but production in bone marrow may be impaired.[224] Functional platelet disorders have also been described, e.g. impaired aggregation due to the presence of circulating HDL with an abnormally high content of apolipoprotein E.[232] Rapid consumption of platelets occurs in disseminated intravascular coagulation.

ALTERATIONS IN CARBOHYDRATE METABOLISM

Hypoglycaemia occurs in a substantial proportion of patients with acute hepatic failure and may be difficult to control.[233,234] This is partly due to hyperinsulinaemia which results from increased synthesis of the hormone rather than from decreased clearance.[235] In those with hepatic failure due to alcoholic liver disease, metabolism of ethanol itself may contribute to hypoglycaemia. Fasting hypoglycaemia is, however, rarely found in chronic liver disease. Indeed, the principal abnormality of carbohydrate metabolism in cirrhosis is glucose intolerance.[236] The precise mechanism of this is uncertain although several factors contribute to it including increased non-esterified fatty acid levels and peripheral insulin resistance.[236]

ALTERATIONS IN XENOBIOTIC METABOLISM

The metabolism of drugs and other xenobiotics may be altered in hepatic failure. There are several possible reasons: uptake of lipophilic compounds in the intestine may be impaired when there is cholestasis, portal-systemic shunting leads to reduced first-pass metabolism, particularly of highly extracted drugs; hypoalbuminaemia and hyperbilirubinaemia alter protein binding and hence levels of free drug in the blood. Intrahepatic metabolism by both phase I and phase II reactions may be impaired, along with many other functions, in both acute and chronic liver disease and there may be decreased excretion at the level of the bile canaliculus. This subject has been reviewed in detail.[237]

ENDOCRINE ABNORMALITIES

Endocrine changes are found in some patients with chronic hepatic failure and are most obvious in males with alcoholic liver disease. They are manifested by gynaecomastia, testicular atrophy and diminished libido. In females, there may also be gonadal atrophy with amenorrhoea. The changes are due partly to diminished clearance and metabolism of sex steroids by the liver because of portal-systemic shunting and partly to the presence of increased sex hormone-binding globulin.[238] However, end-organ sensitivity to hormones may also be altered. Chronic alcohol abuse, for instance, may down-regulate androgen receptors.[239] Increased circulating oestrogens have been implicated in the development of cutaneous spider naevi,[240] although this is more likely due to increased levels of nitric oxide.

IMMUNE FUNCTIONS OF THE LIVER AND ALTERATIONS IN DISEASE

The liver is involved in systemic and mucosal immunity. It contains the largest pool of mononuclear phagocytes and natural killer cells in the body and is involved in the transport of secretory IgA into the biliary and upper gastrointestinal tracts. Impairment of these functions is largely responsible for the development of endotoxaemia, loss of tolerance to gut-derived antigens and increased susceptibility to systemic infection.

KUPFFER CELL FUNCTION

Kupffer cells provide one of the first lines of defence against gut-derived foreign material. They are responsible for the uptake and degradation or sequestration of dietary antigens and bacterial products such as endotoxin.[241] They are also involved in the initiation of immunological responses[242] and the induction of tolerance to antigens absorbed from the gastrointestinal tract.[243] Kupffer cells have an enormous endocytotic capacity for a wide range of endogenous and exogenous substances. The process of phagocytosis is energy-dependent and leads to the generation of superoxide anion, hydrogen peroxide and hydroxyl radicals. These reactive molecules are important for the intracellular degradation of foreign antigen but their release from Kupffer cells following phagocytosis may cause injury to adjacent hepatocytes by lipid peroxidation.[244] A number of arachidonic acid metabolites (eicosanoids) are also produced following phagocytosis. Prostaglandin D_2 is the most abundant but smaller amounts of PGE_2, PGF_2, thromboxane and prostacyclin are also released. The effects of these mediators are complex. Some (e.g. PGE_2) are cytoprotective, while many of the leukotrienes synthesized may be harmful to surrounding hepatocytes. Kupffer cells activated by the uptake of endotoxin also synthesize a number of cytokines including interleukins 1 and 6 and tumour necrosis factor α. Eicosanoids and cytokines derived from Kupffer cells act as mediators of the acute phase response[68,245] but also have other effects on intermediary metabolism in the liver (Table 2.4), and are probably responsible for some of the systemic manifestations of endotoxaemia.[246] Secretory products of activated Kupffer cells act as mediators of fibrogenesis in necro-inflammatory diseases and have been implicated in preservation-reperfusion injury following liver transplantation.[247]

Kupffer cells express MHC class II antigens and are capable of presenting antigen to autologous T-cells, although they appear less efficient at antigen presentation than macrophages at other sites.[248] Intrahepatic interstitial

Table 2.4 Possible effects of Kupffer cell-derived cytokines on intermediary metabolism in the liver

Metabolic function	Cytokine(s) involved
Protein metabolism	
Amino acid uptake	IL-1, IL-6, TNFα
Amino acid degradation	IL-1, IL-6, TNFα
Acute phase protein response	IL-1, IL-6, TNFα
Carbohydrate metabolism	
Glucose release	IL-6
Inhibition of gluconeogenesis	IL-1
Lipid metabolism	
Fatty acid synthesis	IL-1, TNFα
Cholesterol synthesis	IL-1, TNFα

IL = interleukin; TNF = tumour necrosis factor

dendritic cells may also be involved in the stimulation of T-cell responses to antigen.[249]

The capacity of Kupffer cells to clear gut-derived substances is impaired in cirrhosis. This is due largely to the effects of portal-systemic shunting. In alcoholic liver disease, however, a direct inhibitory effect of ethanol on phagocytosis may contribute. In alcoholic cirrhosis, Kupffer cell numbers are normal but their expression of the enzyme lysozyme is diminished.[250] Impaired clearance of endotoxin in liver disease leads to endotoxaemia. This is common in end-stage liver disease and has been implicated in the hepatorenal syndrome. Its role in other complications of hepatic failure is controversial.[251] Further evidence of impaired Kupffer cell function in liver disease is the demonstration of high levels of circulating antibodies to gut-associated bacteria and dietary antigens in cirrhosis. Elevated titres to non-gut-associated bacteria are not found.[243] This abnormality contributes to the hyperglobulinaemia of chronic liver disease.

LIVER-ASSOCIATED LYMPHOCYTES

Originally considered to be a neuroendocrine cell, the liver-associated lymphocyte or pit cell of the sinusoids is now recognized to possess natural killer activity,[252] and cells isolated from rat liver show spontaneous cytotoxicity against YAC1 lymphoma and solid tumour-derived cell lines.[253] It has been postulated that they may be involved in the response of the liver to primary and metastatic tumours.[254] There is little information on the effects of liver disease on their function, and the possible role of impaired natural killer activity in the predisposition to hepatocellular carcinoma in cirrhosis has not been explored. In human liver, liver-associated lymphocytes form a heterogeneous population. The availability of antibodies to cluster differentiation antigens expressed by different subtypes should permit a more detailed study of their population kinetics in different conditions.[252]

IgA AND THE LIVER

IgA is the principal immunoglobulin of mucosal immunity. In some species high concentrations of this protein are found in bile, and an enterohepatic circulation of IgA exists.[255] In rats, only a small proportion of IgA produced by plasma cells of the gastrointestinal tract is released into the bowel lumen. Most of it enters the mesenteric lymph, and subsequently the systemic circulation. IgA is taken up by hepatocytes by secretory component-mediated endocytosis. The protein complex is transported across the cells, and is secreted into the bile canaliculi. There is considerably less enterohepatic circulation of IgA in man, and human hepatocytes are unable to remove it. The majority of IgA in human bile is produced by plasma cells surrounding the biliary ducts and in the wall of the gallbladder. The fraction which is taken up from the gut is cleared via a pathway across periductular capillaries and bile-duct epithelium.

Secretory IgA is considered important for the immunological defence of the biliary and upper gastrointestinal tracts and for the clearance of harmful antigens from the portal circulation in the form of IgA–antigen complexes. Interference with the normal transport of IgA in the biliary tract may explain the elevated levels of serum secretory IgA found in some chronic liver diseases.[256] Impaired clearance of IgA immune complexes by the liver may contribute to the development of IgA nephropathy in cirrhosis.[201,255]

SYSTEMIC INFECTIONS IN HEPATIC FAILURE

Sepsis is common in liver disease, particularly in acute liver failure. Rolando et al[257] found culture-proven bacterial infections in 80% of patients; multiple infections were seen in 14% and bacteraemia was common. All of the late deaths in this series were attributable to infection. Among patients with cirrhosis admitted to hospital, several surveys have reported an incidence of bacterial infections of approximately 40%.[258] Fungal infections also occur, *Candida* and *Aspergillus* species being the most frequent pathogens.[259] While altered Kupffer cell function plays a role in the predisposition to infection, other factors contribute. In alcoholic liver disease, neutrophil polymorphs show impaired phagocytosis and intracellular killing of bacteria.[260] Plasma levels of fibronectin and complement proteins are also reduced and this may interfere with opsonization.[220]

ASSESSMENT OF HEPATIC FUNCTION

A number of blood tests (so-called liver function tests) are commonly used to screen for unsuspected liver disease, to confirm its presence, to estimate severity, assess prognosis and evaluate therapy. These do not provide a specific diagnosis but have a high sensitivity and are inexpensive and easy to perform. Other biochemical tests can be used to establish the presence of specific diseases such as haemochromatosis (serum ferritin, serum and hepatic iron, transferrin saturation),[261] Wilson's disease (caeruloplasmin, serum and hepatic copper, urinary copper excretion),[262] α_1-antitrypsin deficiency (plasma electrophoresis, genotyping using polymerase chain reaction),[263] and hepatocellular carcinoma (α-fetoprotein). Additional methods which can be used to determine the aetiology of liver disease in an individual patient include immunological investigations and imaging techniques.

'CONVENTIONAL' LIVER FUNCTION TESTS

In most centres a battery of 'liver function tests' is used which normally includes serum albumin, bilirubin, amino-transferases, alkaline phosphatase and γ-glutamyltrans-ferase (Table 2.5). Strictly speaking, these do not assess hepatic function but they indicate the presence of hyper-bilirubinaemia, cholestasis and hepatocellular necrosis.[264]

Serum transaminases. Alanine aminotransferase (ALT) and aspartate aminotransferase (AST) are present in high concentrations within hepatocytes. A rise in the plasma levels of these enzymes occurs when there is loss of integrity of hepatocyte membranes, thus providing a useful marker of liver-cell necrosis. AST is also found in extrahepatic tissues including myocardium and kidney; elevated levels of this enzyme are therefore less specific for liver injury.[264] Serum transaminase levels can rise to over ten times the upper limit of normal in acute hepatitis and toxin-induced necrosis. High levels can also be seen in severe venous congestion due to cardiac failure. In chronic hepatitis, the levels are generally less than five times the upper limit of normal. The ratio of AST:ALT is said to be greater than 1 in alcoholic liver disease in contrast to other necro-inflammatory conditions but this is not invariably the case. Serial estimations can be used to monitor pro-gress in an individual patient but correlation is poor between absolute values and the amount of necrosis, and values are often normal in patients with compensated cirrhosis. Other tests which have been used to indicate the presence of hepatocellular necrosis include serum glutathione S-transferases (GST), lactate dehydrogenase (LD5 isoenzyme), ferritin and F protein.[165] Serum GST may be a more sensitive marker of liver-cell necrosis in paracetamol-induced injury[265] but the other investigations offer little advantage over transaminase estimations and are not widely performed.

Alkaline phosphatase. The plasma level of this enzyme rises in cholestasis. Experimental studies have demonstrated that there is increased expression of alkaline phosphatase at the canalicular domain of hepatocytes following bile-duct obstruction.[266] Isoforms of this enzyme are also present in osteoblasts of bone, intestinal enterocytes and the placenta. Distinction between hepatic alkaline phosphatase and other forms is possible but rarely necessary in clinical practice as a hepatic origin can be confirmed by the concomitant elevation of other markers of cholestasis such as 5' nucleotidase or γ-glutamyltrans-ferase. Alkaline phosphatase levels are highest in extrahep-atic biliary obstruction but may be several times the upper limit of normal in chronic cholestatic conditions such as primary biliary cirrhosis. Increased levels of hepatic alka-line phosphatase are also found with intrahepatic space-occupying lesions and, less frequently, in Hodgkin's disease, congestive cardiac failure and some connective tissue disorders. High values are found in the blood of normal children, reflecting osteoblastic activity in growing bones, and this limits the use of this enzyme in paediatric hepatology.

γ-Glutamyltransferase or transpeptidase (γ-GT). This is a membrane-bound glycoprotein which is present in a variety of tissues.[267] In the liver it is predominantly found in bile-duct epithelium. Plasma values are raised in cholestasis but may also be high in necro-inflammatory conditions. Chronic alcohol abuse or regular medication with enzyme-inducing drugs (notably anti-epileptic drugs) leads to induction of this enzyme, and these are further causes of elevated serum γ-GT levels.[268] In contrast to alkaline phosphatase, normal adult levels are found during growth and γ-GT is used as the principal biochemical marker of cholestasis in children.

Serum bilirubin. This is measured using the van den Bergh diazo reaction. Conjugated bilirubin may be esti-mated by a direct reaction at 10 minutes. Total bilirubin levels are determined by the use of an accelerator such as caffeine-benzoate and an approximate value for the amount of unconjugated (indirect) bilirubin is calculated by subtracting conjugated from total bilirubin.

Serum albumin. The measurement of plasma levels of this liver-specific protein[59] provides some indication of the synthetic capacity of the liver. Unfortunately, low levels can be caused by increased loss through the kidneys or gastrointestinal tract, increased catabolism, altered vas-cular permeability and over-hydration. Alterations in the concentration of serum albumin must therefore be inter-preted with caution.

Other tests. Plasma bile acid measurements are used in some centres within the battery of first-line liver function tests. Although serum cholic acid may be useful in screening for hepatic disease,[133] it does not distinguish between cholestatic and hepatitic conditions. Assays have also been developed for the non-invasive assessment of hepatic fibrosis. These are largely based on the detection of extracellular matrix components such as laminin and procollagen type III propeptide.[269,270] These may have a role in monitoring progress during treatment with anti-fibrotic drugs.

Table 2.5 'Conventional' liver function tests: normal ranges. Absolute values vary between different laboratories.

Serum albumin	38–48 g/l
Bilirubin	
Total	5–17 μmol/l
Conjugated	< 5 μmol/l
Serum transaminases	
Alanine aminotransferase (ALT)	5–45 iu/l
Aspartate aminotransferase (AST)	5–30 iu/l
Alkaline phosphatase	3.5–115 iu/l (male)
	25–95 iu/l (female)
γ-glutamyltransferase (γ-GT)	<70 iu/l (male)
	<40 iu/l (female)

DYNAMIC TESTS OF HEPATIC FUNCTION

In view of the limitation of conventional tests, additional methods have been developed which provide a more quantitative assessment of hepatic function. These are of potential value in monitoring disease progression in an individual patient and could be used to indicate the need for transplantation. They are, however, more complex than conventional tests and are not routinely used. Most involve the administration of a test substance which is known to be taken up, metabolized and/or excreted by the liver with the subsequent collection of serum samples or other body fluids to determine clearance rates. Those used most frequently in clinical studies are the *aminopyrine breath test, antipyrene and caffeine clearance tests, galactose elimination* and *indocyanine green extraction*.[271] A recently described method which may be helpful in assessing function prior to transplantation is formation of mono-ethylglycinexylidide (MEGX) after the intravenous administration of low concentrations of lignocaine.[272]

IMMUNOLOGICAL INVESTIGATIONS

Immune reactions are involved in a large number of liver diseases. A T-cell response to viral proteins expressed on hepatocyte membranes in apposition to class I MHC antigens leads to liver-cell necrosis in HBV infection, and an impaired immune response to the virus is associated with chronic hepatitis. Several conditions — in particular primary biliary cirrhosis, primary sclerosing cholangitis and some forms of chronic active hepatitis — are believed to have an autoimmune pathogenesis in which there is loss of tolerance to host antigens.[273] The susceptibility to autoimmune liver disease is associated with specific class II histocompatibility haplotypes. Studies of the immunogenetics of these disorders are being facilitated by the use of rapid methods of genotyping such as sequence-specific oligonucleotide polymerase chain reaction.[274] Cell injury in these conditions is thought to be mediated principally by cytotoxic T-cells. However, B-cell responses lead to the generation of autoantibodies which can be detected in the plasma, and these form the basis of diagnostic tests for autoimmune liver disease. The earliest methods used for the detection of autoantibodies were based on complement fixation or immunofluorescence. The latter is still widely used in screening but, with the identification of the specific epitopes involved, enzyme immunoassay and immunoblotting are used increasingly for the identification of distinct autoantibody subtypes (Fig. 2.13).

Antinuclear antibodies. These are principally associated with type 1 (classic 'lupoid') autoimmune chronic active hepatitis[273] but are also found in a group of patients with primary biliary cirrhosis who are negative for antimitochondrial antibodies ('autoimmune cholangitis')[275] and in some patients with primary sclerosing cholangitis.

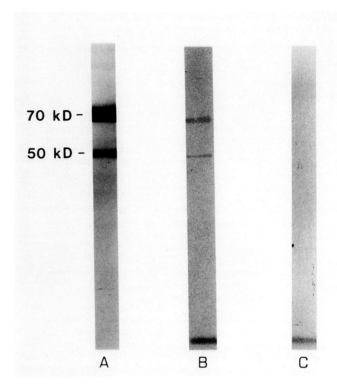

Fig. 2.13 Immunoblot for demonstration of M2 antimitochondrial antibodies. Lane A shows labelling with polyclonal anti-pyruvate dehydrogenase complex antibody. Lane B shows reactivity of serum from a patient with primary biliary cirrhosis against identical epitopes. Lane C is normal human serum.

Antibodies to nuclear envelope proteins have been described in patients with primary biliary cirrhosis, type 1 autoimmune chronic active hepatitis and hepatitis B with HDV co-infection; these are directed against lamins and the lamin B receptor.[276]

Smooth muscle antibodies. These are found in autoimmune chronic active hepatitis types 1 and 4. The principal antigenic determinant is F-actin. They are detected using indirect immunofluorescence.

Liver kidney microsomal (LKM) antibodies.[273] Several distinct types of LKM antibody have been described. The target antigen for LKM-1 has been identified as the enzyme cytochrome P-450 2D6; this auto antibody is characteristic of autoimmune chronic active hepatitis types 2a and 2b. LKM-2 reacts against cytochrome P-450 2C9 and occurs exclusively in patients with drug-induced hepatitis caused by tienilic acid. LKM-3 antibodies have been found in the serum of some Italian patients with HDV infection but the nature of the antigen has not been defined.

Liver membrane antibodies. These were initially identified using immunofluorescence to demonstrate binding of serum IgG to isolated rabbit hepatocytes.[277] They are heterogeneous and have been detected in alcoholic liver disease, autoimmune chronic active hepatitis and acute viral and drug-induced hepatitis.[277,278] Some

LMAs are directed against the so-called liver specific protein (LSP) complex which includes the asialoglycoprotein receptor.[279] Their relevance to the pathogenesis of liver disease is unproven.

Anti-soluble liver antigen. These have been detected using radio-immunoassay in patients with autoimmune chronic active hepatitis type 3 and are directed against cytokeratins.

Antimitochondrial antibodies (AMA). AMAs are readily identified in the plasma using indirect immuno-fluorescence. They are not specific for liver disease and can be found in myocarditis, systemic lupus erythematosus, syphilis, scleroderma and Sjögren's syndrome. There are, however, subtypes of AMA which can be considered specific for primary biliary cirrhosis. These antibodies (designated M2) are directed against epitopes on enzymes of the inner mitochondrial membranes: E2 subunits of the pyruvate dehydrogenase complex, the E2 subunit of the branch chain oxoacid-dehydrogenase and the 2-oxoglutarate-dehydrogenase complex.[280] They can be detected by immunoblotting (Fig. 2.13). Further subtypes (M4, M8 and M9) which may react with components of the outer mitochondrial membranes have been detected by ELISA and complement fixation. It has been suggested that the spectrum of AMA subtypes in an individual patient may relate to the stage of the disease and be of value in prognostication,[281] but recent evidence has cast considerable doubt on this.[282]

IMAGING TECHNIQUES IN CLINICAL HEPATOLOGY

A large number of methods are available which can be used to identify intrahepatic masses, assess liver blood flow and visualize the biliary tract. Because the liver is a large and relatively homogeneous organ, it can be readily studied using most modern imaging techniques but in many cases a combination of methods is required. Plain X-ray films are of limited value although they can detect calcified lesions.

Radionuclide investigations. Sulphur colloid scintigraphy utilizes the phagocytic ability of Kupffer cells. A generalized impairment of uptake is seen in cirrhosis whereas focal defects are observed with most space-occupying lesions. Lubbers et al[283] have shown that Kupffer cells are present within the sinusoids of hepatocellular adenomas and that [99mTc] sulphur colloid is taken up by this tumour; this may be helpful in distinguishing adenomas from carcinomas. Mass lesions are less clearly defined by radionuclide uptake studies than with other imaging modalities but this approach has the advantage of providing information on hepatic function. Radiolabelled iminodiacetic acid derivatives, for example, can be used in the dynamic assessment of biliary excretion (HIDA scanning).

Ultrasonography. This is the most widely used imaging method in clinical hepatology[284] and its use in the management of the jaundiced patient has already been considered. Traditional grey scale sonography assesses the degree of echogenicity of a tissue. Cystic lesions are therefore readily demonstrable. The use of Doppler examination in association with conventional ultrasonography (duplex or colour Doppler) provides additional information on blood flow. This approach can be used to identify collateral vessels in portal hypertension, to evaluate the patency of surgical port-systemic shunts and vascular anastomoses in liver transplants and to examine tumour vascularity (Fig. 2.14). It is also valuable in diagnostic assessment of portal vein thrombosis or Budd–Chiari syndrome. Some centres claim that ultrasonography can provide a guide to likely histology in a patient with homogeneous chronic liver disease (steatosis versus cirrhosis for example).

Computed tomography (CT) and magnetic resonance imaging (MRI).[284-286] The cross-sectional images obtained by CT scanning are derived from differences in density or attenuation between tissues. This can be enhanced by the prior injection of a contrast agent such as iodine. Lipiodol has been used for the delineation of malignant hepatic tumours. This substance is introduced into the hepatic artery following catheterization and is preferentially taken up by hepatocellular carcinomas (Fig. 2.15); CT scanning is carried out 7–10 days later. In plain CT scans, areas of necrosis and fibrosis appear hypodense whereas haemorrhage into the liver parenchyma produces a hyperdense image. Contrast-enhanced CT can provide some information on patency of hepatic vessels but is less sensitive than Doppler ultrasound.

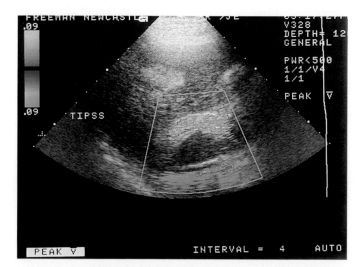

Fig. 2.14 Colour Doppler ultrasonography. In this case the technique has been used to demonstrate patency of a TIPPS stent in a cirrhotic liver (yellow). Flow in the vena cava is seen as a red image. By courtesy of Dr J Rose.

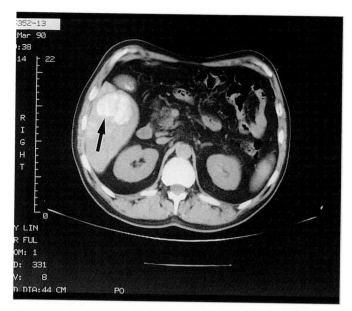

Fig. 2.15 Lipiodal CT scan of a hepatocellular carcinoma. There is selective uptake by the tumour (arrow). By courtesy of Dr J Rose.

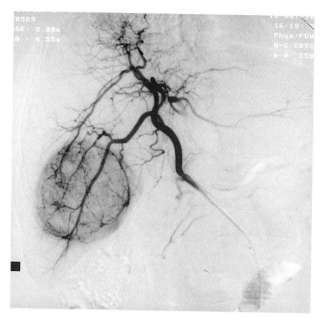

Fig. 2.16 Digital vascular subtraction angiography of tumour depicted in Fig. 2.15. This shows an abnormal vascular pattern within the lesion characteristic of a hepatocellular carcinoma. The tumour was present in segment VI. By courtesy of Dr J Rose.

MRI is the most recent advance in liver imaging. This technique relies upon the detection of energy released from hydrogen protons following forcible alignment in a magnetic field.[286] Resolution is potentially excellent and scans provide important information on the composition of a tissue, such as the amount of steatosis. Intravenous gadolinium compounds and superparamagnetic iron oxide have been used as contrast agents but unenhanced MRI can be used to evaluate hepatic vessels.

Angiography.[287] With the development of Doppler ultrasonography and MRI scanning, diagnostic angiography is now less frequently used in hepatology. It remains, however, an important method for the investigation of liver masses and is being increasingly used in 'interventional radiology' with the chemoembolization of tumours.[288] Contrast is injected under fluoroscopic control following selective catheterization of the hepatic artery. The images can be further enhanced using digital vascular subtraction angiography (Fig. 2.16). Many hepatic tumours have a characteristic angiographic appearance and a distinction can often be made between haemangioma, adenoma and hepatocellular carcinoma.

Choice of imaging technique. The choice of method used is determined by the nature of the clinical problem and by the availability of techniques. As discussed above, real-time ultrasound is the first-line investigation in biliary tract disorders, and in most centres this is the initial examination of choice for the investigation of suspected space-occupying lesions. Several studies have demonstrated that CT and MRI more accurately delineate liver masses than ultrasound[283] but these methods are more expensive; it is as yet unclear whether MRI will prove more effective than CT in routine imaging of the liver.

AGEING AND THE LIVER

Recent studies have documented morphological and functional changes in the livers of elderly individuals without hepatic disease.[289] The liver reaches its maximal size in early adulthood and thereafter there is a steady decline in weight, both in absolute terms and when expressed in relation to body size. The decrease in volume is greater in females than males[6] and by the age of 90 the average liver weight is approximately one-third less than that in the second decade. As discussed earlier, liver blood flow as estimated from indocyanine green clearance studies also declines with age.[6] Macroscopically, the ageing liver assumes a darker colour due to the progressive deposition of lipofuscin pigment in hepatocytes. The liver cells are more frequently binucleate, and flow cytometric studies have shown increased polyploidy in the ageing liver.[290]

Although there are no significant alterations in the results of conventional liver function tests in the elderly, there is some evidence of diminished functional capacity. Drugs dependent on the microsomal mono-oxygenase enzymes are cleared less readily and this effect cannot be fully explained on the basis of decreased blood flow.[291] Studies of a number of enzyme concentrations and specific activities, however, have failed to demonstrate any consistent alterations. Galactose elimination, caffeine clearance, aminopyrines and antipyrine elimination have been shown to decline with age but such decline is explicable on the basis of decreased functional liver-cell mass and/or blood flow.[271] Other experimental data suggest that the ageing liver may be less capable of responding to stress. Old rats are more susceptible than young animals to hepatotoxins such as galactosamine.[292] The effect of ageing on the pattern and severity of liver disease in humans is reviewed elsewhere.[293,294]

REFERENCES

1. Schiff L, Schiff E R, eds. Diseases of the liver, 6th edn. Philadelphia: J B Lippincott, 1987
2. Arias I M, Jakoby W B, Popper H, Schachter D, Shafritz D A, eds. The liver: biology and pathobiology, 2nd edn. New York: Raven Press, 1988
3. McIntyre N, Benhamou J-P, Bircher J, Rizzetto M, Rodes J, eds. Oxford textbook of clinical hepatology. Oxford: OUP, 1991
4. Millward-Sadler G H, Wright R, Arthur M J P, eds. Wright's Liver and biliary disease, 3rd edn. London: W B Saunders, 1992
5. Sherlock S, Dooley J, eds. Diseases of the liver and biliary system, 9th edn. London: Blackwell Scientific, 1993
6. Wynne H A, Cope L H, Mutch E, Rawlins M D, Woodhouse K W, James O F W. The effect of age upon liver blood flow in healthy man. Hepatology 1989; 9: 297–301
7. Orrego J, Mena I, Baraona E, Palma R. Modifications in hepatic blood flow and portal pressure produced by different diets. Am J Dig Dis 1965; 10: 239–248
8. Zeeh J, Lange H, Bosch J et al. Steady-state extrarenal sorbitol clearance as a measure of hepatic plasma flow. Gastroenterology 1988; 95: 749–759
9. Froelich J W, Strauss H W, Moore R H, McKusick K A. Redistribution of visceral blood volume in upright exercise in healthy volunteers. J Nucl Med Allied Sci 1988; 29: 1714–1718
10. Tygstrup N, Winkler K, Melleingaard K et al. Determination of arterial blood flow and oxygen supply in man by clamping the hepatic artery during surgery. J Clin Invest 1962; 41: 447–454
11. Lautt W W. Hepatic vasculature: a conceptual review. Gastroenterology 1977; 73: 1163–1169
12. Bismuth H. Surgical anatomy and anatomical surgery of the liver. World J Surg 1982; 6: 3–9
13. Yamamoto K, Sherman I, Phillips M J et al. Three-dimensional observations of the hepatic arterial terminations in rat, hamster and human liver by scanning electron microscopy of microvascular casts. Hepatology 1985; 5: 452–456
14. Douglas B E, Baggenstoss A H, Hollinshead W H. The anatomy of the portal vein and its tributaries. Surg Gynecol Obst 1979; 91: 562–576
15. Ezzat W R, Lautt W W. Hepatic arterial pressure — flow autoregulation is adenosine mediated. Am J Physiol 1987; 252: H836–H845
16. Myers J D. The hepatic blood flow and splanchnic consumption of man — their estimation from urea production or bromsulphthalein excretion during catheterization of the hepatic veins. J Clin Invest 1947; 26: 1130–1137
17. Lautt W W, Legare D J, D'Almeida M S. Adenosine as putative regulator of hepatic arterial flow (the buffer response). Am J Physiol 1985; 248: H331–338
18. Lautt W W, Greenway C V. Hepatic venous compliance and role of liver as a blood reservoir. Am J Physiol 1976; 231: 292–295
19. Comparini L. Lymph vessels of the liver in man. Angiologia 1969; 6: 262–274
20. Bissell D M. Heme catabolism and bilirubin formation. In: Ostrow J E, ed. Bile pigments and jaundice. New York: Marcel Dekker, 1986: pp 133–156
21. Robinson S H. Formation of bilirubin from erythroid and non-erythroid sources. Semin Hematol 1972; 9: 43–53
22. Fevery J, Vanstapel F, Blackaert N. Bile pigment metabolism. Clin Gastroenterol 1989; 3: 283–312
23. Tiribelli C, Ostrow J D. New concepts in bilirubin chemistry, transport and metabolism: report of the international bilirubin workshop. April 6–8, 1989. Trieste, Italy. Hepatology 1990; 11: 303–313
24. Tiribelli C, Ostrow H D. New concepts in bilirubin chemistry, transport and metabolism: report of the second international bilirubin workshop, April 9–11, 1992, Trieste, Italy. Hepatology 1993; 17: 715–736
25. Tiribelli C. Determinants in the hepatic uptake of organic anions. J Hepatol 1992; 14: 385–390
26. Weissiger R A, Pond S M, Bass L. Hepatic uptake of protein-bound ligands: extended sinusoidal perfusion model. Am J Physiol 1991; 261: G872–G884
27. Ritter J K, Chen F, Sheen Y Y, Tran H M, Kimura S, Yeatman M T, Owens I S. A novel complex locus UGT1 encodes human bilirubin, phenol and other UDP-glucuronosyl transferase isozymes with identical carboxyl termini. J Biol Chem 1992; 267: 3257–3261
28. Kitamura T, Jansen P L M, Hardenbrook C, Kamimoto Y, Gatmaitan Z, Arias I M. Defective ATP-dependent bile canalicular transport of organic anions in mutant (TR) rats with conjugated hyperbilirubinemia. Proc Natl Acad Sci USA 1990; 87: 3557–3561
29. Bernstein R B. Comparison of serum clearance and urinary excretion of mesobilirubinogen-^{3}H in control subjects and patients with liver disease. Gastroenterology 1971; 61: 733–741
30. Hoshita T. Bile alcohols and primitive bile acids. In: Danielsson H, Sjövall J, eds. Sterols and bile acids. Amsterdam: Elsevier Science, 1985: pp 279–302
31. Vlahcevic Z R, Heuman D M, Hyleman P B. Regulation of bile acid synthesis. Hepatology 1991; 13: 590–600
32. Hoffman A F. Overview of bile secretion. In: Schultz S G, ed. Handbook of physiology. Bethesda: American Physiological Society 1989: pp 549–566
33. Bjorkhein I. Mechanism of bile acid biosynthesis in mammalian liver. In: Danielsson H, Sjövall J, eds. Sterols and bile acids. Amsterdam: Elsevier Science, 1985: pp 231–260
34. Jelinek D F, Andersson S, Slaughter C A, Russel D W. Cloning and regulation of cholesterol 7α-hydroxylase, the rate-limiting enzyme in bile acid biosynthesis. J Biol Chem 1990; 265: 8190–8197
35. Pyrek J St, Lester R, Adcock E W, Sanghvi A T. Constituents of human meconium 1. Identification of 3-hydroxy-etianic acids. J Steroid Biochem 1983; 18: 341–351
36. Setchell K D R. Disorders of bile acid synthesis. In: Walker W A, Durie P R, Hamilton J R, Walker-Smith J A, Watkins J A, eds. Pediatric gastrointestinal disease: pathophysiology, diagnosis, management. Toronto: B C Decker, 1990: pp 992–1013
37. Weinman S A, Graft J, Boyer J L. Voltage-driven, taurocholate-dependent secretion in isolated hepatocyte couplets. Am J Physiol 1989; 256: G826–G832
38. Nathanson M H, Boyer F L. Mechanisms and regulation of bile secretion. Hepatology 1991; 14: 551–566
39. Weinburg S L, Burckhardt G, Wilson F A. Taurocholate transport by rat intestinal basolateral membrane vessels. Evidence for the presence of an anion exchange transport system. J Clin Invest 1986; 78: 44–50
40. Caflisch C, Zimmerli B, Reichen J, Meier P J. Cholate uptake in basolateral rat liver plasma membrane vesicles and in liposomes. Biochim Biophys Acta 1990; 1021: 70–76
41. Frimmer M, Ziegler K. The transport of bile acids in liver cells. Biochim Biophys Acta 1988; 947: 75–99
42. McLean J W, Tomlinson J E, Kwang W-J et al. cDNA sequence of human lipoprotein (a) homologous to plasminogen. Nature 1987; 330: 132–137
43. Preiss B, eds. Regulation of HMG CoA reductase. London: Academic Press, 1985
44. Wakil S J, Stoops J K, Joshi V C. Fatty acid synthesis and its regulation. Annu Rev Biochem 1983; 52: 537–579
45. McCarry J D, Foster D W. Regulation of hepatic fatty acid oxidation and ketone body formation. Annu Rev Biochem 1980; 49: 395–420
46. Lazarow P B. Rat liver perioxisomes catalyze the α oxidation of fatty acids. J Biol Chem 1978; 253: 1522–1528

47. Day C P, James O F W, Brown A S I J M, Bennett M K, Fleming I N, Yeaman S J. The activity of the metabolic form of hepatic phosphatidate phosphohydrolase correlates with the severity of alcoholic fatty liver in human beings. Hepatology 1993; 18: 832–838

48. Harry D S, McIntyre N. Plasma lipoproteins and the liver. In: Millward-Sadler G H, Wright R, Arthur M J P, eds. Wright's Liver and biliary disease. London: W B Saunders, 1992: pp 61–78

49. Li W-H, Tanimura M, Luo C-C et al. The apolipoprotein multigene family: biosynthesis, structure, structure-function relationships and evolution. J Lipid Res 1988; 29: 245–271

50. Eisenberg S. High density lipoprotein metabolism. J Lipid Res 1984; 25: 1017–1058

51. Felig P. Amino acid metabolism in man. Annu Rev Biochem 1975; 44: 933–955

52. Christensen H N. Interorgan amino acid nutrition. Physiol Rev 1982; 62: 1193–1233

53. Krebs H A, Hems R, Lund P, Halliday D, Read W W C. Sources of ammonia for mammalian urea synthesis. Biochem J 1978; 176: 733–737

54. Harper A E, Miller R H, Block K P. Branched-chain amino acid metabolism. Annu Rev Nutr 1984; 4: 409–454

55. Powers-Lee S G, Meister A. Urea synthesis and ammonia metabolism. In: Arias I M, Jakoby W B, Popper H, Schacter D, Shafritz D A, eds. The liver: biology and pathobiology, 2nd edn. New York: Raven Press, 1988: pp 317–329

56. Häussinger D. Hepatocyte heterogeneity in glutamine and ammonia metabolism and the role of an intracellular glutamine cycle during ureogenesis in the perfused rat liver. Eur J Biochem 1983; 133: 269–275

57. Sigsaard I, Almdal T, Hansen B A, Vilstrup H. Dexamethasone increases the capacity of urea synthesis dependently and reduces the body weight of rats. Liver 1988; 8: 193–197

58. Häussinger D. Liver glutamine metabolism. J Parent Ent Nutr 1990; 14: 565–625

59. Rothschild M A, Oratz M, Schreiber S S. Serum albumin. Hepatology 1988; 8: 385–401

60. Maniatis T, Goodbourn S, Fischer J A. Regulation of inducible and tissue-specific gene expression. Science 1987; 236: 1237–1245

61. Padgett R A, Grabowski P J, Konaiska M M, Seiler S, Sharp P A. Splicing of messenger RNA precursors. Annu Rev Biochem 1986; 55: 1119–1150

62. Moldave K. Eukaryotic protein synthesis. Annu Rev Biochem 1985; 54: 1109–1149

63. Serfling E, Jasin M, Schaffner W. Enhancers and eukaryotic gene transcription. Trends in Genetics 1985; i: 224–230

64. Pfeffer S R, Rothman J E. Biosynthetic protein transport and sorting by the endoplasmic reticulum and Golgi. Annu Rev Biochem 1987; 56: 829–852

65. Kelly R B. Pathways of protein secretion in eukaryotes. Science 1985; 203: 25–32

66. Chung K N, Walter P, Aponte G W, Moore H-P. Molecular sorting in the secretory pathway. Science 1989; 243: 192–197

67. Tavill A S, McCullough A J. Protein metabolism and the liver. In: Millward-Sadler G H, Wright R, Arthur M J P, eds. Wright's Liver and biliary disease, 3rd edn. London: W B Saunders, 1992: pp 79–106

68. Andus T, Bauer J, Gerok W. Effects of cytokines on the liver. Hepatology 1991; 13: 37–41

69. Peters T. Serum albumin. Adv Clin Chem 1970; 13: 37–41

70. Burt A D, MacSween R N M. Fat, alcohol and iron. In: Wight D G D, ed. Systemic pathology, 3rd edn, volume 11. Liver and pancreas. Edinburgh: Churchill Livingstone, 1993: pp 237–286

71. Bonkovsky H L. Iron metabolism and the liver. Am J Med Sci 1991; 301: 32–45

72. Müller-Eberhard H. Molecular organisation and function of the complement system. Annu Rev Biochem 1988; 57: 321–347

73. Hetland G, Johnson E, Falk R J, Eskeland T. Synthesis of complement components C5, C6, C7, C8 and C9 in vitro by human monocytes and assembly of the terminal complement complex. Scand J Immunol 1986; 24: 421–428

74. Burt A D, Geerts A, MacSween R N M, Whaley K, Wisse E. Synthesis of the complement component C3 by isolated rat Kupffer cells. J Hepatol 1986; 3: 48 (abstr)

75. Matsura S, Nakada H, Sawamura T, Tashiro Y. Distribution of an asialoglycoprotein receptor on rat hepatocyte cell surface. J Cell Biol 1982; 95: 864–875

76. Wileman T, Harding C, Stahl P. Review article: receptor-mediated endocytosis. Biochem J 1985; 232: 1–14

77. Stalmans W. The role of the liver in the homeostasis of blood glucose. Curr Top Cell Regul 1976; 11: 51–97

78. Hue L. Gluconeogenesis and its regulation. Diab Metab Rev 1987; 3: 111–126

79. Alberti K G M, Taylor R, Johnson D G. Carbohydrate metabolism in liver disease. In: Millward-Sadler G H, Wright R, Arthur M J P, eds. Wright's Liver and biliary disease. London: W B Saunders, 1992: pp 43–60

80. Shimazu T. Reciprocal innervation of the liver: its significance in metabolic control. Adv Metab Dis 1983; 10: 355–384

81. Agius L, Peak M, Alberti K G M. Regulation of glycogen synthesis and gluconeogenesis precursors by insulin in periportal and perivenous rat hepatocytes. Biochem J 1990; 266: 91–102

82. Correia M A, Castagnoli N. Pharmacokinetics: II. Drug biotransformation. In: Katzung B G, ed. Basic and clinical pharmacology, 3rd edn. Norwalk: Appleton and Lange, 1987: pp 36–43

83. Tredger J M, Davis M. Drug metabolism and hepatotoxicity. Gut 1991; 32: S34–S39

84. Omura T, Sato R. The carbon monoxide binding pigment of liver microsomes II. Solubilization, purification and properties. J Biol Chem 1964; 239: 2379–2385

85. Gonzalez F J. Molecular genetics of the P-450 superfamily. Pharmacol Ther 1990; 45: 1–38

86. Guengerick F P. Characterization of human microsomal cytochrome P-450 enzymes. Annu Rev Pharmacol Toxicol 1989; 29: 241–264

87. Nebert D W, Nelson Dr, Adesnik M et al. The P-450 superfamily updated listing of all genes and recommended nomenclature for the chromosomal loci. DNA 1989; 8: 1–13

88. Gonzalex F H, Skoda R C, Kimura S et al. Characterization of the common genetic defect in the humans deficient in debrisoquine metabolism. Nature 1988; 331: 442–446

89. Okey A B. Enzyme induction in the cytochrome P-450 system. Pharmacol Ther 1990; 45: 241–298

90. Tephly T R, Burchall B. UDP-glucuronosyl transferases: a family of detoxifying enzymes. Trends Pharm Sci 1990; 7: 276–279

91. Boyer T D. The glutathione S-transferases: an update. Hepatology 1989; 9: 486–496

92. Mannervik B, Alin P, Guthenberg C et al. Identification of three classes of cytosolic glutathione transferase common to several mammalian species: correlation between structural data and enzymatic properties. Proc Natl Acad Sci USA 1985; 82: 7202–7206

93. Mathew J, Cattan A R, Hall A G et al. Glutathione S-transferases in neonatal liver disease. J Clin Pathol 1992; 45: 679–683

94. Harrison D J, May L, Hayes P C, Hague M M, Hayes J D. Glutathione S-transferases in alcoholic liver disease. Gut 1990; 31: 909–912

95. Arias I M. Multidrug resistance genes, p-glycoprotein and the liver. Hepatology 1990; 12: 159–165

96. Vianna A, Hayes P, Moscoso G et al. Normal venous circulation of the gastroesophageal junction. A route to understanding varices. Gastroenterology 1987; 93: 876–889

97. McIndoe A H. Vascular lesions of portal cirrhosis. Arch Pathol Lab Med 1928; 5: 23–45

98. Vianna A. Anatomy of the portal venous system in portal hypertension. In: McIntyre N, Benhamou J-P, Bircher J, Rizzetto M, Rodes J, eds. Oxford textbook of clinical hepatology. Oxford: OUP, 1991: pp 393–399

99. Polio J, Groszmann R J. Hemodynamic factors involved in the development and rupture of oesophageal varices: A pathophysiologic approach to treatment. Semin Liver Dis 1986; 6: 318–329

100. Noda T. Angioarchitectural study of esophageal varices. Virchows Pathol [A] Pathol Anat 1984; 404: 381–392

101. Quintero E, Pique J, Bombi J et al. Gastric mucosal vascular ectasias causing bleeding in cirrhosis. Gastroenterology 1987; 93: 1054–1061

102. McCormack T, Sims I, Eyre-Brook I et al. Gastric lesions in portal hypertension: inflammatory gastritis or congestive gastropathy. Gut 1985; 26: 1226–1232

103. Jabbari M, Cherry R, Lough J O, Daly D S, Kinnear D G, Gorelsky G A. Gastric antral vascular ectasia: the watermelon stomach. Gastroenterology 1984; 87: 1165–1170

104. Choinet B, Hart L M, Reindle F J. Demonstration of esophageal varices by simple technique. Arch Pathol 1960; 69: 185–187

105. Bosch J, Mastai R, Kravetz D, Navasa M, Rodes J. Hemodynamic evaluation of the patient with portal hypertension. Semin Liver Dis 1986; 6: 309–317

106. Valla D, Flejou J F, Lebrec D, Bernau J, Rueff B, Benhamou J P. Portal hypertension and ascites in acute hepatitis. Clinical, hemodynamic and histological correlations. Hepatology 1989; 10: 482–487

107. Barnan J, Degott C, Nouel O, Rueff B, Benhamou J P. Non-fatal acute fatty liver of pregnancy. Gut 1983; 24: 340–344

108. Martini G A. The liver in hereditary haemorrhagic telangiectasia: an inborn error of vascular structure with multiple manifestations. A reappraisal. Gut 1978; 19: 431–437

109. Capron J P, Lebrec D, Degott C, Chivrac D, Coevoet B, Delobel J. Portal hypertension in systemic mastocytosis. Gastroenterology 1978; 74: 595–597

110. Hyun B H, Singer E P, Sharret R H. Esophageal varices and metastatic carcinoma of liver. Arch Pathol 1964; 77: 292–298

111. Popper H, Elias H, Petty D E. Vascular pattern of the cirrhotic liver. Am J Clin Pathol 1952; 22: 717–729

112. Ballet F, Chretien Y, Rey C et al. Differential response of normal and cirrhotic liver to vasoactive agents. A study in the isolated perfused liver. J Exp Pharmacol Ther 1988; 244: 283–289

113. Vorobiioff J, Garcia-Tsao G, Groszmann R et al. Long-term hemodynamic effects of ketanserin, a 5-hydroxytryptamine blocker, in portal hypertensive patients. Hepatology 1989; 9: 88–91

114. Gandhi C R, Stephenson K, Olson M S. Endothelin, a potent peptide agonist in the liver. J Biol Chem 1990; 265: 17432–17435

115. Witte C L, Witte M H. Splanchnic circulatory and tissue fluid dynamics in portal hypertension. Fed Proc 1983; 42: 1685–1689

116. Whittle B J R, Moncada S. Nitric oxide: the elusive mediator of the hyperdynamic circulation of cirrhosis. Hepatology 1992; 42: 1089–1092

117. Freeman J G, Cobden I, Record C O. Placebo-controlled trial of tertypressin (Glypressin) in the management of acute variceal bleeding. J Clin Gastroenterol 1989; 11: 58–60

118. Burroughs A K, McCormack P A, Huges M D, Sprengers D, D'Heygere F, McIntyre N. Randomized, double-blind, placebo-controlled trial of somatostatin for variceal bleeding. Gastroenterology 1990; 99: 1388–1395

119. Paquet K J, Feussner H. Endoscopic sclerosis and esophageal balloon tamponade in acute haemorrhage from esophagogastric varices. Hepatology 1985; 5: 580–583

120. Hayes P C, Davis J M, Leucs J A, Bouchier I A. Meta-analysis of propranolol in prevention of variceal haemorrhage. Lancet 1990; i: 153–156

121. Conn H O. Transjugular intrahepatic portal-systemic shunts: the state of the art. Hepatology 1993; 17: 148–158

122. McIntyre N. Symptoms and signs of liver disease. In: McIntyre N, Benhamou J-P, Bircher J, Rizzetto M, Rodes J, eds. Oxford textbook of clinical hepatology. Oxford: OUP, 1991: pp 273–290

123. Jansen P L M, Onde Elferink R P J. Hereditary hyperbilirubinaemias: a molecular and mechanistic approach. Semin Liver Dis 1988; 8: 168–178

124. Arias I M. Studies of chronic familial non-haemolytic jaundice with conjugated bilirubin in the serum with and without an unidentified pigment in the liver cells. Am J Med 1961; 31: 510–518

125. Becker S D, LaMont J. Postoperative jaundice. Semin Liver Dis 1988; 8: 183–190

126. Lundberg G, Bjorkman A, Hekuers C. A description of diagnostic strategies in jaundice. Scand J Gastroenterol 1983; 18: 257–265

127. Scharschmidt B F, Goldberg H I, Schmid R. Current concepts in diagnosis. Approach to a patient with cholestatic jaundice. N Engl J Med 1983; 308: 1515–1519

128. Malchow-Möller A, Thomsen C, Hatzen P et al. Computer diagnosis in jaundice. Bayes rule founded on 1002 consecutive cases. J Hepatol 1986; 3: 154–163

129. Poynard T. Algorithms and computer-aided diagnosis. In: McIntyre N, Benhamou J-P, Bircher J, Rizzetto M, Rodes J, eds. Oxford textbook of clinical hepatology. Oxford: OUP, 1991: pp 363–367

130. Taylor K J, Rosenfield A T. Greyscale ultrasonography in the differential diagnosis of jaundice. Arch Surg 1977; 112: 820–825

131. Bratlid D. Bilirubin toxicity: pathophysiology and assessment of risk factors. NY State J Med 1991; 91: 489–492

132. Cahalene M J, Neubrand M W, Carey M C. Physical-chemical pathogenesis of pigment gallstones. Semin Liver Dis 1988; 8: 317–328

133. Ferraris R, Florentini T, Galatola G et al. Diagnostic value of serum immunoreactive conjugated cholic or chenodeoxycholic acids in detecting hepatobiliary diseases. Dig Dis Sci 1987; 32: 817–823

134. Murphy G M. Serum bile acids. In: Setchell K D R, Kritchevsky D, Nair P P, eds. The bile acids. Chemistry, physiology and metabolism, vol 4. Methods and applications. New York: Plenum Press, 1988: pp 379–403

135. Bremmelgaard A, Sjövall J. Hydroxylation of cholic, chenodeoxycholic and deoxycholic acids in patients with intrahepatic cholestasis. J Lipid Res 1980; 21: 1072–1081

136. Bartholomew T C, Summerfield J A, Billing B H, Lawson A M, Setchell K D P. Bile acid profiles of human serum and skin interstitial fluid and their relationship to pruritis studied by gas chromatography-mass spectrometry. Clin Sci 1986; 63: 65–73

137. Bergasa N V, Rothman R B, Vergalla J et al. Central mu-opioid receptors are down-regulated in a rat model of cholestasis. J Hepatol 1992; 15: 220–224

138. Jones E A, Bergasa N V. Hypothesis: the pruritis of cholestasis: from bile acids to opiate antagonists. Hepatology 1990; 11: 884–887

139. Gittlen S K, Schuhnan E S, Maddrey W C. Raised histamine concentrations in chronic cholestatic liver disease. Gut 1990; 31: 96–99

140. Seidel D, Gretz H, Ruppert C. Significance of the LP-X test in differential diagnosis of jaundice. Clin Chem 1973; 19: 86–91

141. Crippen J S, Lindor K D, Jorgensen R et al. Hypercholesterolaemia and atherosclerosis in primary biliary cirrhosis: what is the risk? Hepatology 1992; 15: 858–862

142. Mitchison H C, Malcolm A J, Bassendine M F et al. Metabolic bone disease in primary biliary cirrhosis at presentation. Gastroenterology 1988; 94: 463–470

143. Hay J E, Lindor K D, Wiesner R H et al. The metabolic bone disease of primary sclerosing cholangitis. Hepatology 1991; 14: 257–261

144. Compston J E. Hepatic osteodystrophy: vitamin D metabolism in patients with liver disease. Gut 1986; 27: 1073–1090

145. Jung R T, Davie M, Siklos P et al. Vitamin D metabolism in acute and chronic cholestasis. Gut 1979; 20: 840–847

146. Bernuau J, Rueff B, Benhamou J-P. Fulminant and subfulminant liver failure: definitions and causes. Semin Liver Dis 1986; 6: 97–106

147. Lee W M. Acute liver failure. N Engl J Med 1993; 329: 1862–1872

148. O'Grady J G, Scholm S W, Williams R. Acute liver failure: redefining the syndromes. Lancet 1993; ii: 273–275

149. Ede R J, Williams R. Hepatic encephalopathy and cerebral oedema. Semin Liver Dis 1986; 6: 107–118

150. Record C O. Neurochemistry of hepatic encephalopathy. Gut 1991; 32: 1261–1263

151. McDermott M V, Adams R D. Episodic stupor associated with an Eck fistula in the human with particular reference to the metabolism of ammonia. J Clin Invest 1954; 33: 1–9

152. Butterworth R F. Pathogenesis and treatment of portal-systemic encephalopathy. Dig Dis Sci 1992; 37: 321–327

153. Adams R D, Foley J M. The neurological disorder associated with liver disease. In: Merritt H H, Hare C C, eds. Metabolic and toxic diseases of the nervous system. Baltimore: Williams & Wilkins, 1953: pp 198–237

154. Rikkers L, Jenko P, Rudman D, Freides D. Subclinical hepatic encephalopathy: Detection, prevalence and relationship to nitrogen metabolism. Gastroenterology 1978; 75: 426–469

155. Parsons-Smith B G, Summerskill W H J, Dawson A M, Sherlock S. The electroencephalograph in liver disease. Lancet 1957; ii: 867–871

156. Zeneroli M L, Pinelli G, Gollini G et al. Visual evoked potentials: a diagnostic tool for the assessment of hepatic encephalopathy. Gut 1984; 25: 291–299

157. Norenberg M D. The astrocyte in liver disease. In: Federoff S, Hertz L, eds. Advances in cellular neurobiology. London: Academic Press, 1981: pp 304–352

158. Gimson A E S, O'Grady J, Ede R J et al. Late-onset fulminant hepatic failure: clinical, serological and histological features. Hepatology 1986; 6: 288–294

159. Blei A T. Cerebral edema and intracranial hypertension in acute liver failure: distinct aspects of the same problem. Hepatology 1991; 13: 376–379

160. Traber P G, Dal Canto M, Ganger D R, Blei A T. Electron microscopy evaluation of brain edema in rabbits with galactosamine-induced fulminant hepatic failure: ultrastructure and integrity of the blood brain barrier. Hepatology 1987; 7: 1272–1277

161. Torvik A, Lindboc C F, Rogde S. Brain lesions in alcoholics: a neuropathological study with clinical correlations. J Neurol Sci 1982; 56: 233–248

162. Powell E E, Pender M P, Chalk J B et al. Improvement in chronic hepatocerebral degeneration following liver transplantation. Gastroenterology 1990; 98: 1079–1082

163. Polli E, Bianchi-Porro G, Maiolo A T. Cerebral metabolism after portacaval shunt. Lancet 1969; i: 153–156

164. Zimmermann C, Ferenci P, Pifl C et al. Hepatic encephalopathy in thioacetamide-induced acute liver failure in rats: characterization of an improved model and study of amino acid-ergic neurotransmission. Hepatology 1989; 9: 594–601

165. Taylor-Robinson S D, Bell J D, Sargentoni J, Byrant D J, Mallalien R J, Morgan M Y. Cerebral ^{31}P MRS in patients with chronic hepatic encephalopathy. Hepatogastroenterology 1993; 40: 105/0 (abstr)

166. Kreis R, Ross B D, Farrow N A, Ackerman Z. Metabolic disorders of the brain in chronic hepatic encephalopathy detected with H-1 MR spectroscopy. Radiology 1992; 182: 19–27

167. Matthews S A. Ammonia, a causative factor in meat poisoning in Eck fistula dogs. Am J Physiol 1922; 59: 459–460

168. Gabuzda G Jr, Philips G B, Davidson C S. Reversible toxic manifestations in patients with cirrhosis of the liver given cation-exchange resins. N Engl J Med 1952; 246: 124–130

169. Stahl S. Studies of blood ammonia in liver disease; its diagnostic, prognostic and therapeutic significance. Ann Intern Med 1963; 58: 1–24

170. Hindfeldt B, Plum F, Duffy T E. Effect of acute ammonia intoxication on cerebral metabolism in rats with portacaval shunts. J Clin Invest 1977; 59: 386–396

171. Grippon P, Le Ponchin-Lafitte M, Boschat M et al. Evidence for the role of ammonia in the intracerebral transfer and metabolism of tryptophan. Hepatology 1986; 6: 682–686

172. Lavoie J, Giguere J F, Pomier-Layrargues G, Butterworth R F. Amino acid changes in autopsied brain tissue from cirrhotic patients with hepatic encephalopathy. J Neurochem 1987; 49: 692–697

173. Butterworth R F, Lavoie J, Giguere J F, Pomier-Layrargues G, Bergeron M. Cerebral GABA-ergic and glutamatergic function in hepatic encephalopathy. Neurochem Pathol 1987; 6: 131–144

174. Raabe W. Synaptic transmission in ammonia intoxication. Neurochem Pathol 1987; 6: 145–166

175. Lockwood A H, Yap E W H, Wong W-H. Cerebral ammonia metabolism in patients with severe liver disease and minimal hepatic encephalopathy. J Cereb Blood Flow Metab 1991; 11: 337–341

176. Zieve L, Doizaki W M, Zieve F J. Synergism between mercaptanes and ammonia and fatty acids in the production of coma: a possible role for mercaptanes in the pathogenesis of hepatic coma. J Lab Clin Med 1974; 83: 16–28

177. Al Mardini H, Bartlett K, Record C O. Blood and brain concentrations of mercaptans in hepatic and methanethiol induced coma. Gut 1984; 25: 284–290

178. Bergeron M, Swain M S, Reader T A, Grondin L, Butterworth R F. Effect of ammonia on brain serotonin metabolism in relation to function in the portacaval shunted rat. J Neurochem 1990; 55: 222–229

179. Zieve L, Olsen E L. Can hepatic coma be caused by a reduction of brain noradrenaline or dopamine? Gut 1977; 18: 688–691

180. Knell A J, Davidson A R, Williams R et al. Dopamine and serotonin metabolism in hepatic encephalopathy. Brit Med J 1974; ii: 549–551

181. Fischer J E, Baldessarini R J. False neurotransmitters and hepatic failure. Lancet 1971; ii: 75–80

182. Manghani K K, Lunzer M R, Billing B H et al. Urinary and serum octopamine in patients with portal systemic encephalopathy. Lancet 1975; ii: 343–345

183. Cilleret G, Pomier-Layrargues G, Pons F, Cadilhac J, Michel H. Changes in brain catecholamine levels in human cirrhotic hepatic encephalopathy. Gut 1980; 21: 565–569

184. Schafer D F, Jones E A. Hepatic encephalopathy and the γ-aminobutyric acid system. Lancet 1982; i: 18–20

185. Mullen K D, Martin J V, Mendelson W B, Bassett M L, Jones E A. Could an endogenous benzodiazepine ligand contribute to hepatic encephalopathy? Lancet 1988; i: 457–459

186. Scollo-Levizzaire G, Steinmann E. Reversal of hepatic coma by benzodiazepine antagonist (Ro 15-1788). Lancet 1985; i: 1324

187. Mullen K D, Szanter K M, Kaminsky-Russ K. Endogenous benzodiazepine activity in body fluids of patients with hepatic encephalopathy. Lancet 1990; i: 81–83

188. Fischer J E. Portal-systemic encephalopathy. In: Millward-Sadler G H, Wright R, Arthur M J P, eds. Wright's Liver and biliary disease, 3rd edn. London: W B Saunders, 1992: pp 1262–1295

189. Berner C, Fred H L, Riggs S, Davis J S. Diagnostic probabilities in patients with conspicuous ascites. Arch Int Med 1964; 113: 687–690

190. Ratnoff O D, Patek A J. The natural history of Laennec's cirrhosis of the liver: an analysis of 386 cases. Medicine 1942; 41: 207–268

191. Laine G A, Hall J T, Laine S H, Granger H J. Transsinusoidal fluid dynamics in canine liver during venous hypertension. Circ Res 1979; 45: 317–323

192. Jimenez W, Arroyo V. Pathogenesis of sodium retention in cirrhosis. J Hepatol 1993; 18: 147–150

193. Arroyo V, Bosch J, Mauri M et al. Renin, aldosterone and renal haemodynamics in cirrhosis with ascites. Eur J Clin Invest 1979; 9: 69–73

194. Bichet D G, Van Putten V J, Schrier R W. Potential role of increased sympathetic activity in impaired sodium and water excretion in cirrhosis. N Engl J Med 1982; 307: 1552–1557

195. Day C P, James O F W. Digoxin-like factors in liver disease. J Hepatol 1989; 9: 281–284

196. Epstein F H. Underfilling versus overflow in hepatic ascites. N Engl J Med 1982; 307: 1577–1580

197. Lieberman F L, Denison E K, Reynolds T B. The relationship of plasma volume, portal hypertension, ascites and renal sodium retention in cirrhosis. The overfill theory of ascites formation. Ann NY Acad Sci 1970; 170: 202–206

198. Schrier R W, Arroyo V, Bernardi M, Epstein M, Henriksen J H, Rodes J. 'Peripheral arterial vasodilatation hypothesis': a proposal for the initiation of renal sodium and water retention in cirrhosis. Hepatology 1988; 8: 1151–1157

199. Mbopi Keou F-X, Bloch F, Bun Hoi A et al. Spontaneous peritonitis in cirrhotic hospital in-patients: retrospective analysis of 101 cases. Q J Med 1992; 301: 401–407

200. Tito L, Rimol A, Gines P et al. Recurrence and frequency of spontaneous bacterial peritonitis in cirrhosis: frequency and predictive factors. Hepatology 1988; 8: 27–31

201. Eknoyan G. Glomerular abnormalities in liver disease. In: Epstein M, ed. The kidney in liver disease, 3rd edn. Baltimore: Williams & Wilkins, 1988: pp 154–181

202. Epstein M. Hepatorenal syndrome. In: Epstein M, ed The kidney in liver disease, 3rd edn. Baltimore: Williams & Wilkins, 1988: pp 89–118

203. Koppel M H, Coburn T W, Mims M M, Goldstein H, Boyle J D, Rubini M E. Transplantation of cadaveric kidneys from patients with hepatorenal syndrome: evidence for the functional nature of renal failure in advanced liver disease. N Engl J Med 1969; 280: 1367

204. Wilkinson S P, Hurst D, Day D W, Williams R. The spectrum of renal tubular damage in renal failure secondary to cirrhosis and fulminant hepatic failure. J Clin Pathol 1978; 31: 101–107

205. Epstein M, Berk D P, Hollenberg N K et al. Renal failure in the patient with cirrhosis. The role of active vasoconstriction. Am J Med 1970; 49: 175–185

206. Wilkinson S P, Moodie H, Stamatakis J D et al. Endotoxaemia and renal failure in cirrhosis and obstructive jaundice. Brit Med J 1976; ii: 1415–1418

207. Moore K P, Taylor G W, Maltby N et al. Increased production of cysteinyl-leukotrienes in hepatorenal syndrome. J Hepatol 1990; 11: 263–271

208. Zipser R D, Radvan G H, Kronborg I J et al. Urinary thromboxane B2 and prostaglandin E2 in the hepatorenal syndrome: evidence for increased vasoconstrictor factors. Gastroenterology 1983; 84: 697–703

209. Lang F, Tschernko E, Schulze E et al. Hepatorenal reflex regulating kidney functions. Hepatology 1991; 14: 590–594

210. Murray J F, Dawson A M, Sherlock S. Circulating changes in chronic liver disease. Am J Med 1958; 24: 358–367

211. Minuk G T, MacCannell K L. Is the hypotension of cirrhosis a GABA-mediated process? Hepatology 1988; 8: 73–75

212. Wernze H, Tittor W, Goerig M. Release of prostanoids into the portal and hepatic vein in patients with chronic liver disease. Hepatology 1986; 6: 911–919

213. Vallance P, Moncada S. Hypothesis: Hyperdynamic circulation in cirrhosis: a role for nitric oxide. Lancet 1991; i: 776–778

214. Sherlock S. The liver-lung interface. Semin Resp Med 1988; 9: 247–263

215. Stoller J K, Moodie D, Schiavone W A et al. Reduction of intrapulmonary shunt and resolution of digital clubbing associated with biliary cirrhosis after liver transplantation. Hepatology 1990; 11: 54–58

216. Hadengue A, Benhayoun M K, Lebrec D et al. Pulmonary hypertension complicating portal hypertension: prevalence and relation to splanchnic hemodynamics. Gastroenterology 1991; 100: 520–528

217. Morgan M Y, Marshall A W, Milson J P, Sherlock S. Plasma amino acid patterns in liver disease. Gut 1982; 23: 362–370

218. Gerok W, Gross V. Secretory proteins: synthesis, secretion and function. In: McIntyre N, Benhamou J-P, Bircher J, Rizzetto M, Rodes J, eds. Oxford textbook of clinical hepatology. Oxford: OUP, 1991: pp 174–198

219. Rothschild M A, Oratz M, Zimmon D, Schreiber S S, Weiner I, Caneghan A V. Albumin synthesis in cirrhotic subjects with ascites with carbonate-^{14}C. J Clin Invest 1969; 48: 344–350

220. Ellison R T, Horsburgh C R Jr, Curd J. Complement levels in patients with hepatic dysfunction. Dig Dis Sci 1990; 35: 231–266

221. Hansen B A, Vilstrup H. Increased intestinal hydrolysis of urea in patients with alcoholic cirrhosis. Scand J Gastroenterol 1985; 20: 346–350

222. Lab D, Gorbach S L, Levitan R. Intestinal microflora in patients with alcoholic cirrhosis: urea-splitting bacteria and neomycin resistance. Gastroenterology 1972; 62: 275–279

223. Khatra B S, Smith R B, Miliken W J, Sewell C W, Warren W D, Rudman D. Activities of Krebs-Henselert enzymes in normal and cirrhotic human liver. J Lab Clin Med 1974; 84: 708–715

224. Kelly D A, Summerfield J A. Hemostasis in liver disease. Semin Liver Dis 1987; 7: 182–192

225. Pereira L M M B, Langley P G, Hayllar K M et al. Coagulation factor V and VIII/V ratio as predictors of outcome in paracetamol-induced hepatic failure: relation to other prognostic indicators. Gut 1992; 33: 98–102

226. Blanchard R A, Furic B C, Jorgensen M, Kruger S F, Furic B. Acquired vitamin K-dependent carboxylation deficiency in liver disease. N Engl J Med 1981; 305: 242–248

227. Martinez J, Palascak J E, Kavasniak D. Abnormal sialic acid content of the dysfibrinogenesis associated with liver disease. J Clin Invest 1978; 61: 535–538

228. Tsai S-L, Huang G-T, Yang P-M et al. Plasma des-γ-carboxyprothrombin in the early stage of hepatocellular carcinoma. Hepatology 1990; 11: 481–488

229. Knot E, Teu Cate J W, Drujfhout H R et al. Anti-thrombin III metabolism in patients with liver disease. J Clin Pathol 1984; 37: 523–530

230. Carr J M. Disseminated intravascular coagulation in cirrhosis. Hepatology 1989; 10: 103–110

231. Takahashi H, Tatewaki W, Wada K et al. Fibrinolysis and fibrinogenolysis in liver disease. Am J Hematol 1990; 34: 241–245

232. Desai K, Mistry P, Bagget C, Burroughs A K, Bellamy M F, Owens J S. Inhibition of platelet aggregation by abnormal high density lipoprotein particles in plasma from patients with hepatic cirrhosis. Lancet 1989; i: 693–694

233. Record C O, Chase R A, Alberti K G M M, Williams R. Disturbances in glucose metabolism in patients with liver damage due to paracetamol overdose. Clin Sci 1975; 49: 473–479

234. Samson R I, Trey C, Tunme A J, Saunders S J. Fulminant hepatitis with recurrent hypoglycaemia and haemorrhage. Gastroenterology 1967; 53: 291–300

235. Vilstrup H, Iversen J, Tygstrup N. Glucoregulation in acute liver failure. Eur J Clin Invest 1986; 16: 193–197

236. Blancho C D V, Gentile S, Marno R. Alterations of glucose metabolism in chronic liver disease. Diab Res Clin Prac 1990; 8: 29–36

237. Howden C W, Birnie G G, Brodie M J. Drug metabolism in liver disease. Pharmacol Ther 1989; 40: 439–474

238. Johnson P J. Sex hormones and the liver. Clin Sci 1984; 66: 369–376

239. Eagon P K, Willett J E, Seguiti S M et al. Androgen-responsive functions of male rat liver. Effect of chronic alcoholic ingestion. Gastroenterology 1987; 93: 1162–1169

240. Pirovino M, Linder B, Boss C et al. Cutaneous spider nevi in liver cirrhosis: capillary microscopical and hormonal investigations. Klin Wochenschr 1988; 66: 298–304

241. Van Bossuyt H, Desmaretz C, Wisse E. The fate of lipopolysaccharide in cultured rat Kupffer cells. Virchows Archiv [B] Cell Pathol 1989; 58: 89–93

242. Rogoff T M, Lipsky P E. Role of the Kupffer cells in local and systemic immune responses. Gastroenterology 1981; 80: 854–860

243. Thomas H C, MacSween R N M, White R G. Role of the liver in controlling the immunogenicity of commensal bacteria in the gut. Lancet 1973; i: 1288–1291

244. Arthur M J P. Reactive oxygen intermediates and liver injury. J Hepatol 1988; 8: 125–131

245. Brouwer A, Hendricks H F J, Knook D L. The role of eicosanoids in the acute phase response. J Hepatol 1990; 11: 283–286

246. Beutler B, Cerami A. Cachectin, cachexia and shock. Annu Rev Med 1988; 39: 75–83

247. Sheron N, Eddleston A. Preservation-reperfusion injury, primary graft non-function and tumour necrosis factor. J Hepatol 1992; 16: 262–265

248. Rubinstein D, Roska A K, Lipsky P E. Liver sinusoidal lining cells express class II major histocompatibility antigens but are poor stimulators of fresh allogeneic T lymphocytes. J Immunol 1986; 137: 1803–1810

249. Hart D N J, McKenzie J L. Interstitial dendritic cells. Int Rev Immunol 1990; 6: 127–138

250. Kelly P M, Heryet A R, McGee J O'D. Kupffer cell number is normal but their lysozyme content is reduced in alcoholic liver disease. J Hepatol 1990; 8: 173–180

251. Triger D R. Endotoxaemia in liver disease — time for re-appraisal? J Hepatol 1991; 12: 136–138

252. Burt A D, Le Bail B, Balabaud C, Biolac-Sage P. Morphological investigation of sinusoidal cells. Semin Liver Dis 1993; 13: 21–38

253. Bouwens L, Remels L, Baekeland M, Van Bossuyt H, Wisse E. Large granular lymphocytes or 'pit cells' from rat liver: isolation, characterization and natural killer activity. Eur J Immunol 1987; 17: 37–42

254. Martin M, Chauffert B, Caignard A et al. Histoimmunological characterization of the cellular reaction to liver metastasis induced by colon cancer cells in syngeneic rats. Invasion Metastasis 1989; 9: 216–230

255. Brown W R, Kloppel T M. The liver and IgA: immunological, cell biological and clinical implications. Hepatology 1989; 9: 763–784

256. Kutteh W H, Prince B J, Phillips J O et al. Properties of immunoglobulin A in serum of individuals with liver diseases and in hepatic bile. Gastroenterology 1982; 82: 184–193

257. Rolando N, Harvey F, Brahm J et al. Prospective study of bacterial infection in acute liver failure: an analysis of fifty patients. Hepatology 1990; 11: 49–53

258. Rimola A. Infections in liver disease. In: McIntyre N, Benhamou J-P, Bircher J, Rizzetto M, Rodes J, eds. Oxford textbook of clinical hepatology. Oxford: OUP, 1991: pp 1272–1284

259. Rolando N, Harvey F, Brahm J et al. Fungal infection: a common, unrecognised complication of acute liver failure. J Hepatol 1991; 12: 1–9

260. Rajkovic I A, Williams R. Abnormalities of neutrophil phagocytosis, intracellular killing and metabolic activity in alcoholic cirrhosis and hepatitis. Hepatology 1986; 6: 252–260

261. Gordeuk V R, Bacon R B, Brittenham G M. Iron overload: causes and consequences. Ann Rev Nutr 1987; 7: 485–508

262. Walshe J M. Copper: its role in the pathogenesis of liver disease. Semin Liver Dis 1984; 4: 252–263

263. Eriksson S. Alpha-1-antitrypsin deficiency: lessons learned from the bedside to the gene and back again. Chest 1989; 95: 181–183

264. Laker M F. Liver function tests. Brit Med J 1990; 301: 250–251

265. Beckett G J, Foster G R, Hussey A J et al. Plasma glutathione S-transferases and F protein are more sensitive than alanine aminotransferase as makers of paracetamol (acetaminophen)-induced liver disease. Clin Chem 1989; 35: 2186–2189

266. Kaplan M M. Serum alkaline phosphatase — another piece is added to the puzzle. Hepatology 1986; 6: 526–528

267. Rosalki S B. Gamma-glutamyl transpeptidase. Adv Clin Chem 1975; 17: 53–107

268. Gluud C, Andersen I, Dietrichson O et al. Gamma glutamyltransferase, aspartate aminotransferase and alkaline phosphatase as markers of alcohol consumption in out patient alcoholics. Eur J Clin Invest 1981; 11: 171–176

269. Plebani M, Burhina A. Biochemical markers of hepatic fibrosis. Clin Biochem 1991; 24: 219–239

270. Burt A D. Liver fibrosis: better understanding may help diagnosis and treatment. Brit Med J 1992; ii: 537–538

271. Schnegg M, Lauterburg B H. Quantitative liver function in the elderly assessed by galactose elimination capacity, aminopyrine demethylation and caffeine clearance. J Hepatol 1986; 3: 164–171

272. Ollerich M, Burdelski M, Ringe B et al. Lignocaine metabolic formation as a measure of pre-transplant liver function. Lancet 1989; i 640–642

273. Meyer zum Büschenfelde K-H, Lohse A W, Manns M, Poralla T. Autoimmunity and liver disease. Hepatology 1990; 12: 354–363

274. Underhill J, Donaldson P, Bray G, Doherty D, Portmann B, Williams R. Susceptibility to primary biliary cirrhosis is associated with the HLA-DR8-DQB1 *0402 haplotype. Hepatology 1992; 16: 1404–1408

275. Ben-Ari Z, Dhillon A P, Sherlock S. Autoimmune cholangiopathy: part of the spectrum of autoimmune chronic active hepatitis. Hepatology 1993; 18: 10–15

276. Worman J H, Courvalin J-C. Autoantibodies against nuclear envelope proteins in liver disease. Hepatology 1991; 14: 1269–1279

277. Burt A D, Anthony R S, Hislop W S, Bouchier I A D, MacSween R N M. Liver membrane antibodies in alcoholic liver disease. 1. Prevalence and immunoglobulin class. Gut 1982; 23: 221–226

278. Hopf W, Meyer zum Büschenfelde K-H, Arnold W. Detection of a liver membrane autoantibody in HBsAg-negative chronic active hepatitis. N Engl J Med 1976; 294: 574–576

279. Poralla T, Triechel U, Löhr H, Fleischer B. The asialoglycoprotein receptor as target structure in autoimmune liver diseases. Semin Liver Dis 1991; 11: 215–222

280. Bassendine M F, Fussey S P M, Mutimer D J, James O F W, Yeaman S J. Identification and characterization of four M2 mitochondrial autoantigens in primary biliary cirrhosis. Semin Liver Dis 1989; 9: 124–131

281. Berg P A, Klein R, Lindenborn-Fotinos J. Antimitochondrial antibodies in primary biliary cirrhosis. J Hepatol 1986; 2: 123–131

282. Palmer J M, Yeaman S J, Bassendine M F, James O F W. M4 and M9 autoantigens in PBC — a negative study. J Hepatol 1991; 18: 251–254

283. Lubbers P R, Ros P R, Goodman Z D. Accumulation of technetium 99m sulphur colloid by hepatocellular adenoma: scintigraphic-pathologic correlation. Am J Roentgenol 1987; 148: 1105–1108

284. Bennett W F, Bova J G. Review of hepatic imaging and a problem-orientated approach to liver masses. Hepatology 1990; 12: 761–775

285. Foley W D. Dynamic hepatic CT. Radiology 1989; 170: 617–622

286. Ferruci J T. MR imaging of the liver. Am J Roentgenol 1986; 147: 1103–1116

287. Okudo K, Obata H, Jinouchi S et al. Angiographic assessment of gross anatomy of hepatocellular carcinoma: comparison of coeliac angiograms and liver pathology in 100 cases. Radiology 1977; 123: 21–29

288. O'Halpin D, Legge D, MacErlean D P. Therapeutic arterial embolisation: report of five years experience. Clin Radiol 1984; 35: 85–93

289. Popper H. Aging and the liver. In: Popper H, Schaffner F, eds. Progress in liver diseases, vol. 8, Orlando: Grune & Stratton, 1986: pp 659–683

290. Watanabe T, Shimada H, Tanaka Y. Human hepatocytes and aging: a cytophotometrical analysis in 35 sudden death cases. Virchows Archiv [B] Cell Pathol 1978; 27: 307–316

291. Rawlins M D, James O F W, Williams F M, Wynne H, Woodhouse K W. Age and the metabolism of drugs. Q J Med 1987; 64: 545–547

292. Platt D. Age dependent morphological and biochemical studies of the normal and injured rat liver. In: Platt D, ed. Liver and ageing. Stuttgart: F K Schattnauer, 1977: pp 77–83

293. James O F W. Parenchymal liver disease in the elderly. In: Bianchi L, Holt P, James O F W, Butler R N, eds. Aging in liver and gastrointestinal tract. Lancaster: MTP Press, 1988: pp 359–369

294. James O F W. Liver disease in the elderly. In: McIntyre N, Benhamou J-P, Bircher J, Rizetto M, Rodes J, eds. Oxford textbook of clinical hepatology. Oxford: Oxford University Press, 1991: pp 1303–1310

3

Developmental abnormalities and liver disease in childhood*

K. G. Ishak   H. L. Sharp

Anatomical anomalies of the liver
  Agenesis of liver
  Absence of a lobe of the liver
  Hypoplasia of right lobe
  Anomalies of position
  Accessory lobes
  Ectopic hepatic tissue
  Heterotopias of the liver

Hepatic vascular anomalies
  Hepatic artery
  Portal vein
  Hepatic veins
  Hereditary haemorrhagic telangiectasia
    (Osler–Rendu–Weber disease)
  von Hippel-Lindau disease
  Focal nodular hyperplasia

Bile duct anomalies
  Agenesis of the common bile duct
  Agenesis of the common hepatic duct
  Anomalous ('accessory') bile ducts
  Duplication of the bile ducts
  Congenital bronchobiliary and tracheobiliary fistulas
  Ciliated hepatic foregut cyst
  Spontaneous bile duct perforation

Extrahepatic biliary atresia

Neonatal hepatitis

Paucity of the intrahepatic bile ducts

Congenital dilatations of the bile ducts
  Choledochal cyst
  Caroli's disease

Autosomal recessive polycystic kidney disease
  Infantile presentation

  Juvenile and adult presentation (congenital hepatic
    fibrosis)

Autosomal dominant polycystic kidney disease

Solitary (non-parasitic) cyst

Reye's syndrome

Kawasaki's disease

The histiocytoses of childhood
  Langerhans' cell histiocytosis
  Haemophagocytic syndromes (familial, reactive)
  Sinus histiocytosis with massive lymphadenopathy
    (Rosai–Dorfman disease)
  Malignant histiocytosis

Liver disease in Down's syndrome and leukaemia
  Down's syndrome
  Leukaemia

This chapter deals with a variety of developmental abnormalities which may affect the liver, its vasculature and the extra- and intrahepatic biliary system. In addition, some miscellaneous childhood diseases are described, but excluding metabolic disorders many of which manifest themselves in childhood; the congenital cholestatic syndromes are described in chapters 4 and 13, respectively.

ANATOMICAL ANOMALIES OF THE LIVER

AGENESIS OF LIVER

This condition is incompatible with life. It has been reported in stillborn fetuses, usually in association with other severe anomalies.[1]

---

* The opinions or assertions contained herein are the private views of the authors and are not to be construed as official or as reflecting the views of the Department of the Army or the Department of Defense.

ABSENCE (AGENESIS) OF A LOBE OF THE LIVER

A case of absence of the left lobe, diagnosed by computed tomography and ultrasound, was reported by Belton & Van Zandt.[2] Two cases of absence of the right lobe, also detected by imaging studies, have been recorded.[3,4] In total, Radin et al[3] collected 19 cases from the literature. They found that the anomaly may be associated with biliary tract disease, portal hypertension, or other abnormalities including congenital anomalies, or it may be an incidental finding.

HYPOPLASIA OR RIGHT LOBE

This rare anomaly is associated with a supra- or intra-hepatic gallbladder.[5,6]

ANOMALIES OF POSITION

In *situs inversus totalis or abdominalis*, the liver is found in the left hypochondrium, with the falciform ligament coursing from the left anterior margin towards the umbilicus. Varying amounts of hepatic tissue may be displaced into congenital diaphragmatic hernias or omphalocoeles. Hepatic tissue was present in 3 of the 19 omphalocoeles studied by Soper & Green,[7] and in 2 cases reported by Desser & Smith[8] it was the seat of nonparasitic cysts. In the 2 cases of Fock[9] the hepatic tissue within the omphalocoele was detached from the rest of the liver. Several cases of *hepatic herniation* through defects in the diaphragm have been reported.[10] One patient with chest pain related to a hepatic herniation through the diaphragm was cured after surgical repair.[11] Another hepatic herniation through a Morgagni-type foramen was initially thought to be a cardiac tumour but was subsequently correctly diagnosed by hepatic arteriography and isotopic scintiphotography.[12] A unique case of a supradiaphragmatic right liver lobe and gallbladder has been reported.[13] Partial eventration of the right hemidiaphragm is a congenital lesion caused by aplasia or hypoplasia of part of the musculature of the diaphragm with resultant bulging of the affected portion from intra-abdominal pressure.[14] The underlying portion of the liver prolapses into the diaphragmatic pouch where it may become strangulated.

ACCESSORY LOBES

Riedel's lobe is a tongue-like caudal projection from the right lobe of the liver and may be palpable in the right upper quadrant. In the series of 31 cases reported by Reitemeier et al[15] all the patients except one were women, their ages ranging from 31 to 77 years. Supernumerary lobes are relatively frequent findings, particularly on the inferior surface of the liver. They are connected to the liver by hepatic tissue or by a pedicle containing branches of the portal vein, hepatic vein and hepatic artery, and a bile duct.[16] Intrathoracic accessory lobes, with their vascular supply perforating the diaphragm, have been reported.[17,18] Accessory lobes may rarely require surgical intervention because of their large size, torsion of a pedicle, or the presence of other associated defects.[19,20] Radiographically, such cases may mimic intramural gastric or perigastric masses.[21]

ECTOPIC HEPATIC TISSUE

Ectopic hepatic tissue may be found in the suspensory ligaments of the liver, lung, wall of the gallbladder, splenic capsule, retroperitoneal space, adrenal gland and greater omentum.[9,16,22–30] A unique case of ectopic liver in the placenta was reported by Willis.[31] In most instances the hepatic tissue in these ectopic sites is microscopically normal, but when the liver is abnormal (fatty change, chronic hepatitis, cirrhosis) the ectopic liver tissue also reflects the same changes.[32] A unique case of an infantile haemangioendothelioma arising in a heterotopic intrathoracic liver was reported by Shah et al.[24]

HETEROTOPIAS OF THE LIVER

Most of the so-called adrenal heterotopias are actually examples of *adrenal-hepatic fusion*. Dolan & Janovski[33] made a distinction between 'adhesion' and 'fusion' on the basis of presence or absence of a capsule interposed between the two organs. In both types there was a marked diminution or complete absence of medullary tissue. The fusion is unilateral and in no instance has it been associated with any clinical manifestation of adrenal impairment. In a recent report adrenal-hepatic fusion was found in 9.9% of unselected autopsy cases.[34] The incidence was much higher in older age groups, suggesting that the condition may be an ageing phenomenon. In addition to adrenal-hepatic fusion there is one recent example of *hepatolienal fusion*.[35] Two tumours thought to have arisen in *adrenal cell rests* in the liver have been reported.[36,37]

Pancreatic heterotopias in the liver are rare (Fig. 3.1). In the case reported by Ballinger[38] an islet cell carcinoma arose in the aberrant pancreatic tissue. In another case a retention cyst had developed in an obstructed duct.[39] A similar example was reported subsequently by Schaefer et al.[40]

HEPATIC VASCULAR ANOMALIES

HEPATIC ARTERY

Aberrant hepatic arteries occur in a significant proportion of subjects;[41] they are listed and illustrated in Chapter 14.

Anomalous origin of the hepatic artery has been described in 7 children with extrahepatic biliary atresia.[42] Congenital duplication of the gallbladder has been reported in association with an anomalous right hepatic artery.[43] Rupture of

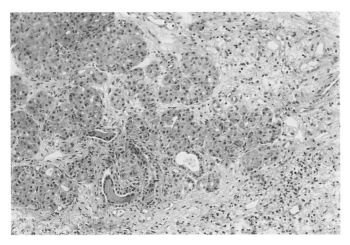

Fig. 3.1 Pancreatic heterotopia. Pancreatic acini and several small ducts are present but there are no islets of Langerhans. H&E.

an aberrant hepatic artery can occur rarely.[44] An example of a congenital hepatoportal arteriovenous fistula occurring in a 5-week-old infant has been reported.[45] The abdominal pain and distension, diarrhoea and guaiac-positive stools were attributed by the authors to mesenteric venous engorgement resulting from acute portal hypertension. A similar case in a 4-month-old girl was clinically manifested by necrotizing enteritis due to portal hypertension.[46] A third case of a congenital arteriovenous fistula (between the right hepatic artery and the ductus venosus) in a 3-year-old girl was successfully treated surgically by Martin et al.[47] A variety of embolization materials, including platinum wire embolization, have been used to treat acquired arterioportal fistulas.[48]

PORTAL VEIN

Preduodenal portal vein is the result of a variation in the normal developmental pattern of the precursors of the portal vein, i.e. the right and left vitelline veins and their three anastomotic channels. It poses a hazard to the surgeon in operations involving the duodenum and biliary tract. Duodenal obstruction was attributed to a preduodenal portal vein by Boles & Smith,[49] but this has been questioned by Esscher.[50] A vascular complex consisting of absence of the inferior vena cava, anomalous origin of the hepatic artery and preduodenal portal vein was reported in 3 children with extrahepatic biliary atresia;[42] it should be sought prior to liver transplantation. Other associated malformations have been reviewed by Esscher.[50]

Obstructing valves within the lumen of the splenic vein, the portal vein or both, may be a rare cause of portal hypertension in children.[51]

A case of *reduplication of the portal vein* was reported by Hsia & Gellis;[51] one branch ran anterior to the pancreas and was obliterated by an old organized thrombus. Another patient reported by Snavely & Breakell[52] died from bleeding oesophageal varices; this patient also had multiple congenital strictures of the portal venous system.

Atresia or hypoplasia of the portal vein has been reported by a number of investigators.[51,53–56] It may involve the entire length of the vessel, be limited to the point of entrance into the liver, or occur just proximal to the division into two branches. Microscopic study of the atretic segments has generally shown no evidence of inflammation.

Congenital absence of the portal vein is rare.[57–60] Thus far only 10 cases have been reported.[60] Other cardiac and inferior vena caval anomalies and polysplenia may occur simultaneously. The patient of Marois et al,[57] a 4½-year-old girl, had an associated hepatoblastoma.

Congenital shunts (portocaval, portohepatic and between the left portal vein and internal mammary veins) have been reported.[61–64]

A congenital *aneurysmal malformation* of the extrahepatic portal vein was described by Thompson et al.[65] Another aneurysm of the left branch of the portal vein was diagnosed in utero by ultrasound examination.[66]

Cavernous transformation of the portal vein (portal cavernoma) is a condition in which the vein is replaced by a spongy trabeculated venous lake which extends into the gastroduodenal ligament.[53–56,67–71] It was once regarded as the major cause of portal hypertension in children.[70] However, with advances in the management of chronic liver disease and the reduced use of aspirin, it is no longer the leading cause of bleeding oesophageal varices in this age group. Haemorrhage is the most common clinical manifestation, but some children present with asymptomatic splenomegaly.[69–71] Children with extrahepatic portal vein obstruction have been reported to show marked growth retardation.[72] Obstructive jaundice is a rare complication.[73] Pancytopenia of varying degree occurs in the majority of cases.[69] Liver function tests show little abnormality. The sonographic findings appear to be characteristic and may obviate the need for splenoportography or angiography.[74–77] Magnetic resonance imaging has also been utilized in diagnosis.[78] The occurrence of serious psychiatric disorders following portosystemic shunts, reported by Voorhees & Price[79], has not been verified by others.

Percutaneous or open liver biopsy specimens are either normal or show minimal fibrosis. Klemperer[67] reported multiple 'adenomas', but the description of the nodules and their designation as 'regenerative formations' suggest that the condition was nodular regenerative hyperplasia.

The pathogenesis of cavernous transformation was discussed by Marks.[56] The theories that have been proposed are that it is a sequel to portal vein thrombosis due to omphalitis, umbilical vein catheterization or intra-abdominal sepsis, or that it represents an angiomatous malformation of the portal vein. Experimental evidence in support of occlusion of the portal vein and the subsequent opening up of adjacent collateral vessels has been reported by Williams & Johnston.[80] In the series of 30 cases studied by Odievre et al,[81] 12 had congenital abnormalities, the most frequent being atrial septal defect, malformation of the biliary tract and anomalous inferior vena cava. It would therefore seem that both mechanisms may operate but more consideration should be given to the rapidly changing portal haemodynamics occurring during birth as the most likely cause, since specific aetiologies are rarely documented.[82]

HEPATIC VEINS

Membranous obstruction of the hepatic portion of the inferior vena cava, which may be associated with occlusion of the hepatic veins, is thought to have a congenital aetiology,[83–85] but this has been disputed.[86,87] Kage et al[87] have demonstrated thrombus formation and occlusion of hepatic vein orifices in 8 cases, suggesting that the condition was acquired. Most cases have been reported from Japan and South Africa.[88,89] Patients present with the Budd–Chiari syndrome and are prone to develop hepatocellular carcinoma without evidence of hepatitis B infection. Symptoms develop mainly in adults but a series of 9 cases in children was reported from Namibia.[90] Rare instances of congenital Budd-Chiari syndrome, attributed to maternal drug abuse[91] or ingestion of herbal tea,[92] have been reported. Cases of veno-occlusive disease in children with cellular and humoral immune deficiency have also been described.[93,94] In the cases of Mellis & Bale[93] consanguinity and early age of onset suggested an inherited cause.

HEREDITARY HAEMORRHAGIC TELANGIECTASIA (OSLER–RENDU–WEBER DISEASE)

The inheritance of the disease is autosomal dominant and the estimated frequency is 1–2 per 100 000.[97] The clinical spectrum of manifestations has been reviewed by several authors.[95–97] It is characterized by telangiectases (skin, mucous membranes), arteriovenous fistulas in the liver (in 30% of cases), lungs and central nervous system, and aneurysms. Hepatic involvement is indicated by pain in the right upper quadrant of the abdomen, and enlargement of the organ which is sometimes pulsatile. High output cardiac failure may result from arteriovenous shunting in the liver. Portal hypertension and encephalopathy may develop.[98,99]

The hepatic lesions can be demonstrated by angiography, ultrasound[100,101] and colour doppler ultrasound,[102] and are readily visualized during laparoscopy.[103] Arterial embolization has been used successfully in treatment of the disease.[104,105]

Cases with morphological descriptions of the liver have been reported.[98,106–110] Macroscopically, the liver is nodular, fibrotic or rarely cirrhotic. Spider-like arrange-

ments of minute blood vessels may be noted on the surface. Microscopically, three fibrovascular patterns were described by Daly & Schiller.[109] One pattern comprised a honeycomb meshwork of dilated sinusoidal channels lined by endothelial cells set either directly upon hepatocyte plates or amid a loose fibrous stroma (Fig. 3.2a); the distribution of these foci was haphazard. A second pattern consisted of tortuous thick-walled veins flanked by numerous wide-calibre arteries that coursed randomly through the parenchyma amid variable amounts of fibrous tissue. A third pattern was evident in the enlarged portal areas in which numerous dilated vessels (veins, arteries and lymphatics) showed prominently against a background of fibrous tissue (Fig. 3.2b). Regenerative nodules (nodular transformation) were described in the cases reported by Zelman[107] and Wanless & Gryfe.[110] One 69-year-old woman treated with ethinyloestradiol, multiple blood transfusions and iron-dextran developed hepatocellular carcinoma and acquired hepatocerebral degeneration.[108]

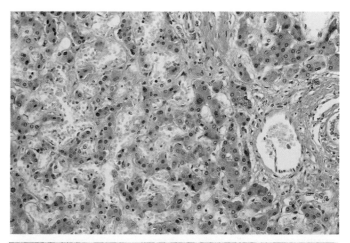

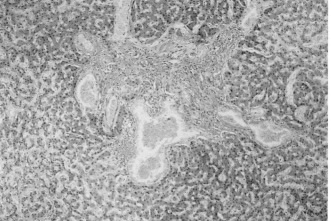

Fig. 3.2 Hereditary haemorrhagic telangiectasia. (a) Dilated anastomosing sinusoidal channels, lined by endothelial cells with some subendothelial fibrous tissue. Masson's trichrome. (b) Same case as (a) showing dilated vessels within a portal tract; foci of dilated sinusoidal vessels are also present (left and upper right). Masson's trichrome.

VON HIPPEL–LINDAU DISEASE

This disease rarely involves the liver. Multiple cavernous haemangiomas were reported by Zeitlin,[111] and multiple haemangioblastomas were described by Rojiani et al[112] and McGrath et al.[113] Occasionally, pancreatic cysts may lead to jaundice from common bile-duct obstruction.[114]

FOCAL NODULAR HYPERPLASIA

Wanless et al[115] have shown that focal nodular hyperplasia is a hyperplastic response of the hepatic parenchyma to a pre-existing arterial malformation. Multiple lesions may be associated with haemangioma of the liver, meningioma, astrocytoma, telangiectases of the brain, berry aneurysm, dysplastic systemic arteries and portal vein atresia.[116] It was proposed by Wanless et al[116] that this new syndrome is the result of an underlying systemic abnormality of unknown nature. Components of the syndrome (berry aneurysms, cerebral telangiectases) were reported in 3 patients who had only a solitary focal nodular hyperplasia.[117]

BILE DUCT ANOMALIES

Congenital abnormalities of the biliary tract are best demonstrated and studied by radiographic methods. In a series of 3845 operative cholangiograms, Puente & Bannura[118] demonstrated anatomical variations (defined as those having no pathological significance) in 24%, and congenital abnormalities (defined as pathologically significant deviations from the normal pattern) in 18.4%. The latter included left-sided cystic duct (9.5%), aberrant hepatic ducts (4.6%) and accessory hepatic ducts (1.7%).

AGENESIS OF THE COMMON BILE DUCT

In this very rare anomaly the common hepatic duct empties directly into the gallbladder, while the latter drains by a long cystic duct into the second part of the duodenum.[119]

AGENESIS OF THE COMMON HEPATIC DUCT

Three patients with this anomaly were reported by Stellin et al.[120] They presented with obstructive jaundice and at operation were found to have no proximal biliary tree. There were no ductal structures in the hepatic hilus.

ANOMALOUS ('ACCESSORY') BILE DUCTS

These are found in about 15% of cases when the bile ducts are dissected.[121] Anomalous hepatic ducts which pass beyond the porta hepatis almost invariably arise from the right lobe and frequently from a dorsal segment. The mode of termination is variable and final entry may be into the gallbladder, cystic duct, right or common hepatic ducts, junction of the cystic and common hepatic ducts or even the common bile duct.[122] A rare case of an anomalous right posterior segmental hepatic duct associated with a stricture and hepatolithiasis was reported by Cullingford et al.[123] Cholecystohepatic ducts are rare and occur when there is persistence of the fetal connections between the gallbladder and liver parenchyma, with no recanalization of the right and left hepatic ducts.[124] Failure to recognize their presence at cholecystectomy may lead to a persistent biliary fistula, bile peritonitis, stricture or death.[125] Cholangiography is mandatory whenever there is any doubt about the anatomy of the biliary tree in order to avoid the increased morbidity and mortality of re-operation.[126] Anomalous bile ducts may occur in association with biliary cystadenoma of the liver.[127] Recently, two examples of a long accessory hepatic duct were found in 23 cases of congenital dilatation of the common bile duct.[128] A unique case of atresia of the common hepatic duct with an accessory duct has been reported.[129] Accessory hepatic ducts may occasionally contain calculi.[130]

DUPLICATION OF THE BILE DUCTS

These have been reviewed by Boyden[131] and by Swartley & Weeder.[132] One duct may empty into the pylorus or both may drain into the duodenum. One patient also had a choledochal cyst.[123] Patients are usually free of symptoms until obstruction by stone or infection occurs. A case of congenital duplication of the cystic duct and common hepatic duct with a gastric mucosal lining was reported by Lee.[133] The patient, a 13-year-old boy, suffered from bouts of severe epigastric pain apparently due to extrinsic compression of the common hepatic duct.

CONGENITAL BRONCHOBILIARY AND TRACHEOBILIARY FISTULAS

A number of cases of bronchobiliary and tracheobiliary fistula have been reported.[134–141] One patient had a bronchobiliary fistula, as well as a tracheo-oesophageal fistula and oesophageal atresia.[142] The patient reported by Chan et al[140] had a bronchobiliary fistula with biliary atresia. The bronchobiliary fistula typically arises from the proximal part of the right main stem bronchus a short distance below the carina and generally joins the biliary system at the level of the left hepatic duct. The proximal part of the fistula resembles a bronchus while the distal part is lined by columnar and/or squamous epithelium. The presentation is in early infancy with aspiration pneumonia and atelectasis. The diagnosis is established by bronchoscopy or bronchography.

CILIATED HEPATIC FOREGUT CYST

Three examples were described by Terada et al,[143] who also reviewed three previously published cases. The cysts are solitary, unilocular and small (less than 4 cm in diameter). Histologically, the cyst wall consists of four layers: pseudostratified ciliated columnar epithelium with mucous cells, subepithelial connective tissue, bundles of smooth muscle and an outermost fibrous capsule. They are believed to arise from the embryonic foregut, and to differentiate towards bronchial structures in the liver.

SPONTANEOUS BILE DUCT PERFORATION

In the first few months of life, spontaneous bile peritonitis may occur from leakage of bile at the junction of the cystic and common bile ducts. In patients without other structural bile duct lesions, the aetiology is unknown, although congenital weakness of the bile duct walls, mucous plugs and gallstones have been suggested as possible causes.[144-148] The clinical presentation consists of jaundice, ascites, failure to thrive, variable abdominal pain and signs of peritoneal irritation. The diagnosis can be suspected by finding bile on abdominal paracentesis and confirmed by ^{99m}Tc-labelled hepatobiliary scanning.[149] Sonographic findings in 5 patients included ascites in 3, a loculated fluid collection around the gallbladder in 2, and both findings in 1; there was no dilatation of the biliary tree in any of the patients.[147] Treatment is surgical and the prognosis is excellent. Histological descriptions of the liver are sparse but are usually consistent with obstruction, with bile-duct proliferation and oedematous portal tracts, in addition to cholestasis.[145]

EXTRAHEPATIC BILIARY ATRESIA

Fifty per cent of the infants presenting with prolonged cholestasis in infancy have extrahepatic biliary atresia, the overall incidence being approximately 1 in 8000 live births.[150] Rarely is an aetiology for this malformation discovered or recurrence within a family found. Recently, two sisters, one with atresia and the other with congenital dilatation of the biliary tree, were reported by Ando et al.[151] Multiple causes are possible, judging from the reported associations with simple or composite vascular anomalies,[42] anomalous choledocho-pancreatic ductal junction,[152] polysplenia,[153] Turner's syndrome,[154] trisomy 17-18,[155,156] trisomy21,[157] small bowel atresia,[158] occurrence in one of non-identical or identical[159-162] twins, and viral infections such as cytomegalovirus,[163,164] rubella,[165,166] and non-A, non-B hepatitis.[167] Reovirus 3 has been suggested as a cause of extrahepatic biliary atresia and neonatal hepatitis on the basis of clinical and experimental studies,[168-172] but the association has been refuted by two groups of investigators.[173,174]

The aetiopathogenetic heterogeneity of the condition was made obvious recently by a study of 237 children by Silveira et al.[175] Forty seven of the children (20%) had associated congenital anomalies (28 cardiovascular, 22 digestive and 19 splenic). The splenic malformations included 13 with polysplenia syndrome and 2 with asplenia. Karyotypic abnormalities were found in 2 of 8 children who were studied. Silveira et al[175] proposed that extrahepatic biliary atresia could be divided into four distinct subgroups, three involving a congenital form that could arise through a malformation, a disruption or a chromosomal abnormality, while the fourth, the acquired form, could be attributed to agents active in the perinatal period.

The atresia may involve the whole of the extrahepatic biliary tree or only proximal or distal segments. The intrahepatic bile ducts are rarely affected early, but they are gradually destroyed with progression of the disease. Most infants have a raised serum bilirubin from birth but may remain clinically anicteric for several weeks.[176] Jaundice is obstructive in type, with dark urine and pale stools. The infants are not ill and have hepatomegaly with little splenomegaly. Later, progressive fibrosis and subsequent cirrhosis lead to all the complications of portal hypertension. Death usually occurs by 1 or 2 years of age if the lesion cannot be corrected surgically.[177] The median age of death is 12 months if the condition is not diagnosed and treated.[178]

The following diseases should be included in the differential diagnosis of extrahepatic biliary atresia: 'inspissated bile syndrome' associated with severe haemolytic anaemia[179] and bacterial infection (either systemic or urinary),[180] idiopathic perforation of the biliary tract,[144-148] viral infections (rubella, cytomegalovirus, herpes simplex and hepatitis B), toxoplasmosis and, finally, inherited diseases (particularly galactosaemia, α_1-antitrypsin deficiency and cystic fibrosis). The clinical aspects of cholestasis during infancy have been reviewed.[181-183]

Pre-operative diagnosis relies on demonstrating the presence or absence of bile secretion in the intestine. The value of radionuclide imaging is hotly debated and can only be interpreted by positive results, usually aided by the prior use of choleretics. A modification has been reported by El Tami et al.[184] Direct demonstration of bile or bile products is more accurate.[185-187] Recently, endoscopic retrograde cholangiopancreatography (ERCP) has been utilized for duct visualization.[188] Percutaneous liver biopsy may be accurate in the range of 60-95%, depending on the expertise of the interpreter.[189,190]

Histological studies of the extrahepatic bile ducts removed at surgery have been carried out by several groups of investigators.[191-197] In a study of 98 cases, Gautier & Eliot[196] classified the biliary remnants into three types:

- type 1 — absence of any lumen lined by biliary epithelium, with few or no inflammatory cells in the connective tissue.

• type 2 — presence of lumens lined by cuboidal epithelium, these being sometimes very numerous and usually having a diameter less than 50 μm. Periluminal neutrophilic infiltration is characteristic; cellular debris, and less often bile, may be found in the lumen. Epithelial necrosis is evident in ducts with a diameter exceeding 300 μm.

• type 3 — presence of a central altered bile duct incompletely lined by columnar epithelium, in addition to smaller epithelial structures resembling those in Type 2.

The three histological types were evaluated by the authors at three levels — porta hepatis, junction of the cystic and common hepatic ducts and an intermediate level; type 1 becomes increasingly more frequent from the porta hepatis to the junction of the hepatic duct and cystic ducts. Correlations between the size and number of residual ducts and establishment of bile flow after surgery have yielded conflicting results. Two groups of investigators suggested that bile flow is most likely to occur when the diameter of the residual ducts exceeds 150 μm.[194,198] A completely atretic common bile duct is illustrated in Fig. 3.3.

The prognosis for a good long-term result from hepatic porto-enterostomy (the Kasai procedure) depends primarily on operation before 60 days of age and the absence of cholangitis.[199–203] It may be better in the presence of gallbladder drainage of the liver because of the lack of cholangitis. Results of porto-enterostomy have been variable and liver transplantation has become the treatment of choice even for children under one year of age who have a failed porto-enterostomy.[204] The safety and results of liver transplantation with the use of livers from living related donors and cadaveric donors are excellent. One-year survival is greater than 90%, with better results obtained under elective conditions[205–207] and in children who are over 10 kg in weight.

The macroscopic appearance of the liver varies according to the stage of the disease. At first it enlarges and is dark green in colour, becoming finely nodular as cirrhosis develops. In untreated cases cirrhosis may take between 1 and 6 months from birth to develop. Histologically, dilated bile ducts filled with inspissated bile may be seen in sections of large portal areas (Fig. 3.4) and these may resemble Caroli's disease.[208] They are seen only after the age of 3 months and are not amenable to surgical drainage procedures. Portal lymphadenopathy may be evident: the median maximum node dimension in 6 cases studied by Hubscher & Harrison[209] was 14 mm. These lymph nodes are brown in colour and full of lipofuscin-laden macrophages (Fig. 3.5).

The main histological features include cholestasis, periportal ductular proliferation and the presence of bile plugs in cholangioles and interlobular bile ducts (Figs. 3.6–3.8). Giant cell transformation of hepatocytes is seen in approximately 15% of cases.[210] Fibrosis is

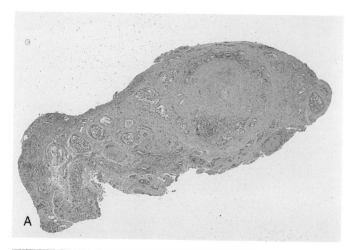

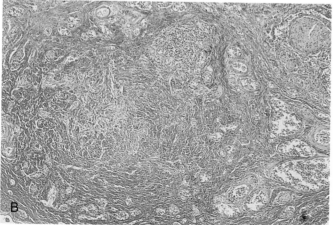

Fig. 3.3 Extrahepatic biliary atresia. (a) Section of common bile duct reveals complete fibrous occlusion of the lumen. The artretic duct is surrounded by inflammatory cells. H&E. (b) The atretic duct lacks a lumen and is well vascularized. A lymphoid aggregate is present in the wall (bottom). Note absence of muscle fibres. Masson's trichrome.

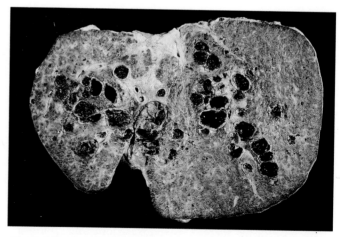

Fig. 3.4 Section of liver from patient with extrahepatic biliary atresia Multiple, dilated bile ducts are filled with black bilirubin casts. Some of the ducts have thick fibrous walls. The hepatic parenchyma is green and fibrotic.

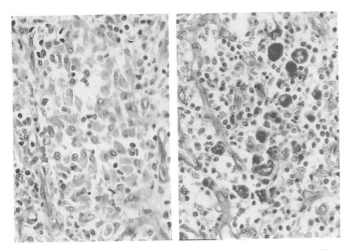

Fig. 3.5 Section of lymph node from hilum of liver from a patient with extrahepatic biliary atresia. Sinus histiocytes are hypertrophied and full of brown ceroid pigment (left) H&E. The pigment is strongly PAS positive (right). PAS after diastase digestion.

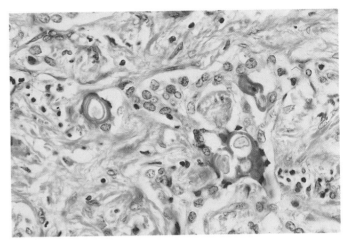

Fig.3.7 Extrahepatic biliary atresia. Bile plugs in cholangioles are inspissated and laminated. The epithelium of the cholangioles is atrophic. A few neutrophils infiltrate the supporting fibrous tissue. H&E.

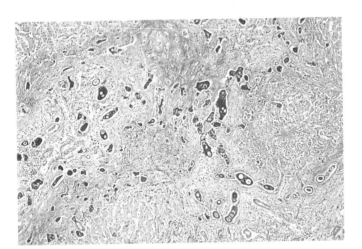

Fig. 3.6 Biliary fibrosis and cholangiolar proliferation. Many of the cholangioles are dilated and contain inspissated bile plugs. PAS after diastase digestion.

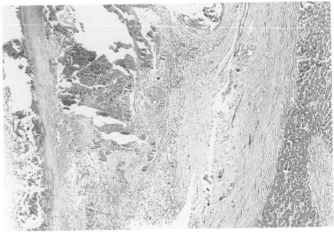

Fig. 3.8 Extrahepatic biliary atresia. A large hilar bile duct contains inspissated bile, has a fibrous, chronically inflamed wall, and lacks a lining epithelium. H&E.

progressive and periportal/periacinar in location, with linkage of portal areas and eventual development of a secondary biliary cirrhosis (Fig. 3.9). A study of the extracellular and cellular components of the connective tissue matrix was reported by DeFreitas et al.[211] Activation of a connective tissue clone by the proliferated ductules may be responsible for the portal fibrosis. Ho et al[212] have reported an arteriopathy (hyperplasia and hypertrophy) of the common hepatic artery and its peripheral branches supplying the entire biliary tree in 11 cases of biliary atresia; the possible pathogenetic significance of their findings remains to be established by future studies. In addition to severe cholestasis, the cirrhotic stage is characterized by marked pseudoxanthomatous transformation, the presence of bile lakes, Mallory bodies in some cases, and variable copper accumulation in liver cells (Figs. 3.10–3.12). In one study, copper concentrations

were increased in over two-thirds of liver samples obtained during porto-enterostomy and decreased in some patients after successful biliary drainage.[213] Acute and chronic inflammation is noted in portal/periportal areas in both precirrhotic and cirrhotic stages, and bile duct degeneration and inflammation may be evident (Fig. 3.13). Phenotypic characterization of the mononuclear infiltrates at the time of transplantation has shown a similarity to normal adult liver.[214] Bile lakes are seen after the age of 3 months, by which time irreversible hepatic damage has occurred.[215] Landing et al[216] and Sung & Stadlan[217] have shown that increasing fibrosis is associated with progressive loss of bile ducts beginning at the age of 8 or 9 months. Interlobular bile ducts become few in number as early as the fourth or fifth month after birth (Fig. 3.14).[218]

In addition to paucity of ducts, Raweily et al[219] identified concentric tubular ductal structures in 21.6% of

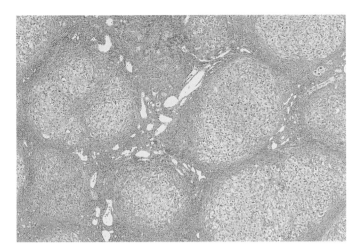

Fig. 3.9 Extrahepatic biliary atresia. Micronodular cirrhosis, with moderate portal and septal inflammation. H&E.

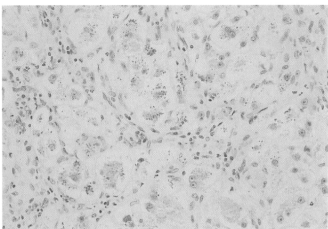

Fig. 3.12 Extrahepatic biliary atresia. Same case as illustrated in Figs 3.9–3.11. Marked copper accumulation in liver cells (red granules). Rhodanine.

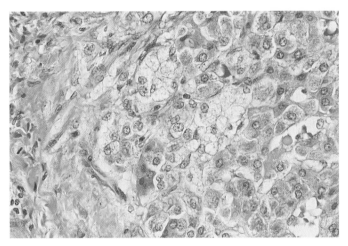

Fig. 3.10 Extrahepatic biliary atresia. Same case as illustrated in Fig. 3.9. Pseudoxanthomatous transformation at edge of cirrhotic septum. Note bile plug (lower right). H&E.

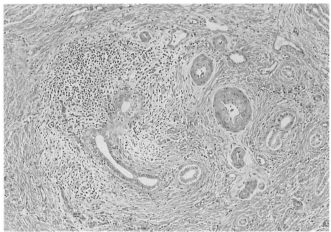

Fig. 3.13 Extrahepatic biliary atresia. One of a few residual bile ducts shows epithelial degeneration and is surrounded and infiltrated by lymphocytes and plasma cells. H&E.

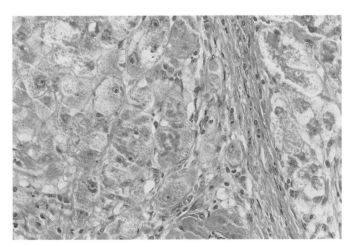

Fig. 3.11 Extrahepatic biliary atresia. Same case as illustrated in Figs 3.9 and 3.10. Mallory bodies in ballooned periseptal hepatocytes. H&E.

cases of extrahepatic biliary atresia; these were similar to those seen in ductal plate malformations. Similar observations had been made earlier by Desmet & Callea[220] who coined the term 'early severe' for this subgroup. It is of interest that such children reveal a histopathological picture resembling that of congenital hepatic fibrosis four or five years after porto-enterostomy[220,221] (Figs 3.15 and 3.16)

It is important to emphasize that interlobular bile ducts continue to disappear and that cirrhosis can develop despite satisfactory bile drainage after porto-enterostomy.[222] The loss of bile ducts has been attributed to recurrent or persistent obstruction of bile flow, recurrent cholangitis or continuation of the initial insult (e.g. viral) that caused the condition. A recent study by Nietgen et al[223] provides evidence that the vanishing intrahepatic bile ducts are due to an unpredictable and uneven obliteration of bile ducts in the porta hepatis during wound healing and scarring after porto-enterostomy.

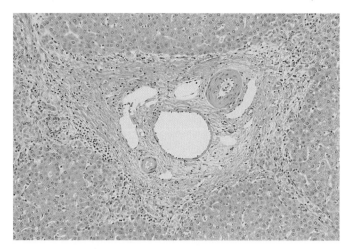

Fig. 3.14 Extrahepatic biliary atresia. A portal area is bereft of bile ducts. There is periportal cholangiolar proliferation with an associated neutrophilic response. H&E.

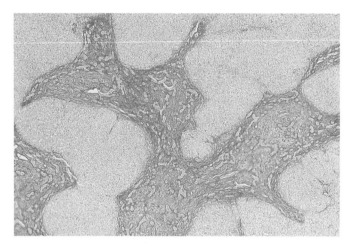

Fig. 3.15 Extrahepatic biliary atresia. Liver resection one year after porto-enterostomy. Pattern of fibrosis and proliferated small bile ducts is reminiscent of congenital hepatic fibrosis. There were only minimal chronic cholestatic features in this liver. PAS after diastase digestion.

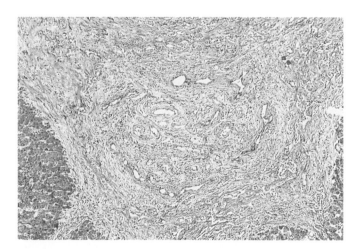

Fig. 3.16 Extrahepatic biliary atresia. Same liver as illustrated in Fig. 3.15. Ductal plate malformation. Note absence of an interlobular bile duct. Masson's trichrome.

Ultrastructural degenerative changes affecting the intrahepatic bile ducts and ductules in biliary atresia have been described in detail by Ito et al.[224] The degree of obstruction of the lumen of these ducts appears to be an important determinant of prognosis following corrective surgery.[224] A number of malignant epithelial tumours (hepatocellular carcinoma, cholangiocarcinoma and a mixed type) have developed in cirrhosis secondary to extrahepatic biliary atresia.[225]

The various theories of the pathogenesis of extrahepatic biliary atresia have been discussed by a number of authors.[182,183,195,216,226–229] Landing et al[216] first proposed that neonatal hepatitis, extrahepatic biliary atresia, choledochal cyst (at least in infants) and possibly some instances of 'intrahepatic biliary atresia' are all manifestations of a single basic disease process that he named 'infantile obstructive cholangiopathy'. They consider that biliary atresia (and choledochal cyst) is the result of an inflammatory rather than a maldevelopmental process and have postulated that the most probable cause is a viral infection. A few cases of extrahepatic biliary atresia have been attributed to congenital rubella, cytomegalovirus or reovirus 3 infection (see earlier section). A viral aetiology is not incompatible with the various chromosomal abnormalities that occur since both may be due to such a cause.[156] On the basis of experiments in rats given the drug 1,4-phenylenediiso-thiocyanate at different developmental stages, it has been proposed that the various manifestations of infantile obstructive cholangiopathy may depend on the timing of the insult.[230] Thus, rats given the drug during fetal life developed stenotic or atretic bile ducts due to thickening and fibrosis, whereas those given the drug after birth had dilatation of the ducts with inflammation.[230] Discordance in twins, however, supports a postnatal event being of primary importance in the pathogenesis of this disorder.[162]

NEONATAL HEPATITIS

Neonatal 'hepatitis' is a term that was coined for presumed viral infections of the liver in early infancy. Other diseases such as galactosaemia, hereditary fructose intolerance,[231] cystic fibrosis[232] and the conditions discussed under extrahepatic biliary atresia and paucity of the intrahepatic bile ducts may also present with pathological changes in the liver that resemble an infectious process. For example, giant cell transformation, a frequent histological component of neonatal hepatitis, has been seen in all cholestatic conditions in infancy including pure haemolytic anaemia and endotoxic injury.[233]

More than half the cases of neonatal hepatitis have no known aetiology. The incidence of such idiopathic cases in two series was 53.7%[234] and 59.3%.[235] For the rest, a number of infectious agents have been implicated. They include cytomegalovirus, rubella virus, hepatitis B virus, herpes simplex, varicella, the Coxsackie and Echo viruses, toxoplasma and *Treponema pallidum*.[236] Diseases caused by these agents are discussed in Chapter 7. An unusually high incidence of cytomegalovirus infection (49%) was first reported in a series of 45 cases from Taiwan.[237] An association with hypopituitarism was reported in 2 infants by Herman et al,[238] and more recently Sheehan et al[239] reported 5 more cases and reviewed all those previously published.

Neonatal hepatitis may be familial or non-familial. The familial form may be progressive, with or without the development of cirrhosis, or the course may be characterized by recurrent cholestasis.[240-243] The pattern of inheritance is considered to be autosomal recessive. A hereditary form with giant cell transformation and lymphoedema resulting from abnormal deep lymphatics has been reported.[244,245] Liver biopsies are characterized by varying degrees of cholestasis (with or without pseudoglandular structures), giant cell transformation, ballooning, sinusoidal apoptotic (acidophilic) bodies, extramedullary haemopoiesis, active fibroblastic proliferation and parenchymal and portal tract inflammation.

The pathological aspects of giant cell transformation, a frequent and often dominant finding in neonatal hepatitis, have been reviewed extensively.[236,246] It is seen throughout the hepatic acinus but zone 3 is often more strikingly affected. The giant cells contain four or more nuclei, and sometimes many have ill-defined outlines and may be detached from other cells in the hepatic plate (Figs 3.17 and 3.18). The cytoplasm may contain remnants of cell membranes. It is partially rarefied and often contains bile and/or haemosiderin. The cells may have more glycogen than normal hepatocytes and a greater activity of a variety of enzymes, such as glucose-6-phosphatase, acid phosphatase and succinic dehydrogenase. Death of the giant cells is associated with a neutrophilic inflammatory response (Fig. 3.19). Their number decreases as patients grow older, and they are rare after the age of one year. Formation of giant cells is considered to be a characteristic change resulting from mitotic inhibition of the young, growing liver tissue by a number of agents such as viruses, drugs, or hereditary abnormalities,[247] or to dissolution of cell membranes, as suggested by Craig & Landing[248] who first described this phenomenon.

Survival in neonatal hepatitis depends on the aetiology. Long-term follow-up studies have shown surprisingly different results in two series. Thus, 2 of the 29 patients with cryptogenic neonatal hepatitis reported by Dick & Mowat[234] died, and only a further 2 had signs of persisting liver disease. They concluded that the prognosis of the hepatitis syndrome without known associated factors is good, and that every effort should be made to minimize the short-term effects of cholestasis. Deutsch et al,[235] on the other hand, found a high mortality (25%) in their 73

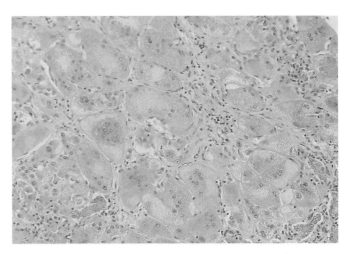

Fig. 3.17 Neonatal hepatitis, idiopathic, with giant cell transformation. H&E.

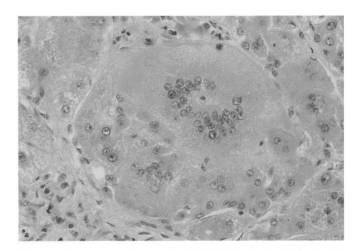

Fig. 3.18 Same case as illustrated in Fig. 3.17. Detail of multinucleated giant hepatocyte. Periphery of cell (left) suggests fusion with several smaller cells. H&E.

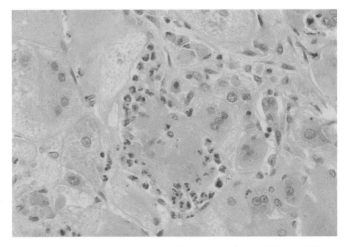

Fig. 3.19 Same case as illustrated in Figs 3.17 and 3.18. Neutrophilic satellitosis of degenerated giant cell. H&E.

babies with idiopathic neonatal cholestasis. Deaths resulted from liver failure, septicaemia or associated developmental defects. Progression to chronic liver disease occurred in 7.5% of the children surviving beyond one year of age.

PAUCITY OF THE INTRAHEPATIC BILE DUCTS

The term 'paucity of the intrahepatic bile ducts' is less confusing and more accurate than the formerly used one of 'intrahepatic biliary atresia'. The disease has also been referred to as 'hepatic ductular hypoplasia'.[249] The entity has been associated with α_1-antitrypsin deficiency,[250] chromosomal defects such as 45X[251,252] and trisomy 17–18,[229] Down's syndrome,[253] prune belly syndrome[254] and a metabolic block in the catabolism of trihydroxy-coprostanic acid.[255,256] Three comprehensive reviews of paucity of intrahepatic bile ducts in childhood are recommended for further reading.[257–259]

The majority of patients with this syndrome, excluding those with the above associations, can be divided into two groups, syndromatic and non-syndromatic. Patients in the *syndromatic* group may be easily recognized by their characteristic facies. Comprehensive descriptions have been published by Alagille and associates[249,257] and Henriksen et al.[260] Synonyms for the syndrome are arteriohepatic dysplasia, first coined by Watson & Miller,[216] and 'Alagille's syndrome'. The facies consists of slight hypertelorism, deeply set eyes, cheek bones that are wide apart and a broad forehead. The specificity of this appearance has been questioned.[262] All patients have a systolic murmur which is usually related to stenosis of the pulmonary arterial system. Up to 15% of patients may have life-threatening cardiac complications.[257] Vertebral anomalies are common and include hemivertebrae, clefts in the vertebrae, and unsegmented or wedge-shaped vertebral bodies.

Other associated anomalies and conditions include posterior embryotoxon, retinal pigmentary lesions, Axenfeld's anomaly, cataracts, short distal phalanges, a small flat face on lateral X-ray, mild conductive hearing loss and various renal abnormalities such as tubulo-interstitial nephropathy, membranous nephropathy, congenital single kidney and renovascular hypertension.[263–270] Abnormalities of the biliary tract include hypoplasia of the extrahepatic bile ducts,[271–275] hypoplasia of the gallbladder[273] and cholelithiasis.[271] Endoscopic retrograde cholangiopancreatography has demonstrated narrowing of the intrahepatic ducts, reduced arborization and focal areas of dilatation, as well as narrowing of the extrahepatic ducts.[271–274]

Most of the patients are growth-retarded prior to adolescence,[270] and some are mentally retarded. All patients have pruritus, although it may be mild, with elevated serum bile acids, the levels of cholic acid being greater than those of chenodeoxycholic acid. No abnormal bile acids have been found in the serum. The usual signs of cholestasis are always present. Variable hyperlipidaemia is frequent and sometimes severe, with xanthomas. An autosomal dominant genetic basis for this disorder, initially proposed by Henriksen et al,[260] is strongly supported by the studies of LaBrecque et al.[267] Diet and either cholestyramine or phenobarbitone lower the blood lipid levels, decrease the intensity of the cardiac murmur (apparently by decreasing the atherosclerotic plaques in the pulmonary vessels), diminish the pruritus, and lower the serum bile acid levels.

Long-term complications of arteriohepatic dysplasia have been reported.[270,275] In one series, 5 of 6 patients who survived beyond 16 years of age had complications that resulted in severe morbidity in 3 and death in 2.[275] These complications included hepatic failure (2), renal failure (1), cerebellar herniation (1) and hepatocellular carcinoma (1). Other cases of hepatocellular carcinoma complicating this syndrome have been reported.[276–279] One 17-year-old patient with cirrhosis had an incidental focal nodular hyperplasia.[280]

Liver transplantation has been undertaken in patients with arteriohepatic dysplasia and end-stage liver disease. Tzakis et al[281] reported 23 patients who underwent liver transplantation; 57% of the children were still alive 2–9 years (mean 4.4 years) after surgery. Three of the fatalities were related to cardiovascular failure. The mortality was higher among patients who had more severe cardiac disease or who had previously undergone a Kasai procedure.

The second, *non-syndromatic*, group of patients with paucity of intrahepatic bile ducts presents with persistent cholestasis and severe pruritus, but without significant elevation of serum lipids. No associated aetiological agent, defined genetic factors or congenital anomalies have been found in this group. No abnormal bile acids have been demonstrated, although again the serum level of cholic acid is higher than that of chenodeoxycholic acid. Growth retardation is common. This group responds well to cholestyramine therapy in doses which reduce the serum bile acid levels to normal. Liver function tests return to normal values except for a persistently raised alkaline phosphatase activity. Pruritus is relieved, hepatomegaly improves along with the pathological changes in the liver, and the weight and height increase towards normal levels. A possible relationship between non-syndromatic paucity of bile ducts in infancy and idiopathic adulthood ductopenia was suggested by Bruguera et al.[282]

Pathological aspects of the syndromatic form of paucity of the intrahepatic bile ducts are covered in reports of several series and review articles.[249,257,260,271,273,281,283–291] The major finding is absence of bile ducts from portal areas (Figs 3.20 and 3.21). According to Alagille,[289] the ratio of interlobular bile ducts to the number of portal

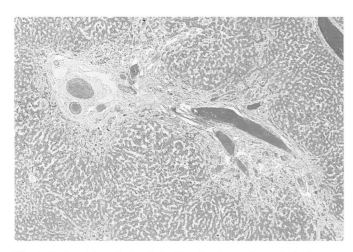

Fig. 3.20 Arteriohepatic dysplasia. Two fused portal areas lack bile ducts. H&E.

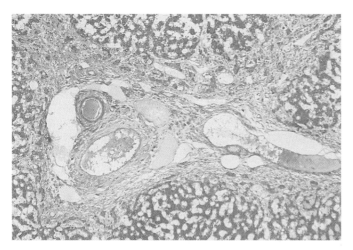

Fig. 3.21 Same case as illustrated in Fig. 3.20. Portal area contains vessels but no ducts. There is patchy periportal fibrosis but no cholangiolar proliferation. Masson's trichrome.

areas is between 0 and 0.4 compared with 0.9 and 1.8 in normal children. A reduced number of portal areas has been noted by Hadchouel et al.[286] The loss of bile ducts is progressive from early infancy to childhood.[273,290,291] Cholangiodestructive lesions have been observed in infants between 3 and 6 months of age.[273,291] The degree of cholestasis is variable in intensity and is especially prominent in the first 12 months of life. Giant cell transformation may be seen in early infancy.[273,290,291] There is usually patchy pseudoxanthomatous transformation of hepatocytes and Kupffer cells,[284,290] and slight accumulation of histologically demonstrable copper in periportal hepatocytes.[273,290,291] Copper accumulation has also been demonstrated by quantitative methods in both syndromatic and non-syndromatic types of paucity of the intrahepatic bile ducts.[283,292] Periportal fibrosis, when present, remains unchanged in long-term follow-up studies.[249] Cirrhosis is rare,[271,281,283,284] but it may develop in

occasional patients (Fig. 3.22). Portal inflammation and periportal cholangiolar proliferation, when present, are seen mainly in early infancy.[273,291] Unicellular hepatocytic degeneration (ballooning, acidophilic bodies) has been noted in some studies.[284,290]

Ultrastructural studies of the syndromatic type of paucity of the intrahepatic bile drugs have been reported.[284,290,291,293] Bile canalicular changes, although described,[290,291] are considered to be an infrequent finding by others.[284] Valencia-Mayoral et al,[284] who studied 12 biopsies from 10 patients, noted distinctive ultrastructural changes. Bile pigment retention was found in the cytoplasm of liver cells, especially in lysosomes and in vesicles of the outer convex face of the Golgi apparatus (*cis*-Golgi), but only rarely in bile canaliculi or the immediate pericanalicular region. Valencia-Mayoral et al[284] suggested that the basic defect in arteriohepatic dysplasia involves the bile secretory apparatus, possibly the Golgi apparatus of liver cells. The pathogenesis of the cholangiodestructive lesions described histopathologically[273,291] and ultrastructurally[291] remains to be elucidated, but the possibility of 'disuse atrophy' has been raised by two groups of investigators.[284,291]

A histopathological and ultrastructural study of 17 children with non-syndromatic paucity of bile ducts was reported by Kahn et al.[294] Before 90 days of age there was paucity of ducts and periportal fibrosis as well as non-specific intra-acinar changes (cholestasis, giant cell transformation, perisinusoidal fibrosis and haemopoiesis). After 90 days the duct paucity and fibrosis persisted. Cholestasis was mild or no longer apparent. Ultrastructural studies revealed bile duct destruction characterized by undulation and breaks in the basal lamina, and infiltration of the epithelium by lymphocytes. It is the opinion of Khan et al[294] that the paucity in non-syndromatic cases may result from a primary ductal insult leading to destruction and disappearance of the ducts.

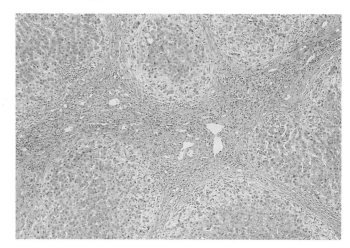

Fig. 3.22 Arteriohepatic dysplasia. Micronodular cirrhosis. Note ductopenia, moderate septal inflammation and 'cholate' stasis. H&E.

CONGENITAL DILATATIONS OF THE BILE DUCTS

Congenital dilatations of the bile ducts were originally classified into three types by Alonso-Lej et al.[295] That classification has been replaced by one with five types, both extrahepatic and intrahepatic:[296,297]

- type I — a dilatation of the common bile duct which may present three anatomical variations:
  a. large saccular,
  b. small localized, and
  c. diffuse fusiform;
- type II — diverticulum of the common bile duct or the gallbladder;
- type III — choledochocoele;
- type IV — multiple intrahepatic and extrahepatic dilatations (Caroli's disease); and
- type V — fusiform intrahepatic and extrahepatic dilatations.

Types IV and V appear to be the most common, especially in the Orient where the disease occurs more frequently.

CHOLEDOCHAL CYST

The classic clinical triad of pain, a mass in the right upper quadrant and jaundice occurs in less than one third of patients with choledochal cyst.[298,299] In children, jaundice is the most common presentation, while in adults the signs and symptoms are those of ascending cholangitis.[300] Although the lesion is congenital, less than 60% are diagnosed in patients under 20 years of age and some cases may present for the first time in the sixth decade of life. Several cases have been diagnosed antenatally.[301] Eighty per cent of the patients are female. The pre-operative diagnosis can be made in the majority of patients by cholangiographic studies, ultrasound and isotope scanning.[297,302–306] Complications include perforation, liver abscesses, stone formation, secondary biliary cirrhosis, pancreatitis, amyloidosis and carcinoma of the biliary tree.[299,300,303,307–312] A case of regression of biliary cirrhosis following drainage of a choledochal cyst has been reported.[313]

A variety of biliary tract anomalies, summarized by Crittenden & McKinley,[298] have been reported in association with choledochal cyst. They include double common bile duct, double gallbladder, absent gallbladder, annular pancreas, biliary atresia or stenosis[310] and anomalies of the pancreatico-biliary junction.[314–317] In the series of choledochal cysts reported by Barlow et al,[310] patients under one year of age had a higher incidence of atresia or stenosis of the biliary tree associated with cirrhosis and portal hypertension, as well as a higher mortality rate, than did patients between 3 and 20 years of age. Malformation of the pancreatico-biliary ductal system is considered the most plausible pathogenetic mechanism for choledochal cyst,[318] and is supported by experimental studies.[319]

Treatment usually involves drainage of the cystic structure by choledocho-cysto-jejunostomy, but ascending cholangitis often continues to be a problem. Total excision has been successful in some hands,[303,320–322] and is advocated as a preventive measure for the subsequent development of carcinoma by Kagawa et al[311] and Nagorney et al.[300] Surgeons from several centres in Japan[323,324] and the USA[325] believe that the treatment of choice is excision of the dilated common bile duct along with the gallbladder and hepato-enterostomy. Surgical procedures have reduced the mortality rate from 97 to 3 or 4%.[309]

Choledochal cysts vary greatly in size, with some of the larger ones containing 5–10 litres in bile (Figs 3.23 and 3.24). Histopathologically, the wall is usually thickened by inflammation and fibrosis, and is bile stained. Smooth muscle fibres may be identified in the lower portion of the cyst but not in the narrow (intrapancreatic) portion.[326] There is generally no epithelial lining but islets of cylindrical or columnar epithelium may be preserved (Fig. 3.25).[295] Intestinal metaplasia with mucous gland proliferation, as well as the presence of goblet and Paneth cells and neuroendocrine differentiation, have been reported.[327–329] According to Komi et al,[328] intestinal metaplasia increases with age, so that cysts from almost all patients over 15 years of age show it. Kusunoki et al[330] noted the absence of ganglion cells in the narrow portion of a choledochal cyst, and suggested that the cyst could be the result of postganglionic neural dysfunction.

The majority of malignant tumours arising in congenital cystic dilatation of the bile ducts are adenocarcinomas, but some anaplastic and a few squamous carcinomas have been reported.[311,331,332] The overall incidence of carcinomas arising in all cystic dilatations of the bile ducts is about 3%.[311] Analysis of the literature indicates that the

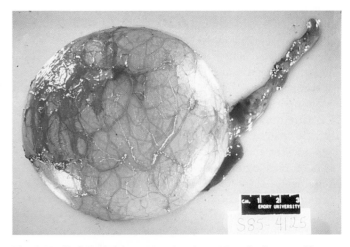

Fig. 3.23 Choledochal cyst measuring about 10 cm in diameter. Note numerous vessels over the surface.

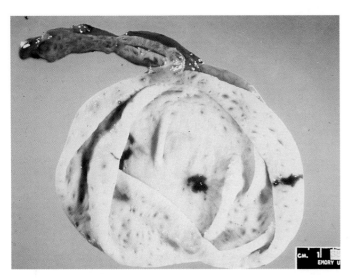

Fig. 3.24 Same cyst as illustrated in Fig. 3.23. Opened, collapsed cyst has a smooth inner lining. It did not contain bile.

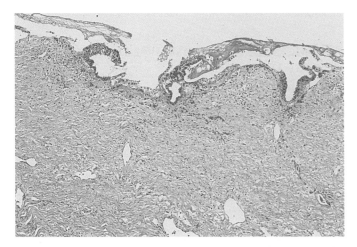

Fig. 3.25 Segment of wall of choledochal cyst shows inflammation and focal epithelial ulceration. H&E.

incidence of carcinoma in choledochal cysts is age related. The risk increases from 0.7% in the first decade to 6.8% in the second decade and 14.3% in later decades.[332] Reveille et al[333] found that stasis of bile in choledochal cysts contributes to bacterial overgrowth and the generation of unconjugated secondary bile acids; they proposed this as a possible cause of the development of biliary metaplasia and carcinoma.

CAROLI'S DISEASE

While this condition generally involves the entire liver, it may be segmental or lobar. It was first described by Caroli.[334] The inheritance is autosomal recessive. By 1982 some 99 cases had been reported.[335] Ten other personally studied cases were analysed with the 99 cases of Mercadier et al.[335] Since then many other case reports, as well as small series,[336,337] have appeared. Clinically, patients

suffer from bouts of recurrent fever and pain. Jaundice occurs only when a stone blocks the common bile duct. Leucocytosis is observed typically when acute cholangitis develops. Liver function tests are generally normal except during episodes of obstructive jaundice. The diagnosis is established by cholangiography, (intravenous or transhepatic), ERCP, ultrasonography and computed tomography.[334,338–341] Selective hepatic arteriography provides useful information prior to surgical intervention.[335] The complications of Caroli's disease resemble those of choledochal cyst and include recurrent cholangitis, abscess formation, septicaemia or pyaemia, intrahepatic lithiasis and amyloidosis. Adenocarcinomas, including some arising in cases with a lobar distribution, have also been reported.[342–347] Hepatocellular carcinoma occurs rarely.[348] Surgical treatment consists of internal or external drainage procedures.[335] Transhepatic decompression has been advocated.[349] Segmental or lobar forms of Caroli's disease can be treated by partial hepatectomy.[335,350–352] Extra corporeal shock wave lithotripsy has been utilized for disintegration of intrahepatic bile-duct stones.[353]

Macroscopically, the intrahepatic cystic dilatations are round or lanceolate, 1.0–4.5 cm in diameter, and may be separated by stretches of essentially normal duct[334] (Fig. 3.26). Inspissated bile or soft and friable bilirubin calculi may be noted in the lumen. Microscopically, the dilated ducts usually show severe chronic inflammation, with or without superimposed acute inflammation, and varying degrees of fibrosis (Fig. 3.27). The epithelium may appear normal (cuboidal to tall columnar), may be partly or completely ulcerated, or may be focally hyperplastic; all of these changes can be found in different ducts in the same case (Fig. 3.28). Mucous glands (sometimes in abundance) may be present in the fibrotic and inflamed wall. Areas of severe epithelial dysplasia or carcinoma in situ are seen rarely.[354,355] The lumen contains admixtures of inspissated mucin and bile, calcareous material, or

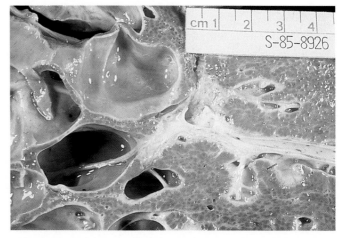

Fig. 3.26 Caroli's disease. Section of liver shows cystically dilated bile ducts. The lining of the ducts is bile stained.

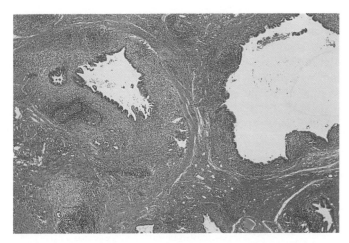

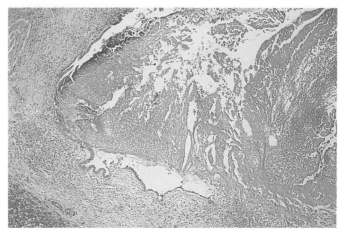

Fig. 3.27 Caroli's disease. Dilated bile ducts have thickened walls due to marked chronic inflammation. Note lymphoid follicles in the wall of one duct (left). H&E.

Fig. 3.29 Caroli's disease. Markedly dilated duct contains golden-yellow inspissated bile. It shows marked inflammation, as well as ulceration (bottom). H&E.

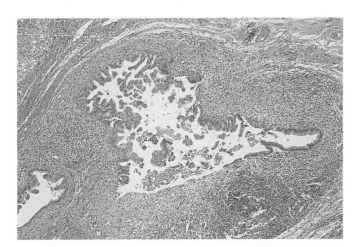

Fig. 3.28 Caroli's disease. The thickened bile duct wall reveals marked chronic inflammation. The lining epithelium is hyperplastic, except for a small segment of the duct (right). There is an area of ulceration (bottom). H&E.

frank pus during bouts of acute cholangitis (Fig. 3.29). Caroli's disease can be associated with congenital hepatic fibrosis and, rarely, with infantile polycystic disease[356] and even adult polycystic disease.[357]

According to Desmet,[358] the pathogenesis of Caroli's disease seems to involve total or partial arrest of remodelling of the ductal plate of the larger intrahepatic bile ducts. In Caroli's 'syndrome' (Caroli's disease with congenital hepatic fibrosis), the hereditary factor causing the arrest of remodelling seems to exert its influence, not only during the early period of bile duct embryogenesis, but also later on during development of the more peripheral biliary ramifications (the interlobular bile ducts).

A unique case of Marfan's syndrome associated with diffuse ectasia of the entire biliary tract has been reported.[359] It was suggested by the authors that the defect of connective tissue in that disease could have led to weakness of the wall of the bile ducts with resultant ectasia.

AUTOSOMAL RECESSIVE POLYCYSTIC KIDNEY DISEASE

INFANTILE PRESENTATION

This disease is inherited in an autosomal recessive manner. The prevalence is estimated to be between 1/10000 and 1/60 000.[360] The gene for this disorder has not been mapped. There is an equal sex incidence. Depending on the age of presentation and the degree of renal involvement, it has been divided into four types by Blyth & Ockenden[361] — perinatal, neonatal, infantile and juvenile. These authors proposed that four different mutant alleles are responsible and that there may be a fifth group in which the onset of symptoms is later than juvenile. The subject has been reviewed by a number of authors.[362–368]

The *perinatal* type is the most severe form of this condition. Some affected patients are stillborn. In the series of Blyth & Ockenden[361] no infant survived beyond 6 weeks of age. The majority of patients were admitted with signs of respiratory distress from various forms of pulmonary insufficiency and had marked abdominal distension due to huge symmetrical renal masses. Liver function test abnormalities were uncommon. Surviving patients with the *neonatal* type of the disease develop gradually increasing renal insufficiency and hypertension. Pyelonephritis is common. Portal fibrosis and cystic dilatation of bile ducts are more marked, and cholangitis is a frequent complication. In the *infantile* group the clinical picture is either of chronic renal failure or of increasing portal hypertension. Portal fibrosis is moderate. The *juvenile* group[361] typically includes children (1–5 years old) who present with portal hypertension. Liver changes are marked. It is likely that this group represents cases of congenital hepatic fibrosis, as suggested by Landing et al.[364] Gang & Herrin[369] have found that there is a spectrum of phenotype expression with prognostic implications, but feel that all cases do not fit into the sharply defined subgroups of Blyth & Ockenden.[361] In their study of 11 patients, 4 had 90% or more renal cystic change; these patients did not survive beyond 20 days of birth. In contrast, 5 of the 7 less severely diseased patients with a 20–75% range of cystic changes in the kidneys were all alive at 6–21 years of age.

The liver in autosomal recessive polycystic kidney disease does not appear abnormal macroscopically, although it may be enlarged and firm; rarely, this feature may be more marked in the left lobe.[370] Histologically, there is a striking increase in the number of biliary channels that arise in portal areas and these extend irregularly and deeply into the acini (Figs. 3.30 and 3.31). They appear to branch or 'anastomose'[371] and often show polypoid projections (Fig. 3.31). A circular, often interrupted, appearance (ductal plate malformation) is thought to represent arrested development of the bile ducts (Fig. 3.30).[372] Normal interlobular ducts with corresponding arteries are not seen. According to Witzleben,[366] the biliary channels are in continuity with the rest of the biliary system (communicating cystic disease), in contrast to the non-communicating autosomal dominant form of the disease. The supporting connective tissue is scanty and, in the intralobular extensions, the basement membrane of the epithelium appears to be in direct contact with the liver cell plates. The epithelial lining consists of a single layer of low columnar to cuboidal cells. Cyst formation is uncommon. The dilated channels may contain a small quantity of a pink or orange-coloured material or, rarely, pus. According to Potter & Craig,[373] the blood vessels and lymphatics in portal areas are unusually prominent. Reconstruction studies of a portal tract by

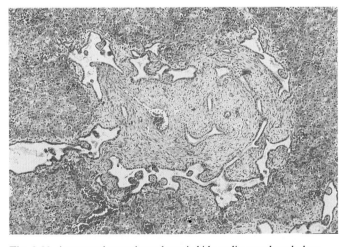

Fig. 3.30 Autosomal recessive polycystic kidney disease: ductal plate malformation. The bile ducts form an interrupted ring at the periphery of what should eventually become a portal area. There is no interlobular bile duct. Note branch of portal vein, as well as smaller vessels. H&E.

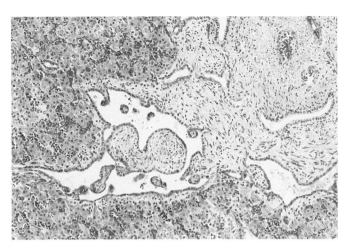

Fig. 3.31 Same case as illustrated in Fig. 3.30. Higher magnification of part of the ductal plate showing irregularity in outline of the ducts with polypoid projections into a dilated lumen. The lining epithelium is low cuboidal. H&E.

Adams et al[371] showed irregularly dilated ducts running longitudinally at the periphery of the portal tract and anastomosing so extensively that they formed a single annular channel; no main interlobular duct could be identified. A stereological study of 10 cases by Jörgensen[374] showed ductal structures that could be divided into two groups: one consisted of irregular tubular structures shaped like circular cylinders, and the other of elliptical cylinders (the ductal plates). These were dilated but cysts were rare. In patients who survive for months or years there is progressive fibrosis of the liver and kidney lesions.[363]

JUVENILE AND ADULT PRESENTATION — CONGENITAL HEPATIC FIBROSIS

This condition occurs predominantly in children and adolescents. The inheritance pattern is not a simple autosomal recessive one. It may be associated with dilatation of the intra- or extrahepatic bile ducts.[375–378] An unusual association with adult-type polycystic disease, an autosomal dominant disease, has been reported.[379] Infants present with abdominal distension from enlarged organs, respiratory distress and hypertension. Older patients come to medical attention because of hepatosplenomegaly or bleeding from oesophageal varices secondary to portal hypertension that is usually presinusoidal,[380] but asymptomatic cases have been reported.[381] Infants may have evidence of systemic hypertension and/or renal failure. Cholangitis has been emphasized as a manifestation by Fauvert & Benhamou.[382] They recognized four clinical forms — portal hypertensive, cholangitic, mixed portal hypertensive-cholangitic, and latent. The pure cholangitic form is rare. In the mixed form patients suffer from recurrent bouts of cholangitis, with or without jaundice, in addition to the manifestations of portal hypertension. A number of associated conditions and diseases have been reported occasionally. They include familial congenital heart disease,[383] pulmonary arteriovenous fistulas,[384] multiple gastric ulcers,[385] protein-losing enteropathy and recurrent thrombosis,[386] and the Laurence–Moon–Biedl syndrome.[387]

The usual kidney disease, when present, is medullary tubular ectasia, a fusiform or cystic dilatation of tubules, particularly the collecting ducts, that may be detected by intravenous pyelography and renal angiography. Some patients may have cystic kidneys resembling those of adult polycystic disease and others may have nephronophthisis.[380,388,389] The organ most affected, be it kidney or liver, may vary within the same family. Routine liver function tests are usually normal, but the serum alkaline phosphatase activity may be increased.

The combination of a patent portal vein and well-preserved liver function makes patients with congenital hepatic fibrosis ideal candidates for portosystemic shunt surgery. Follow-up examination of 16 patients who underwent portosystemic shunt surgery by Alvarez et al[390] revealed no impairment of liver function or signs of hepatic encephalopathy in any. Of 75 published cases reviewed by Sommerschild et al,[380] 50% had died; the major causes of death were renal failure and uncontrollable haemorrhage. One complication that should be noted is the rare development of cholangiocarcinoma.[391–393]

Pathological descriptions have been published by many authors.[366,380,382,389,394–397] Grossly, the liver is enlarged, has a firm to hard consistency, and shows a fine reticular pattern of fibrosis; no cysts are visible to the naked eye. Although the entire liver is usually involved, occasional lobar cases are on record.[390] Microscopically, there is diffuse periportal fibrosis, the bands of fibrous tissue varying in thickness. Irregularly shaped islands of hepatic tissue, some incorporating several acini, may be seen (Fig. 3.32). When the bands of fibrous tissue are thick, terminal hepatic venules may be encroached upon and these become incorporated within the fibrous tissue; thus, portal hypertension in this condition may not always be presinusoidal.[398] The fibrous bands may encircle single acini or groups of them; occasionally, a small islet of hepatic tissue becomes separated. Numerous uniform and generally small bile ducts are scattered in the fibrous tissue (Fig. 3.33). An interrupted circular arrangement of the ducts (ductal plate malformation) may be recognizable (Fig. 3.34). The ducts are lined by cuboidal to low columnar epithelium and may contain bile or traces of mucin. They may be slightly dilated and irregular in outline. Cholestasis is not a feature of the uncomplicated case. Paucity of portal vein branches has been noted in some studies,[380,396] and has usually been invoked as the cause of portal hypertension. In one study the portal vein branches were dilated and hepatic arterial branches showed marked medial hypertrophy, suggesting excessive arteriovenous anastomoses as another possible mechanism.[399] The ultra-

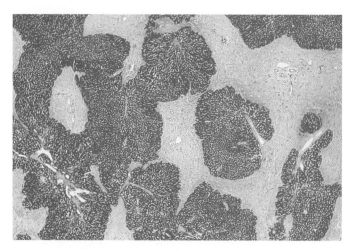

Fig. 3.32 Congenital hepatic fibrosis. Jigsaw pattern of hepatic parenchyma and fibrous tissue. PAS.

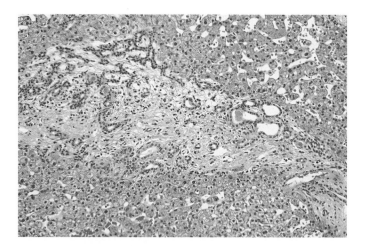

Fig. 3.33 Congenital hepatic fibrosis. Fibrous tissue contains small bile ducts, a few of which are dilated and contain bile. Note absence of inflammation. The adjacent hepatic parenchyma shows no evidence of cholestasis. H&E.

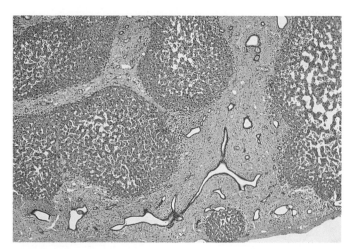

Fig. 3.34 Congenital hepatic fibrosis. Same case as illustrated in Fig. 3.33. Appearance of ducts suggests part of a ductal plate malformation. H&E.

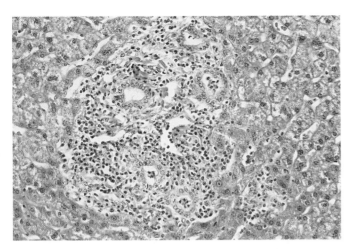

Fig. 3.35 Congenital hepatic fibrosis, 'cholangitic type.' The ducts are involved by an acute cholangitis. H&E

structural studies of Albukerk & Duffy[400] suggest that compression of the intrahepatic portal vein branches by progressive expansion of the fibro-epithelial growth could also contribute to the portal hypertension. There is generally little inflammation except in cases associated with cholangitis, when numerous neutrophils infiltrate the ducts and surrounding connective tissue (Fig. 3.35); rupture of the ducts can result in microabscess formation. The latter cases may be difficult to differentiate from extrahepatic biliary obstruction with ascending infection, particularly since there may be associated parenchymal cholestasis. The correct diagnosis must be based on the history, clinical findings and the results of radiographic studies. It is important to reiterate at this juncture that congenital hepatic fibrosis may be associated with Caroli's disease or, rarely, with choledochal cyst.[401]

A number of malformation syndromes, characterized by hepatic morphological changes which resemble those of congenital hepatic fibrosis, can be differentiated by the associated findings. They include: *Meckel's syndrome* with encephalocoele, polydactyly and cystic kidneys;[402] *Ivemark's syndrome* with dysplasia of the pancreas, liver and kidneys, together with cysts in the pancreas and liver in some cases;[403,404] *Ellis–van Creveld syndrome or chondro-ectodermal dysplasia;*[405] *nephronophthisis–congenital hepatic fibrosis syndrome* with retinal lesions, mental retardation, cerebellar hypoplasia and osseous abnormalities;[406] *Jeune syndrome* — skeletal dysplasia, pulmonary hypoplasia and retinal lesions[407,408] — in which one of two siblings with the syndrome had cirrhosis;[408] *vaginal atresia syndrome;*[364] *tuberous sclerosis;*[364] and *medullary cystic disease.*[364]

AUTOSOMAL DOMINANT POLYCYSTIC KIDNEY DISEASE

The abnormal gene is on the short arm of chromosome 16, closely linked to the α haemoglobin and phosphogly-colate phosphatase genes,[409–411] and can be identified by a DNA probe, 16S4, when there are two other affected family members. The incidence of this mutant (still to be identified) gene is 1 in 1000 and comprises 90% of cases. In adults, the other 10% of patients present with a milder form of polycystic disease. The spontaneous mutation rate may be less than 10%.[412] The autopsy incidence from one large hospital was 1 per 687 autopsies.[413] In one series of 173 autopsies of individuals with polycystic kidneys, one to several liver cysts were found in 16%, and numerous cysts were present in 21%.[414] The renal disease can be present at birth but hepatic manifestations are rare before 16 years of age.[415]

In the series of Henson et al[416] the average age at first admission for liver-related problems was 52.8 years, with an average duration of symptoms of three years. The symptoms included a gradually enlarging abdominal mass, upper abdominal pain or discomfort, and rare episodes of severe pain with or without nausea, vomiting and fever in an occasional patient. The most frequent physical finding is hepatomegaly, which can be massive.[417] Liver function tests are often normal. Jaundice is unusual[418,419] and portal hypertension is rare.[420–423] Rarely is treatment needed by a combination of excision and fenestration.[424–427] Liver or combined liver and renal transplantation has been performed successfully in several patients.[428,429]

The incidence of liver involvement and its complications has been reviewed in a large series including 132 patients on, and 120 patients not on haemodialysis.[428] Liver cysts were found by non-invasive radiological procedures in 85 of 124 patients on dialysis; sex distribution was equal. In contrast, the non-dialysed population demonstrated a 75% incidence of liver cysts in females and a 44% incidence in males, the peak incidence occurring 10 years sooner in females. The cysts were larger and greater in number in that population, and there was a correlation with the number of pregnancies. Nineteen autopsies were reported in which 5 deaths were liver related. Risk factors for the development of hepatic cysts were also examined in a large series (39 patients and 189 unaffected family members) by Gabow et al.[412] The hepatic expression of the disease was found to be modulated by age, female gender, pregnancy, severity of the renal lesion and kidney function.

The leading hepatic complication is infection of liver cysts, with cholangiocarcinoma the second most common. A recent study examining hepatic cyst infection suggests that the incidence increases from 1 to 3% during end-stage renal failure.[430] Enterobacteriaceae were cultured from the infected cysts in 9 out of 12 patients.[430] In the case of Ikei et al,[431] *Pseudomonas aeruginosa* was cultured from the infected cysts. Treatment recommended by Telenti et al[430] includes antibiotics plus drainage.

Hepatic cysts are rarely detected before puberty and increase in incidence with age (ultimately to 75%) in

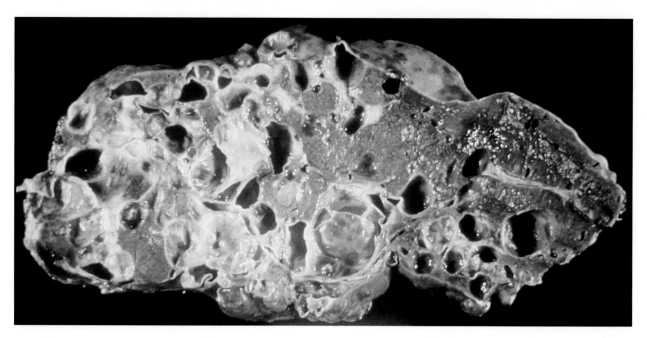

Fig. 3.36 Autosomal dominant polycystic kidney disease. Numerous cysts of varied size are studded throughout the liver. They contained clear fluid.

individuals over 70 years.[432] Associated conditions include colonic diverticula (70%), cardiac valve complications (25%), ovarian cysts (40%), inguinal hernia (15%), and intracranial aneurysms (10%), suggesting a diffusely abnormal matrix. High-resolution computed tomography has been recommended as a screening test for intracranial aneurysms.[433] Prior to the availability of a genetic probe, the criteria for identification of this disorder in children included a positive paternal history, cysts in any portion of the renal tubule or Bowman's space, macroscopic cysts in the liver and cerebral aneurysms.[434]

Grossly, the liver is enlarged and diffusely cystic, the cysts varying from less than a millimetre to 12 cm or more in diameter (Fig. 3.36). The liver of one patient reported by Kwok & Lewin[417] weighed 7.7 kg. Occasionally one lobe, usually the left, is affected. Diffuse dilatation of the intra- and extrahepatic bile ducts has been reported in some cases.[435,436] The cysts contain a clear, colourless or light yellow fluid. Analysis of cyst fluid in one case showed similarities to the 'bile salt-independent' fraction of human bile and suggests that such cysts are lined by a functioning secretory bile-duct epithelium.[437]

Microscopically, the cysts are lined by columnar or cuboidal epithelium, but the larger cysts have a flat epithelium (Fig. 3.37). Collapsed cysts resemble corpora atretica of the ovary (Fig. 3.38). The supporting connective tissue is scanty except in relation to von Meyenburg's complexes, a frequently associated lesion, where it may be dense and hyalinized. A small number of inflammatory cells, usually lymphocytes, may infiltrate the supporting stroma. Infected cysts contain pus and may rupture

(Fig. 3.39). Calcification of the wall of hepatic and renal cysts has been reported.[438]

Von Meyenburg complexes are considered part of the spectrum of adult polycystic disease, and Melnick[413] was of the opinion that polycystic disease of the liver develops progressively over the years by gradual cystic dilatation of these complexes. This view is supported by a recent study of 28 cases of autosomal dominant polycystic kidney disease reported by Ramos et al.[439] Keda et al[440] have suggested that cystic dilatation of peribiliary glands may also contribute to the cysts. von Meyenburg complexes are small (less than 0.5 cm in diameter) and

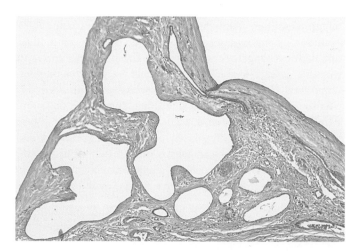

Fig. 3.37 Autosomal dominant polycystic kidney disease. Section of liver shows multiple cysts of varied size that are lined by a flattened epithelium. H&E.

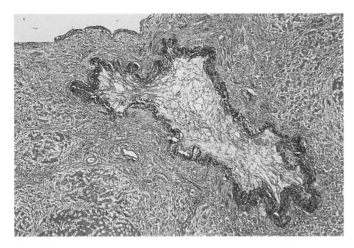

Fig. 3.38 Autosomal dominant polycystic kidney disease. Collapsed cyst has a corrugated wall and the lumen is filled in with a loose connective tissue. Masson's trichrome.

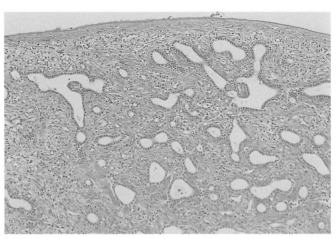

Fig. 3.40 von Meyenburg complex. Small bile ducts are embedded in a fibrous stroma. Note irregular shape of two of the ducts, each of which contains a polypoid projection. H&E.

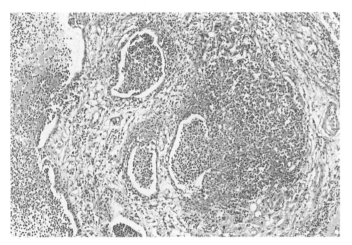

Fig. 3.39 Autosomal dominant polycystic kidney disease. Infected cysts are filled with pus. The cyst to the right has ruptured with formation of a small cholangitic abscess. H&E.

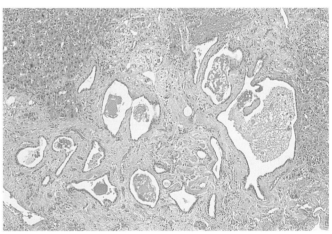

Fig. 3.41 von Meyenburg complex. The ducts are variably dilated and contain altered bile. H&E.

usually scattered in both lobes. Their colour is greyish white or green.[441] They are occasionally associated with cavernous haemangiomas and have an abnormal vascular pattern in angiographic studies.[442] Microscopically, the lesions are discrete, round to irregular in shape and periportal in location. The constituent ducts are embedded in a collagenous stroma and are often round but may be irregular in shape and have slightly dilated lumens (Fig. 3.40). They are lined by low columnar or cuboidal epithelium and contain pink amorphous material that may be bile-stained, or actual bile (Fig. 3.41). Cholangiocarcinoma has been reported in association with von Meyenburg complexes,[443–446] as well as with multiple hepatic cysts considered part of the spectrum of autosomal dominant polycystic kidney disease.[447–450]

SOLITARY (NON-PARASITIC) CYST

This is usually subdivided into unilocular (95%) and multilocular (biliary cystadenoma) varieties. Another type of solitary cyst, the ciliated foregut cyst, is discussed on page 88. The aetiology and pathogenesis of solitary cysts remain undetermined. The evidence favouring a developmental origin is discussed elsewhere.[127] They have been referred to as cystadenomas, although the evidence for their being neoplastic is equivocal. Reported cases of both types have been the subject of several reviews.[127,451,454] For the purposes of this discussion the two are considered together, though unilocular cysts are more likely to be developmental and multilocular cysts neoplastic, with an enhanced potential for malignant change. They occur at all ages, though the majority present in the fourth to sixth decades of life. A unique congenital cyst presenting as a congenital diaphragmatic hernia was reported by Chu et al.[455] Another solitary cyst was associated with the Peutz–Jeghers syndrome.[456] The multilocular biliary cystadenoma is rare in children. The female to male ratio in two reviews of solitary cysts was 4:1[451] and 5.25:1.[452] Cysts less than 8–10 cm rarely cause symptoms[296] and may be found incidentally at laparotomy for some other disease.[415] Symptoms, when present, include an upper abdominal mass with fullness, nausea and occasional vomiting. Rapid enlargement has been reported in infancy.[457] An acute abdominal crisis may result from torsion, strangulation, haemorrhage into the cyst or rupture.[458–465]

Jaundice is an infrequent complication.[452,466–470] Diagnosis is established by ultrasonography or computed tomography. In the past the treatment of choice was excision,[471] but aspiration and injection of sclerosing solutions such as alcohol,[472,473] polidocanol[474] or minocycline chloride[475] have obviated the need for surgery in many cases.

Solitary cysts involve the right lobe twice as often as the left. Rarely, they can arise in the falciform ligament.[476,477] The cysts are round to oval and well encapsulated, and they may rarely be pedunculated. They can contain up to 17 litres of fluid and fill the abdominal cavity. The fluid may be clear, opalescent, milky, mucoid, purulent, or rarely bloody or bile-stained. Individual loculi of some multilocular cysts may contain different types of fluid. The cyst fluid may contain albumin, protein and non-protein nitrogen, mucin, chlorides, bilirubin, cholesterol, diastase, sugar and epithelial debris.

The lining of the cysts usually consists of a single layer of flat, cuboidal or columnar epithelium, but it may be ciliated[478] or squamous in type. The cells rest on a basement membrane and are supported by a fibrous stroma. A mesenchymal stroma that resembles ovarian stroma is found in some of the multilocular cystadenomas of females. The wall may contain lipofuscin-laden macrophages, cholesterol crystals with an associated foreign body giant-cell reaction, and varying numbers of inflammatory cells.[127] The occurrence of smooth muscle, together with a lining of ciliated, pseudostratified columnar epithelium, has been cited as evidence of origin of some solitary hepatic cysts from the embryonic foregut.[478] Malignant tumours may arise in both unilocular and multilocular cysts. These are usually adenocarcinomas,[127,331,479,480] but occasional squamous cell carcinomas[481–483] and even a carcinoid tumour[484] have been reported.

REYE'S SYNDROME

The syndrome of fatty liver and encephalopathy was described over 30 years ago by Reye et al,[485] based on post-mortem findings in 17 children from Australia. The disease is now known to have a worldwide distribution.[486] With few exceptions,[487,488] Reye's syndrome occurs almost exclusively in children, has no sex predilection, and is usually preceded by a resolving viral illness, particularly influenza B or varicella. Initial symptoms include vomiting (usually repetitive), lethargy and changes in mental status. Hepatic dysfunction can be overlooked since the liver is minimally enlarged, and there is no jaundice or splenomegaly. Subsequent symptoms and signs are predominantly neurological and terminate in coma. Seizures may develop, particularly in younger children with hypoglycaemia. Most patients had received multiple medications, including aspirin, for the symptoms of the viral illness. Initial laboratory screening tests show elevation of serum aminotransferase levels, hyperammonaemia and hypoprothrombinaemia. Although the liver disease is benign and transient, the encephalopathy (secondary to a hypoxic/metabolic insult resulting in cerebral oedema) may be life-threatening and can result in permanent neurological disability.[486] Early diagnosis based on clinical findings and liver biopsy, along with closely monitored supportive care, have resulted in improved mortality and morbidity figures.

Grossly, liver biopsy or autopsy specimens from patients with Reye's syndrome are yellow. The major histopathological finding is panacinar steatosis. This change was first reported by Reye et al,[485] but the first allusion to the microvesicular nature of the accumulated lipid was made by Becroft.[489] The most complete account of the hepatic changes, based on sequential biopsies from 49 children, was published by Bove et al.[490] In the typical case the hepatocytes are swollen and packed with multiple small vacuoles (Fig. 3.42); neutral lipid can be demonstrated in frozen sections stained with oil red O or Sudan black B (Fig. 3.43). The lipid droplets are consistently smaller in acinar zone 3 than in zones 2 or 1.[490] It is important to emphasize that vacuolization may not be evident in biopsy

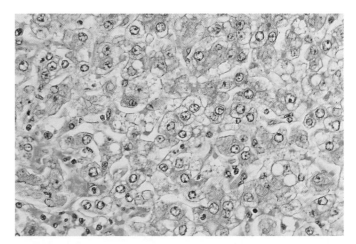

Fig. 3.42 Reye's syndrome. Liver cells show microvesicular steatosis. H&E.

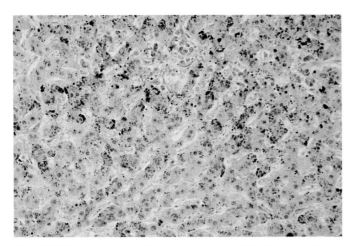

Fig. 3.43 Reye's syndrome. Microvesicular steatosis is shown in this frozen section stained with Sudan black B.

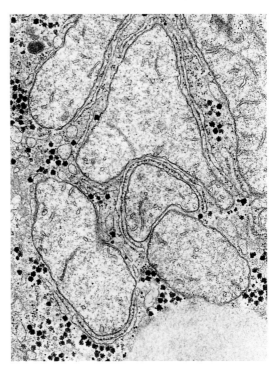

Fig. 3.44 Reye's syndrome. Mitochondria are swollen, and show loss of matrical density with fragmentation and reduction in the number of cristae. Note absence of dense granules in the mitochondria. × 20 000. Courtesy of Dr Cynthia C Daugherty, Children's Hospital Medical Center, Cincinnati, Ohio, USA

material obtained less than 24 hours after the onset of encephalopathy, even though appropriately stained frozen sections will reveal an abundance of fat.[490] Nuclei of the liver cells are enlarged and centrally located. Mitotic activity of variable degree may be seen. Hepatocellular necrosis is generally absent or is mild and spotty. Periportal necrosis, first noted in 2 of the 17 cases described by Reye et al,[485] has been observed subsequently in several other cases.[453,491,492] It is preceded by ballooning degeneration of cells in acinar zone 1. Variation in the severity of glycogen depletion of liver cells in early biopsies correlates with other histological measures of severity, and with the occurrence of hypoglycaemia, severity of encephalopathy at the time of admission, and the mortality rate.[490] Portal inflammation is either minimal or absent. Cholestasis is rarely observed but in some instances it may be related to an associated pancreatitis.[493] Reduction of succinic dehydrogenase and cytochrome oxidase activities (and other mitochondrial enzymes) has been demonstrated by enzymatic stains and is helpful in confirming the diagnosis.[490,494]

At the ultrastructural level, the most dramatic changes are seen in liver cell mitochondria[494,495] which are enlarged and misshapen. The degree of enlargement correlates to some extent with the stage of encephalopathy.[495] The severity of the disease may also be correlated with lucency of the mitochondrial matrix and loss of matrical dense bodies (Fig. 3.44). Other mitochondrial changes in initial hepatic biopsy specimens from patients who die or have severe neurological sequelae include a decrease in size and number of mitochondrial cristae (Fig. 3.44). There may be an increase in the amount of smooth endoplasmic reticulum with varying degrees of dilatation, and 50% of hepatic biopsy specimens reveal flocculent peroxisomes.[496] For a more detailed description of the ultrastructural findings in Reye's syndrome the reader is referred to Phillips et al.[494]

Although a number of diseases can clinically simulate Reye's syndrome, the presence of microvesicular steatosis has only been reported in some of the urea cycle defects, systemic carnitine deficiency, and as an effect of certain drugs and toxins such as tetracycline, anti-emetics, aflatoxin, pyrrolizidine, margosa oil, hypoglycin A, pentenoic acid and valproic acid.[486,497,498] Aspirin toxicity may mimic Reye's syndrome.[499,500] At the light microscopic level, the hepatic pathology findings in children with fatal salicylate intoxication resemble those of Reye's syndrome,[501] but hepatic ultrastructural changes appear to be different.[495] More recently, anti-emetics have also been incriminated in Reye's syndrome.[502]

Since the original observation of Starko et al[501] of an association between aspirin and Reye's syndrome, further retrospective studies have been confirmatory.[503,504] Based on these studies, the Surgeon General of the United States[505] advised that the use of salicylates be avoided in children suffering from influenza or varicella. A pilot prospective study suggested similar results.[506,507] Since then, the incidence of Reye's syndrome has continued to decline.[508] At the present time, all patients presenting with Reye's-like syndrome are presumed to have an inherited metabolic disorder.[509–511] One report suggests that a controversy still exists in Australia where up to one third of parents continue to treat children with aspirin, even though over 50% are aware of the association.[512]

Animal models of Reye's syndrome with encephalomyocarditis virus[513] and influenza B,[514] treatment with 4-pentenoic acid[515] and the spontaneous Reye's-like syndrome in BALB/c ByJ mice,[516] have been developed.

KAWASAKI'S DISEASE

Kawasaki first described an acute febrile mucocutaneous lymph node syndrome in 1967.[517] Contributions to our understanding of the disease have been made by numerous investigators.[518–524] According to Melish & Hicks,[524] the principal diagnostic criteria are; fever, conjunctival injection; oral changes (erythema, fissuring and crusting of the lips; diffuse oropharyngeal erythema, and strawberry tongue); changes in the extremities (induration of the hands and feet, erythema of the palms and soles, desquamation of the tips of the fingers and toes) about two weeks after the onset, and transverse grooves across the fingernails two to three months after the onset; an erythematous rash; and an enlarged lymph node mass (>1.5 cm in diameter). A typical cases not fulfilling these criteria have a much higher mortality rate, perhaps because of the lack of therapy.[525] Gastrointestinal complications include abdominal tenderness, vomiting, diarrhoea, bloody stools, mild jaundice, hepatosplenomegaly, mild ascites, hydrops of the gallbladder and elevated serum aminotransferases. The laboratory data include abnormal electrocardiograms, neutrophil leucocytosis with a shift to the left, thrombocytosis and an increased erythrocyte sedimentation rate. Mortality is twice the normal rate in boys during the first two months of the illness.[526] Coronary aneurysms and myocarditis occur in 10–20% of patients, with a higher incidence in boys.[527,528] Mitral insufficiency occurs in 1% of patients.[529] Early therapy with intravenous γ-globulin and perhaps aspirin has proved beneficial.[530]

The hepatobiliary complications of Kawasaki's disease have been underestimated in the past. The most common problem results from an enlarged and inflamed gallbladder and patients have right upper quadrant pain sometimes associated with vomiting. A majority have hepatomegaly and, at times, a palpable gallbladder. Ultrasound detects hydrops of the gallbladder, usually without cystic duct obstruction. The incidence of this complication ranges from 2.5 to 13.7%.[530] Non-interventional resolution usually occurs in four weeks. Perforation is a rare complication.[531] Laparotomy has been performed in 17 cases, with pathological findings found in 10.[532] Inflammation was observed in 7 cases and vasculitis in 4; 3 cases had cystic duct obstruction (2 because of inflammation and oedema, and 1 by lymph node compression). In another case, obstructive jaundice with marked dilatation of the intrahepatic bile ducts and hydrops of the gallbladder was attributed to arteritis.[533] The serum alanine aminotransferase value is elevated in approximately one third of patients, with values over 100 IU in 18%.[534]

Inflammation has been noted in autopsy cases in the oral cavity (including ductal structures), small bowel, liver (including the large ducts), and the pancreas (including the pancreatic ducts).[535] An acute cholangitis or bile-duct damage has also been observed.[536–538] Portal and sinusoidal infiltrates with proliferation and swelling of Kupffer cells are commonly seen. γ-Glutamyl transpeptidase activities are significantly elevated. Slight bile ductular proliferation has been noted but, to date, decreased bile ducts have not been described.

Similarities between this condition and leptospirosis have been pointed out by several authors.[539,540] Although the Weil–Felix reaction may be positive, tests for leptospirosis are negative.[540] The close resemblance of fatal cases to infantile periarteritis nodosa has also been emphasized in several studies.[364,519,535,541,542] Affected vessels include the larger coronary arteries, splenic, renal, pulmonary, pancreatic, spermatic, peri-adrenal, hepatic and mesenteric vessels. Microscopically, the vessels show peri-arterial inflammation, necrosis and destruction of the media, and intimal inflammation. Lesions of varying stages can be observed in different vessels in the same patients and in different areas of the same type of vessel (e.g. coronary arteries), suggesting that the inflammatory process continues over a period of time during the course of the disease. Aneurysmal dilatation of coronary and other vessels (brachial, iliac, renal and pulmonary) may occur.[519,535] A case of a 4-year-old boy with a hepatic artery aneurysm that caused obstructive jaundice was reported by Marks et al.[536] High-dose intravenous γ-globulin seems to reduce the frequency of coronary artery abnormalities.[531,543]

Other than leptospirosis, duct mites,[544] *Propionobacterium acnes*,[545] a retroviral agent,[546] EBV,[547] and an unusual response in a susceptible individual to an infectious agent such as measles virus[548] have all been proposed as the cause of Kawasaki's disease; none has been confirmed.

THE HISTIOCYTOSES OF CHILDHOOD

The classification for these disorders used in this chapter is one recommended by the Histiocyte Society:[549]

Class I. Langerhans' cell histiocytosis
Class II. Histiocytoses of mononuclear phagocytes other than Langerhans' cells:
1. Haemophagocytic lymphohistiocytosis (familial haemophagocytic reticulosis)
2. Infection-associated (reactive) haemophagocytic syndrome
3. Other histiocytosis syndromes:
   a. sinus histiocytosis with massive lymphadenopathy (Rosai–Dorfman disease),
   b. juvenile xanthogranuloma,
   c. reticulohistiocytoma,
   d. miscellaneous/other/unclassified.

Class III. Malignant histiocytic disorders:
1. Monocytic leukaemia (FAB M5)
2. Malignant histiocytosis (includes forms featuring ordinary histiocytes, interdigitating dendritic cells, and Langerhans' cells).
3. True histiocytic lymphoma (also theoretically divisible into forms featuring ordinary histiocytes, interdigitating cells, and Langerhans' cells).

Characteristics of cells of the mononuclear phagocyte system are compared and contrasted in Table 3.1.

LANGERHANS' CELL HISTIOCYTOSIS

In 1953, Lichtenstein[550] integrated the disorders eosinophilic granuloma of bone, Hand–Schuller–Christian disease and Letterer–Siwe disease under the term histiocytosis X. The prognosis depends on the degree of organ involvement and is usually related to the age of onset. Younger children can have fatal disease while adolescents and adults may have a more benign disorder. Nezelof et al[551] prompted the current terminology by noting that these disorders resulted from a non-malignant, localized or widespread proliferation of Langerhans' cells. These cells have a pale, bean-shaped nucleus and an eosinophilic cytoplasm.[552-554] Identification can be confirmed by histochemical and ultrastructural techniques listed in Table 3.1, although each confirmatory feature is not present in every cell. During the active, potentially treatable phase, poorly formed granulomas contain other cells including eosinophils (92%), multinucleated giant cells (84%), lymphocytes (75%), necrotic cells (61%), and neutrophils (49%)[553] (Figs 3.45–3.47). Later stages no longer responsive to therapy reveal foamy or lipid-laden histiocytes and fibrosis.[555] Patients are primarily seen by the oncology service, and the range of therapies is extensive and at times questionable. Most children present between the ages of 1 and 16 years of age, the mean being 6½ years. No genetic predisposition has been noted.

The incidence of this disorder is estimated to be 1 in 200 000 children.[556] The liver is considered by some to be the most useful organ in ante-mortem diagnosis.[557] In adults, usually only one to three organs are involved. Pulmonary histiocytosis X (eosinophilic granuloma) in adults, which contains increased neuroendocrine cells and is clearly related to smoking, should be considered a separate entity.[558,559] The aetiology of Langerhans' cell histiocytosis is unknown. Table 3.2 lists the incidence of organ involvement in generalized cases from four large series.[560-563]

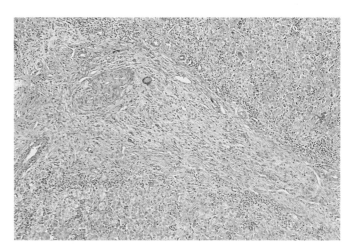

Fig. 3.45 Langerhans' cell histiocytosis. Expanded portal area contains a granulomatoid infiltrate of Langerhans' cells, as well as one giant cell near the artery (left). H&E.

Table 3.1 Comparison of characteristics of Langerhans' cell histiocytes and other cells of the mononuclear phagocytic system

Characteristics	Langerhans' cells	Interdigitating reticulum cells	Dendritic reticulum cells	Macrophages	Monocytes
Phagocytic capacity	0	0	0	+	+
Surface antigens					
OKT6	++	0	0	0	0
Ia	++	++	++	+	+
ATPase	+	+	+	0	0
S-100 protein	+	+	0	+/0	0
Lysozyme	0	0	0	+/0	+
FcIgG	+	+	+	+	+
C3 receptors	0	0	+	+	+
Mixed lymphocyte response	++	++	++	+/0	+/0
Birbeck granules (EM)	+	0	0	0	0
Clinical expression	Langerhans' cell histiocytosis (histiocytosis X)	Dermatopathic lymphadenitis; interdigitating reticulum cell sarcoma	Dendritic reticulum cell sarcoma	Sinus histiocytosis with massive lymphadenopathy; virus-associated haemophagocytic syndrome; familial haemophagocytic lymphohistiocytosis	Acute monocytic leukaemia; malignant histiocytosis; true histiocytic lymphoma

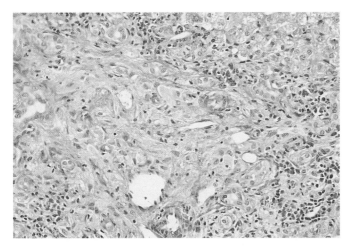

Fig. 3.46 Same case as illustrated in Fig. 3.45. Higher magnification of Langerhans' cells. Note the eosinophils. H&E.

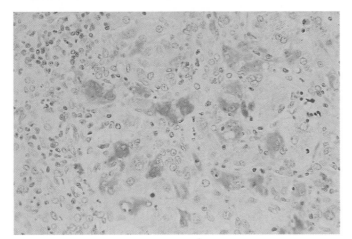

Fig. 3.47 Same case as illustrated in Figs 3.45 and 3.46. Langerhans' cells are immunoreactive for S-100 protein.

The first clue to understanding the primary pathogenesis of liver involvement in this disease was the report on cholestatic problems in 6 children which implicated damage to the intrahepatic bile ducts producing lesions resembling those of primary sclerosing cholangitis.[564] Five had already developed portal hypertension and, therefore, were no longer responsive to the best systemic therapy of prednisone and/or vinblastine.[552,565] Two patients progressed to complete loss of intrahepatic bile ducts. Three

adults were described in 1984 with sclerosing cholangitic lesions, which inlcuded strictures in the hepatic and common bile ducts.[566] Subsequent patients have been documented with strictures at the porta hepatis (Klatskin-tumour-like lesions)[567] and in the pancreatic ducts.[568] In early cases, affected livers are studded with fine white nodules which can often be missed by a percutaneous needle biopsy. The usual finding in a needle biopsy is a non-specific triaditis.[569] Other reported lesions include bile duct proliferation, variable fibrosis with histiocytic infiltration, cirrhosis, parenchymal and portal granulomas, portal hepatic nodal infiltrates, and Langerhans' cell infiltration of the sinusoids with dilatation.[569–571] In addition, both the large and small bowel may be involved with this disorder, which particularly leads to destruction of crypt cells.[572]

Systemic chemotherapy appears to be clinically beneficial. The prognosis is unpredictable and the mortality rate may be as high as 33%. The more extensively the liver, spleen and lymph nodes are involved, the worse the prognosis, especially in infants. Liver transplantation for end-stage liver disease has been successful in a number of cases.[573–575]

THE HAEMOPHAGOCYTIC SYNDROMES

Haemophagocytic lymphohistiocytosis (familial haemophagocytic reticulosis)

This disorder can usually be distinguished from other infantile causes of histiocytosis by the absence of skin lesions and the high incidence of central nervous system involvement. The disease is characterized by fever, anorexia, irritability and pallor in infancy and early childhood. Jaundice and hepatosplenomegaly may develop later.[576] Markedly abnormal results of coagulation studies reflect low fibrinogen levels and thrombocytopenia, but other coagulation factors are normal. Neurological symptoms may develop from histiocytic involvement of the brain. Although clinical manifestations may remit temporarily, the disease is eventually fatal. The diagnosis is based on identifying erythrophagocytosis by histiocytes in bone marrow biopsy material. The hereditary pattern is usually autosomal recessive.[577] Reviews of this inherited disorder

Table 3.2 Incidence of organ involvement in generalized Langerhans' cell histiocytosis

	Lahey[560]	Nezelof et al[561]	Raney & D'Angio[562]	Nesbit[563]
Number of patients	69	50	31	24
Bone lesions	57 (82%)	41 (83%)	22 (71%)	24 (100%)
Skin lesions	42 (61%)	40 (80%)	17 (55%)	21 (87%)
Hepatomegaly	30 (43%)	18 (35%)	9 (29%)	17 (71%)
Splenomegaly	30 (43%)	15 (30%)	4 (13%)	6 (25%)
Pulmonary	35 (51%)	30 (60%)	3 (10%)	13 (54%)
Lymphadenopathy	not available	23 (46%)	10 (32%)	10 (42%)
Diabetes insipidus	20 (29%)	20 (40%)	2 (6%)	6 (25%)

by Janker[578] and Favara[579] are recommended for further reading.

Hepatic involvement is common. Microscopically, there is hypertrophy of Kupffer cells and portal macrophages which manifest striking erythrophagocytosis,[577] but this may be inconspicuous or even absent.[579] Portal areas show lymphohistiocytic infiltrates with a predominance of T-lymphocytes, in a pattern reminiscent of chronic hepatitis.[579] In some cases there is striking enlargement of endothelial cell nuclei and perivenous erythropedesis resembling graft rejection in graft-versus-host disease.[579] Other changes include mild hepatocellular damage in the vicinity of the lymphohistiocytic infiltrates, variable cholestasis and epithelioid granulomas.[579]

Infection-associated (reactive) haemophagocytic syndrome

In this condition there is proliferation of morphologically non-malignant histiocytes showing phagocytosis of haemopoietic cells, with associated fever and pancytopenia. It was first described in patients secondary to EBV infection (virus-associated haemophagocytic syndrome),[580] but has since been reported in association with many other viruses, as well as virtually any infectious agent.[581] There is infiltration of the portal tracts with normal-appearing histiocytes, lymphocytes and plasma cells, together with marked hypertrophy of Kupffer cells displaying prominent haemophagocytosis. The Kupffer cells are only weakly stained with PAS, a feature helpful in distinguishing this change from a response to necro-inflammatory conditions, in which the Kupffer cells are often strongly PAS positive.[582] Additionally, Kupffer cells frequently show siderosis, possibly related to the erythrophagocytosis itself or to blood transfusions.[582] There is a lack of correlation between the degree of peripheral cytopenia and the degree of hepatic haemophagocytosis.[582]

SINUS HISTIOCYTOSIS WITH MASSIVE LYMPHADENOPATHY (ROSAI–DORFMAN DISEASE)

This disorder was first reported by Rosai & Dorfman[583] and has been reviewed recently by Foucar et al.[584] It usually affects patients between the ages of 10 and 20 years. In addition to massive enlargement of cervical and other lymph nodes, there is fever, leucocytosis, an elevated sedimentation rate and hyperglobulinaemia. The course is protracted, lasting from 3 to 9 months, but the prognosis is usually excellent. The disease can involve extranodal sites, including soft tissues, the oral cavity, lower respiratory tract, genitourinary system, and the liver. Involvement of the last three organs is associated with a poor prognosis.[584]

In the review of Foucar et al,[584] hepatomegaly was noted in 27 of 157 cases. Four patients had histopathological evidence of hepatic involvement. The hallmark of the disease is the proliferation of histiocytes which have an abundant cytoplasm and normal-appearing nuclei (Fig. 3.48 and 3.49). The cells display avid leucophagocytosis, but can also phagocytose red cells. According to Eisen et al,[585] the cells express: S-100 protein (Fig. 3.50); pan-macrophage antigens such as EBM11, HAM56, and Leu-M3; antigens functionally associated with phagocytosis (Fc receptor for IgG and complement receptor); antigens functionally associated with lysosomal activity (lysozyme, α_1-antitrypsin and α_1-antichymotrypsin; antigens associated with early inflammation (Mac-387, 27E10); antigens commonly found on monocytes, but not tissue macrophages (OKM5, Leu-M1); and activation antigens (Ki-1 and receptors for transferrin and interleukin-2). The cells thus appear to be true, functionally activated macrophages derived recently from circulating monocytes.[585]

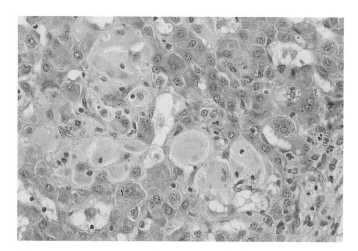

Fig. 3.48 Rosai–Dorfman disease. Sinusoids are filled with large histiocytes showing leucophagocytosis. H&E.

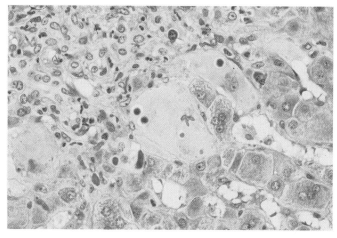

Fig. 3.49 Same case as illustrated in Fig. 3.48. Histiocytes display both erythro- and leucophagocytosis. H&E.

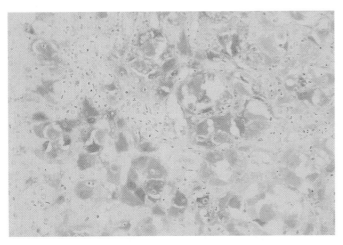

Fig. 3.50 Same case as illustrated in Figs 3.48 and 3.49. Histiocytes are immunoreactive for S-100 protein

MALIGNANT HISTIOCYTOSIS

The existence of this entity has been questioned since the advent of monoclonal antibodies for the characterization of B- and T-cell lymphomas. Cases morphologically consistent with malignant histiocytosis have been found to be malignant lymphomas by immunohistochemical and enzymatic techniques.[586-589] Recently, Oka et al[589] reported 3 cases of malignant histiocytosis that were biphenotypic (positive with both T-cell and macrophage markers). According to Nezelof et al,[590] a chromosomal translocation involving 5q35 argues in favour of an authentic malignancy of the mononuclear phagocyte system. These investigators have pointed out that paediatricians have long been aware of the existence of a disease characterized by fever, wasting, generalized lymphadenopathy and hepatosplenomegaly and, in its final stages, by jaundice, purpura, anaemia and profound leucopenia. The discrepancy between the clinical manifestations of a severe blood disease, and the absence or late occurrence of abnormal cells in the blood or bone marrow, provides important clues to the diagnosis of malignant histiocytosis in children.[590]

Histopathologically, the disease is characterized by proliferation of large (10–20 μm) atypical, pleomorphic cells with an abundant, finely vacuolated cytoplasm.[590] In routine stains the nuclei are amphophilic with irregular, grooved or scalloped borders. There is clumping of the chromatin and large, irregular and dense nucleoli are present. Multi-lobated nuclei and mitotic figures, sometimes atypical, are frequently seen. Erythrophagocytosis may or may not be present. Ultrastructurally, the cells contain primary lysosomes and phagolysosomes. In the liver the malignant histiocytic cells are found in portal areas (together with lymphocytes and plasma cells) as well as in sinusoids.[591-594] Beaugrand et al[594] have suggested that jaundice and hepatic abnormalities may be a con-

sequence of Kupffer cell dysfunction (e.g. lack of clearance of endotoxin) rather than an effect of the infiltrates.

In the series studied by Nezelof et al,[590] the malignant histiocytic cells showed acid phosphatase, α-naphthyl acetate esterase and α_1-antichymotrypsin activity, and reacted to antibodies directed against EMA, HLA-DR, CD25, CD30, CD68 and CD71. No B- and T-cell antigens were detected, except in 1 of their 20 cases.

LIVER DISEASE IN DOWN'S SYNDROME AND LEUKAEMIA

DOWN'S SYNDROME

Severe liver disease can occur in Down's syndrome. Ten cases were described by Ruchelli et al,[595] who also reviewed 8 that had been previously reported. Other cases not included in that review have also been described.[596-598] Patients may present with severe liver disease at or within a few weeks of birth. There is diffuse intra-acinar fibrosis surrounding proliferating ductules and residual hypatocytes.[595] In most of the cases a large number of megakaryocytes or megakaryoblasts, as well as other haematopoietic elements, are present in the sinusoids.[595,596] Parenchymal iron deposition of variable degree was noted in most of the cases studied by Ruchelli et al,[595] who felt that these represented a subset of perinatal haemochromatosis.

It has been postulated that fibrosis-promoting factors and/or metabolic factors, such as those resulting from a gene dosage effect, could play a role in the genesis of the liver disease in Down's syndrome.[595] However, at least in one reported case, there was extensive hepatic necrosis and the patient had a severe bleeding diathesis.[596] The question of whether the megakaryoblastic leukaemoid reaction of Down's syndrome is leukaemic or the result of abnormal regulation of myelopoiesis is unresolved; the reader is referred to the paper of Becroft et al[597] for a discussion of this issue.

LEUKAEMIA

Extensive fibrosis has been reported in childhood leukaemia, both acute and chronic.[599-602] In one of the early reports on acute leukaemia the hepatic fibrosis was postulated to be due to a combination of factors related to therapy with folic acid antagonists; tests for hepatitis B and C were not available at that time.[599] In a later study, hepatitis B markers were noted in 48.3% of 103 children with acute leukaemia in long-term remission after chemotherapy.[600] Liver changes in that series included chronic lobular hepatitis, chronic persistent hepatitis and chronic active hepatitis. The serum HBV markers correlated significantly with both the severity of histological changes and the persistent biochemical abnormalities for over 6 months after cessation of therapy.

Hepatic fibrosis has also been described in chronic lymphocytic and chronic granulocytic leukaemia.[601,602] Shcwartz & Shamsuddin[601] studied 47 cases of chronic lymphocytic leukaemia; in 44% of the cases, hepatic fibrosis was attributed to the leukaemic infiltrates. Changes in the liver included expansion of portal tracts, bridging infiltration, and fibrosis and cirrhosis. Mikel et al[602] also attributed the fibrosis in their 3 cases of chronic granulocytic leukaemia to the leukaemic infiltrates rather than to chemotherapy or other aetiologies.

REFERENCES

1. Grosfeld J L, Clatworthy H W. Hepatic agenesis. In: Bergsma D, ed. Birth defects. Atlas and compendium, 2nd edn. New York: Alan R Liss, 1973: p 517
2. Belton R L, Van Zandt T F. Congenital absence of the left lobe of the liver: A radiologic diagnosis. Radiology 1983; 147: 184
3. Radin D R, Colletti P M, Ralls P W, Boswell W D, Halls JM. Agenesis of the right lobe of the liver. Radiology 1987; 164: 639–642
4. Morphett A, Adam A. Agenesis of the right lobe of the liver: diagnosis by computed tomography. Australas Radiol 1992; 36: 68–69
5. Faintuch J, Machado M C C, Raia A A. Suprahepatic gallbladder with hypoplasia of the right lobe of the liver. Arch Surg 1980; 115: 658–659
6. Van Gansbeke D, de Toeuf J, Cremer M, Engelholm L, Struyven J. Intrahepatic gallbladder: a rare congenital anomaly. Gastrointest Radiol 1984; 9: 341–343
7. Soper R T, Green E W. Omphalocele. Surg Gynecol Obstet 1961; 113: 501–508
8. Desser P L, Smith S. Nonparasitic liver cysts in children. J Pediatr 1956; 49: 297–305
9. Fock G. Ectopic liver in omphalocele. Acta Paediatrica 1963; 52: 288–292
10. Rendina E A, Venuta F, Pescarmona E O, Martelli M, Ricci C. Intrathoracic lobe of the liver: case report and review of the literature. Eur J Cardio Thorac Surg 1989; 3: 75–78
11. Feist J H, Lasser E C. Identification of uncommon liver lobulations. JAMA 1959; 169: 1859–1862
12. Korobkin M T, Miller S W, deLorimier A A, Gordon L S, Palubinskas A J. Hepatic herniation through the Morgagni foramen. Am J Dis Child 1973; 126: 117–219
13. Organ C H, Hayes D F. Supradiaphragmatic right liver lobe and gallbladder. Arch Surg 1980; 115: 989–990
14. Vogel A, Small A. Partial eventration of the right diaphragm (congenital diaphragmatic herniation of the liver). Ann Intern Med 1955; 43: 63–82
15. Reitemeier R J, Butt H R, Baggenstoss A H. Riedel's lobe of the liver. Gastroenterology 1958; 34: 1090–1095
16. Cullen TSL. Accessory lobes of the liver. Arch Surg 1925; 11: 718–764
17. Hansbrough E T, Lipin R J. Intrathoracic accessory lobe of the liver. Ann Surg 1957; 145: 564–567
18. Naganuma H, Ishida H, Niizawa M, Morikawa P, Masamune O, Kato T. Intrathoracic accessory lobes of the liver. J Clin Ultrasound 1993; 21: 143–146
19. Johnstone G. Accessory lobe of liver presenting through a congenital deficiency of anterior abdominal wall. Arch Dis Child 1965; 40: 541–544
20. Peter H. Strohm W D. Torquierter akzessorischer Leberlappen als Ursache eines akuten abdomens. Leber Magen Darm 1980; 4: 203–206
21. Battle W M, Laufer I, Moldofsky P J, Trotman B W. Anomalous liver lobulations as a cause of perigastric masses. Am J Dig Dis 1979; 24: 65–69
22. Heid G J, Von Hamm E. Hepatic heterotopy in the splenic capsule. Arch Pathol 1948; 46: 377–379
23. Mendoza A, Voland J, Wolf P, Benirschke K. Supradiaphragmatic liver in the lung. Arch Pathol Lab Med 1986; 110: 1085–1086
24. Shah K D, Beck A R, Jhaveri M K, Keohane M, Weinberg B, Gerber M A. Infantile hemangioendothelioma of heterotopic intrathoracic liver associated with diaphragmatic hernia. Hum Pathol 1987; 18: 754–756
25. Fellbaum C, Beham A, Schmid C. Isolierte Neben leber (Hepas succerturatium) am Gallenblasenhals Fallbericht mit Literaturubersicht. Wien Klin Wochkenschr 1987; 99: 825–827
26. Buck F S, Koss M N. Heterotopic liver in an adrenal gland. Pediatr Pathol 1988; 8: 535–540
27. Tejada E, Danielson C. Ectopic or heterotopic liver (choristoma) associated with the gallbladder. Arch Pathol Lab Med 1989; 113: 950–952
28. Shapiro J L, Metlay L A. Heterotopic supradiaphragmatic liver formation in association with congenital cardiac anomalies. Arch Pathol Lab Med 1991; 115: 238–240
29. Boyle L, Gallivan M V E, Chan B, Lack E E. Heterotopia of gastric mucosa and liver involving the gallbladder. Arch Pathol Lab Med 1992; 116: 138–142
30. Ikoma A, Tanaka K, Hamada N et al. Left-sided gallbladder with accessory liver accompanied by intrahepatic cholangiocarcinoma. J Jpn Surg Soc 1992; 93: 434–436
31. Willis R A. Some unusual developmental heterotopias. Br Med J 1968; 2: 267–272
32. Lieberman M K. Cirrhosis in ectopic liver tissue. Arch Pathol 1966; 82: 443–446
33. Dolan M F, Janovski N A. Adreno-hepatic union (adrenal dystopia). Arch Pathol 1960; 86: 22–24
34. Honma K. Adreno-hepatic fusion: an autopsy study. Zentralbl Allg Pathol 1991; 137: 117–122
35. Cotelingam J D, Saito R. Hepatolienal fusion: case report of an unusual lesion. Hum Pathol 1978; 9: 234–236
36. Mason J R, Speese J. Tumor of the liver of adrenal origin. Ann Surg 1933; 97: 150–153
37. Wilkins L, Ravitch M M. Adrenocortical tumor arising in the liver of a three-year-old boy with signs of virilism and Cushing's syndrome. Report of a case and cure after partial resection of the right lobe of the liver. Pediatrics 1952; 9: 671–681
38. Ballinger J. Hypoglycemia from metastasizing insular carcinoma of aberrant pancreatic tissue in liver. Arch Pathol 1941; 32: 277–285
39. Mobini J, Krouse T B, Cooper D R. Intrahepatic pancreatic heterotopia. Review and report of a case presenting as an abdominal mass. Am J Dig Dis 1974; 19: 64–70
40. Schaefer B, Meyer G, Arnholdt H, Hohlbach G. Heterotope Pankreaspseudocyste in der Leber. Chirurg 1989; 60: 556–558
41. Michels N. The hepatic, cystic and retroduodenal arteries and their relation to the biliary ducts. Ann Surg 1951; 133: 503–524
42. Lilly J R, Starzl T E. Liver transplantation in children with biliary atresia and vascular anomalies. J Pediatr Surg 1974; 9: 707–714
43. Udelsman R, Sugarbaker P H. Congenital duplication of the gallbladder associated with an anomalous right hepatic artery. Am J Surg 1985; 149: 812–815
44. Perea A, Tinsley E A, Mason L B. Abdominal apoplexy due to spontaneous rupture of an aberrant accessory hepatic artery. South Med J 1982; 75: 234–235
45. Helikson M A, Shapiro D L, Seashore J H. Hepatoportal arteriovenous fistula and portal hypertension in an infant. Pediatr 1977; 60: 921–924
46. Housegger K A, Fotter R, Sorantin E, Flückiger F. Kongenitale intrahepatische arterioportale Fisteln als Ursache einer nekrotisicrerden Enteritis — dopplersonographische und angiographische Erfassung. Ultraschall Med 1991; 12: 193–196
47. Martin L W, Benzing G, Kaplan S. Congenital intrahepatic arteriovenous fistula. Report of a successfully treated case. Ann Surg 1965; 161: 209–212
48. Bilbao J L, Longo J M, Aquerreta J D, Rodriguez-Cabello J, Fernandez A. Platinum wire embolization of an intrahepatic arterioportal fistula. Am J Gastroenterol 1990; 85: 859–860
49. Boles E T Jr, Smith B. Preduodenal portal vein. Pediatrics 1978; 28: 805–809

50. Esscher T. Preduodenal portal vein — A cause of intestinal obstruction? J Pediatr Surg 1980; 15: 609–612

51. Hsia D Y Y, Gellis S S. Portal hypertension in infants and children. Am J Dis Child 1955; 90: 290–298

52. Snavely J G, Breakell E S. Fatal hemorrhage from esophageal varices; due to malformations and congenital stenoses in portal venous system. Am J Med 1954; 16: 459–464

53. Marks C. Developmental basis of the portal venous system. Am J Surg 1969; 117: 671–681

54. Bell J W. Portal-vein hypoplasia with inferior mesenteric hypertension. N Engl J Med 1970; 282: 1149–1150

55. Raffensperger J G, Shkolnik A A, Boggs J D, Swenson O. Portal hypertension in children. Arch Surg 1972; 105: 249–254

56. Marks C. The portal venous system. Springfield: Charles C Thomas, 1973

57. Marois D, van Heerden J A, Carpenter H A, Sheedy P F. Congenital absence of the portal vein. Mayo Clin Proc 1979; 54: 55–59

58. Nakasaki H, Tanaka Y, Ohta M et al. Congenital absence of the portal vein. Ann Surg 1989; 210: 190–193

59. Woodle E S, Thistlewaite J R, Emond J C et al. Successful hepatic transplantation in congential absence of recipient portal vein. Surgery 1990; 107: 475–479

60. Matsuoka Y, Ohtomo K, Okubo T, Nishikawa J, Mine T, Ohno S. Congenital absence of the portal vein. Gastrointest Radiol 1992; 17: 31–33

61. Gouin B, LeGal J, Duprey J, Sanson J. Congenital portacaval intrahepatic shunt: analysis of revealing glucose metabolism disorders. Gastroenterol Clin Biol 1984; 8: 464–468

62. Shawker T H, Chang R, Garra B, Edelstein R A, Barton NW, Filling-Katz M R. An unusual anomalous intrahepatic connection between the left portal vein and internal mammary veins. J Clin Ultrasound 1988; 16: 425–435

63. Lewis A M, Aquino N M. Congenital portohepatic vein fistula that resolved spontaneously in a neonate. Am J Roentgenol 1992; 159: 837–838

64. Fiane A E, Gjestvang F T, Smevik B. Hepatoportal arteriovenous fistula and bleeding oesophageal varices in a child. Eur J Surg 1993; 159: 185–186

65. Thompson P B, Oldham K T, Bedi D G, Guice K S, Davis M. Aneurysmal malformation of the extrahepatic portal vein. Am J Gastroenterol 1986; 81: 695–697

66. Gallagher D M, Leiman S, Hux C H. In utero diagnosis of a portal vein aneurysm. J Clin Ultrasound 1993; 21: 147–151

67. Klemperer P. Cavernous transformation of the portal vein. Arch Pathol 1928; 6: 353–377

68. Clatworthy H W Jr, Boles E T. Extrahepatic portal bed block in children. Pathogenesis and treatment. Ann Surg 1959; 150: 371–383

69. Voorhees A B Jr, Harris R D, Britton R C, Price J B, Santulli TV. Portal hypertension in children: 98 cases. Surg 1965; 58: 540–549

70. Myers N A, Robinson M J. Extrahepatic portal hypertension in children. J Pediatr Surg 1973; 8: 467–473

71. Berdon W E, Baker D H, Casarella W. Liver disease in children: portal hypertension, hepatic masses. Semin Roentgenol 1975; 10: 207–214

72. Sarin S K, Bansal A, Sasan S, Nigem A. Portal-vein obstruction in children leads to growth retardation. Hepatology 1992; 15: 229–233

73. Choudhuri G, Tandon R K, Nundy S, Misra N K. Common bile duct obstruciton by portal cavernoma. Dig Dis Sci 1988; 33: 1626–1628

74. Braun V B, Börner N, Majdandzic J, Dormeyer H H, Reuss J, Schild H. Diagnostik der kavernomatösen Pfortadertransformation. Z Gastroenterol 1984; 22: 244–249

75. Kauzlaric D, Petrovic M, Barmeir E. Sonography of cavernous transformation of the portal vein. Am J Radiol 1984; 142: 383–384

76. Philips R L. Cavernous transformation of the portal vein. Australas Radiol 1988; 32: 239–241

77. Frider B, Marin A M, Goldberg A. Ultrasonographic diagnosis of portal vein cavernous transformation in children. J Ultrasound 1989; 8: 445–449

78. Ros P R, Viamonte M, Soila K, Sheldon J, Tobias J, Cohen B. Demonstration of cavernomatous transformation of the portal vein by magnetic resonance imaging. Gastrointest Radiol 1986; 11: 90–92

79. Voorhees A B Jr, Price J B Jr. Extrahepatic portal hypertension. A retrospective analysis of 127 cases and associated clinical implications. Arch Surg 1974; 108: 338–341

80. Williams A O, Johnston G V. Cavernous transformation of the portal vein in rhesus monkeys. J Pathol Bacteriol 1965; 90: 613–618

81. Odievre M, Pige G, Alagille D. Congenital abnormalities associated with extrahepatic portal hypertension. Arch Dis Child 1977; 52: 383–385

82. Meyer W W, Lind J. Postnatal changes in the portal circulation. Arch Dis Child 1966; 41: 606–612

83. Schaffner F, Gadboys H L, Safran A P, Baron M G, Ausses AH Jr. Budd–Chiari syndrome caused by a web in the inferior vena cava. Am J Med 1967; 42: 838–843

84. Yamamoto S, Yokoyama Y, Takeshige K, Iwatsuki S. Budd–Chiari syndrome with obstruction of the inferior vena cava. Gastroenterology 1968; 54: 1070–1084

85. Takeuchi J, Takada A, Hasumura Y, Matsuda Y, Ikegami F. Budd–Chiari syndrome associated with obstruction of the inferior vena cava. Am J Med 1971; 51: 11–20

86. Terabayashi H, Okuda K, Nomura F, Ohnishi K, Wong P. Transformation of inferior vena caval thrombosis to membranous obstruction in a patient with the lupus anticoagulant. Gastroenterology 1986; 91: 219–224

87. Kage M, Arakawa M, Kojiro M, Okuda K. Histopathology of membranous obstruction of the inferior vena cava in the Budd–Chiari syndrome. Gastroenterology 1992; 102: 2081–2090

88. Okuda K. Membranous obstruction of the inferior vena cava: etiology and relation to hepatocellular carcinoma. Gastroenterology 1982; 82: 376–379

89. Simson I W. Membranous obstruction of the inferior vena cava and hepatocellular carcinoma in South Africa. Gastroenterology 1982; 82: 171–178

90. Hoffman H D, Stockland B, von der Heyden U. Membranous obstruction of the inferior vena cava with Budd–Chiari syndrome in children: a report of nine cases. J Pediatr Gastroenterol Nutr 1987; 6: 878–884

91. Jaffe R, Yunis E J. Congenital Budd–Chiari syndrome. Pediatr Pathol 1983; 1: 187–192

92. Roulet M, Laurini R, Rivier L, Calame A. Hepatic veno-occlusive disease in newborn infant of a woman drinking herbal tea. J Pediatr 1988; 112: 433–436

93. Mellis C, Bale P M. Familial hepatic veno-occlusive disease with probable immune deficiency. J Pediatr 1976; 88: 236–242

94. Etzioni A, Benderly A, Rosenthal E et al. Defective humoral and cellular immune functions associated with veno-occlusive disease of the liver. J Pediatr 1987; 110: 549–554

95. Martini G A. Cirrhosis of the liver in hereditary hemorrhagic telangiectasia. Proceedings of the First World Congress of Gastroenterology. Baltimore: Williams & Wilkins, 1959: vol 2, pp 857–858

96. Reilly P J, Nostrant T T. Clinical manifestations of hereditary hemorrhagic telangiectasia. Am J Gastroenterol 1984; 79: 363–367

97. Peery W H. Clinical spectrum of hereditary hemorrhagic telangiectasia (Osler–Weber–Rendu disease). Am J Med 1987; 82: 989–997

98. Feizi O. Hereditary hemorrhagic telangiectasia presenting with portal hypertension and cirrhosis of the liver. Gastroenterology 1972; 63: 660–664

99. Fagel W J, Perlberger R, Kauffmann R H. Portosystemic encephalopathy in hereditary hemorrhagic telangiectasia. Am J Med 1988; 85: 858–860

100. Thomas M L, Carty H. Hereditary hemorrhagic telangiectasia of the liver demonstrated angiographically. Acta Radiol 1974; 15: 433–438

101. Cloogman H M, DiCapo R D. Hereditary hemorrhagic telangiectasia: Sonographic findings in the liver. Radiology 1984; 1505: 521–522

102. Ralls P W, Johnson M B, Radin R, Lee K P, Boswell W D. Hereditary hemorrhagic telangiectasia: findings in the liver with color Doppler sonography. Am J Roentgenol 1992; 159: 59–61

103. Solis-Herruzo J A, Garcia-Cabezudo J, Santalla-Pecina F, Duran-Aguado A, Olmedo-Camacho J. Laparoscopic findings in hereditary haemorrhagic telangiectasia (Osler–Weber–Rendu disease). Endoscopy 1984; 16: 137–139

104. Gothlin J H, Nordgard K, Jonsson K, Nyman U. Hepatic telangiectasia in Osler's disease treated with arterial embolization. Eur J Radiol 1982; 2: 27–30

105. Derauf B J, Hunter D W, Sirr S A, Cardella J F, Castaneda-Zuniga W, Amplatz K. Peripheral embolization of diffuse hepatic arteriovenous malformations in a patient with hereditary hemorrhagic telangiectasia. Cardiovasc Intervent Radiol 1987; 10: 80–83

106. Smith J L, Lineback M L. Hereditary hemorrhagic telangiectasia: 9 cases in one Negro family, with special reference to hepatic lesions. Am J Med 1954; 17: 41–49

107. Zelman S. Liver fibrosis in hereditary hemorrhagic telangiectasia. Fibrosis of diffuse insular character. Arch Pathol 1962; 74: 66–72

108. Sussman E B, Sternberg S S. Hereditary hemorrhagic telangiectasia, a case with hepatocellular carcinoma and acquired hepatocerebral degeneration. Arch Pathol 1975; 99: 95–100

109. Daly J J, Schiller A L. The liver in hemorrhagic telangiectasia (Osler–Weber–Rendu disease). Am J Med 1976; 60: 723–726

110. Wanless I R, Gryfe A. Nodular transformation of the liver in hereditary hemorrhagic telangiectasia. Arch Pathol Lab Med 1986; 110: 331–335

111. Zeitlin H. Hemangioblastomas of the meninges and their relationship to Lindau's disease. J Neuropathol Exp Neurol 1942; 1: 14–23

112. Rojiani A M, Owen D A, Berry K et al. Hepatic hemangioblastoma; an unusual presentation in a patient with von Hippel–Lindau disease. Am J Surg Pathol 1991; 15: 81–86

113. McGrath F P, Gibney R G, Morris D C, Owen D A, Erb SR. Case report: multiple hepatic and pulmonary hemangioblastomas — a new manifestation of von Hippel–Lindau disease. Clin Radiol 1992; 45: 37–39

114. Deboever G, Dewulf P, Maerteus J. Common bile duct obstruction due to pancreatic involvement in the von Hippel–Lindau syndrome. Am J Gastroenterol 1992; 87: 1866–1868

115. Wanless I R, Mawdsley C, Adams R. On the pathogenesis of focal nodular hyperplasia of the liver. Hepatology 1985; 5: 1194–1200

116. Wanless I R, Albrecht S, Bilbao J et al. Multiple focal nodular hyperplasia of the liver associated with vascular malformations of various organs and neoplasia of the brain: a new syndrome. Mod Pathol 1989; 3: 456–462

117. Goldin R D, Rose D S C. Focal nodular hyperplasia of the liver associated with intracranial vascular malformations. Gut 1990; 31: 554–555

118. Puente S G, Bannura G C. Radiological anatomy of the biliary tract: Variations and congenital abnormalities. World J Surg 1983; 7: 271–276

119. Markle G B. Agenesis of the common bile duct. Arch Surg 1981; 116: 350–352

120. Stellin G P, Karner F M, Toyama W M, Lilly J R. Biliary agenesis. Hepatology 1986; 6: 1218 (abstract)

121. Dowdy G S, Waldron G W, Brown W G. Surgical anatomy of the pancreaticobiliary system: observations. Arch Surg 1962; 84: 229–246

122. Hand B H. Anatomy and function of the extrahepatic biliary system. Clin Gastroenterol 1973; 2: 3–29

123. Cullingford G, Davidson B, Dooley J, Habit N. Hepatolithiasis with anomalous biliary anatomy and a vascular compression. HPB Surgery 1991; 3; 129–137

124. Jackson J B, Kelly T B. Cholecystohepatic ducts: case report. Ann Surg 1964; 159: 581–584

125. Stokes T L, Old L. Cholecystohepatic duct. Ann Surg 1978; 135: 703–705

126. Benson M D. Aberrant hepatic ducts. Australas Radiol 1988; 32: 348–355

127. Ishak K G, Willis G W, Cummins S D, Bullock A A. Biliary cystadenoma and cystadenocarcinoma. Report of 14 cases and review of the literature. Cancer 1977; 39: 322–338

128. Ng J W T, Wong M K, Kong C K. Long accessory hepatic duct with congenital dilation of the common bile duct. Am J Gastroenterol 1993; 88: 619–621

129. Nygren E J, Barnes W A. Atresia of the common hepatic duct with shunt via an accessory duct: report of a case. Arch Surg 1954; 68: 337–343

130. Walters W. Surgical lesions of the biliary tract. Arch Surg 1960; 81: 1–13

131. Boyden E A. The problem of the double ductus choledochus (an interpretation of an accessory bile duct found attached to the pars superior of the duodenum). Anat Recod 1932; 55: 71–93

132. Swartley W B, Weeder S D. Choledochus cyst with a double common bile duct. Ann Surg 1935; 101: 912–920

133. Lee C M Jr. Duplication of the cystic and common hepatic ducts, lined with gastric mucosa: a rare congenital anomaly. N Engl J Med 1957; 256: 927–931

134. Neuhauser E B D, Elkin M, Landing B. Congenital direct communication between biliary and respiratory tract. Am J Dis Child 1952; 83: 654–659

135. Enjoji M, Watanabe H, Nakamura Y. A case report: congenital biliotracheal fistula with trifurcation of bronchi. Ann Paediatr 1963; 200: 321–332

136. Stigol L C, Traversaro J, Trigo E R. Carinal trifurcation with congenital tracheobiliary fistula. Pediatrics 1966; 37: 89–91

137. Weitzman J J, Cohen S R, Woods L O, Chadwick D L. Congenital bronchobiliary fistula. J Pediatr 1968; 73: 329–334

138. Wagget J, Stoll S, Bishop H C, Kurtz M B. Congenital broncho-biliary fistula. J Pediatr Surg 1970; 5: 566–569

139. Sane S, Sieber W K, Girdany B R. Congenital bronchopulmonary fistula. Surg 1971; 69: 599–608

140. Chan Y T, Ng W D, Mak W P, Kwong M L, Chow C B. Congenital bronchobiliary fistula associated with biliary atresia. Br J Surg 1984; 71: 240–241

141. Levasseur P, Navajas M. Congenital tracheobiliary fistula. Ann Thorac Surg 1987; 44: 318–319

142. Kalayoglu M, Olcay I. Congenital bronchobiliary fistula associated with esophageal atresia and tracheoesophageal fistula. J Pediatr Surg 1976; 11: 463–464

143. Terada T, Nakanuma Y, Kono N, Ueda K, Kadoya M, Matsui O. Ciliated hepatic foregut cyst. A mucus histological, immunohistochemical, and ultrastructural study in three cases in comparison with normal bronchi and intrahepatic bile ducts. Am J Surg Pathol 1990; 14: 356–363

144. Lilly J R, Weintraub W H, Altman R P. Spontaneous perforation of extrahepatic bile ducts and bile peritonitis in infancy. Surgery 1974; 75: 664–669

145. Howard E R, Johnston D I, Mowat A P. Spontaneous perforation of the common bile duct in infants. Arch Dis Child 1976; 51: 883–886

146. Stringel G, Mercer S. Idiopathic perforation of the biliary tract in infancy. J Pediatr Surg 1983; 18; 546–550

147. Haller J O, Condon V R, Berdon W E et al. Spontaneous perforation of the common bile duct in children. Radiology 1989; 172: 621–624

148. Davenport M, Heaton N D, Howard E R. Spontaneous perforation of the bile duct in infants. Br J Surg 1991; 78: 1068–1070

149. So S K S, Lindahl J, Sharp H L, Cook A M, Leonard AS. A case report of bile ascites during infancy diagnosed by Tc-99m-disofenin sequential scintiphotography. Pediatrics 1983; 71: 402–405

150. Rickham R P, Lee E Y C. Neonatal jaundice; surgical aspects. Clin Pediatr 1964; 3: 197–208

151. Ando K, Miyano T, Kimura K, Shimmura H, Ohya T. Congenital biliary atresia and congenital biliary dilatation in siblings. J Pediatr Surg 1991; 26: 1399–1400

152. Miyano T, Siruga K, Kimura K et al. A histopathologic study of the region of the ampulla of Vater in congenital biliary atresia. Jpn J Surg 1980; 10: 34–38

153. Chandra R S. Biliary atresia and other structural anomalies in the congenital polysplenic syndrome. J Pediatr 1974; 85: 649–655

154. Kasai M, Watanabe I, Ohi R. Follow-up studies of long-term survivors after hepatic portoenterostomy for 'non-correctable' biliary atresia. J Pediatr Surg 1975; 10: 173–182

155. Weichsel M E, Luzzatti L. Trisomy 17-18 syndrome with congenital extrahepatic biliary atresia and congenital amputation of the left foot. J Pediatr 1965; 67: 324–327

156. Alpert L I, Strauss L, Hirschorn K. Neonatal hepatitis and biliary atresia associated with trisomy 17-18. N Engl J Med 1969; 280: 16–20

157. Danks D M. Prolonged neonatal obstructive jaundice. A survey of modern concepts. Clin Pediatr 1965; 4: 499–510

158. Le Coultre C, Cuendet A, Berclaz J-P. An unusual association of small bowel atresia and biliary atresia: a case report. J Pediatr Surg 1983; 18: 136–137

159. Werlin S L. Extrahepatic biliary atresia. Acta Paediatr Scand 1981; 70: 943–944

160. Moore T C, Hyman P E. Extrahepatic biliary atresia in one human leukocyte antigen identical twin. Pediatrics 1985; 76: 604–605

161. Strickland A D, Shannon K, Coln C D. Biliary atresia in two sets of twins. J Pediatr 1985; 107: 418–420

162. Hyams J S, Glaser J H, Leichtner A M, Morecki R. Discordance for biliary atresia in two sets of monozygotic twins. J Pediatr 1985; 107: 420–422

163. Lang D J, Marshall W C, Pincott J R, Stern H. Cytomegalovirus: association with neonatal hepatitis and biliary atresia. In: Javitt M B, ed. Neonatal hepatitis and biliary atresia. Washington, D C: US Government Printing Press, 1979: pp 33–41

164. Hart M H, Kaufman S S, Vanderhoof J A et al. Neonatal hepatitis and extrahepatic biliary atresia associated with cytomegalovirus infection in twins. Am J Dis Child 1991; 145: 302–305

165. Strauss L, Bernstein J. Neonatal hepatitis in congenital rubella; a histopathological study. Arch Pathol 1968; 86: 317–327

166. Rosenberg H S, Oppenheimer E H, Esterly J R. Congenital rubella syndrome; the late effects and their relation to early lesions. Perspect Pediatr Pathol 1981; 6: 183–202

167. Scotto J M, Alvarez F. Biliary atresia and non-A, non-B hepatitis? Gastroenterology 1982; 82: 393

168. Bangaru S, Morecki R, Glaser L M, Horwitz M S. Comparative studies in the human newborn and reovirus-induced cholangitis in weanling mice. Lab Invest 1980; 43: 456

169. Morecki R, Glaser J H, Cho S, Balistreri W F, Horwitz M S. Biliary atresia and reovirus type 3 infection. N Engl J Med 1982; 307: 481–484

170. Rosenberg D P, Morecki R, Lollini L O, Glaser J, Cornelius C E. Extrahepatic biliary atresia in a Rhesus monkey (Macaca mulatta). Hepatology 1983; 3: 577–580

171. Glaser J H, Balisteri W F, Morecki R. Role of reovirus type 3 in persistent infantile cholestasis. J Pediatr 1984; 105: 912–915

172. Morecki R, Glaser J H, Johnson A B, Kress Y. Detection of Reovirus type 3 with extrahepatic biliary atresia: Ultrastructural and immunocytochemical study. Hepatology 1984; 4: 1137–1142

173. Dussaix E, Hadchonel M, Tardieu M, Alagille D. Biliary atresia and reovirus type 3 infection. N Engl J Med 1984; 310: 658

174. Brown W R, Sokol R J, Levin M J et al. Lack of correlation between infection with reovirus 3 and extrahepatic biliary atresia and neonatal hepatitis. J Pediatr 1988; 113: 670–676

175. Silveira T R, Salzano F M, Howard E R, Mowat A P. Congenital structural abnormalities in biliary atresia: evidence for etiopathogenic heterogeneity and therapeutic implications. Acta Paediatr Scand 1991; 80: 1192–1199

176. Thaler M M. Biliary disease in infancy and childhood. In: Sleisinger M H, Fordtran J S, eds. Gastrointestinal disease; pathophysiology, diagnosis, management. Philadelphia: Saunders, 1973: pp 1087–1098

177. Hays D M, Snyder W H. Life-span in untreated biliary atresia. Surgery 1963; 54: 373–375

178. Adelman S. Prognosis of uncorrected biliary atresia: an update. J Pediatr Surg 1978; 13: 389–391

179. Harris L E, Farrell F J, Shorter R G, Banner E A, Mathieson D R. Conjugated serum bilirubin in erythroblastosis fetalis: an analysis of 38 cases. Staff Meetings of the Mayo Clinic 1962; pp 574–581

180. Lloyd D A, Mikel R E. Spontaneous perforation of the extrahepatic bile ducts in neonates and infants. Br J Surg 1980; 67: 621–623

181. Freese D. Intracellular cholestatic syndromes of infancy. Semin Liver Dis 1982; 2: 255–270

182. Mowat A P. Pediatric liver disease. In Arias I M, Frenkel M, Wilson J H P, eds. The liver. Annual 2/1982. Amsterdam: Excerpta Medica, 1982: pp 262–304

183. Mowat A P. Biliary disorders in childhood. Semin Liver Dis 1982; 2: 271–281

184. El Tami M A, Clarke M D, Barett J T, Mowat H P. Ten minute radiopharmaceutical test for biliary atresia. Arch Dis Childh 1987; 62: 180–184

185. Greene H L, Helinek G L, Moran R, O'Neill J. A diagnostic approach to prolonged obstructive jaundice by 24-hour collection of duodenal fluid. J Pediatr 1979; 95: 412–414

186. Rosenthal P, Liebman, Sinatra R R et al. String test in evaluation of cholestatic jaundice in infancy. J Pediatr 1985; 107: 253

187. Fawega A G, Akinjunka O, Sodeende O. Duodenal intubation and aspiration test; utility in the differential diagnosis of infantile cholestasis. J Pediatr Gastroenterol Nutr 1991; 13: 290–292

188. Wilkinson M L, Mieli-Vergani G, Ball C, Portmann B, Mowat A P. Endoscopic retrograde cholangiopancreatography in infantile cholestasis. Arch Dis Child 1991; 66: 121–123

189. Brough A J, Bernstein J. Conjugated hyperbilirubinemia in early infancy. A reassessment of liver biopsy. Hum Pathol 1974; 5: 507–516

190. Manolaki A G, Larcher V F, Mowat A P, Barrett J J, Portmann B, Howard E R. The prelaparotomy diagnosis of extrahepatic biliary atresia. Arch Dis Child 1983; 58: 591–594

191. Gautier M, Jehan P, Odievre M. Histologic study of biliary fibrous remnants in 48 cases of extrahepatic biliary atresia: correlation with post-operative bile flow restoration. J Pediatr 1976; 89: 704–709

192. Miyano T, Suruga K, Suda K. Abnormal choledocho-pancreatico ductal junction related to the etiology of infantile obstructive jaundice diseases. J Pediatr Surg 1979; 14: 16–26

193. Scotto J M, Stralin H C. Congenital extrahepatic biliary atresia. Arch Pathol Lab Med 1977; 101: 416–419

194. Chandra R S, Altman R P. Ductal remnants in extrahepatic biliary atresia: a histopathological study with clinical correlation. J Pediatr 1978; 93: 196–200

195. Witzleben C L, Buck B E, Schnaufer L, Brzosko W J. Studies on the pathogenesis of biliary atresia. Lab Invest 1978; 38: 525–532

196. Gautier M, Eliot N. Extrahepatic biliary atresia. Morphological study of 98 biliary remnants. Arch Pathol Lab Med 1981; 105: 397–402

197. Ohi R, Shikes R H, Stellin G P, Lilly J R. In biliary atresia duct histology correlates with bile flow. J Pediatr Surg 1984; 19: 467–470

198. Kasai M, Watanabe I, Ohi R. Follow-up studies of long term survivors after hepatic portoenterostomy for 'noncorrectible' biliary atresia. J Pediatr Surg 1975; 10: 173–182

199. Kasai M. Advances in treatment of biliary atresia. J Pediatr Surg 1983; 13: 265–276

200. Ohkohchi N, Chiba T, Ohi R, Mori S. Long-term follow-up study of patients with cholangitis after successful Kasai operation in biliary atresia: selection of recipients for liver transplantation. J Pediatr Gastroenterol Nutr 1989; 9: 416–420

201. Ohi R, Nio M, Chiba T, Endo N, Goto M, Ibrahim M. Long-term follow-up after surgery for patients with biliary atresia. J Pediatr Surg 1990; 442: 445

202. Houwen R H J, Zwierstra R P, Severijnen R S V M et al. Prognosis of extrahepatic biliary atresia. Arch Dis Childh 1989; 64: 214–218

203. Tagge D U, Tagge E R, Drongowski R A, Oldhanik T, Coran A G A long-term experience with biliary atresia. Reassessment of prognostic tests. Am J Surg 1991; 214: 590–598

204. Sokol E M, Veyekemans F, de Ville da Goye J et al. Liver transplantation in children less than 1 year of age. J Pediatr 1990; 117: 205–210

205. Shimahara Y, Awane M, Yamaoka Y et al. Safety and operative stress for donors in living-related partial liver transplantation. XIV International Congress of the Transplantation Society, August 16–21, 1992

206. Edmond J, Heffron T G, Kortz E O, Gonzalez-Vallina R, Contis J C, Black D D, Whitington P. Improved results of living-related liver transplantation (LRT) with routine application in a pediatric program. XIV International Congress of the Transplantation Society, August 16–21, 1992

207. Tanaka K, Uemoto S, Sano K et al. Liver transplantation in children from living-related donors. XIV International Congress of the Transplantation Society, August 16–21, 1992

208. Fain J S, Lewin K J. Intrahepatic biliary cysts in congenital biliary atresia. Arch Pathol Lab Med 1989; 113: 1383–1386

209. Hubscher S G, Harrison R F. Portal lymphadenopathy associated with lipofuscin in chronic cholestatic liver disease. J Clin Pathol 1989; 42: 1160–1165

210. Landing B H, Wells T R, Reed G B, Natayan M S. Diseases of the bile ducts in children. In: Gall E A, Mostofi F K, eds. The liver. Baltimore, M D: Williams & Wilkins, 1973: pp 480–509

211. DeFreitas L A R, Chevallier M, Louis D, Grimand J A. Human extrahepatic biliary atresia: portal connective tissue activation related to ductular proliferation. Liver 1986; 6: 253–261

212. Ho C-W, Shioda K, Shirasaki K et al. The pathogenesis of biliary atresia; a morphological study of the hepatobiliary system and the hepatic artery. J Pediatr Gastroenterol Nutr 1993; 16: 53–60

213. Ohi R, Lilly J R. Copper kinetics in infantile hepatobiliary disease. J Pediatr Surg 1980; 15: 509–512

214. Chan K, Gavaler J S, Van Thiel D H, Whiteside T. Phenotypic characterization of mononuclear infiltrate present in liver of biliary atresia. Dig Dis Sci 1989; 34: 1564–1570

215. Fonkelsrud E W, Arima E. Bile lakes in congenital biliary atresia. Surgery 1975; 77: 384–390

216. Landing B H, Wells T R, Reed G B, Natayan M S. Neonatal hepatitis, biliary atresia and choledochal cyst. The concept of infantile obstructive cholangiopathy. Prog Pediatr Surg 1974; 6: 113–119

217. Sung J H, Stadlan E M. Neuro-axonal dystrophy in congenital biliary atresia. J Neuropathol Exp Neurol 1966; 25: 341–361

218. Kasai M. Intra- and extrahepatic bile ducts in biliary atresia. In: Javitt N B, ed. Neonatal hepatitis and biliary atresia. Washington, D C: US Government Printing Press, 1979: pp 351–364

219. Raweily E A, Gibson A A M, Burt A D. Abnormalities of intrahepatic bile ducts in extrahepatic biliary atresia. Histopathology 1990; 17: 521–527

220. Desmet V J, Callea F. Cholestatic syndromes of infancy and childhood. In: Zakim D, Boyer T D, eds. Hepatology: a textbook of liver disease, vol. 2, 2nd edn. Philadelphia: W B Saunders, 1990: pp 1355–1395

221. Callea F, Facchetti F, Lucini L et al. Liver morphology in anicteric patients at long-term follow-up after Kasai operation: a study of 16 cases. In: Ohi R, ed. Biliary atresia. Tokyo: Professional Postgraduate Services, 1987: pp 304–310

222. Alagille D. Extrahepatic biliary atresia. Hepatology 1984; 4: 7S–10S

223. Nietgen G W, Vacanti J P, Perez-Atayde A R. Intrahepatic bile duct loss in biliary atresia despite portoenterostomy: a consequence of ongoing obstruction? Gastroenterology 1992; 102: 2126–2133

224. Ito T, Horisawa M, Ando H. Intrahepatic bile ducts in biliary atresia — a possible factor determining prognosis. J Pediatr Surg 1983; 18: 124–130

225. Kulkarni P B, Beatty E C. Cholangiocarcinoma associated with biliary cirrhosis due to congenital biliary atresia. Am J Dis Child 1977; 131: 442–444

226. Witzleben C L. The pathogenesis of biliary atresia. In: Javitt N B, ed. Neonatal hepatic and biliary atresia. Washington, D C: US Government Printing Press, 1979: pp 339–350

227. Desmet V J. Cholangiopathies: past, present and future. Semin Liver Dis 1987; 7: 67–76

228. Desmet V J. Embryology of the liver and intrahepatic biliary tract and an overview of malformations of the bile duct. In: McIntyre N, Benhamou J-P, Bircher J, Rizzetto M, Rodes J, eds. Oxford textbook of clinical hepatology. Oxford: Oxford University Press, 1991: pp 496–519

229. Desmet V J. Congenital diseases of intrahepatic bile ducts: variations on the theme 'ductal plate malformation'. Hepatology 1992; 16: 1069–1083

230. Ogawa T, Suruga K, Kojima Y, Kitahara T, Kuwabara N. Experimental study of the pathogenesis of infantile obstructive cholangiography and its clinical evaluation. J Pediatr Surg 1983; 18: 131–135

231. Finegold M J. Cholestatic syndromes in infancy. In: Rosenberg H S, Bolande R B, eds. Perspectives in pediatric pathology. Chicago: Year Book Medical Publishers, 1976: vol 3, pp 41–84

232. Rosenstein B, Oppenheimer E. Prolonged obstructive jaundice and giant cell hepatitis in an infant with cystic fibrosis. J Pediatr 1977; 91: 1022–1023

233. Campbell L V Jr, Gilbert E F. Experimental giant cell transformation in the liver induced by E. coli endotoxin. Am J Pathol 1967; 51: 855–864

234. Dick M C, Mowat A P. Hepatitis syndrome in infancy — an epidemiological survey with 10 year follow-up. Arch Dis Childh 1985; 60: 512–516

235. Deutsch J, Smith A L, Danks D M, Campbell P E. Long term prognosis for babies with neonatal liver disease. Arch Dis Childh 1985; 60: 447–451

236. Montgomery C K, Ruebner B H. Neonatal hepatocellular giant cell transformation: a review. In: Rosenberg H S, Bolande R P, eds. Perspectives in pediatric pathology. Chicago: Year Book Medical Publishers, 1976: vol 3, pp 85–101

237. Chang M-H, Hsu H-C, Lee C-Y, Wang T-R, Kao C-L. Neonatal hepatitis: a follow-up study. J Pediatr Gastroenterol Nutr 1987; 6: 203–207

238. Herman S P, Baggenstoss A H, Cloutier M D. Liver dysfunction and histological abnormalities in neonatal hypopituitarism. J Pediatr 1975; 87: 892–895

239. Sheehan A G, Martin S R, Stephure D, Scott R B. Neonatal cholestasis, hypoglycemia, and congenital hypopituitarism. J Pediatr Gastroenterol Nutr 1992; 14: 426–430

240. Gray O P, Saunders R A. Familial intrahepatic cholestatic jaundice in infancy. Arch Dis Childh 1966; 41: 320–328

241. Clayton R J, Iber F L, Ruebner B H, McKusick V A. Byler disease. Am J Dis Child 1969; 117: 112–124

242. Greco M A, Finegold M J. Familial giant cell hepatitis. Arch Pathol 1973; 95: 240–244

243. Lawson E E, Boggs J D. Long-term follow-up of neonatal hepatitis: safety and value of surgical exploration. Pediatrics 1974; 53: 650–655

244. Sharp H L, Krivit W. Hereditary lymphedema and obstructive jaundice. J Pediatr 1971; 78: 491–496

245. Aägenaes O, Henriksen T, Sorland S. Hereditary neonatal cholestasis with vascular malformations. In: Berenberg S R, ed. Liver diseases in infancy and childhood. Baltimore: Williams & Wilkins, 1976: pp 198–206

246. Ruebner B, Thaler M M. Giant cell transformation in infantile liver disease. In: Javitt N B, ed. Neonatal hepatitis and biliary atresia. Washington, D C: US Government Printing Press, 1979: pp 299–311

247. Oledzka-Slotwinska H, Desmet V. Morphologic study on neonatal liver 'giant' cell transformation. Exp Mol Biol 1969; 10: 162–175

248. Craig J M, Landing B H. Form of hepatitis in neonatal period simulating biliary atresia. Arch Pathol 1952; 54: 321–333

249. Alagille D, Odievre M, Gautier M, Dommergues J P. Hepatic ductular hypoplasia associated with characteristic facies, vertebral malformations, retarded physical, mental and sexual development, and cardiac murmur. J Pediatr 1975; 86: 63–71

250. Odievre M, Martin J P, Hadchouel M, Alagille D. Alpha$_1$-antitrypsin deficiency and liver disease in children: phenotypes, manifestations and prognosis. Pediatrics 1976; 57: 224–231

251. Gardner L J. Intrahepatic bile stasis in 45/x Turner's syndrome. N Engl J Med 1974; 290: 406
252. Mulland E A, Purcell M. Biliary atresia and the Dandy–Walker anomaly in a neonate with 45, X Turner's syndrome. J Pathol 1975; 115: 227–230
253. Puri P, Guiney E J. Intrahepatic biliary atresia in Down's syndrome. J Pediatr Surg 1975; 10: 423–424
254. Aanpreung P, Beckwith B, Galansky S H, Koyle M A, Sokol R J. Association of paucity of interlobular bile ducts with prune belly syndrome. J Pediatr Gastroenterol Nutr 1993; 16: 81–86
255. Eyssen H, Paramentier G, Compernolle F, Boon J, Eggermont C. Trihydroxycoprostanic acid in the duodenal fluid of two children with intrahepatic bile duct anomalies. Biochim Biophys Acta 1972; 273: 212–221
256. Hanson R F, Isenberg J N, Williams G C et al. The metabolism of 3x, 7x, 12x trihydroxy-5 cholestan-26-oic acid in two siblings with cholestasis due to intrahepatic bile duct anomalies: an apparent inborn error of cholic acid synthesis. J Clin Invest 1975; 56: 577–587
257. Alagille D, Estrada A, Hadchouel M, Gautier M, Odievre M, Dommengues J-P. Syndromatic paucity of interlobular bile ducts Alagille syndrome or arteriohepatic dysplasia: review of 80 cases. J Pediatr 1987; 110: 195–200
258. Kahn E. Paucity of interlobular bile ducts: arteriohepatic dysplasia and nonsyndromatic duct paucity. Perspect Pediatr Pathol 1991; 14: 168–215
259. Hadchouel M. Paucity of interlobular bile ducts. Semin Diag Pathol 1992; 9: 24–30
260. Henriksen N T, Langemark F, Sorland S J, Fausa O, Landaas S, Aegenaes O. Hereditary cholestasis combined with peripheral pulmonary stenosis and other anomalies. Acta Paediatr Scand 1977; 66: 7–15
261. Watson G H, Miller V. Arteriohepatic dysplasia: familial pulmonary arterial stenosis with neonatal liver disease. Arch Dis Child 1973; 48: 459–466
262. Sokol R J, Heubi J E, Ballistreri W F. Intrahepatic 'cholestasis facies': Is it specific for Alagille syndrome? J Pediatr 1983; 103: 205–208
263. Riely C A. Familial intrahepatic cholestasis: an update. Yale J Biol Med 1979; 52: 89–98
264. Riely C A, Collier E, Jensen P S, Klatskin G. Arteriohepatic dysplasia: a benign syndrome of intrahepatic cholestasis with multiple organ involvement. Ann Intern Med 1979; 91: 520–527
265. Rosenfield N S, Kelley M J, Jensen P S, Cotlier E, Rosenfield A T, Riely C A. Arteriohepatic dysplasia: radiologic features of a new syndrome. Am J Roentgenol 1980; 135: 1217–1223
266. Levin S E, Zarvos P, Milner S, Schmaman A. Arteriohepatic dysplasia: association of liver disease with pulmonary arterial stenosis as well as facial and skeletal abnormalities. Pediatrics 1980; 66: 876–883
267. LaBrecque D R, Mitros F A, Nathan R J, Romanchuk K G, Judisch G F, El-Khoury G H. Four generations of arteriohepatic dysplasia. Hepatology 1982; 2: 467–474
268. Hyams J S, Berman M M, Davis B H. Tubulointerstitial nephropathy associated with arteriohepatic dysplasia. Gastroenterology 1983; 85: 430–434
269. Russo P A, Ellis E, Hashida Y. Renal histopathology in Alagille's syndrome. Pediatr Pathol 1987; 7: 557–568
270. Deprettere A, Portmann B, Mowat A P. Syndromic paucity of the intrahepatic bile ducts: diagnostic difficulty; severe morbidity throughout early childhood. J Pediatr Gastroenterol Nutr 1988; 6: 865–871
271. Gorelick F S, Dobbins J W, Burrell M, Reily C A. Biliary tract abnormalities in patients with arteriohepatic dysplasia. Dig Dis Sci 1982; 27: 815–820
272. Markowitz J, Daum F, Kahn F I et al. Arteriohepatic dysplasia. I. Pitfalls in diagnosis and management. Hepatology 1983; 3: 74–76
273. Kahn E I, Daum F, Markowitz J et al. Arteriohepatic dysplasia. II. Hepatobiliary morphology. Hepatology 1983; 3: 77–84
274. Morelli A, Pelli A A, Vedovelli A, Narducci F, Solinas A, De Benedictis F M. Endoscopic retrograde cholangiopancreatography study in Alagille's syndrome: first report. Am J Gastroenterol 1983; 78: 241–244
275. Schwartzenberg S J, Grothe R M, Sharp H L, Snover D C, Freese D. Long-term complications of arteriohepatic dysplasia. Am J Med 1992; 93: 171–176
276. Ong E, Williams S M, Anderson J C et al. MR imaging of a hepatoma associated with Alagille's syndrome. J Comp Assist Tomogr 1986; 10: 1047–1049
277. Rabinovitz M, Imperial J C, Schade R R, Van Thiel D H. Hepatocellular carcinoma in Alagille's syndrome: a family study. J Pediatr Gastroenterol Nutr 1989; 8: 26–30
278. Kauffmann S S, Wood P, Shaw B W, Markin R S, Gridelli B, Vanderhoof J A. Hepatocarcinoma in child with the Alagille's syndrome. Am J Dis Child 1987; 141: 698–700
279. Bach N, Kahn H, Thung S N, Schaffner F, Klion F M, Miller CM. Hepatocellular carcinoma in a long-term survivor of intrahepatic biliary hypoplasia. Am J Gastroenterol 1991; 86: 1527–1530
280. Nishikawa A, Mori H, Takahashi M, Ojima A, Shimakawa K, Furuta T. Alagille's syndrome: A case with a hematomatous nodule of the liver. Acta Pathol Jpn 1987; 37: 1319–1326
281. Tzakis A G, Reyes J, Tepetes K, Tzoracoleftherakis V, Todo S, Starzl T E. Liver transplantation for Alagille's syndrome. Arch Surg 1993; 128: 337–339
282. Bruguera M, Llach J, Rodes J. Nonsyndromatic paucity of intrahepatic bile ducts in infancy and idiopathic ductopenia in adulthood: the same syndrome? Hepatology 1992; 15: 830–834
283. Perrault J. Copper overload in paucity of interlobular bile ducts syndrome. Gastroenterology 1980; 75: 875–878
284. Valencia-Mayoral P, Weber J, Cutz E, Edwards V D, Phillips MJ. Possible defect in the bile secretory apparatus in arteriohepatic dysplasia (Alagille's syndrome): a review with observations on the ultrastructure of the liver. Hepatology 1984; 4: 691–698
285. Alagille D, Thomasin N. L'atrésie des voies biliares intrahepatiques avec voeis biliares extrahepatiques permeables chez l'enfant. Rev Med Chir Mal Foie 1970; 45: 93–104
286. Hadchouel M, Hugon R N, Gautier M. Reduced ratio of portal tracts to paucity of intrahepatic bile ducts. Arch Pathol Lab Med 1978; 102: 402–403
287. Witzleben C L. Bile duct paucity ('intrahepatic atresia'). Perspect Pediatr Pathol 1982; 7: 185–201
288. Hashida Y, Yunis E J. Syndromatic paucity of inter-lobular bile ducts: hepatic histopathology of the early and endstage liver. Pediatr Pathol 1988; 8: 1–15
289. Alagille D. Intrahepatic biliary atresia (hepatic ductular hypoplasia). In: Berenberg S R, ed. Liver diseases in infancy and childhood. Baltimore: Williams & Wilkins, 1976: pp 129–142
290. Berman M D, Ishak K G, Schaefer E J, Barnes S, Jones E A. Syndromatic hepatic ductular hypoplasia (arteriohepatic dysplasia): a clinical and hepatic histologic study of three patients. Dig Dis Sci 1981; 26: 485–497
291. Dahms B B, Petrelli M, Wyllie R et al. Arteriohepatic dysplasia in infancy and childhood: a longitudinal study of six patients. Hepatology 1982; 2: 350–358
292. Perrault J. Paucity of interlobular bile ducts: getting to know it better. Dig Dis Sci 1981; 26: 481–484
293. Witzleben C L, Finegold M, Piccoli D A, Treem WR. Bile canalicular morphometry in arteriohepatic dysplasia. Hepatology 1987; 7: 1262–1266
294. Kahn E, Daum F, Markowitz J et al. Nonsyndromatic paucity of interlobular bile ducts: light and electron microscopic evaluation of sequential liver biopsies in early childhood. Hepatology 1986; 6: 890–901
295. Alonso-Lej F, Rever W B, Pessagno D J. Congenital choledochal cyst, with a report of two, and an analysis of 94 cases. Surg Gynecol Obstet 1959; 108: 1–30
296. Longmire W P, Mandiola S A, Gordon H E. Congenital cystic disease of the liver and biliary system. Ann Surg 1971; 174: 711–724
297. Hadad A R, Estbrook K C, Campbell F T, Morris W D. Congenital dilatation of the bile ducts. Am J Surg 1976; 132: 799–804
298. Crittenden S L, McKinley M J. Choledochal cyst — clinical features and classification. Am J Gastroenterol 1985; 80: 643–647

252. Mulland E A, Purcell M. Biliary atresia and the Dandy–Walker anomaly in a neonate with 45, X Turner's syndrome. J Pathol 1975; 115: 227–230

253. Puri P, Guiney E J. Intrahepatic biliary atresia in Down's syndrome. J Pediatr Surg 1975; 10: 423–424

254. Aanpreung P, Beckwith B, Galansky S H, Koyle M A, Sokol R J. Association of paucity of interlobular bile ducts with prune belly syndrome. J Pediatr Gastroenterol Nutr 1993; 16: 81–86

255. Eyssen H, Paramentier G, Compernolle F, Boon J, Eggermont C. Trihydroxycoprostanic acid in the duodenal fluid of two children with intrahepatic bile duct anomalies. Biochim Biophys Acta 1972; 273: 212–221

256. Hanson R F, Isenberg J N, Williams G C et al. The metabolism of 3x, 7x, 12x trihydroxy-5 cholestan-26-oic acid in two siblings with cholestasis due to intrahepatic bile duct anomalies: an apparent inborn error of cholic acid synthesis. J Clin Invest 1975; 56: 577–587

257. Alagille D, Estrada A, Hadchouel M, Gautier M, Odievre M, Dommengues J-P. Syndromatic paucity of interlobular bile ducts Alagille syndrome or arteriohepatic dysplasia: review of 80 cases. J Pediatr 1987; 110: 195–200

258. Kahn E. Paucity of interlobular bile ducts: arteriohepatic dysplasia and nonsyndromatic duct paucity. Perspect Pediatr Pathol 1991; 14: 168–215

259. Hadchouel M. Paucity of interlobular bile ducts. Semin Diag Pathol 1992; 9: 24–30

260. Henriksen N T, Langemark F, Sorland S J, Fausa O, Landaas S, Aegenaes O. Hereditary cholestasis combined with peripheral pulmonary stenosis and other anomalies. Acta Paediatr Scand 1977; 66: 7–15

261. Watson G H, Miller V. Arteriohepatic dysplasia: familial pulmonary arterial stenosis with neonatal liver disease. Arch Dis Child 1973; 48: 459–466

262. Sokol R J, Heubi J E, Ballistreri W F. Intrahepatic 'cholestasis facies': Is it specific for Alagille syndrome? J Pediatr 1983; 103: 205–208

263. Riely C A. Familial intrahepatic cholestasis: an update. Yale J Biol Med 1979; 52: 89–98

264. Riely C A, Collier E, Jensen P S, Klatskin G. Arteriohepatic dysplasia: a benign syndrome of intrahepatic cholestasis with multiple organ involvement. Ann Intern Med 1979; 91: 520–527

265. Rosenfield N S, Kelley M J, Jensen P S, Cotlier E, Rosenfield A T, Riely C A. Arteriohepatic dysplasia: radiologic features of a new syndrome. Am J Roentgenol 1980; 135: 1217–1223

266. Levin S E, Zarvos P, Milner S, Schmaman A. Arteriohepatic dysplasia: association of liver disease with pulmonary arterial stenosis as well as facial and skeletal abnormalities. Pediatrics 1980; 66: 876–883

267. LaBrecque D R, Mitros F A, Nathan R J, Romanchuk K G, Judisch G F, El-Khoury G H. Four generations of arteriohepatic dysplasia. Hepatology 1982; 2: 467–474

268. Hyams J S, Berman M M, Davis B H. Tubulointerstitial nephropathy associated with arteriohepatic dysplasia. Gastroenterology 1983; 85: 430–434

269. Russo P A, Ellis E, Hashida Y. Renal histopathology in Alagille's syndrome. Pediatr Pathol 1987; 7: 557–568

270. Deprettere A, Portmann B, Mowat A P. Syndromic paucity of the intrahepatic bile ducts: diagnostic difficulty; severe morbidity throughout early childhood. J Pediatr Gastroenterol Nutr 1988; 6: 865–871

271. Gorelick F S, Dobbins J W, Burrell M, Reily C A. Biliary tract abnormalities in patients with arteriohepatic dysplasia. Dig Dis Sci 1982; 27: 815–820

272. Markowitz J, Daum F, Kahn F I et al. Arteriohepatic dysplasia. I. Pitfalls in diagnosis and management. Hepatology 1983; 3: 74–76

273. Kahn E I, Daum F, Markowitz J et al. Arteriohepatic dysplasia. II. Hepatobiliary morphology. Hepatology 1983; 3: 77–84

274. Morelli A, Pelli A A, Vedovelli A, Narducci F, Solinas A, De Benedictis F M. Endoscopic retrograde cholangiopancreatography study in Alagille's syndrome: first report. Am J Gastroenterol 1983; 78: 241–244

275. Schwartzenberg S J, Grothe R M, Sharp H L, Snover D C, Freese D. Long-term complications of arteriohepatic dysplasia. Am J Med 1992; 93: 171–176

276. Ong E, Williams S M, Anderson J C et al. MR imaging of a hepatoma associated with Alagille's syndrome. J Comp Assist Tomogr 1986; 10: 1047–1049

277. Rabinovitz M, Imperial J C, Schade R R, Van Thiel D H. Hepatocellular carcinoma in Alagille's syndrome: a family study. J Pediatr Gastroenterol Nutr 1989; 8: 26–30

278. Kauffmann S S, Wood P, Shaw B W, Markin R S, Gridelli B, Vanderhoof J A. Hepatocarcinoma in child with the Alagille's syndrome. Am J Dis Child 1987; 141: 698–700

279. Bach N, Kahn H, Thung S N, Schaffner F, Klion F M, Miller CM. Hepatocellular carcinoma in a long-term survivor of intrahepatic biliary hypoplasia. Am J Gastroenterol 1991; 86: 1527–1530

280. Nishikawa A, Mori H, Takahashi M, Ojima A, Shimakawa K, Furuta T. Alagille's syndrome: A case with a hematomatous nodule of the liver. Acta Pathol Jpn 1987; 37: 1319–1326

281. Tzakis A G, Reyes J, Tepetes K, Tzoracoleftherakis V, Todo S, Starzl T E. Liver transplantation for Alagille's syndrome. Arch Surg 1993; 128: 337–339

282. Bruguera M, Llach J, Rodes J. Nonsyndromatic paucity of intrahepatic bile ducts in infancy and idiopathic ductopenia in adulthood: the same syndrome? Hepatology 1992; 15: 830–834

283. Perrault J. Copper overload in paucity of interlobular bile ducts syndrome. Gastroenterology 1980; 75: 875–878

284. Valencia-Mayoral P, Weber J, Cutz E, Edwards V D, Phillips M J. Possible defect in the bile secretory apparatus in arteriohepatic dysplasia (Alagille's syndrome): a review with observations on the ultrastructure of the liver. Hepatology 1984; 4: 691–698

285. Alagille D, Thomasin N. L'atrésie des voies biliares intrahepatiques avec voeis biliares extrahepatiques permeables chez l'enfant. Rev Med Chir Mal Foie 1970; 45: 93–104

286. Hadchouel M, Hugon R N, Gautier M. Reduced ratio of portal tracts to paucity of intrahepatic bile ducts. Arch Pathol Lab Med 1978; 102: 402–403

287. Witzleben C L. Bile duct paucity ('intrahepatic atresia'). Perspect Pediatr Pathol 1982; 7: 185–201

288. Hashida Y, Yunis E J. Syndromatic paucity of inter-lobular bile ducts: hepatic histopathology of the early and endstage liver. Pediatr Pathol 1988; 8: 1–15

289. Alagille D. Intrahepatic biliary atresia (hepatic ductular hypoplasia). In: Berenberg S R, ed. Liver diseases in infancy and childhood. Baltimore: Williams & Wilkins, 1976: pp 129–142

290. Berman M D, Ishak K G, Schaefer E J, Barnes S, Jones E A. Syndromatic hepatic ductular hypoplasia (arteriohepatic dysplasia): a clinical and hepatic histologic study of three patients. Dig Dis Sci 1981; 26: 485–497

291. Dahms B B, Petrelli M, Wyllie R et al. Arteriohepatic dysplasia in infancy and childhood: a longitudinal study of six patients. Hepatology 1982; 2: 350–358

292. Perrault J. Paucity of interlobular bile ducts: getting to know it better. Dig Dis Sci 1981; 26: 481–484

293. Witzleben C L, Finegold M, Piccoli D A, Treem WR. Bile canalicular morphometry in arteriohepatic dysplasia. Hepatology 1987; 7: 1262–1266

294. Kahn E, Daum F, Markowitz J et al. Nonsyndromatic paucity of interlobular bile ducts: light and electron microscopic evaluation of sequential liver biopsies in early childhood. Hepatology 1986; 6: 890–901

295. Alonso-Lej F, Rever W B, Pessagno D J. Congenital choledochal cyst, with a report of two, and an analysis of 94 cases. Surg Gynecol Obstet 1959; 108: 1–30

296. Longmire W P, Mandiola S A, Gordon H E. Congenital cystic disease of the liver and biliary system. Ann Surg 1971; 174: 711–724

297. Hadad A R, Estbrook K C, Campbell F T, Morris W D. Congenital dilatation of the bile ducts. Am J Surg 1976; 132: 799–804

298. Crittenden S L, McKinley M J. Choledochal cyst — clinical features and classification. Am J Gastroenterol 1985; 80: 643–647

299. Sherman P, Kolster E, Davies C, Stringer D, Weber J. Choledochal cysts: heterogeneity of clinical presentation. J Pediatr Gastroenterol Nutr 1986; 5: 867–872

300. Nagorney D M, McIlrath D C, Adson M A. Choledochal cysts in adults: clinical management. Surgery 1984; 96: 656–663

301. Howell C G, Templeton J M, Weiner S, Glassman M, Betts JM, Witzleben C L. Antenatal diagnosis and early surgery for choledochal cyst. J Pediatr Surg 1983; 18: 387–393

302. Kobayashi A, Ohbe Y. Choledochal cyst in infancy and childhood: analysis of 16 cases. Arch Dis Childh 1977; 52: 121–128

303. Kim S H. Choledochal cyst; Survey by the surgical section of the American Academy of Pediatrics. J Pediatr Surg 1981; 16: 402–407

304. Venu R P, Geenen J E, Hogan W J et al. Role of endoscopic retrograde cholangiopancreatography in the diagnosis and treatment of choledochocele. Gastroenterology 1984; 87: 1144–1149

305. Shemesh E, Gernick A, Klein E, Avigad I. The role of endoscopic retrograde cholangiopancreatography in the diagnosis and treatment of adult choledochal cyst. Surg Gynecol Obstet 1988; 167: 423–426

306. Camponovo E, Buck J L, Drane W E. Scintigraphic features of choledochal cyst. J Nucl Med 1989; 30: 622–628

307. Fevery T, Tanghe W, Kerremans R, Desmet V, DeGroote J. Congenital dilatation of the intrahepatic bile ducts associated with the development of amyloidosis. Gut 1972; 13: 604–609

308. Chen W J, Chang W H, Hung W T. Congenital choledochal cyst: with observations on rupture of the cyst and intrahepatic ductal dilatation. J Pediatr Surg 1973; 8: 529–538

309. Flanigan D P. Biliary cysts. Ann Surg 1975; 182: 635–643

310. Barlow B, Tabor E, Blanc W A, Santulli T V, Harris R C. Choledochal cyst: a review of 19 cases. J Pediatr 1976; 89: 934–940

311. Kagawa Y, Kashihara S, Kuramoto S, Maetani S. Carcinoma arising in a congenitally dilated biliary tract. Report of a case and review of the literature. Gastroenterology 1978; 74: 1286–1294

312. Robertson J F R, Raine P A M. Choledochal cyst: a 33-year review. Br J Surg 1988; 75: 799–801

313. Yeong M L, Nicholson G I, Lee S P. Regression of biliary cirrhosis following choledochal cyst drainage. Gastroenterology 1982; 82: 332–335

314. Nagata E, Sakai K, Konoshita H, Herohashi K. Choledochal cyst: complications of anomalous connection between the choledochus and pancreatic duct and carcinoma of the biliary tract. World J Surg 1986; 10: 102–110

315. Oguchi Y, Okada A, Nakamura T et al. Histopathologic studies of congenital dilatation of the bile duct or related to an anomalous junction of the pancreaticobiliary ductal system: clinical and experimental studies. Surgery 1988; 103: 168–173

316. Okada A, Nakamura T, Higaki J, Okumura K, Kamata S, Oguchi Y. Congenital dilatation of the bile duct in 100 instances and its relationship with anomalous junction. Surgery 1990; 171: 291–298

317. Young W T, Thomas G V, Blethyn A J, Lawrie B W. Choledochal cyst and congenital anomalies of the pancreatico-biliary junction: the clinical findings, radiology and outcome in nine cases. Br J Radiol 1992; 65: 33–38

318. Babbitt D P, Starshak R J, Clemett A R. Choledochal cyst: a concept of etiology. Am J Roentgenol 1973; 119: 57–62

319. Yamashiro Y, Mijano T, Suruga K, et al. Experimental study of the pathogenesis of choledochal cyst and pancreatitis, with special reference of the role of bile acids and pancreatic enzymes in the anomalous choledocho-pancreatico ductal junction. J Pediatr Gastroenterol Nutr 1984; 3: 721–727

320. Jones P G, Smith F D, Clarke A M, Kent M. Choledochal cysts: experience with radical excision. J Pediatr Surg 1971; 6: 112–120

321. Kimura K, Tsugawa C, Ogawa K et al. Choledochal cyst. Etiological considerations and surgical management in 22 cases. Arch Surg 1978; 113: 159–163

322. Filler R M, Stringel G. Treatment of choledochal cyst by excision. J Pediatr Surg 1980; 15: 437–442

323. Okada A, Nakamura T, Okumura K, Oguchi Y, Kamata S. Surgical treatment of congenital dilatation of bile duct (choledochal cyst) with technical considerations. Surgery 1987; 101: 239–243

324. Chijiiwa K, Koga A. Surgical management and long-term follow-up of patients with choledochal cysts. Am J Surg 1993; 165: 238–242

325. Cosentino C M, Luck S R, Raffensperger J G, Reynolds M. Choledochal duct cyst: resection with physiologic reconstruction. Surgery 1992; 112: 740–748

326. Ando H, Ito T, Sugito T. Histological study of the choledochal cyst wall. Jap J Gastroenterol 1987; 84: 1797–1801

327. Kozuka S, Kurashima M, Tsubone M, Hachisuka K, Yasui A. Significance of intestinal metaplasia for evolution of cancer in the biliary tract. Cancer 1984; 54: 2277–2285

328. Komi N, Tamura T, Tsuge S, Miyoshi Y, Udaka H, Takehara H. Relation of patient age to premalignant changes in choledochal cyst epithelium: histochemical and immunohistochemical studies. J Pediatr Surg 1986; 21: 430–433

329. Case Records of the Massachusetts General Hospital: Case 52-1988. N Engl J Med 1988; 319: 1718–1725

330. Kusunoki M, Yamamura T, Takahashi T, Kantoh M, Ishikawa M, Utsunomiya J. Choledochal cyst: its possible autonomic involvement in the bile duct. Arch Surg 1987; 122: 997–1000

331. Gallagher P J, Mills R R, Mitchinson M J. Congenital dilatation of the intrahepatic bile ducts with cholangiocarcinoma. J Clin Pathol 1972; 25: 804–808

332. Voyles C R, Smadja C, Shands C, Blumgart L H. Carcinoma in choledochal cysts: age-related incidence. Arch Surg 1983; 118: 986–988

333. Reveille R M, Van Stiegmann G, Everson G T. Increased secondary bile acids in a choledochal cyst. Possible role in biliary metaplasia and carcinoma. Gastroenterology 1990; 99: 525–527

334. Caroli J. Diseases of the intrahepatic biliary tree. Clin Gastroenterol 1973; 2: 147–161

335. Mercadier M, Chigot J P, Clot J P, Langlois P, Lansieux P. Caroli's disease. World J Surg 1984; 8: 22–29

336. Nagusue N. Successful treatment of Caroli's disease by hepatic resection. Ann Surg 1984; 200: 718–723

337. Tandon R K, Grewal H, Amand A C, Vashisht S. Caroli's syndrome: a heterogeneous entity. Am J Gastroenterology 1990; 85: 170–173

338. Moreno A J, Parker A L, Spicer M J, Brown T J. Scintigraphic and radiographic findings in Caroli's disease. Am J Gastroenterol 1984; 79: 299–303

339. Marchal G J, Desmet V J, Proesmans W C et al. Caroli's disease: high-frequency US and pathologic findings. Radiology 1986; 158: 507–511

340. Hopper K D. The role of computed tomography in the evaluation of Caroli's disease. Clin Imag 1989; 13: 68–73

341. Choi B I, Mo-Yeon K, Kim S H, Han M C. Caroli disease: central dot sign in CT. Radiology 1990; 174: 161–163

342. Leroy J P, Charles J F, Diveres B, Bettet M. Carcinome biliaire développé sur maladie de Caroli: á propos d'un cas. Sem Hôp 1980; 56: 5–6

343. Phinney P R, Austin G E, Kadell B M. Cholangiocarcinoma arising in Caroli's disease. Arch Pathol Lab Med 1981; 105: 194–197

344. Chen K T K. Adenocarcinoma of the liver: association with congenital hepatic fibrosis and Caroli's disease. Arch Pathol Lab Med 1981; 105: 294–295

345. Dayton M T, Longmire W P, Tompkins R K. Caroli's disease: a premalignant condition? Am J Surg 1983; 145: 41–48

346. Chevillotte G, Sastre B, Sahel J, Payan H, Michotey G, Sarles H. Maladie de Caroli localisée et associée à un adenocarcinome papillaire mucosécrétant: intérêt de la résection hépatique. Presse Méd 1984; 13: 1137–1139

347. Etienne J C, Bouillot J L, Alexandre J H. Cholangiocarcinome développé au maladie de Caroli: à propos d'un cas. Revue de la littérature. J Chir (Paris) 1987; 124: 168–171

348. Kchir N, Haouet S, Boubaker S et al. Maladie de Caroli associée à un hépatocarcinome: à propos d'une observation et revue de la littérature. Semin Hôp (Paris) 1990; 66: 1962–1966

349. Witlin L T, Gadacz TR, Zuidema G D, Kridelbaugh WW.

Transhepatic decompression of the biliary tree in Caroli's disease. Surgery 1982; 91: 205–209

350. Ramond M-J, Huguet C, Danan G, Rueff B, Benhamou JP. Partial hepatectomy in the treatment of Caroli's disease. Dig Dis Sci 1984; 29: 367–370

351. Boyle M J, Doyle E D, McNulty J G. Monolobar Caroli's disease. Am J Gastroenterol 1989; 84: 1437–1444

352. Guntz P, Coppo B, Lorimier G, Crouier P, Guntz M. La maladie de Caroli unilobaire. J Chir (Paris) 1991; 128: 167–181

353. Lointier P H, Kauffmann P, Francannet P, Dezet D, Chipponi J. Management of intrahepatic calculi in Caroli's disease by extracorporeal shock wave lithotripsy. Br J Surg 1990; 77: 987–988

354. Fozard J B J, Wyatt J I, Hall R I. Epithelial dysplasia in Caroli's disease. Gut 1989; 30: 1150–1153

355. Joly I, Choux R, Baroui J L et al. Carcinome in situ sur maladie de Caroli localisée. Gastroenterol Clin Biol 1990; 14: 90–92

356. Hussman K L, Friedwald J P, Gollub M J, Melamed J. Caroli's disease associated with infantile polycystic kidney disease: prenatal sonographic appearance. J Ultrasound 1991; 10: 235–237

357. Jordon D, Harpaz N, Thung S N. Caroli's disease and adult polycystic kidney disease: a rarely recognized association. Liver 1989; 9: 30–35

358. Desmet V J. What is congenital hepatic fibrosis? Histopathology 1992; 20: 465–477

359. Merza A P, Raiser M W. Biliary tract manifestations of the Marfan syndrome. Am J Gastroenterol 1987; 82: 779–782

360. McDonald R A, Avner E A. Inherited polycystic kidney disease in childhood. Semin Nephrol 1991; 11: 632–642

361. Blyth H, Ockenden B G. Polycystic disease of kidneys and liver presenting in childhood. J Med Genet 1971; 81: 257–284

362. Bradford W D, Bradford J W, Porter F S, Sidbury J B Jr. Cystic disease of liver and kidney with portal hypertension. A cause of sudden unexpected hematemesis. Clin Pediatr 1968; 7: 249–306

363. Lieberman E, Salinas-Madrigal L, Gwinn J L, Brenman L P, Fine R N, Landing B H. Infantile polycystic disease of the kidneys and liver. Medicine 1971; 50: 227–318

364. Landing B H, Walls T R, Claireaux A E. Morphometric analysis of liver lesions in cystic diseases of childhood. Hum Pathol 1980; 11: 549–560

365. Bernstein J, Chandra M, Creswell J et al. Renal–hepatic–pancreatic dysplasia: a syndrome reconsidered. Am J Med Genet 1987; 26: 391–403

366. Witzleben C L. Cystic diseases of the liver. In: Zakim D, Boyer T D, eds. Hepatology. A textbook of liver disease, 2nd edn. Philadelphia: W B Saunders, 1990: pp 1395–1411

367. Kaplan I, Bingol N, Kaplan BS. Kidney, polycystic disease, recessive. In: Buyse M L, ed. Birth defects encyclopedia. Dover, M A: Center for Birth Defects Information Services, 1990: pp 1010–1011

368. Desmet V J. Congenital diseases of intrahepatic bile ducts: variations on the theme 'ductal plate malformation'. Hepatology 1992; 16: 1069–1083

369. Gang D L, Herrin J T. Infantile polycystic disease of the liver and kidneys. Clin Nephrol 1986; 25: 28–36

370. Lathrop D B. Cystic disease of the liver and kidney. Pediatrics 1959; 24: 215–224

371. Adams C M, Danks D M, Campbell P E. Comments upon the classification of infantile polycystic diseases of the liver and kidney, based upon three dimensional reconstruction of the liver. J Med Genet 1974; 11: 234–243

372. Jörgensen M J. The ductal plate malformation. APMIS (suppl) 1977; 257: 1–88

373. Potter E L, Craig J M. Pathology of the fetus and the infant, 3rd edn. Chicago: Year Book Medical Publishers, 1975: pp 393–425

374. Jörgensen M. A stereological study of intrahepatic bile ducts. 3. Infantile polycystic disease. APMIS 1973; 81A: 670–675

375. Fujiwara Y, Ohizumi T, Kakizaki G, Fujiwara T. Congenital dilatation of intrahepatic and common bile ducts with congenital hepatic fibrosis. J Pediatr Surg 1976; 11: 273–274

376. Kerr D N S, Warrick C K, Hart-Mercer J. A lesion resembling medullary sponge kidney in patients with congenital hepatic fibrosis. Clin Radiol 1962; 13: 85–91

377. Nakanuma Y, Terada T, Ohta G. Caroli's disease in congenital hepatic fibrosis and infantile polycystic disease. Liver 1982; 2: 346–354

378. Summerfield J A, Nagafuchi Y, Sherlock S et al. Hepatobiliary fibropolycystic diseases. A clinical and histological review of 51 patients. J Hepatol 1986; 2: 141–156

379. Lee F I, Paes A R. Congenital hepatic fibrosis and adult-type autosomal dominant polycystic kidney disease in a child. Postgrad J Med 1985; 61: 641–642

380. Sommerschild H C, Langmark F, Maurseth K. Congenital hepatic fibrosis: report of two new cases and review of the literature. Surgery 1973; 73: 53–58

381. Averback P. Congenital hepatic fibrosis. Asymptomatic adults without renal anomaly. Arch Pathol Lab Med 1977; 101: 260–261

382. Fauvert R, Benhamou J P. Congenital hepatic fibrosis. In: Schaffner F, Sherlock S J, Leevy C M, eds. The liver and its diseases. New York: Intercontinental Medical Book, 1974: pp 283–288

383. Naveh Y, Roguin N, Ludatscher R, Auslaender L, Schramek A, Maharon M. Congenital hepatic fibrosis with congenital heart disease. Gut 1980; 21: 799–807

384. Maggiore G, Borgana-Pignatti C, Marni E, Abbati G, Magrini U. Pulmonary arteriovenous fistulas: an unusual complication of congenital hepatic fibrosis. J Pediatr Gastroenterol 1983; 2: 183–186

385. Bogomoletz W V, Lefaucher C C. Congenital hepatic fibrosis (asymptomatic and latent forms) and multiple gastric ulcers. Dig Dis Sci 1979; 24: 887–890

386. Pedersen P S, Tygstrup I. Congenital hepatic fibrosis combined with protein-losing enteropathy and recurrent thrombosis. Acta Paediatr Scand 1980; 69: 571–574

387. Nakamura F, Sasaki H, Kajihara H, Yamanoue M. Laurence–Moon–Biedl syndrome accompanied by congenital hepatic fibrosis. J Gastroenterol Hepatol 1990; 5: 206–210

388. Boichis H, Passwell J, David R, Miller H. Congenital hepatic fibrosis and nephronophthisis. Q J Med 1973; 42: 221–233

389. Kerr D N S, Harrison C V, Sherlock S, Walker R M. Congenital hepatic fibrosis. Q J Med 1960; 30: 91–117

390. Alvarez F, Bernard O, Brunelle O et al. Congenital hepatic fibrosis in children. J Pediatr 1981; 99: 370–375

391. Daroca P J, Tuthill R, Reed R J. Cholangiocarcinoma arising in congenital hepatic fibrosis. Arch Pathol 1975; 99: 592–595

392. Scott J, Shousha S, Thomas H C, Sherlock S. Bile duct carcinoma: a late complication of congenital hepatic fibrosis. Am J Gastroenterology 1980; 73: 113–119

393. Chen K T K. Adenocarcinoma of the liver: association with congenital hepatic fibrosis and Caroli's disease. Arch Pathol Lab Med 1981; 105: 294–295

394. Bernstein J. Hepatic and renal involvement in malformation syndromes. Mt Sinai J Med 1986; 53: 421–428

395. De Vos B F, Cuvelier C. Congenital hepatic fibrosis. J Hepatol 1988; 6: 222–228

396. McCarthy L J, Baggenstoss A H, Logan G B. Congenital hepatic fibrosis. Gastroenterol 1966; 49: 27–36

397. Nathan M, Batsakis J G. Congenital hepatic fibrosis. Surg Gynecol Obstet 1969; 128: 1033–1041

398. Foulk W T. Congenital malformations of the intrahepatic biliary tree in the adult. Gastroenterology 1970; 58: 253–256

399. Ehrlich J C, Goodfriend A J, Shinohara Y, Seki M. Fetal ascites and portal dysplasia of the liver (polycystic disease without cysts). Pediatrics 1964; 33: 216–226

400. Albukerk J, Duffy J L. Fibrogenesis in congenital hepatic fibrosis. An electron and light microscopic study. Arch Pathol 1971; 92: 126–135

401. Lake D N W, Smith P M, Wheeler M H. Congenital hepatic fibrosis and choledochus cyst. Br Med J 1977; 2: 1259–1260

402. Case records of the Massachusetts General Hospital: Case 11–1983. N Engl J Med 1983; 308: 642–648

403. Strayer D S, Kissane J M. Dysplasia of the kidneys, liver, and pancreas: report of a variant of Ivemark's syndrome. Hum Pathol 1979; 10: 228–234

404. Bernstein J, Chandra M, Creswell J et al. Renal–hepatic–pancreatic dysplasia: a syndrome reconsidered. Am J Med Genet 1987; 26: 391–403

405. Böhm N, Fukuda M, Staudt R, Helwig H. Chondroectodermal dysplasia (Ellis–van Creveld syndrome) with dysplasia of the renal medulla and bile ducts. Histopathology 1978; 2: 267–281

406. Witzleben C L, Sharp A R. 'Nephronophthisis — congenital hepatic fibrosis': an additional hepatorenal disorder. Hum Pathol 1982; 13: 728–733

407. Langer L O. Thoracic–pelvic–pharyngeal dystrophy. Radiology 1968; 91: 447–456

408. Hudgins L, Rosengren S, Treem W, Hyams J. Early cirrhosis in survivors with Jeune thoracic dystrophy. J Pediatr 1992; 120: 754–756

409. Reeders S T, Breuning M H, Davies K E et al. A highly polymorphic DNA marker linked to adult polycystic kidney disease on chromosome 16. Nature 1985; 317: 542–544

410. Parfrey P S, Bear J C, Morgan J et al. The diagnosis and prognosis of autosomal dominant polycystic kidney disease. N Engl J Med 1990; 323: 1085–1090

411. Kimberling W J, Pieke-Dahl S A, Kumar S. The genetics of cystic diseases of the kidney. Sem Nephrol 1991; 11: 596–606

412. Gabow P A. Autosomal dominant polycystic kidney disease: more than a renal disease. Am J Kidney Dis 1990; 16: 403–413

413. Melnick P J. Polycystic liver. Arch Pathol 1955; 59: 162–172

414. Dalgaard O Z. Bilateral polycystic disease of the kidneys. A follow-up of 284 patients and their families. Acta Med Scand 1957; Suppl 328: 13–255

415. Fick G M, Johnson A M, Strain J D et al. Characteristics of very early onset autosomal dominant polycystic kidney disease. J Am Soc Nephrol 1993; 3: 1863–1876

416. Henson S W Jr, Gray H K, Dockerty M B. Benign tumours of the liver III. Solitary cysts. Surg Gynecol Obstet 1956; 103: 607–612

417. Kwok M K, Lewin K J. Massive hepatomegaly in adult polycystic liver disease. Am J Surg Pathol 1988; 12: 321–324

418. Howard R J, Hanson R F, Delaney J P. Jaundice associated with polycystic liver disease: relief by surgical decompression of the cysts. Arch Surg 1976; 111: 816–817

419. Lerner M E, Roshkow J E, Smithline A, Ng C. Polycystic liver disease with obstructive jaundice: treatment with ultrasound-guided cyst aspiration. Gastrointest Radiol 1992; 17: 46–48

420. Katzen N G. Fatal hepatic polycystic disease. Br Med J 1964; 1: 839–840

421. Del Guercio E, Greco J, Kim K E, Chintz J, Swartz C. Esophageal varices in adult patients with polycystic kidney and liver disease. N Engl J Med 1973; 289: 678–679

422. Ratcliffe P J, Reeders S, Theaker J M. Bleeding oesophageal varices and hepatic dysfunction in adult polycystic kidney disease. Br Med J 1984; 288: 1330–1331

423. van Erpecum K J, Janssens A R, Tyon A, Tham R T O. Highly symptomatic adult polycystic disease of the liver: a report of 15 cases. J Hepatol 1987; 5: 109–117

424. Armetage N C, Blumgart L H. Partial resection and fenestration in the treatment of polycystic liver disease. Br J Surg 1984; 71: 742–744

425. Newman K D, Torres V E, Rakela J, Nagorney D M. Treatment of highly symptomatic polycystic liver disease. Ann Surg 1990; 212: 30–37

426. Sanchez H, Ganer M, Rossi R L et al. Surgical management of nonparasitic cystic liver disease. Am J Surg 1991; 161: 113–119

427. Vauthey J-N, Maddern G J, Kolbinger P, Baer H U, Blumgart L H. Clinical experience with adult polycystic liver disease. Br J Surg 1992; 79: 562–565

428. Starzl T E, Reyes J, Tzakis A, Mieles L, Todo S, Gordon R. Liver transplantation for polycystic liver disease. Arch Surg 1990; 125: 575–577

429. Taylor J E, Calne R Y, Stewart W K. Massive cystic hepatomegaly in a female patient with polycystic kidney disease treated by combined hepatic and renal transplantation. Q J Med 1991; 80: 771–775

430. Telenti A, Torres V E, Gross J B Jr, Van Scoy R E, Brown M L, Hattery R R. Hepatic cyst infection in autosomal dominant polycystic kidney disease. Mayo Clin Proc 1990; 65: 933–942

431. Ikei S, Yamaguchi Y, Mori K. Infection of hepatic cysts with Pseudomonas aeruginosa in polycystic liver disease. Dig Surg 1990; 7: 117–121

432. Kachney W P, Everson G T. Extrarenal manifestations of autosomal dominant polycystic kidney disease. Sem Nephrol 1991; 11: 661–670

433. Chapman A B, Rubinstein D, Hughes R et al. Intracranial aneurysms in autosomal dominant polycystic kidney disease. N Engl J Med 1992; 327: 916–920

434. Cole B R, Conley S B, Stapleton F B. Polycystic kidney disease in the first year of life. J Pediatr 1987; 111: 693–699

435. Terada T, Nakanuma Y. Congenital biliary dilatation in autosomal dominant adult polycystic disease of the liver and kidneys. Arch Pathol Lab Med 1988; 112: 1113–1116

436. Grateau G, Hospitel S, Charbonneau R et al. Dilatation des voies biliares au cours de la polykystose rénale de l'adulte. Presse Méd 1990; 19: 1669–1671

437. Patterson M, Gonzalez-Witale J C, Fagan C J. Polycystic liver disease: a study of cyst fluid constituents. Hepatology 1982; 2: 475–478

438. Coffin B, Hadengue A, Gegos F, Benhamou J-P. Calcified hepatic and renal cysts in adult dominant polycystic kidney disease. Dig Dis Sci 1990; 35: 1172–1175

439. Ramos M, Torres V E, Holley K E, Offord K P, Rakela J, Ludwig J. The liver in autosomal dominant polycystic kidney disease. Arch Pathol Lab Med 1990; 114: 180–184

440. Keda T, Nakanuma Y, Terada T. Cystic dilatation of peribiliary glands in livers with adult polycystic disease and livers with solitary nonparasitic cysts: an autopsy study. Hepatology 1992; 16: 334–340

441. Chung E B. Multiple bile-duct hamartomas. Cancer 1970; 25: 287–296

442. McLaughlin M J, Phillips M J. Angiographic findings in multiple bile-duct hamartomas of the liver. Radiology 1975; 116: 41–43

443. Homer L W, White H J, Reed R C. Neoplastic transformation of von Meyenburg complexes of the liver. J Pathol Bacteriol 1968; 96: 499–502

444. Bonfors M. The development of cholangiocarcinoma from multiple bile-duct adenomas. Acta Pathol Microbiol Immunol Scand Sect (A) 1984; 92: 285–289

445. Honda N, Cobb C, Lechago J. Bile duct carcinoma associated with multiple von Meyenburg complexes in the liver. Hum Pathol 1986; 17: 1287–1290

446. Bruns C D, Kuhms J G, Wieman J. Cholangiocarcinoma in association with multiple biliary microhamartomas. Arch Pathol Lab Med 1990; 114: 1287–1289

447. Azizah N, Paradinas F J. Cholangiocarcinoma coexisting with developmental liver cysts: a distinct entity different from liver cystadenocarcinoma. Histopathology 1980; 4: 391–400

448. Imamura M, Miyashita T, Tani T et al. Cholangiocellular carcinoma associated with multiple liver cysts. Am J Gastroenterol 1984; 79: 790–795

449. Rossi R L, Silverman M L, Braasch J W, Munson J L, Remine S G. Carcinomas arising in cystic conditions of the bile ducts. Ann Surg 1987; 205: 377–384

450. Thiese N, Miller F, Worman H J et al. Biliary cystadenocarcinoma arising in a liver with fibropolycystic disease. Arch Pathol Lab Med 1993; 117: 163–165

451. Geist D C. Solitary nonparasitic cyst of the liver. Arch Surg 1955; 71: 867–880

452. Flagg R S, Robinson D W. Solitary nonparasitic hepatic cysts. Arch Surg 1967; 95: 964–973

453. Wheeler D A, Edmondson H A. Cystadenoma with mesenchymal stroma (CMS) in the liver and bile ducts: a clinicopathologic study of 17 cases, 4 with malignant change. Cancer 1985; 56: 1434–1445

454. Akwari O E, Tucker A, Seigler H F, Itani K M F. Hepatobiliary cystadenoma with mesenchymal stroma. Ann Surg 1990; 211: 18–27

455. Chu D Y, Olson A L, Mishalany H G. Congenital liver cyst presenting as congenital diaphragmatic hernia. J Pediatr Surg 1986; 21: 897–899

456. Thrasher S, Adelman S, Chang C-H. Hepatic cyst association with Peutz–Jeghers syndrome. Arch Pathol Lab Med 1990; 114: 1278–1280

457. Byrne W J, Forkalsrud E W. Congenital solitary nonparasitic cyst of the liver: a rare cause of a rapidly enlarging abdominal mass in infancy. J Pediatr Surg 1982; 17: 316–317

458. Morgenstern L. Rupture of solitary nonparasitic cyst of the liver. Ann Surg 1959; 150: 167–171

459. Sanfelippo P M, Beahrs D H, Weiland L H. Cystic disease of the liver. Ann Surg 1974; 179: 922–925

460. Sood S C, Watson A. Solitary cyst of the liver presenting as an abdominal emergency. Postgrad Med J 1974; 50: 48–50

461. Coutsoftides T, Hermann R E. Nonparasitic cysts of the liver. Surg Gynecol Obstet 1974; 138: 906–910

462. March J L, Dahms B, Longmire W P. Cystadenoma and cystadeno-carcinoma of the biliary system. Arch Surg 1974; 109: 41–43

463. Ayyash K, Haddad J. Spontaneous rupture of a solitary nonparasitic cyst of the liver. Acta Chir Scand 1988; 154: 241–243

464. Akriviadis E A, Steindel H, Ralls P, Redeker AG. Spontaneous rupture of nonparasitic cyst of the liver. Gastroenterology 1989; 97: 213–215

465. Shipley P, Bayles B, Hershfield N, Lui R, Wong N C W. Spontaneous rupture of a nonparasitic hepatic cyst associated with peritonitis. Can J Gastroenterol 1991; 5: 171–173

466. Dardik H, Glotzer P, Silver C. Congenital hepatic cyst causing jaundice. Ann Surg 1964; 159: 585–592

467. Santman F W, Thigs L G, Van der Veen E A, den Otter G, Blok P. Intermittent jaundice: a rare complication of a solitary nonparasitic liver cyst. Gastroenterology 1977; 72: 325–328

468. Morin M E, Baker D A, Vanagunas A, Tass A, Sue H K. Solitary nonparasitic hepatic cyst causing obstructive jaundice. Am J Gastroenterology 1980; 73: 434–436

469. Clinkscales N B, Trigg L P, Poklepvovic J. Obstructive jaundice secondary to benign hepatic cyst. Radiology 1985; 154: 643–644

470. Cappell M S. Obstructive jaundice from benign nonparasitic hepatic cysts: identification of risk factors and percutaneous aspiration for diagnosis and treatment. Am J Gastroenterol 1988; 83: 93–96

471. Deziel D J, Rossi R J, Munson J L, Braasch J W, Silverman M L. Management of bile duct cysts in adults. Arch Surg 1986; 121: 410–415

472. Bean W J, Rodan B A. Hepatic cysts: treatment with alcohol. Am J Roentgenol 1985; 144: 237–241

473. Furuta T, Yoshida Y, Saku M et al. Treatment of symptomatic non-parasitic liver cysts — surgical treatment versus alcohol injection therapy. HPB Surgery 1990; 2: 269–279

474. Lingenfelser T, Overkamp D, Koveker G, Lauchart W. Giant, symptomatic nonparasitic hepatic cyst: successful treatment with aspiration and sclerotherapy. Eur J Gastroenterol Hepatol 1992; 4: 465–466

475. Hagiwara H, Kasahara A, Hayashi N et al. Successful treatment of a hepatic cyst by one-shot instillation of minocycline chloride. Gastroenterology 1992; 103: 675–677

476. Enterline D S, Rauch R E, Silverman P M, Korofkin M, Adwan O E. Cyst of the falciform ligament of the liver. Am J Roentgenol 1984; 142: 327–328

477. Brock J S, Pachter H L, Schreiber J, Hofstetter S R. Surgical diseases of the falciform ligament. Am J Gastroenterol 1992; 67: 757–758

478. Wheeler D A, Edmondson H A. Ciliated hepatic foregut cyst. Am J Surg Pathol 1984; 8: 467–470

479. Huguier M, Cherqui D, Houry S, Roland J, Lacaline F. Kystes biliaires du foie. Presse Med 1966; 15: 827–829

480. Kashima S, Asanuma Y, Nwa M, Koyama K. A case of true hepatic cyst with malignant change. Acta Hepatol Jpn 1988; 29: 1265–1268

481. Greenwood N, Orr W McN. Primary squamous-cell carcinoma arising in a solitary nonparasitic cyst of the liver. J Pathol 1972; 107: 145–148

482. Bloustein P A, Silverberg S G. Squamous cell carcinoma originating in a hepatic cyst: case report with a review of the hepatic cyst–carcinoma association. Cancer 1976; 38: 2002–2005

483. Pliskin A, Cualing H, Stenger R J. Primary squamous cell carcinoma originating in congenital cysts of the liver. Arch Pathol Lab Med 1992; 116: 105–107

484. Ueyama T, Ding J, Hashimoto H, Tsneyoshi M, Enjoji M. Carcinoid tumor arising in the wall of a congenital bile duct cyst. Arch Pathol Lab Med 1992; 116: 291–293

485. Reye R D K, Morgan G, Baral J. Encephalopathy and fatty degeneration of the viscera, a disease entity in childhood. Lancet 1963; 2: 749–752

486. Crocker J F S. Reye's syndrome. Semin Live Dis 1982; 2: 340–352

487. Varma R R, Riedel D R, Komorowski R A, Harrington G J, Norwak T V. Reye's syndrome in nonpediatric age groups. JAMA 1979; 242: 1373–1375

488. Stillman A, Gitter H, Shillington D et al. Reye's syndrome in the adult: case report and review of the literature. Am J Gastroenterol 1983; 78: 365–368

489. Becroft D M O. Syndrome of encephalopathy and fatty degeneration of viscera in New Zealand children. Br Med J 1966; 2: 135–140

490. Bove K E, McAdams A J, Partin J C, Partin J S, Hug G, Schubert W K. The hepatic lesion in Reye's syndrome. Gastroenterology 1975; 69: 605–697

491. Brown R E, Ishak K G. Hepatic zonal degeneration and necrosis in Reye syndrome. Arch Pathol Lab Med 1976; 100: 123–126

492. Benz M S, Cohen C. Periportal necrosis in Reye's syndrome: one case in a review of eight patients. Am J Gastroenterol 1980; 73: 49–53

493. Ellis G H, Mirkin D, Mills M C. Pancreatitis and Reye's syndrome. Am J Dis Child 1979; 133: 1014–1016

494. Phillips M J, Poucell S, Patterson J, Valencia P. The liver. An atlas and text of ultrastructural pathology. New York: Raven Press, 1987

495. Partin J C, Schubert W K, Partin J S. Mitochondrial ultrastructure in Reye's syndrome (encephalopathy and fatty degeneration of the viscera). N Engl J Med 1971; 285: 1339–1343

496. Bradel E J, Reiner C B. The fine structure of hepatocytes in Reye's syndrome. In: Pollack J D, ed. Reye's syndrome. New York: Grune & Stratton, 1975: pp 147–158

497. De Vivo D C. Do animals develop Reye syndrome? Lab Invest 1984; 51: 367–372

498. Zimmerman H J, Ishak K G. Valproate-induced hepatic injury: analyses of 23 fatal cases. Hepatology 1982; 2: 591–597

499. Temple A R. Pathophysiology of aspirin overdosage toxicity, with implications for management. Pediatrics Suppl 1978; 62: 873–876

500. Baboolal R, Monaghan H, Ward O C. Reye's syndrome in a boy treated with salicylates for Reiter's disease. Irish Med J 1986; 79: 289–291

501. Starko K M, Ray C G, Dominguez L B, Stromberg W L, Woodall D F. Reye's syndrome and salicylate use. Pediatrics 1980; 66: 859–864

502. Casteels-Van Daele M. Reye syndrome or side-effects of anti-emetics? Eur J Pediatr 1990; 150: 456–459

503. Waldman R J, Hall W N, McGee H et al. Aspirin as a risk factor in Reye's syndrome. JAMA 1982; 247: 3089–3094

504. Halpin T J, Hultzhauer M S, Campbell J R et al. Reye's syndrome and medication use. JAMA 1982; 248: 687–691

505. Surgeon General's advisory on the use of salicylates and Reye's syndrome. MMWR 1982; 31: 289–290

506. Hurwitz E S, Barrett M J, Bregman D et al. Public Health Service study on Reye's syndrome and medications: report of the pilot phase. N Engl J Med 1985; 313: 849–857

507. Hurwitz E S, Barrett M J, Bergman D et al. Public Health Service study of Reye's syndrome and medications: report of the main study. JAMA 1987; 257: 1905–1911

508. Barrett M J, Hurwitz E S, Schonberger L B et al. Changing epidemiology of Reye syndrome in the United States. Pediatrics 1986; 77: 598–602

509. Greene C L, Blitzer M G, Shapira E. Inborn errors of metabolism and Reye syndrome: differential diagnosis. J Pediatr 1988; 113: 156–159

510. Rowe P C, Valle D, Brusilow S W. Changing trends of inborn errors in Reye's syndrome: rarity is relative. JAMA 1988; 260: 3167–3170

511. Elpeleg O N, Christensen E, Hurvitz H, Branski D. Recurrent, familial Reye-like syndrome with a new complex amino and organic aciduria. Eur J Pediatr 1990; 149: 709–712

512. Hancock L, Henry D A, Sanson-Fisher R W. Aspirin use in children: heeding the warning. Newcastle, New South Wales. Aust J Publ Hlth 1992; 16: 35–37

513. Hug G, Bosken J, Bove K, Linnemann C C, McAdams L. Reye's syndrome simulacra in liver of mice after treatment with chemical agents and encephalomyocarditis virus. Lab Invest 1981; 45: 89–109

514. Davis L E, Cole L L, Lockwood S J, Kornfeld M. Experimental influenza B virus toxicity in mice. Lab Invest 1983; 48: 140–147

515. Sakaida N, Senzaki H, Shikata N. Microvesicular fatty liver in rats resembling Reye's syndrome induced by 4-pentanoic acid. Acta Pathol Jpn 1990; 40: 633–642

516. Brownstein D G, Johnson E A, Smith A L. Spontaneous Reye's-like syndrome in BALB/c ByJ mice. Lab Invest 1984; 51: 386–395

517. Kawasaki T. Acute febrile mucocutaneous syndrome with lymphoid involvement with specific desquamation of the fingers and toes in children. Arerugi 1967; 16: 178–222

518. Kawasaki T, Kosaki F, Okawa S, Shigematsu I, Yamagawa H. A new infantile acute febrile mucocutaneous lymph node syndrome (MLNS) prevailing in Japan. Pediatrics 1974; 54: 273–276

519. Kato H, Koike S, Yamamoto M, Ito Y, Yano E. Coronary aneurysms in infants and young children with acute febrile mucocutaneous lymph node syndrome. J Pediatr 1975; 86: 892–898

520. Darby C P, Kyong C V. Mucocutaneous lymph node-syndrome. JAMA 1976; 236: 2295–2297

521. Melish M E, Hicks R M, Larson E J. Mucocutaneous lymph node syndrome in the United States. Am J Dis Child 1976; 130: 599–607

522. Morens D M, O'Brien R J. Kawasaki disease in the United States. J Infect Dis 1978; 137: 91–93

523. Melish M E. Kawasaki syndrome (the mucocutaneous lymph node syndrome). Ann Rev Med 1982; 33: 569–585

524. Melish M E, Hicks R V. Kawasaki syndrome clinical features, pathophysiology, etiology and therapy. J Rheumatol 1990; Suppl 24: 2–8

525. Levy M, Koren G. Atypical Kawasaki disease; analysis of clinical presentation and diagnostic clues. Pediatr Infect Dis J 1990; 9: 122–126

526. Nakamura Y, Yanagawa H, Kawasaki T. Mortality among children with Kawasaki disease in Japan. N Engl J Med 1992; 326: 1246–1249

527. Nakamura Y, Fujita J, Nagai M et al. Cardiac sequelae of Kawasaki disease in Japan: statistical analysis. Pediatrics 1991; 88: 1144–1149

528. Shylman S T, McAuley J B, Pachman L M, Miller M L, Ruschhaupt D G. Epidemiology of Kawasaki syndrome in an urban U.S. area with a small Asian population. Am J Dis Child 1987; 141: 420–425

529. Akaji T, Kato H, Inoue O, Sato N, Imamura K. Valvular heart disease in Kawasaki syndrome: incidence and natural history. Am Heart J 1990; 120: 366–372

530. Suddleson E A, Reid B, Woolley M M, Takahashi M. Hydrops of the gallbladder associated with Kawasaki syndrome. J Pediatr Surg 1987; 22: 956–959

531. Newburger J W, Takahashi M, Burns J C et al. The treatment of Kawasaki syndrome with intravenous gamma-globulin. N Engl J Med 1986; 315: 341–347

532. Choi C P T, Sharma B. Gallbladder hydrops in mucocutaneous lymph node syndrome. South Med J 1989; 82: 397–398

533. Luzzatto C, Chiesura-Corona M, Zancan L, Guglielmi M. Obstructive jaundice in Kawasaki disease. Z Kinderchir 1990; 45: 50–51

534. Burns J C, Mason W H, Glode M P et al. Clinical and epidemiologic characteristics of patients referred for evaluation of possible Kawasaki disease. J Pediatr 1990; 118: 680–686

535. Amano S, Hazama F, Kubagawa H, Tasaka K, Haebara H, Hamashima Y. General pathology of Kawasaki disease. Acta Pathol Jpn 1980; 30: 681–694

536. Marks W H, Coran A G, Wesley J R, et al. Hepatic artery aneurysm associated with the mucocutaneous lymph node syndrome. Surgery 1985; 98: 598–601

537. Edwards K M, Glick A D, Greene H L. Intrahepatic cholangitis associated with mucocutaneous lymph node syndrome. J Pediatr Gastroenterol Nutr 1985; 4: 140–142

538. Ohshio G, Furukawa F, Fujiwara H, Hamashima Y. Hepatomegaly and splenomegaly in Kawasaki disease. Pediatr Pathol 1985; 4: 257–264

539. Wong M L, Kaplan S, Dunkle L M, Stechenberg B W, Feigin RD. Leptospirosis: a childhood disease. J Pediatr 1977; 90: 532–537

540. Bergeson P S, Serlin S P, Corman L I. Mucocutaneous lymph-node syndrome with positive Weil–Felix reaction but negative leptospira studies. Lancet 1978; i: 720–721

541. Yanagisawa M, Kobayashi N, Matsuya S. Myocardial infarction following acute febrile mucocutaneous lymph node syndrome (MLNS) in an infant. Pediatrics 1974; 54: 277–281

542. Ahlström H, Lundström N, Mortensson W, Östberg G, Lantorp K. Infantile periarteritis nodosa or mucocutaneous lymph node syndrome. Acta Paediatr Scand 1977; 66: 193–198

543. Furusho K, Kamiya T, Nakano H et al. High dose intravenous gammaglobulin for Kawasaki disease. Lancet 1984; ii: 1055–1058

544. Furusho K, Ohba T, Soeda T et al. Possible role for mite antigen in Kawasaki disease [letter]. Lancet 1981; ii: 194–195

545. Kato H, Fujimoto T, Inoue O et al. Variant strain of Propionobacterium acnes; a clue to the aetiology of Kawasaki disease. Lancet 1983; ii: 1383–1388

546. Shulman S T, Rawley A H. Does Kawasaki disease have a retroviral aetiology? Lancet 1986; ii: 545–546

547. Kikuta H, Taguchi Y, Tomizawa K et al. Epstein–Barr virus genome-positive T-lymphocytes in a boy with chronic active EBV infection associated with Kawasaki-like disease. Nature 1988; 333: 455–457

548. Whitby D, Hoad J G, Tizard E J et al. Isolation of measles virus from child with Kawasaki disease. Lancet 1991; 338: 1215

549. Writing Group of the Histiocyts Society. Histiocytosis syndromes in children. Lancet 1987; i: 208–209

550. Lichtenstein L. Histiocytosis X integration of eosinophilic granuloma of bone, Letterer–Siwe disease, and Schuller–Christian disease as related manifestations of a single nosologic entity, Arch Pathol 1953; 56: 86–102

551. Nezelof C, Basset F, Rousseau M F. Histiocytosis X; histogenetic arguments of a Langerhans cell origin. Biomed 1973; 18: 365–371

552. Egeler R M, Nesbit M E. In: Voute P A, Barrett A, Lemerle J, eds. Current concepts and treatment of Langerhans cells histiocytes. Cancer in children: clinical management, 3rd edn. Heidelberg: Springer-Verlag, 1992: pp 162–172

553. Risdall R J, Dehner L P, Duray P, Kobrinsky N, Robison L, Nesbit M E. Histiocytosis X (Langerhans' cell histiocytosis): prognostic role of histopathology. Arch Pathol Lab Med 1983; 107: 59–63

554. Van Heerde P, Egeler R M. The cytology of Langerhans cell histiocytosis (histiocytosis X). Cytopathology 1991; 2: 149–158

555. Engelbreth-Holm J, Tulin G, Christensen E. Eosinophilic granuloma of bone–Schuller–Christian disease. Acta Med Scand 1984; 118: 292–318

556. Jurco S, Starling K, Hawkins E P. Malignant histiocytosis in childhood: Morphologic considerations. Hum Pathol 1983; 14: 1059–1065

557. Grundy P, Ellis R. Histiocytosis X: a review of the etiology, pathology, staging and therapy. Med Pediatr Oncol 1986; 14: 664–671

558. Von Essen S, West W, Sitorius M, Rennard S I. Complete resolution of roentgenographic changes in a patient with pulmonary histiocytosis X. Chest 1990; 98: 765–767

559. Aguayo S M, King T E Jr, Waldron J A Jr, Sherritt K M, Kane M A, Miller Y E. Increased pulmonary neuroendocrine cells with

bombesin-like immunoreactivity in adult patients with eosinophilic granuloma. J Clin Invest 1990; 86: 838–844

560. Lahey M E. Prognosis in reticuloendotheliosis in children. J Pediatr 1962; 60: 664–671

561. Nezelof C, Frileux-Herbet F, Cronier-Sachet J. Disseminated histiocytosis X: analysis of prognostic factors based on a retrospective study of 50 cases. Cancer 1979; 44: 1824–1838

562. Raney R B, D'Angio G J. Langerhans' cell histiocytosis (histiocytosis X); experience at the Children's Hospital of Philadelphia, 1970–1984. Med Pediatr Oncol 1989; 17: 20–28

563. Nesbit M E. Current concepts and treatment of histiocytosis X (Langerhans' cell histiocytosis). In: Voute P A, Barret A, Bloom H J G, Lamerle J, Neidhardt M K, eds. Cancer in children, 2nd edn. New York: Springer, 1986: 1: 176–184

564. Le Blanc A, Hadchouel M, Jehan D, Odievre M, Alagille D. Obstructive jaundice in children with histiocytosis X. Gastroenterology 1981; 80: 134–139

565. Sharp H L, White J G, Krivit W. 'Histiocytosis X' treated with vinblastine sulfate (NSC-4942). Cancer Chemother Rep 1964; 39: 53–59

566. Thompson H H, Pitt H A, Lewin K J, Longmire W P Jr. Sclerosing cholangitis and histiocytosis X. Gut 1984; 25: 526–530

567. Pirovino M, Jeanneret C, Lang R H, Lusier J, Bianch L, Spichtin H. Liver cirrhosis in histiocytosis X. Liver 1988; 8: 293–298

568. Iwai M, Kashewadani M, Okuno T, Takino T, Koshikawa T. Cholestatic liver disease in a 20 year old woman with histiocytosis X. Am J Gastroenterol 1988; 83: 164–168

569. Heyn R M, Hamoudi A, Newton W A Jr. Pretreatment liver biopsy in 20 children with histiocytosis X: a clinicopathologic correlation. Med Pediatr Oncol 1990; 18: 110–118

570. Favara B E. The pathology of 'histiocytosis'. Am J Pediatr Hematol Oncol 1981; 3: 45–56

571. Favara B E, McCarthy R C, Meirau G W. Histiocytosis X. Hum Pathol 1983; 14: 663–676

572. Lee R G, Braziel R M, Stenzel P. Gastrointestinal involvement in Langerhans cell histiocytosis (histiocytosis X): diagnosis by rectal biopsy. Mod Pathol 1990; 3: 154–157

573. Steiber A C, Sever C, Starzl T E. Liver transplantation in patients with Langerhans cell histiocytosis. Transplantation 1990; 50: 338–340

574. Mahmond H, Gaber O, Wang W et al. Successful orthotopic liver transplantation in a child with Langerhans cell histiocytosis. Transplantation 1991; 51: 278–280

575. Concepcion W, Esquivel C O, Terry A et al. Liver transplantation in Langerhans cell histiocytosis (histiocytosis X). Semin Oncol 1991; 18: 24–28

576. Koto A, Morecki R, Santorineou M. Congenital hemophagocytic reticulosis. Am J Clin Pathol 1976; 65: 495–503

577. Hsu T S, Komp D M. Clinical features of familial histiocytosis. Am J Pediatr Hematol Oncol 1981; 3: 61–65

578. Janker G E. Familial hemophagocytic lymphohistiocytosis. Eur J Pediatr 1983; 140: 221–230

579. Favara B E. Hemophagocytic lymphohistiocytosis: a hemophagocytic syndrome. Semin Diagn Pathol 1992; 9: 63–74

580. Risdall R J, McKenna R W, Nesbit M E et al. Virus-associated hemophagocytic syndrome: a benign histiocytic proliferation distinct from malignant histiocytosis. Cancer 1979; 44: 993–1002

581. Woda B A, Sullivan J L. Reactive histiocytic disorders. Am J Clin Pathol 1993; 99: 459–463

582. Tsui W M S, Wong K F, Tse C C H. Liver changes in reactive haemophagocytic syndrome. Liver 1992; 12: 363–367

583. Rosai J, Dorfman R F. Sinus histiocytosis with massive lymphadenopathy: a newly recognized benign clinicopathological entity. Arch Pathol 1969; 87: 63–70

584. Foucar E, Rosai J, Dorfman R. Sinus histiocytosis with massive lymphadenopathy (Rosai–Dorfman disease): review of the entity. Semin Diag Pathol 1990; 7: 19–73

585. Eisen R N, Buckley P J, Rosai J. Immunophenotypic characterization of sinus histiocytosis with massive lymphadenopathy (Rosai–Dorfman disease). Semin Diag Pathol 1990; 7: 74–82

586. Turner R R, Colby T V, Wood G S, Horning S J, Beckstead J H, Warnke R A. Histiocytic malignancies: morphologic, immunologic, and enzymatic heterogeneity. Am J Surg Pathol 1984; 8: 485–500

587. Delsol G, Al Saati T, Gatter K C et al. Coexpression of epithelial membrane antigen (EMA), Ki-1, and interleukin-2 receptor by anaplastic large cell lymphomas: diagnostic value in so-called malignant histiocytosis. Am J Pathol 1988; 130: 59–70

588. Wilson M S, Weiss L M, Gatter K C et al. Malignant histiocytosis: a reassessment of cases previously reported in 1975 based on paraffin section immunophenotyping studies. Cancer 1990; 66: 530–536

589. Oka K, Mori N, Yatabe Y, Kojima M. Malignant histiocytosis: a report of three cases. Arch Pathol Lab Med 1992; 116: 1228–1233

590. Nezelof C, Barbey S, Gogusen J, Terrier-Lacombe M-J. Malignant histiocytosis in childhood: a distinctive CD30-positive clinicopathological entity associated with a chromosomal translocation involving 5q35. Semin Diag Pathol 1992; 9: 75–89

591. Colby T V, La Brecque D R. Lymphoreticular malignancy presenting as fulminant hepatic disease. Gastroenterology 1982; 82: 339–345

592. Jurco S, Starling K, Hawkins E P. Malignant histiocytosis in childhood: morphologic considerations. Hum Pathol 1985; 14: 1059–1065

593. Ducatman B S, Wick M R, Morgan T W, Banks P M, Pierre R V. Malignant histiocytosis: a clinical, histologic, and immunohistochemical study of 20 cases. Hum Pathol 1984; 15: 368–377

594. Beaugrand M, Trinchet J C, Callard P, Ferrier J P. Malignant histiocytosis presenting as a fulminant hepatic disease. Gastroenterology 1983; 84: 447–448

595. Ruchelli E D, Uri A, Dimmick J E et al. Severe perinatal liver disease and Down syndrome: an apparent relationship. Hum Pathol 1991; 22: 1274–1280

596. Tsuda T, Komiyama A, Aonuma K, Akabane T, Nakayama M. Transient abnormal myelopoiesis and diffuse hepatic necrosis in Down's syndrome with bleeding diathesis. Acta Paediatr Scand 1990; 79: 241–244

597. Becroft D M O, Zwi J. Perinatal visceral fibrosis accompanying the megakaryoblastic leukemoid reaction of Down syndrome. Pediatr Pathol 1990; 10: 397–406

598. Gilson J P, Bendon R W. Megakaryocytosis of the liver in a trisomy 21 stillbirth. Arch Pathol Lab Med 1993; 117: 738–739

599. Colsky J, Greenspan E M, Warren T N. Hepatic fibrosis in children with acute leukemia after therapy with folic acid antagonists. Arch Pathol 1955; 59: 198–206

600. Locasciulli A, Vergani G M, Uderzo C et al. Chronic liver disease in children with leukemia in long-term remission. Cancer 1983; 52: 1080–1087

601. Schwartz J B, Shamsuddin A M. The effects of leukemic infiltrates in various organs in chronic lymphocytic leukemia. Hum Pathol 1981; 12: 432–440

602. Mikel J J, Owen G, Lewis I J. Hepatic fibrosis in juvenile chronic granulocytic leukemia: an unusual finding in three cases. Pediatr Pathol 1990; 10: 385–395

4

Metabolic errors and liver disease

K. G. Ishak   H. L. Sharp

Disorders of porphyrin metabolism
Acute intermittent porphyria and porphyria cutanea tarda
Erythropoietic protoporphyria

Disorders of carbohydrate metabolism and related conditions
Glycogen storage diseases
Galactosaemia
Hereditary fructose intolerance
Myoclonus epilepsy with Lafora bodies (Lafora's disease)

Disorders of glycoprotein and protein metabolism
Mucopolysaccharidoses
Aspartylglucosaminuria
Mannosidosis
Fucosidosis
Mucolipidoses

Endoplasmic reticulum storage diseases
α_1-Antitrypsin deficiency
α_1-Antichymotrypsin deficiency
Afibrinogenaemia and hypofibrinogenaemia
Antithrombin III deficiency

Disorders of amino acid metabolism
Tyrosinaemia (hereditary tyrosinaemia, tyrosinaemia type I)
Congenital hyperammonaemia syndromes and urea cycle disorders
Cystinosis
Cystathionine β-synthase deficiency (homocystinuria)

Disorders of lipoprotein and lipid metabolism
Beta lipoprotein deficiency
Familial high density lipoprotein deficiency (Tangier disease)
Familial hypercholesterolaemia
Familial hyperlipoproteinaemias

GM_1 gangliosidosis
GM_2 gangliosidoses
Glycosphingolipid lipidosis (Fabry's disease)
Sulphatide lipidosis (metachromatic leucodystrophy)
Glycosylceramide lipidosis (Gaucher's disease)
Sphingomyelin-cholesterol lipidosis (Niemann–Pick disease)
Wolman's and cholesterol ester storage diseases
Cerebrotendinous xanthomatosis
Fatty acid oxidation disorders
Ceramidase deficiency (Farber's lipogranulomatosis)

Peroxisomal disorders
Primary hyperoxaluria
Disorders of peroxisomal beta oxidation

Mitochondrial cytopathies

Diseases of metal metabolism
Wilson's disease (hepatolenticular degeneration)

Miscellaneous disorders
Chronic granulomatous disease
Cystic fibrosis of the pancreas
Shwachman's syndrome
Alpers' disease
Aarskog's syndrome
Congenital total lipodystrophy
Familial hepatosteatosis
Leprechaunism (Donohue's syndrome)
Albinism

123

Over 400 inherited metabolic diseases have been described, most having immediate or eventual relevance to the liver. For example, liver histology is usually normal in primary hyperoxaluria while the kidneys and other organs may be irreparably damaged; however, despite medical management, dialysis, and repetitive kidney transplants, cure is only obtained with a liver transplant.[1] In other inherited disorders, the liver disease is often asymptomatic until precipitous acute liver failure develops. The classic example is Wilson's disease, in which again the only cure is liver transplantation.[2] In this instance, the screening of family members will prevent those affected from developing further liver injury by the utilization of a number of medical therapies. In many instances, the clinical diagnosis of an inherited disorder may not be evident and thus, diagnosis becomes the responsibility of the histopathologist, who may save not only the life of the patient but that of other family members. Pertinent examples are Reye's syndrome and the sudden infant death syndrome which simulate many disorders, including those that affect the urea cycle or beta oxidation of fatty acids.[3,4] Since the last edition of this book, both medical therapy and transplantation procedures have altered the natural course of many inherited disorders, and by the time the next edition is published, somatic gene therapy may no longer be experimental.

The advanced techniques now required for precision in the study of inherited diseases are summarized in the latest edition of *The Metabolic Basis of Inherited Disease*,[5] and screening has been reviewed in two recent chapters.[6,7] Along with mapping the chromosome of the gene defect, DNA probes and restriction fragment length polymorphism (RFLP) techniques can now not only identify the various types of diseases that have been described clinically, but are also beginning to explain the variability within a single clinical type that enzyme analysis could not previously distinguish.

The effect of the inherited metabolic disorders on the liver may be considered *primary*, i.e. due to the accumulation of a metabolite resulting from an enzyme defect (e.g. sphingomyelin in Niemann–Pick disease), or *secondary*, when the major changes are the result of the extrahepatic manifestations or complications (e.g. fatty change of the liver secondary to pancreatic insufficiency in Schwachman's syndrome).

Unfortunately, many metabolic disorders of divers aetiologies manifest similar morphological findings. Thus, fat accumulation in the hepatocyte is one of the most frequent abnormalities, either alone (e.g. in the urea cycle disorders, homocystinuria, lipoprotein disorders, Refsum's disease, primary carnitine deficiency and Schwachman's syndrome) or in combination with other changes such as cholestasis, pesudoglandular transformation and fibrosis (e.g. in galactosaemia, tyrosinaemia and hereditary fructose intolerance). Furthermore, neutral lipid may be stored in combination with other metabolites such as cholesterol (e.g.

in Wolman's disease, cholesterol ester storage disease) or glycogen (e.g. in type I glycogenosis). While most of the disorders of lipid metabolism are expressed morphologically by 'foam' cells (e.g. in Niemann–Pick disease and the gangliosidoses),[8] the ultimate diagnosis is dependent on the clinical and laboratory data and identification of the specific enzyme defect. The ultrastructural features of some of the disorders of lipid metabolism are distinctive but require experience in their interpretation. Some diseases show no or minimal light microscopic changes yet may demonstrate highly characteristic if not pathognomonic ultrastructural features (e.g. Wilson's disease, Chediak–Higashi syndrome, cerebrotendinous xanthomatosis). In occasional diseases, such as erythropoietic protoporphyria, α_1-antitrypsin deficiency, type IV glycogenosis and cystic fibrosis, both the light and electron microscopical changes are highly characteristic.

Disappointingly, the pathogenesis of hepatic disease in inherited disorders remains poorly understood. It is assumed that the cause of progressive injury results from 'storage' of a particular substance (e.g. copper, cholesterol, protoporphyrin). End-stage liver disease may be manifested by hepatic failure, the complications of portal hypertension, or both. Portal hypertension may be the consequence of established cirrhosis (e.g. in galactosaemia, type IV glycogenosis, Wilson's disease and haemochromatosis), or the result of severe intra-acinar ('pericellular') fibrosis in the absence of a true cirrhosis (e.g. in Gaucher's disease).

The histopathologist has at his disposal many special stains and techniques, both at the light microscopic and ultrastructural level. The best all-round fixative for light microscopy is 10% buffered formalin, but some metabolic diseases (e.g. the mucopolysaccharidoses, cystinosis and the glycogenoses) may require special fixatives to prevent leaching of the metabolites that are water soluble. Special stains for lipid, cholesterol and sphingomyelin (e.g. oil red O, Schultz modification of the Lieberman–Burchard reaction, Baker's acid haematin with pyridine extraction) must be performed on frozen sections cut from formalin-fixed or fresh material since routine processing will extract the lipid material from the cells. Familiarity is required with the many special stains that can be used on formalin-fixed and routinely processed material for the demonstration of uroporphyrin, haemosiderin, copper, bile, 'lipofuscin', lipomelanin (the pigment in the Dubin–Johnson syndrome), carbohydrates, mucopolysaccharides and other substances that need to be identified. Special microscopy should be utilized whenever necessary. The porphyrins can be demonstrated by their autofluorescence in frozen sections made from unfixed hepatic biopsy or autopsy material. Polarizing microscopy is especially useful for the identification of various crystals such as cholesterol, cystine, calcium oxalate, uroporphyrin and protoporphyrin.

Immunohistochemical stains are useful in a limited number of diseases, for example in the identification of catalase, α_1-antitrypsin, α_1-antichymotrypsin and fibrinogen, and in patients with peroxisomal diseases. Recently, a monoclonal antibody to the PiZ gene of α_1-antitrypsin deficiency was used to distinguish PiZ gene carriers from other subjects in the absence of serum protein analysis.[9]

Transmission electron microscopy is very important in the diagnosis of many inherited metabolic diseases.[10–12] According to Phillips et al,[12] the findings are diagnostic in α_1-antitrypsin deficiency, Farber's disease, glycogenoses types II and IV, hereditary fructose intolerance, Gaucher's disease, metachromatic leucodystrophy, gangliosidosis type I, Tay–Sachs disease, the Dubin–Johnson syndrome, erthropoietic protoporphyria, Wilson's disease, Zellweger's syndrome and infantile Refsum's disease. In other disorders, electron microscopy, although not diagnostic, can help to categorize the disease (e.g. as a glycogenosis, phospholipidosis, or oligosaccharidosis) or to suggest the correct diagnosis (e.g. Rotor's disease, arteriohepatic dysplasia, cholesterol ester storage disease). The role of scanning electron microscopy is much more limited.[13]

DISORDERS OF PORPHYRIN METABOLISM

The porphyrias are disorders of the biosynthesis of porphyrins and haem. The majority are inherited in an autosomal dominant pattern, with the possible exception of porphyria cutanea tarda, which can be acquired. They are usually divided into hepatic and erythropoietic types, depending on the major site where the error of metabolism expresses itself by increased accumulation of porphyrins and their precursors. While only liver injury is discussed in this chapter, all the porphyrias are listed in Table 4.1, together with their salient clinical manifestations, principal biochemical abnormalities, and enzyme defects. The

clinical, biochemical, diagnostic and therapeutic aspects of the porphyrias have been extensively reviewed.[14–17] All the hepatic porphyrias are characterized by neurological lesions leading to severe colicky abdominal pain, constipation, peripheral neuropathy and neuropsychiatric attacks. These are frequently precipitated by drugs such as barbiturates, oestrogens, oral contraceptives, griseofulvin and alcohol.[18] All the porphyrias, except acute intermittent porphyria, are also associated with photosensitivity. The symptoms include itching and burning or stinging of the skin exposed to sunlight. This is followed by erythema and oedema, with bullous lesions in porphyria cutanea tarda and erythropoietic porphyria. Chronic changes include milia, hirsutism, areas of hyperpigmentation or depigmentation and thickening and scarring of the skin. The diagnosis rests upon the demonstration of increased amounts of the porphyrins or their precursors in the urine, faeces and/or blood and is confirmed by the appropriate enzyme assay.

ACUTE INTERMITTENT PORPHYRIA (AIP) AND PORPHYRIA CUTANEA TARDA (PCT)

Liver biopsy specimens from 7 patients with PCT and 4 with AIP were studied cytochemically and ultrastructurally by Biempica et al.[19] The changes were similar in both diseases, but the damage was more severe in patients with PCT. Comparable degrees of iron overload and fat deposition were present in all specimens regardless of the clinical severity of the disease. Mitochondria showed a wide range of abnormalities, but the most consistent finding was the presence of large electron-dense granules measuring up to $200\,\mu m$ in diameter. Autophagic vacuoles were more numerous than in normal human liver, and myelin-like figures were common. Lipofuscin bodies were large, increased in number and contained extensive ferritin

Table 4.1 The porphyrias

Disease classification	Symptoms	Inheritance	Porphyrin	Enzyme defect
Hepatic				
Acute intermittent porphyria	N	D	↑PBG & ALA in urine	Porphobilinogen deaminase in RBC, skin fibroblasts and amniotic cells
Variegate porphyria	N,S	D	↑Protoporphyrin and porphyrin–peptide complexes in faeces	Protoporphyrinogen oxidase
Hereditary coproporphyria	N,S	D	↑Coproporphyrin in urine and faeces	Coproporphyrinogen oxidase in leucocytes, lymphocytes, and fibroblasts
Porphyria cutanea tarda	S,H	D (in familial form)	↑Uroporphyrin & hepatocarboxylic porphyrin in urine	Uroporphyrinogen decarboxylase (in liver only in sporadic form)
Erythropoietic				
Congenital erythropoietic porphyria	S,A	R	↑Uroporphyrin I in urine and RBC	Uroporphyrinogen cosynthetase in PB, RBC and fibroblasts
Erythropoietic protoporphyria	S,H	D	↑Protoporphyrin IX in RBC, liver, faeces, plasma, and fibroblasts	Ferrochelatase in RBC

Abbreviations: N=neurological; S=skin; H=hepatic; A=anaemia; PBG=porphobilinogen; ALA= δ-aminolaevulinic acid; D=dominant; R=recessive; RBC=red blood cell; PB=peripheral blood deposits. Giant misshapen mitochondria containing fila-mentous material and showing decreased density of the matrix were reported in hepatocytes in AIP by Jean et al.[20] Needle-shaped cytoplasmic inclusions have been identified in liver cells by light, fluorescent and electron microscopy in biopsy specimens from patients with PCT; the crystals are also birefringent under polarizing light.[21-23] According to Cortes et al,[23] the inclusions are best seen by light microscopy in unstained paraffin sections. The crystals can be specifically stained in paraffin sections by the ferric ferri-cyanide reduction test (Fig. 4.1).[22] They have been induced experimentally in mice by iron overload.[24] Ultra-structurally, they reveal alternating areas of different electron density. The crystals may be a mixture of por-phyrinogens and porphyrins surrounding uroporphyrin crystals.[25]

Histopathological findings in liver biopsy specimens from patients with PCT have been described in several series.[23,26,27] They include fatty change, variable haemo-

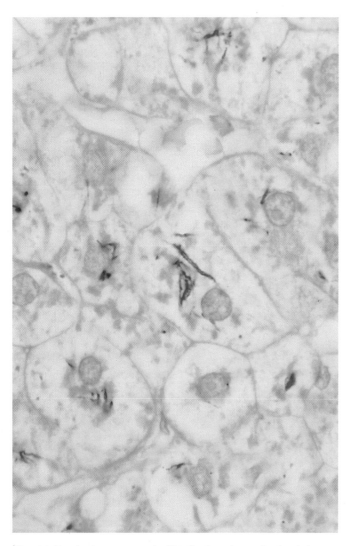

Fig. 4.1 Porphyria cutanea tarda. Needle-shaped crystals of varied length are present in the cytoplasm of liver cells. Ferric ferricyanide.

siderosis in periportal hepatocytes and fibrosis. Cortes et al[23] found periductal lymphoid aggregates in 43% of their cases. The incidence of cirrhosis in two series was 33% and 34%.[23,28] Factors related to an increased risk of hepatocellular carcinoma in PCT are a long symptomatic period before start of therapy, and the presence of chronic active hepatitis and/or advanced fibrosis or cirrhosis.[29] There appears to be a direct relationship between increasing age and extent of liver damage, with fibrosis present at a mean of 48 years, cirrhosis at 57 years and hepatocellular carcinoma at 66 years.[23] Hepatocellular carcinoma has been reported not only in association with PCT,[23,29,30] but also with AIP and variegate porphyria.[31-34] The possible role of alcohol and iron accumulation in hepatic disease in PCT was discussed by Turnbull et al[28] and by Bloomer.[14] A recently described pedigree study lends support to the hypothesis that a single allele for HLA-linked hereditary haemochromatosis is responsible for the hepatic siderosis in sporadic PCT.[35]

As already noted, experimental porphyria can be induced by iron overload alone.[25] There is a high incidence (40%, 57% and 70.7% in three series) of hepatitis B serological markers in PCT,[36-38] and hepatitis B is considered to play a pathogenetic role in the liver disease in this condition.[37,38] Recently, hepatitis C has emerged as an even more important cause of liver disease in PCT.[36,39] Of 74 Italian patients studied by Fargion et al,[36] hepatitis C virus antibodies were detected in 82% by recombinant immunoblot assay. Hepatitis C antibody was detected in 100% of patients with PCT who had chronic active hepatitis and in about 80% of other patients with chronic persistent hepatitis, fibrosis, or cirrhosis. In the series of 75 patients with PCT studied by Herrero et al,[39] 75% of patients with sporadic PCT but none of 5 patients with familial PCT were positive for antibodies to hepatitis C. These studies implicate hepatitis C as the main pathogenetic factor of liver disease in patients with PCT. Note should also be made of the occasional associa-tion of PCT with HIV infection.[40-42]

ERYTHROPOIETIC PROTOPORPHYRIA (EPP)

Macroscopically, the liver affected by EPP is generally black. The first description of the characteristic, if not pathognomonic, changes was published by Cripps & Scheuer.[43] Sections from percutaneous hepatic biopsy specimens from 5 patients showed focal accumulations of dense, dark brown pigment in canaliculi, interlobular bile ducts, connective tissue and Kupffer cells (Fig. 4.2). The pigment had an intense red autofluorescence in frozen sections examined by fluorescence microscopy with an iodine tungsten quartz light source. Two of the patients had portal and periportal fibrosis and, in one case, the portal areas were infiltrated by mononuclear cells. Cholelithiasis occurs in some patients with EPP, and the

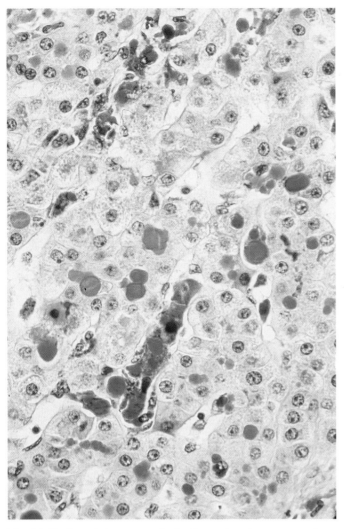

Fig. 4.2 Erythropoietic protoporphyria. Brown deposits are present in canaliculi, liver and Kupffer cells. H&E.

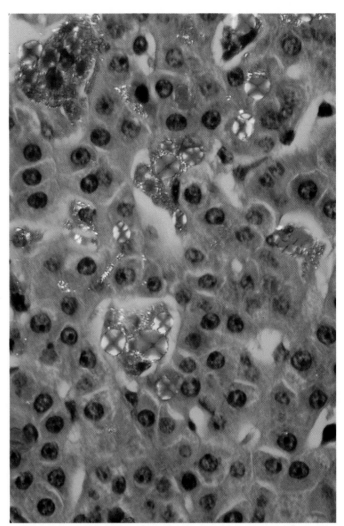

Fig. 4.3 Protoporphyrin deposits have a red to yellow birefringence with a maltese cross configuration. H&E.

calculi contain protoporphyrin.[43] Crystals isolated from the liver in one case of EPP had the same fluorescence spectrum as protoporphyrin.[44]

The deposits in canaliculi, bile ducts and Kupffer cells in EPP display bright red birefringence with a centrally-located dark maltese cross (Fig. 4.3).[45] Some of the larger deposits and most of the smaller ones in the cytoplasm of hepatocytes and Kupffer cells appear as clusters of brilliantly illuminated granules on polarizing microscopy.

Transmission electron microscopic studies by a number of investigators[12,45–50] have demonstrated that the deposits of protoporphyrin in EPP consist of numerous, slender, electron-dense crystals arranged singly in sheaves or in a 'star-burst' pattern (Fig. 4.4). The crystals are straight or slightly curved and are 43–646 nm in length and 6.1–22.0 nm in width. The crystalline accumulations in the cytoplasm of liver cells are not surrounded by a membrane, but in Kupffer cells they are intralysosomal.

Non-membrane-bound crystals of protoporphyrin have also been demonstrated in the cytoplasm of bile-duct cells.[51] The protoporphyrin casts in canaliculi are readily visualized by scanning electron microscopy (Fig. 4.5).

The liver disease in EPP may progress to cirrhosis, although the overall incidence of significant hepatic disease is probably small.[52–54] Cases of EPP with death from hepatic failure have been reviewed by several authors.[51,52,55–57] The youngest patient reported to date was an 11-year-old boy, described by Cripps et al.[55] Hepatic failure may be precipitated by viral infection (e.g. EBV),[58] or by alcohol. A direct toxic effect of protoporphyrin in the pathogenesis of liver disease in EPP is suggested by the experimental studies of Lee et al.[59] The occurrence of cirrhosis in two sisters with EPP raises also the possibility of a genetic predisposition for hepatic disease.[60] A unique association of two rare diseases, histiocytosis X and EPP, has been reported.[61]

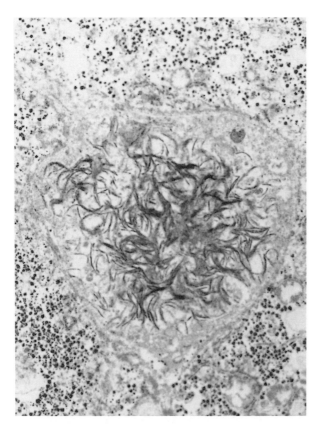

Fig. 4.4 Erythropoietic protoporphyria. Electron micrograph showing a mass of radiating, hair-like pigment crystals in a dilated canaliculus. × 1800. Courtesy of the late Dr G Klatskin

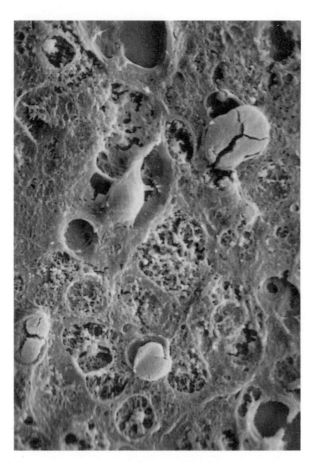

Fig. 4.5 Erythropoietic protoporphyria. Rounded protoporphyrin casts in canaliculi show fracture lines. Casts are solid and have a granular structure at higher magnifications. Hypertrophied Kupffer cell (upper left) probably contains phagocytosed protoporphyrin. Scanning electron micrograph, × 1250

DISORDERS OF CARBOHYDRATE METABOLISM AND RELATED CONDITIONS

GLYCOGEN STORAGE DISEASE (GSD) (Table 4.2)

The glycogenoses are inherited in an autosomal recessive manner, with the exception of one or two sex-linked subtypes of type IX.[62-64] Glycogen storage disease should be considered in any child presenting with hepatomegaly, hypoglycaemia, growth failure, excessive fat in the face and buttocks (doll-like appearance), hyperlipidaemia, and only mild serum transaminase elevations. The liver is always the most instructive organ to biopsy because variant subtypes may not involve other tissues, and standards for substrate and enzyme analysis often are better defined. As a screening procedure, a needle biopsy should at least be processed for light and electron microscopic study after a prolonged fast, if possible, i.e. without the patient developing severe hypoglycaemia. A portion of the specimen should be quick frozen for biochemical analysis. The ultrastructural appearance of types II and IV is virtually pathognomonic. If types Ib, VI, IX or X are being seriously considered, then arrangements should be made for fresh tissue analysis. For definitive subtype determination, biopsies of skeletal and/or cardiac muscle

Table 4.2 The hepatic glycogen storage diseases

Type	Enzyme defect	Affected tissues
Ia	Glucose-6-phosphatase	Liver, gastrointestinal mucosa, kidney
Ib	Glucose-6-phosphatase translocase-1	Liver, gastrointestinal mucosa, kidney, neutrophils
II	Lysosomal α-1,4-glucosidase (acid maltase)	Generalized
III	Amylo-1-6 glucosidase (debrancher enzyme)	Liver, muscle, leucocytes
IV	α-1,4-Glucan; α-1,4-glucan-6-glycosyl	Generalized
VI	Liver phosphorylase	Liver, leucocytes
IXa	Phosphorylase b kinase	Liver
IXb	Phosphorylase b kinase	Liver, muscle (?), leucocytes
IXc	Phosphorylase b kinase	Liver, muscle, leucocytes
X	Cyclic AMP dependent kinase	Liver, muscle

should be considered, particularly in types II, IV, and IX. Care should be taken to avoid extraneous contamination by starch from surgical glove powder.[65]

The hepatic light microscopic and ultrastructural

changes of the glycogenoses involving the liver are described together after the clinical and biochemical findings have been discussed.

Type I glycogen storage disease

Type Ia GSD (von Gierke's disease) results from the impairment of hepatic glucose production, either from glycogenolysis or gluconeogenesis secondary to the virtual absence of glucose-6-phosphatase activity.[66] Patients usually present during the first year of life with fasting hypoglycaemia and seizures, if the brain supply of lactate is inadequate. Metabolic acidosis and massive hepatomegaly are also present. Other symptoms include bleeding (usually epistaxis) related to platelet abnormalities. The kidneys are enlarged. Stunted growth is noticeable by 1 year of age,[67] along with the characteristic adiposity noted above.

Results of serum laboratory tests not already alluded to include abnormal hepatocellular enzyme levels, a normal bilirubin, elevations of cholesterol and triglyceride and later of uric acid.[68] Usually, the patient survives into adulthood if death does not occur in the first year of life. The adult complications include marked shortness of stature (50%), hepatomegaly, hepatocellular adenomas (33%), hepatocellular carcinoma (4–5%), osteoporosis, uric acid nephropathy or gout, glomerulonephritis, and amyloidosis.[69–80] Although hyperlipidaemia may persist and xanthomas have been reported, premature atherosclerosis is poorly documented.

In *type Ib GSD*, the enzyme is present on the inner surface of the endoplasmic reticulum, but a transmembrane transport protein, translocase 1, is defective. Consequently, the substrate glucose-6-phosphate cannot gain access to the enzyme.[81–84] Patients have a similar presentation to those with type Ia, and also endure complications related to neutropenia and neutrophil dysfunction.[85] Thus, they are predisposed to infections, including unique lesions of the gastrointestinal tract resembling those of Crohn's disease.[86–88]

Medical therapies for type I GSD include nasogastric drip feedings[89] or, more recently, uncooked cornstarch four to five times a day.[90] Granulocyte colony stimulating factor has altered the infectious course of type Ib patients.[91] Liver or liver–kidney transplants have been performed in adults primarily because of concern about the possible development of hepatocellular carcinoma or poor metabolic control.[76,78,92,93]

By mapping, the wild type gene for type I GSD is located on chromosome 17q23.[94] Prenatal diagnosis is possible.[95]

Type II glycogenosis (Pompe's disease)

Three varieties of the disease, with onset in infancy, childhood and adulthood, are known; the most severe is the infantile form.[96,97] The disease has been diagnosed before birth by electron microscopy of fresh amniotic fluid cells.[98] Infants present with hypotonia, firm skeletal musculature, respiratory distress, marked cardiomegaly and mild hepatomegaly. The disease is not accompanied by hypoglycaemia or hepatic dysfunction. Death usually results from respiratory or cardiac failure in the first year of life. Children who present with a muscular dystrophy-like disease have glycogen accumulation in muscle but not in the liver, though both organs are deficient in acid maltase.[99] Adults present with skeletal muscle weakness in the third to the fifth decades of life but do not show manifestations of hepatic or cardiac involvement.[100–102] While acid maltase activity is absent in muscle in the infantile and adult forms, neutral maltase is only reduced in the former.

Vacuolated lymphocytes are found in the peripheral blood and bone marrow. All organs show vacuolated cells due to enlarged lysosomes containing glycogen. In liver cells, the vacuoles are particularly prominent in autopsy material as a result of the disappearance of extralysosomal glycogen.[103] Muscle fibres in voluntary and smooth muscle and in the heart contain glycogen-filled vacuoles; they may be displaced and destroyed.[104] In the kidneys, glycogen accumulation is primarily in the loops of Henle and collecting tubules, a location that distinguishes this variety from type I.[105]

Type III glycogen storage disease (Forbes' disease, limit dextrinosis).

There are a number of subtypes for amylo-1-6-glucosidase deficiency that are based on enzyme levels in liver and muscle.[106] Presentation is usually within the first year of life, with 50% showing complications of hypoglycaemia. Liver adenomas occur in 10–25% of patients.[79] Approximately two-thirds of patients have muscle weakness with elevated serum enzymes from that tissue. Growth failure is less severe than in type I, often with improvement during puberty. Hepatomegaly can still be found in adults, 50% of whom have normal liver function tests. Cardiac failure and sudden death can occur at any age. Most patients with muscle involvement have abnormal ECGs and EMGs although significant disease of just one organ is possible. A high protein diet has been advocated in the past,[107] but more recently uncooked cornstarch feeds were found to be more beneficial.[108]

Type IV glycogen storage disease (brancher deficiency, amylopectinosis, Anderson's disease)

Bannayan et al[109] reported a case and referred to 13 (possibly 15) previously published cases. The enzyme deficiency results in a less soluble form of glycogen with decreased branch points. The enzyme deficiency can be measured in multiple tissues in classic early onset patients.[110,111] Such patients present with hepatosplenomegaly and failure to thrive, with death from complications of cirrhosis before 4 years of age, and later from cardiac failure.[108,112] Unusual variants without evidence of progressive disease were reviewed recently by Greene et al.[113] Since 1984, Selby et al[114] have performed liver transplantation in 7 patients without evidence of disease progression in other tissues. However, a recent report has documented the occurrence of progressive cardiac failure following liver transplantation in a 15-month-old child with type IV glycogenosis.[115]

Types VI and IX glycogen storage diseases

Patients present with hepatomegaly because of enzyme defects in converting glycogen to glucose-1-phosphate. Analysis of fresh tissue is required for an accurate diagnosis. Type VI (liver phosphorylase deficiency)[116] patients have a good prognosis but may have mild hypoglycaemia. Type IX (phosphorylase B kinase deficiency) has at least 3 subtypes, with IXa resembling type VI because of exclusive liver involvement. Type IXb has a sex-linked inheritance pattern. Van den Berg & Berger[117] have suggested more subtypes based, in part, on patterns of organ involvement. Rarely, severe liver disease is found, but it responds to uncooked starch therapy.[118] In patients without significant muscle involvement, the usual presentation again includes hepatomegaly, growth retardation, some delay in motor development, and hyperlipidaemia. Most adults are asymptomatic.[119] The gene encoding liver phosphorylase maps to chromosome 14.[120] Phosphorylase B kinase contains four subunits. The alpha subunit locus has been assigned to Xq12–q13.1 for muscle. The beta subunit has been mapped to 16q12–q13.[121] The gamma subunit has been assigned to chromosome 7 and delta is a member of the calmodulin family.[117]

Gross, light microscopic and ultrastructual features of the glycogenoses

Grossly, the liver in the glycogenoses is enlarged, smooth and paler than normal. A reticular pattern of fibrosis or, rarely, a micronodular or mixed type of cirrhosis may be seen in some types, for example types III and IV. Tumour nodules of varied size (representing either adenomas or carcinoma) may be visible macroscopically in glycogenosis type I.

The diagnosis of a specific type of glycogen storage disease requires biochemical determination of the enzyme defect. Although subtle differences have been described by McAdams et al,[104] the pathological features are distinctive in only a few of the glycogenoses, e.g., the light micro-

scopic appearance of the liver in glycogenosis type IV, and the ultrastructural features of types II and IV.

In the majority of the glycogenoses, hepatocytes are two to several times the normal size and are rarefied, with wisps of pinkish material in an otherwise empty cytoplasm (Fig. 4.6). Cell membranes appear thickened due to peripheral displacement of organelles by the stored glycogen. The overall appearance of hepatocytes has been likened to that of plant cells. The presence of sharply defined vacuoles in the cytoplasm, particularly in glycogenosis type I, indicates the simultaneous accumulation of neutral lipid. Nuclei of liver cells are centrally placed, and those in zone 1 may be glycogenated. The excess cytoplasmic glycogen is readily stained with PAS, even in formalin-fixed and routinely processed tissue; it is readily digested by diastase (Fig. 4.7). The absence of glucose-6-phosphatase activity in glycogenosis type Ia, in contrast to

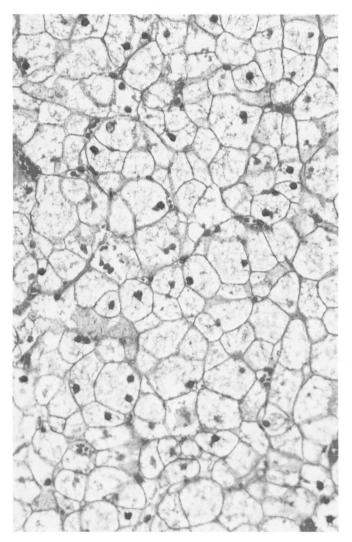

Fig. 4.6 Glycogenosis type III. Liver cells are swollen and have pyknotic centrally or eccentrically-located nuclei. The cytoplasm is rarefied. H&E.

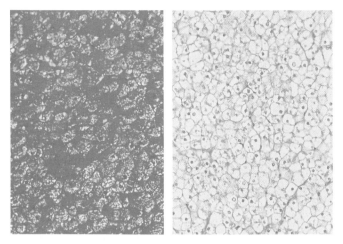

Fig. 4.7 Glycogenosis type III. A large quantity of glycogen in liver cells (left) has been digested by diastase (right). PAS before and after diastase.

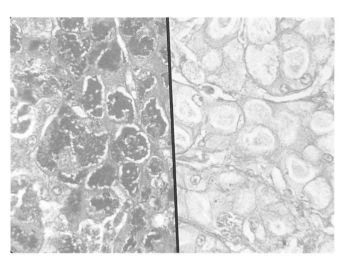

Fig. 4.9 Glycogenosis type IV. Cytoplasmic inclusions, intensely stained with PAS (left), have been digested by pectinase (right). PAS before and after pectinase.

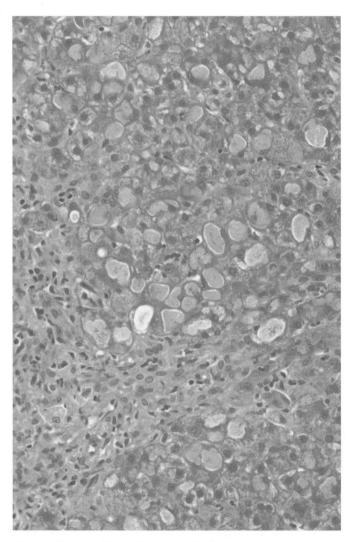

Fig. 4.8 Glycogenosis type IV. Rounded or irregular cytoplasmic inclusions are lightly eosinophilic; some are surrounded by an artefactual empty space. H&E.

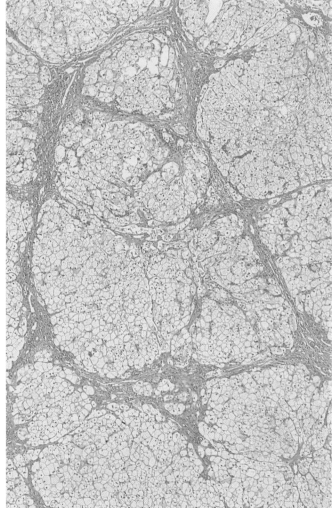

Fig. 4.10 Glycogenosis type III. Micronodular cirrhosis. Note absence of inflammation and piecemeal necrosis. H & E.

its presence in type Ib, has been demonstrated by histochemical staining.[122] Mallory bodies in zone 3 and periportal fibrosis have been reported in glycogenosis type Ia.[123] Another unusual finding was the occurrence of localized peliosis hepatis in an adult patient with glycogenosis type I.[124]

The histopathology of the liver in glycogenosis type IV is markedly different from that of the other glycogenoses.[109,125,126] The changes closely resemble those of Lafora's disease,[127] but in that disease progression to cirrhosis does not occur. Typically, hepatocytes in glycogenosis type IV are enlarged and contain colourless or lightly eosinophilic ground-glass inclusions that are round, oval or bean-shaped (Fig. 4.8). An artefactual space may surround the inclusions. They are most heavily concentrated in zone 1, but can be found in other zones.

Both the inclusions and the rest of the hepatocytic cytoplasm in type IV glycogenosis are stained deeply with PAS (Fig. 4.9); diastase treatment removes the normal glycogen but not the abnormal amylopectin-like material in the inclusions. The latter can, however, be digested by pectinase (Fig. 4.10) and α- or β-amylase.[128,129] The inclusions can be nonspecifically stained with colloidal iron (green), Best's carmine (red) and Lugol's iodine (mahogany brown to violet).[128]

Fibrosis, which can progress to cirrhosis, is a frequent finding in glycogenosis type IV, but can also occur in glycogenosis types III and VI (Fig. 4.10). As already noted, patients with glycogenosis type I may develop hepatocellular adenoma or carcinoma. The hepatocellular adenomas are often multiple and arise in a non-cirrhotic parenchyma. Unusual histological features in the adenomas have been described in 2 cases by Poe & Snover.[78] They included marked steatosis, Mallory bodies, lamellar fibrosis and, in one case, amyloidosis.

The ultrastructural features of the glycogenoses are quite comparable, with the exception of types II and IV. In the cytoplasm of liver cells there are large pools of glycogen rosettes that displace organelles, such as mitochondria and the endoplasmic reticulum, to the periphery of the cell. The glycogen may be associated with vesicles of smooth endoplasmic reticulum or it may assume a starry-sky

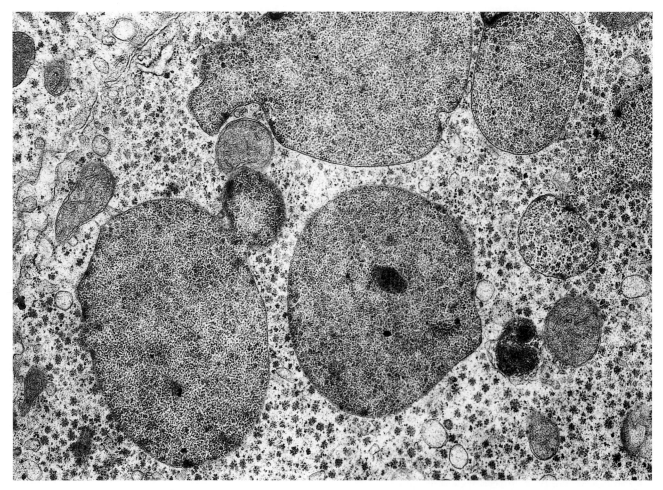

Fig. 4.11 Glycogenosis type II. Electron micrograph reveals accumulation of monoparticulate glycogen in enlarged lysosomes. Note glycogen rosettes between the lysosomes. × 15 000

pattern, as observed in glycogenosis types III, VI and IX.[12] Morphometric analysis in glycogenosis type I has shown an increased volume of glycogen per unit volume of the hepatocytic cytoplasm.[129] Additionally, there is marked reduction (by 50%) of the rough endoplasmic reticulum per unit volume of liver tissue.[129] Double-contoured vesicles in the endoplasmic reticulum are characteristic of glycogenosis type I.[129] Lipid droplets of varied size are seen in most of the glycogenoses, but appear to be more prominent in types I, II and VI.[11] Nuclear glycogenation is minimal or absent in glycogenosis type Ib in comparison to type Ia.[130] Increased collagen deposition in the space of Disse is observed in the glycogenoses types I, III, IV, VI and XI.[12]

Glycogenosis type II differs from the other types in the accumulation of monoparticulate glycogen in lysosomes that vary from 1–8 μm in diameter (Fig. 4.11).[131] Increased accumulation of glycogen rosettes may also be noted in the cytoplasm.[12] According to Phillips et al,[12] the ultrastructural features of glycogenosis type IV are pathognomonic. The inclusions noted by light microscopy consist ultrastructurally of undulating, randomly-oriented, delicate fibrils that measure up to 5 nm in diameter; these accumulations are not membrane bound (Fig. 4.12).

GALACTOSAEMIA

Galactosaemia is an autosomal recessive disease which primarily presents in infancy following galactose exposure via lactose. The principal defective enzyme is galactose-1-phosphate uridyl transferase.[132] A number of variants of this enzyme exist which result in the accumulation of galactose-1-phosphate.[133] The 'classical' disease may also be secondary to UDP-galactose-4 epimerase, the subsequent enzyme in the galactose metabolic pathway.[133] However, this enzyme deficiency must be extreme to result in clinical manifestations. Deficiency of galactokinase, the initial enzyme for galactose metabolism, leads to the formation of cataracts, and cerebral oedema occurs occasionally during infancy; no liver injury has ever been documented.[134]

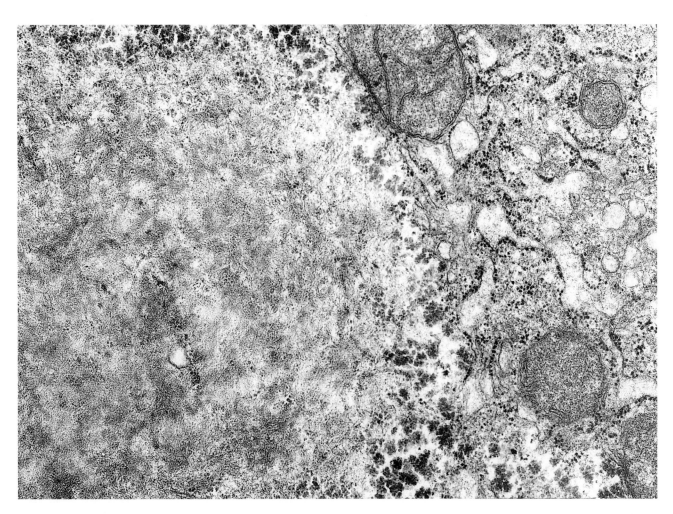

Fig. 4.12 Glycogenosis type IV. Electron micrograph shows segment of inclusion (left) consisting of non-membrane-bound fibrillar material; some glycogen rosettes are present between the inclusion and the hepatocyte cytoplasm (right). × 21130

This section relates primarily to the transferase deficiency disease, which has an incidence of 1 in 62 000 live births. This disease is screened for in the newborn by detection of erythrocyte galactose-1-phosphate level elevation. The diagnosis is most simply made by demonstrating deficiency of the transferase in red cells, although other tissues including chorionic villi are as reliable prenatally.[133] The gene for this enzyme is mapped to chromosome 9, p13, but the basic defect is unknown.

All the clinical manifestations are related directly to the ingestion of galactose. The frequencies of symptoms and signs in the series of 55 patients reported by Nadler et al[135] were failure to thrive (87.3%), vomiting (72.7%), diarrhoea (80.0%), jaundice (84.3%), and ascites (34.1%). Renal findings include galactosuria in all patients and, in some, albuminuria and generalized aminoaciduria as well. About 10% of patients have a documented episode of normochromic normocytic haemolytic anaemia.[135] The clinical course can be fulminant in some cases with early fatal infections, inanition or hepatic failure.[136] Haemorrhagic manifestations occur in 5% of patients.[136] Mature cataracts, which develop in 48.9% of patients, generally do so by the age of six months.[135] Inexplicable infantile cataracts may be due to marginal maternal deficiency of either galactokinase, galactose-1-phosphate uridyl transferase or both, in the presence of substantial lactose intake during pregnancy.[137] A long-term follow-up of 60 galactosaemic children maintained on a galactose-low diet has shown that mental development was below that of the average population and that there was a significant incidence of psychological disturbances.[138] A late complication not related to diet is partial or complete failure of secondary sexual development due to ovarian involvement.[139]

Of the pathological changes, those in the liver are the most distinctive, although they are not pathognomonic.[140,141] The earliest, which may appear within 10 or 11 days of birth, is marked steatosis and periportal cholangiolar proliferation; the cholangioles usually contain bile plugs and may be surrounded and infiltrated by neutrophils (Fig. 4.13). The next change, which begins as early as 2 weeks and is fully developed by 4–6 weeks, is the striking pseudoglandular (pseudoacinar) transformation of the hepatic plates. The hepatocytes surround a dilated canaliculus that is either empty or contains bile or some other pink or orange-coloured material. During this and the preceding phase, variable degrees of extramedullary haemopoiesis and haemosiderosis may be seen. Fibrosis, beginning by the age of 6 weeks and culminating in cirrhosis in 3–6 months, spreads from portal areas. As this progresses, the portal areas become linked together and fibrous septa reach in to connect them to terminal hepatic venules. Hyperplasia of segments of pre-existing acini, carved out by the fibrous septa, leads to a micronodular cirrhosis. While it is doubtful that established cirrhosis is ever reversible, Appelbaum & Thaler[142] have documented

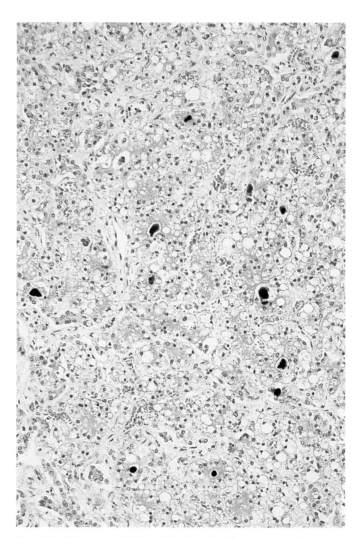

Fig. 4.13 Galactosaemia. Marked cholestasis with pseudogland formation and steatosis. Note periportal cholangioles (top, corners). H&E.

the regression of extensive liver damage in an infant 5 months after the institution of a galactose-free diet. One patient who survived to the age of 52 years with established cirrhosis has been reported.[143] Occasional findings in the liver in galactosaemia include giant cell transformation[144] and hepatocellular adenoma.[145] In today's terminology, the 'adenomas' would be called macrogenerative nodules since they occurred in a cirrhotic liver and measured 2.9, 1.5 and 1.0 cm in diameter.

The pathogenesis of the lesions in the liver and other organs in galactosaemia is discussed in detail by Sidbury.[146] It appears that neither galactose-1-phosphate nor galactitol is likely to be the cause of the hepatic lesions. It is possible that an as yet unknown metabolite is responsible for liver damage. The cataracts are due to accumulation of galactitol in the lens. This leads to inactivation of glutathione peroxidase which allows toxic levels of hydrogen peroxide to accumulate and the peroxide in turn denatures the lens protein.

HEREDITARY FRUCTOSE INTOLERANCE

Two hereditary disorders of fructose metabolism involve the liver. The more common one, which may result acutely in liver failure or chronically in cirrhosis, is characterized by a deficiency of fructose-1-phosphate aldolase (aldolase B, EC 4.1.2.13).[147] The less common one, which presents with hypoglycaemia, is characterized by a deficiency of fructose-1,6-biphosphatase (EC 3.1.3.11).[148,149] Both disorders are autosomal recessive in inheritance. Details of other rare variants have been reviewed by Gitzelmann et al.[150]

Aldolase B deficiency is the more common form of the disease, estimated to occur in 1 in 20 000 births,[150] and it was first documented by Hers & Joassin in 1961.[151] The presentation is quite variable, with severe liver disease appearing in infants upon introduction of fructose in the diet at the time of weaning.[152,153] The predominant symptoms are poor feeding, vomiting and failure to thrive.[153,154] Other findings include hepatomegaly, pallor, haemorrhages, trembling and jerkiness, shock, jaundice, oedema, tachypnoea, ascites, splenomegaly, fever, and rickets, in that order of frequency. Laboratory tests reveal fructosaemia and fructosurea after recent fructose administration, together with hypophosphataemia, metabolic acidosis and abnormal liver tests. A generalized aminoaciduria with excretion of organic acids, as well as elevated serum levels of tyrosine and methionine, can simulate the findings in tyrosinaemia. Aversion to sweets often develops as the affected child grows.

Inasmuch as diagnostic tests are not simple or readily available, the diagnosis usually is made after removal of fructose from the diet. An intravenous fructose tolerance test rapidly lowers inorganic phosphorus, following which there is hypoglycaemia with elevation of serum levels of lactate, urate and magnesium. Analysis of liver tissue for both enzymes confirms the diagnosis.[150] In future, diagnostic testing may include nuclear magnetic resonance with unlabelled fructose to document phosphorus and ATP depletion, or the use of labelled fructose with detection of a greater than threefold lowering of fructose conversion to glucose.[155,156] Treatment is dietary restriction of fructose but hepatomegaly may take years to resolve. The aldolase B gene was located on chromosome 9q22 by Tolan & Penhoet in 1986.[157] In a limited number of patients, the mutation is a G to C base change in exon 5 that results in the substitution of alanine by a proline residue at position 149 of the protein.[158]

The symptoms of patients with fructose-1,6-biphosphatase deficiency relate to severe ketotic hypoglycaemia, and 50% of patients present at 1–4 days of age.[143] Half of the remainder present before 6 months of age; only one individual has been diagnosed after 4 years of age. Hepatomegaly is present as well as muscle hypotonia. Illnesses which prevent oral intake of food can cause recurrent symptoms of hypoglycaemia and severe metabolic acidosis. Failure to thrive and liver function abnormalities are rare and there is no aversion to sweets. Treatment is aimed at avoidance of fasting, and less restriction is needed for fructose and sucrose.

Pathological findings in hereditary fructose intolerance include neonatal hepatitis with giant cell transformation,[159] steatosis,[152,153,159,160] fibrosis and cirrhosis.[152,153,161–164] Quantification of the amount of glycogen showed a high level in one case, but microscopic findings were not documented.[165] The resemblance of the lesions to those of galactosaemia has been noted.[152,166] As pointed out by Hardwick & Dimmick,[167] most descriptions of the pathology of the liver in hereditary fructose intolerance refer to changes consistent with the early phases of cirrhosis rather than with established cirrhosis. Hepatocellular carcinoma has been reported in a 49-year-old man suspected of having hereditary fructose intolerance.[168]

Ultrastructural changes in hepatic biopsy material were reported by Phillips et al.[160] Concentric and irregularly disposed membranous arrays are present in the glycogen areas of most hepatocytes and are associated with marked rarefaction of the hyaloplasm (Fig. 4.14). Many of the membranous formations resemble cytolysosomes. It has been suggested that these changes are related to the intracellular accumulation of substrates.[160] Similar ultrastructural changes have been reproduced in rats whose livers were infused with fructose via the portal vein.[169] Survival of injured cells is thought to be dependent on the sequestration of damaged areas (cytolysosome formation), as might occur with minimal or mild exposure to fructose. Larger quantities of fructose, particularly if repeated, may lead to more severe liver injury with necrosis and, ultimately, to cirrhosis.

MYOCLONUS EPILEPSY WITH LAFORA BODIES (LAFORA'S DISEASE)

This disease is discussed in this section because of morphological and immunohistochemical similarities of the liver changes to those of glycogenosis type IV. It starts in adolescence with epileptic seizures (grand mal attacks being the most common) followed by myoclonus (beginning in the face and extremities, but progressively involving other muscles), and mental changes.[170–173]

Atypical cases without myoclonus or epilepsy have been reported.[174] Routine clinical laboratory investigations on urine, blood and CSF reveal nonspecific findings. Skin biopsy is the simplest and least invasive diagnostic procedure, inclusion bodies are reliably found in eccrine sweat gland duct cells.[173] Most patients die between the ages of 16 and 24. Inheritance is autosomal recessive. The underlying biochemical defect has not been elucidated. A canine model for the disease has been reported.[175]

The histological hallmark of the disease is the presence

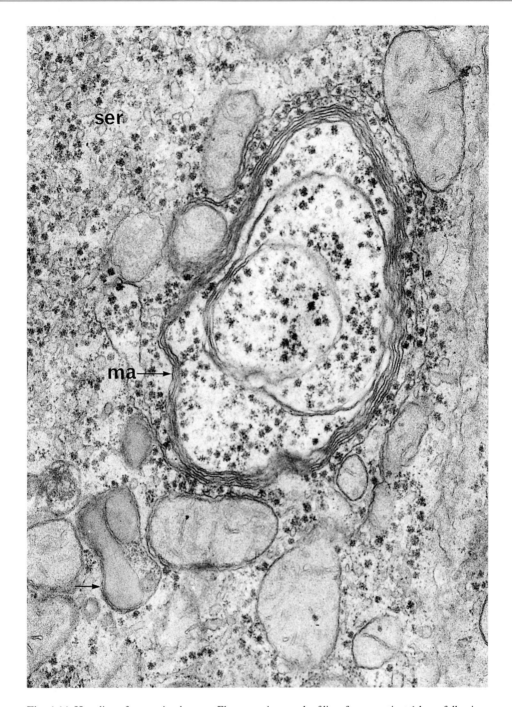

Fig. 4.14 Hereditary fructose intolerance. Electron micrograph of liver from a patient 1 hour following the ingestion of a fructose load. Note the prominence of the smooth endoplasmic reticulum (ser) and the formation of membranous arrays (ma). Glycogen particles are aligned between the layers of the smooth membranes, and the enclosed cytoplasm is rarefied and watery. A cytolysosome (arrow) is also illustrated. × 28 200. Courtesy of Dr M J Phillips

of distinctive intraneuronal inclusions (Lafora bodies) which are most frequently found in the substantia nigra, globus pallidum, dentate nucleus, parts of the reticular system and cerebral cortex. Lafora bodies vary in size from dot-like to as large as 35 μm. They stain positively with PAS, Best's carmine, Lugol's iodine (dark brown), colloidal iron and methenamine silver nitrate.[176–180] Three types

have been described by Van Hoof & Hageman-Bal.[181] With the PAS stain, type I bodies (the most common) are granular and red, type II bodies have a densely-stained, bright red core and radiating lines in a more faintly stained peripheral zone, and type III bodies (the least common) are homogeneously bright red.[181] The bodies are digested by α-amylase, amyloglucosidase and pectinase. On the basis of histochemical and chemical studies, Yokoi et al[178] have concluded that Lafora bodies are composed predominantly of an unusual branched polyglucosan. Ultrastructurally, they are not membrane-bound and are composed of varying proportions of fibrillar and granular material. The core is usually granular while the fibrils, which measure from 6–13 nm, radiate outwards and branch repeatedly.[171,179–183]

Extraneural deposits of abnormal material are frequently found when searched for. The histochemical and ultrastructural characteristics of these deposits in skeletal and smooth muscle, myocardium, liver and other organs are similar to those of Lafora bodies in the brain, with only minor differences.[171,174] Hepatic involvement has been reported by a number of investigators.[127,174,184–188] In haematoxylin and eosin preparations, liver cells contain round, oval or kidney-shaped inclusions that are sharply circumscribed, homogeneous or finely granular and lightly eosinophilic; they may be surrounded by a 'halo' that is probably artefactual[127] (Fig. 4.15). The nuclei of hepatocytes are frequently displaced to the periphery.

Affected cells in Lafora's disease are predominantly periportal in location. They resemble those seen in type IV glycogenosis and show identical staining reactions, with the exception of the colloidal iron stain; the cytoplasm in Lafora's disease is homogeneous (Fig. 4.16) while the stained material in type IV glycogenosis is coarse and clumped. Hepatocytes not harbouring Lafora bodies contain a large quantity of glycogen. According to Yokota et al,[188] antibodies prepared against Lafora bodies are immunoreactive to deposits of glycogenosis type IV. The inclusions also bear a resemblance to ground-glass hepatocytes of hepatitis B antigen carriers (but do not stain with the orcein, Victoria blue or aldehyde fuchsin stains), as well as to liver cells injured by cyanamide, a drug used in alcohol aversion therapy. Lafora body-like inclusions were

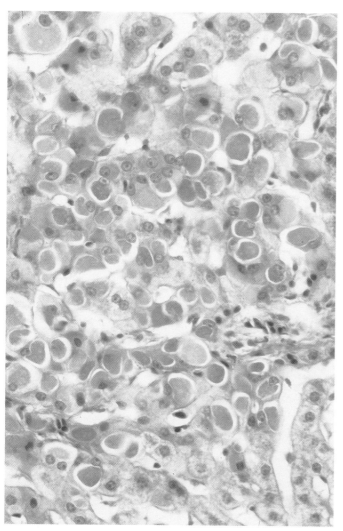

Fig. 4.15 Lafora's disease. More or less rounded pink inclusions in the cytoplasm of zone 1 hepatocytes; note artefactual 'halo' around the inclusions. H&E.

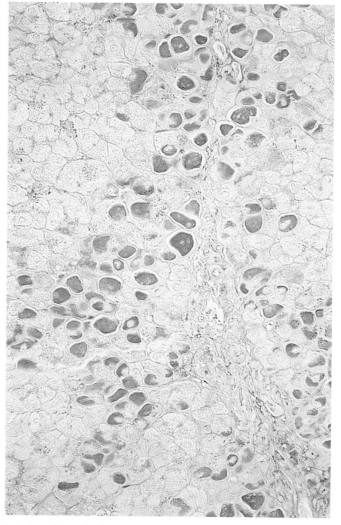

Fig. 4.16 Lafora bodies are positively stained with colloidal iron. Note varied shapes and location in liver cells in zone 1. Rinehart–Abul Haj stain.

also reported by Ng et al[189] in two patients who did not have myoclonus or epilepsy. Cirrhosis has not been reported in myoclonus epilepsy, but there may be slight periportal fibrosis.[127,176]

DISORDERS OF GLYCOPROTEIN AND PROTEIN METABOLISM

MUCOPOLYSACCHARIDOSES

This is a group of six different disorders, each with its own set of distinctive clinical features.[190] They represent systemic disorders that result from deficient activity of various enzymes involved in the catabolism of glycosaminoglycans. Excessive amounts of mucopolysaccharides accumulate in the somatic and visceral tissues and their partial degradation products are excreted in the urine; in addition, there may be accumulation of gangliosides. The various mucopolysaccharidoses are distinguished by their clinical manifestations and the specific enzyme deficiency which can be estimated in white blood cells or fibroblasts. Five of the mucopolysaccharidoses (Hurler's syndrome, Hunter's syndrome, Sanfilippo's syndrome,

Maroteaux–Lamy syndrome and type VII β-glucuronidase deficiency) are associated with enlargement of the liver and spleen. The major clinical findings, enzyme defects and the type of mucopolysaccharide excreted in the urine in the mucopolysaccharidoses are shown in Table 4.3. Only those that affect the liver are discussed in this chapter.

Mucopolysaccharidosis type I (MPS I), Hurler (H), Scheie (S), Hurler–Scheie (H/S)

This autosomal recessive disorder is characterized by deficiency of the degradative lysosomal enzyme α-L-iduronidase in multiple tissues. Obligate heterozygotes have about half the mean specific activity of normal controls of the enzyme in their leucocytes.[191] The gene is located on chromosome 4p16.3. Diagnosis of the three MSP I types depends on the clinical presentation because of lack of correlation with enzyme levels.

MPS I (H) patients manifest developmental delay by 12–14 months. Features not listed in Table 4.3 include macroglossia, a prominent forehead and stiff joints. Death occurs by 10 years of age because of obstructive airway

Table 4.3 Classification of the mucopolysaccharidoses

Number	Eponym	Clinical manifestations	Enzyme defects	Urinary mucopolysaccharide excretion
MPS I H	Hurler	Corneal clouding, dysostosis multiplex, organomegaly	α-L-Iduronidase	Dermatan sulphate, heparan sulphate
MPS I S	Scheie	Corneal clouding, stiff joints, normal intelligence and life span	α-L-Iduronidase	Dermatan sulphate, heparan sulphate
MPS I H/S	Hurler–Scheie	Phenotype intermediate between IH and IS	α-L-Iduronidase	Dermatan sulphate, heparan sulphate
MPS II	Hunter (severe)	Dysostosis multiplex, organomegaly, no corneal clouding, mental retardation, death before 15 years	Iduronate sulphatase	Dermatan sulphate, heparan sulphate
MPS II	Hunter (mild)	Normal intelligence, short stature, survival to 20s to 60s	Iduronate sulphatase	Dermatan sulphate, heparan sulphate
MPS IIIA	Sanfilippo A	Profound mental deterioration, hyperactivity, relatively mild somatic manifestations	Heparan N-sulphatase	Heparan sulphate
MPS IIIB	Sanfilippo B	Phenotype similar to IIIA	α-N-Acetylglucosaminidase	Heparan sulphate
MPS IIIC	Sanfilippo C	Phenotype similar to IIIA	Acetyl-CoA: α-glucosaminide acetyltransferase	Heparan sulphate
MPS IIID	Sanfilippo D	Phenotype similar to IIIA	N-Acetylglucosamine 6-sulphatase	Heparan sulphate
MPS IVA	Morquio A	Distinctive skeletal abnormalities, corneal clouding, odontoid hypoplasia; milder forms known to exist	Galactose 6-sulphatase	Keratan sulphate, chondroitin 6-sulphate
MPS IVB	Morquio B	Spectrum of severity as in IV A	β-Galactosidase	Keratan sulphate
MPS VI	Maroteaux–Lamy	Dysostosis multiplex, corneal clouding, normal intelligence, survival to teens in severe forms; milder forms known to exist	N-Acetylgalactosamine 4-sulphatase (arylsulphatase B)	Dermatan sulphate
MPS VII	Sly	Dysostosis multiplex, hepatosplenomegaly; wide spectrum of severity	β-Glucuronidase	Dermatan sulphate, heparan sulphate

disease, respiratory infection or cardiac complications. Bone marrow transplantation continues to be evaluated since it was first used in 1981.[192–194] Prenatal diagnosis by amniocentesis is now routine, and in utero therapy has been attempted.

MPS I (H/S) is an intermediate form of this disorder. Early mortality results either from cardiac involvement or from upper airway obstruction. A canine model exists which responds to bone marrow transplantation,[195] including reduction of brain glycosaminoglycan comparable to that seen in the liver. Aortic valve disease complicates MPS I (S).

Mucopolysaccharidosis type II (MPS II), Hunter's syndrome

MPS II is caused by a deficiency of α-L-iduronidase sulphatase and is the only X-linked mucopolysaccharidosis. The gene has been localized to Xq28.1. Affected children have a coarse facies, deafness, mental deficiency, failure to grow, joint contractures, hepatosplenomegaly and chronic diarrhoea by 4 years of age. A milder form of this disease exists with complications that include hearing impairment, and papilloedema resulting from local infiltration in the eye. Death is usually from airway obstruction or cardiac failure. Bone marrow transplantation has not been vigorously pursued.[196]

Mucopolysaccharidosis type III (MPS III), Sanfilippo's disease

This comprises four phenotypically identical forms with different enzyme defects. Type A results from deficiency of heparan sulphatase and type B from deficiency of N-acetyl α-D-glucosidase; types C and D, with different enzyme defects, are now also known. All forms are characterized by coarse features, hepatomegaly, variable splenomegaly and mental retardation; there is no corneal clouding. The milder somatic complaints include recurrent diarrhoea.

Mucopolysaccharidosis type VI (MPS VI), Maroteaux–Lamy syndrome

MPS VI also has three clinical types (infantile, intermediate and adult) which vary in severity but without alterations of intellect. The infantile form is characterized by growth retardation, coarse facial features, restricted movement, hepatosplenomegaly and corneal involvement. Death in the second and third decades is the result of cardiac failure. The intermediate type has been found to have a valine for glycine substitution at position 137 of arylsulphatase.[197] Bone marrow transplantation has been helpful in this disorder.[198]

Mucopolysaccharidosis type VII (MPS VII), Sly syndrome

MPS VII is due to a deficiency of ß-glucuronidase. This rare disorder is characterized by dysostosis multiplex, hepatosplenomegaly, mental retardation, and frequent pulmonary infections. It is one of the storage disorders that can present with hydrops foetalis. The gene has been localized to chromosome 7q22.

Pathological changes in the mucopolysaccharidoses

Macroscopically, the liver in the mucopolysaccharidoses is enlarged, firm or hard and has a pale, slightly yellowish or greyish colour.[199] There may be extensive fibrosis or cirrhosis. Microscopically, both hepatocytes and Kupffer cells are swollen and have an empty or faintly vacuolated cytoplasm. Since much of the stored acid mucopolysaccharide is leached out by aqueous fixatives, other methods of fixation, such a Lindsay's dioxane picrate solution,[200] are preferable. Alternatively, addition of a 10% solution of acetyl trimethylammonium bromide to the formalin fixative is said to preserve acid mucopolysaccharide in the cells.[201]

The stored acid mucopolysaccharide is best demonstrated by a colloidal iron stain, and most of it can be digested with hyaluronidase (Fig. 4.17). It is weakly positive with the PAS stain but cannot be digested by diastase. Acid mucopolysaccharide is metachromatic when stained with toluidine blue. Little or no neutral lipid can be demonstrated in frozen sections of the liver stained with the sudanophilic dyes.

When fibrosis is present in the mucopolysaccharidoses it is diffuse, with heavy deposition of collagen bundles in the space of Disse and gradual microdissection of the parenchyma into nodules (Fig. 4.18). Periportal bridging fibrosis has been emphasized by Parfrey & Hutchins.[202] The type of cirrhosis associated with the mucopolysaccharidoses may be macronodular or micronodular.[203] When it supervenes, it generally does so in older children and adults.[200,203–206]

Ultrastructural studies of the liver in MPS I, MPS II and MPS III have demonstrated the presence of vacuoles of varied size in both hepatocytes and Kupffer cells; these are bounded by a single membrane and contain some electron-dense, poorly structured material.[199,207,208] It is now generally accepted that the clear vacuoles represent lysosomes filled with acid mucopolysaccharide. It has been suggested that cytoplasmic vacuoles may form by mitochondrial 'budding' in the hepatocytes of patients with MPS I and MPS III.[209] A peculiar crystalloid structure has been described in mitochondria of hepatocytes in MPS III.[210] In MPS IV Kupffer cells but not hepatocytes contain clear vacuoles.[211] The ultrastructural changes in MPS V are similar to those of MPS I and MPS II.[212] In MPS VI there is moderate storage of electron-lucent

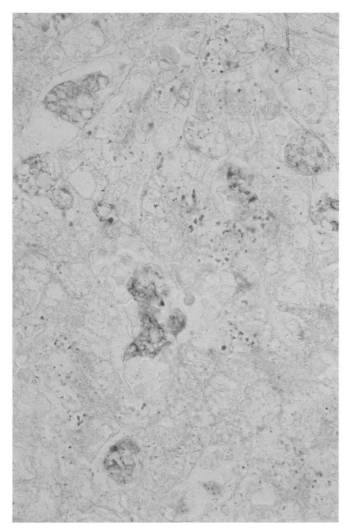

Fig. 4.17 Hurler's disease. Greenish-blue, punctate mucopolysaccharide is present in the cytoplasm of hepatocytes and Kupffer cells. Rinehart–Abul Haj stain.

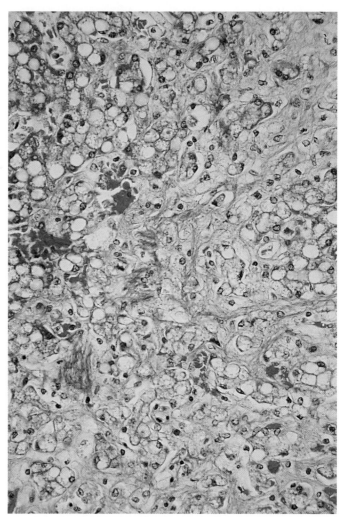

Fig. 4.18 Hurler's disease. Perisinusoidal fibrosis deep within a hepatic acinus. Note also the swollen vacuolated appearance of the hepatocytes. Masson's trichrome.

material in lysosomes of hepatocytes, but Kupffer cells and hepatic fibroblasts contain as much acid mucopolysaccharide as in MPS I.[211]

ASPARTYLGLUCOSAMINURIA

Aspartylglucosaminuria is an autosomal recessive disorder that was first reported by Jenner & Pollitt in 1967.[213] This disease, which causes mental retardation, is most frequently seen in Finland where the estimated incidence is approximately 1 : 26 000.[214] It is the only lysosomal storage disease caused by an amidase deficiency, aspartyl-glucosaminidase (AGA, EC 3.5.26). The structural gene is assigned to chromosome 4q23–q27. Prenatal diagnosis is possible and pathological changes at this stage are found in the liver but not in the brain.[215] The predominant gene defect in Finland is a G^{448}—7C alteration located in exon 4 which results in a serine substitution of cysteine

163.[216–218] Three patients have been reported from the United States including an African-American.[219] One patient has a GT to TT transversion at the splice donor site of intron 8, resulting in its deletion.[220] It is proposed that both defects affect conformational folding which results in the accumulation of the enzyme in the endoplasmic reticulum and/or Golgi apparatus. That in turn leads to loss of enzyme tracking to the lysosome for cleavage of asparagine from the residual N-acetyl-glucosamines of glycoprotein.

A diagnosis of aspartyglucosaminuria should be considered in children who present with a mucopolysaccharide-like disorder but are not excreting mucopolysaccharides in their urine.[221] The patients are usually investigated because of psychomotor retardation in early childhood.[222] They have coarse facial features, clear corneas, and no rhinorrhoea. The abdomen is protuberant with an umbilical defect. Hepatosplenomegaly is an early manifestation but regresses with age. A heart murmur of mitral insufficiency may be present. Some patients have mild diarrhoea. There may be generalized growth retardation. Other minor features may include acne, photosensitivity, crystal-like lens opacities, joint laxity, macroglossia, hoarseness and short stature. IQ values below 40, with uncontrollable behaviour, are reported in adults.

Radiological examination reveals dysostosis multiplex. Cardiac investigation results are consistent with mitral insufficiency. Peripheral blood and bone marrow examinations show vacuolated lymphocytes that do not stain with Best's carmine or PAS. The urine contains large quantities or 2-acetamido-1(B-L-aspartamido)-1,2-dideoxy B-D-glucose.[213] Aspartylglucosaminidase is markedly deficient in white blood cells as well as in the brain and liver. Heterozygotes can be identified be deficiency of the enzyme in cultured fibroblasts.

Histopathologically, liver cells contain large and small vacuoles that stain variably with PAS.[221] Kupffer cell vacuoles do not react with PAS. There is no increase in connective tissue. Ultrastructurally, enlarged lysosomes are present in hepatocytes and Kupffer cells.[221,223] The fine matrix background is similar to that of the mucopolysaccharidoses. Membranous structures are found in these large lysosomes as well as electron-lucent lipid droplets. Round, electron-dense structures and, less frequently, single membranous structures of varied sizes are also present.

MANNOSIDOSIS

This is a rare autosomal recessive disease that is characterized by the tissue accumulation and abnormally high urinary excretion of mannose-rich oligosaccharides. The primary metabolic defect is a deficiency of acidic α-mannosidase A and B in various tissues and leucocytes. Prenatal diagnosis is now feasible.[224] The gene has been localized to chromosome 19p13.2–q12. Several reviews of this disease have been published.[225–230] Two types are recognized. Type I is the more severe infantile type with death between 3 and 10 years of age, while type II is a milder disease with a juvenile or adult onset. Patients present with psychomotor retardation. They have a distinctive coarse facies, corneal and lenticular opacities, hearing loss, hepatosplenomegaly (usually early in the course of the disease) and symptoms and signs of recurrent infection. Dysostosis multiplex is demonstrated by skeletal radiology in the majority of patients. Vacuolated lymphocytes are seen in the peripheral blood. About half the patients have decreased values of serum IgG. The susceptibility to infection may be a direct consequence of impaired leucocyte membrane recognition processes which result from defective catabolism of substrates with α-D-mannose residues.[225] There is no known treatment but, despite recurrent infections, some patients may survive into adulthood.[231]

Hepatocytes in mannosidosis contain PAS-negative vacuoles in the cytoplasm. Ultrastructurally, they are bounded by a single membrane and contain amorphous and occasionally membranous and/or filamentous material.[224,232] Vacuoles may also be present in sinusoidal lining cells.[232] Light microscopic changes, which are nonspecific, include vacuolization of liver cells, steatosis and perisinusoidal fibrosis.[232]

FUCOSIDOSIS

This inherited autosomal recessive metabolic disorder is characterized by storage of fucose-containing glycolipids, glycoproteins and polysaccharides or oligosaccharides. It is caused by a total or profound deficiency of α_1-fucosidase in all tissues tested, including liver, kidney, lung, brain, leucocytes and skin fibroblasts. The gene has been localized to chromosome 1p34. Some 40 cases have been reported.[233] There appear to be two variants of the disease.[211,233,234] Type I is rapidly progressive and ends fatally between 4 and 6 years of age; type II follows a much slower course with survival into adolescence and beyond. Common to both variants are psychomotor retardation, neurological deficits and skeletal abnormalities. Hurler's syndrome-like features, hepatosplenomegaly, thickness of the skin, tendency to herniae and cardiomegaly are often present. Almost all patients experience repeated bouts of respiratory infection. The cases with the slower evolution are characterized by angiokeratoma corporis diffusum. No biochemical difference in α_1-fucosidase has been detected between types I and II.[235]

The gross and light microscopic changes are similar to those of Hurler's disease. Both hepatocytes and Kupffer cells are vacuolated. Ultrastructurally, hepatocytes show membrane-bound vacuoles representing lysosomes that contain granular or reticulogranular material suggesting polysaccharide, as well as lamellar bodies which indicate the accumulation of complex lipids.[236,237] Kupffer cells contain similar material but the vacuoles are smaller and are poor in lipid content. Bile-duct cells are markedly vacuolated by light microscopy and contain numerous clear vacuoles by electron microscopy.[236]

MUCOLIPIDOSES

These are a group of diseases with features overlapping those of the mucopolysaccharidoses and sphingolipidoses. They are lysosomal storage diseases with evidence of multiple primary defects of mucopolysaccharide, lipid and glycoprotein metabolism in various combinations.[238]

Mucolipidosis I (ML I, sialidosis)

The following account of the disease is based on the studies of Van Hoof,[211] Spranger,[238] Legum et al,[239]

Lowden & O'Brien[240] and Kelly.[241] It is a rare syndrome characterized by moderate developmental retardation by late infancy, and gargoyle-like facial dysmorphism and dysostosis by 4 or 5 years of age. Peripheral neuropathy develops subsequently, with muscular weakness and difficulties in coordination. Vacuolated lymphocytes are found in all cases. Inconstant findings include corneal opacities, a cherry-red macular spot and impaired hearing. Lowden & O'Brien[240] have proposed two major forms of the disease, dysmorphic (Hurler-like) and nondysmorphic (non-Hurler-like). An increased amount of bound sialic acid is excreted in the urine, a finding that can be used as a simple screening test. Definitive diagnosis is established by demonstration of a deficiency of neuraminidase (sialidase) in peripheral leucocytes or cultured fibroblasts.

Light microscopy of the liver reveals marked enlargement of portal macrophages and Kupffer cells, both of which have a foamy cytoplasm.[12,238,242] Ultrastructurally, hepatocytes contain membrane-bound vacuoles that are electron lucent.[11] The vacuoles frequently contain numerous osmiophilic droplets as well as a reticulogranular or flocculent material.[12,211,238] Riches & Smuckler[242] also described multilamellar bodies and fragments of membrane-like material in the vacuoles. Phillips et al[12] found vacuoles similar to those of hepatocytes in Kupffer cells, and to a lesser extent in endothelial cells, Ito cells and biliary epithelial cells.

Mucolipidosis II (ML II, I-cell disease)

Mucolipidosis II (ML II, I-cell disease) is an autosomal recessive disease in which clinical manifestations appear in the first year of life. These include severe psychomotor retardation, early growth retardation, facial dysmorphism with characteristic gingival hyperplasia, equivocal or absent corneal clouding, mild hepatomegaly, skeletal dysplasia and severe dysostosis multiplex.[211,243–245] Fibroblasts cultured from patients with ML II contain numerous dense inclusions (hence the term 'I-cell') which are best seen on phase contrast microscopy; their ultrastructural appearance was reviewed by Van Hoof.[211] In a recently reported autopsy case, vacuolated lymphocytes of B-cell lineage in lymph nodes, spleen, and kidney were found to contain large amounts of hexosamine.[246] Cytoplasmic vacuoles were also noted in Kupffer cells, fibroblasts in the myocardium, renal podocytes and acinar cells of the pancreas. The vacuolated cells stained positively with Hale's colloidal iron method.

Light microscopy of the liver may show no changes in hepatocytes but enlargement of Kupffer cells, portal macrophages with foamy cytoplasm and granulomas in portal areas that are composed of finely vacuolated epithelioid cells.[247] The vacuoles are limited by single membranes and contain either fibrillo-granular material, membranous lamellae or lipid globules.[247] Hepatocytes are generally only slightly affected but may contain different types of dense polymorphic inclusions.[211,243,248] Vacuoles in hepatocytes correspond to triglyceride droplets and membranous inclusions, as well as enlarged lysosomes containing granular material by electron microscopy. Kupffer cells contained electron-dense membranous lamellae.

The basic defect in mucolipidosis II is abnormal enzyme transport in cells of mesenchymal origin.[249] In normal cells, targeting of lysosomal enzymes to lysosomes is mediated by receptors that bind mannose-6-phosphate recognition markers on the enzymes. The recognition marker is synthesized in a two-step reaction in the Golgi complex. The enzyme that catalyses the first step in this process, UDP-N-acetylglucosamine: lysosomal enzyme N-acetyglucosaminyl-1-phosphotransferase, is defective.[249] Diagnosis can be made by measurement of the activity of the enzyme, or by demonstration of elevated levels of serum lysosomal enzyme. Prenatal diagnosis is also possible.

Mucolipidosis III (ML III, pseudo-Hurler polydystrophy)

This disease is biochemically related to ML II, but is milder and presents later. Survival into adulthood is possible. Diagnosis is also established by clinical findings, demonstration of ten- to twenty-fold elevations of lysosomal enzymes (β-hexosaminidase, iduronate sulphatase and arylsulphatase A) in plasma, and deficiency of the phosphotransferase enzyme.[250]

Vacuolated cells (leucocytes and bone marrow cells) similar to those of ML I are present. Cultured fibroblasts show inclusions resembling those of the I-cells of ML II. Ultrastructural findings in the liver include slightly enlarged secondary lysosomes without storage of any abnormal material, while Kupffer cells are relatively rich in unstructured osmiophilic material.[211]

Mucolipidosis IV (ML IV, sialolipidosis)

This is the most recently delineated mucolipidosis.[239] Some 20 cases have been reported.[251] It appears to be confined to Ashkenazi Jews and is characterized by an early onset of corneal opacification and psychomotor retardation; a small head circumference is frequent.[251–253] Gargoyle-like facies, skeletal deformities and organomegaly are absent. Biochemically, the disease is characterized by the accumulation of gangliosides, phospholipids and acidic mucopolysaccharides.[251] Ultrastructural studies of conjunctival biopsies from four patients have shown two types of abnormal inclusion bodies, both in stromal fibroblasts and in epithelial cells: (i) single membrane-limited cytoplasmic vacuoles containing both fibrillo-granular material and membranous lamellae, and (ii) lamellar and concentric bodies similar to those found in Tay–Sachs disease.[254] In liver biopsy material, Berman et al[251] have shown that hepatocytes contain inclusions composed predominantly of concentric lamellae, whereas vacuoles in Kupffer cells have clear contents. The prenatal diagnosis of ML IV was reported by Kohn et al.[255] A partial ganglioside sialidase deficiency has been found in cultured fibroblasts, but it is doubtful that that is the primary enzyme defect.[256]

ENDOPLASMIC RETICULUM STORAGE DISEASES

The endoplasmic reticulum storage diseases are defined as a group of inborn errors of metabolism affecting secretory proteins that result in hepatocytic storage and deficiency of the corresponding protein in the plasma.[257,258] The storage results from a molecular abnormality of the protein hindering its transfer from the rough to the smooth endoplasmic reticulum.[257] No abnormality of the endoplasmic reticulum itself has been uncovered. The most important of this group of diseases is α_1-antitrypsin deficiency. Three other diseases—α_1-anti-chymotrypsin deficiency, 'fibrinogen storage' disease and possibly antithrombin III deficiency—are also included in this section. The accumulation of various components of complement in liver cells, reported by Storch,[259,260] does not appear to have a clinical manifestation.

α_1-ANTITRYPSIN DEFICIENCY

α_1-Antitrypsin (α_1-AT) is a plasma glycoprotein of approximately 52 kD which is synthesized primarily by hepatocytes,[261] although several other tissues produce small amounts of it.[262,263] Interstitial tissue levels relate to its molecular size, which is similar to that of albumen, while plasma acute response levels depend significantly on secretion from macrophages and monocytes.[264,265] α_1-AT is a competitive inhibitor of leucocyte elastase with reaction kinetics favouring elastase complexing with α_1-AT rather than with its substrate elastin.[261,266] It also inhibits human activated protein C, an antithrombotic enzyme.[267] α_1-AT also inhibits many other serine proteases in vitro but the rate of action may be too slow for physiological significance in vivo.[268] Elastase is inhibited when it attempts to cleave the reaction centre (met[358]-ser[359]) of α_1-AT. A stable enzyme–inhibitor complex is formed, together with a terminal fragment which is the proteolysis product that can act as a neutrophil chemoattractant.[266,269,270] The plasma half-life is shortened (from 5–7 days to 10–90 minutes) when α_1-AT is complexed and taken up by a serine protease inhibitor receptor on macrophages and hepatocytes.[264,271,272]

Because of its association with the immunoglobulin heavy chain gene locus at 14q32.3,[273] the α_1-AT gene is also located on the long arm of chromosome 14 at

14q31–32.3.[274] The transcriptional start site of α_1-AT varies, as reflected by a longer mRNA from macrophages than from hepatocytes.[275,276] Serum levels of α_1-AT in humans are increased by hormonal influences, inflammatory stimuli and most liver diseases.[277–279]

The phenotypic expression of α_1-AT involves both alleles, i.e. it is codominant. Most allelic variants are the result of an amino acid substitution in the polypeptide chain. Protease inhibitor (Pi) typing is based on this variation which produces different charges that can be detected by isoelectric focusing in polyacrylamide gels. To date, more than 70 allelic variants of α_1-AT have been described.[280] The most common deficiency alleles are PiZ and PiS. Hepatic pathology is predominantly seen in individuals carrying the Z allele. The substitution of Lys[342] for Glu[342] directly affects secretion of α_1-AT which accumulates in the rough endoplasmic reticulum.[281,282]

The association of panlobular emphysema with α_1-AT

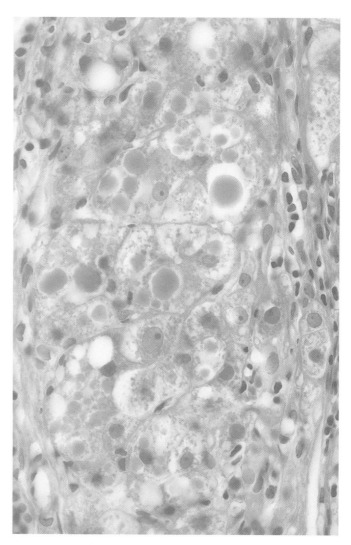

Fig. 4.19 Homozygous α_1-antitrypsin (α_1-AT) deficiency. Eosinophilic globules of varied size are present in the cytoplasm of periportal liver cells. H&E.

deficiency was first recognized by Laurell & Eriksson.[283] Sharp et al[279] reported cirrhosis in 10 children from 6 different kindreds with α_1-AT deficiency. Characteristic eosinophilic, PAS-positive, diastase-resistant, globular inclusions are found in hepatocytes (Figs 4.19 and 4.20). These globules can be demonstrated to contain α_1-AT antigen by immunohistochemical methods (Fig. 4.21) and have a characteristic amorphous appearance in the lumen of the rough endoplasmic reticulum by electron microscopy (Fig. 4.22).[282] Immunoelectron microscopic studies have confirmed the localization of α_1-AT to the endoplasmic reticulum.[284] Globules have subsequently been found in homozygous and heterozygous PiZ individuals with no liver disease,[282] in those with emphysema without liver disease, and in chronic liver disease in all age groups.[128] Similar globules have also been seen in patients without the Z allele, such as PiMalton,[285] and PiMi/

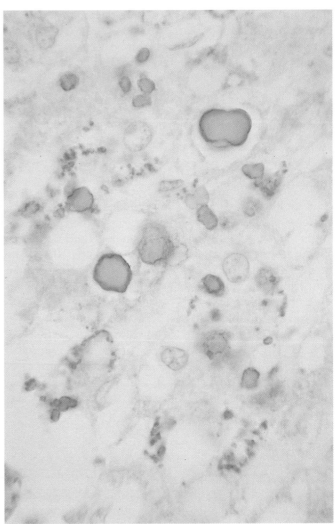

Fig. 4.21 The presence of α_1-AT in the globules is confirmed by a PAP immunohistochemical technique. Note that the periphery of the larger globules is more intensely stained than the centre

PiMDuarte.[286-288] In conditions of clinical stimulation, large areas of hepatic parenchyma may be immunopositive for α_1-AT in PiMZ persons.[289] The positivity appears in the form of crescents or rectilinear arrays in the cytoplasm of liver cells. These patients also have the usual globular inclusions. It should be noted that α_1-AT globules, in the absence of the Z allele, may be found in elderly patients who are severely ill and have high plasma concentrations of the enzyme.[290]

Liver disease in children with α_1-AT deficiency

There is only one prospective study on the incidence of liver disease in PiZ individuals. Identified at birth by Sveger[291] in Sweden, 127 homozygous PiZ children and 54 PiSZ children have been now followed into adolescence by physical examinations and routine serum liver

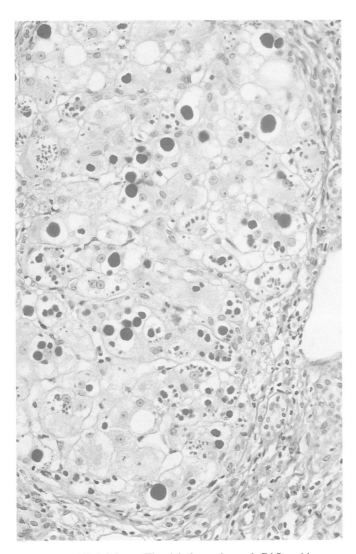

Fig. 4.20 α_1-AT deficiency. The globules are intensely PAS-positive. PAS after diastase digestion.

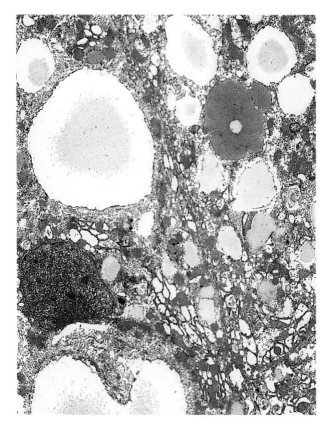

Fig. 4.22 α_1-AT deficiency. Electron micrograph showing moderately electron-dense amorphous material in the cisterns of the dilated endoplasmic reticulum of a hepatocyte. The larger deposits have a serrated edge. Note the 'halo' surrounding the deposits. × 6500

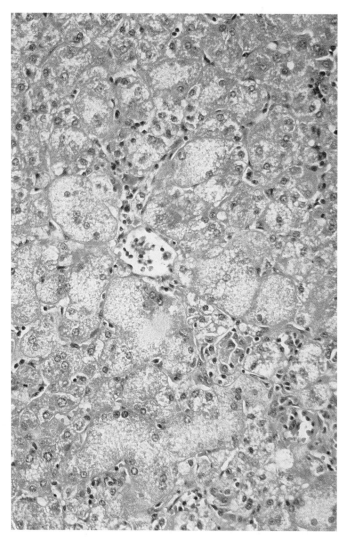

Fig. 4.23 Neonatal 'hepatitis' in an infant with homozygous α_1-AT deficiency. Note giant hepatocytes in zone 3 and focus of necrosis (top) H&E.

tests. Because of its rarity,[292] no PiQO (null) children were detected in this series. Initially, symptomatic liver disease was found in 11% of infants. Follow-up revealed the development of chronic liver disease leading to death in only 2.5% by age 12.[291,293] Despite the absence of clinical liver disease, 75% of all PiZ infants had an elevated serum alanine transferase (ALT). By the age of 12 years, only 33% of infants presenting with any signs of liver disease had an ALT elevation, while 14% of normal appearing infants had an elevated ALT. Thus, evidence of hepatic cell injury decreased as the children approached the teenage years. In contrast, PiSZ children who had serum α_1-AT levels that were 40% of normal did not have abnormal ALT levels.[294]

The most common presentation of α_1-AT-associated liver disease is cholestasis during infancy.[291,295,296] α_1-AT deficiency is a frequent cause of neonatal cholestasis (Figs 4.23 and 4.24). In one study, more than 30% of infants with undefined neonatal hepatitis had abnormal Pi phenotypes.[296] For practical purposes, the presence of a serum α_1-AT level that is 10–40% of normal excludes the consideration of laparotomy for conditions like extrahepatic biliary atresia.

Cholestasis usually resolves by 6 months of age without

therapy except when paucity of the intrahepatic ducts is present. Up to 10% of infants with α_1-AT deficiency may have paucity of the intrahepatic bile ducts with prolongation of cholestasis and the development of pruritus (Figs 4.25–4.27) In these patients, the prognosis is related to the development of cirrhosis. Persistence of an elevated bilirubin after 1 year of age suggests a poor prognosis.[295] Rarely, cirrhosis without clinical evidence of cholestasis may be present at birth.[297] An example of cirrhosis in a 6-year-old homozygous PiZ boy with α_1-AT deficiency is illustrated in Figures 4.28–4.30. This patient had no other risk factors for chronic liver disease.

A recent retrospective review of 98 children with α_1-AT deficiency, of whom 85 presented with liver disease, evaluated prognostic parameters.[295] While only 45% in that series were female, their ultimate outcome was worse, in part because of a higher incidence of lung and kidney

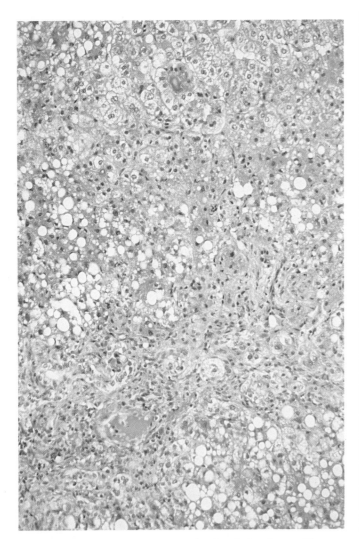

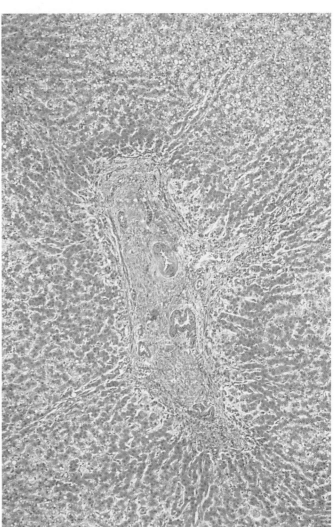

Fig. 4.24 Case illustrated in Fig. 4.28 showing similar changes. Note cholestasis and mild portal inflammation. H&E.

Fig. 4.25 Homozygous α_1-AT deficiency with paucity of intrahepatic bile ducts. Portal area is bereft of bile ducts. H&E.

complications. Approximately 50% of patients died or were transplanted, 10% were anticipated to need a transplant, and 40% were asymptomatic. In about 20% of the 85 patients, physical examinations and liver tests returned to normal. Similar results were reported in a review of α_1-AT liver disease in children from the United Kingdom.[298] An ALT greater than 260 U/l, a prothrombin time greater than 16 seconds, and a trypsin inhibitory capacity less than 0.25 mg/ml were associated with an elevenfold increase in the probability of a poor outcome. On follow-up, serum bilirubin elevations and abnormal coagulation tests associated with factor V levels below normal predicted death within one year and were used as criteria for liver transplant evaluation.[295] Occult hepatocellular carcinoma has not been a clinical problem in children, though it has been found at the time of liver transplantation.

Renal complications. Glomerulonephritis occurs in

about 17% of patients with liver disease but may be subtle in its presentation. The clinical hallmarks of proteinuria and haematuria may not be present, particularly if the serum albumin is below 20 g/l. Immunofluorescence studies of α_1-AT deficiency-associated membranoproliferative glomerulonephritis reveal the presence of immunoglobulins, complement, and α_1-AT in the subendothelial region of the glomerular basement membrane.[299]

Liver disease in adults with α_1-AT deficiency

α_1-AT-deficient individuals who escape severe liver disease in childhood generally are free of clinical liver disease until late in life. Liver disease primarily affects the elderly,[300] in contrast to emphysema which occurs in young adults. From the ages of 20–40, the incidence of liver disease in the α_1-AT-deficient population is approximately 2%.[301] From 41–50 years of age, the incidence

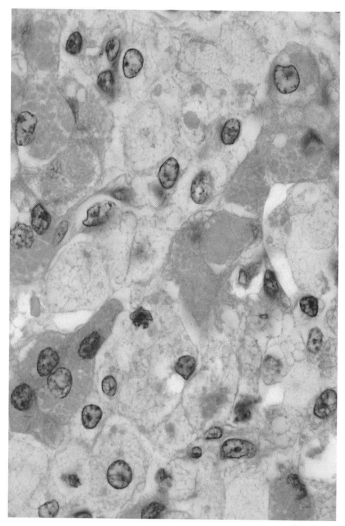

Fig. 4.26 Same case as illustrated in Figs 4.30 and 4.31. Higher magnification of pseudoxanthomatous cells, some of which contain bile particles. H&E.

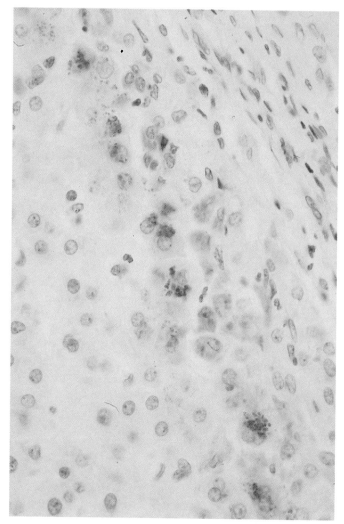

Fig. 4.27 Same as illustrated in Figs 4.30–4.32. Abundant copper accumulation (red granules) in periseptal liver cells. Rhodanine.

increases to approximately 5%, with a 2:1 male predominance. Between 51 and 60 years of age, there is a 15% incidence in males and 0% in females. In an autopsy series of 246 Swedish PiZ patients, the incidence of cirrhosis was 12%, but this increased to 19% in individuals over 50 years of age.[300] There was no known association with alcoholism. Death usually occurred within two years of the clinical diagnosis of cirrhosis. Rare cases of liver disease have been reported in adults with PiMalton and PiMDuarte.[286,302]

A high prevalence of hepatotropic viral infection in predominantly heterozygote patients with α_1-AT deficiency and chronic liver disease has been documented recently by Propst et al.[303] In patients with cirrhosis, 62% of patients were anti-HCV-positive and 33% had HBV infection. Also, 41% of the patients had a history of alcoholism, and 12% had features of autoimmune liver disease. Only 9% of patients with cirrhosis and α_1-AT

deficiency had no other risk factor for chronic liver disease. Among the patients with chronic active hepatitis, 80% were anti-HCV-positive, 30% had HBV infection, 18% had autoimmune hepatitis and 8% had abused alcohol. Among patients with steatosis, 5% were anti-HCV-positive, 18% had serological evidence of past HBV infection and 28% had abused alcohol. Based on their study, Propst et al[303] concluded that the high prevalence of viral infection, rather than the α_1-AT deficiency per se, may be the cause of the chronic liver disease. These findings of hepatitis C in adults are not confirmed in homozygous children.[304]

Swedish investigators have documented an increased incidence of malignancy with or without cirrhosis in adult homozygous PiZ patients. They have determined that the odds ratio in α_1-AT deficiency for cirrhosis was 7.8 and that for hepatocellular carcinoma was 20, compared to age-matched control subjects.[305] According to a recent study from the United States, heterozygosity for α_1-AT Pi types is not associated with an increased risk for hepatocellular carcinoma or bile-duct carcinoma.[306]

Heterozygote risk for disease

Heterozygotes (PiMZ) may be at increased risk for both liver and lung disease as evidenced by retrospective specialist surveys. Fortunately, this incidence must be low because prospective, non-disease-oriented population surveys do not confirm the risk.[307] Liver disease population studies in England, Sweden, and Norway have shown an increased frequency of the PiMZ phenotype in patients with cryptogenic cirrhosis.[308–310]

Liver pathology

The finding of PAS-positive, diastase-resistant globules in periportal hepatocytes is the hallmark of Z-type α_1-AT. They represent the retention of the abnormal enzyme within the rough endoplasmic reticulum or its transition zone.[282] Only a small number of very rare alleles produce a similar picuture (PiMalton, MDuarte). In some instances, PiM associated with an acute inflammatory lesion has produced typical globules.[311] This is thought to be due to overproduction of α_1-AT, exceeding the capacity of the endoplasmic reticulum to process the protein for secretion.

In one case, hepatocyte globules were acquired in a 60-year-old man with the Pi Elemberg M phenotype and primary biliary cirrhosis. This phenotype is not associated with very low serum α_1-AT levels.[312] Globules of α_1-AT may be seen in cells of hepatocellular carcinoma, but the majority of these patients have a normal phenotype for α_1-AT.

The eosinophilic globules of α_1-AT may not be readily apparent with haematoxylin and eosin staining. They can be difficult to detect in the infant less than 12 weeks of age.[313] Immunoperoxidase staining for α_1-AT can be helpful in ambiguous cases; it has been found to be positive as early as 19 weeks of gestation.[314] While immunostaining is more sensitive it can be misleading, particularly when the material is non-zonal in distribution. Non-zonal distribution of α_1-AT is not associated with abnormal Pi phenotypes. Liver biopsies have rarely been performed in patients with the PiQO (null) phenotype. Presumably, individuals producing no A1AT would have no globules, while those producing truncated but unsecreted forms of α_1-AT (e.g. PiQO Hong Kong) might have globules.[315]

The histopathological features of α_1-AT deficiency in cholestatic infants may resemble extrahepatic biliary atresia as the most common findings are bile ductular proliferation and varying degrees of fibrosis or cirrhosis (Fig. 4.28). This emphasizes the need for screening for

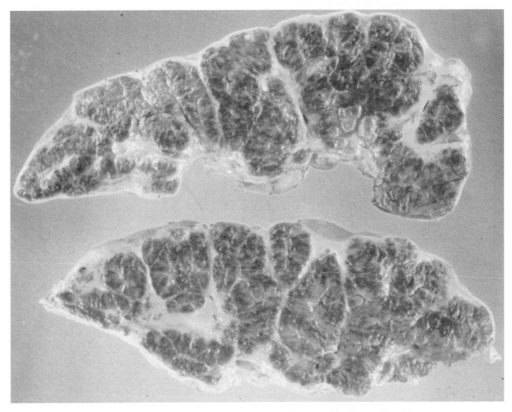

Fig. 4.28 Cirrhotic liver of a 6-year-old-boy with homozygous α_1-AT deficiency.

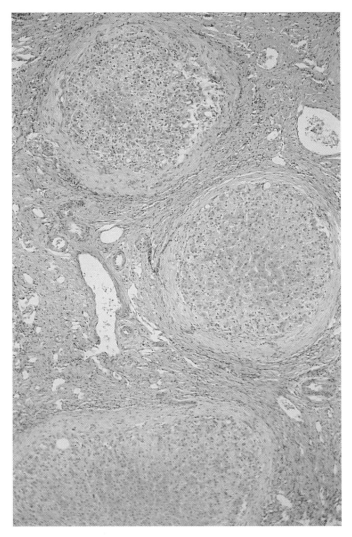

Fig. 4.29 Cirrhotic nodules are surrounded by a ring of dense collagen and separated by loose fibrous tissue. Note lack of piecemeal necrosis and significant inflammation (same case as illustrated in Fig. 4.28. H&E.

α_1-AT deficiency before a patient is subjected to a Kasai procedure. The distinction is made more difficult by the often small size of the external biliary tree in these patients. Inexperienced surgeons may misinterpret operative cholangiograms from these patients as showing biliary atresia and perform an unnecessary Kasai procedure. Bile stasis can be seen in hepatocytes, canaliculi, and even bile ducts. Hepatoytes vary in size with some tendency for acinar formation, but giant cell transformation is usually absent to minimal. Hepatocytes may show mild steatosis in zone 1 (Fig. 4.23) and haemosiderosis. Necrosis, if present, is minimal. Macrophages and Kuppffer cells containing large lysosomes are frequently seen. Residual extramedullary haematopoiesis may be present depending on the timing of the biopsy, and is often confused with inflammation. Up to 10% of patients may have paucity of the intrahepatic bile ducts. Globules have occasionally been found in biliary epithelial cells.[316,317]

As the disease progresses during childhood, hepatocyte necrosis remains minimal except in the end stage. Mild steatosis is fairly common, but inflammation is rarely a prominent feature. The cirrhosis is mixed macro- and micronodular in type, with asymptomatic gradual disappearance of bile ducts with time (Figs 4.28–4.30). A patent but narrow extrahepatic biliary tree is often found during infancy or at the time of liver transplantation. A Roux-en-Y procedure, rather than a duct to duct anastomosis, may be necessary at transplantation.

Other than the globules, the histopathological findings in homozygous adults remain nonspecific and are usually termed cryptogenic. They include fibrosis and variable portal inflammation with predominance of lymphocytes. Bile-duct proliferation is only obvious when cirrhosis is present, and piecemeal necrosis is present occasionally. Mild fat accumulation is usually seen in the hepatocytes but ballooning, bile stasis and iron accumulation are less

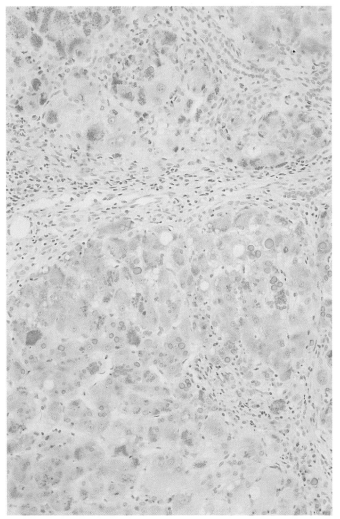

Fig. 4.30 Many α_1-antitrypsin globules are present in liver cells throughout the cirrhotic nodules in case illustrated in Figs 4.28 and 4.29. Peroxidase–antiperoxidase.

common. In one series, 2 patients died from rupture of a non-neoplastic liver nodule. Mallory bodies have been reported.[318,319] The α_1-AT globules can also be detected in heterozygotes, although less frequently than in homozygotes.

The pathogenesis of emphysema in α_1-AT deficiency is reasonably explained by protease-inhibitor imbalance.[320] Two hypotheses have been suggested to explain the liver disease in α_1-AT deficiency—the globule hypothesis[313] and the protease-inhibitor imbalance hypothesis.[321] Neither hypothesis is adequate on its own. Transgenic mice constructed using either the M or the Z types of α_1-AT human genomic clones express these proteins in the liver as well as in several other organs. Unfortunately, abnormalities were noted in both types of transgenic mice. One mouse lineage with multiple copies of the Z α_1-AT gene developed runting with a liver disease characterized by hepatocyte necrosis, microcyst formation, peliosis and microabscesses.[322] Another group reported increased chronic lobular inflammation, small foci of necrosis, and mild fibrosis with damage in M mice but more in Z mice.[323] In one study, mild fibrosis was seen in older mice at 9–12 months of age.[324] The globules are present in all acinar zones and require a high number of copies of the α_1-AT gene. Recent studies suggest that the serum mouse α_1-AT is deficient in this model.[325]

Recent studies have documented that the secretory defect is a direct consequence of the replacement of a negatively charged amino acid Glu with a positively charged amino acid Lys.[326] As a result Z α_1-AT is more aggregable not only in the hepatocyte, where it would stimulate the synthesis of heat shock proteins (particularly BIP), but also in the serum.[327] This defect persists, regardless of the status of the usual salt bridge with an amino acid 290, suggesting that it is due to a crucial B sheet curve alteration. Thus, it is not surprising to find that heat shock proteins are elevated in PiZ individuals with liver disease.[328] Interestingly, similar findings are found in their monocytes, in contrast to PiZ individuals with no liver disease and PiSS individuals.

The diagnosis of α_1-AT deficiency should be sought in all patients with undefined liver disease by measuring the serum level and confirming it with the Pi type of the patient and of the parents if they are available. Medical therapy is mainly supportive. Breast milk should be encouraged in infants although there are no prospective studies to validate its value in the prevention of chronic liver disease.[295,329,330] Liver transplantation corrects the genetic defect and cures the patient.[331] To date, 742 children with liver disease have been reported, of whom 113 subsequently underwent liver transplantation. This establishes α_1-AT deficiency as the second most frequent indication for this procedure in children and the most common inherited disease for which liver transplantation is performed.[321]

α_1-ANTICHYMOTRYPSIN (α_1-ACT) DEFICIENCY

Low levels of α_1-AT and α_1-ACT were found in 4 adult patients with cryptogenic chronic active hepatitis by Lindmark & Erikkson.[332] Subsequently, Eriksson et al[333] estsblished the familial nature of heterozygous α_1-ACT deficiency which has a gene frequency of 0.003 and a heterozygote prevalence of 1/200–300 in Sweden. The inheritance is autosomal dominant. The deficiency occurs independently of α_1-AT deficiency. Among relatives with the α_1-ACT deficiency, there is an increased incidence of cryptogenic liver and lung disease.[333]

Liver biopsy from a patient with α_1-ACT deficiency disclosed cirrhosis with chronic active hepatitis.[334] Granular α_1-ACT inclusions were identified in periportal/periseptal liver cells. A 'fluffy' material was present in dilated cisterns of the endoplasmic reticulum. Further patients need to be evaluated to define this entity more clearly.

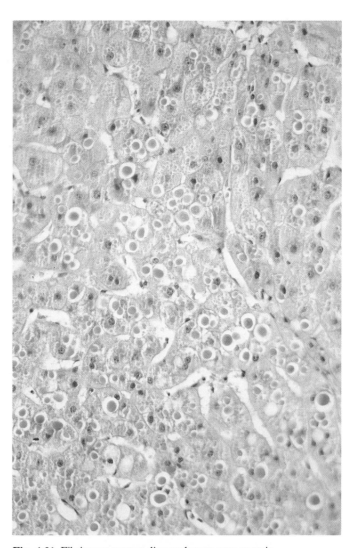

Fig. 4.31 Fibrinogen storage disease: hepatocytes contain eosinophilic globules of varied size. H&E.

AFIBRINOGENAEMIA AND HYPOFIBRINOGENAEMIA

The fibrinogen gene is located on chromosome 4. The inheritance of afibrinogenaemia is autosomal recessive, but hypofibrinogenaemia may be either autosomal recessive or dominant. Over 150 cases of each disorder have been reported. Afibrinogenaemia usually presents with umbilical bleeding. Other complications include intracranial haemorrhage following mild trauma, severe epistaxis, gingival and gastrointestinal bleeding, ecchymoses, and spontaneous splenic rupture. Mild thrombocytopenia may be present. Complications in females include menorrhagia, recurrent abortions and postpartum haemorrhage.[335]

Hypofibrinogenaemia can be divided into cases with levels below 50 and cases with levels between 0.5 and 1.0 g/l of plasma. Symptoms depend on the fibrinogen levels. Thrombosis has been reported. Treatment consists of administration of fibrinogen or cryoprecipitate.

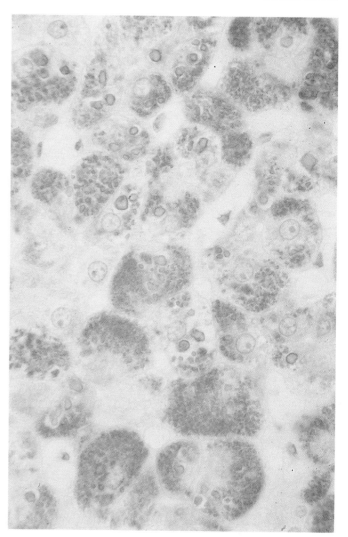

Fig. 4.33 Same case as illustrated in Figs 4.31 and 4.32. Globules are immunoreactive to fibrinogen antibodies. PAP technique.

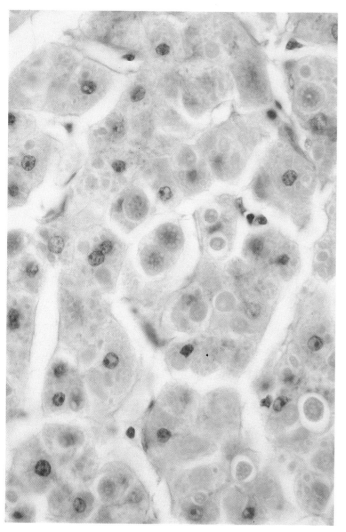

Fig. 4.32 Same case as illustrated in Fig. 4.31. Some globules are vacuolated and others have a dark core. PAS after diastase digestion.

Round and elongated inclusions may be present in the liver in patients with familial hypofibrinogenaemia (Figs 4.31–4.33).[257,336–339] In our experience, the small inclusions in 'fibrinogen storage disease' are irregular in outline, while the large inclusions are spherical and often vacuolated. They are strongly positive with the phosphotungstic acid–haematoxylin stain but are only weakly PAS-positive. Immunoreactivity to fibrinogen antibody can be demonstrated. Ultrastructurally, the cisterns of the rough endoplasmic reticulum are filled with densely packed, curved tubular structures arranged in a fingerprint-like pattern[336,338,339] (Fig. 4.34). However, in the two cases reported by Ng et al,[257] the stored fibrinogen was described as granular by electron microscopic study. In some patients, cirrhosis may occur.

ANTITHROMBIN III DEFICIENCY

This uncommon disorder has an autosomal dominant

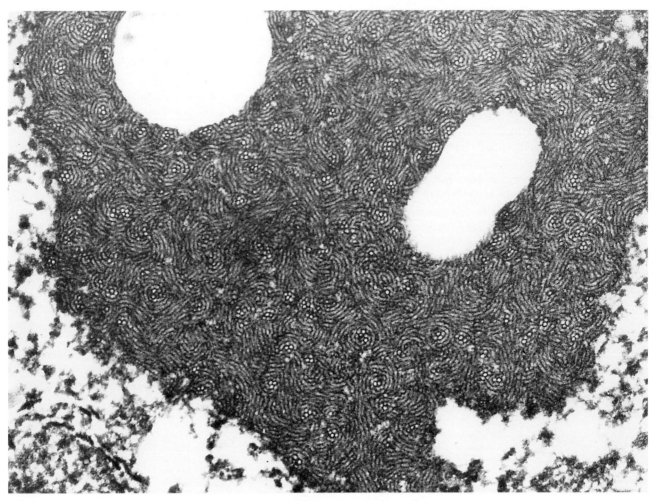

Fig. 4.34 Electron micrograph of the same case as illustrated in Figs 4.31–4.33. The fibrinogen inclusion in the liver cell has a fingerprint-like pattern. × 31 700.

inheritance with complete penetrance. There is a propensity for venous thromboembolism ranging from superficial thrombophlebitis to pulmonary embolism.[340,341] The deficiency may be complicated by the Budd–Chiari syndrome.[342,343] An 8-month-old infant with antithrombin III deficiency reported by Mendelsohn et al[344] developed multiple large venous and arterial thromboses and *E. coli* sepsis. He had a micronodular cirrhosis, and liver cells contained multiple, eosinophilic, PAS-positive globules resembling those of α_1-AT deficiency. However, the globules failed to react with anti-α_1-AT or with anti-antithrombin antisera.

DISORDERS OF AMINO ACID METABOLISM

TYROSINAEMIA (HEREDITARY TYROSINAEMIA, TYROSINAEMIA TYPE I)

This is a disorder of amino acid metabolism which is transmitted as an autosomal recessive trait. It has a worldwide distribution with a high prevalence in Quebec, Canada,

France and Scandinavia. Acute and chronic forms are recognized.[345–347] In the *acute* form, with onset within a few weeks or months of birth, there is failure to thrive, anaemia, vomiting, diarrhoea, hepatosplenomegaly, bleeding diathesis, and rickets. Death results from liver failure associated with infection or bleeding, or both, by the end of the first year of life. A variant, characterized by bilateral idiopathic keratitis and unexplained skin lesions without evidence of liver damage or the Fanconi syndrome, has been reported by Buist et al.[348] The *chronic* form is generally manifested in the first year of life by growth retardation, gastrointestinal symptoms, hepatic failure, and multiple renal tubular defects with secondary rachitic changes. Episodes of acute intermittent porphyria have been reported.[349–351] Death usually occurs within the first decade.

Biochemical determinations in both forms of the disease show elevated plasma levels of tyrosine (above 30 mg/l) and constant hyperexcretion of tyrosyl compounds (p-hydroxyphenylpyruvic acid and p-hydroxyphenylacetic acid) in the fasting stage. Other features include hypoglycaemia, hypermethioninaemia, hypophosphataemia, generalized aminoaciduria of a distinct type, glycosuria, protein-uria and hyperphosphaturia. Radiological examination demonstrates the characteristic changes of rickets.

Liver function tests show hyperbilirubinaemia, usually less than 135 μmol/l (8 mg/100 ml), normal or slightly elevated alkaline phosphatase values, hypoproteinaemia (affecting both albumin and globulin), diminished pro-thrombin levels and slightly increased transaminase values.[352] There may be significant elevation of serum α-fetoprotein levels.[353] Prenatal diagnosis and detection of the carrier state are discussed by Kvittingen et al[354] in a recent review.

The basic biochemical defect in tyrosinaemia is now postulated to be a deficiency of fumarylacetoacetate hydro-lase (fumarylacetoacetase).[355,356] The gene for the deficient enzyme has been mapped to chromosome 15q23–q25.[357] Deficiencies of glutathione and of mixed function oxidases may play a significant role in the carcinogenic potential of this disorder.[358] These and other enzyme deficiencies (S-amino levulinic acid dehydratase, methionine adenosyl transferase) are considered secondary to the primary deficiency of fumarylacetoacetate hydrolase.[356]

Pathological aspects of tyrosinaemia have been reported by a number of authors.[167,359–368] About 50% of patients have hyperplasia of the islets of Langerhans.[361] Renal changes include interstitial oedema, tubular dilatation with vacuolar and granular degeneration, loss of glomeruli,[346,348] and hypertrophy and hyperplasia of the juxtaglomerular complex.[363] The liver at autopsy is slightly to moderately enlarged, yellow, firm and nodular (Fig. 4.35).[361] The microscopic features include fatty change, cholestasis, pseudoacinar transformation of hepatic plates, pericellular and periportal fibrosis, variable haemosiderosis and extra-medullary haemopoiesis, and varying-sized foci of nodular regeneration with some qualifying as macroregenerative nodules (Figs 4.36 and 4.37). The regenerating nodules, which appear as high attenuation foci on CT scans, are difficult to differentiate from multifocal hepatocellular carcinoma.[369] In our experience, the nodules often show much more fat accumulation than the adjacent liver, a finding also previously noted by Prive (Fig. 4.36).[361] Periportal cholangiolar proliferation, although present, is usually not striking. Cirrhosis may be micronodular, macronodular or mixed.[359,362] Transition from a micro-nodular to a macronodular cirrhosis has been documented by Dehner et al.[365] Liver-cell dysplasia, both the large and small cell varieties, has been reported by three groups of investigators.[365–367]

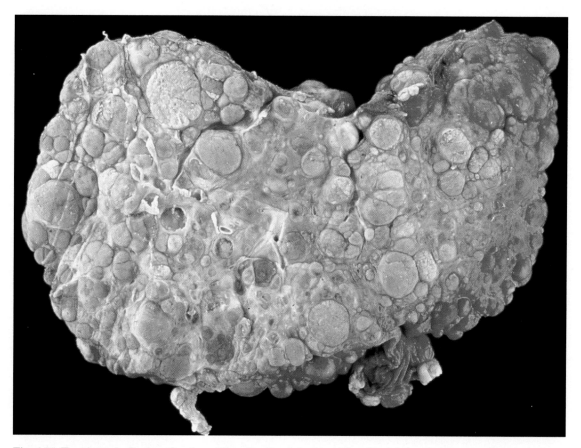

Fig. 4.35 Tyrosinaemia. Section of explanted liver showing cirrhotic nodules of varied size, that are tan, yellow or green in colour.

Cytogenetic studies on skin fibroblasts from a patient with tyrosinaemia type I and hepatocellular carcinoma have demonstrated chromosome breakage in 71% of cells.[370] Recently, DNA ploidy abnormalities were detected in 3 cases by Zerbini et al.[368] These authors suggested that DNA ploidy may be a useful marker for early malignant transformation in this disease.

Ultrastructural studies have confirmed the presence of fat in hepatocytes and the cholestasis, as well as a number of non-specific changes.[12,359,363] In the case studied by Jevtic et al,[363] hepatocytes surrounded a central canaliculus forming tubules; the cells were joined by many desmosomes. The basal portions of the cells were not covered by microvilli or a space of Disse, and basement membrane-like material was present. Mitochondria of liver cells can be markedly increased in number in tyrosinaemia, and may

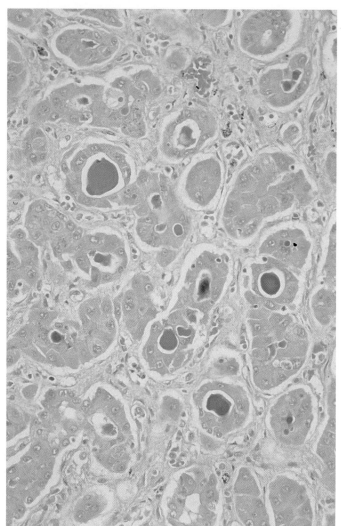

Fig. 4.37 Tyrosinaemia. Marked cholestasis in neocholangioles. H&E.

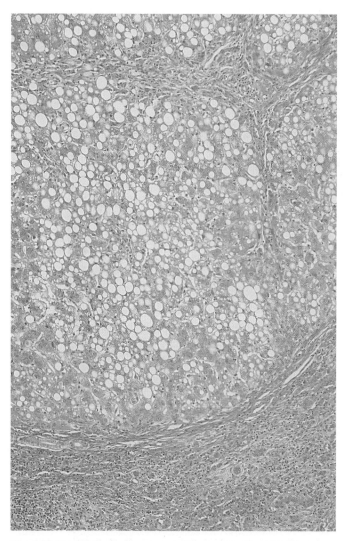

Fig. 4.36 Tyrosinaemia. Same case as illustrated in Fig. 4.35. The patient had developed cirrhosis; a segment of a macroregenerative nodule shows marked steatosis. H&E.

show mild to moderate pleomorphism with randomly oriented cristae.[12] Peroxisomes are frequently enlarged and may contain nucleoids or small lipid droplets.[12]

Hepatocellular carcinoma is a recognized complication of tyrosinaemia. Weinberg et al,[371] who reported a case and reviewed the previous literature, found 16 (37%) cases amongst 43 patients who had survived beyond 2 years of age. Females and males are equally at risk.

Liver transplantation is the ultimate therapy in tyrosinaemia and may even cure hepatocellular carcinomas,[367,372] but some renal tubular dysfunction persists, suggesting a contribution of extrahepatic tissues to the biochemical abnormalities of this disease.[373] Recently, medical therapy aimed at preventing the formation of maleylacetoacetate and fumarylacetoacetate and their saturated derivatives has been found to prevent the development of cirrhosis and to abolish or diminish the risk of development of hepatocellular carcinoma.[374]

The basic injury in hereditary tyrosinaemia has in the past been attributed to toxicity from defective tyrosine degradation. A study by Hostetter et al[375] throws doubt on this hypothesis; these investigators found that the liver disease began before birth in 3 infants, but that hypertyrosinaemia and hypermethioninaemia occurred after birth. Nevertheless, recent data confirm four phenotypic variants of the deficiency of fumarylacetoacetate hydrolase.[376]

CONGENITAL HYPERAMMONAEMIA SYNDROMES AND THE UREA CYCLE DISORDERS

Hyperammonaemia secondary to an hepatocyte enzyme defect, rather than due to liver failure as in cirrhosis, can present at any age but is disastrous to the central nervous system of children, especially in the newborn period. This group of disorders is extremely important to recognize since failure to do so has not only grave consequences for the patient but also prevents a chance of treatment for present and future family members.[377] Medical treatment should begin at birth and can prevent serious damage to the central nervous system. The patients are normal at birth. After 24 hours, however, irritability, poor feeding, vomiting, lethargy, and respiratory distress develop. This is quickly followed by hypotonia, seizures, coma and respiratory arrest. The diagnosis can be arrived at by relatively simple plasma and urine tests, as listed below.[378] Possible misdiagnoses include respiratory distress syndrome, sepsis or intraventricular haemorrhage in the newborn period, or Reye's syndrome when presenting later.

Clues and tests for the neonatal diagnosis of hyperammonaemia:

1. Respiratory distress before or after 24 hours of age

2. Acidosis and/or ketosis (methylmalonate or propionate)

3. Normal plasma glycine level

4. Carbamyl phosphate synthetase: absent/trace plasma citrulline, low urine orotate

5. Ornithine transcarbamylase: absent/trace plasma citrulline, high urine orotate

6. Argininosuccinate aciduria: plasma citrulline = 100 – 300 μM/l

7. Citrullinaemia: plasma citrulline > 1000 μM/l.

Carbamyl phosphate synthetase (CPS) deficiency

This liver mitochondrial enzyme is located on the short arm of chromosome 2. Inheritance of the deficiency is autosomal recessive. The diagnosis can be confirmed by liver biopsy, in which enzyme levels range from

0–22%.[379,380] Prenatal diagnosis is facilitated by three different types of restriction patterns following digestion with BgII. When the affected allele is transmitted from a heterozygous parent, 50% of cases can be diagnosed; the rest require fetal or day one liver biopsy.[377] Light and electron microscopic appearances have been reported to be normal.[381] Medical therapy has improved survival, especially when started form birth. Liver transplantation has been successful late in the course of the disease, but needs to be performed as early as feasible.

Ornithine transcarbamylase (OTC) deficiency

OTC is also a liver mitochondrial enzyme.[382] The most reliable studies have been performed in the liver, although the enzyme is also present in the small intestine. The enzyme maps to band p21.2 of the X chromosome just proximal to the Duchenne muscular dystrophy gene.[383] In hemizygous males, the residual enzyme activity ranges from 0–30%. Prior to birth, 90% of patients can be identified by chorionic biopsy if three RFLP enzymes are utilized, and the carrier state has been identified in the mother.[377] This can be achieved by finding elevated levels of orotidine following oral allopurinol administration. The drug blocks the final enzymatic step in pyrimidine biosynthesis via its metabolite oxipurinal ribonucleotide at the level of orotidine monophosphate decarboxylase.[384] The disease can be symptomatic in females, is most commonly diagnosed as Reye's syndrome in children and, most recently, has been identified as a cause of postpartum coma in adults.[385]

Pathological studies of the liver in males have generally been normal. Occasional case reports suggest some mitochondrial and peroxisomal changes.[386] Acquired abnormalities, more likely to be seen with the passage of time, are documented in females. At the light microscopic level, the mild changes include fat accumulation, inflammation, piecemeal necrosis and mild periportal fibrosis.[387,387a] Organelles in the hepatocytes usually are normal. The results of medical and surgical treatment are similar to those of CPS deficiency.[377]

Argininosuccinate synthetase deficiency (citrullinaemia)

The enzyme is located on chromosome 9, q34. Homozygotes may be hard to distinguish from heterozygotes except by studies of citrulline incorporation into acid-precipitable protein using cultured fibroblasts.[388]

Argininosuccinic lyase deficiency (argininosuccinicaciduria)

The enzyme is located on chromosome 7.[389] Absence of the enzyme protein has been documented in the liver.[390]

Enzyme levels can also be measured in red blood cells, fibroblasts, and amniotic cells, with substrate accumulation occurring in the fluid of cultured cells. This is the only urea cycle enzyme defect in which significant liver disease is also present, as evidenced by hepatomegaly, elevations of serum alanine transferase, and severe fibrosis on liver biopsy.[391] Marked macrovesicular steatosis was described in a case reported by Jorda et al.[392] Ultrastructural changes include dilatation of the rough or smooth endoplasmic reticulum,[391–393] and the presence of megamitochondria in zones affected by steatosis.[392] Despite the structural changes, survival figures in these patients and in those with argininosuccinate synthetase deficiency are much better than in those with OTC and CPS deficiencies.

N-acetylglutamate synthetase deficiency

Three cases of partial deficiency have been reported in one family.[394] All patients presented at around one year of age. Citrulline was undetectable in the plasma. Orotic acid secretion was normal. The activity of the arginine-activated enzyme in the liver was 33% of control values. Liver cells contained both small and large droplet fat. Mitochondria were small with an electron-dense matrix and reduced cristae. Two other reported patients were newborns;[395,396] they presumably presented earlier because of liver enzyme levels of only 2–3%. The data so far suggest that the disease is inherited in an autosomal recessive mode.

CYSTINOSIS

Cystinosis has been reviewed recently in detail by Gahl et al.[397] It is a rare autosomal recessive disease (1 in 100 000 – 200 000 live births) characterized by the accumulation of L-cystine crystals in lysosomes that is secondary to a defective carrier-mediated transport system for cystine. As a result, cystine accumulates in the eye, reticuloendothelial system, kidney, and other internal organs. Three clinical forms are recognized.

Nephrogenic (infantile) cystinosis. Patients are normal at birth. Symptoms of renal tubular dysfunction of Fanconi type develop by 6–12 months and progress to renal failure by 10 years of age. The tubular defect accounts for the presenting symptoms of polyuria, polydipsia and failure to thrive. Affected children are often hospitalized because of vomiting, dehydration, electrolyte imbalance and acidosis resulting from potassium and bicarbonate urinary loss. Phosphaturia ultimately leads to vitamin D resistant rickets. Mental development is normal. Patients develop photophobia secondary to deposition of the crystals in the cornea and conjunctiva, where their detection by slit lamp examination is diagnostic of the disease.[398] Hot weather accentuates the symptoms because of a decreased ability to sweat. Crystal accumulation in the thyroid leads to hypothyroidism.[399]

Dialysis or renal transplantation is initiated between 6 and 12 years of age. Although the defect is corrected in the kidney following renal transplantation, storage continues in other organs resulting in blindness, corneal erosions, diabetes, and neurological deterioration between 13 and 30 years of age. Medical therapy consists of medications for the renal tubular defects plus carnitine. Cysteamine has been given both systemically and also applied topically to the eyes. Significant toxic effects in the gastrointestinal tract and a case of veno-occlusive disease of the liver have been reported.[400] The best results have been obtained in siblings treated early after diagnosis of the index case.

Massive hepatomegaly has been reported in this disorder;[397] its incidence may be as high as 42% in patients over 10 years of age. However, most patients do not have significant liver dysfunction. Up to 50% of dialysis and kidney transplant patients may have depatomegaly and elevated liver enzymes but the aetiology is unclear.[401] The majority of these patients also have splenomegaly. Bleeding varices were reported in 2 patients despite little evidence of significant liver disease.[401] The diagnosis is usually made by detection of elevated cystine levels in cells. Prenatal diagnosis is accomplished by measuring cystine levels in the chorionic villi, or by pulse labelling studies with cystine, utilizing amniotic cells.

Late onset (intermediate or adolescent) cystinosis. Late onset (intermediate or adolescent) cystinosis is an attenuated form of the disease not associated with symptoms before the fifth year of life, and is compatible with survival well into the second decade. Clinical manifestations include retinal depigmentation, rickets, mild renal failure, and accumulation of cystine crystals in the conjunctiva and bone marrow.

Benign cystinosis. Patients are asymptomatic and have a normal life expectancy, presumably because substantially less cystine accumulates within cells than in the nephropathic or intermediate form.[402] This form of the disease is diagnosed only by slit lamp examination of the eyes.

Pathological findings

The diagnosis of cystinosis is established by visualization of the rectangular and hexagonal crystals in bone marrow aspirates, in conjunctival, rectal or renal biopsy tissue, or by ophthalmological examination. Phase contrast and polarizing microscopy are especially useful in searching for the crystals in biopsy material. Because of the solubility of the crystals in water, all tissues should be fixed in alcohol, and aqueous stains should be avoided.[403] The crystals are therefore best seen in unstained frozen sections or in sections made from alcohol-fixed tissue, and examined by phase or polarizing microscopy. Electron microscopy is a useful method of diagnosis if light microscopic examination of biopsy tissue fails to reveal the crystals.[404] The

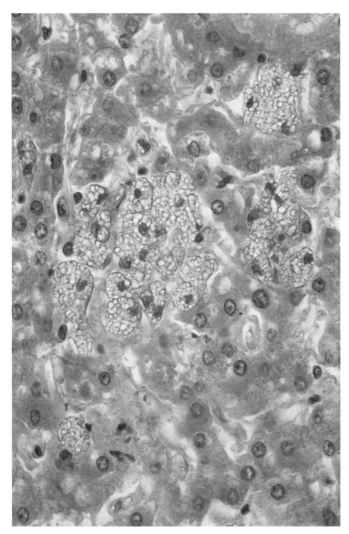

Fig. 4.38 Cystinosis. Cystine crystals are packed in the cytoplasm of hypertrophied Kupffer cells. H&E.

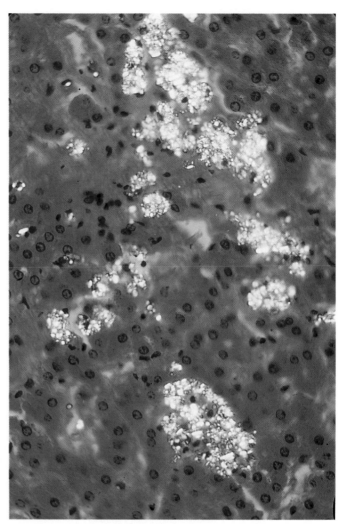

Fig. 4.39 Same case as illustrated in Fig. 4.38. Cystine crystals display brilliant silvery birefringence. H&E.

diagnosis has been made before birth by light and electron microscopic examination of fetal tissues.[405,406] Other methods of diagnosis include the determination of the amount of cystine in white blood cells or in cultured skin fibroblasts. A non-invasive method of diagnosis based on infra-red spectroscopy of hair, was reported by Lubec et al.[407]

The cystine crystals accumulate within lysosomes.[408,409] The most severely affected organ is the kidney.[403,410] Most of the cells containing the crystals are of reticuloendothelial origin. Crystals in many organs, such as the cornea, conjunctiva, bone marrow, spleen and liver, excite little or no reaction. In the liver, markedly hypertrophied Kupffer cells packed with cystine are located mainly in acinar zone 3 (Fig. 4.38). They have a brilliant silvery birefringence under polarized light (Fig. 4.39). The spaces made by the crystals in Kupffer cells can be seen by electron microscopy[411,412] (Fig. 4.40) and the crystals

have a characteristic appearance by scanning electron microscopy (Fig. 4.41).

CYSTATHIONINE ß-SYNTHASE DEFICIENCY (HOMOCYSTINURIA)

This deficiency, inherited as an autosomal recessive trait, is the most frequent cause of homocystinuria. More than 600 cases have been studied.[413] Methionine and other metabolites of homocysteine also accumulate in the body and are excreted in the urine.

The clinical features include ocular abnormalities (ectopia lentis and its complications), skeletal manifestations (osteoporosis, genu valgum, pes cavus, kyphoscoliosis and others), neurological signs and symptoms (mental retardation, that is usually progressive), and the multiple and varied effects of thrombosis of arteries such as the coronary, renal, subclavian, iliac and carotid.

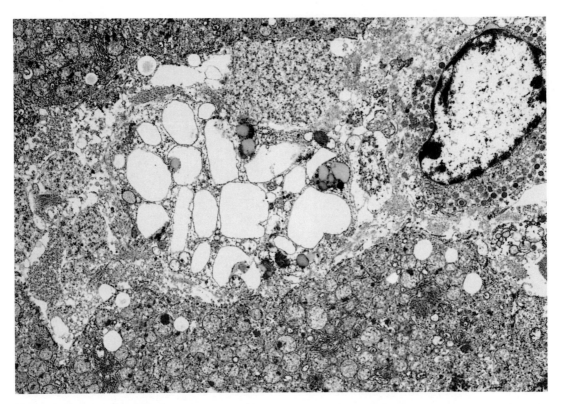

Fig. 4.40 Electron micrograph shows spaces created by cystine crystals that were dissolved during processing. Several have rectangular shapes. × 32 000.

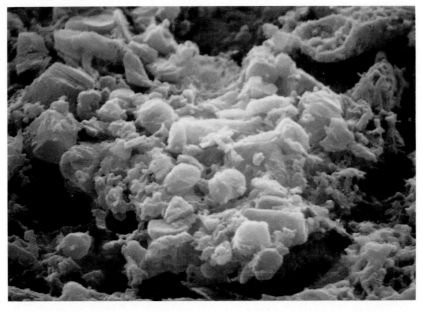

Fig. 4.41 Three-dimensional appearance of cystine crystals, some having a hexagonal shape. Scanning electron micrograph, × 5000.

Hyperhomocysteinaemia has been identified as an important risk factor for occlusive vascular disease in adults.[414] Hepatomegaly may be present, but liver function tests are usually normal.[415]

Light microscopic studies of the liver in homocystinuria have shown steatosis, more prominent in acinar zone 3.[415–417] Mild to moderate portal fibrosis and thickened arterioles with intimal hyperplasia or fibrosis have been observed in some patients.[416] Ultrastructural studies have demonstrated mitochondria with unusual shapes, increased smooth endoplasmic reticulum and numerous pericanalicular lysosomes.[418,419]

DISORDERS OF LIPOPROTEIN AND LIPID METABOLISM

BETA LIPOPROTEIN DEFICIENCY

There are two species of apolipoprotein B in plasma lipoprotein. Apolipoprotein B100 (Apo B100) is synthesized primarily in the liver and is secreted in low density lipoportein (LDL) and very low density lipoprotein (VLDL). Apolipoprotein B48 (Apo B48) is synthesized exclusively in the intestine and is transported from its epithelial cells in chylomicrons and chylomicron remnants.[420] Apo B48 is homologous from the amino acid terminus through amino acid 2152, i.e. 47% of Apo B100.[421] This protein is translated from mRNA containing a single base substitution which produces a stop codon corresponding to residue 2153 of the larger glycoprotein Apo B100.[422,423] Only Apo B100 contains a binding domain for the LDL receptor.[424]

The gene for apolipoprotein B has been mapped to chromosome 2. However, recent investigators suggest that the defect in abetalipoproteinaemia is not related to the gene product by RFLP analysis.[425,426] Microsomal triglyceride transfer protein (MTP) is present in the liver and intestine microsomes to mediate transport of cholesterol ester, triglyceride, and phosphatidyl choline between membranes. Recently, it has been found to be absent in 4 patients with abetalipoproteinuria, suggesting that this protein disulphide isomerase is required for lipoprotein assembly.[427] This is consistent with the absence of VLDL, LDL, and chylomicronaemia in patients with abetalipoproteinaemia.

Abetalipoprotein deficiency was described by Bassen & Kornzweig[428] in 1950, with the deficiency of betaglobulin detected by Jampel & Falls in 1958.[429] It is an autosomal codominant disorder.[425] The disease has five basic features: abetalipoproteinaemia, malabsorption of fat, acanthocytosis, retinitis pigmentosa, and an ataxic neuropathic disease.[430-434] Symptoms begin during infancy with steatorrhoea resulting in failure to thrive. Acanthocytes are evident by 12 months of age. Neurological abnormalities causing an unsteady gait develop between 2 and 17 years of age. Degenerative changes affect the posterior and lateral columns of the spinal cord, spinocerebellar pathways and peripheral nerves. The diagnosis is suspected by the aforementioned features, a serum cholesterol level of less than 1.3 mmol/l (50 mg/dl) and an extremely low triglyceride value. The diagnosis is confirmed by determination of beta lipoprotein using electrophoresis, ultracentrifugation, or immunochemical methods. Small bowel biopsies reveal fat droplets in the epithelium (Fig. 4.42). Treatment consists of a low fat diet and supplements of vitamins A

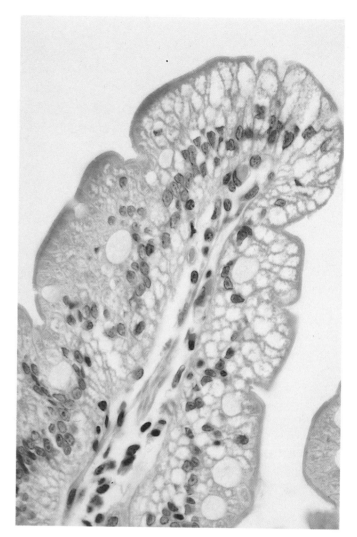

Fig. 4.42 Abetalipoproteinaemia. Intestinal microvillus reveals marked vacuolization of epithelial cells. H&E.

and E.[435] Late manifestations include essential fatty acid deficiency and peripheral vascular disease.

Histological studies of several cases of abetalipoproteinaemia have shown variable fatty change in the liver.[417,422-425] The patient studied by Partin et al[436] underwent biopsies prior to and after 2, 14 and 20 months of therapy with medium chain triglycerides. Before treatment, hepatocytes contained large fat droplets which had ruptured to form 'fatty lakes' in acinar zone 3. Ultrastructurally, the Golgi apparatus was nearly completely deficient in trans-Golgi vacuole formation. Endogenous triglyceride particles could not be found and the circum-Golgi smooth endoplasmic reticulum was absent. During the 14 months of dietary treatment, the fat droplets in hepatocytes became smaller and less numerous, but there was progression of initially mild hepatic fibrosis to a micronodular cirrhosis. Mallory bodies were identified in hepatocytes of the cirrhotic liver by electron microscopy. Clinically, the patient had substantial hepatomegaly and a

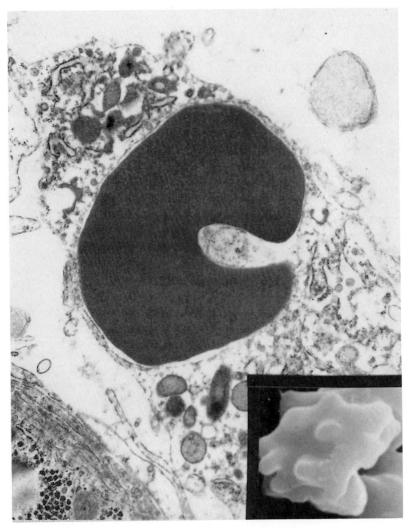

Fig. 4.43 Abetalipoproteinaemia. Transmission electron micrograph shows Kupffer cell with phagocytosed acanthocyte. × 40 000. Scanning electron micrograph (inset) shows a sinusoidal acanthocyte. × 5000.

persistent increase of serum aminotransferase activity. Whether the hepatic lesions were part of the natural course of the disease or related to therapy remains undetermined. The ultrastructural findings of one reported case included fatty change, a normal Golgi apparatus and endoplasmic reticulum, acanthocytes in sinusoids, and phagocytosis of deformed erythrocytes by Kupffer cells[437] (Fig. 4.43). An ultrastructural study of another case by Collins et al[438] demonstrated striking changes in hepatocellular peroxisomes.

Recently, a 20-year-old black woman with abetalipoproteinaemia but without therapy with medium chain triglycerides developed cirrhosis and underwent liver transplantation.[439] She also had a polyclonal gammopathy. Postoperatively, the cholesterol rose from 0.69 to 2.89 μmol/l (27–112 mg/dl), triglycerides from 0.31 to 3.88 μmol/l (28–344 mg/dl), and a barely measurable Apo B (<1) rose to 76. Apo B100 was found in VLD and LDL but Apo B48 was never detected in this patient. In the resected liver and intestine, reduced quantities of Apo B were present in the cytosol supernatant. Apo B mRNA in the intestine was four times the normal control value. Approximately 10–15% of Apo B is synthesized in the small intestinal mucosa.[440] Apo B messenger RNA levels are markedly elevated in abetalipoproteinaemia.[440,441]

Variants of abetalipoproteinaemia have been described. Homozygous hypobetalipoproteinaemia produces the same clinical findings but the parents have intermediate levels as would be expected in an autosomal recessive disorder. In contrast, liver Apo B mRNA is only 8–14% normal.[442] Malloy et al[443] in 1981 described normotriglyceridaemic abetalipoproteinaemia in which cholesterol levels remained low; lipid did not accumulate in the small intestine but some fat malabsorption persisted. No normal-sized Apo B100 is present in these patients.[444] Steinberg et al[445] described a patient who subsequently was found to have a truncated Apo B37 resulting in hypobetalipoproteinaemia.[446,447] Anderson et al[448] documented steatorrhoea and failure to thrive in a 7-month-old girl. Serum alpha and beta lipoprotein levels were 50% of the normal ranges. Recently, 7 cases from five kindreds have been described by Bouma et al;[441] and 8 other infants were reported by Roy et al.[449] Selective deletion of Apo B48 was found. Lipid droplets were found in the intestinal mucosa. Neurological problems were of later onset. MTP levels were normal.

FAMILIAL HIGH DENSITY LIPOPROTEIN DEFICIENCY (TANGIER DISEASE)

This autosomal recessive disease, named after the island in Chesapeake Bay, United States, where the first two cases were reported,[450] is characterized by the absence of normal alpha or high density lipoprotein (HDL) in the plasma, low plasma cholesterol levels and the accumulation of esterified cholesterol in reticuloendothelial cells.[451–453] The basic defect is thought to be a mutation in an allele regulating the synthesis of one of the major apoproteins of alpha lipoprotein, which results in a reduction of the concentration of alpha lipoprotein.[454] The disease may involve a defect in the formation of circulating high density lipoproteins or their enhanced catabolism.[453]

The clinical findings include tonsillar enlargement with a striking orange discolouration, lymphadenopathy, hepatosplenomegaly and peripheral neuropathy. Thrombocytopenia, corneal opacities and xanthomas are less frequent. Occasional patients may have hyperbilirubinaemia.[455,456]

The pathological aspects of the disease are comprehensively discussed in the publications of Bale et al[452] and Ferrans & Fredrickson.[455] Deposition of cholesterol esters is widespread, with involvement of tonsillar and adenoidal tissue, liver, spleen, lymph nodes, bone marrow, thymus, intestinal mucosa, skin and cornea. The foam cells contain birefringent, needle-shaped cholesterol crystals, are sudanophilic and PAS-negative, and stain positively with the Schultz modification of the Lieberman–Burchard reaction. Involvement of the liver by clusters of cholesterol-containing cells has been noted in patients studied by a number of investigators.[451,436,456–459] The differential diagnosis from other cholesterol storage diseases is discussed by Bale et al.[452]

FAMILIAL HYPERCHOLESTEROLAEMIA

This disease is characterized clinically by an elevated concentration of low density lipoprotein (LDL)—the major cholesterol transport lipoprotein in plasma), and deposition of cholesterol in tendons and skin (xanthomas) and in arteries (atheroma). It is inherited as an autosomal dominant trait with a gene dosage effect, i.e. homozygotes are more severely affected than heterozygotes.[460] Hetero-

zygotes, who number about 1 in 500 persons, have twofold elevations of plasma cholesterol from birth. Tendon xanthomas and coronary atherosclerosis develop after the age of 20. Homozygotes, who number 1 per million persons, have severe hypercholesterolaemia. Xanthomas appear in the first four years of life. Coronary heart disease begins in childhood and frequently leads to death before the age of 20. The primary defect is a mutation in the gene, located on the short arm of chromosome 19, which specifies the receptor for plasma LDL.

Reported pathological findings in homozygous familial hypercholesterolaemia have been reviewed by Buja et al.[461] Therapy is discussed in detail by Goldstein & Brown.[460] The role of portacaval shunt and liver transplantation is reviewed by Bilheimer.[462] Liver transplantation should be reserved for those patients who cannot produce functioning LDL receptors and who do not respond to more conservative forms of therapy.[462] In addition to atherosclerosis of the aorta and coronary vessels there in neutral lipid accumulation in extravascular sites that include the skin, tendons, spleen, thymus and other organs.[461] In the liver, there is accumulation of lipid in hepatocytes and Kupffer cells. Ultrastructurally, accumulation of both neutral lipid and cholesterol has been observed in hepatocytes.[12] Some liver cells may show proliferation of the smooth endoplasmic reticulum.[12]

FAMILIAL HYPERLIPOPROTEINAEMIAS

These are disorders of lipid metabolism characterized by increased secretion and elevated blood levels of various lipoproteins. Five abnormal lipoprotein patterns are recognized.[463,464] Histological studies in the hyperlipoproteinaemias have shown lipid-laden foam cells in the bone marrow, spleen and liver.[465–467] Hepatocytes may also be vacuolated.[466] Ultrastructural studies in patients with types IV and V have disclosed lipid droplets, giant mitochondria with paracrystalline inclusions and various changes in the rough endoplasmic reticulum, e.g. dilatation, vesiculation, disruption and degranulation.[468]

GM₁ GANGLIOSIDOSIS

GM_1 or generalized gangliosidosis is characterized by the accumulation of GM_1 ganglioside in neural and visceral cells resulting from deficient activity of the lysosomal isoenzymes of GM_1-ß galactosidase.[469,470] The inheritance is autosomal recessive.

The infantile form, type I, manifests itself during the first 6 months of life. Clinically, patients present with progressive psychomotor retardation, seizures, hepatosplenomegaly, oedema of the extremities and failure to thrive. The appetite is poor and suckling is weak. By the first year of life, the patients are blind, deaf and in decerebrate rigidity. Death usually supervenes from broncho-

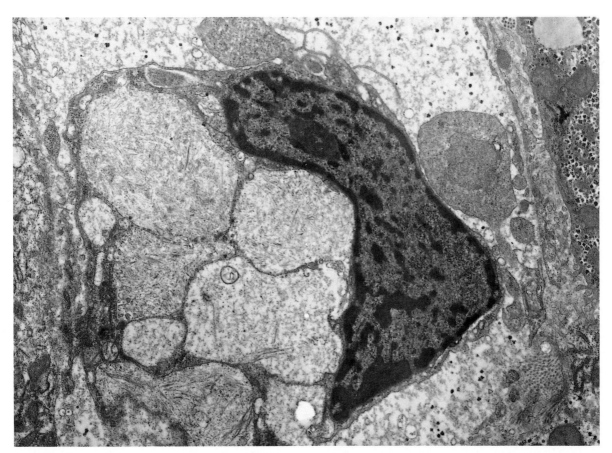

Fig. 4.44 GM₁ gangliosidosis, type I. The cytoplasm of a Kupffer cell is replaced by single membrane-bound vacuoles. Some of the vacuoles contain amorphous material, while others are filled with irregularly arranged fibrillar material. × 9300. Courtesy of Dr M Petrelli

pneumonia by 2 years of age. Physical examination reveals a dull-looking, hypoactive and hypotonic infant with facial and peripheral oedema. Facial abnormalities include frontal bossing, a depressed nasal bridge, large low-set ears, increased distance between the nose and upper lip, and downy hirsutism of the forehead and neck. The gums are hypertrophied and there is mild to moderate macroglossia. The corneas are clear. Cherry-red spots are present in the macula in half the patients.

Foam cells are seen in bone marrow preparations. Lymphocytes are vacuolated. Mild radiological abnormalities consist of inferior beaking of the lumbar vertebrae and proximal pointing of the metacarpal bones. Neurons are ballooned and contain cytoplasmic membranous inclusions similar to those of Tay–Sachs disease. Lipid-laden histiocytes are found throughout the reticulo-endothelial system. Renal glomerular epithelial cells, hepatocytes and Kupffer cells are finely vacuolated. Ultrastructurally, the vacuoles contain amorphous material. A few Kupffer cells may also contain membrane-bound fibrillary structures[471] (Fig. 4.44). Enzyme analysis indicates almost complete absence of β-galactosidase A, B and C in skin fibroblasts and leucocytes.

The juvenile form, type II, presents at about 1 year of age. Clinical findings are primarily neurological and include seizures, spasticity, ataxia and mental retardation. Radiological changes are minimal. Facial abnormalities, visceromegaly and macular cherry-red spots are absent. Death occurs between 3 and 8 years of age.[469] The enzyme defect is similar to that of type I, except that iso-enzyme A is present. An accurate prenatal diagnosis can be made from amniotic cells.

In common with type I, there is neuronal storage and foamy histiocytes are present in various organs (Fig. 4.45). Hepatocytes are only slightly vacuolated and Kupffer cells stain intensely with the PAS reagent (Fig. 4.46). Ultrastructurally, the Kupffer cells contain a distinctive granulofibrillar material[471] (Fig. 4.47), or membrane-bound inclusions may be seen in both Kupffer cells and hepatocytes.[472] Two canine models of GM₁ gangliosidosis have been described.[473]

GM₂ GANGLIOSIDOSES

The GM₂ gangliosidoses have become a diverse group of

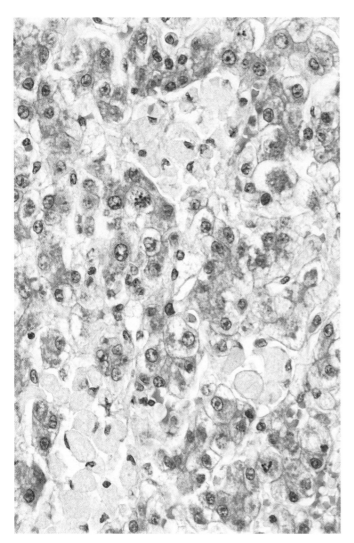

Fig. 4.45 GM$_1$ gangliosidosis, type II. Clusters of pale-staining foamy Kupffer cells that have eccentric nuclei. H&E.

diseases which primarily present with neurological manifestations.[474] The various disorders reflect defects in the lysosomal enzyme β-hexosaminidase, resulting in the accumulation of glycolipids, particularly ganglioside GM$_2$ as well as oligosaccharides from glycoproteins in Sandhoff's disease. The enzyme β-hexosaminidase consists of two major isoenzymes, hexosaminidase A composed of an alpha and beta subunit, and hexosaminidase β composed of two beta subunits. The alpha subunit has been localized to chromosome 15 and the beta subunit to chromosome 5. A lysosomal enzyme, GM$_2$ activator protein, also localized to chromosome 5, complexes with the lipid substrate to present β-hexosaminidase for cleavage hydrolysis. Inheritance of all the variants is autosomal recessive. Prenatal diagnosis is available though there is no therapy. The disease variants reflect the activity of available enzyme and all can be characterized by utilizing natural or synthetic substrates.

Hexosaminidase alpha subunit defect or deficiency (variant B, Tay–Sachs disease), infantile Tay–Sachs disease

Patients with this best known variant usually first present at 3–6 months of age with motor weakness, apathy and feeding problems. The most common initial sign is the startle response to sound that is characterized by upper and lower extremity extension, often associated with a myoclonic jerk. Progressive weakness and hypotonia develop with neurological regression by 10–12 months of age. The mental and motor deterioration continue and death occurs from bronchopneumonia, usually by 4 years of age. The typical, but not specific, cherry-red spot is observed in the macula in the early stages of the disease. Degeneration of the optic nerve is common and results in blindness. Megalocephaly may develop during the second year of life. Tay–Sachs disease has a carrier frequency of 1:30 for Ashkenazi Jews and 1:300 for non-Jewish persons.[469]

In Tay–Sachs disease, hexosaminidase A is nearly

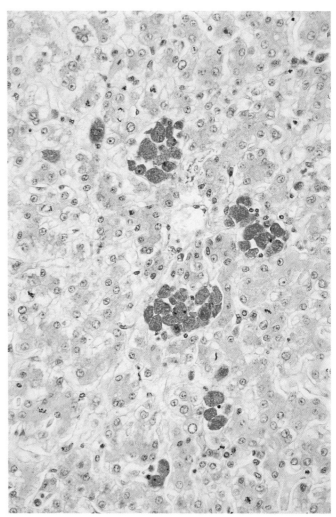

Fig. 4.46 Same case as illustrated in Fig. 4.45. Ganglioside-laden Kupffer cells are intensely PAS-positive. PAS after diastase digestion.

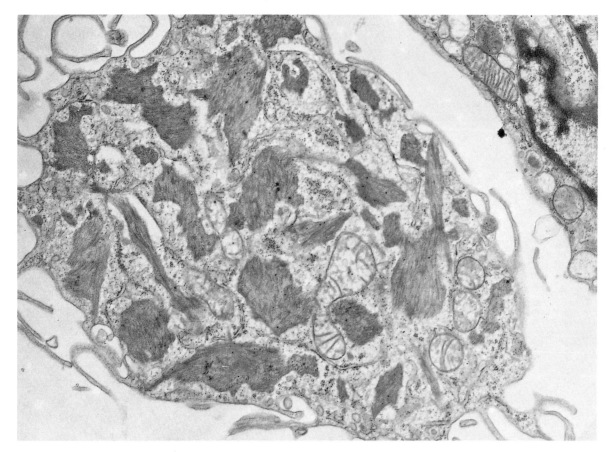

Fig. 4.47 GM$_1$ gangliosidosis, type II. A Kupffer cell contains several angulated and focally membrane-bound inclusions. The inclusions are composed of granulofibrillar material and a few osmiophilic granules. × 13 500. Courtesy of Dr M Petrelli

absent and the diagnosis is made on the basis of serum or cell culture enzyme assays. Akli et al[475] have reviewed the multiple gene defects in this disorder. The essentially complete hexosaminidase A deficiency allows massive accumulation of GM$_2$ ganglioside and asialo-GM$_2$ in enlarged cerebral neurones, retinal ganglion cells and the autonomic ganglia. Electron microscopy shows concentrically laminated inclusions or membranous cytoplasmic bodies in affected neurons, and somewhat more pleomorphic inclusions in the glia. Although hepatocytes appear normal by light microscopy, they may contain such bodies by electron microscopic examination.[472]

Juvenile GM$_2$ gangliosidosis

This disorder presents with motor ataxia between 2 and 6 years of age followed by progressive dementia. Optic atrophy and retinitis pigmentosa occur late in the course of the disease and cherry-red spots do not appear. Decerebrate rigidity is present by 10–12 years of age and death from infection occurs between 10 and 15 years of age.

Chronic GM$_2$ gangliosidosis

Patients present with abnormal gait and posture between

2 and 5 years of age. This is followed by progressive spinocerebellar degeneration. Vision and mentation remain good and patients have been reported as surviving into their 30s.

Adult onset GM$_2$ gangliosidosis

Patients usually present with symptoms of spinocerebellar and lower motor neuron dysfunction. Up to a third develop hebephrenic schizophrenia. Vision and intellect remain intact. By light microscopy, swollen neurones are seen with nuclei and Nissl substance pushed to the periphery. The cytoplasm contains membranous bodies. This late onset disease can be detected on rectal biopsy by swollen ganglia which contain the characteristic bodies, together with membranous structures and granular or amorphous material within lysosomes.

Hexosaminidase B subunit deficency or defect (variant O, Sandhoff's disease), infantile Sandhoff's disease

This disease results from deficient activity of both hexosaminidase A and B. It is characterized by the neural and visceral deposition of GM$_2$ ganglioside, its asialo derivative, and tetrahexosyl ceramide.[476] Previously, affected infants were misdiagnosed as having Tay–Sachs disease because the clinical features and course are similar. The disease shows no ethnic predilection. During the first few months of life subtle signs of delayed motor development are noted. Cardiovascular symptoms may be observed early in the course of the disease and the liver and spleen may be slightly enlarged. During the second six months of life, little if any progress is made in motor or mental development. Cherry-red spots and early optic atrophy are evident. By 12 months of age, the patients no longer use their pincer grasp and develop bilateral pyramidal tract abnormalities, including increased tendon reflexes, spasticity and positive Hoffman's and Babinski's signs. In addition, there is regression in sitting, smiling, and laughing appropriately. The psychomotor deterioration is progressive, with death resulting from aspiration pneumonia, usually between 22 and 36 months of age.

There are mild skeletal abnormalities, and ECG changes range from those of mild left ventricular hypertrophy to severe abnormalities compatible with endocardial fibroelastosis. Vacuolated lymphocytes may be present in the peripheral blood. Markedly increased levels of globoside in the urinary sediment and plasma differentiate Sandhoff's from Tay–Sachs disease. Decreased activities of hexosaminidase A and B are found in biopsy specimens, peripheral leucocytes, platelets, cerebrospinal fluid, cultured skin fibroblasts and plasma. Heterozygosity of the parents is more reliably established by examination of tissue specimens than of serum.[477] In utero, the diagnosis of Sandhoff's disease can be made by demonstration of deficient hexosaminidase levels in amniotic fluid.[478]

Patients with Sandhoff's disease were previously missed at autopsy because routine formalin fixation of tissues obscures the visceral lipid accumulation. However, 1 mm sections of Epon-embedded material reveal the lipid deposition when studied by light microscopy. Lysosomal lipid accumulation in the liver progresses with age; the lysosomes are twice the normal size at 3 months of age, and by 1 year many are distended by membranous lipid deposits to a diameter equal to that of the liver cell nucleus[477,479] (Fig. 4.48). The extent, size and variation of the membranous deposits within lysosomes are characteristic but not pathognomonic of Sandhoff's disease.

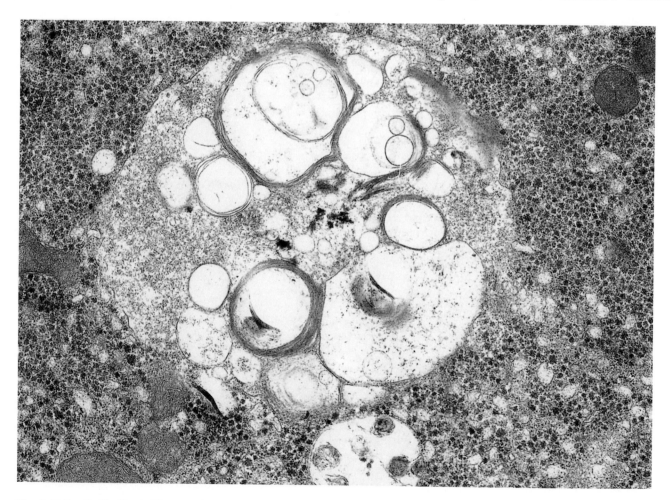

Fig. 4.48 Sandhoff's disease. Electron micrograph showing a large cytoplasmic lysosome containing single and laminated membranous structures within a finely particulate matrix. Note the size of the lysosome in comparison to the other cytoplasmic organelles. × 13 500.

Kupffer cells are also involved and stain positively with the PAS reagent. Periportal fibrosis has been reported.[480] The acinar cells of the pancreas are markedly involved. Electron microscopy reveals membranous and zebra body hybrids.

A juvenile form of this disease exists. It is more protracted than the other forms and commences from 2–6 years of age. Usually, the initial symptoms are locomotor ataxia, impairment of speech and loss of intellectual abilities. Extrapyramidal rigidity, muscular twitching and a persistent startle response to sound are also common. Grand mal seizures, decerebrate rigidity and somnolence characterize the final stage of the disease, some 4–9 years after the presenting symptoms. Cherry-red spots are absent and blindness occurs late in the course of the disease or not at all.[477] Hepatosplenomegaly, bony deformities, lymphocyte vacuolization and histiocytosis of the bone marrow have not been observed. The diagnosis can be made by demonstration of a partial deficiency of hexosaminidase A in serum or skin fibroblasts.[469] The genetic defects have been reviewed by Neote et al.[481].

GM₂ activator deficiency (variant AB)

This disease also resembles Tay–Sachs disease, with similar pathological findings. Normal enzyme levels are observed using synthetic substrates but no activity is found using ganglioside GM₂.[474]

GLYCOSPHINGOLIPID LIPIDOSIS (FABRY'S DISEASE)

Fabry's disease is an X-linked disorder of glycosphingolipid metabolism[482] that is due to the deficiency of the lysosomal hydrolase, α-galactosidase.[483] The defect results in the accumulation of globotriaosylceramide in tissue. The gene for this enzyme is located on chromosome Xq21.33–q22. The enzyme defect shows molecular heterogeneity. The diagnosis can be confirmed by enzyme assay in plasma, leucocytes, chorionic villi and cultured amniotic cells.

Clinical disease usually begins during childhood or adolescence in hemizygous males and rarely in heterozygous females.[482,484] The usual onset is characterized by pain and paraesthesias in the extremities secondary to vascular substrate accumulation that affects peripheral nerves. Hypohidrosis results from similar vascular changes in the autonomic nervous system. Skin signs of the disease are angiokeratomas.

Renal lipid deposition leads to proteinuria, isosthenuria and gradual deterioration of renal function. In the cardiovascular system, the deposition of glycosphingolipid is associated with hypertension, left ventricular hypertrophy, myocardial ischaemia or infarction, and cerebral vascular disease. Other clinical features include lymphoedema and

mild anaemia. Nausea, vomiting and diarrhoea are common gastrointestinal symptoms. Death is usually from renal or cardiovascular complications. Recently, an atypical variant of the disease, with manifestations confined to the myocardium, was reported by von Scheidt et al.[485]

The diagnosis may be suspected by the combined findings of corneal dystrophy, lipid-laden and PAS-positive macrophages in the bone marrow, and birefringent maltese crosses in the urinary sediment. Therapy includes phenytoin or carbamazepine for the presenting symptoms and renal transplantation for kidney failure.[486] Trials of enzyme replacement therapy are in progress.[480]

The substance that accumulates in the blood vessels, myocardium, kidney, liver, spleen and other organs is ceramide trihexoside. Pathological findings in Fabry's disease have been reviewed in detail by Brady & King.[487] In the liver there is accumulation of the glycolipid and cholesterol in Kupffer cells and portal macrophages and the endothelial cells of blood vessels. The phagocytic cells of the liver are swollen and light tan in colour in H & E

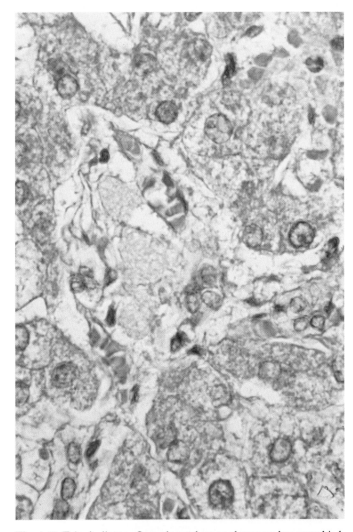

Fig. 4.49 Fabry's disease. Several portal macrophages are hypertrophied and have a tan-coloured cytoplasm. H&E.

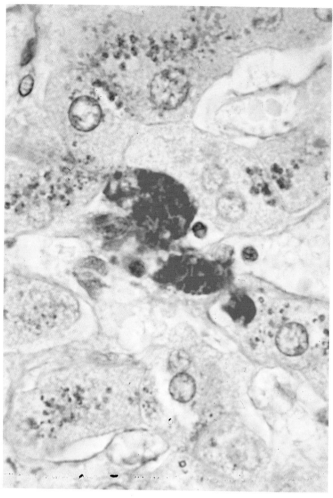

Fig. 4.50 Fabry's disease. Kupffer cells contain a granular material that stains intensely with PAS after diastase digestion.

preparations (Fig. 4.49). They contain birefringent crystals in frozen sections, and the Schultz modification of the Lieberman–Burchard reaction is moderately positive. The stored material is intensely PAS-positive and resists diastase digestion (Fig. 4.50). Two peroxidase-labelled lectins, known to have affinity for α- and β-D-galactose, have been found to be strongly reactive with the storage material of Fabry's disease.[488] This observation has important diagnostic implications since lectin binding is more specific than any other histochemical method. Ultrastructurally, the stored material in Fabry's disease consists of concentrically laminated inclusions with a periodicity of 5–6 nm (Figs 4.51 and 4.52). Lipid accumulations consisting of amorphous material as well as stacks of lamellar leaflets may be seen in hepatocytes, Kupffer cells and portal tract macrophages.[489]

SULPHATIDE LIPIDOSIS (METACHROMATIC LEUCODYSTROPHY)

Metachromatic leucodystrophy (MLD) is a glycosphingo-lipidosis with accumulation of cerebroside 3-sulphate in the nervous system, kidney and gallbladder as a result of deficient activity of arylsulphatase A.[490] Six variants are now known.[491] Inheritance is autosomal recessive. Aryl-sulphatase A is located on chromosome 22 in the region of q13. One variant lacks a sphingolipid activator protein (SAP-1) located on chromosome 10. Another variant is deficient in arylsulphatase A, B, and C, plus four other sulphatases involved in mucopolysaccharide metabolism.

Late infantile MLD presents between 1 and 2 years of age with developmental delay. Signs of neurological deterioration include progressive mental retardation, optic atrophy, loss of speech, hypertonic quadriplegia, ataxia and absent tendon reflexes. Pain in the extremities and unexplained fever are common. In the terminal stages of the disease, the patient loses sensory contact with his surroundings. Death results from infection or hyperpyrexia.

Early juvenile MLD presents at 4–6 years of age with mental confusion. The above neurological progression occurs at a slower rate. *Late juvenile MLD* presents at 6–12 years of age with cognitive difficulties. The progressive deterioration includes gait disturbances with pyramidal and extrapyramidal signs. *Cerebroside sulphate sulphatase activator deficiency* has a similar presentation to that of the juvenile forms. All variants are characterized by elevated spinal fluid protein, slow nerve conduction velocity, and elevated urinary sulphatide excretion.

The adult form of MLD presents after 16 years of age, the average being 29 years. Mean duration of the disease is 15 years.[492] Most patients present with psychological problems, dementia or paralysis. Progressive neurological abnormalities develop during the course of the disease and include incoordination, ataxia, spastic paresis, visual disorders, tremors, skeletal muscle rigidity, athetotic movements and spastic dysuria. Spinal fluid protein and nerve conduction velocity may be normal. Hydrocephalus has been reported. The causes of death include cachexia and pneumonia. In contrast, *multiple sulphatase deficiency MLD* presents before one year of age like the late infantile form; patients may also have coarse facies, deafness, ichthyosis, hepatosplenomegaly and skeletal abnormalities. Increased mucopolysaccharides are present in the urine, and Alder–Reilly granules are found in the white blood cells. More than 40 cases have been reported.[491]

Excessive sulphatide may be detected in peripheral nerves, urinary sediment and the gallbladder. The latter organ loses concentrating ability with the accumulation of the substrate. A deficiency of arylsulphatase A is found in leucocytes, cultured skin fibroblasts and amniotic cells.[493,494]

Histologically, sulphatide accumulation has been demonstrated in the central nervous system, the liver, gallbladder, pancreas, kidneys, adrenals and other organs.[495,496] The gallbladder is small and fibrotic and may show multiple polyps or papillomas.[497–504] Microscopic examination reveals large foamy macrophages in the tunica propria that

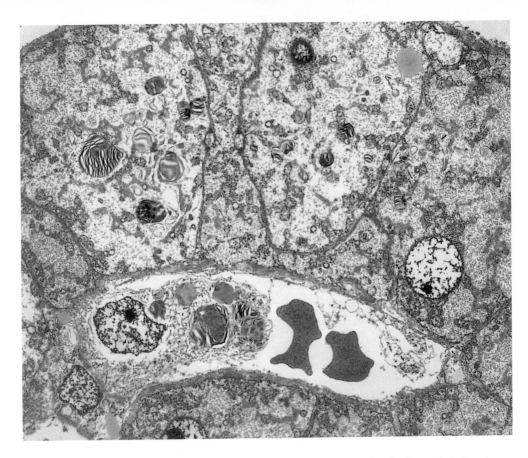

Fig. 4.51 Fabry's disease. Electron micrograph showing multiple dense and often laminated inclusions in hepatocytes and in a Kupffer cell. × 8800.

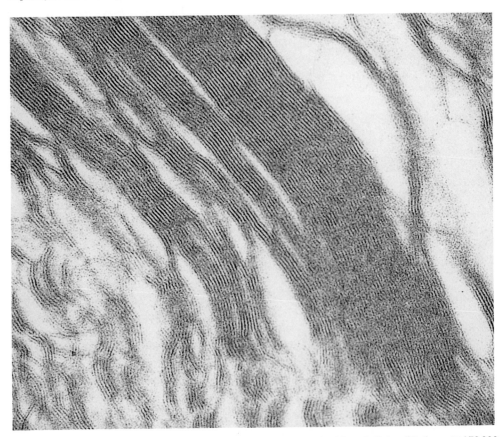

Fig. 4.52 Fabry's disease. Concentric lamination of inclusion material, with periodicity of 5–6 nm. × 170 000.

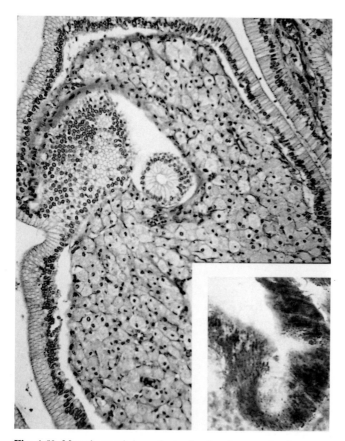

Fig. 4.53 Metachromatic leucodystrophy. Lamina propria of gallbladder is packed with large macrophages with a lightly stained cytoplasm. H&E. Inset shows positive staining (metachromasia) of epithelium. Hirsch–Pfeiffer stain.

stain positively with cresyl voilet, toluidine blue and the PAS reaction (Fig. 4.53). In frozen section they contain sudanophilic material that is anisotropic and can also be stained with the Schultz modification of the Lieberman–Burchard reaction; these properties are thought to be due to the simultaneous accumulation of cholesterol.[499] Metachromatic granules can be demonstrated in epithelial cells of the gallbladder and to a lesser extent in those of the intrahepatic bile ducts.[497] In the liver, metachromatic granules may be seen in some portal macrophages and less often Kupffer cells and hepatocytes.[495] Ultrastructurally, prismatic lysosomal are found in epithelial cells of the gallbladder and reticuloendothelial cells of the liver.[12] They are composed of periodic leaflets which appear tubular in cross section.[12]

GLUCOSYLCERAMIDE LIPIDOSIS (GAUCHER'S DISEASE)

Gaucher's disease is the commonest lysosomal storage disease. Three clinical variants of this autosomal recessive disorder, which cannot be distinguished by cellular enzyme levels, have been decribed .[505,506]

The onset of *type I* (chronic non-neuronopathic) usually occurs in late childhood or adolescence, with an incidence of 1/2500, predominantly in individuals of Ashkenazi Jewish descent. Patients present with hepatosplenomegaly, and over half have thrombocytopenia associated with mild haemorrhagic phenomena.[507] Pancytopenia has responded to splenectomy in the past, but only partial splenectomy has been recommended by one group of investigators because of post-splenectomy acceleration of the disease in bones, liver and lungs.[508] Another group, however, has shown that partial splenectomy can only be regarded as a temporary solution for the treatment of hypersplenism, and that total splenectomy may be required eventually.[509] On X-ray examination, 60% have abnormal bones, usually an expansion of the distal femur (Erlenmeyer flask); 10% of patients suffer skeletal symptoms such as bone pain, spontaneous fractures, degenerative hip disease or pseudo-osteomyelitis. The latter is classically seen in adolescents with aseptic necrosis of metaphyseal areas.

Type II disease is usually manifested at 2–3 months of age by neurological signs. Late manifestations include laryngeal stridor and pulmonary infiltrates. Physical findings include hepatosplenomegaly, lymphadenopathy, opisthotonic posturing, spasticity and cranial nerve involvement. Death usually occurs by 2 years of age. Hydrops fetalis has been reported.[510,511] Recently, Sidaransky et al[512] and Sidransky & Ginns[513] have drawn attention to a subset of children with type II disease who manifest a particularly devastating clinical course. In addition to hydrops fetalis, these infants have ichthyosis.

Type III disease presents in adulthood. Initially, it has a similar presentation to that of type I disease but later is complicated by the gradual onset of mental deterioration, often signalled by supranuclear ophthalmoplegia. Death usually occurs in the second to fourth decades.

Patients can present with fibrosis or cirrhosis of the liver with the typical complications of portal hypertension including ascites, and oesophageal bleeding.[514] Sclerotherapy can transiently prevent or control haemorrhagic episodes. Hepatic calcification is rare.[515] Pulmonary arteriovenous shunts causing hypoxia and cyanosis have been documented mainly in patients with liver disease,[516] but infiltration with storage cells can also be present in the lungs. The pulmonary arteriovenous shunts may improve immediately after liver transplantation.[517]

Two independent reports[518,519] documented a defect of the enzyme, variously termed acid α-glucosidase and acid glucocerebrosidase (D-glucosyl-acyl sphingosine glucohydrolase EC 3.2.1.45), which cleaves the α-glucoside linkage of glucosylceramide (glucocerebroside). Although the enzyme can be measured in all affected tissues, white blood cells or cultured fibroblasts are the usual sources for diagnostic purposes. A small acidic protein, SAP-2, is required for optimal hydrolytic rates. One patient has been described with glucosylceramide storage and normal in vitro enzyme activity but a deficiency of SAP-2 cross-reacting immunological material in multiple organs.[520] The major source of the accumulated substrate is from degradation of leucocyte membranes.[521]

The human B-glucosidase structural gene and its pseudogene are localized to chromosome 1 (q21 → 31).[522,523] Two major mutations have been found in over 50% of homozygotes and heterozygotes. A mutation in Exons 9 (5841G, Asn[370] → Ser) can identify type I disease.[524,525] A mutation in Exon 10 (6533c, Leu[444] → Pro) is found in both types II and III.[524,526,527]

At the present time, the treatment of choice is the available enzyme itself injected intravenously.[528,529] It is obtained from human placentas and sequentially deglycosylated of its secondary branch carbohydrates. This exposes mannose of the primary branched carbohydrates and allows preferential uptake by macrophages, via a mannose receptor.[528] Enzyme replacement is very costly; its use must be weighed against the natural history of Gaucher's disease, which is a rather stable disorder in adults.[507] Bone marrow transplantation is also successful, but it has a higher mortality and morbidity risk.[530,531] Orthotopic liver transplantation has been performed successfully in Gaucher's disease.[532,533] In the case of Smanik et al,[532] there was a 61% increase in hepatic glucocerebrosidase activity after transplantation. In the patient of Starzl et al,[533] lymph node deposits of glucocerebroside were dramatically reduced after transplantation; systemic microchimerism was documented in this patient and resulted in improved metabolism in enzyme-deficient tissues.

Pathological features

Histiocytes containing glucocerebroside (Gaucher cells) are dispersed throughout the reticuloendothelial system. A

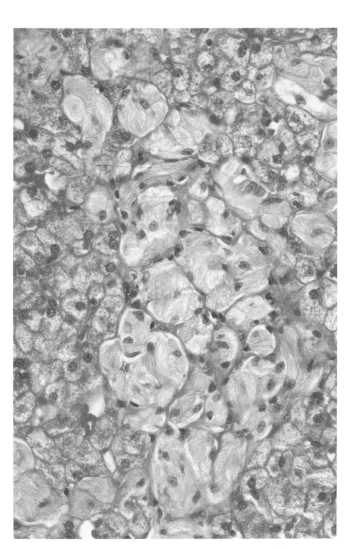

Fig. 4.54 Pale-staining Gaucher cells have a faintly striated cytoplasm. H&E.

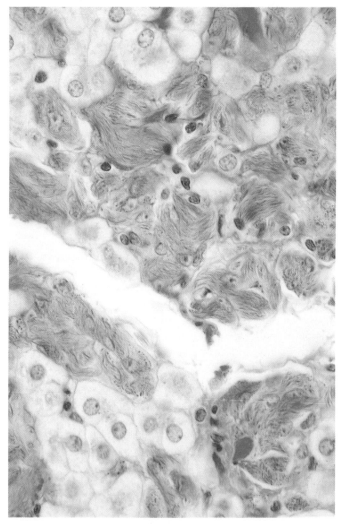

Fig. 4.55 Gaucher's disease. Striations are well visualized in a PAS-stained preparation.

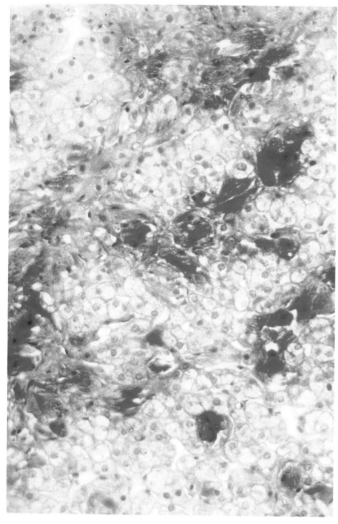

Fig. 4.56 Gaucher cells exhibit marked acid phosphatase activity (red). Phenylphosphate Mx acid phosphatase reaction.

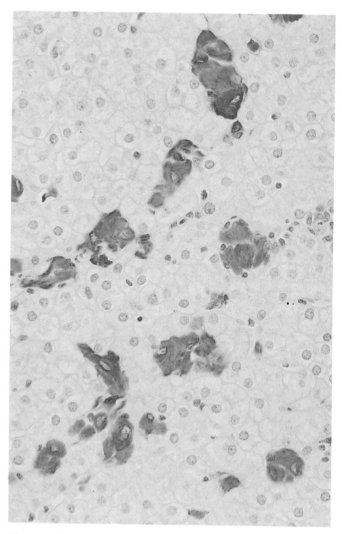

Fig. 4.57 Gaucher cells are strongly immunoreactive to KP-1 antibody.

full surface marker study of the splenic storage cells in a case of Gaucher's disease has largely substantiated the monocyte/histiocyte nature of Gaucher cells.[534] Scanning electron microscopy reveals microvilli, ruffles, ridges and blebs of varying number and shape on their surface.[535] In the liver, Kupffer cells and portal macrophages are primarily affected. The distribution may be focal or zonal, with acinar zone 3 being mainly affected.[514] The cells, which can measure up to 100 μm, are lightly stained with eosin, have a faintly striated or crinkled cytoplasm and pyknotic, eccentric or centrally located nuclei (Fig. 4.54). The striations are best demonstrated with the Masson trichrome or a PAS stain (Fig, 4.55). Intense acid phosphatase (Fig. 4.56) and lysozyme activity are found by histochemical or immunohistochemical methods respectively. They are also strongly immunoreactive to KP-1 (Fig. 4.57). The cells usually contain a small amount of iron that is derived both from ingested erythrocytes and

from the labile plasma pool.[536] Other staining reactions of Gaucher cells are described in several reviews.[536–538]

Gaucher cells in the liver may enlarge to such an extent that they completely block sinusoidal spaces. They also compress hepatocytes with progressive atrophy and disruption of the hepatic plates. There ia a variable increase in the number of reticulin and collagen fibres in the space of Disse. Pericellular fibrosis and mechanical blockage of sinusoidal spaces are presumed to be the cause of portal hypertension, but the pathogenesis of tissue injury in Gaucher's disease is complex. It may be related to the toxic effect of the storage cell itself, or could result from failure of the lipid-laden macrophages to detoxify a circulating toxin.[505] Severe fibrosis, formation of septa and cirrhosis (Fig. 4.58) have been reported.[167,514,532,539–541] One case report described coexistent autoimmune chronic active hepatitis.[542]

The ultrastructural aspects of the Gaucher cell have

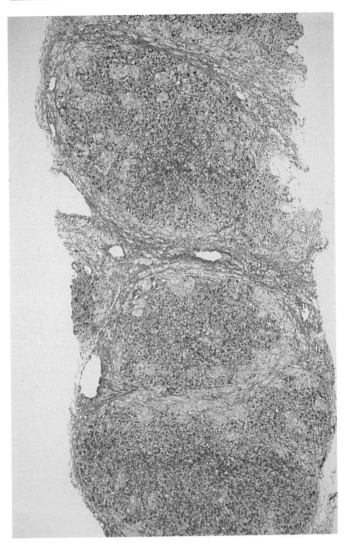

Fig. 4.58 Gaucher's disease. Section of needle biopsy specimen reveals established cirrhosis. Masson's trichrome.

been described in detail.[536–538] The cytoplasm is filled with spindle or rod-shaped inclusion bodies bounded by a limiting membrane; these measure 0.6–4 μm in diameter (Fig. 4.59). In cross section the inclusions contain numerous small tubules, 13–75 μm in diameter. Acid phosphatase activity has been localized to the inclusions by electron microscopic histochemistry.[537] Freeze-fracture and X-ray diffraction analysis of the purified deposits have shown them to consist of twisted membranous bilayers 6 μm in thickness.[543] The iron in the Gaucher cell is dispersed as individual micelles of ferritin.[544]

SPHINGOMYELIN-CHOLESTEROL LIPIDOSIS (NIEMANN-PICK DISEASE)

There are at least two major forms of Niemann–Pick disease with multiple variants.[545] Types A and B are characterized by massive accumulation of sphingomyelin secondary to a severe deficiency of sphingomyelinase.[546]

Type C and its variants have much less sphingomyelin accumulation. Cholesterol accumulates in all types but fibroblast studies in type C suggest various possible defects in its intracellular metabolism, including the accumulation of non-esterified cholesterol.[545,547,548] An update on current theories is summarized by Bowler et al.[549] All types appear to be inherited as autosomal recessive disorders. Types A and B are usually detected because of the typical tissue foam cells and type C because of sea-blue histiocytes, although both cells may be present in the same type. The diagnosis of types A and B depends on sphingomyelinase levels of 10% or less of normal in fibroblasts, leucocytes, liver, or spleen. The gene for this lysosomal enzyme has been mapped to chromosome 11p15.1–p.15.4.[550] Initial studies of the gene defects have so far revealed an arginine to leucine point mutation in position 496 in type A,[551] and removal of arginine from position 608 in type B.[552] Type C can be diagnosed by metabolic or histochemical studies of cholesterol non-esterification in cultured fibroblasts, amniocytes or chorionic villus cells. No therapy is presently available. Bone marrow and liver transplantation have led to detrimental results,[533–555] except for a recently reported case.[532] No long-term success has been achieved by furnishing cells with the missing enzymes.[556]

All three types usually present with massive hepatosplenomegaly. Type A can be detected in utero, by pancreatic enlargement from foam cell accumulation, in addition to hepatosplenomegaly.[557] Both types A and non-neurological B present during infancy. In type A, neurological symptoms are evident by 3 months, with clear regression by 1 year of age. Late subtle manifestations of nervous system involvement have occasionally been seen in type B.

Patients with **type A** develop feeding problems and fail to thrive, and death occurs by 4–5 years of age. Lung infiltration with storage cells is common, and contributes to infectious complications. Macular degeneration with a cherry-red spot is seen in 30–50% of patients.[558]

Type B disease also begins in infancy or early childhood with massive hepatosplenomegaly; however, neurological abnormalities are absent or subtle and late in onset. Manifestations of liver disease, including cholestasis or cirrhosis, are usually seen in either types B or C. Recently, fatal liver failure has been documented in two children with type B disease,[559] and cirrhosis with portal hypertension has been reported in a 33-year-old adult.[560] A 42-year-old woman with Niemann–Pick disease type B underwent successful orthotopic liver transplantation.[532] Six to 14 months after transplantation she had above normal hepatic sphingomyelinase activity and lower than normal hepatic sphingomyelin and cholesterol content.

Patients with type C (non-A, non-B variants) of Niemann–Pick disease present at any time from birth to adulthood with hepatosplenomegaly, followed by moder-

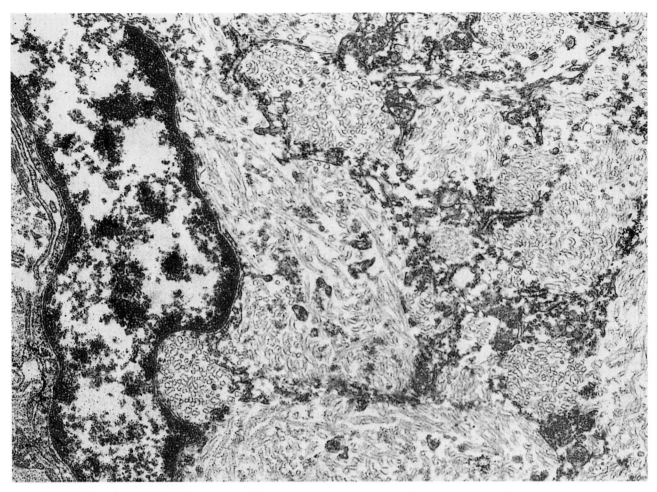

Fig. 4.59 Electron micrograph showing cytoplasm of Gaucher cell that is packed with tubules cut tangentially or in cross section. × 8475.

ately progressive neurological impairment. During infancy, they can present with cholestasis, which may or may not resolve. The pathology of the liver has been variable, with some livers showing features of 'neonatal hepatitis'.[561,562] Rarely, the biliary system may be involved, with paucity of the intrahepatic bile ducts that is manifested clinically by pruritus.[561–566] One patient developed hepatocellular carcinoma.[567]

Veritcal supranuclear ophthalmoplegia without evidence of brain stem involvement should alert physicians to the juvenile form of type C disease.[568,569] Over 50% of patients have sea-blue histiocytes in the bone marrow; the cells are best visualized by a Wright stain. Neurological abnormalities develop between 5 and 9 years of age. Poor school performance resulting from a decline in intelligence may be the initial presentation in 80% of patients. Other findings include lack of coordination and gait disturbances (70%) slurred speech and dysarthria (53%), seizures (40%), jaundice (25%), hepatomegaly (50%) and splenomegaly (90%).[570]

This disorder has been diagnosed in adults of 20–40 years of age.[571] Fink et al[572] have subdivided the presenta-

tion into C_1 with onset in infancy including hepatic and neurological signs, C_2 presenting in early childhood with slower onset of neurological signs, and C_3 with onset during adolescence or adulthood with slower progression. It is important to note that splenomegaly is more impressive than hepatomegaly and that there is an overlap between the three types in affected families. The lack of hepatosplenomegaly in the least severe cases has been noted by Vanier et al.[573]

Pathological features

Both the liver and the spleen are enlarged in Niemann–Pick disease. The characteristic finding is the presence of large foam cells in the reticuloendothelial system. These are least conspicuous in type C.[563] In the liver, Kupffer cell are hypertrophied and show a vacuolated cytoplasm (Fig. 4.60). They often have a light tan colour due to their content of lipofuscin (ceroid). A single small eccentric or centrally placed nucleus is generally found in each cell. Hepatocytes also contain sphingomyelin, and their cytoplasm shows progressive loss of eosinophilia with

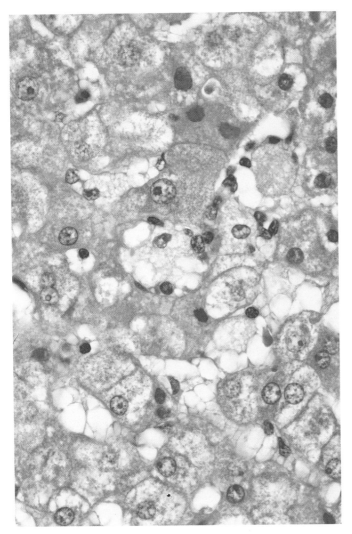

Fig. 4.60 Niemann–Pick disease. Kupffer cells storing sphingomyelin are foamy. H&E.

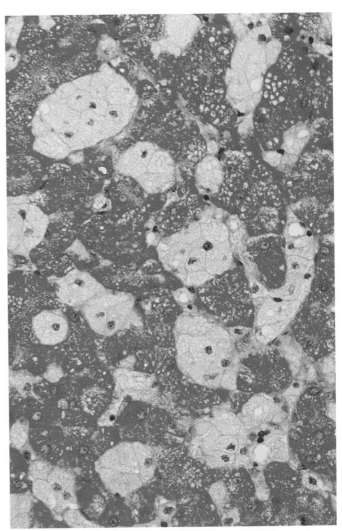

Fig. 4.61 Niemann–Pick disease. Pale-staining clusters of foam cells containing sphingomyelin stand out in sharp contrast to glycogen-containing (purple) liver cells. PAS after diastase digestion.

increasing vacuolization, until they become indistinguishable from affected Kupffer cells. Intrahepatic cholestasis is found in some infants, and a number of cases with giant cell transformation have been reported in both type C[562] and type B Niemann–Pick disease.[561,566,574] As is the case in Gaucher's disease and other metabolic disorders, there may be varying degrees of atrophy of hepatic plates and intra-acinar fibrosis. A true cirrhosis has been reported in both children and adults.[557,560,575]

The foam cells in Niemann–Pick disease are auto-fluorescent but have a nodular pattern, in contrast to the uniform fluorescence of Gaucher cells.[576] The cells are positively stained with oil red O, Luxol fast blue and Baker's acid haematin stain in frozen sections; the latter stain becomes negative after pyridine extraction. The cytoplasm is variably PAS-positive or negative, depending on the quantity of lipofuscin (Fig. 4.61). Cholesterol is usually present in the foam cells and can be specifically

demonstrated in frozen sections by the Schultz modification of the Lieberman–Burchard reaction. In addition to foam cells, some patients with variant types of Niemann–Pick disease may have 'sea-blue' histiocytes in the bone marrow, lymph nodes and spleen [577,578]

Ultrastructurally, the foam cells contain dense mixed lipid inclusions or lipid cytosomes; these are polymorphic and range from less than 1 μm to 5 μm in diameter.[576] The inclusions consist of concentrically laminated myelin-like figures with a periodicity of roughly 5 μm (Fig. 4.62).[12,579] Typical lipofuscin bodies, lipid droplets and cholesterol clefts may also be observed.[12]

WOLMAN'S AND CHOLESTEROL ESTER STORAGE DISEASES

The disorders of Wolman's and cholesterol ester storage disease (CESD) are presented together because of the

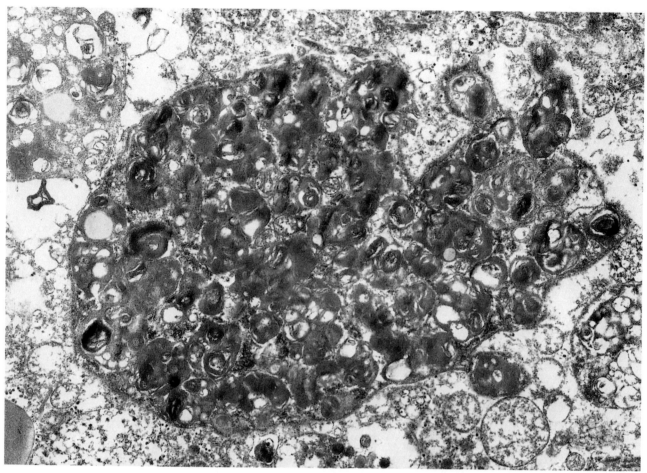

Fig. 4.62 Niemann–Pick disease. Electron micrograph showing electron-opaque laminated inclusions densely packed in the cytoplasm of a Kupffer cell. × 7900.

overlap in the clinical findings and the underlying enzyme deficiency. Patients with Wolman's disease may present with hydrops fetalis or congenital ascites.[580] However, the disease is usually manifested by progressive pallor, failure to thrive, abdominal distension, vomiting, and severe diarrhoea with steatorrhoea.[581] Death occurs within the first year of life,[582,583] but one patient has been reported to live to the age of 10 years.[584] Physical findings include hepatosplenomegaly, ascites, severe malnutrition, and mild lymphadenopathy. No xanthomas are present. Abdominal X-ray films reveal enlarged adrenals with calcification. Peripheral blood smears show vacuolated lymphocytes. Bone marrow examination discloses foam cells which stain positively for cholesterol and neutral fat or triglyceride. Markedly increased levels of cholesterol esters are present in the serum. Liver function tests reveal mild increases in the aminotransferases but plasma lipid levels are usually normal. The laboratory diagnosis is based on finding greatly reduced acid lipase levels in the liver, white blood cells and fibroblasts.[585–587] Heterozygotes have intermediate acid lipase levels.[588–590] The low levels of acid esterase activity can also be demon-

strated by histochemical staining methods.[591] Inheritance is autosomal recessive.

Cholesterol ester storage disease (CESD) is a milder disease presenting during childhood with hepatomegaly and, in some patients, with splenomegaly.[587,592] Children tend to be short and diarrhoea may be present. Jaundice suggests the development of cirrhosis. There have been reports of premature atherosclerosis, pulmonary vascular obstruction, and mesenteric lipodystrophy.[593,594] Liver function tests show elevated serum bile acids, serum lipids (including cholesterol and its esters), triglycerides and phospholipids. There may be mild aminotransferase elevations. The adrenals are not abnormal.

Acid lipase levels in tissues, white blood cells, cultured fibroblasts, amniotic cells and chorionic villi are low.[587,595] The inheritance is autosomal recessive and the gene is located on chromosome 10q24–q25. The exact genetic defect has not been defined. Attempts at medical treatment of the hyperlipidaemia have shown mixed results but are encouraging.[596–600] Liver transplantation for CESD has been reported.[601]

The adrenal glands in Wolman's disease are grossly

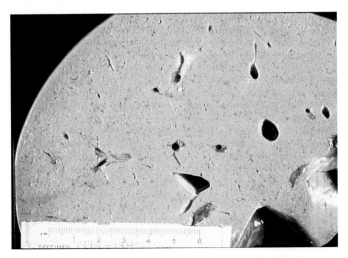

Fig. 4.63 Cholesterol ester storage disease. This section of liver has a yellow colour and is faintly nodular.

enlarged, hard and bright yellow. They cut with a gritty sensation and have a yellow cortex and an inner calcified zone. The surface of the small intestine, particularly the duodenum and ileum, shows a yellow velvety appearance. The liver is enlarged, yellow-orange and greasy (Fig. 4.63). All affected organs, particularly the liver (Figs 4.64 and 4.65), spleen, adrenals, haemopoietic system and the intestines, are infiltrated by numerous foamy histiocytes that contain cholesterol and/or cholesterol esters.[585,586,602,603] Stains for lipid (oil red O, Sudan black) are positive, as is the Schultz modification of the Lieberman–Burchard reaction for cholesterol; these stains must be performed on frozen sections, either of fresh or of formalin-fixed tissue. Frozen sections examined by polarizing microscopy show numerous anisotropic acicular crystals in the foamy histiocytes (Fig. 4.66). In the liver, cholesterol and cholesterol ester are mainly stored in Kupffer cells and portal macrophages, while hepatocytes

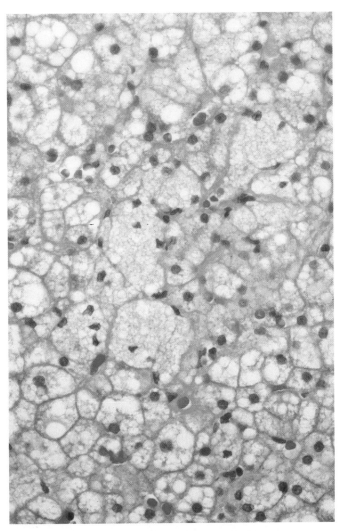

Fig. 4.64 Cholesterol ester storage disease. Kupffer cells are markedly hypertrophied and have a foamy, light tan-coloured cytoplasm; their nuclei are pyknotic. Hepatocytes show microvesicular steatosis. H&E.

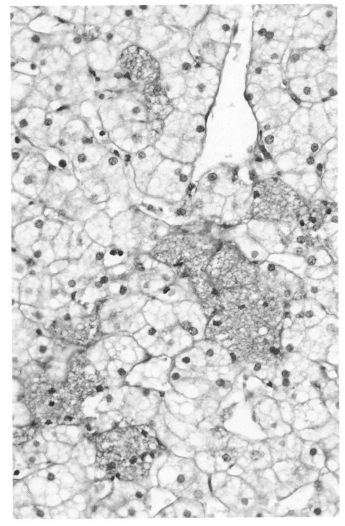

Fig. 4.65 Cholesterol ester storage disease. Foamy Kupffer cells in zone 3 are PAS-positive. PAS after diastase digestion.

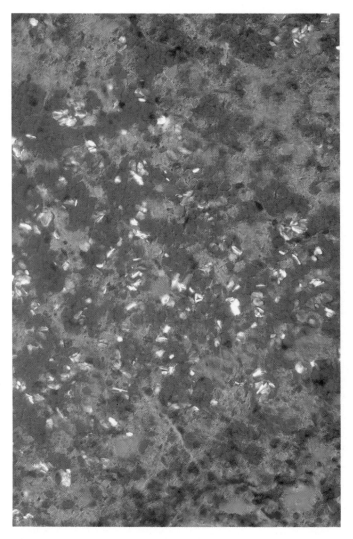

Fig. 4.66 Cholesterol ester storage disease. Cholesterol crystals display brilliant silvery birefringence. There is a large amount of fat (red) in liver cells. Oil red O stain of frozen section.

contain increased neutral lipid. Reticuloendothelial cells may also contain free fatty acids.[604] There may be marked pericellular fibrosis and varying degrees of periportal cholangiolar proliferation and fibrosis.[604] Ultrastructurally, the enlarged Kupffer cells contain peripheral vacuoles, sometimes within lysosomes, and large central crystal clefts of cholesterol ester.[605] Lake & Patrick[604] have observed that the crystals are membrane-bound. Hepatocytes contain many lipid droplets but only occasional crystal clefts.[604] It has been suggested that the cholesterol esters are discharged from the hepatic parenchymal cells in an insoluble form and then taken up by the Kupffer cells where crystallization occurs.[605]

The light microscopic and ultrastructural changes in the liver of patients with CESD are similar to those of Wolman's disease.[592,594,598] A highly characteristic feature of CESD is the presence of markedly hypertrophied

Kupffer cells and portal macrophages with a foamy, tan-coloured cytoplasm that stains strongly with PAS (Fig. 4.65).[598] Periportal fibrosis of varied degree is present in most of the cases but cirrhosis is rare.[594,598,606] Ultrastructurally, triglyceride droplets are noted in abundance in hepatic and reticuloendothelial cells; most are surrounded by a single membrane. Many of the lysosomal lipid droplets have a 'moth-eaten' appearance due to the inclusion of cholesterol within them (Fig. 4.67). Cholesterol crystals are also seen lying free in the cytoplasm.

CEREBROTENDINOUS XANTHOMATOSIS

Cerebrotendinous xanthomatosis was first described in 1973.[607] Since then, approximately 150 cases have been reported, with the highest incidence in Japan.[608] The disease results from excessive deposition of cholestanol and cholesterol in tissues but only cholestanol is elevated in the serum. A deficiency of mitochondrial C^{27}-steroid 26-hydroxylase on the inner mitochondrial membrane was first reported in 1980 and confirmed in fibroblasts in 1986.[609,610] This defect results in low bile-acid concentrations in bile and high bile alcohol levels in bile and urine. The disorder is autosomal recessive and heterozygotes can be detected by measurement of urinary bile alcohol levels following administration of cholestyramine.[611] The diagnosis is usually made by the clinical features and elevated serum cholestanol levels in patients without significant liver disease.

A recent report suggests the occurrence of chronic diarrhoea from infancy.[612] The most diagnostically helpful signs during childhood are juvenile cataracts and tuberous xanthomas, particularly over the achilles tendons. The neurological manifestations vary from mental retardation during adolescence to normal intelligence at the age of 60. Spasticity and ataxia are usually detected in the second and third decades. Progression results in dementia, spinal cord paresis and peripheral neuropathy; microscopic examination shows diffuse infiltration by cholesterol associated with demyelination. Xanthomas are rare in the central nervous system.[613] Less frequent findings include seizures, gallstones and osteoporosis. Death in the fourth to sixth decades is usually related to neurological deterioration; however, approximately 10% of patients have heart disease and/or atheroma. Liver specimens from 2 patients revealed intracellular inclusions that appeared either as amorphous pigment or had a crystalloid form.[614] The pigment is usually found in association with the smooth endoplasmic reticulum but ocassionally lies free in the cytosol. An ultrastructural study of 4 cases revealed perisinusoidal fibrosis, bile canalicular changes (dilatation, distortion and loss of microvilli and an increase in microfilaments), fatty change, proliferation of smooth endoplasmic reticulum, accumulation of lipofuscin, focal cytoplasmic degeneration, proliferation of microbodies

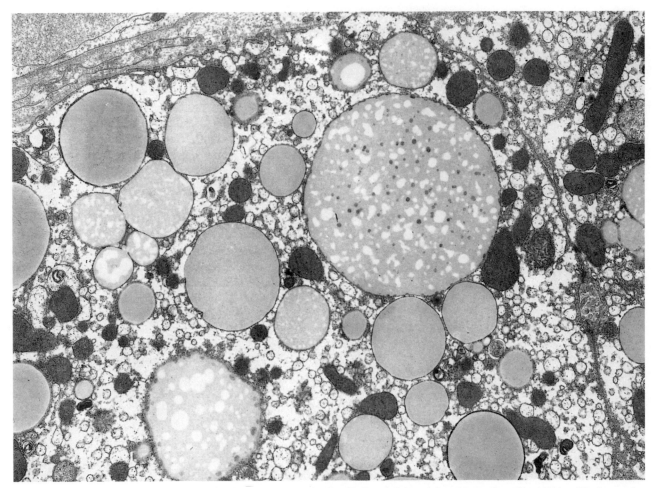

Fig. 4.67 Cholesterol ester storage disease. Electron micrograph of liver cell containing triglyceride droplets of varied size. 'Moth-eaten' appearance of several droplets is due to the presence of cholesterol crystals within them. × 10 000.

and prominent mitochondrial changes.[615] One patient had crystalloid cores in microbodies that disappeared after therapy.[615] Salen et al[614] suggested that the accumulated material may indicate the presence of non-metabolizable bile alcohols resulting from a defect of bile-acid synthesis. Long-term therapy with chenodeoxycholic acid may correct the progression of the disease.[616]

FATTY ACID OXIDATION DISORDERS

Much recent progress has been made in the understanding of fatty acid oxidation enzymatic and transport defects. Most of these inborn errors of metabolism are characterized by secondary carnitine deficiency; they include some of the previously reported cases of 'primary' carnitine deficiency. Over nine enzyme defects are now documented and these have been reviewed by Hale & Bennett[617] and Vockley.[617a]

Many patients, previously thought to have Reye's syndrome or sudden infant death syndrome (SIDS), have inherited defects of fatty acid oxidation. Unfortunately, the clinical presentation may be similar for many of these disorders, yet dissimilar even within the same family. There are certain clinical findings[617] that should alert physicians to these disorders particularly in newborns, infants and children:

1. Metabolic decompensation during fasting (often caused by a viral illness) with features of Reye-like syndrome or SIDS, especially if recurrent or familial.

2. Involvement of tissues that depend on fatty acid metabolism including the liver and/or heart and skeletal muscle. Usually, these tissues demonstrate fatty infiltration.

3. Hypoketotic hypoglycaemia accompanied by elevation of serum free fatty acids without evidence of hyperinsulinism or hypopituitarism.

4. Decreased total plasma or tissue carnitine concentrations (seen in all carnitine deficiencies) with an increased esterified carnitine concentration, except in carnitine palmitoyl transferase I (CPT I) deficiency.

Common abnormal laboratory findings include hyperammonaemia, hyperuricaemia, dicarboxylic aciduria, metabolic acidosis, and increased aminotransferase and creatinine kinase activities in the serum. Crucial studies that should be performed when the patient is admitted (prior to glucose administration) include serum glucose and plasma carnitine and ketones; urine should be saved for analysis for ketones and organic acids.

Carnitine (3-hydroxy-4N-trimethylamine butyric acid) shuttles long chain fatty acids, activated acetate, end products of peroxisomal fatty acid oxidation, and alpha ketoacids derived from branched chain amino acids, from the cytoplasm into the mitochondria. Carnitine esters are normally less than 25% of the total plasma concentration; therefore the esterified to free ratio is usually less than 0.33. The main source of carnitine is dietary.

Systemic carnitine deficiency

The first case, thoroughly described only 18 years ago,[618] was a patient who presented with neuromuscular weakness. The most affected tissue in this disease is muscle, and cardiomyopathy eventually develops.[619,620] Twenty reported cases were reviewed by Stanley et al.[621] The initial presentation was cardiomyopathy in 12, hypoglycaemia in 9, and skeletal muscle weakness in 4. Subsequently, more patients developed cardiomyopathy and muscle weakness. Physical findings included hepatomegaly, hypotonia with weak atrophic muscles and failure to thrive. Patients with hypoglycaemia presented at an earlier age.

Hepatic abnormalities may be reflected by elevated serum aminotransferase levels, hyperammonaemia, and hypoglycaemia which does not respond well to glucagon during carbohydrate deprivation. Hepatomegaly and hypotonia may be present during the acute illness but may not be noticeable when the patient is asymptomatic. Liver tissue obtained following an infection may show fat accumulation in the cytoplasm of hepatocytes (Fig. 4.68); however, tissue obtained during a steady state demonstrates fat accumulation only in sinusoidal lining cells. Mild portal fibrosis has been reported. Hepatocyte mitochondria may have bizarre shapes and a dense matrix.[620] Microscopic examination of muscle always reveals lipid accumulation. Muscle enzymes and EMG may be normal despite the presence of structural abnormalities. Patients with only the muscle carnitine palmitoyl transferase deficiency may experience recurrent attacks of myoglobinuria, which are usually precipitated by prolonged exercise and/or fasting. During these attacks the muscles are swollen, tender and weak, and serum creatinine kinase activity may be increased.

Inheritance is autosomal recessive. The parents are almost always carnitine deficient. The diagnosis depends on finding low tissue carnitine concentrations in liver and muscle and on the demonstration of a carnitine transport

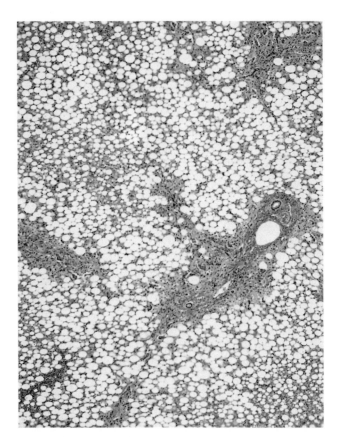

Fig. 4.68 Systemic carnitine deficiency. The liver shows marked steatosis (medium-sized vacuoles), as well as periportal fibrosis. H&E.

defect utilizing cultured fibroblasts *in vitro*.[621,622] This sodium-dependent plasma membrane transport system can be inhibited by acylcarnitine.[623,624] Urinary dicarboxylic acids are normal. L-carnitine is the treatment of choice, despite high urinary losses. It prevents severe hypoglycaemia, elevation of free fatty acids, hypoketonaemia, hyperammonaemia and triglyceride accumulation in tissues when plasma carnitine levels approach normal. Cardiac and muscle diseases respond well despite persistence of low levels in muscle. Liver carnitine levels return to normal because of a different transport system.[621]

Hepatic carnitine palmitoyl transferase I (CPT I) deficiency

CPT I esterifies long chain fatty acids to carnitine at the outer mitochondrial membrane. Patients with the deficiency present with seizures and coma from hypoglycaemia and hypoketonaemia during fasting. Hepatomegaly is present with normal or abnormal liver function tests and ammonia levels. Few cases have been reported to date.[625,626] A recent one was documented to have renal tubular acidosis with bilateral cystic changes.[627] In this disorder, plasma carnitine studies are normal. CPT I levels are low in liver or cultured skin fibroblasts. Liver biopsy reveals microvesicular fat. Muscle tissues are involved.

Further episodes can be prevented by the administration of medium chain triglycerides which also improves the renal tubular acidosis.

Carnitine palmitoyl transferase II (CPT II) deficiency

The first patient was documented by DiMauro & Di-Mauro in 1973.[628] Since then, most patients observed have presented during adolescence or adulthood with episodic muscle necrosis and paroxysmal myoglobinuria after vigorous exercise or prolonged fasting. Two cases with an hepatic presentation were described in 1991.[629,630] Muscle was also involved, as was the case in previously reported patients. Clarification of CPT deficiency may be forthcoming since the gene has been cloned, sequenced, analysed and located on chromosome 1q 12–1pter.[631]

Carnitine–acylcarnitine translocase deficiency

This enzyme carries the product of CPT I (acylcarnitine) across the inner mitochondrial membrane. CPT II releases free carnitine and converts acylcarnitine to acyl-CoA for beta oxidation and ketone synthesis. The first case of this mitochondrial translocase deficiency has been reported recently.[632] Presentaton was at 36 hours of age with a seizure, severe apnoea, and bradycardia upon fasting. Cardiac arrhythmias complicated the initial course. A sibling had died of a similar illness at 2 days of age. Recurrent hospitalization was required for vomiting, lethargy and coma despite a high medium chain, low long chain fat formula diet. Hyperammonaemia remained a clinical problem. The child had muscle, cardiac, and liver dysfunction until death at 3 years of age. The plasma acylcarnitine level was high. The low plasma free carnitine changed very little following oral carnitine. The low plasma β-hydroxybutyrate level responded to medium chain triglycerides. Both parents were carriers.

Long chain acyl-CoA dehydrogenase (LCAD) deficiency

Approximately 20 cases of this deficiency have been reported. The first cases were described by Hale et al in 1985.[632] LCAD is a mitochondrial enzyme which catalyses the initial reactions in beta oxidation of C_{18}–C_{12} acyl-CoA esters. Patients present with the classic symptoms of fatty acid oxidation defects between 2 and 6 months of age.[633] These symptoms include those of a Reye- or SIDS-like syndrome, hypoketotic hypoglycaemia, hepatomegaly, cardiomegaly, hypotonia and failure to thrive. Examination of the heart may or may not reveal cardiomyopathy. Hepatocellular enzymes and the ammonia level may or may not be elevated and coagulation tests and bilirubin levels are usually normal. Acute respiratory or cardiac arrest is not uncommon. Chronic cases may develop muscle cramps and myoglobinuria.[634] Hypotonia with normal reflexes may persist. Central nervous system insults resulting from the acute events can result in microcephaly and delayed development even though these diseases do not primarily involve the brain.

The liver reveals pansteatosis, predominantly macrovesicular, regardless of when the biopsy is obtained during the course of the disease.[633] Prominent fibrosis with portal inflammation was noted at initial presentation in one patient, with a subsequent liver biopsy being compatible with cirrhosis; residual microvesicular fat was present. Electron microscopic findings are limited to the non-acute state in 2 patients. Only one patient had abnormalities of mitochondria which included widening of the intracristal spaces and irregular separation of the double limiting membrane. The matrix contained dense bodies.

The inheritance is autosomal recessive. Prenatal testing has not been verified due to the small number of cases. Possible screening tests obtained during the acute stage include a low plasma carnitine with high esterification, and abnormalities in urine organic acids (increased medium chain dicarboxylic acids and decreased ketones). The diagnosis can be confirmed by demonstration of LCAD activity that is less than 10% of normal in cultured fibroblasts, leucocytes, or liver cells. Preventive measures include avoidance of fasting, and the use of intravenous glucose when oral feeding is not possible. High caloric feedings (containing high carbohydrate and low long chain fat supplemented with medium chain triglycerides) should be given frequently.

Medium chain acyl-coenzyme A dehydrogenase (MCAD) deficiency

MCAD deficiency was first reported in 1982[635] and the enzyme deficiency was documented the following year.[636] Estimates of the incidence of this autosomal recessive disorder range from 1 in 10 000 to 1 in 18 500 births,[637,638] which suggests that it is the most common inherited fatty acid oxidation defect. Approximately 100 cases have been reported in which the initial diagnosis was Reye's syndrome, SIDS or carnitine deficiency. MCAD is a tetrameric mitochondrial flavoprotein that catalyses the dehydrogenation of acyl-CoA esters containing 6–12 carbons.[639] The gene has been localized to the short arm of chromosome 1,[640] and in 90% of cases the defect results from a point mutation involving a glutamine instead of a lysine at residue 304.

Patients usually present in the first two years of life during an intercurrent illness resulting in poor oral intake. Up to a third of them may die during the first episode.[636] They may present with recurrent episodes of vomiting and lethargy progressing to hypoketonaemic hypoglycaemic coma. Hepatomegaly, abnormal liver function tests and hyperammonaemia may or may not be present.

Urine organic acids during the acute episode demonstrate elevated C_6–C_{12} dicarboxylic acids and acyl carnitine profiles plus other abnormalities.[641] Usually, the total carnitine in the plasma is decreased with increased acetyl carnitine except when the infant is breast fed. Carnitine challenge tests may be a good screening test during the asymptomatic period.[642] The diagnosis is confirmed by measurement of MCAD activity in mononuclear leucocytes, cultured fibroblasts, or liver. Prenatal diagnosis is possible. Therapy again includes the avoidance of fasting. The diet should be high in carbohydrates and low in fat. Oral L-carnitine may decrease the number of episodic attacks. Death results from cerebral oedema.

On light microscopy, the liver may be found to contain macro- or microvesicular steatosis.[623] It is not usual for any fibrosis to be present. Mitochondria demonstrate a dense matrix with occasional widening of intracristal spaces.

Short chain acyl-coenzyme A dehydrogenase (SCAD) deficiency

This disease is not well-defined since only 5 cases with variable clinical manifestations have been reported.[637] Infants have had acute episodes of poor feeding, lethargy, hypoglycaemia, hyperammonaemia, and metabolic acidosis.[643,644] Children fail to thrive and have muscle weakness, and one adult presented with proximal muscle weakness. The location of the gene is on chromosome 12 q 22 qter,[645] and the diagnosis is confirmed by measuring muscle SCAD activity; cultured fibroblasts contain less than 11% SCAD activity.[646] Variable defects have been demonstrated.[646,647] Lipid is stored in the muscle and liver; liver mitochondrial changes are similar to those of MCAD deficiency.

Long chain 3-hydroxyacyl coenzyme A dehydrogenase deficiency

Approximately 20 cases of this disorder have been documented.[648–651] All three major organs are involved and manifestations are accentuated by fasting. Presentation may range from a Reye's-like illness to episodes of muscle weakness with myoglobinuria. Cardiomyopathy is common. Sensorimotor neuropathy may be present. Fat accumulates in tissues. Ultrastructurally, mitochondria do not appear abnormal. Screening tests reveal the usual abnormalities in altered carnitine levels and increased dicarboxylic aciduria. Both muscle and liver enzymes may be elevated. Unique 3-hydroxy intermediates can be found in the urine. Enzyme assays are not readily available.

Short chain 3-hydroxyacyl-CoA dehydrogenase (SCHAD) deficiency

Only 3 cases have been reported. The best documented was a 16-year-old girl who presented with recurrent myoglobinuria, hypoketotic hypoglycaemia, encephalopathy and cardiomyopathy following viral infections.[652] Severe muscle involvement resulted in facial diplegia, dysarthria, dysphagia, mild ptosis, hypotonia and leg weakness. Acidosis and hyperammonaemia were not a problem. Death resulted from the cardiomyopathy. Fat was not found in skeletal muscle, and mitochondria appeared normal ultrastructurally. The liver demonstrated zone 3 changes related to cardiac failure and mild microvesicular steatosis. The enzyme defect could be demonstrated in muscle but not in fibroblasts.

CERAMIDASE DEFICIENCY (FARBER'S LIPOGRANULOMATOSIS)

Forty patients with this disease have recently been reviewed by Moser et al.[653] The mode of inheritance is autosomal recessive. The presentation is variable, resulting in a classification of five types. Patients with Type I, the most common 'classic' form of the disease, present between 2 weeks and 4 months of age with the usual triad of joint disease, subcutaneous nodules, and a hoarse cry which may progress to aphonia. The last manifestation is secondary to swelling and granuloma formation in the epiglottis and larynx. Other symptoms include difficulties with feeding and respiration, resulting in poor weight gain, fever, and pneumonia.

Severely affected patients have generalized lymphadenopathy, an enlarged tongue, cardiac valve granulomas and hepatomegaly. Nerve involvement is common, particularly in the lower motor neurons, and the spinal fluid protein level may be elevated. Excess gangliosides are found in the granulomatous lesions and neurons of the cerebral cortex while lymph nodes, liver, kidney, and lung (as well as the subcutaneous nodules) contain very high levels of free ceramide.[653] The diagnosis depends on demonstration of the deficiency of acid ceramidase (less than 8% of normal) in cultured skin fibroblasts, white blood cells, or amniocytes.[653,654] No therapy is available.

Types II and III are milder forms of the disease and there is significant liver, lung or brain involvement in the latter. Type IV presents like a histiocytic disorder with neonatal hepatosplenomegaly progressing to systemic involvement with death by 6 months of age. Other classic symptoms and findings may vary even within the same family.[655] Type V presents with psychomotor deterioration at 1–2 years of age but the viscera are spared. Findings include subcutaneous nodules, joint disease and macular cherry-red spots.

Histological studies have shown granulomatous infiltrates in the subcutaneous nodules, periarticular and synovial tissues, lymph nodes, and to a lesser extent in the lungs, liver, spleen and other viscera.[653] These consist of lymphocytes, histiocytes and foam cells which contain PAS-positive material. Necrosis and dense fibrosis may develop in older lesions.[656] In one case, a liver biopsy revealed numerous atypical histiocytes with cytoplasmic vacuolization which filled the sinusoids and distorted the liver architecture. Post-mortem examination revealed massive histiocytic infiltration of the liver, spleen, lymph nodes, thymus and lungs.[655]

The granulomatous lesions of Farber's disease have been reproduced experimentally by injection of ceramide from a patient with the disease and by commercial ceramide.[653] Neurons of the central and autonomic nervous systems of patients with the disease are distended with PAS-positive cytoplasmic material.[657] Abul-Haj et al[656] considered the stored material to be a mucopolysaccharide–polypeptide complex to which lipid was later added. Ultrastructurally, the histiocytes contain rectilinear and curvilinear structures in the cytoplasmic inclusions that are sometimes referred to as Farber bodies.[654,658–660] Cross sections strongly suggest a tubular disposition of the stored material, the diameter being 20–23 nm.[654] The Farber bodies have also been reproduced experimentally in mice by injection of ceramides and related sphingolipids.[661] Van Hoof & Hers[658] described dense bodies and clear vacuoles in hepatocytes in a case studied by electron microscopy. The former were generally round, osmiophilic deposits that surrounded electronlucent material in a dense granular matrix. The clear vacuoles, which were also noted in cells lining intrahepatic bile ducts, resembled those seen in the mucopolysaccharidoses. Banana-like bodies have been seen in Schwann cells ultrastructurally.[662] They resemble miniature bananas and seem to arise from needle-like, membrane-bound inclusions. On average, they are about 1.6 µm long and have a diameter of 0.23 µm.

PEROXISOMAL DISORDERS

Peroxisomes contain enzymes pre-packaged elsewhere in the cell. They perform multiple functions including catabolism of glyoxylate, oxidation of prostaglandins, biosynthesis of bile acids, biosynthesis of ether phospholipids and beta oxidation of very long chain fatty acids.

Numerous clinical syndromes result from the pathological consequences of decreased enzymatic activity of this organelle. Primary acatalasia and adult Refsum's disease will not be discussed in this chapter as they do not affect the liver.

PRIMARY HYPEROXALURIA

This disease results from the deficiency of either of two known peroxisomal enzymes. Type I disease, first described by LePoutre in 1925,[663] is caused by a deficiency of alanine-glyoxylate aminotransferase (AGAT, EC 2.6.1.44) and was recently reviewed by Latta.[664] Deficiency of this enzyme allows accumulation of glyoxylate, which in turn forms oxalate. The primary source of glyoxylate in humans, however, remains unclear. An even more rare variant, type II, was initially described by Williams & Smith,[665] with defective D-glycerate dehydrogenase activity (EC 1.1.1.29) uncovered.[666] Only 16 type II cases have been published,[667] in contrast to 330 patient with type I.[668] Although both types present with urinary complications of calcium oxalate stones, only type I is usually associated with renal failure, particularly during childhood.

Both variants are inherited as autosomal recessive traits. AGAT is an enzyme found almost exclusively in liver peroxisomes and requires pyridoxal phosphate as a coenzyme. The onset and course of the disease depend on the amount of functional enzyme. Most patients present before 5 years of age with a range from 1–40 years and over.[669] End stage renal failure usually develops within two years after impaired renal function is first detected.[670] Since liver transplantation is only proposed for type I, this description deals primarily with this variant.

The presenting symptoms are haematuria and renal pain from calcium oxalate stones. Failure to thrive begins when renal failure develops. Other manifestations relate to calcium oxalate accumulation in the heart, bones, and arteries. Signs of overwhelming oxalate accumulation include cardiac arrhythmias, peripheral vascular disease, and bone fractures in patients with renal failure. Massive hepatosplenomegaly can develop because of extramedullary haemopoiesis secondary to bone marrow obliteration by calcium oxalate.[671] Liver function is always normal except when vascular involvement results in zone 3 hepatic necrosis.[672]

In early onset disease, discrete, white, pinhead-size lesions (flecked retina) can be seen by funduscopic examination; they are more dense towards the equator and initially spare the macula. The calcium oxalate infiltration is in the retinal pigment epithelium. Eventually, detachment can occur in the macular area followed by scarring.[673,674] Ultrasound studies include intense echogenicity of the renal parenchyma with a distinct corticomedullary junction; the kidneys are of normal size.[675] Routine X-rays reveal nephrolithiasis and nephrocalcinosis. Dense calcifications can be seen in arteries. The bones reveal abnormal densities with signs of renal osteodystrophy and pathological fractures. A characteristic metaphyseal lesion consists of a wide translucent zone with a sclerotic zone adjacent to the diaphysis and metaphyseal wasting.[676]

Danpure & Jennings[677] defined the enzyme defect in 1986 when they found that activity of AGAT was virtually absent in most individuals. A milder disease course correlates with residual enzyme activity.[678] Subtypes include functional enzyme only in mitochondria and functionally inactive protein.[679] The diagnosis can only be confirmed by liver biopsy in patients in whom secondary hyperoxaluria has been excluded, such as that due to the short bowel syndrome. However, urinary excretion of oxalate over 70 mg/day per 1/73 m² patient surface area is pathological. Antenatal diagnosis can only be made by liver biopsy.[677,680] Type II disease is better detected by L-glyceric aciduria rather than oxalaturia. D-glycerate dihydrogenase also is a reductase for glyoxalate and it can be detected in many patients in leucocytes as well as in the liver.[667]

The liver demonstrates non-specific changes by light microscopy including lipofuscin and aggregates of iron, probably secondary to dialysis.[681] Peroxisomes were smaller in size and number when compared to normal-sized mitochondria at the ultrastructural level. Similar findings have been reported in Menkes' syndrome, analbuminaemia, and occasionally in Wilson's disease. Oxalate crystals do not accumulate in the liver parenchyma and have only been seen in the media of the arteries and connective tissue in portal areas.[682]

Medical therapy includes a large fluid intake and restriction of oxalate-rich foods. When residual enzyme activity exists, pyridoxine can reduce the production of oxalate.[683] Thiazides which decrease calcium excretion in the urine are the diuretics of choice.[670] Haemodialysis is superior to peritoneal dialysis but neither can cope with the oxalate production in type I.[684]

Renal transplantation offers only temporary relief.[670] Watts et al[685] reported that liver transplantation corrects the metabolic lesion when combined with renal transplantation. This group has recently summarized the results of transplantation in 9 patients from three centres.[1] There are 4 long-term survivors who are asymptomatic with resolution of systemic oxalosis. They propose that better results will be obtained when hepatic transplantation is performed prior to end stage renal failure. The same applies to cardiac involvement since this is also reversed following liver–kidney transplantation.[1,686]

DISORDERS OF PEROXISOMAL BETA OXIDATION

Trihydroxycoprostanic acid (THCA), a bile acid, is converted to Δ^{24}-THCA by microsomal THCA-CoA synthetase and THCA-Co oxidase. Very long chain fatty acids (VLCFA) are converted to Δ^2-VLCFA-CoA by peroxisomal VLCFA-CoA synthetase and acyl-CoA oxidase. Subsequent beta oxidation steps within the peroxisomes accommodate the above substrates via enol-CoA hydratase and 3-OH-acyl-CoA dehydrogenase (a bifunctional enzyme) and 3-oxo-acyl-CoA thiolase. Liver disease only occurs in patients in whom the bile acid pathway is altered.

Disorders with peroxisomes and predominantly one enzyme defect

X-linked adrenoleucodystrophy

A 7-year-old boy was described by Siemerling & Creutz-feldt in 1923.[687] He became hyperpigmented at 3 years of age with neurological symptoms at $6\frac{1}{2}$ years. Post-mortem examination at 7 years of age revealed atrophy and extensive demyelination of the central nervous system. Biochemical studies of his adrenal glands and cerebral white matter disclosed C_{23}–C_{30} long chain fatty acids in cholesterol esters and gangliosides.[688] Over 300 patients have been described. Psychomotor development is normal up to 3 years of age. Early signs of nervous system involvement include emotional lability with auditory and visual impairment, later progressing to optic atrophy and dementia. In cases with an early onset during childhood, these signs precede the pigmentation from adrenal insufficiency. In adult cases, pigmentation may have been present since early childhood. Rare cases just have Addison's disease.[689] It is postulated that the adrenal membranes are unresponsive to ACTH.[690] The biochemical characteristics are listed in Table 4.4, which is based on the publication of Wanders et al.[691] Liver problems have not been noted. The defect has been demonstrated in fibroblast peroxisomes to be at the level of VLCFA-CoA synthetase (the initial enzymate reaction) but the mechanism is unclear.[692,693]

Pseudo-neonatal adrenoleucodystrophy

Two cases from the same family have been described.[694] They were hypotonic at birth with psychomotor regression by 2 years of age accompanied by sensorineural hearing loss and optic atrophy. Cholesterol levels were low and ACTH levels were high. The liver contained large fat droplets with trilaminar leaflets of VLCFA at their edges. Mitochondria had a clear matrix. Peroxisomes were triangular and elongated. The biochemical findings are listed in Table 4.4. Deficiency of acyl-CoA oxidase was documented.

Bifunctional protein deficiency

One case has been reported which combined the features found in Zellweger's syndrome and neonatal adrenoleucodystrophy.[695] The patient was not dysmorphic but was hypotonic with no developmental progress. Adrenal atrophy, renal microcysts, and chondrodysplasia punctata were present. In addition to VLCFA, THCA was also elevated. The liver was mildly enlarged and fibrosis was present. No abnormalities in phytanic acid, L-pipecolic acid, and plasmalogen were found. Peroxisomal enzymes prior to and after this enzymatic step were found in the fibroblast peroxisomal fraction. The mRNA coding for the bifunctional enzyme was present by Northern blot analysis in the patient's fibroblasts. A second patient had the protein for this enzyme and, presumably, the mutation affects the active site of the enzymes.[691]

Table 4.4 Biochemical characteristics of the inborn errors of peroxisomal beta oxidation (after Wanders et al[691])

Parameter measured	Peroxisome deficiency disorders	X-linked ALD	Pseudo-neonatal ALD	Bifunctional protein deficiency	Pseudo-Zellweger syndrome	'Zellweger-like' syndrome
Metabolites in body fluids						
Very long chain fatty acids	Elevated	Elevated	Elevated	Elevated	Elevated	Elevated
Bile acid intermediates	Elevated	Normal	Normal	Elevated	Elevated	Elevated
Pipecolic acid	Elevated+	Normal	Normal	Normal	Normal	Normal
Phytanic acid	Elevated+	Normal	Normal	Normal	Normal	Normal
Plasmalogen synthesis						
DHAPAT	Deficient	Normal	Normal	Normal	Normal	Deficient
Alky DHAP synthesis	Deficient	Normal	Normal	Normal	Normal	—
De novo synthesis	Impaired	Normal	Normal	Normal	Normal	Impaired
Peroxisomes						
Hepatic peroxisomes	(Virtually absent)	Present	Present	Present	Present	Present
Particle-bound catalase	< 5	> 65	> 65	> 65	n.d.	> 65
Peroxisomal beta oxidation						
Activity with C26:0	Deficient	Deficient	Deficient	Deficient	Deficient	Deficient
Enzyme proteins						
Acyl-CoA oxidase	Deficient	Normal	Deficient	Normal	Normal	Deficient
Bifunctional protein	Deficient	Normal	Normal	Deficient	Normal	Deficient
Peroxisomal thiolase	Deficient	Normal	Normal	Normal	Deficient	Deficient

ALD = adrenal leucodystrophy; n.d. = not done; + = age dependent

Pseudo-Zellweger's syndrome

One child was reported who had all the features of Zellweger's syndrome including hepatosplenomegaly.[696] Liver biopsy revealed abundant and enlarged peroxisomes. Large fat droplets were present in the hepatocytes which were often birefringent, and the characteristic lamellae were found in the cytoplasm at the periphery of the fat droplets. Post-mortem examination of the liver at 11 months of age revealed slight stellate portal fibrosis. Lamellar inclusions were present in both the cytoplasm and lysosomes of hepatocytes and Kupffer cells. The single enzyme defect was deficiency of 3-oxacyl-CoA thiolase.

'Zellweger-like' syndrome

One of the patients with this syndrome died of liver failure at 5 months of age; however, no fibrosis or cirrhosis was present.[697] Peroxisomes were normal in size but the mitochondria were slightly enlarged. Other findings included zonal necrosis, extramedullary haemopoiesis and small amounts of lipid and iron. The multiple deficient enzymes are listed in Table 4.4.

Rhizomelic chondrodysplasia punctata[698]

This disorder has no abnormality of VLCFA and no liver disease. Patients present with severe shortening and disturbed ossification of the proximal limbs. Psychomotor retardation, failure to thrive, microcephaly and cataracts are other characteristics. Inheritance is autosomal recessive and death usually occurs in the first year of life.

Defects are found in phytanic acid oxidation and ether lipid (plasmalogen) biosynthesis.

Impaired assembly of peroxisomes—Zellweger's syndrome, neonatal adrenoleucodystrophy, and infantile Refsum's disease

Zellweger's syndrome was originally described in 1964.[699] Peroxisomes could not be identified in the liver of classic patients by Goldfisher et al in 1973.[700] Incidence figures range from 1/25 000 to 1/100 000 births.[701] The clinical features include facial dysmorphia, severe hypotonia, hepatomegaly, renal cysts, optic atrophy, seizures, and severe neurological impairment. A more complete listing of the clinical features with examples is found in the review by Martinez et al.[701] Milder variants of classic Zellweger's syndrome have been described including neonatal adrenoleucodystrophy and infantile Refsum's disease. There is no unanimity on whether hyperpipecolic acidaemia should also be included in this list.[702] Neonatal adrenoleucodystrophy was first described in 1978.[703] The dysmorphic features are less striking than those of classic Zellweger's syndrome, and the peroxisomes in the liver are not as severely diminished.[704] Chondrodysplasia punctata and renal cysts are not observed in these patients. Infantile Refsum's disease was first described by Scotto et al in 1982.[705] All patients have sensorineural hearing loss and pigmentary degeneration of the retina along with moderate dysmorphic features and early hypotonia. Hepatomegaly with abnormal liver function is routinely found and may progress to cirrhosis. Again, chondrodysplasia punctata and renal cysts are not observed.

Fibroblast complementation studies indicate that at least seven different genes account for these disorders.[702,706,707] They are characterized by an impairment in the assembly of peroxisomes, but ghost remnants of these organelles remain.[708] A recent case has been documented to be a point mutation resulting from premature termination of peroxisome assembly factor 1.[709] To date, no treatment has been of any help.

Morphological findings in the peroxisomal disorders

The autopsy findings in Zellweger's syndrome include cerebral anomalies (abnormal convolutional pattern, heterotopic cortex, olivary dysplasia), renal glomerular microcysts, cardiovascular defects (patent ductus and patent foramen ovale), thymic anomalies and pancreatic islet cell hyperplasia.[710]

The hepatic histopathological findings in Zellweger's syndrome have not been consistent, and some cases have shown no or only minimal non-specific alterations. Portal inflammation, periportal fibrosis, focal necrosis with progression to intra-acinar fibrosis, cholestasis and haemosiderosis have been recorded.[710–715] In a survey of the literature, Gilchrist et al[711] found reduction of 'cholangioles' in 23% of cases. Cases with severe fibrosis with disruption of the parenchyma,[714–718] and even cirrhosis[719,720] have also been described.

The absence of peroxisomes in liver cells, first described by Goldfischer et al,[700] has been a consistent finding in subsequent ultrastructural studies.[12,714,715] In some cases, however, small bodies resembling incompletely developed peroxisomes could be found.[12] A variant of the disease with detectable hepatic peroxisomes has also been reported.[697] Another ultrastructural feature is the occurrence within macrophages of large angulate lysosomes filled with fine double lamellae.[715] Mitochondria show disarrangement and twisting of their cristae and have a dense matrix.[12,721,722] Mooi et al[715] demonstrated the absence of colatase, a peroxisomal enzyme, at the ultrastructural level in a liver biopsy from a patient with Zellweger's syndrome. It is also possible to demonstrate several other peroxisomal enzymes by immunogold labelling.[723]

In adrenoleucodystrophy, there is variable fibrosis and irregular nodularity of the hepatic parenchyma.[724,725] Cirrhosis was reported in one case.[726] PAS-positive macrophages and Kupffer cells were identified in another.[724]

Ultrastructurally, hepatic peroxisomes are reported to be either absent or markedly reduced in number and size[704,726] and may contain electron-dense cores.[727] Lamellar cytoplasmic inclusions are found in Kupffer cells and hepatocytes.[724,727] Mitochondria with crystalline inclusions and/or abnormal cristae have also been noted.[727]

Accentuated 'lobular' architecture, with fibrous bands linking portal areas together, has been observed in Refsum's disease.[728] A micronodular cirrhosis was found in a patient who died at the age of 12 years.[729] A deficiency of hepatic peroxisomes has been detected ultrastructurally and cytochemically.[728,730,731] Phillips et al[12] believe that, while some hepatocytes totally lack peroxisomes, others contain very small underdeveloped ones that sometimes have a very dense matrix. They have also noted the presence of numerous angulate lysosomes in Kupffer cells in this disorder.

MITOCHONDRIAL CYTOPATHIES

Mitochondrial myopathies constitute a clinically heterogeneous group of disorders that can affect multiple systems besides skeletal muscle (mitochondrial encephalomyopathies or cytopathies), and are usually defined by morphological abnormalities of muscle mitochondria.[732,733] They all represent disorders of oxidative phosphorylation. Because mitochondria have their own DNA and their own translation and transcription apparatuses, mitochondrial myopathies can be due to defects of either a nuclear or mitochondrial genome, and can be transmitted by mendelian or maternal inheritance.[732]

Hepatic involvement has been reported in the mitochondrial cytopathies.[734–736a] The first report by Boustany et al[734] described two infant cousins with a similar fatal mitochondrial disorder, the cytochrome deficiency being limited to skeletal muscle in one infant and to liver in the other. The infant with hepatopathy had clinical manifestations of liver disease at 5 months of age and died at the age of 9 months. Electron microscopy revealed liver cells packed with large, rounded mitochondria. The second cousin with myopathy died at 18 weeks of age; her liver was enlarged and fatty, but the mitochondria were normal in size and number. Two of the three patients reported by Cormier et al[735] had steatosis (panacinar in one and confined to zone 3 in the other), and one also had cholestasis.

The patient studied by Fayon et al[736] had ascites, which was diagnosed prenatally, and severe liver failure; death from multisystem failure occurred on the fourth day of life. Light microscopy revealed an incomplete cirrhosis, microvesicular steatosis, marked cholestasis and proliferation of neocholangioles, which often contained bile plugs. Electron microscopy showed abnormal mitochondria in numerous hepatocytes with occasional cristae in a fluffy matrix; some contained dense inclusions. A defect of cytochrome C oxidase (complex IV) was demonstrated in muscle and liver. Fayon et al[736] pointed out that the association of neonatal liver failure with hyperlacticacidaemia warrants investigation of oxidative phosphorylation.

DISEASES OF METAL METABOLISM

Hereditary haemochromatosis is discussed in Chapter 5.

WILSON'S DISEASE (HEPATOLENTICULAR DEGENERATION)

Wilson's disease is the result of tissue injury caused by copper overload in the liver and other organs. The prevalence of this disorder is 1 in 30 000 and inheritance is autosomal recessive.[737] A linkage to red cell esterase D has localized the gene mutation for Wilson's disease to chromosome 13q 14–21.[738,739] A test may soon be available: (a) to better distinguish homozygotes from heterozygotes; (b) perhaps to explain the current variability in the clinical course of the liver disease; and (c) to explain why children predominantly present with hepatic disease while adults present with neurological manifestations. Since caeruloplasmin maps to chromosome 3, this glycoprotein can no longer be considered the product of the Wilsons' disease gene, even though it is useful in establishing the diagnosis in 95% of patients. As is the case in the neonate, the low serum caeruloplasmin level in Wilson's disease appears to be the result of faults in both transcriptional and post-transcriptional processing.[740,741]

Overt clinical manifestations of liver disease are never seen before the age of 5 years. It may be manifested in one of four ways:[742]

1. Acute hepatitis, which occurs in about a quarter of the cases, may be mistaken for acute viral hepatitis or infectious mononucleosis. It may be associated with a transient haemolytic anaemia, unconjugated hyperbilirubinaemia or hypouricaemia.

2. Fulminant hepatitis, with severe haemolytic anaemia, hepatic insufficiency, marked clotting abnormalities (including intravascular coagulopathy), renal insufficiency and death.[742–745] It has been suggested that an alkaline phosphatase–total bilirubin ratio of <2.0 provides 100% sensitivity and specificity in identifying the fulminant hepatic failure of Wilson's disease from other causes of hepatic failure.[746] However, a subsequent report of a larger series with younger patients did not confirm the ratio to be diagnostic and advocated reliance on urine copper excretion.[747]

3. Chronic active hepatitis that is clinically indistinguishable from that due to viral and other aetiologies. The prognosis of this form of presentation is good after treatment with D-penicillamine and/or trientine.[748]

4. Cirrhosis is the initial presentation in about half of the cases.

Hepatocellular carcinoma is a rare complication.[742,749] Cholelithiasis can occur in both children and adults.[750] Wilson's disease may coexist with other genetically determined conditions such as thalassaemia minor[751] or Gilbert's disease.[742]

According to Sternlieb,[752] the diagnosis of Wilson's disease requires demonstration of a low level of serum caeruloplasmin—less than 1.3 mmol/l (20 mg/100ml), and an increased quantity of copper in the liver (greater than 250 µg/g dry weight). However, 5% of patients have a normal caeruloplasmin. Kayser–Fleischer rings appear late in the course of the disease.

In the presymptomatic stage, the serum aminotransferase levels may be the best biochemical indicator of liver damage; increased levels correlate well with abnormal hepatic histology.[753] The diagnostic value of radiocopper studies has been reviewed by Scheinberg & Sternlieb.[742] Screening of asymptomatic family members for Wilson's disease has been reviewed by Lindahl & Sharp.[754] Prenatal diagnosis, carrier detection and presymptomatic diagnosis have been accomplished by analysis of restriction fragment length polymorphism.[755–757]

The pathological effects of Wilson's disease are considered to be directly related to the accumulation of copper in the brain, cornea, liver and kidneys. Patients presenting with acute hepatitis are rarely biopsied. According to Scheinberg & Sternlieb,[742] their livers show ballooning of hepatocytes, acidophilic bodies, cholestasis and a sparse lymphocytic infiltration. Usually, the biopsy in the precirrhotic stage is characterized by moderate anisonucleosis, focal necrosis, scattered sinusoidal acidophilic bodies and moderate to marked fatty change.[758] Variable numbers of glycogenated nuclei are a constant finding in periportal

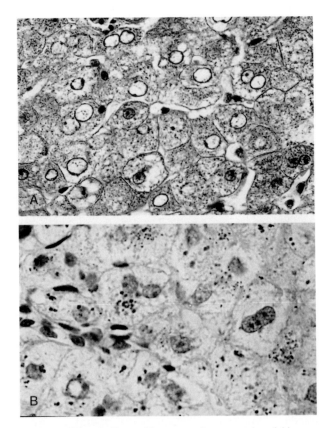

Fig. 4.69 (a) Wilson's disease. Numerous glycogenated nuclei in periportal hepatocytes. (b) Periportal hepatocytes contain many varying-sized lipofuscin granules that are irregularly dispersed in the cytoplasm. (a) H&E; (b) Fontana.

hepatocytes (Fig. 4.69). Lipofuscin accumulates in periportal areas and some of the granules are large, irregular in shape and vacuolated[758] (Fig. 4.69). Kupffer cells may be slightly enlarged and laden with haemosiderin, presumably as a result of the acute haemolytic crises that may complicate the disease. There is a progressive increase in periportal cholangiolar proliferation and fibrosis. Variable numbers of inflammatory cells, chiefly lymphocytes and plasma cells, are seen in the connective tissue of portal areas. Changes indistinguishable from those of chronic active hepatitis due to other aetiologies may be seen (Figs 4.70–4.72).[748–761] In our experience, helpful differential clues in the diagnosis of Wilson's disease include the presence of steatosis, glycogenated nuclei, moderate to marked copper storage (Fig. 4.72) and the presence of Mallory bodies in periportal liver cells.

Cytochemically demonstrable copper is usually confined to hepatocytes in acinar zones 1 in the precirrhotic stage of Wilson's disease. With the use of special stains and electron probe microanalysis, Goldfischer & Sternlieb[762] have shown that in young asymptomatic patients copper is diffusely distributed in the cytoplasm of hepatocytes. In slightly older patients who exhibit early symptoms or signs of the disease, the metal is both diffusely distributed and intralysosomal, while in patients with advanced disease all the copper is confined to lysosomes (Fig. 4.72). The various staining methods for the demonstration of copper in tissue sections have been reviewed by Lindquist[763] and Irons et al.[764] In our experience and that of others[764] the p-dimethylaminobenzylidene rhodanine method gives the most reproducible results (Fig. 4.72); both it and the rubeanic acid method are specific for copper. There is a linear relationship between microscopical evaluation of the stain and actual tissue copper levels.[764] Copper-binding protein can be stained by orcein in Wilson's disease and other conditions (e.g. chronic cholestatic disorders),[765–767]

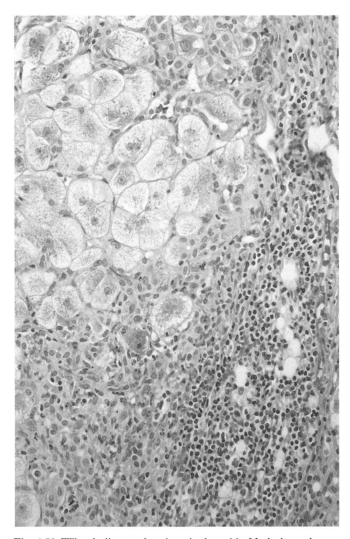

Fig. 4.70 Wilson's disease, chronic active hepatitis. Marked portal inflammation and piecemeal necrosis. H&E.

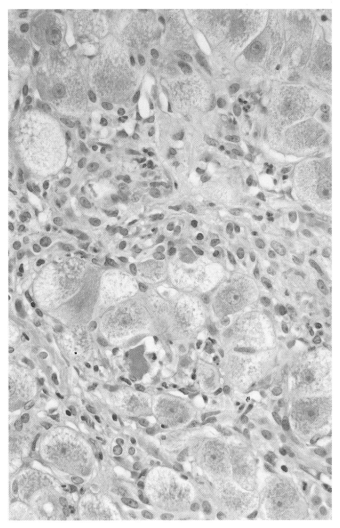

Fig. 4.71 Wilson's disease, chronic active hepatitis. Ballooning and apoptotic bodies in area of piecemeal necrosis. H&E.

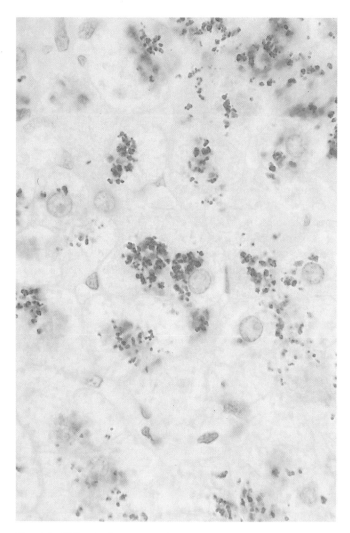

Fig. 4.72 Wilson's disease, chronic active hepatitis. Marked copper accumulation (red granules) in periportal liver cells. Rhodanine.

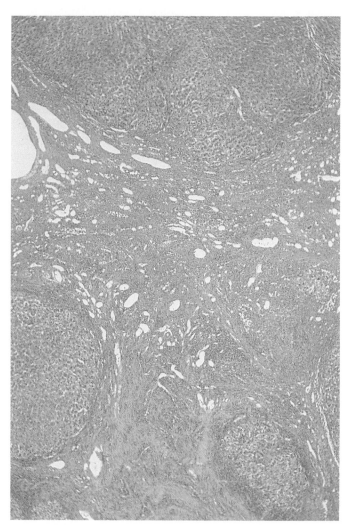

Fig. 4.73 Wilson's disease. Cirrhotic nodules are separated by wide bands of fibrous tissue with many vessels and chronic inflammation. H&E.

as well as by aldehyde fuchsin and Victoria blue. The granules also stain with a variety of stains for lipofuscin that is presumably aggregated in the same lysosomes.[742]

Both caeruloplasmin and metallothionein have been demonstrated immunohistochemically in the liver in Wilson's disease. Graul et al[768] found no difference in the pattern of staining of caeruloplasmin in the livers of patients with Wilson's disease and normal adults or neonates. The distribution of metallothionein in Wilson's disease was studied by Nartey et al.[769] In sections with minimal tissue damage, there was intense cytoplasmic staining for metallothionein in liver cells, whereas in sections with extensive necrosis and fibrosis there was both nuclear and cytoplasmic staining.

The cirrhosis of Wilson's disease is usually macronodular, but can be mixed or even micronodular in type.[742] Microscopically, it is characterized by varying-sized nodules separated by fibrous septa that may be wide or very thin, with minimal cholangiolar proliferation and variable

inflammation (Fig. 4.73). All changes in the precirrhotic stage are also seen in the cirrhotic liver. In addition, Mallory bodies can be identified frequently at the periphery of the cirrhotic nodules (Fig. 4.74). Variable numbers of acidophilic bodies may be present. Occlusive venous lesions have been described in some cases.[758] The distribution of copper is quite variable, with some of the cirrhotic nodules containing a lot and others containing little or none. The patterns of copper distribution have been described in detail by Stromeyer & Ishak[758] in a series of 34 cases. Copper is rarely demonstrable in Kupffer cells or portal macrophages in the cirrhotic stage, but is frequently encountered in cases of submassive or massive necrosis in patients who present with fulminant liver failure (Figs 4.75 and 4.76). Davies et al[770] also noted the presence of copper in hepatic parenchymal and mononuclear phagocytic cells in 11 cases of Wilson's disease presenting as fulminant hepatic failure.

Ultrastructural findings in the precirrhotic stage of

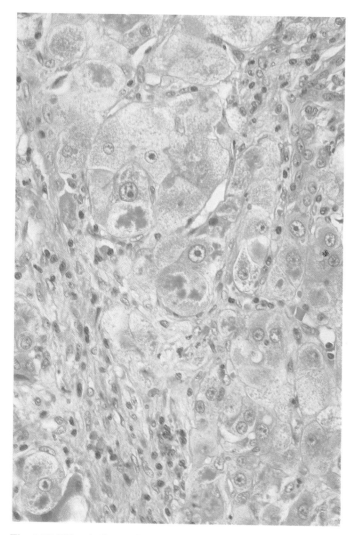

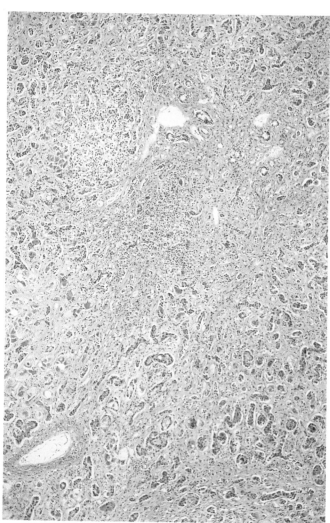

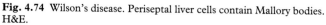

Fig. 4.74 Wilson's disease. Periseptal liver cells contain Mallory bodies. H&E.

Fig. 4.75 Wilson's disease. Massive necrosis. H&E.

Wilson's disease have been described in detail by a number of investigators.[12,742,752] Of these, the mitochondrial changes are the most distinctive and pathogenetically significant; they include heterogeneity of size and shape, increased matrix density, separation of inner from outer membranes, enlarged intercristal spaces and various types of inclusions (Fig. 4.77). In a recent study, Sternlieb[771] described three distinct patterns of structural abnormalities of the mitochondria in hepatocytes of 40 of 42 asymptomatic and 8 of 32 symptomatic patients with Wilson's disease prior to therapy. There was no correlation between the type of abnormality and the patient's age, hepatic copper concentration, degree of hepatic steatosis or the serum aminotransferase levels. There was, however, a high degree of fraternal concordance, indicating that the structural changes are genetically determined. Alterations in Wilson's disease other than those affecting mitochondria include an increase in the number of peroxisomes (which

may appear heterogeneous and denser and larger than normal), lipofuscin granules and multivesicular bodies. Mallory bodies appear as masses of randomly oriented and densely packed fibrils (each about 15 μm in diameter) which are partially rimmed by bundles of finer filaments, but not limited by membranes.[752] Lipolysosomes, which constitute 1–2% of the lipid droplets in hepatocytes in Wilson's disease, may represent a non-specific alternate route for the mobilization of excess lipid from hepatocytes.[772] An ultrastructural study of liver tissue from a family of 9 siblings has demonstrated that this method is not useful in distinguishing the presymptomatic affected person from the homozygous one.[773]

The long-term effects of D-penicillamine therapy on the structure and function of the liver in patients with Wilson's disease were reported by Sternlieb & Feldmann.[774] Liver biopsy specimens from 7 patients, obtained before and after 3–5 years of therapy, were studied by electron

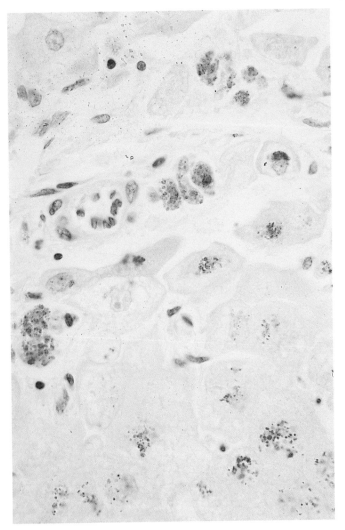

Fig. 4.76 Wilson's disease. Same case as illustrated in Fig. 4.75 showing accumulation of copper in Kupffer cells as well as in liver cells. Rhodanine.

microscopy and stereology. The characteristic mitochondrial abnormalities encountered in the hepatocytes of untreated patients were less pronounced or disappeared after treatment in 5 of the 7 patients. Simultaneously, relative mitochondrial volume, surface density of the external mitochondrial membranes, and the number of these profiles per unit area increased, whereas abnormal elevations of serum aminotransferases returned to normal.

The basic hepatic defect in Wilson's disease remains to be determined. The current treatment of choice is D-penicillamine. Neurological symptoms may worsen before improvement is noted.[775] The rationale for this therapy has been to chelate unbound copper for urinary excretion. It has been assumed that this would result in a decrease in hepatic copper concentration. However, serial liver biopsies in selected patients have shown a stable, or a slightly increased, hepatic copper concentration despite clinical improvement.[776] The possibility exists that a therapeutic

effect is obtained by the induction of metallothionein (demonstrated in rats) which prevents copper toxicity by its preferential binding capacity.[777]

Zinc has been effective both in patients with neurological and/or hepatic manifestations.[778,779] The proposed mechanism of action is to increase both intestinal cell and hepatocyte metallothionein, which acts as a ligand preventing copper absorption as well as its cell toxicity. Compliance can be monitored by urinary zinc levels.[780] Haemofiltration and penicillamine may stabilize moribund patients prior to liver transplantation.[781] Liver transplantation has been successful in patients diagnosed too late for effective medical therapy.[782,783,783a,783b]

MISCELLANEOUS DISORDERS

CHRONIC GRANULOMATOUS DISEASE (CGD)

This disease was originally referred to as pigmented-lipid histiocytosis[784] or fatal granulomatous disease of childhood.[785] It is characterized by recurrent purulent infections caused by bacteria (usually catalase-positive) or fungi. The clinical findings in 168 patients are summarized in Table 4.5 and the usual organisms are listed in Table 4.6.[786] Although hepatic abscesses are the most common gastrointestinal manifestation, the disease can mimic Crohn's disease.[787-794] The white cells can phagocytose bacteria and fungi but are unable to kill them.[795] While the disease usually presents in infancy, milder defects may only be manifested in adulthood; a recent report documented initial presentation in a 69-year-old man.[796] The most common inheritance pattern is X-linked, but an autosomal recessive inheritance has been reported in a substantial number of patients.

The disease results from decreased neutrophil production of oxidants by NADPH and four different defective oxidase peptides. The X-linked variants are all related to the gp 91-phox subunit of cytochrome B which usually results in no detectable level of phagocyte cytochrome B. In contrast, the aforementioned 69-year-old man had normal levels of cytochrome B but markedly reduced NADPH oxidase activity.[796] This was the result of an abnormally spliced gp 91-phox mRNA caused by an A-G substitution which deleted 10 amino acids in the C-terminal portion. Table 4.7 summarizes the most recent classification of chronic granulomatous disease.[797] The most reliable method for prenatal diagnosis is the nitroblue tetrazolium test on cord blood.[786] Treatment in the past has consisted of antibiotics for active disease and prophylactic antibiotics to decrease the incidence of infections. Abscesses often require surgical intervention. Corticosteroids have been used rarely for acute strictures of the gastrointestinal or genitourinary tracts.[798] Bone marrow transplantation has been attempted rarely.[799] The latest beneficial treatment to decrease serious infectious compli-

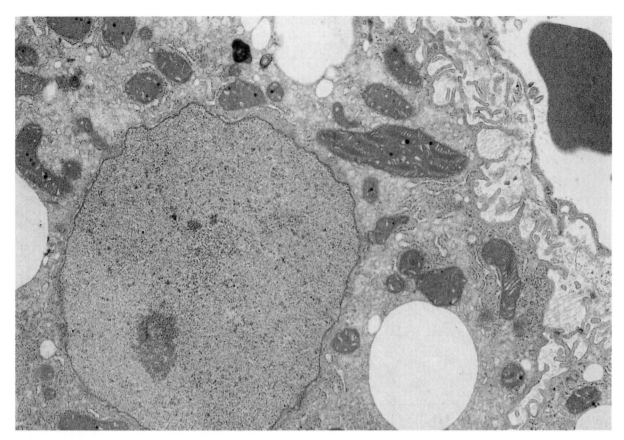

Fig. 4.77 Wilson's disease. Mitochondria show a denser than normal matrix, enlarged and occasionally vacuolated granules, vacuoles with granular contents, crystalline inclusions and separation of the outer from the inner membranes. × 16 275.

Table 4.5 Clinical findings in 168 patients with chronic granulomatous disease (see Forehand et al[786])

Clinical findings	Number of patients
Marked lymphadenopathy	137
Pneumonia	134
Dermatitis	120
Hepatomegaly	114
Onset by 1 year of age	109
Suppuration of nodes	104
Splenomegaly	95
Hepatic/perihepatic abscess	69
Osteomyelitis	54
Onset with dermatitis	42
Onset with lymphadenitis	38
Facial/periorifacial dermatitis	35
Persistent diarrhoea	34
Septicaemia or meningitis	29
Perianal abscess	28
Conjunctivitis	27
Death from pneumonia	26
Persistent rhinitis	26
Ulcerative stomatitis	26

Table 4.6 Major microorganisms in 168 patients with chronic granulomatous disease (see Forehand et al[786])

Microorganism	Number of patients
Staphylococcus aureus	87
Klebsiella-aerobacter	29
Escherichia coli	26
Serratia marcescens	16
Pseudomonas	15
Staphylococcus albus	13
Aspergillus	13
Candida albicans	12
Salmonella	10

cations has been subcutaneous γ-interferon. However, the mechanism of action is unclear since bacterial killing and superoxide production are unaffected.[800]

The characteristic pathological features are the granulo-matous response to infection and the presence of lipo-fuscin pigment in reticuloendothelial cells.[784,785,801,802] The small granulomas consist of rings of mononuclear cells which surround an area of homogeneous eosinophilic material, and are associated with many plasma cells and a few giant cells.[785] Confluent granulomas may show larger areas of necrosis and suppuration (Fig. 4.78). Palisading granulomas with central necrosis and associated giant cells were reported in 4 of 7 cases by Nakhleh et al.[802] Special stains for microorganisms are usually negative, unless the granulomas are caused by fungi.[803] The pigmented histio-cytes have a light tan colour (Fig. 4.79) and are PAS-

Table 4.7 Classification of chronic granulomatous disease (see Smith & Curneitte[797])

Type of disease	Inheritance	CytB spectrum (% normal)	NBT score (% pos)	Intact cell O^2 production (% normal)	Frequency (% of cases)	Activity in cell-free system (% of normal) Membrane	Cytosol
			Defects in membrane located components				
Defects in gp 91-phox							
Absent protein	X	0	0	<1	52	0	100
Non-functioning protein	X	100	0	<1	3	0	1000
Partial deficieny	X	8–15	80–100 (weak)	1–10	2	0.6	100
Kim defect	X	0	60–90 (weak)	1–10	5 cases	0	100
Defects in 22-phox							
Absent protein	AR	0–4	0	<1	5	0	100
Non-functional protein	AR	100	0	<1	1 case	0	100
			Defects in cytosolic components				
Defects in p67-phox							
Absent protein	AR	100	0	<1	33	100	0.2–2.0%
Defects in p67-phox							
Absent protein	AR	100	0	<1	5	100	2–22
			Unclassified cystolic components				
Kim variant	AR	100	85	1–4	1 case	100	0.6

X = X-linked; AR = autosomal recessive; CytB = cytochrome B; NBT = nitroblue tetrazolium

positive, argentaphilic, sudanophilic (in frozen section), and autofluorescent. The accumulation of the pigment is thought to be a secondary phenomenon.[804] In the liver, most of the lipofuscin is found in clusters of markedly hypertrophied portal macrophages of Kupffer cells. Portal areas are infiltrated with plasma cells and lymphocytes and there may be minimal to moderate fibrosis. A hepar lobatum-like cirrhotic process was described by Carson et al[805] in one of their patients. Varying numbers of granulomas and/or microabscesses may be scattered within hepatic acini, and there may be slight to moderate fatty change.

CYSTIC FIBROSIS

Cystic fibrosis (CF), initially described by Andersen in 1938,[806] is inherited as an autosomal recessive trait. The incidence in Caucasian populations approximates 1 in 2000 to 3000.[807] The CF gene is on chromosome 7q31.3–q32. One mutation which involves the deletion of three nucleotides is found in approximately 70% of patients. This mutation causes the omission of a single amino acid, phenylalanine, in position 508 and has been termed F508. The cloned gene is termed the Cystic Fibrosis Transmembrane Conductance Regulator (CFTR),[808-810] and is thought to be intimately associated with the epithelial cell cAMP-dependent chloride channel.[811] Ninety-nine percent of patients homozygous for F508 have severe pancreatic insufficiency.[812] In contrast, 72% of patients heterozygous for F508, and only 36% of patients with other mutations, have severe pancreatic insufficiency. Thus, the genotype correlates with the severity of the pancreatic disease. The CF gene is present in pancreatic duct epithelium but has not so far been demonstrated in bile-duct epithelium. Inhibition of the expression of the wild type CFTR gene in normal, untransvected sweat duct cells results in an inhibition of chloride permeability.[813] An animal model based on gene targeting has recently been created.[814]

Cystic fibrosis is best known for pulmonary and pancreatic disease followed by the gastrointestinal complications, and is least well-known as a cause of chronic liver disease.[815-819] Other manifestations include nasal polyposis, pansinusitis, and non-ketotic insulin-dependent hyperglycaemia.[818] Approximately 50% of CF patients have impaired glucose tolerance.[818] Overt diabetes has been found in 6–10% of CF patients.[819,820] Recent findings suggest that it is secondary to exocrine disease-related islet cell injury. An impaired pancreatic polypeptide response to hypoglycaemia is an excellent marker of exocrine pancreatic function in young adults.[821] Approximately 15% of CF patients do not have exocrine dysfunction but do have pancreatic duct fluid and electrolyte disturbances.

Both the distal intestinal obstruction syndrome[819] and rectal prolapse[822] occur in 20% of patients. Meconium ileus occurs in 5–10% of newborns with CF.[807] Neonatal jaundice is common.[823,824] Other complications include distal intestinal atresia, intrauterine perforation and meconium peritonitis.[815-817] In newborns without intestinal obstruction, intrinsic and extrinsic causes for jaundice have been identified. Idiopathic giant cell hepatitis and cytomegalovirus infection have been reported.[824-826] 'Focal biliary cirrhosis' is present in 25–30% of CF patients, with progression to multinodular cirrhosis in

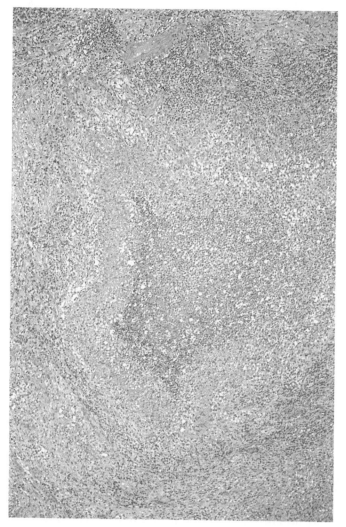

Fig. 4.78 Chronic granulomatous disease. Necrotizing granuloma with purulent material in centre and a serpiginous, palisaded periphery. H&E.

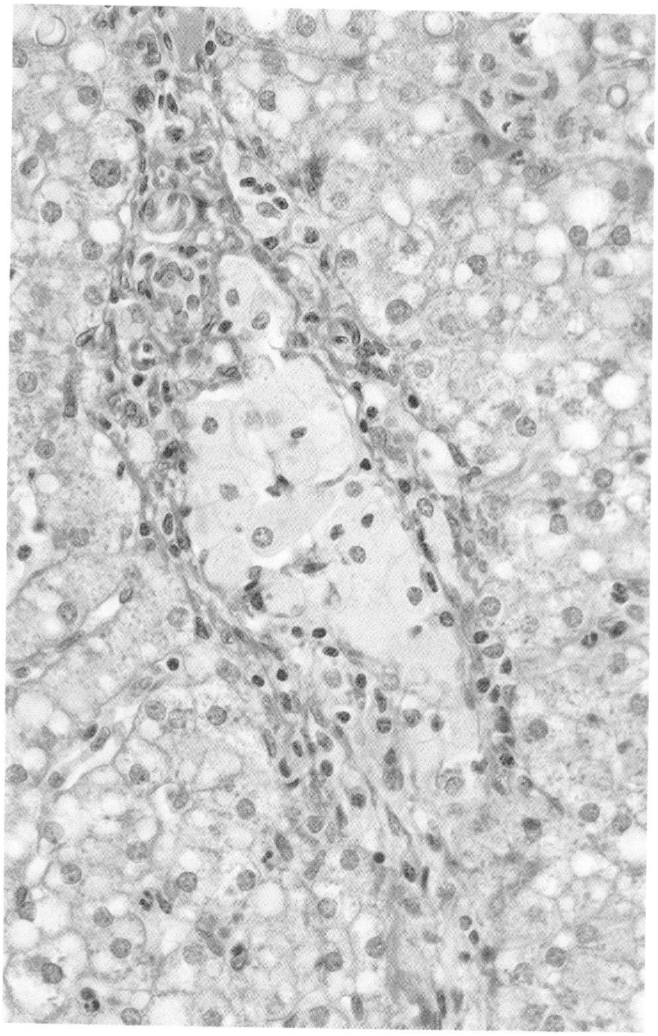

Fig. 4.79 Chronic granulomatous disease. Cluster of hypertrophied, light tan coloured portal macrophages. H&E.

5–10% of cases.[817] Approximately 25% of adults with CF have abnormal liver tests. Endoscopic retrograde cholangiography reveals lesions similar to those of intrahepatic sclerosing cholangitis.[827–829] Partial obstruction of the distal common duct as a consequence of pancreatic fibrosis is certainly seen, but not perhaps with the frequency reported recently.[828–830]

The earliest abnormalities of liver function tests may reflect biliary disease; however, up to 20% of patients with histopathological evidence of liver disease may have normal tests. Pathological abnormalities were detected in about half of the 150 patients reported by Isenberg et al.[831] Cholestasis may be the result of intrahepatic sludge, stones and/or thick bile and mucus in the bile ducts.[832,833]

Cholesterol gallstones are a complication in 8% of patients with cystic fibrosis.[817,831,832,834,835] The risk of developing gallstones increases with age. Lithogenic bile is associated with a contracted bile acid pool.[836] Partial

correction may be achieved by the administration of pancreatic enzymes. Ileal reabsorption of bile salts may be defective.[837] However, the underlying systemic membrane, water and electrolyte defect and inspissation of mucus remain the main pathogenetic mechanisms. A recent study has challenged the above data and concluded that the radiolucent stones are not of the usual cholesterol type.[838]

A report of 29 adults dying after 24 years of age indicates that liver disease is progressive.[839] Four of the patients had shunt operations and 2 developed terminal hepatic encephalopathy. Sclerotherapy has been suggested as an alternative to the various shunting procedures.[826] Thirty-eight percent of non-shunted patients reported by Psacharopoulos et al[826] also had cirrhosis and 72% had focal biliary changes. Two had cardiac cirrhosis while 4 had no changes related to cystic fibrosis.

As a result of increased longevity, a number of complications have come to light in adult patients with cystic fibrosis. They include pancreatitis as the initial presentation,[840] obstructive jaundice due to severe pancreatic fibrosis,[841] intrahepatic bile-duct abnormalities,[828,842] findings consistent with sclerosing cholangitis,[827-829] common bile-duct stenosis,[830] carcinoma of the extrahepatic biliary tree[843] and secondary amyloidosis.[844-846]

Pathological studies of the liver have been reported by several investigators.[847-851] The changes include steatosis, periportal fibrosis with cholangiolar proliferation (with or without inspissation of secretions) (Fig. 4.80), focal biliary fibrosis ('cirrhosis') and multinodular biliary fibrosis ('cirrhosis'). Steatosis is probably the most frequent lesion. It was present in 121 of 198 cases reported by Craig et al.[848] The fat was located most frequently in acinar zone 1, but was distributed throughout the acinus when it was of marked severity. No positive correlations could be made between the presence of fat in the liver and the general nutritional status of the patient.

An incidental finding in infant livers in CF is the deposition of haemosiderin in the parenchymal cells.[851] The pigment accumulation is heaviest in periportal liver cells.[852] This finding is presumably related to the increased iron transport from the gut in pancreatic insufficiency.[853]

The characteristic if not pathognomonic lesion in the liver is focal biliary fibrosis, originally described by Bodian,[847] who found it in 25% of his series of 62 patients. The incidence in the series of de Sant'Agnese et al[849] was 22%, while a third of the patients reported by Isenberg et al[831] had the lesion. Oppenheimer & Esterly[851] found an increasing frequency with duration of survival. Thus, it was found at post-mortem examination in 10.6% of infants younger than 3 months, in 15.6% of infants from 3–12 months, and in 26.9% of children older than 1 year.

Macroscopically, the liver with focal biliary fibrosis shows multiple, depressed, greyish-white scars that are triangular or stellate in shape.[848,849] Microscopically, there is variable cholangiolar proliferation and periportal fibrosis (Fig. 4.80). The cholangioles are generally dilated and show varying degrees of atrophy of the lining cells (Figs 4.81 and 4.82). The lumen is filled by pink to light orange rounded masses (concretions) or amorphous material (Fig. 4.82). The inspissated secretion in the cholangioles stains intensely with PAS and resists diastase digestion; it does not stain positively with mucicarmine or Alcian blue, but there may be some mucin in the interacinar bile ducts. Some greatly dilated cholangioles eventually rupture with extrusion of their contents and induction of an acute inflammatory response.[849] The cholangitis is thus 'chemical' but it may be complicated by bacterial infection.[854] Chronic inflammatory cells may also be present in the fibrous tissue. It is important to emphasize that periportal fibrosis may occur in the absence of cholangiolar proliferation and inspissation of secretions.[848,850] In the series of Oppenheimer & Esterly,[851] this non-specific change was only found in infants less than 3 months of age.

With the passage of time the focal biliary lesions may coalesce, with extension of fibrosis, atrophy of the intervening parenchyma and entrapment and encirclement of groups of hepatic acini.[849] This type of lesion, referred to as 'multilobular biliary cirrhosis with concretions' or 'multilobular cirrhosis', occurs in 6% of patients who are over 1 year of age.[850] Large irregular nodules are produced and the deep clefts between the nodules may impart to the liver the appearance of hepar lobatum.[849]

In addition to the presence of excessive mucus in extrahepatic bile ducts in occasional patients, there may be excessive mucus accumulation in intrahepatic bile ducts, particularly those adjacent to the porta hepatis.[850] This change occurs in 23.4% of infants under 3 months of age and in 12.5% of patients from 3–12 months of age. In the series of Oppenheimer & Esterly[851] more than two-thirds of the patients who were less than 3 months of age and with ductal mucus had histological cholestasis, often with a history of jaundice. The gallbladder in up to 30% of

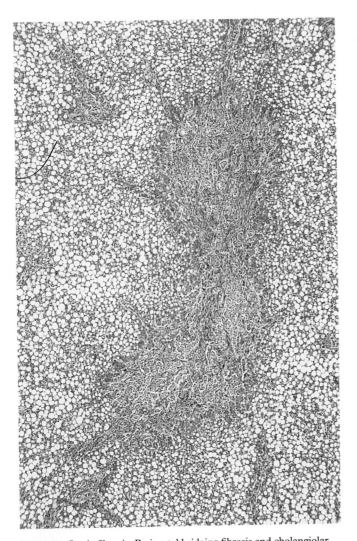

Fig. 4.80 Cystic fibrosis. Periportal bridging fibrosis and cholangiolar proliferation. Note marked steatosis. Masson's trichrome.

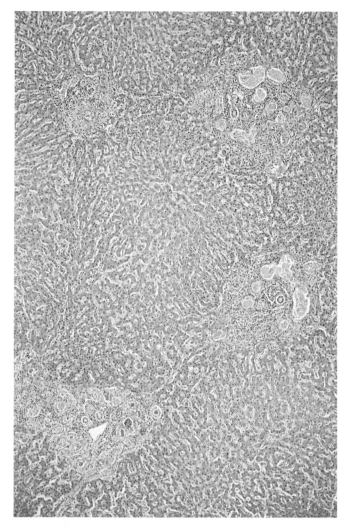

Fig. 4.81 Cystic fibrosis. Portal areas are expanded and there is cholangiolar proliferation and moderate portal inflammation. Many of the cholangioles are dilated and contain a pink secretion. H&E.

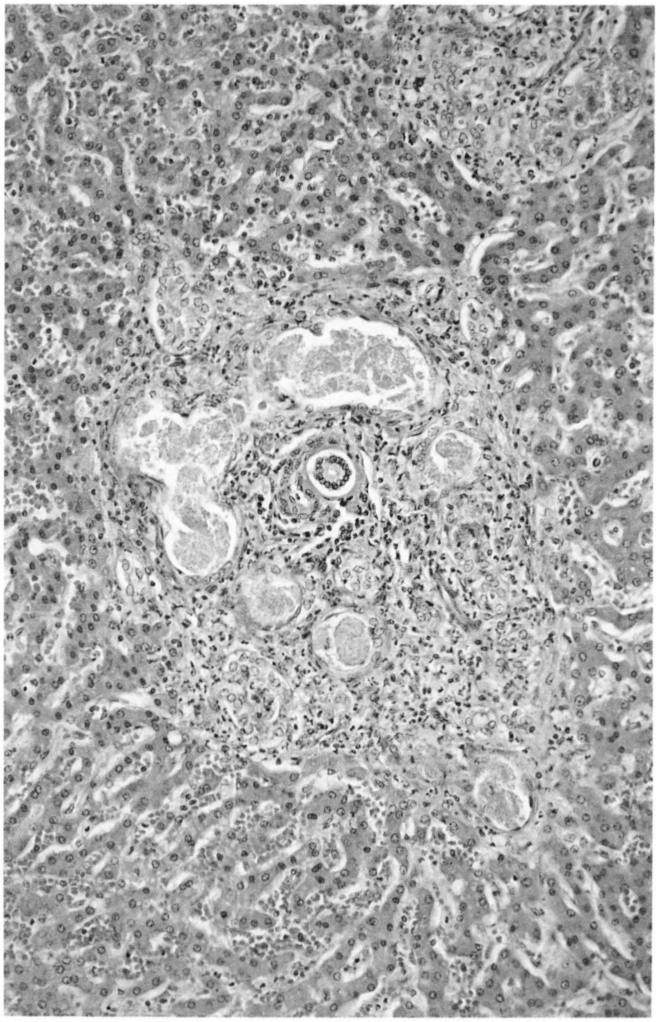

Fig. 4.82 Cystic fibrosis. Dilated cholangioles contain an amorphous, pink secretion. Note absence of lining cells. H&E.

patients is hypoplastic, and contains mucoid material and a small amount of viscid bile. Mucous cysts are seen in the wall and stones may be present in the lumen.[855]

Liver biopsy material from 11 patients with cystic fibrosis was examined ultrastructurally by Arends et al.[856] A finding unique to this disease was the presence of filamentous material, with an average diameter of 15 nm, in the lumen of bile ductules and ducts. Bile granules were scattered between the filaments. A reaction product of carbohydrates was found in the filaments by histochemical techniques. It was suggested that the typical mucus deposits in bile ducts are built up from these filaments. Similar ultrastructural findings have been observed by Dominick,[854] Bradford et al[857] and Phillips et al.[12] Bile-duct cells with irregular shapes, protruding into the lumen, and necrosis of cells have been observed.[842] Bradford et al[857] studied the ultrastructure of liver cells in detail and described the presence of membrane-bound deposits of

electronlucent material containing electron-dense cores that resembled mucus. An increase in the number of perisinusoidal cells around portal areas, with deposition of collagen around bile ducts and ductules, has been noted.[842,858]

The gold standard for the diagnosis of CF remains the pilocarpine iontophoresis sweat test. Accuracy requires 50 mg of sweat and not testing newborns in the first 2 days of life. Levels of sweat chloride over 60 mmol/l in children and 80 in adults are abnormal. Other diseases which rarely are seen with this elevation are listed by Boat et al.[807] Rarely, patients with CF have been documented in the 40–60 mmol/l range or even lower.[822] In such patients, abnormal bioelectric potential and the presence of eosinophilic concretions on biopsy can confirm the diagnosis.[859,860] Newborn screening tests have been advocated for many years and have been funded both in the past and present, but they clearly do not fulfill the economic criterion that present therapy can alter the course of the disease. One such test is measurement of immunoreactive trypsinogen on dried blood spots.[861,862] Only 6.1% of infants with a positive first test are ultimately found to have abnormal sweat chlorides. This assay may detect 85% of CF patients but only 42% of patients with meconium ileus. Thus, its accuracy resembles the cumbersome intraluminal pancreatic insufficiency testing. DNA testing is not diagnostic since all the mutations are not known, but certainly can be utilized if both parent phenotypes are known. Monitoring patients for hepatobiliary complications can best be accomplished by the use of ultrasound with doppler. Other liver diseases such as α_1-AT deficiency and vitamin A toxicity need to be considered in the differential diagnosis of CF.

Supportive therapy (antibiotics, pancreatic enzymes, provision of adequate nutrition and physiotherapy) has extended the life expectancy into adulthood. Bile acid and accompanying taurine deficiency have been documented in CF.[863,864] Taurine supplementation may improve fat digestion and absorption[865,866] by making the circulating bile acid pool more hydrophilic.[867] When taurine was combined with ursodeoxycholic acid in 10–15 mg/kg doses, improvement of liver function tests was noted.[868]

Clinical studies have been initiated with a combination of aerosolized amiloride and UTP or nucleotide analogues as therapeutic agents to correct the sodium and chloride defect in the lungs.[869] This is a potential route for gene therapy in the future. Heart–lung transplantation corrects the abnormal bioelectric potential.[870] Donor shortage makes it unlikely that this procedure will benefit many patients. Liver transplantation for CF is successful if a Roux-en-Y anastomosis is performed to prevent recurrent biliary problems;[871] criteria need to be established for this procedure. N-acetylcysteine (2%) infused into the biliary tree has relieved the obstruction by the thick inspissated bile.[872]

SHWACHMAN'S SYNDROME

Shwachman's syndrome is the second most common form of inherited pancreatic insufficiency in childhood. Over 100 cases have been reported.[873] The inheritance is autosomal recessive. Symptoms of malabsorption are secondary to the pancreatic insufficiency. The follow-up studies of Hill et al[874] have shown that most patients ultimately absorb fat normally, possibly because of a marginal increase in pancreatic lipase secretion. Stunting of growth after pancreatic enzyme replacement and/or medium chain triglycerides in the diet is related to metaphyseal dysostosis. Susceptibility to pulmonary and systemic infections is caused by neutropenia. Eczema occurs in 50% of patients.

Patients with Shwachman's syndrome present with failure to thrive. The finding of normal sweat chloride levels distinguishes them from patients with cystic fibrosis.

The pancreozymin-secretin test shows reduced enzyme and bicarbonate concentrations but, in contrast to cystic fibrosis, normal volume secretion. Neutropenia may be inconsistent, cyclic or constant, being somewhat dependent on the age of the patient and the development of bone marrow hypoplasia. In some patients, granulopoiesis is normal in vitro, whereas in others there appears to be a defect at stem cell level.[875] Anaemia, thrombocytopenia and, rarely, immunoglobulin deficiency may subsequently develop.[876,877] Several cases of leukaemia have been reported.[878] Hepatic dysfunction is rare.[879,880] Death results from pulmonary or systemic bacterial infections.[881,882]

The pancreas in Shwachman's syndrome shows replacement of exocrine tissue by fat.[879,883] According to Burke et al,[884] the degeneration of pancreatic exocrine tissue is progressive. Cardiomegaly and testicular fibrosis were reported in one case.[885] The liver shows variable steatosis.[879,883] Some of the patients in the series of Bodian et al[879] also had portal fibrosis or 'cirrhosis', but detailed histological descriptions of the hepatic changes were not reported.

ALPERS' DISEASE

Synonyms for this disease include 'familial progressive poliodystrophy with cirrhosis of the liver', and 'infantile diffuse cerebral degeneration with hepatic cirrhosis'.[886–890] The onset of the neurological disorder is between 1 and 3 years of age; none of the affected children survive beyond 3 years. There are characteristic EEG changes, progressive brain atrophy on CT scan, absent or reduced visual evoked responses, hepatomegaly and abnormal liver tests.[888,890] Liver disease in the series of Narkewicz et al[890] was noted at a mean age of 35 months; death in liver failure occurred within a mean interval of 4–6 weeks. The inheritance is autosomal recessive.

Early morphological changes include acinar disarray, microvesicular steatosis, unicellular necrosis and portal/periportal acute and chronic inflammation.[890] Later changes are characterized by massive microvesicular steatosis, submassive to massive necrosis, ductular proliferation and fibrous scarring.[888,890]

AARSKOG'S SYNDROME

The salient features of this 'faciodigitogenital syndrome' include shortness of stature and facial, digital and genital malformations.[891–893] More than 100 cases have been reported.[893]

The inheritance is thought to be X-linked recessive. The gene has been mapped to Xq13. One reported case had a slightly elevated total serum bilirubin and needle biopsy of the liver revealed haemosiderosis and a micronodular cirrhosis.[892]

CONGENITAL TOTAL LIPODYSTROPHY

This disease is characterized by total absence of adipose tissue, insulin-resistant diabetes mellitus, hyperlipidaemia, hepatosplenomegaly, muscular hypertrophy, hypertrichosis, and acanthosis nigricans. Inheritance is believed to be autosomal recessive.

The liver is enlarged and grossly yellow or light yellow-brown in colour. Light microscopic changes in the liver have been described in a number of case reports.[894–900] They include steatosis and periportal fibrosis, with portal to portal bridging. Ductular proliferation was described in several cases.[897] Cirrhosis is present in some patients.[896,898,899] Hepatocytes in one case were described as 'plant-like' with prominent cell walls, a pale vacuolated cytoplasm and pale, centrally placed nuclei; the presence of fat and glycogen was demonstrated in the cytoplasm of liver cells by special stains.

Ultrastructural abnormalities have been described in several reports.[12,899,901] In addition to numerous lipid droplets, there are many lysosomes containing variable quantities of lipofuscin and lipolysosomes.[12] Peroxisomes are said to be increased[847,849] or reduced in number[11] and they contain dense matrix granules. Mitochondria are misshapen and, according to Phillips et al,[12] contain distinctive, elongated, crystal-like matrical inclusions that adopt various geometric configurations. They possibly represent cholesterol or other lipid material. Klar et al[899] described partial lysis of swollen and irregular mitochondria in a case.

FAMILIAL HEPATOSTEATOSIS

This disorder is characterized by jaundice, kernicterus, fatty change of the liver (as well as other organs and viscera) and death in the neonatal period.[902–906] Since all affected patients have been males, a sex-linked inheritance has been suggested.[905] The liver shows fatty change in all acinar zones, mainly in the form of large vacuoles which displace the nuclei. Chemical analysis in one case demonstrated a striking increase in the concentration of total lipids and fatty acids.[905] In addition to hepatosteatosis, Suprun & Freundlich[906] described steatosis of the myocardium and kidney in 3 siblings. The biochemical defect has not been determined, and it is not certain that all reported cases represent a single entity. It is worth noting that steatosis and steatohepatitis, with or without fibrosis or cirrhosis, can occur in obese and/or diabetic children.[907–909] Recently, hepatosteatosis was reported in a child with the immotile cilia syndrome.[910]

LEPRECHAUNISM (DONOHUE'S SYNDROME)

This is a rare disorder characterized by a grotesque elfin facies (with a flat nasal bridge and flaring nostrils, thick lips, and large, low set ears), hirsutism, enlargement of the breasts and external genitalia, motor and mental retardation, failure to thrive, progressive marasmus and death before 2 years of age.[911–920] Liver function tests were reported as normal in some patients.[913,914,917] The condition is inherited as an autosomal recessive trait. It is due to mutations in the insulin receptor gene.[921]

A consistent pathological feature of the syndrome in females is follicular maturation of the ovaries with cyst formation. Some patients have hyperplasia of the islets of Langerhans and severe malformations of the brain and heart. Other associated findings have been reviewed by Rosenberg et al.[919] The liver has been reported to be histologically normal in some patients,[912,917] or to show non-specific changes such as an increased glycogen content,[912,913] mild fatty change[913] or haemosiderosis.[915,916] Haemosiderosis, both hepatocellular and reticuloendothelial, was also present in the cases reported by Donohue & Uchida[911] and Ordway & Stout,[918] in combination with other changes. Both these reports described multiple small nodules in the liver that were composed of large pale foamy hepatocytes containing a large quantity of glycogen and a little fat, with occasional fusion of cells and formation of syncytial masses. Ordway & Stout[918] interpreted these foci as regenerating nodules. An example is illustrated in Figures 4.83 and 4.84. Intrahepatic cholestasis has been reported in several cases[919] and bile-duct proliferation in one.[918]

Patients with leprechaunism have become the subjects of investigations to study insulin resistance and exemplify multiple defects in the insulin receptor. Insulin binds to the alpha subunit of its receptor and activates tyrosine kinase intrinsic to the beta subunit of this receptor which results in autophosphorylation. The exact mechanisms of

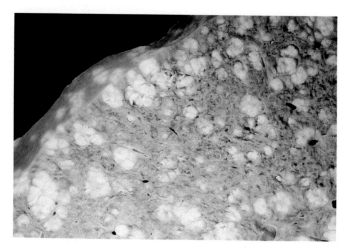

Fig. 4.83 Leprechaunism. This section of liver is green and studded with pale, white nodules of varied size.

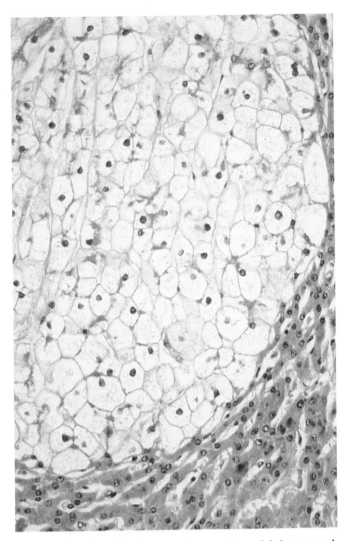

Fig. 4.84 Leprechaunism. Segment of regenerative nodule is composed of large, empty hepatocytes. A PAS-stained section (not shown) confirmed the presence of glycogen in these cells. H&E.

these actions are not clear, and multiple gene defects are being found in this disorder that are associated with insulin binding abnormalities in the liver, lymphocytes and fibroblasts.[922] Those reported include substitution of glutamic acid for lysine at position 460 in the alpha subunit, premature chain termination after amino acid 671 in the alpha subunit[923] and a leucine to proline mutation at position 233 of the alpha subunit.[924]

ALBINISM

Two general forms are recognized—oculocutaneous albinism and ocular albinism. Ten types of oculocutaneous albinism are known, of which two—Hermansky–Pudlak syndrome and Chediak–Higashi syndrome—can involve the liver.

Hermansky–Pudlak syndrome

This autosomal recessive disorder is characterized by oculocutaneous albinism, a mile bleeding diathesis due to a storage pool platelet defect, and widespread deposition of ceroid pigment in cells of the reticuloendothelial system.[925-927] Complications of the syndrome include pulmonary fibrosis, renal failure, cardiomyopathy and granulomatous colitis.

Involvement of the liver in this syndrome is limited to the presence of a light tan, granular pigment in hypertrophied Kupffer cells and portal macrophages (Fig. 4.85). The pigment has all the characteristics of ceroid or lipofuscin, being PAS-positive and diastase-resistant, sudanophilic and argentaphilic, and it reveals bright yellow autofluorescence when viewed by ultraviolet microscopy (Fig. 4.86). Ultrastructurally, the pigment is granular, intermingled with lipid and bounded by a single

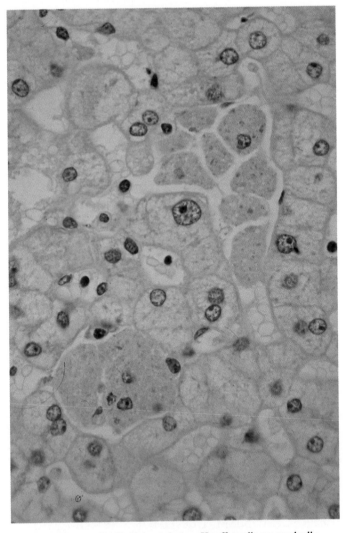

Fig. 4.85 Hermansky–Pudlak syndrome. Kupffer cells are markedly hypertrophied and contain a light tan pigment. H&E.

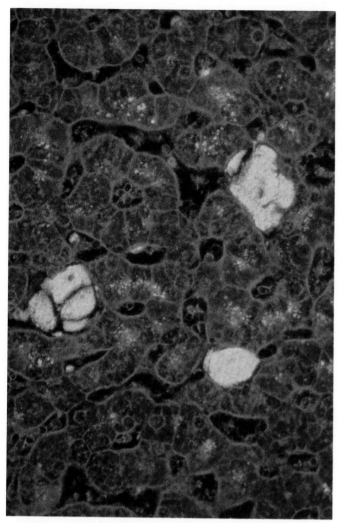

Fig. 4.86 Hermansky–Pudlak syndrome. Pigment in Kupffer cells displays bright yellow autofluorescence. Unstained section, examined under ultraviolet light.

membrane. Occasionally, it shows a finger-print pattern of concentric light and dark bands which have a periodicity of approximately 20 nm.[927]

Chediak–Higashi syndrome

Chediak–Higashi syndrome is an autosomal recessive disorder involving lysosomes throughout the body. Symptoms, which appear in early childhood, are related to partial oculocutaneous albinism that is secondary to fusion of melanocytic granules, and to recurrent infections. Subsequent difficulties include peripheral neuropathies, haemorrhages, and malignant lymphomas in patients who survive the early infections.[928,929] Cases are recognized by the presence of giant cytoplasmic granulations (lysosomes) in their leucocytes. Hepatosplenomegaly is present in all patients.

Ultrastructually, abnormal inclusions are found in circulating leucocytes,[930] as well as in hepatocytes and Kupffer cells.[931,932] The inclusions are bounded by a unit membrane and contain electron-dense spherical structures of various sizes.[932] A lymphohistiocytic portal/periportal infiltrate has been reported.[932,933]

REFERENCES

1. Watts R W S, Morgan S H, Dampure C J et al. Combined hepatic and renal transplantation in primary hyperoxaluria type I: Clinical report of nine cases. Am J Med 1991; 90: 179–188
2. Sternlieb I. Wilson's disease: Indications for liver transplants. Hepatology 1984; 4: 155–175
3. Yokoi T, Honke K, Funabashi T et al. Partial ornithine transcarbamylase deficiency simulating Reye syndrome. J Pediatr 1981; 99: 929–931
4. Roe C R, Mullington D S, Maltby D A, Kinnebrew P. Recognition of medium-chain acyl-CoA dehydrogenase deficiency in asymptomatic siblings of children dying of sudden infant death or Reye-like syndrome. J Pediatr 1986; 108: 13–18
5. Scriver C R, Beaudet A L, Sly W S, Valle D, eds. The metabolic basis of inherited disease, 6th edn. New York: McGraw-Hill, 1989
6. Tuchman M, Sharp H L. An approach to the diagnosis and management of inherited metabolic liver disorders. In: Lebinthal E ed. Textbook of gastroenterology and nutrition in infancy, 2nd edn. 1988: New York: Raven Press, 1989: pp 969–1003
7. Sharp H L. Approach to the child with metabolic liver disease. In: Suchy F J, ed. Textbook of liver disease in children. St. Louis Mosby Yearbook; (in press)
8. Ishak K G. Hepatic morphology in the inherited metabolic diseases. Semin Liver Dis 1986; 6: 246–258
9. Callea F, Brisigotti, Faa G, Lucine L, Eriksson S. Identification of PiZ gene products in liver tissue by a monoclonal antibody specific for the Z mutant of α-1-antitrypsin. J Hepatol 1991; 12: 372–276
10. Tanikawa K. Ultrastructural aspects of the liver and its disorders, 2nd edn., Tokyo: Igaku-Shoin, 1979
11. Spycher M A. Electron microscopy: A method for the diagnosis of inherited metabolic storage diseases. Electron microscopy in diagnosis. Pathol Res Pract 1980; 167: 118–135
12. Phillips M J, Poucell S, Patterson J, Valencia P. The liver. An atlas and text of ultrastructural pathology. New York: Raven Press, 1987
13. Ishak K G. Pathology of inherited metabolic disorders. In: Balistreri W F, Stocker J T, eds. Pediatric hepatology. New York: Hemisphere Publishing, 1990; pp 77–181
14. Bloomer J R. The hepatic porphyrias. Pathogenesis, manifestations, and management. Gastroenterology 1976; 71: 689–701
15. Kappas A, Sassa S, Galbraith R A, Nordmann Y. The porphyrias. In: Scriver C R, Beaudet A L, Sly W S, Valle D, eds. The metabolic basis of inherited disease, 6th edn. New York, McGraw-Hill, 1989; pp 1305–1365
16. Rank J M, Straka J G, Bloomer J R. Liver in disorders of porphyrin metabolism. J Gastroenterol Hepatol 1990; 5: 573–585
17. Bonkovsky H L. Porphyrin and heme metabolism and the porphyrias. In: Zakim D, Boyer T D, eds. Hepatology. A textbook of liver disease, 2nd edn. Philadelphia. Saunders, 1990: pp 378–424
18. Cripps D J. Diet and alcohol effects on the manifestations of hepatic porphyrias. Fed Proc 1987; 5: 1894–1900
19. Biempica L, Kosower N, Ma H H, Goldfischer S. Hepatic porphyrias. Cytochemical and ultrastructural studies of liver in acute intermittent porphyria and porphyria cutanea tarda. Arch Pathol 1974; 98: 336–343
20. Jean G, Lambertenghi G, Ranzi T. Ultrastructural study in hepatic porphyria. J Clin Pathol 1968; 21: 501–507
21. Everback L, Lundvall O. Properties and distribution of liver fluorescence in porphyria cutanea tarda (PCT). Virchows Arch (A) 1970; 350: 293–302

22. Waldo E D, Tobias H. Needle-like cytoplasmic inclusions in the liver in porphyria cutanea tarda. Arch Pathol 1973; 96: 368–371

23. Cortes J M, Oliva H, Paradinas F J, Hernandez-Guio C. The pathology of the liver in porphyria cutanea tarda. Histopathology 1980; 4: 471–485

24 Fakan F, Chlumska A. Demonstration of needle-shaped hepatic inclusions in porphyria cutanea tarda using the ferric ferricyanide reduction test. Virchows Arch A 1987; 411: 365–368

25. Siersema P D, Van Helvoirt R P, Ketelaars D A M et al. Iron and uroporphyrin in hepatocytes of inbred mice in experimental porphyria: a biochemical and morphological study. Hepatology 1991; 14: 1179–1188

26. Lefkowitch J H, Grossman M E. Hepatic pathology in porphyria cutanea tarda. Liver 1983; 3: 19–29

27. Campo E, Bruguera M, Rodes J. Are there diagnostic histologic features of porphyria cutanea tarda in liver biopsy specimens? Liver 1990; 10: 185–190

28. Turnbull A, Baker H, Vernon-Roberts B, Magnus I A. Iron metabolism in porphyria cutanea tarda and in erythropoietic protoporphyria. Q J Med, New Series 1973; 42: 341–355

29. Salata H, Cortes J M, de Salamanca R E et al. Porphyria cutanea tarda and hepatocellular carcinoma. Frequency of occurrence and related factors. J Hepatol 1985; 1: 477–487

30. Siersema P D, Kate F J W, Mulder P G H, Wilson J H P. Hepatocellular carcinoma in porphyria cutanea tarda: frequency and factors related to its occurrence. Liver 1992; 12: 56–61

31. Lithner F, Wetlerberg L. Hepatocellular carcinoma with acute intermittent porphyria. Acta Med Scand 1984; 215: 271–274

32. Hardell L, Bengtsson N O, Jonsson U, Eriksson S, Larsson L G. Aetiological aspects on primary liver cancer with special regard to alcohol, organic solvents and acute intermittent porphyria—an epidemiological investigation. Br J Cancer 1984; 50: 389–397

33. Kauppinen R, Mustajoki P. Acute hepatic porphyria and hepatocellular carcinoma. Br J Cancer 1988; 57: 117–120

34. Tidman M J, Higgins E M, Elder G H, Macdonald D M. Variegate porphyria associated with hepatocellular carcinoma. Br J Dermatol 1989; 121: 503–505

35. Kushner J P, Edwards C A, Dadone M M, Skolnick M H. Heterozygosity for HLA-linked hemochromatosis as a likely cause of the hepatic siderosis associated with sporadic porphyria cutanea tarda. Gastroenterology 1985; 88: 1232–1238

36. Fargion S, Piperno A, Capellini M D et al. Hepatitis C virus and porphyria cutanea tarda: evidence of a strong association. Hepatology 1992; 16: 1322–1326

37. Valls V, de Salamanca R E, Lapena L et al. Hepatitis B serum markers in porphyria cutanea tarda. J Dermatol 1986; 15: 24–29

38. Rocchi E, Gibertini P, Cassanelli M, Pietrangelo A, Jensen J, Ventura E. Hepatitis B virus infection in porphyria cutanea tarda. Liver 1986; 6: 153–157

39. Herrero C, Vicente A, Bruguera M et al. Is hepatitis C virus infection a trigger of porphyria cutanea tarda. Lancet 1993; 341: 288–289

40. Wissel P S, Sordillo P, Anderson K E, Sassa S, Savillo R L, Kappas A. Porphyria cutanea tarda associated with the acquired immune deficiency syndrome. Am J Hematol 1987; 25: 107–113

41. Lobato M N, Berger T G Porphyria cutanea tarda associated with the acquired immunodeficiency syndrome. Arch Dermatol 1988; 124: 1009–1010

42. Boisseau A-M, Couzigou P, Forestier J-F et al. Porphyria cutanea tarda associated with human immunodeficiency virus infection. Dermatologica 1991; 182: 155–159

43. Cripps D J, Scheuer P J. Hepatobiliary changes in erythropoietic protoporphyria. Arch Pathol 1965; 80: 500–508

44. Bloomer J R, Enriquez R. Evidence that hepatic crystalline deposits in a patient with protoporphyria are composed of protoporphyrin. Gastroenterology 1982; 82: 569–572

45 Klatskin G, Bloomer J R. Birefringence of hepatic pigment deposits in erythrohepatic protoporphyria. Gastroenterology 1974; 67: 294–302

46. Matilla A, Molland E A. A light and electron microscopic study of the liver in case of erythrohepatic protoporphyria and in griseofulvin-induced porphyria in mice. J Clin Pathol 1974; 27: 698–709

47. Bloomer J R, Phillips M J, Davidson D L, Klatskin G. Hepatic disease in erythropoietic protoporphyria. Am J Med 1975; 58: 869–882

48. Wolff K, Wolff-Schreiner E, Gschnait F. Liver inclusions in erythropoietic protoporphyria. Eur J Clin Invest 1975; 5: 21–26

49. Bruguera M, Esquerada J E, Mascaro J M, Pinol J. Erythropoietic protoporphyria. A light and electron microscopical study of the liver in three patients. Arch Pathol Lab Med 1976; 100: 587–589

50. Rademakers L H P M, Cleton M I, Kooijman C, de la Faille H B, Van Hattum J. Early involvement of hepatic parenchymal cells in erythrohepatic protoporphyria? An ultrastructural study of patients with and without overt liver disease and the effect of chenodeoxycholic acid treatment. Hepatology 1990; 11: 449–457

51. Nakanuma Y, Wada M, Kono N, Miyamura H, Ohta G. An autopsy case of erythropoietic protoporphyria with cholestatic jaundice and hepatic failure, and a review of the literature. Virchows Arch Pathol Anat 1981; 393: 123–132

52. Bloomer J R. Protoporphyria. Semin Liver Dis 1982; 2: 143–153

53. Bonkovsky H L, Schned A R. Fatal liver failure in protoporphyria. Synergism between ethanol excess and the genetic defect. Gastroenterology 1986; 90: 191–201

54. Wagner S, Doss M O, Wittekind C, Backer U, Meassen D, Schmidt F W. Erythrohepatische Protoporphyrie mit rasch progredienter Leberzirrhose. Dtsch Med Wschr 1989; 114: 1837–1841

55. Cripps D J, Gilbert L A, Goldfarb S S. Erythropoietic protoporphyria. Juvenile protoporphyrin hepatopathy, cirrhosis and death. J Pediatr 1977; 91: 744–748

56. Singer J A, Plant A G, Kaplan M M. Hepatic failure and death from erythropoietic protoporphyria. Gastroenterology 1978; 74: 588–591

57. DeLeo V A, Mathews-Roth M, Harber L C. Erythropoietic protoporphyria. 10 years experience. Am J Med 1976; 60: 8–22

58. Poh-Fitzpatrick M B, Whitlock R T, Lefkowitch J H. Changes in protoporphyrin distribution dynamics during liver failure and recovery in a patient with protoporphyria and Epstein-Barr viral hepatitis. Am J Med 1986; 80: 943–950

59. Lee R G, Avner D L, Berenson M M. Structure-function relationship of protoporphyrin-induced liver injury. Arch Pathol Lab Med 1984; 108: 744–746

60. Thompson R P H, Molland E A, Nicholson D A, Gray C H. Erythropoietic protoporphyria and cirrhosis in sisters. Gut 1973; 14: 934–938

61. Graham-Brown R A C, Scheuer P J, Sarkany I. Histiocytosis X and erythropoietic protoporphyria. J Roy Soc Med 1984; 77: 238–240

62 Huijing F, Fernandes J. X-chromosomal inheritance of liver glycogenosis with phosphorylase kinase deficiency. Am J Hum Genet 1969; 21: 275–284

63. Keating J P, Brown B I, White N H, DiMauro S. X-linked glycogen storage disease: a cause of hypotonia, hyperuricemia, and growth retardation. Am J Dis Child 1985; 139: 609–613

64. Moses S W. Pathophysiology and dietary treatment of glycogen storage diseases. J Pediatr Gastroenterol Nutr 1985; II: 155–174

65. Ryman B E. The glycogen storage diseases. J Clin Pathol 1975; 28: 106–121

66. Cori G T, Cori D F. Glucose-6-phosphatase of the liver in glycogen storage disease. J Biol Chem 1952; 199: 661–667

67. Dunger D B, Leonard J V, Preece M A. Patterns of growth in hepatic glycogenoses. Arch Dis Child 1984; 59: 657–660

68. Wakid N W, Bitar J G, Allan C K. Glycogen storage disease type I: laboratory data and diagnosis. Clin Chem 1987; 33: 2008–2010

69. Zangeneh F, Livibrick G A, Brown B I et al. Hepatorenal glycogenosis (Type I glycogenosis) and carcinoma of the liver. J Pediatr 1968; 74: 773–783

70. Howell R R, Stevenson R E, Ben-Menachem Y. Hepatic adenomata with type I glycogen storage disease. JAMA 1976; 236: 1481–1484

71. Greene H L, Wilson F A, Hefferan P et al. ATP depletion, a possible role in the pathogenesis of hyperuricemia in glycogen storage disease type I. J Clin Invest 1978; 62: 321–328

72. Miller J H, Gates G F, Landing B H et al. Scintigraphic

abnormalities in glycogen storage disease. J Nucl Med 1978; 19: 354–358

73. Grossman H, Ram P C, Coleman R A et al. Hepatic ultrasonography in type I glycogen storage disease (von Gierke disease): Detection of hepatic adenoma and carcinoma. Radiology 1981; 141: 753–756

74. Cohen J L, Vinik A, Faller J, Fox I H. Hyperuricemia in glycogen storage disease type I: contributions by hypoglycemia and hyperglucagonemia to increased urate production. J Clin Invest 1985; 75: 251–257

75. Fink A S, Appleman H D, Thompson N W. Hemorrhage into a hepatic adenoma and type Ia glycogen storage disease: a case report and review of the literature. Surgery 1985; 97: 117–124

76. Coire C F, Qizilbash A H, Castelli M F. Hepatic adenomata in type Ia glycogen storage disease. Arch Pathol Lab Med 1987; 111: 166–169

77. Baker L, Dahlen S, Goldfarb S et al. Hyperfiltration and renal disease in glycogen storage disease type I. Kidney Internat 1989; 35: 1345–1350

78. Poe R, Snover D C. Adenomas in glycogen storage disease type I: Two cases with unusual histological features. Am J Surg Pathol 1988; 12: 477–483

79. Smit G P A, Fernandes J, Leonard J V et al. The long-term outcome of patients with glycogen storage diseases. J Inherit Dis 1990; 13: 411–418

80. Conti J A, Kemeny N. Type Ia glycogenosis associated with hepatocellular carcinoma. Cancer 1992; 69: 1320–1322

81. Bialek D S, Sharp H L, Kane W J, Elders J, Nordlie R C. Latency of glucose-6-phosphatase in Type 1B glycogen storage disease. J Pediatr 1977; 91: 838

82. Narisawa K, Igarashi Y, Otomo H, Tada K. A new variant of glycogen storage disease type 1 probably due to a defect in the glucose-6-phosphate transport system. Biochem Biophys Res Commun 1978; 83: 1360–1364

83. Lange A L, Arion W J, Beaudet A L. Type 1B glycogen storage disease is caused by a defect in the glucose-6-phosphate translocase of the microsomal glucose-6-phosphatase system. J Biol Chem 1980; 155: 8381–8384

84. Kuzuya T, Matsuda A, Yoshida S et al. An adult case of type Ib glycogen-storage disease: enzymatic and histochemical studies. N Engl J Med 1983; 308: 566–569

85. Ambruso D R, McCabe E R B, Anderson D et al. Infectious and bleeding complications in patients with glycogenosis Ib. Am J Dis Child 1985; 139: 691–697

86. Roe T F, Thomas D W, Gilsanz V, Isaacs A, Atkinson J B. Inflammatory bowel disease in glycogen storage disease Ib. J Pediatr 1986; 109: 55–59

87. Sanderson I R, Bisset W M, Milla P J, Leonard J V. Chronic inflammatory bowel disease type in glycogen storage disease type I B. J Inherit Metab Dis 1991; 14: 771–776

88. Couper R, Kapelushknik J, Griffiths A M. Neutrophil dysfunction in glycogen storage disease Ib: association with Crohn's-like colitis. Gastroenterology 1991; 100: 549–554

89. Greene H L. Glycogen storage disease. Semin Liver Dis 1982; 2: 291–301

90. Chen Y T, Cornblath M, Sidbury J. Cornstarch therapy in type I glycogen storage disease. N Engl J Med 1984; 310: 171–175

91. Schroten H, Roesler J, Breidenbach T et al. Granulocytes and granulocyte-macrophage colony-stimulating factors for treatment of neutropenia in glycogen storage disease type 1b. J Pediatr 1991; 119: 748–754

92. Malatack J J, Iwatsuki S, Gartner J C et al. Liver transplantation for Type I glycogen storage disease. Lancet 1983; 1: 1073–1075

93. Kirshner B S, Baker A L, Thorp F K. Growth in adulthood after liver transplantation for glycogen storage disease type I. Gastroenterology 1991; 101: 238–241

94. Martinuik F, Ellenbogen A, Hirschhorn K, Hirschhorn R. Further regional localization of the genes for human acid alpha glucosidase (GAA), peptidase D (PEPD) and alpha-mannosidase (MANB) by somatic cell hybridization. Human Genet 1985; 69: 109

95. Hers H-G, Van Hoof F, de Barsy T. Glycogen storage diseases. In: Scriver C R, Beaudet A L, Sly W S, Valle D, eds. The metabolic basis of inherited disease, 6th edn. New York: McGraw-Hill, 1989, pp 425–452

96. Hers H G, DeBarsy T. Type II glycogenosis (acid maltase deficiency). In: Hers H G, Van Hoof: eds. Lysosomes and storage disease. New York: Academic Press, 1973: pp 197–216

97. Gerson B, Hemphill J M, Rock R C. Creatine kinase and lactate dehydrogenase in type II glycogenosis (Pompe disease). Arch Pathol Lab Med 1977; 101: 213–215

98. Hug G, Soukup S, Ryan M, Chuck G. Rapid prenatal diagnosis of glycogen-storage type II by electron microscopy of uncultured amniotic fluid cells. N Engl J Med 1984; 310: 1014–1022

99. Sharp H L, Desnick R J, Krivit W. The liver in inherited metabolic diseases of childhood. In: Popper H, Schaffner F, eds. Progress in liver diseases. New York: Grune & Stratton, 1972: pp 463–488

100. Engel A G, Acid maltase deficiency in adults. Studies in four cases of a syndrome which may mimic muscular dystrophy or other myopathies. Brain 1970; 93: 599–616

101. Angelini C, Engel A G. Comparative study of acid maltase deficiency. Biochemical differences between infantile, childhood and adult types. Arch Neurol 1972; 26: 344–349

102. Askanas V, Engel W K, Dimauro S, Brooks B R, Mehler M. Adult-onset acid maltase deficiency. Morphologic and biochemical abnormalities reproduced in cultured muscle. N Engl J Med 1976; 294: 573–578

103. McAdams A J, Wilson H E. The liver in generalized glycogen storage disease. Am J Pathol 1966; 49: 99–111

104. McAdams A J, Hug C, Bove K E. Glycogen storage disease, types I to X. Criteria for morphologic diagnosis. Hum Pathol 1974; 5: 463–487

105. Potter E L, Craig J M. Pathology of the fetus and the infant, 3rd edn. Chicago: Year Book Medical, 1975

106. Van Hoof F, Hers H G. The subgroups of type III glycogenosis. Eur J Biochem 1967; 2: 265–270

107. Slomin A E, Weisberg C, Benke P, Evans O B, Burr I M. Reversal of debrancher deficiency myopathy by use of high protein nutrition. Ann Neurol 1982; 11: 420–422

108. Borowitz S M, Green H L. Cornstarch therapy in a patient with type III glycogen storage disease. J Pediatr Gastroenterol Nutr 1987; 6: 631–634

109. Bannayan G A, Dean W J, Howell R R. Type IV glycogen storage disease. Light-microscopic, electron microscopic, and enzymatic study. Am J Clin Pathol 1976; 66: 702–709

110. Howell R R, Kaback M M, Brown B I. Type IV glycogen storage disease. Branching enzyme deficiency in skin fibroblasts and possible heterozygote detection. J Pediatr 1971; 78: 638–642

111. Servidei S, Rieke R E, Langston C et al. Severe cardiopathy in branching enzyme deficiency. J Pediatr 1987; 111: 51–56

112. Krivit W, Sharp H L, Lee J C, Larner J, Edstrom R. Low molecular weight glycogen as a cause of generalized glycogen storage disease. Am J Med 1973; 54: 88–97

113. Greene H L, Brown B I, McClenathan D T, Agostini R M Jr, Taylor S R. A new variant of Type IV glycogenosis: deficiency of branching enzyme activity without apparent progressive liver disease. Hepatology 1988; 8: 302–306

114. Selby R, Starzl T E, Yunis E, Brown B I, Kendall R S, Tzakis A. Liver transplantation for Type IV glycogen storage disease. N Engl J Med 1991; 324: 39–42

115. Sokal E M, Van Hoof E, Alberti D, deVille de Groyet J, deBarry T, Otte J B. Progressive cardiac failure following orthotopic liver transplantation for type IV glycogenosis. Eur J Pediatr 1992; 131: 200–203

116. Hug G, Schubert W K, Chuck G. Phosphorylase kinase of the liver: deficiency in a girl with increased hepatic glycogen. Science 1966; 21: 275–284

117. Van den Berg I E T, Berger R. Phosphorylase 6 kinase deficiency in man: a review. J Inherit Metab Dis 1990; 13: 442–451

118. Tuchman M, Brown B I, Burke B A, Ulstrom R A. Clinical and laboratory observations in a child with hepatic phosphorylase deficiency. Metabolism 1986; 35: 627–633

119. Willems P J, Gerver W J M, Berger R, Fernandes J. The natural history of liver glycogenosis due to phosphorylase kinase deficiency: a longitudinal study of 41 patients. Eur J Pediatr 1990; 149: 268–271

120. Newgard C B, Fletterick R J, Anderson L A, Lebo R V. The polymorphic locus for glycogen storage disease VI (liver glycogen phosphorylase) maps to chromosome 14. Am J Hum Genet 1987; 40: 351–364

121. Francke U, Darras B T, Zander N F, Killmann M W. Assignment of human genes for polyphorylase kinase subunits (PHKA) to Xq12-q13 and (PHKB) to 16q12q13. Am J Hum Genet 1989; 45: 276–282

122. Kuzuya T, Matsuda A, Yoshida S et al. An adult case of type Ib glycogen storage disease. Enzymatic and histochemical studies. N Engl J Med 1983; 308: 566–569

123. Itoh S, Ishida Y, Matsuo S. Mallory bodies in a patient with type Ia glycogen storage disease. Gastroenterology 1987; 92: 520–523

124. Eising E G, Auffermann W, Peters P E, Schmidt H, Ullrich K. Fokale peliosis der Leber im Erwachsenenalter in Kombination mit Glycogenose Typ II (V. Gierke). Radiologie 1990; 30: 428–432

125. Ishihara T, Yokota T, Yamashita Y et al. Comparative study of the intracytoplasmic inclusions in Lafora disease and type IV glycogenosis of electron microscopy. Acta Pathol Jpn 1987; 37: 1591–1601

126. Reed G B, Dixon J E P, Neustein H B, Donnell G N, Landing B H. Type IV glycogenosis. Lab Invest 1968; 19: 546–557

127. Nishimura R N, Ishak K G, Reddick R, Porter R, James S, Barranger J A. Lafora disease: Diagnosis by liver biopsy. Ann Neurol 1979; 8: 409–415

128. Ishak K G, Sharp H L. Metabolic errors and liver disease. In: MacSween R N M, Anthony P J, Scheuer P J, eds. Pathology of the liver, 2nd edn. Edinburgh: Churchill Livingstone, 1987: pp 99–180

129. Riede U N, Spycher M A, Gitzelmann R. Glycogenosis type I (glucose G-phosphatase deficiency). I. Ultrastructural morphometric analysis of juvenile liver cells. Pathol Res Pract 1980; 167: 136–150

130. Buchino J J, Brown B I, Volk D M. Glycogen storage disease type I B. Arch Pathol Lab Med 1983; 107: 283–285

131. Bandhuin P, Hers H G, Loeb H. An electron microscopic and biochemical study of type II glycogenosis. Lab Invest 1964; 13: 1139–1152

132. Isselbacher K J, Anderson E R, Kurakoski K, Kalckar H M. Congenital galactosemia, a single enzymatic block in galactose metabolism. Science 1956; 123: 635

133. Segal S. Disorders of galactose metabolism. In: Scriver C R, Beaudet A L, Sly W S, Valle D, eds. The metabolic basis of inherited disease, 6th edn. New York: McGraw-Hill, 1989: pp 453–480

134. Gitselman R. Hereditary galactokinase deficiency, a newly recognized cause of juvenile cataracts. Pediatr Res 1967; 1: 14–23

135. Nadler H L, Inouye T, Hsia D Y Y. Classical galactosemia. A study of fifty-five cases. In: Hsia D Y Y, ed. Galactosemia. Springfield: Charles C. Thomas, 1969: pp 127–132

136. Donnell G N, Bergen W R. Galactosemia. In: Bergsma D, ed. Birth defects. Atlas and compendium. Baltimore: Williams & Wilkins, 1973: p 422

137. Harley J D, Mutton P, Irvine S, Guta J D. Maternal enzymes of galactose metabolism and the 'inexplicable' infantile cataract. Lancet 1974; 11: 259–261

138. Komrower G M, Lee D H. Long-term follow-up of galactosemia. Arch Dis Childh 1970; 45: 367–373

139. Xu Y-K, Ng W G, Kaufman F R, Lobo R A, Donnell G N. Galactose metabolism in human ovarian tissue. Pediatr Res 1989; 25: 151–155

140. Smetana H F, Olen E. Hereditary galactose disease. Am J Clin Pathol 1962; 38: 3–25

141. Buyssens N. Cholestasis and regeneration of the liver in congenital galactosemia. Tijdschr Gastroenterol 1964; 76: 125–132

142. Appelbaum N M, Thaler M M. Reversibility of extensive liver damage in galactosemia. Gastroenterology 1975; 69: 496–502

143. Gitzelman R. Galactosaemia and other inherited disorders of galactose metabolism. In: Bianchi L, Gerok W, Landmann L, Sicking K, Stalder G A, eds. Liver in metabolic diseases. Lancaster: MTP Press, 1983: pp 235–238

144. Suzuki H, Gilberg E F, Anido V, Jones B, Klingeberg W G. Galactosemia: a report of two fatal cases with giant cell transformation of the liver in one. Arch Pathol 1966; 82: 602–609

145. Edmonds A M, Hennigar C R, Crooks R. Galactosemia. Pediatrics 1952; 10: 40–47

146. Sidbury J R. Investigations and speculations on the pathogenesis of galactosemia. In: Hsia D Y Y, ed. Galactosemia. Springfield: Charles C. Thomas, 1969: pp 13–19

147. Froesch E R, Wolf H P, Baitsch H. Hereditary fructose intolerance. An inborn defect of hepatic fructose-1-phosphate splitting aldolase. Am J Med 1963; 34: 151–167

148. Baker L, Winegard A I. Fasting hypoglycemia and metabolic acidosis associated with deficiency of hepatic fructose-1, 6-diphosphatase activity. Lancet 1970; 11: 13–16

149. Hopwood N J, Holzman I, Drash A L. Fructose-1, 6-diphosphatase deficiency. Am J Dis Child 1977; 131: 418–421

150. Gitzelmann R, Steinman R, van den Berghe G. Disorders of fructose metabolism. In: Scriver R C, Beaudet A L, Sly W S, Valle D, eds. The metabolic basis of inherited diseases, 6th edn. New York: McGraw-Hill, 1989: pp 399–424

151. Hers H G, Joassin G. Anomalie de l'aldolasce hepatique dans l'intolerance un fructose. Enzymol Biol Clin 1961; 1: 4–14

152. Levin B, Snodgrass G J, Oberholzer V G, Brugess E A, Dobbs R H. Fructosemia. Am J Med 1968; 45: 826–838

153. Odievre M, Gertil C, Gautier M, Alagille D. Hereditary fructose intolerance in childhood: diagnosis, management and course in 55 patients. Am J Dis Child 1978; 132: 605–608

154. Baerlocher K, Gitzelmann R, Steinmann B, Gitzelmann-Cumarasamy N. Hereditary fructose intolerance in early childhood: a major diagnostic challenge. Helv Paediat Acta 1979; 33: 465–487

155. Oberhaenski R D, Taylor D J, Rajagophalen B et al. Study of hereditary fructose intolerance by use of 31p magnetic resonance spectroscopy. Lancet 1987; ii: 931–934

156. Gopher A, Vaisman N, Mandel H, Lapidot A. Determination of fructose metabolic pathways in normal and fructose intolerant children: 12C NMR study using (U-13C) fructose. Proc Natl Acad Sci USA 1990; 87: 5449–5453

157. Tolan D R, Penhoet E E. Characterization of the human aldolase B gene. Mol Biol Med 1986; 3: 245–264

158. Cross N C P, Tolan D R, Cox T M. Catalytic deficiency of human aldolase B in hereditary fructose intolerance caused by a common massive mutation. Cell 1988; 53: 881–885

159. Black J A, Simpson K. Fructose intolerance. Br Med J 1967; 2: 138–141

160. Phillips M J, Little J A, Ptak T W. Subcellular pathology of hereditary fructose intolerance. Am J Med 1968; 44: 910–921

161. Jeune M, Planson E, Cotte J, Bonnefoy S, Nivelon J L, Skosowsky J. L'intolerance hereditaire au fructose. A propos d'un cas. Pediatrie 1961; 16: 605–613

162. Lelong M, Alagille D Gentil J et al. Cirrhose hepatique et tubulopathic par absence congenitale de l'aldolase hepatique. Bull Mem Soc Med Hop Paris 1962; 113: 58–72

163. Lelong M, Alagille D Gentil J et al. L'intolerance hereditaire au fructose. Arch Franc Pediatr 1962; 19: 841–866

164. Perheentupa J, Pitkanen E, Nikkila E A, Somersalo O, Hakosalo J. Hereditary fructose intolerance: a clinical study of four cases. Ann Pediatr Fenn 1962; 8: 221–235

165. Cain A R R, Ryman B E. High liver glycogen in hereditary fructose intolerance. Gut 1971; 12: 929–932

166. Royer P, Lestradet H, Habib R, Lardinosis R, Debuquois B. L'intolerance hereditaire au fructose. Bull Mem Soc Med Hop Paris 1964; 115: 805–823

167. Hardwick D F, Dimmick J E. Metabolic cirrhosis of infancy and early childhood. Persp Pediatr Pathol 1976; 3: 103–144

168. See G, Marchal G, Odievre M. Hepatocarcinome chez un adulte suspect d'une intolerance hereditaire au fructose. Ann Pediatr 1984; 31: 49–51

169. Phillips M J, Hetenyi G, Adachi F. Ultrastructural hepatocellular alterations induced by in vivo fructose infusion. Lab Invest 1970; 22: 370–379

170. Van Heycop ten Ham M W. Lafora disease: a form of progressive myoclonus epilepsy. In: Vinken P J, Bruyn G W, eds. Handbook of clinical neurology, vol 15. Amsterdam: North Holland Publishing, 1974: pp 382–422

171. Austin J H, Sakai M. Disorders of glycogen and related macromolecules in the nervous system. In: Vinkin P J, Bruyn G W, eds. Metabolic and deficiency diseases of the nervous system, Part I. Amsterdam: North Holland Publishing, 1976: pp 169–219

172. Berkovic S F, Andermann F, Carpenter S, Wolfe L S. Progressive myoclonus epilepsies: specific causes and diagnosis. N Engl J Med 1986; 315: 296–305

173. Andermann E, Andermann F. Seizures, progressive myoclonic, Lafora type. In: Buyse M L, ed. Birth defects encyclopedia. Dover, M A: Center for Birth Defects Information Services, 1990: pp 1522–1523

174. Suzuki K, David E, Kutschman B. Presenile dementia with 'Lafora-like' intraneuronal inclusions. Arch Neurol 1971; 25: 69–80

175. Holland J M, Davis W C, Prieur D J, Collins G H. Lafora's disease in the dog. Am J Pathol 1970; 58: 509–529

176. Schwarz G A, Yanoff M. Lafora's disease. Distinct clinicopathologic forms of Univerricht's syndrome. Arch Neurol 1965; 12: 172–188

177. Janeway R, Ravens J R, Pearce L A, Odar D L, Suzuki K. Progressive myoclonus epilepsy with Lafora inclusion bodies. Arch Neurol 1967; 16: 565–582

178. Yokoi S, Austin J, Witmer F, Sakai M. Studies on myoclonus epilepsy (Lafora body form). Arch Neurol 1968; 19: 15–33

179. Gambetti P, DiMauro S, Hirt L, Blume R P. Myoclonic epilepsy with Lafora bodies. Some ultrastructural, histochemical, and biochemical aspects. Arch Neurol 1971; 25: 483–493

180. Ota T, Hisatomi Y, Kashiwamura K et al. Histochemistry and substructure of atypical myoclonus body (type II). Acta Neuropathol 1974; 28: 45–54

181. Van Hoof F, Hageman-Bal M. Progressive familial myoclonic epilepsy with Lafora bodies. Electronmicroscopic and histochemical study of a cerebral biopsy. Acta Neuropathol 1967; 7: 315–326

182. Jenis E H, Schochet S S, Earle K M. Myoclonus epilepsy with Lafora bodies. Case report with electron microscopic observations. Milit Med 1970; 135: 116–119

183. Ishihara T, Yokota T, Yamashita Y et al. Comparative study of the intracytoplasmic inclusions in Lafora disease and type IV glycogenesis by electron microscopy. Acta Pathol Jpn 1987; 37: 1591–1601

184. Harriman D G F, Miller J H D. Progressive familial myoclonus epilepsy in three families. Its clinical features and pathological basis. Brain 1955; 78: 325–349

185. Edgar G W F. Progressive myoclonus epilepsy as an inborn error of metabolism comparable to storage disease. Epilepsia 1963; 4: 120–137

186. Collins G H, Cowden R R, Nevis A H. Myoclonus epilepsy with Lafora bodies. Arch Pathol 1968; 86: 239–254

187. Seitelberger F. Myoclonus body disease. In: Minckler J, ed. Pathology of the nervous system. New York: McGraw-Hill, 1968: pp 1121–1134

188. Yokota T, Ishihara T, Kawano H et al. Immunological homogeneity of Lafora bodies, corpora amylacea, basophilic degeneration in heart, and intracytoplasmic inclusions of liver and heart in type IV glycogenosis. Acta Pathol Jpn 1987; 37: 941–946

189. Ng I O L, Sturgess R P, Williams R, Portmann B. Ground-glass hepatocytes with Lafora body like inclusions — histochemical, immunohistochemical and electron microscopic characterization. Histopathology 1990; 17: 109–115

190. Neufeld E F, Muenzer J. The mucopolysaccharidoses. In: Scriver C R, Beaudet A L, Sly W S, Valle D, eds. The metabolic basis of inherited disease, 6th edn. New York: McGraw-Hill, 1989: pp 1565–1587

191. Dulaney J T, Milunsky A, Moser H W. Detection of the carrier state of Hurler's syndrome by assay of L-iduronidase in leukocytes. Clin Chem Acta 1976; 69: 305–310

192. Hobbs J R, Hugh-Jones K, Barrett A J et al. Reversal of clinical features of Hurler's diseases and biochemical improvement after treatment by bone marrow transplantation. Lancet 1981; ii: 709–712

193. Whitley C B, Ramsay N K C, Hersey J H, Krivit W. Bone marrow transplantation for Hurler syndrome: assessment of metabolic correction. Birth Defect Orig Artic Ser 1986; 22: 7–24

194. Hobbs J R. Correction of 34 genetic diseases by displacement bone marrow transplantation. Plasma Ther Transfus Technol 1985; 6: 221–246

195. Shull R M, Hastings N E, Selcer R R, Jones J B, Smith J R, Cullen W C, Constantopoulos G. Bone marrow transplantation in canine mucopolysaccharidosis I: effects within the central nervous system. J Clin Invest 1987; 79: 435–443

196. Wicker G, Prill V, Brooks D et al. Mucopolysaccharidosis VI. Maroteaux-Lamy syndrome. J Biol Chem 1991; 266: 1386–1391

197. Krivit W, Pierpoint M E, Ayaz K et al. Bone-marrow transplantation in the Maroteaux-Lamy syndrome (Mucopolysaccharidosis type VI). N Engl J Med 1984; 311: 1606–1611

198. Petushkova N A. First trimester diagnosis of an unusual case of α-mannosidosis. Prenatal Diagnosis 1991; 11: 279–283

199. Van Hoof F. Mucopolysaccharidoses. In: Hers H A, Van Hoof F, eds. Lysosomes and storage disease. New York: Academic Press, 1973: pp 217–259

200. Lindsay S, Reilly W A, Gotham T J, Skahen R. Gargoylism. II. Study of pathologic lesions and clinical review of twelve cases. Am J Dis Child 1948; 76: 239–306

201. Wolfe H J, Blennerhauser J B, Young G F, Cohen R B. Hurler's syndrome. A histochemical study. New techniques for localization of very water soluble acid mucopolysaccharides. Am J Pathol 1964; 45: 1007–1027

202. Parfrey N A, Hutchins G M. Hepatic fibrosis in the mucopolysaccharidoses. Am J Med 1986; 81: 825–829

203. Schwarz H, Cagne R. A case of gargoylism. Can Med Anoc 1952; 66: 375–377

204. Strauss R, Merlin R, Reiser R. Gargoylism. Review of the literature and report of the sixth autopsied case with chemical studies. Am J Clin Pathol 1947; 17: 671–691

205. Strauss L. The pathology of gargoylism. Report of a case and review of the literature. Am J Pathol 1948; 24: 855–888

206. Henderson J L, MacGregor A P, Thanhauser S J, Holden R. The pathology and biochemistry of gargoylism. A report of three cases with a review of the literature. Arch Dis Childh 1952; 27: 230–253

207. Callahan W P, Lorincz A E. Hepatic ultrastructure in the Hurler syndrome. Am J Pathol 1966; 48: 277–298

208. Loeb H, Jonniaux G, Resibois A et al. Biochemical and ultrastructural studies in Hurler's syndrome. J Pediatr 1968; 72: 860–874

209. Haust M D. Mitochondrial budding and morphogenesis of cytoplasmic vacuoles in hepatocytes of children with Hurler's syndrome and Sanfilippo disease. Exper Mol Biol 1968; 9: 242–257

210. Haust M D. Crystalloid structure of hepatic mitochondria in children with heparitin sulfate mucopolysaccharidosis (Sanfilippo type). Exper Mol Biol 1968; 8: 123–134

211. Van Hoof F. Mucopolysaccharidoses and mucolipidoses. J Clin Pathol 1974; 27, Suppl 8: 64–93

212. Dekaban A S, Constantopoulos G, Herman M M, Stensing J K. Mucopolysaccharidosis type V (Scheie syndrome). Arch Pathol Lab Med 1976; 100: 237–245

213. Jenner F A, Pollitt R J. Large quantities of 2-acetamido-1-(B-L-aspartamido)-1,2-dideoxyglucose in the urine of mentally retarded siblings. Biochem J 1967; 103: 48–49

214. Aula P, Renlund M, Raivio K O, Koskela S-L. Screening of inherited oligosaccharidurias among mentally retarded patients in northern Finland. J Ment Defic Res 1986; 30: 365–368

215. Aula P, Rapola J, von Koskull H, Ammala P. Prenatal diagnosis and fetal pathology of aspartylglucosaminuria. Am J Med Genet 1984; 19: 359

216. Ikonen E, Baumann M, Gron K et al. Aspartylglycosaminuria: cDNA encoding human aspartylglycosaminidase and the missense mutation causing the disease. EMBO J 1991; 10: 41–48

217. Fisher K J, Aronson Jr N N. Characterization of the mutation responsible for aspartylglucosaminuria in three Finnish patients. J Biol Chem 1991; 266: 12105–12113

218. Mononen I, Heiserkamp N, Kaartinen V et al. Aspartylglycosaminuria in the Finnish population: Identification of

two point mutations in the heavy chain of glycoasparaginase. Proc Natl Acad Sci USA 1991; 88: 2941–2945

219. Hreidarsson J, Thomas G H, Valle D L et al. Aspartylglucosaminuria in the United States. Clin Genet 1983; 23: 427–435

220. Fisher K J, Aronson Jr N N. Deletion of exon 8 causes glycosylasparaginase deficiency in an African-American aspartylglycosaminuria (AGU) patient. FEBS Letters 1991; 288: 173–178

221. Isenberg J N, Sharp H L. Aspartylglucosaminuria. Biochemical and ultrastructural characteristics unique to this visceral storage disease. Hum Pathol 1976; 7: 469–481

222. Isenberg J N, Sharp H L. Aspartylglycosaminuria: psychomotor retardation masquerading as a mucopolysaccharidosis. J Pediatr 1975; 86: 713–717

223. Palo J, Rickkinen P, Arstila A, Autio S. Biochemical and fine structural studies on brain and liver biopsies in aspartylglucosaminuria. Neurology 1971; 21: 1198–1204

224. Petushkova N A. First-trimester diagnosis of an unusual case of ß-mannosidosis. Prenatal Diagnoses 1991; 11: 279–283

225. Desnick R J, Sharp H L, Grabowski G A et al. Mannosidosis: clinical, morphologic, immunologic, and biochemical studies. Pediatr Res 1976; 10: 985–995

226. Yunis J J, Lewandowski R C, Sanfilippo S J, Tsai M Y, Foni I, Bruhl H H. Clinical manifestations of mannosidosis. A longitudinal study. Am J Med 1976; 61: 841–848

227. Kistler J P, Lott I T, Kolodny E H et al. Mannosidosis. New clinical presentation, enzyme studies and carbohydrate analysis. Arch Neurol 1977; 34: 45–51

228. Milla P J, Black I E, Patrick A D, Hugh-Jones K, Oberholzer V. Mannosidosis: clinical and biochemical study. Arch Dis Childh 1977; 52: 937–942

229. Irons M. Mannosidosis. In Buyse M L, ed. Birth defects encyclopedia. Dover, M A: Center for Birth Defects Information Services, 1989: pp 1101–1102

230. Beaudet A L, Thomas G H. Disorders of glycoprotein degradation: Mannosidosis, fucosidosis, sialidosis, and aspartylglycosaminuria. In: Scriver C R, Beaudet A L, Sly W S, Valle D. eds. The metabolic basis of inherited disease, 6th edn. New York: McGraw-Hill, 1989: pp 1603–1621

231. Montgomery T R, Thoms G H, Valle D L. Mannosidosis in an adult. Johns Hopkins Med J 1982; 151: 113–121

232. Gordon B A, Carson R, Haust M D. Unusual clinical and ultrastructural features in a boy with biochemically typical mannosidosis. Acta Paediatr Scand 1980; 69: 787–792

233. Kornfeld M, Snyder R D, Wenger D A. Fucosidosis with angiokeratoma. Electron microscopic changes in the skin. Arch Pathol Lab Med 1977; 101: 478–485

234. Koussef B G, Beratis N G, Strauss L et al. Fucosidosis type II. Pediatrics 1976; 57: 205–213

235. Peratis N G, Turner B M, Labadie G, Kirschorn K. L-fucosidase in cultured skin fibroblasts from normal subjects and fucosidosis patients. Pediatr Res 1977; 11: 862–866

236. Freitag F, Kuchemann K, Flumcke S. Hepatic ultrastructure in fucosidosis. Virchows Arch (A) 1971; 7: 99–113

237. Van Hoof F. Fucosidosis. In: Hers H G, Van Hoof F, eds. Lysosomes and storage diseases. New York: Academic Press, 1973: pp 277–290

238. Spranger J. Mucolipidosis I. In: Bergsma D, ed. Disorders of connective tissue. New York: Stratton Intercontinental, 1975: pp 279–282

239. Legum C P, Schorr S, Berman E R. The genetic mucopolysaccharidoses and mucolipidoses. Review and comment. In Schulman I, ed. Advances in pediatrics, vol 22. Chicago: Year Book Publishers, 1976: pp 305–347

240. Lowden J A, O'Brien J S. Sialidosis: a review of human neuraminidase deficiency. Am J Hum Genet 1979; 31: 1–18

241. Kelly T E. Mucolipidosis I. In: Buyse M L, ed. Birth defects encyclopedia. Dover, M A: Center for Birth Defects Information Services, 1989: pp 1155–1157

242. Riches W G, Smuckler E A. A severe infantile mucolipidosis: clinical, biochemical and pathologic features. Arch Pathol Lab Med 1983; 107: 147–152

243. Leroy J G, Martin J J. Mucolipidosis II. In: Bergsma D, ed. Disorders of connective tissue. New York: Stratton Intercontinental, 1975: pp 283–293

244. Patriquin H B, Kaplan P, Kind H P, Giedion A. Neonatal mucolipidosis II (I-cell disease). Clinical and radiologic features in three cases. Am J Roentgenol 1977; 129: 37–43

245. Amato R S S. Mucolipidosis II. In Buyse M L, ed. Birth defects encyclopedia. Dover, M A: Center for Birth Defects Information Services, 1989: pp 1157–1158

246. Kitagawa H, Toki J, Morimoto T et al. An autopsy case of I-cell disease. Ultrastructural and biochemical analyses. Am J Clin Pathol 1991; 96: 262–266

247. Kenyon K R, Sensenbrenner J A, Wyllie R G. Hepatic ultrastructure and histochemistry in mucolipidosis II (I-cell disease). Pediatr Res 1973; 7: 560–568

248. Tondeur M, Vamos-Hurwitz E, Mockel-Pohl S et al. Clinical, biochemical and ultrastructural studies in a case of chondrodystrophy presenting the I-cell phenotype in tissue culture. J Pediatr 1971; 79: 366–378

249. Nolan C M, Sly W S. I-cell disease and pseudo-Hurler polydystrophy: disorders of lysosomal enzyme phosphorylation and localization. In: Scriver C R, Beaudet A L, Sly W S, Valle D, eds. The metabolic basis of inherited disease, 6th edn. New York: McGraw-Hill, 1989: pp 1589–1601

250. Kelly T, Thomas G H, Taylor H A, McKusick V A. Mucolipidosis III. Clinical and laboratory findings. In: Bergsma D, ed. Disorders of connective tissue. New York: Stratton Intercontinental, 1975: pp 295–299

251. Berman E R, Livni N, Shapira E, Merin S, Levy I S. Congenital corneal clouding with abnormal systemic storage bodies. A new variant of mucolipidosis. J Pediatr 1974; 84: 519–526

252. Trujillo-Bottero C J. Mucolipidosis III. In: Buyse M L ed. Birth defects encyclopedia. Dover, M A: Center for Birth Defects Information Services, 1989: pp 1158–1159

253. Amir N, Zlotogora J, Bach G. Mucolipidosis type IV: clinical spectrum and natural history. Pediatrics 1987; 79: 953–959

254. Merin S, Livni N, Berman E R, Yatziv S. Mucolipidosis IV. Ocular, systemic and ultrastructural findings. Invest Ophthalmol 1975; 14: 437–448

255. Kohn G, Livni N, Onoy A et al. Prenatal diagnosis of mucolipidosis IV by electron microscopy. J Pediatr 1977; 90: 62–66

256. Crandall B, Philipart M. Mucolipidosis IV. In: Buyse M L, ed. Birth defects encyclopedia. Dover, M A: Center for Birth Defects Information Services, 1989: pp 1159–1160

257. Ng I O L, Ng M, Lai E C S, Wu P C. Endoplasmic storage disease of liver: characterization of intracytoplasmic hyaline inclusions. Histopathology 1989; 15: 473–481

258. Callea F, Brisigotti M, Fabbretti G, Bonino F, Desmet V J. Hepatic endoplasmic reticulum storage diseases. Liver 1992; 12: 357–362

259. Storch W, Riedel H, Trautmann B, Justus J, Hiemann D. Storage of the complement components C_4, C_3 and C_3-activator in the human liver as PAS-negative globular hyaline bodies. Exp Pathol 1982; 21: 199–203

260. Storch W. Immunohistological investigations of PAS-negative intracisternal hyaline in human liver biopsy specimens. Virchows Arch (A) 1985; 48: 155–165

261. Carrell R W, Jeppsson J O, Laurell C B et al. Structure and variation of human α_1-antitrypsin. Nature 1982; 298: 329–334

262. Carlson J A, Rogers B B, Sifers R N, Hawkins H K, Finegold M J, Woo S L C. Multiple tissues express alpha-1-antitrypsin in transgenic mice and men. J Clin Invest 1988; 82: 26–36

263. Kelsey G D, Povey S, Bygrave A E, Lovell-Badge R H. Species- and tissue-specific expression of human α_1-antitrypsin in transgenic mice. Genes and Develop 1987; 1: 161–171

264. Perlmutter D H, Schlesinger M J, Pierce J A, Punsal P I, Schwartz A L. Synthesis of stress proteins is increased in individuals with homozygous PiZZ alpha-1-antitrypsin deficiency and liver disease. J Clin Invest 1989; 84: 1555–1561

265. van Furth R, Kramps J A, Disselhoff-Den Dulk M M C. Synthesis of α_1-antitrypsin by human monocytes. Clin Exp Immunol 1983; 51; 551–557

266. Johnson D A, Travis J. Human alpha-1-proteinase inhibitor

mechanism of action: Evidence for activation by limited proteolysis. Biochem Biophys Res Commun 1976; 72; 33–39

267. Heeb M J, Griffin J H. Physiologic inhibition of human activated protein C by α_1-antitrypsin. J Biol Chem 1988; 263: 11613–11616

268. Travis J, Salvesen G S. Human plasma proteinase inhibitors. Ann Rev Biochem 1983; 52: 655–709

269. Loebermann H, Tokuoka R, Deisenhofer J, Huber R. Human α_1-proteinase inhibitor: Crystal structure analysis of two crystal modifications, molecular model and preliminary analysis of the implications for function. J Mol Biol 1984; 177: 531–556

270. Banda M J, Rice A G, Griffin G L, Senior R M. α_1-proteinase inhibitor is a neutrophil chemoattractant after proteolytic inactivation by macrophage elastase. J Biol Chem 1988; 263: 4481–4484

271. Makino S, Reed C E. Distribution and elimination of exogenous alpha-1-antitrypsin. J Lab Clin Med 1970; 75: 742–746

272. Ohlsson K, Laurell C-B. The disappearance of enzyme-inhibitor complexes from the circulation of man. Clin Sci Mol Med 1976; 51: 87–92

273. Cox D W, Markovic V D, Teshima I E. Genes for imunoglobulin heavy chains and for alpha-1-antitrypsin are localized to specific regions of chromosome 14q. Nature 1982; 297: 428–430

274. Schroeder W T, Miller M F, Woo S L C, Saunders G F. Chromosomal localization of the human alpha-1-antitrypsin gene (Pi) to 14q31–32. Am J Hum Genet 1985; 37: 868–872

275. Perlmutter D H, Cole F S, Kilbridge P, Rossing T H, Colten H R. Expression of the α_1-protease inhibitor gene in human monocytes and macrophages. Proc Natl Acad Sci 1985; 82: 795–799

276. Perlino E, Cortese R, Ciliberto G. The human alpha-1-antitrypsin gene is transcribed from two different promoters in macrophages and hepatocytes. EMBO J 1987; 6: 2767–2771

277. Gadek J E, Crystal R G. Alpha-1 antitrypsin deficiency. In: Stanbury J B, Wyngaarden J B, Fredrickson D S, Goldstein J L, Brown M S, eds. Metabolic basis of inherited disease. New York: McGraw-Hill, 1983: pp 1450–1467

278. Schwarzenberg S J, Sharp H L. Alpha-1-antitrypsin deficiency. In: Schiff L, Schiff E R, eds. Diseases of the liver. New York: Lippincott, 1993: pp 692–706

279. Sharp H L, Bridges R A, Krivit W, Freier E F. Cirrhosis associated with alpha-1-antitrypsin deficiency. A previously unrecognized inherited disorder. J Lab Clin Med 1969; 73: 934–939

280. Brantly M T, Nukiwa T, Crystal R G. Molecular basis of α_1-1-antitrypsin deficiency. Am J Med 1988; 84 (Suppl 6A): 13–31

281. Jeppsson J-O. Amino acid substitution Glu → Lys in α_1-1-antitrypsin PiZ. FEBS Lett 1976; 65: 195–197

282. Sharp H L. Alpha-1-antitrypsin deficiency. Hosp Pract 1971; 6: 83–96

283. Laurell C B, Eriksson S. The electrophoretic α_1-globulin pattern of serum alpha-1-antitrypsin deficiency. Scand J Clin Lab Invest 1963; 15: 132–140

284. Feldman G, Bignon J, Chahinian P, Degott C, Benhamou J P. Hepatocyte ultrastructural changes in alpha-1-antitrypsin deficiency. Gastroenterology 1974; 67: 1214–1224

285. Roberts E A, Cox D W, Medline A, Wanless I R. Occurrence of alpha-1-antitrypsin deficiency in 155 patients with alcoholic liver disease. Am J Clin Pathol 1984; 82: 424–427

286. Crowley J J, Sharp H L, Frier E, Ishak K G, Schow P. Fatal liver disease associated with alpha-1-antitrypsin deficiency, PIM_1/PiM_{Duarte}. Gastroenterology 1987; 93: 242–244

287. Lieberman J, Gaidulis L, Klotz S D. A new deficient variant of α_1-antitrypsin (MDuarte): inability to detect the heterozygous state by antitrypsin phenotyping. Am Rev Resp Dis 1976; 113: 31–36

288. Fabbretti G, Sergi S, Consales G et al. Genetic variants of alpha-1-antitrypsin. Liver 1992; 12: 296–301

289. Callea F, Fevery J, Massi G, Lievens C, DeGroote J, Desmet V J. Alpha-1-antitrypsin (AAT) and its stimulation in the liver of PiMZ phenotype individuals. A "recruitment-secretory block" ("R-SB") phenomenon. Liver 1984; 4: 325–337

290. Carlson J, Eriksson S, Hagerstrand I. Intra- and extracellular alpha-1-antitrypsin in liver disease with special reference to Pi phenotype. J Clin Pathol 1981; 34: 1020–1025

291. Sveger T. Liver disease in alpha-1-antitrypsin deficiency detected

292. Burn J, Dunger D, Lake B. Liver damage with alpha-1-antitrypsin deficiency due to phenotype PiZ null (Z-). Arch Dis Childh 1981; 3: 311–313

293. Sveger T. Prospective study of children with α_1-antitrypsin deficiency: eight-year-old follow-up. J Pediatr 1989; 104: 91–94

294. Sveger T. The natural history of liver disease in α_1-antitrypsin deficient children. Acta Pediatr Scand 1988; 77: 847–851

295. Ibarguen E, Gross C, Savik K, Sharp H L. Liver disease in alpha$_1$-antitrypsin deficiency: prognostic indicators. J Pediatr 1990; 117: 864–870

296. Moroz S P. Liver disease associated with alpha-1-antitrypsin deficiency in childhood. J Pediatr 1976; 88: 19–25

297. Ghishan F K, Gray G F, Greene H L. α_1-antitrypsin deficiency presenting with ascites and cirrhosis in the neonatal period. Gastroenterology 1983; 85: 435–438

298. Psacharopoulos H T, Mowat A P, Cook P J L, Carbile P A, Portmann B, Rodeck C H. Outcome of liver disease associated with alpha-1-antitrypsin deficiency. Arch Dis Childh 1983; 58: 882–887

299. Davis I D, Burke B, Freese D K, Sharp H L, Kim Y. The pathologic spectrum of the nephropathy associated with alpha-1-antitrypsin deficiency. Hum Pathol 1992; 23: 57–62

300. Larsson C. Natural history and life expectancy in severe alpha-1-antitrypsin deficiency, PiZ. Acta Med Scand 1978; 204: 345–351

301. Cox D W, Smyth S. Risk for liver disease in adults with alpha-1-antitrypsin deficiency. Am J Med 1983; 74: 221–227

302. Reid C L, Wiener G J, Cox D W, Richter J E, Geisinger K R. Diffuse hepatocellular dysplasia and carcinoma associated with Mmalton variant of alpha$_1$-antitrypsin. Gastroenterology 1987; 93: 181–187

303. Propst T, Propst A, Dietze O et al. High prevalence of viral infection in adults with homozygous and heterozygous alpha-1-antitrypsin deficiency and chronic liver disease. Ann Intern Med 1992; 117: 641–645

304. Demedina M, Li X, Schiff E R, Cleary K, Sharp H L. The liver disease in children associated with alpha-1-antitrypsin (A1AT) deficiency is not related to hepatitis C virus. Hepatology 1992; 16: 230A

305. Eriksson S, Carlson J, Velez R. Risk of cirrhosis and primary liver cancer in alpha-1-antitrypsin deficiency. N Engl J Med 1986; 314: 736–739

306. Berkowitz M, Gavalier J S, Kelly R H, Prieto M, Van Thiel D H. Lack of increased heterozygous alpha-1-antitrypsin deficiency phenotypes among patients with hepatocellular and bile duct carcinoma. Hepatology 1992; 15: 407–410

307. Morse J O. Alpha$_1$-antitrypsin deficiency. N Engl J Med 1978; 299: 1099–1105

308. Bell H, Schrumpf E, Farhol M K. Heterozygous M Z alpha-1-antitrypsin deficiency in adults with chronic liver disease. Scand J Gastroenterol 1990; 25: 788–792

309. Carlson J, Eriksson S. Chronic "cryptogenic" liver disease in malignant hepatoma in intermediate alpha-1-antitrypsin deficiency identified by PiZ specific monoclonal antibody. Scand J Gastroenterol 1985; 20: 835–842

310. Hodges J R, Millward-Sadler G H, Barbatis C, Wright R. Heterozygous MZ alpha-1-antitrypsin deficiency in adults with chronic hepatitis and cryptogenic cirrhosis. N Engl J Med 1981; 304: 557–560

311. Bradfield J W B, Blenkinsopp W K. Alpha-1-antitrypsin globules in the liver and PiM phenotype. J Clin Pathol 1977; 30: 579–584

312. Berninger R W, DeLellis R A, Kaplan M M. Liver disease and the Pi Elemberg M phenotype of alpha-1-antitrypsin. Am J Clin Pathol 1983; 83: 503–506

313. Talbot I C, Mowat A P. Liver disease in infancy: histological features and relationship to α_1-antitrypsin phenotype. J Clin Pathol 1975; 28: 559–563

314. Malone M, Mieli-Vergani G, Mowat A P, Portmann B. The fetal liver in PiZZ α_1-antitrypsin deficiency: A report of five cases. Pediatr Pathol 1989; 9: 923–931

315. Takahashi H, Crystal R G. Alpha-1-antitrypsin Null$_{isola}$ di

by screening in 200,000 infants. N Engl J Med 1976; 294: 1316–1321 procida: an alpha-1-antitrypsin deficiency allele caused by deletion of all alpha-1-antitrypsin coding exons. Am J Hum Genet 1990; 47: 403–413

316. Robert P F. PiZZ alpha-1-antitrypsin deficiency in a 20-week fetus. Hum Pathol 1985; 16: 188–190

317. Sharp H L. Relationship between alpha$_1$-antitrypsin deficiency and liver disease. In: Bernberg S R, ed. Liver disease in infancy and childhood. The Hague: Martinus Nijhoff, 1976: pp 52–76

318. Triger D K, Milward-Sadler G H, Czaykowski A A, Trowell J, Wright R. Alpha-1-antitrypsin deficiency and liver disease in adults. Quart J Med 1976; 45: 351–372

319. Rubel L R, Ishak K G, Benjamin S B, Knuff T E. α_1-antitrypsin deficiency and hepatocellular carcinoma: association with cirrhosis, copper storage and Mallory bodies. Arch Pathol Lab Med 1982: 106: 678–681

320. Crystal R A. Alpha-1-AT deficiency, emphysema, and liver disease. J Clin Invest 1990; 85: 13413–13452

321. Schwarzenberg S J, Sharp H L. Pathogenesis of alpha-1-antitrypsin deficiency-associated liver disease. J Pediatr Gastroenterol Nutr 1990; 10: 5–12

322. Dycaico M J, Grant S G N, Felts K et al. Neonatal hepatitis induced by alpha-1-antitrypsin: a transgenic mouse model. Science 1988; 242: 1409–1412

323. Carlson J A, Rogers B B, Sifers R N et al. Accumulation of PiZ alpha-1-antitrypsin causes liver damage in transgenic mice. J Clin Invest 1989; 83: 1183–1190

324. Geller S A, Nichols W S, Dycaico M J, Felts K A, Sorge J A. Histopathology of alpha-1-antitrypsin liver disease in a transgenic mouse model. Hepatology 1990; 12: 40–47

325. Sifers R N, Hardick C P, Woo S L C. Disruption of the 290–342 salt bridge is not responsible for the secretory defect of the PiZ alpha-1-antitrypsin variant. J Biol Chem 1989; 264: 2997–3001

326. McCracken A A, Kruse K B, Brown J L. Molecular basis for defective secretion of the Z variant of human alpha-1-proteinase inhibitor. Secretion of variants having altered potential for salt bridge formation between amino acids 290 and 342. Mol Cel Biol 1989; 9: 1406–1414

327. Cox D W, Billingsley G D, Callahan J W. Aggregation of plasma Z type alpha-1-antitrypsin suggests basic defect for the deficiency. FEBS Lett 1986; 205: 255–260

328. Perlmutter D H, Schlesinger M J, Pierce J A, Punsal P I, Schwatz A L. Synthesis of stress proteins is increased in individuals with homozygous PiZZ α_1-antitrypsin deficiency and liver disease. J Clin Invest 1989; 84: 1555–1561

329. Udall J, Dixon M, Newman A P, Wright J A, James B, Bloch K J. Liver disease in alpha-1-antitrypsin deficiency. A retrospective analysis of the influence of early breast-vs bottle-feeding. JAMA 1985; 253: 2679–2682

330. Sveger T. Breast-feeding, alpha-1-antitrypsin deficiency, and liver disease? JAMA 1985; 254: 3036

331. Esquivel C O, Vicente E, Van Thiel D et al. Orthotopic liver transplantation for alpha-1-antitrypsin deficiency: an experience in 29 children and 10 adults. Transplant Proc 1987; 19: 3798–3802

332. Lindmark B E, Erikkson S G. Plasma α_1-antichymotrypsin in liver disease. Clin Chim Acta 1985; 152: 261–269

333. Eriksson S, Lindmark B, Lilja H. Familial alpha$_1$-antichymotrypsin deficiency. Acta Med Scand 1986; 220: 447–453

334. Lindmark B, Millward-Sadler H, Callea F, Eriksson S. Hepatocyte inclusions of α_1-antichymotrypsin in a patient with partial deficiency of α_1-antichymotrypsin and chronic liver disease. Histopathology 1990; 16: 211–225

335. Grech H, Majamdar G, Lawril A S, Savidge G F. Pregnancy in congenital afibrinogenemia: Report of a successful case and review of the literature. Br J Haematol 1991; 78: 571–572

336. Pfeifer U, Ormanns W, Klinge O. Hepatocellular fibrinogen storage in familial hypofibrinogenemia. Virchows Arch Cell Pathol 1981; 36: 247–225

337. Wehinger H, Klinge O, Alexandrakis E, Schurman J, Witt J, Seydewitz H H. Hereditary hypofibrinogenemia with fibrinogen storage in the liver. Eur J Pediatr 1983; 141: 109–112

338. Callea F, De Vos R, Tagni R, Tardanico R, Vanstapel M J, Desmet V J. Fibrinogen inclusions in liver cells: a new type of ground-glass hepatocyte. Immune light and electron microscopic characterization. Histopathology 1986; 10: 65–73

339. Callea F, De Vos R, Pinackay J et al. Hereditary hypofibrinogenaemia with hepatic storage of fibrinogen. Ital J Gastroenterol 1987; 19: 304–305

340. Sharon B I. Antithrombin III deficiency. In: Buyse M L, ed. Birth defects encyclopedia. Dover, MA: Center for Birth Defects Information Services, 1990: pp 152–154

341. Demers C, Ginsberg J S, Hirsch J, Henderson P, Blajchman M A. Thrombosis in antithrombin-III-deficient persons. Report of a large kindred and literature review. Ann Intern Med 1992; 116: 754–761

342. McClure S. Dincsoy H P, Glueck H. Budd-Chiari syndrome and antithrombin III deficiency. Am J Clin Pathol 1982; 78: 236–241

343. Das M, Carroll S F. Antithrombin III deficiency: an etiology of Budd-Chiari syndrome. Surgery 1985; 97: 242–245

344. Mendelsohn G, Gomperts E D, Gurwitz D. Severe antithrombin III deficiency in an infant associated with multiple arterial and venous thrombosis. Thromb Haemost 1976; 36: 495–502

345. Goldsmith L A, Laberge C. Tyrosinemia and related disorders. In: Scriver C R, Beaudet A L, Sly W S, Valle D, eds. The metabolic basis of inherited disease, 6th edn. New York: McGraw-Hill, 1989: pp 547–562

346. Shear C S, Nyhan W L. In: Buyse M L, ed. Birth defects encyclopedia. Dover, MA: Center for Birth Defects Information Services, 1990: pp 1722–1724

347. Kvittingen E A. Tyrosinaemia type I — an update. J Inher Metab Dis 1991; 14: 554–562

348. Buist N R M, Kennaway N G, Burns R P. Eye and skin lesions in tyrosinaemia. Lancet 1973; i: 620–621

349. Strife F. Tyrosinemia with acute intermittent porphyria: aminolevulinic acid dehydratase deficiency related to elevated urinary aminolevulinic acid levels. J Pediatr 1977; 90: 400–404

350. Mitchell G, Larochelle J, Lambert M et al. Neurological crises in hereditary tyrosinemia. N Engl J Med 1990; 322: 432–437

351. Rank J M, Pascual-Leone A, Payne W et al. Hematin therapy for neurologic crises of tyrosinemia. J Pediatr 1991; 118: 136–199

352. LaRochelle J, Mortezai A, Belanger M, Tremblay M, Clavean J C, Aubin G. Experience with 37 infants with tyrosinemia. Can Med Assoc J 1967; 97: 1051–1054

353. Alpert E. Human alpha-1-fetoprotein. In: Okuda K, Peters R L, eds. Hepatocellular carcinoma. New York: Wiley 1976: pp 353–384

354. Kvittingen E A, Halvorsen S, Jellum E. Deficient fumarylacetoacetate fumarylhydrolase activity in lymphocytes and fibroblasts from patients with hereditary tyrosinaemia. Pediatr Res 1983; 17: 541–544

355. Linblad B, Lindstedt S, Stein G. On the enzymatic defects in hereditary tyrosinemia. Proc Natl Acad Sci USA 1977; 74: 4641

356. Berger R, Van Faassen H, Smith G P A. Biochemical studies on the enzymatic deficiencies in hereditary tyrosinaemia. Clin Chem Acta 1983; 134: 129–141

357. Berube D, Phaneuf D, Tanguay R M, Gagne R. Assignment of the fumarylacetoacetate hydrolase gene to chromosome 15q23-15q25. Cytogenet Cell Genet 1989; 51: 962 (abstract)

358. Stoner E, Starkman H, Wellner D et al. Biochemical studies of a patient with hereditary tyrosinaemia: evidence of glutathione deficiency. Pediatr Res 1984; 18: 1332–1336

359. Partington M W, Haust M D. A patient with tyrosinemia and hypermethioninemia. Can Med Assoc J 1967; 97: 1059–1067

360. Perry T L. Tyrosinemia associated with hypermethioninemia and islet cell hyperplasia. Can Med Assoc J 1967; 97: 1067–1072

361. Prive L. Pathological findings in patients with tyrosinemia. Can Med Assoc J 1967; 97: 1054–1056

362. Scriver C R, Silverberg M, Clow C L. Hereditary tyrosinemia and tyrosyluria: clinical report of four patients. Can Med Assoc J 1967; 97: 1047–1050

363. Jevtic M M, Thorp F K, Hruban Z. Hereditary tyrosinemia with hyperplasia and hypertrophy of juxtaglomerular apparatus. Am J Clin Pathol 1974; 61: 423–437

364. Carson N A J, Biggart J D, Bittles A H, Donovan D. Hereditary tyrosinaemia. Clinical, enzymatic, and pathological study of an infant with the acute form of the disease. Arch Dis Childh 1976; 51: 106–113

365. Dehner L P, Snover D C, Sharp H L, Ascher N, Nakhleh R, Day D L. Hereditary tyrosinemia type I (chronic form): pathologic findings in the liver. Hum Pathol 1989; 20: 149–159

366. Manowski Z, Silver M M, Roberts E A, Superina R A, Phillips M J. Liver cell dysplasia and early liver transplantation in hereditary tyrosinemia. Mod Pathol 1990; 3: 694–701

367. Mieles L A, Esquivel C O, Van Thiel D H et al. Liver transplantation for tyrosinemia. A review of 10 cases from the University of Pittsburgh. Dig Dis Sci 1990; 35: 153–157

368. Zerbini C, Weinberg D S, Hollister K A, Perez-Atayde A R. DNA ploidy abnormalities on the liver of children with hereditary tyrosinemia type I. Correlation with histopathologic features. Am J Pathol 1992; 140: 1111–1119

369. Day D L, Letourneau J G, Allan B T et al. Hepatic regenerating nodules in hereditary tyrosinemia. Am J Roentgenol 1987; 149: 391–393

370. Gilbert-Barness E, Barness L A, Meisner L F. Chromosomal instability in hereditary tyrosinemia type I. Pediatr Pathol 1990; 10: 243–252

371. Weinberg A G, Mize C E, Worthen H G. The occurrence of hepatoma in the chronic forms of hereditary tyrosinemia. J Pediatr 1976; 88: 434–438

372. Van Thiel D H, Gartner L M, Thorp F K et al. Resolution of the clinical features of tyrosinemia following orthotopic liver transplantation for hepatoma. J Hepatol 1986; 3: 42–48

373. Tuchman M, Freese D K, Sharp H L, Ramnaraine M L R, Ascher N, Bloomer J R. Contribution of extrahepatic tissue to biochemical abnormalities in hereditary tyrosinemia type I: study of three patients after liver transplantation. J Pediatr 1987; 110: 399–403

374. Lindstedt S, Holme E, Lock E A, Hjalmarson O, Strandvik B. Treatment of hereditary tyrosinaemia type I by inhibitor of 4-hydroxyphenylpyruvate dioxygenase. Lancet 1992; 813–817

375. Hostetter M K, Levy H L, Winter H S, Knight G J, Hadlow J E. Evidence for liver disease preceding amino acid abnormalities in hereditary tyrosinemia. N Engl J Med 1983; 308: 1265–1267

376. Phaneu F D, Lambert M, LaFramboise R, Mitchell G, Lettre F, Tanguay R M. Type I hereditary tyrosinemia. J Clin Invest 1992; 90: 1185–1192

377. Brusilow S W, Horwich A L. Urea cycle enzymes. In: Scriver C R, Beaudet A L, Sly W S, Valle D, eds. The metabolic basis of inherited disease. New York: McGraw-Hill, 1989: pp 629–670

378. Tuchman M, Sharp H L. An approach to the diagnosis and management of inherited metabolic liver disorders. In: Lebinthal E, ed. Textbook of gastroenterology and nutrition in infancy, 2nd edn. New York: Raven Press, 1989: pp 969–1003

379. Mantagos S, Tsagaraki S, Burgess E A. Neonatal hyperammonemia with complete absence of liver carbamylphosphate synthetase activity. Arch Dis Childh 1978; 53: 230–234

380. Freeman J M, Nicholson J P, Schinke R T, Rowland L P, Carter S. Congenital hyperammonemia: association with hyperglycinemia and decreased levels of carbamylphosphate synthetase. Arch Neurol 1970; 23: 430–437

381. LaBrecque D R, Latharn P S, Riely C A, Hoia Y E, Klatskin G. Heritable urea cycle enzyme deficiency — liver disease in 16 patients. J Pediatr 1979; 76: 262–266

382. Briand P, Francois B, Rabier D, Cathelineau L. Ornithine trans-carbamylase deficiencies in human males: Kinetic and immuno-chemical classification. Biochem Biophys Acta 1982; 704: 100–106

383. Lindgrin V, de Martinville B, Horwich A L, Rosenberg L E, Franke U. Human ornithine transcarbamylase locus mapped at band x 21.2 near Duchenne muscular dystrophy locus. Science 1984; 226: 698–700

384. Hauser E R, Finkelstein J E, Valle D, Brusilow S W. Allopurinol-induced orotidinurea: a test for mutations at the ornithine carbamoyl transferase locus in women. N Engl J Med 1990; 322: 1641–1645

385. Arn P A, Hauser E R, Thomas G H, Herman G, Hess D, Brusilow S W. Hyperammonemia in women with a mutation at the ornithine carbamoyl transferase locus: A cause for post-partum coma. N Engl J Med 1990; 322: 1652–1655

386. Tallen H, Schaffner F, Taffet S, Schneidman K, Gaul G. Ornithine carbamoyl transferase deficiency in an adult male patient: significance of hepatic ultrastructure in clinical diagnosis. Pediatric Res 1983; 71: 224–232

387. Aida S, Ogata T, Kamota T, Nakamura N. Primary ornithine transcarbamylase deficiency. A case report and electron microscopic study. Acta Pathol Jpn 1989; 39: 451–456

387a. Capistrano-Estrada S. Marsden D L. Nyhan W L. Histopathological findings in a male with late-onset ornithine transcarbamylase deficiency. Pediatr Pathol 1994; 14: 235–243

388. Beaudet A L, O'Brien W E, Bock H G O, Freytag S O, Su T S. The human argininosuccinate synthetase locus and citrullinaemia. In: Harris H, Hirshhorn K, eds. Advances in human genetics. New York: Plenum, 1986: p 161

389. Naylor S L, Klebe R S, Shows T B. Argininosuccinic aciduria: Assignment of the argininosuccinate lyase gene to the pter-q-22 region of human chromosome 7 by bioautography. Proc Natl Acad Sci USA 1978; 75: 6159–6162

390. Kobayashi K, Itakura Y, Saheki T et al. Absence of argininosuccinate lyase protein in the liver of two patients with argininosuccinic aciduria. Clin Chim Acta 1986; 159: 59–67

391. Zimmerman A, Bachmann C, Baumgartner R. Severe liver fibrosis in argininosuccinic aciduria. Arch Pathol Lab Med 1986; 110: 136–140

392. Jorda A, Portoles M, Rubio V. Liver fibrosis in arginase deficiency. Arch Pathol Lab Med 1987; 111: 691–692

393. Travers H, Reed J S, Kennedy J A. Ultrastructural study of the liver in argininosuccinase deficiency. Pediatr Pathol 1986; 5: 307–318

394. Elpeleg O N, Colombo J P, Amir N, Bachmann C, Hurvitz H. Late-onset form of partial N-acetyl-glutamate synthetase deficiency. Eur J Pediatr 1990; 149: 634–636

395. Bachman C, Krahenbuhl S, Colombo J P, Schubiger G, Jaggi K H, Tonz O. N-acetylglutamate synthetase deficiency: a disorder of ammonia detoxification. N Engl J Med 1981; 304: 543

396. Bachman C, Brandis M, Weissenbarth-Reidel E, Bughard R, Colombo J P N-acetylglutamate synthetase deficiency. A second case. J Inherit Metabol Dis 1988; 11: 191–193

397. Gahl W A, Renlund M, Thoenev G. Lysosomal transport disorders: Cystinosis and sialic acid storage disorders. In: Scriver C R, Beaudet A L, Sly W S, Valle D, eds. The metabolic basis of inherited disease, 6th edn. New York: McGraw-Hill, 1989: pp 2619–2647

398. Wong V G. The eye in cystinosis. In: Schulman J D, ed. Cystinosis. Washington, DC: Government Printing Office, 1973: pp 23–35

399. Chan A M, Lynch M J G, Bailey J D, Ezrin C, Fraser D. Hypothyroidism in cystinosis. Am J Med 1970; 48: 673–692

400. Avner E D, Ellis D, Jaffe R. Veno-occlusive disease of the liver associated with cysteamine treatment of nephropathic cystinosis. J Pediatr 1983; 102: 793–796

401. Broyer M, Guillot M, Gubler M C, Habib R. Infantile cystinosis: a reappraisal of early and late symptoms. Adv Nephrol 1981; 8: 127–131

402. Brubaker R F, Wong V G, Schulman J D, Seegmiller J E, Kawabare T. Benign cystinosis. The clinical, biochemical and morphological findings in a family with two affected siblings. Am J Med 1970; 49: 546–550

403. Seegmiller J E. Cystinosis. In: Hers H G, Van Hoof, eds. Lysosomes and storage diseases. New York: Academic Press, 1973: pp 485–513

404. Witzleben C L, Monteleone J A, Rejent A J. Electron microscopy in the diagnosis of cystinosis. Arch Pathol 1972; 94: 362–365

405. Haynes M E, Carter R F, Pollard A C, Carey W F. Light and electron microscopy of infants and foetal tissues in cystinosis. Micron 1980; 11: 443–444

406. Boman H, Schneider J A. Prenatal diagnosis of nephropathic cystinosis. Acta Paediatr Scand 1981; 70: 389–393

407. Lubec G, Nauer G, Pollack A. Non-invasive diagnosis of cystinosis by infra-red spectroscopy of hair. Lancet 1983; 1: 623

408. Schulman J D, Wong V, Olson W H, Seegmiller J E. Lysosomal site of crystalline deposits in cystinosis as shown by ferritin uptake. Arch Pathol 1970; 90: 259–284

409. Harms E. Cystinosis and liposomal free amino acids. In: Bianchi L, Gerok W, Landmann L, Sickinger K, Stalder G A, eds. Liver in metabolic diseases. Lancaster: MTP Press, 1983; pp 129–136

410. Spears G S. Pathology of the kidney in cystinosis. Pathol Annu 1974; 9: 81–92

411. Roels H. Pathology of aminoacidurias. In: Beckman L, Hauge M, eds. Monographs in human genetics. Basel: Karger, 1972: pp 79–80

412. Scotto J M, Stralin H G. Ultrastructure of the liver in a case of childhood cystinosis. Virchows Arch A Pathol Anat Histol 1977; 377: 43–48

413. Mudd S H, Levy H L, Flemming S. Disorders of transsulfuration. In: Scriver C R, Beaudet A L, Sly W S, Valle D, eds. The metabolic basis of inherited disease, 6th edn. New York: McGraw-Hill, 1989: pp 693–734

414. Clarke R, Daly L, Robinson K et al. Hyperhomocysteinemia: an independent risk for vascular disease. N Engl J Med 1991; 324: 199–200

415. Schimke R N, McKusick V A, Huang T, Pollack A D. Homocystinuria. Studies of 20 families with 38 affected members. JAMA 1963; 193: 711–719

416. Gibson J B, Carson N A J, Neill D W. Pathological findings in homocystinuria. J Clin Pathol 1964; 17: 427–437

417. Carson N A J, Dent C E, Field C M B, Gaull G E. Homocystinuria; clinical and pathological review of ten cases. J Pediatr 1965; 66: 565–583

418. Gaull G E, Sturman J A, Schaffner F. Homocystinuria due to cystathionine synthase deficiency: enzymatic and ultrastructural studies. J Pediatr 1974; 84: 381–390

419. Gaull G E, Schaffner F. Electron microscopic changes in hepatocytes of patients with homocystinuria. Pediatr Res 1971; 5: 23–32

420. Kane J B, Apolipoprotein B, structural and metabolic heterogeneity. Annu Rev Physiol 1983; 45: 637–650

421. Innerarity T L, Yough S G, Poksay K S et al. Structural relationship of human apolipoprotein B48 to apolipoprotein B100. J Clin Invest 1987; 80: 1794–1798

422. Hospattankur A V, Higuchi K, Law S W, Meglin N, Brewer H B. Identification of a novel in-frame translational stop codon in human intestine apo B mRNA. Biochem Biophys Res Commun 1987; 148: 279–285

423. Chen S-H, Habib G, Yang G-Y et al. Apolipoprotein B-48 is the product of a messenger RNA with an organ-specific in frame stop codon. Science 1987; 238: 363–366

424. Olofsson S-O, Bjursell G, Bostrom K et al. Apolipoprotein B: structure, biosynthesis, and the role in the lipoprotein assembly process. Atherosclerosis 1987; 68: 1–17

425. Talmud P J, Lloyd J K, Muller D P R, Collins D R, Scott J, Humphries S. Genetic evidence from two families that the B gene is not involved in abetalipoproteinemia. J Clin Invest 1988; 82: 1803–1806

426. Huang L S, Janne P A, DeGraaf J et al. Exclusion of linkage between the human apolipoprotein B. Am J Hum Genet 1990; 46: 1141–1148

427. Wetterau J R, Aggerbeck L P, Bouma M-E, Eisenberg C. Triglyceride transfer protein in individuals with abetalipoproteinemia. Science 1992; 258: 999–1001

428. Bassen F A, Kornzweig A L. Malformation of the erythrocytes in a case of a typical retinitis pigmentosa. Blood 1950; 5: 381–387

429. Jampel R S, Falls H F. Atypical retinitis pigmentosa, acanthocytosis, and heredodegenerative neuromuscular disease. Arch Ophthalmol 1958; 59: 818–820

430. Salt H B, Wolf O H, Lloyd J K, Fosbrook A S, Cameron A H, Hubble D V. On having no beta-lipoprotein: a syndrome comprising a-beta-lipoproteinaemia, acanthocytosis, and steatorrhoea. Lancet 1960; ii: 325–329

431. Isselbacher K J, Scheig R, Plotkin G R, Caulfield J B. Congenital beta-lipoprotein deficiency: an hereditary disorder involving a defect in the absorption and transport of lipids. Medicine 1964; 41: 347–361

432. Gotto A M, Levy R I, John K, Fredrickson D S. On the protein deficit in abetalipoproteinemia. N Engl J Med 1971; 284: 813–878

433. Lloyd J K. Hypolipoproteinaemia. J Clin Pathol 1973; 26 (Suppl) 5: 53–58

434. Kane J P, Havel R J. Disorders of the biogenesis and secretion of lipoproteins containing the beta-lipoproteins. In: Scriver C R, Beaudet A L, Sly W S, Valle D, eds. The metabolic basis of inherited disease, 6th edn. New York: McGraw-Hill, 1989: pp 1139–1164

435. Bieri J G, Hoeg J M, Schafer J, Zech L A, Brewer H B. Vitamin A and vitamin E replacement in abetalipoproteinemia. Ann Intern Med 1984; 100: 238–239

436. Partin J S, Partin J C, Schubert W K, McAdams J. Liver ultrastructure in abetalipoproteinemia: Evolution of micronodular cirrhosis. Gastroenterology 1974; 67: 107–118

437. Avigan M I, Ishak K G, Gregg R E, Hoofnagle J H. Morphologic features of the liver in abetalipoproteinemia. Hepatology 1984; 4: 1223–1226

438. Collins J C, Scheinberg H, Giblin D R, Sternlieb I. Hepatic peroxisomal abnormalities in abetalipoproteinemia. Gastroenterology 1989; 97: 766–770

439. Black D D, Hay R V, Rohwer-Nutter P L et al. Intestinal and hepatic apolipoprotein 13 gene expression in abetalipoproteinemia. Gastroenterology 1991; 101: 520–528

440. Glickman R M, Glickman J N, Magnum A, Brin M. Apolipoprotein synthesis in normal and abetalipoproteinemia intestinal mucosa. Gastroenterology 1991; 101: 749–755

441. Bouma M E, Beucler I, Pessah M et al. Description of two different patients with abetalipoproteinemia: synthesis of a normal-sized apolipoprotein B-48 in intestinal organ culture. J Lipid Res 1990; 31: 1–15

442. Ross R S, Gregg R E, Law S W et al. Homozygous hypobetalipoproteinemia: A disease distinct from abetalipo-proteinemia at the molecular level. J Clin Invest 1988; 81: 590–595

443. Malloy M J, Kane J P, Hardman D A, Hamilton R J, Dalal K B. Normotriglyceridemic abetalipoproteinemia: absence of the B-100 apolipoprotein. J Clin Invest 1981; 67: 1441–1450

444. Herbert P N, Hyams J S, Bernier D N et al. Apolipoprotein B-100 deficiency: intestinal steatosis despite apolipoprotein B48 synthesis. J Clin Invest 1985; 76: 403–412

445. Sternberg D, Grundy S M, Mok H I et al. Metabolic studies in an unusual case of asymptomatic familial hypobetalipoproteinemia and hypoalphahypoproteinemia and fasting chylomicronemia. J Clin Invest 1979; 64: 292

446. Young S G, Bertics S J, Curtise L K, Witzum J L 1987 Characterization of an abnormal species of apolipoprotein B, Apolipoprotein B-37, associated with familial hypobetalipoproteinemia. J Clin Invest 1987; 79: 1831–1841

447. Young S O, Bertics S J, Curtise L K, Dubois B W, Witztum J L. Genetic analysis of a kindred with familial hypobetalipoproteinemia. J Clin Invest 1987; 79: 1842–1851

448. Anderson C M, Townley R R W, Freeman J P. Unusual causes of steatorrhea in infancy and childhood. Med J Aust 1961; 11: 619–621

449. Roy C C, Levy E, Green P H R et al. Malabsorption, hypocholesterolemia, fat-filled enterocytes with increased intestinal apoprotein B: chylomicron retention disease. Gastroenterology 1987; 92: 390

450. Fredrickson D S, Altrocchi P H, Avioli L V, Goodman W S, Goodman H C. Tangier disease. Ann Intern Med 1961; 55: 1016–1031

451. Hoffman H N, Fredrickson D S. Tangier disease (familial high density lipoprotein deficiency). Clinical and genetic features in two adults. Am J Med 1965; 39: 582–593

452. Bale P M, Clifton-Bligh P, Benjamin B N P, Whyte H M. Pathology of Tangier disease. J Clin Pathol 1971; 24: 609–616

453. Assmann G, Schmitz G, Brewer H B. Familial high density lipoprotein deficiency: Tangier disease. In: Scriver C R, Beaudet A L, Sly W S, Valle D, eds. The metabolic basis of inherited disease, 6th edn. New York: McGraw-Hill, 1989: pp 1139–1164

454. Lux S E, Levy R I, Gotton A M, Fredrickson D S. Studies on the protein defect in Tangier disease. Isolation and characterization of an abnormal high density lipoprotein. J Clin Invest 1972; 51: 2505–2519

455. Ferrans V J, Fredrickson D S. The pathology of Tangier disease. Am J Pathol 1975; 78: 101–136

456. Brook J G, Lees R S, Yules J H, Cusack B. Tangier disease (alpha-lipoprotein deficiency). JAMA 1977; 238: 332–334

457. Kummer H, Laissue J, Spiess H, Pflugshaupt R, Bucher U.

Familiale Analphalipoproteinamie (Tangier-Krankheit). Schweitz Med Woch 1963; 98: 406–412

458. Dechelotte P, Kantelip B, de Laguillamie B V. Tangier disease. A histological and ultrastructural study. Pathol Res Pract 1985; 180: 424–430

459. Labbe A, Dechelotte P, Meyer M, Dubray C, Jouanel P. La maladie de Tangier. Une thesaurismose rare. Presse Med 1985; 14: 1189–1192

460. Goldstein J L, Brown M S. Familial hypercholesterolemia. In: Scriver C R, Beaudet A L, Sly W S, Valle D, eds. The metabolic basis of inherited disease, 6th edn. New York: McGraw-Hill, 1989: pp 1215–1250

461. Buja M, Kovanen P T, Bilheimer D W. Cellular pathology of homozygous familial hypercholesterolemia. Am J Pathol 1979; 327 –345

462. Bilheimer D W. Portacaval shunt and liver transplantation in treatment of familial hypercholesterolemia. Arteriosclerosis Suppl 1 1989; 9: 1-158–1-163.

463. Fredrickson D S, Gotto A M, Levi R. Familial lipoprotein deficiency. In: Stanbury J B, Wyngarden J B, Fredrickson D S, eds. The metabolic basis of inherited disease. New York: McGraw-Hill, 1972: pp 493–530

464. Schaefer E J, Levy R I. Pathogenesis and management of lipoprotein disorders. N Engl J Med 1985; 312: 1300–1310

465. Bruton O C, Kanter A J. Idiopathic familial hyperlipemia. Am J Dis Child 1951; 82: 153–159

466. Tanaka Y, Brecher G, Fredrickson D S. Cellules de la maladie de Niemann-Pick et de quelques autres lipoidoses. Nouv Rev Franc Hematol 1963; 3: 2–16

467. Roberts W C, Levy R I, Fredrickson D S. Hyperlipoproteinemia: A review of the five types with first report of necropsy findings in Type 3. Arch Pathol 1970; 90: 46–56

468. Kovacs K, Lee R, Little J A. Ultrastructural changes of hepatocytes in hyperlipoproteinemia. Lancet 1972; i: 752–753

469. O'Brien J S. Ganglioside-storage diseases. N Engl J Med 1971; 284: 893–896

470. O'Brien J S. B-galactosidase deficiency (G_1M_1 gangliosidosis, galactosialidosis, and Morguio syndrome type B); ganglioside sialidase deficiency (mucolipidosis IV). In: Scriver C R, Beaudet A L, Sly W S, Valle D, eds. The metabolic basis of inherited disease, 6th edn. New York: McGraw-Hill 1989: pp 1797–1806

471. Petrelli M, Blair J D. The liver in GM gangliosidosis types 1 and 2. Arch Pathol 1975; 99: 111–116

472. Volk B W, Wallace B J. The liver in lipidosis. An electron microscopic and histochemical study. Am J Pathol 1966; 49: 203–225

473. Alroy J, Orgad U, DeGasperi R et al. Canine G_1M_1-gangliosidosis: a clinical, morphologic, histochemical, and biochemical comparison of two different models. Am J Pathol 1992; 140: 675–689

474. Sandhoff K, Conzelmann E, Neufeld M, Kabach M M, Suzuki K. The GM_2 gangliosidoses. In: Scriver C R, Beaudet A L, Sly W S, Valle D, eds. The metabolic basis of inherited disease II, 6th edn. New York: McGraw-Hill, 1989: pp 1807–1842

475. Akli S, Chelly J, LaCorte J M, Poenaru L, Kahn A. Seven novel Tay-Sachs mutations detected by clinical mismatch cleavage of PCR-amplified cDNA fragments. Genomics 1991; 11: 124–134

476. Sandhoff K, Andreae V, Jatzkesvitz H. Deficient hexosaminadase activity in an exceptional case of Tay-Sachs disease with additional storage of kidney globoside in visceral organs. Life Sciences 1968; 7: 283–288

477. Desnick R J, Snyder P D, Desnick S J, Krivit W, Sharp H L. Sandhoff's disease: ultrastructural and biochemical studies. In: Volk R W, Aronson S M, eds. Sphingolipids, sphingolipidoses and allied disorders. New York: Plenum, 1972: pp 351–371

478. Desnick R J, Krivit W, Sharp H L. In utero diagnosis of Sandhoff's disease. Biochem Biophys Res Comm 1973; 51: 20–26

479. Krivit W, Desnick R J, Lee J et al. Generalized accumulation of neutral glycosphingolipid with GM_1 ganglioside accumulation in the brain, Sandhoff's disease (variant of Tay-Sach's disease). Am J Med 1972; 52: 763–770

480. Hadfield M G, Mammes P, David P B. The pathology of Sandhoff's disease. J Pathol 1977; 123: 137–144

481. Neote K, McInnes B, Mahuran D J, Gravel R A. Structure and distribution of an Alu-type deletion mutation in Sandhoff disease. J Clin Invest 1990; 86: 1524–1531

482. Desnick R J, Bishop D F. Fabry disease; alpha-galactosidase deficiency; Shindler Disease; alpha-N-alpha-N-acetylgalactosaminidase deficiency. In: Scriver C R, Beaudet A, Sly W S, Valle D, eds. The metabolic basis of inherited disease, 6th edn. New York: McGraw-Hill, 1989: pp 1751–1796

483. Brady R O, Gal A E, Bradley K M, Martenson E, Warshaw A L, Lester L. Enzymatic defect in Fabry's disease: ceramide trihexoside deficiency. N Engl J Med 1967; 276: 1163–1167

484. Rodriquez F H, Hoffman E O, Ordinario A T, Baliga M. Fabry's disease in a heterozygous woman. Arch Pathol Lab Med 1985; 109: 89–91

485. von Scheidt W, Eng C M, Fitzmaurice T F et al. An atypical variant of Fabry's disease with manifestations confined to the myocardium. N Engl J Med 1991; 324: 395–399

486. Desnick R J, Allen K Y, Simmonds L. Correction of enzymatic deficiencies by renal transplantation: Fabry's disease. Surgery 1972; 72: 203–211

487. Brady R O, King F M. Fabry's disease. In: Dyck P J, Thomas P K, Lambert E H, eds. Peripheral neuropathy, vol II. New York: Saunders, 1975: pp 914–927

488. Faraggiana T, Churg J, Grishman E et al. Light- and electron-microscopic histochemistry of Fabry's disease. Am J Pathol 1981; 103: 247–262

489. Meuwissen S G M, Dingemans K P, Stryland A, Taer J M, Ooms B C M. Ultrastructural and biochemical liver analyses in Fabry's disease. Hepatology 1982; 2: 263–268

490. Austin J H, Balasubramian A S, Habiraman T M, Sarawattir S, Basu D K, Bachhaut B K. A controlled study of enzyme activities on three human disorders of glycolipid metabolism. J Neurochem 1963; 70: 805–816

491. Kolodny E H. Metachromatic leukodystrophy and multiple sulfatase deficiency: Sulfatide lipidosis. In: Scriver C R, Beaudet A L, Sly W S, Valle D, eds. The metabolic basis of inherited diseases. New York: McGraw-Hill, 1989: pp 1721–1750

492. Muller D, Pilz H, Meulen V. Studies on adult metachromatic leukodystrophy. I. Clinical morphological and histochemical observations in two cases. J Neurol Sci 1969; 9: 567–584

493. Kaback M M, Howell R R. Infantile metachromatic leukodystrophy; deficiency of arylsulfatase A in fibroblasts. N Engl J Med 1970; 282: 1336–1340

494. Rattazi M C, Davidson R G. Prenatal diagnosis of metachromatic leukodystrophy by electrophoretic and immunologic techniques. Pediatr Res 1977; 11: 1030–1035

495. Wolfe H J, Pietra G G. The visceral lesions of metachromatic leukodystrophy. Am J Pathol 1964; 44: 921–930

496. Austin J. Metachromatic leukodystrophy (sulfatide lipidosis). In: Hers H G, Van Hoof F, eds. Lysosomes and storage diseases. New York: Academic Press, 1973: pp 411–437

497. Hagberg B, Sourander P, Svennerholm L. Sulfatide lipidosis in childhood. Am J Dis Child 1962; 104: 644–656

498. Dalinka M K, Rosen R A, Kurth R J, Hemming V G. Metachromatic leukodystrophy, a cause of cholelithiasis in childhood. Am J Dig Dis 1969; 14: 603–606

499. Dische M R. Metachromatic leukodystrophic polyposis of the gallbladder. J Pathol Bacteriol 1969; 97: 388–390

500. Kohn R. Papillomatosis of the gallbladder in metachromatic leukodystrophy. Am J Clin Pathol 1969; 52: 737–740

501. Warfel K A, Hull M T. Villous papilloma of the gallbladder in association with leukodystrophy. Hum Pathol 1984; 15: 1192–1194

502. Burgess J H, Kalfayan B, Shingaard R K, Gilbert E. Papillomatosis of the gallbladder associated with metachromatic leukodystrophy. Arch Pathol Lab Med 1985; 109: 79–81

503. Tesluk H, Munn R J, Schwartz M Z, Ruebner B H. Papillomatous transformation of the ballbladder in metachromatic leukodystrophy. Pediatr Pathol 1989; 9: 741–746

504. Siegel E G, Lucke H, Schauer W, Creutzfeldt W. Repeated upper gastrointestinal hemorrhage caused by metachromatic leukodystrophy of the gall bladder. Digestion 1992; 51: 121–124

505. Barranger J A, Ginns E I. Glucosylceramide lipidosis: Gaucher

disease. In: Scriver C R, Beaudet A L, Sly W S, Valle D, eds. The metabolic basis of inherited disease, 6th edn. New York: McGraw-Hill, 1989; pp 1677–1698

506. Beaudet A L. Gaucher's disease. N Engl J Med 1987; 316: 619–620

507. Zimran A, Kay A, Gelbart T et al. Gaucher's disease. Clinical, laboratory, radiologic, and genetic features of 53 patients. Medicine 1992; 71: 337–353

508. Rubin M, Yampolski F, Lambrozo R, Zaizov R, Dintsman M. Partial splenectomy in Gaucher's disease. J Pediatr Surg 1986; 21: 125–128

509. Cohen I J, Katz K, Freud E, Zer M, Zaigov R. Long-term follow-up of partial splenectomy in Gaucher's disease. Am J Surg 1992; 164: 345–347

510. Ginsburg H N, Groll M. Hydrops fetalis due to infantile Gaucher's disease. J Pediatr 1973; 82: 1046–1048

511. Sun C C, Panny S. Combs J, Gutberlett R. Hydrops fetalis associated with Gaucher disease. Pathol Res Pract 1984; 179: 101–104

512. Sidransky E, Sherer D M, Ginns E L. Gaucher disease in the neonate: a distinct Gaucher phenotype is analogous to a mouse model created by targeted disruption of the glucocerebrosidase gene. Pediatr Res 1992; 32: 494–498

513. Sidransky E, Ginns E I. Clinical heterogeneity among patients with Gaucher's disease. JAMA 1993; 269: 1154–1157

514. James S P, Stromeyer F W, Chang C, Barranger J A. Liver abnormalities in patients with Gaucher's disease. Gastroenterology 1981; 80: 126–133

515. Stone R, Benson J, Tronic B, Brennan T. Hepatic calcification in a patient with Gaucher's disease. Am J Gastroenterol 1982; 77: 95–98

516. Schneider E L, Epstein C J, Kaback M J, Brandes D. Severe pulmonary involvement in adult Gaucher's disease. Report of three cases and review of the literature. Am J Med 1977; 63: 475–480

517. Carlson D E, Busuttil R W, Giudici T A, Barranger J A. Orthotopic liver transplantation in the treatment of complications of Type I Gaucher disease. Transplantation 1990; 49: 1192–1194

518. Brady R O, Kanfer J N, Shapiro D. Metabolism of glucocerebrosides. II. Evidence of enzymatic deficiency in Gaucher's disease. Biochem Biophys Res Commun 1965; 18: 221–225

519. Patrick A D. A deficiency of glucocerebrosidase in Gaucher's disease. Biochem J 1965; 97: 17C–18C

520. Christomanou H, Aignesberger A, Linke R P. Immunochemical characterization of two activator proteins simulating enzymatic sphingomyelin degradation in vitro. Absence of one of them in a human Gaucher disease variant. Biol Chem Hoppa Seyler 1986; 367: 879–890

521. Kattlove H E, Williams J C, Gaynor E, Spivak M, Bradley R M, Brady R O. Gaucher cells in chronic myelocytic leukemia, an acquired abnormality. Blood 1969; 334: 379–390

522. Barneveld R A, Keijzer W, Tegelaers F P W et al. Assignment of the gene coding for human B-glucocerebrosidase to the region of q21-q31 of chromosome 1 using monoclonal antibodies. Hum Genet 1983; 64: 227

523. Horowitz M, Wilder S, Horowitz Z, Reiner O, Gelbart T, Beutler E. The human glucocerebrosidase gene and pseudogene structure and evolution. Genomics 1989; 4: 87–96

524. Theophilus B D M, Latham T, Grabowski G A, Smith F I. Comparison of RNase A, chemical cleavage, and GC-clamped denaturing gradient gel electrophoresis for the detection of mutations in exon 9 of the human acid B-glucosidase gene. Nucleic Acid Res 1989; 17: 7707–7722

525. Zimran A, Sorge J, Gross E, Kubitz M, West C, Bentler E. Prediction of severity of Gaucher's disease by identification of mutations at DNA level. Lancet 1989; ii: 349–352

526. Tsuji S, Choudary P V, Martin B M et al. A mutation in the human glucocerebrosidase gene in neuronopathic Gaucher disease. N Engl J Med 1987; 316: 570

527. Feron N, Kolodny E, Eyal W, Horowitz M. Mutation specific genotyping in Gaucher disease by selective amplification of the active glucocerebrosidase gene. Am J Hum Genet 1990; 46: 527

528. Barton N W, Brady R O, Dumbrosia J M et al. Replacement therapy for inherited enzyme deficiency-macrophage-targeted glucocerebrosidase for Gaucher's disease. N Engl J Med 1991; 324: 1464–1470

529. Mistry P K, Davies S, Corfield A, Dixon A K, Cox T M. Successful treatment of bone marrow failure with low-dose modified glucocerebrosidase. Q J Med 1992; 83: 541–546

530. Rappaport J M, Ginns E I. Bone-marrow transplantation in severe Gaucher's disease. N Engl J Med 1984; 311: 84–88

531. Tsai P, Lipton J M, Sahdev I et al. Allogenic bone marrow transplantation in severe Gaucher disease. Pediatr Res 1992; 31: 503–507

532. Smanik E J, Tavill A S, Jacobs G H et al. Orthotopic liver transplantation in two adults with Niemann-Pick and Gaucher's disease: implications for the treatment of inherited metabolic diseases. Hepatology 1993; 17: 42–49

533. Starzl T E, Demetris A J, Trucco M et al. Chimerism after liver transplantation for type IV glycogen storage disease and type I Gaucher's disease. N Engl J Med 1993; 328: 745–749

534. Burns G F, Cawley J C, Flemans R J et al. Surface marker and other charaterics of Gaucher's cells. J Clin Pathol 1977; 30: 981–983

535. Djaldetti M, Fishman P, Bessler H. The surface ultrastructure of Gaucher cells. Am J Clin Pathol 1979; 71: 146–150

536. Peters S P, Lee R E, Glen R H. Gaucher's disease. A review. Medicine 1977; 56: 425–442

537. Hibbs R G, Ferrans V J, Cipriano P R, Tardiff K J. A histo-chemical and electron microscopic study of Gaucher cells. Arch Pathol 1970; 89: 137–153

538. Brady R O, King F M. Gaucher's disease. In: Hers H G, Van Hoof F, eds. Lysosomes and storage diseases. New York: Academic Press, 1973: pp 381–394

539. Gall E A, Landing B H. Hepatic cirrhosis and hereditary disorders of metabolism. Am J Clin Pathol 1956; 26: 1398–1426

540. Cadaval R L, Gonzalez-Campora R, Davidson H G, Vicente A M. Cirrosis hepatica en la enfermedad de Gaucher. Gastroenterol Hepatol 1983; 6: 299–301

541. Benita Leon V, Garcia Cabezudo J, Gomex Tabera C et al. Enfermedad de Gaucher con cirrosis y gammapetia monoclonal benigna. Gastroenterol Hepatol 1985; 8: 354–357

542. Patel S C, Davis G L, Barranger J A. Gaucher's disease in a patient with chronic active hepatitis. Am J Med 1986; 80: 523–525

543. Lee R L. The bilayer nature of deposits occurring in Gaucher's disease. Arch Biochem Biophys 1973; 159: 259–266

544. Lorber M, Niemes J L. Identification of ferritin within Gaucher cells. An electron microscopic and immunofluorescent study. Acta Haematol 1967; 37: 18

545. Spence M W, Callahan J W. Sphingomyelin-cholesterol lipidoses: the Neimann-Pick group of diseases. In: Scriver R C, Beaudet A L, Sly W S, Valle D, eds. The metabolic basis of inherited disease, 6th edn. New York: McGraw-Hill, 1989: pp 1655–1676

546. Brady R O, Kanfer J N, Mock M D, Fredrickson D S. The metabolism of sphingomyelin II. Evidence of an enzymatic deficiency in Niemann-Pick disease. Proc Natl Acad Sci USA 1966; 55: 366–369

547. Butler J D, Comly M E, Kruth H S et al. Niemann-Pick variant disorders: Comparison of errors in cellular cholesterol homeostatis in group D and group C fibroblasts. Proc Natl Acad Sci USA 1987; 84: 556–560

548. Liscum L, Faust J R. Low-density lipoprotein (LDL)-mediated suppression of cholesterol synthesis and LDL uptake is defective in Niemann-Pick type C fibroblasts. J Biol Chem 1987; 262: 17002–17008

549. Bowler L M, Shankaran R, Das I, Callahan J W. Cholesterol esterification and Niemann-Pick disease. An approach to identifying the defect in fibroblasts. J Neurosci Res 1990; 27: 505–511

550. Pereira L, Desnick R J, Heller D, Disteche C M, Schuckman E H. Regional assignment of the human acid sphingomyelinase gene (5 MPD1) by PCR analysis of somatic cell hybrids and in situ hybridization to 11p15.1–15.4. Genomics 1987; 9: 229–234

551. Levran O, Desnick R J, Schuchman E H. Niemann-Pick disease: a frequent massive mutation in the acid sphingomyelinase gene of

Ashkenazi type A & B patients. Proc Natl Acad Sci USA 1991; 88: 3748–3752

552. Levran O, Desnick R J, Schuchman E H. Niemann-Pick type B disease. Identification of a single codon deletion in the acid sphingomyelinase gene and genotypic/phenotypic correlations in type A & B patients. J Clin Invest 1991; 88: 806–810

553. Vellodi A, Hobbs J R, O'Donnell N M et al Treatment of Niemann-Pick disease type B by allogeneic bone marrow transplantation. Br Med J 1987; 295: 1375–1376

554. Gartner J C Jr, Bergman I, Malatack J J et al. Progression of neurovisceral storage disease with supranuclear ophthalmoplegia following orthotopic liver transplantation. Pediatrics 1986; 77: 104–106

555. Duloze P, Delvin E E, Glorieaux F H, Corman J L, Bettez P, Toussi T. Replacement therapy for inherited enzyme deficiency. Liver orthotopic transplantation in Niemann-Pick disease type A. Am J Med Genet 1977; 1: 229–239

556. Scaggianle B, Pineschi A, Sustersich M, Anbolina M, Agosti E, Romea D. Successful therapy of Niemann-Pick disease by implantation of human amniotic membrane. Transplantation 1987; 44: 59–61

557. Schoenfeld A, Abramovici A, Kilbanski C, Ovadia J. Placental ultra-sonographic biochemical and histochemical studies in human fetuses affected with Niemann-Pick type A. Placenta 1985; 6: 33–44

558. Crocker A C, Farber S. Niemann-Pick disease: a review of 18 patients. Medicine 1958; 37: 1–95

559. Lebrune P, Bedossa P, Huguet P, Roset F, Vanier M T, Odievre M. Fatal liver failure in two children with Niemann-Pick disease type B. J Pediatr Gastroenterol Nutr 1991; 13: 104–109

560. Tassoni J P, Fawaz K A, Johnston D E. Cirrhosis and portal hypertension in a patient with adult Niemann-Pick disease. Gastroenterology 1991; 100: 567–569

561. Ashkenazi A, Yarom R, Gutman A, Abrahamov A, Russell A. Niemann-Pick disease and giant cell transformation of the liver. Acta Paediatr Scand 1971; 60: 285–294

562. Rutledge J C. Case 5 Progressive neonatal liver disease due to Type C Niemann-Pick disease. Pediatr Pathol 1989; 9: 779–784

563. Elleder M, Smid F, Hymova H. Liver findings in Niemann-Pick disease Type C. Histochem J 1984; 16: 1147–1170

564. Ivemark B I, Svennerholm I, Thoren C et al. Niemann-Pick disease in infancy: report of two siblings with clinical, histologic and biochemical studies. Acta Paediatr Scand 1963; 52: 391–404

565. Jaeken J, Proesmans W, Eggermont E et al. Niemann-Pick type C disease and early cholestasis in three brothers. Acta Paediatr Belg 1980; 33: 43–46

566. Semeraro L A, Riely C A, Kolodny E H, Dickerson G R, Gryboski J D. Niemann-Pick variant lipidosis presenting as "neonatal hepatitis". J Pediatr Gastroenterol Nutr 1986; 5: 492–500

567. Gartner J C, Bergman I, Malatack J J et al. Progression of neurovisceral storage disease with supranuclear ophthalmoplegia following orthotopic liver transplantation. Pediatrics 1986; 77: 104–106

568. Grover W D, Naiman J L. Progressive paresis of vertical gaze in lipid storage disease. Neurology 1971; 21: 896–899

569. Neville B G R, Lake B D, Stephens R, Sanders M D. A neurovisceral storage disease with vertical supranuclear ophthalmoplegia, and its relationship to Niemann-Pick disease. A report of nine patients. Brain 1973; 96: 97–120

570. Breen L, Morris H H, Alperin J B, Schochet S S Jr. Juvenile Niemann-Pick disease with vertical supranuclear ophthalmoplegia. Arch Neurol 1981; 38: 388–390

571. Yan-Go F I, Yanagihara T, Pierre R V, Goldstein N P. A progressive neurologic disorder with supranuclear vertical gaze paresis and distinctive bone marrow cells. Mayo Clin Proc 1984; 59: 404–410

572. Fink J K, Filling-Katz M R, Sokol J et al. Clinical spectrum of Niemann-Pick disease type C. Neurology 1989; 39: 1040–1049

573. Vanier M T, Rousson R M, Mandom G, Choiset A, Lake B D, Pentchev R G. Diagnosis of Niemann-Pick disease type C on chorionic villus cells. Lancet 1989; i: 1014–1015

574. Tamaru J, Iwasaki I, Horie H et al. Niemann-Pick disease associated with liver disorders. Acta Pathol Jpn 1985; 35: 1267–1272

575. Witzleben C L, Palmieri M J, Watkins J B, Hogan P. Sphingomyelin lipidosis variant with cirrhosis in the pediatric age group. Arch Pathol Lab Med 1986; 110: 508–512

576. Brady R O, King F M. Niemann-Pick disease. In: Hers H G, Van Hoof F, eds. Lysosomes and storage diseases. New York: Academic Press, 1973: pp 439–452

577. Wenger D A, Bartha G, Githens J H. Nine cases of sphingomyelin lipidosis, a new variant in Spanish-American children. Juvenile variant of Niemann-Pick disease with foamy and sea-blue histiocytes. Am J Dis Child 1977; 131: 955–961

578. Long R G, Lake R D, Pettit J E, Scheuer P J, Sherlock S. Adult Niemann-Pick disease. Its relationship to the syndrome of the sea-blue histiocyte. Am J Med 1977; 62: 627–635

579. Lynn R, Terry R D. Lipid histochemistry and electron microscopy in adult Niemann-Pick disease. Am J Med 1964; 37: 987–994

580. Machim G A. Hydrops revisited. Literature review of 1414 cases published. Am J Med Genet 1989; 34: 366–390

581. Abramov A, Schorr S, Wolman M. Generalized xanthomatosis with calcified adrenals. Am J Dis Child 1956; 91: 282–286

582. Meyers W F, Hoeg J M, DeMosky S J, Herbst J J, Brewer H B. The use of parenteral hyperalimentation and elemental formula feeding in the treatment of Wolman disease. Nutr Res 1988; 5: 423–429

583. Kikuchi M, Igarashi K, Noro T, Fgarashi Y, Hirokka M, Tada K. Evaluation of jejunal function in Wolman's disease. J Pediatr Gastroenterol Nutr 1991; 12: 65–69

584. Philippart M, Durand P, Borrone C. Neutral lipid storage with acid lipase deficiency: a new variant of Wolman's disease with features of the Senior syndrome. Pediatr Res 1982; 16: 954–959

585. Wolman M, Sterk V V, Gatt S, Frenkel M. Primary familial xanthomatosis with involvement and calcification of the adrenals. Pediatrics 1961; 28: 742–745

586. Crocker A C, Vawter G W, Neuhauser E B D, Bonkowsky A. Wolman's disease: three new patients with a previously described lipidosis. Pediatrics 1965; 35: 627–640

587. Schmitz G, Assman G. Acid lipase deficiency: Wolman disease and cholesteryl ester storage disease. In: Scriver C R, Beaudet A, Sly W S, Valle D, eds. The metabolic basis of inherited disease. New York: McGraw-Hill, 1989: pp 1623–1654

588. Lake B D, Patrick A D. Wolman's disease: deficiency of E600 resistant acid esterase with storage of lipids in lysosomes. J Pediatr 1970; 76: 262–266

589. Burge J A, Schubert W K. Deficient activity of hepatic lipase in cholesterol ester storage disease. Science 1972; 176: 309

590. Suzuki Y, Sakoe K, Kobayashi A, Ohbe Y, Endo H. Partial deficiency of acid lipase with storage of triglyceride and cholesterol esters in liver. Genetic variant of Wolman's disease? Clin Chim Acta 1976; 69: 219–224

591. Lake B D. Histochemical detection of the enzyme deficiency in blood films in Wolman's disease. J Clin Pathol 1971; 24: 617–620

592. Schiff L, Schubert W K, McAdams A J, Spiegel E L, O'Donnell J F. Hepatic cholesterol ester storage disease: a familial disorder. Am J Med 1968; 44: 538–546

593. Michels V V, Driscoll D J, Ferry G D et al. Pulmonary vascular obstruction associated with cholesteryl ester storage disease. J Pediatr 1979; 94: 621–623

594. Dincsoy H P, Rolfes D B, McGraw C A, Schubert W K. Cholesterol ester storage disease and mesenteric lipodystrophy. Am J Clin Pathol 1984; 81: 263–269

595. Patrick A D, Lake B D. Deficiency of acid lipase in Wolman's disease. Nature 1969; 222: 1067–1068

596. Tarantino M D, McNamara D J, Grandstone F, Ellefson R D, Fluger E C, Udall J W. Lovastatin therapy for cholesterol ester storage disease in two sisters. J Pediatr 1991; 118: 131–135

597. Ginsberg H N, Le N A, Short P, Ramakrishnan R, Desnick R J. Suppression of apolipoprotein production during treatment of cholesteryl ester storage disease with lovastatin. J Clin Invest 1987; 80: 1692–1697

598. DiBisceglie A M, Ishak K G, Rabin L, Hoeg J M. Cholesteryl ester storage disease: hepatopathology and effects of therapy with lovastatin. Hepatology 1990; 11: 764–772

599. Leone L, Ippolitti P E. Use of simvastatin plus cholestyramine in

the treatment of lysosomal lipase deficiency. J Pediatr 1991; 119: 1008–1109

600. Glueck C J, Lichtenstein P, Tracy T, Speirs J. Safety and efficacy of treatment of pediatric cholesterol ester storage disease with lovastatin. Pediatr Res 1992; 32: 559–565

601. Ferry G D, Whisennand H H, Finegold M J, Alpert E, Glombick A. Liver transplantation for cholesteryl ester storage disease. J Pediatr Gastroenterol and Nutr 1991; 12: 376–378

602. Marshall W C, Ockenden B G, Fosbrooke A S, Cumings J N. Wolman's disease. A rare lipidosis with adrenal calcification. Arch Dis Childh 1969; 46: 331–341

603. Miller R, Bialer M G, Rogers F, Johnson H T, Allen R V, Hennigar G R. Wolman's disease: report of a case with multiple studies. Arch Pathol Lab Med 1982; 106: 41–45

604. Lake B D, Patrick A D. Wolman's disease: deficiency of E600 resistant acid esterase with storage of lipids in lysosomes. J Pediatr 1970; 76: 262–266

605. Lough J, Fawcett J, Wiegensberg B. Wolman's disease. An electron microscopic, histochemical and biochemical study. Arch Pathol 1970; 89: 103–110

606. Beaudet A L, Ferry G D, Nichols B L, Rosenberg H S. Cholesterol ester storage disease: clinical, biochemical and pathological studies. J Pediatr 1977; 90: 910–914

607. Von Bogaert L, Scherer H J, Epstein E. Une forme cerebrale de cholesterinose generalisee. Paris: Masson, 1937

608. Bjorkhem I, Skrede S. Familial diseases with storage of sterols other than cholesterol. Cerebrotendinous xanthomatosis and phytosterolemia. In: Scriver C R, Beaudet A L, Sly W S, Valle D, eds. The metabolic basis of inherited disease, 6th edn. New York: McGraw-Hill, 1989: pp 1283–1302

609. Oftebro H, Bjorkhem I, Skrede S, Schreiner A, Pedersen J I. Cerebro-tendinous xanthomatosis: a defect in mitochondrial 26-hydroxylation required for normal biosynthesis of cholic acid. J Clin Invest 1980; 65: 1418–1430

610. Skrede S, Bjorkhem I, Kvittingen E A et al Demonstration of 26-hydroxylation of C_{27}-steroid in human skin fibroblasts, and a deficiency of this activity in cerebrotendinous xanthomatosis. J Clin Invest 1986; 78: 729–735

611. Koopman B J, Waterreus F J, Van Den Brekel H W C, Wolthers B G. Detection of carriers of cerebrotendinous xanthomatosis. Clin Chem Acta 1986; 158: 179–186

612. Cruyberg J R M, Webers R A, Tolboom J J M. Juvenile cataract associated with chronic diarrhea in pediatric cerebrotendinous xanthomatosis. Am J Ophthalmol 1991; 119: 606–607

613. Arlazoroff A, Roitberg B, Werber F, Shield R, Berginer V M. Epileptic seizure as a presenting symptom of cerebrotendinous xanthomatosis. Epilepsia 1991; 32: 657–661

614. Salen G, Zaki G, Sobesin S, Boehme D, Shefer S, Mosbach E H. Intrahepatic pigment and crystal forms in patients with cerebrotendinous xanthomatosis (CTX). Gastroenterology 1978; 74: 82–89

615. Boehme D H, Sobel H J, Marquet E, Salen G. Liver in cerebro-tendinous xanthomatosis (CTX): a histochemical and EM study of four cases. Pathol Res Pract 1980; 170: 192–201

616. Berginer V M, Salen G, Shefer S. Long-term treatment of cerebrotendinous xanthomatosis with chenodeoxycholic acid. N Engl J Med 1984; 311: 1649–1652

617. Hale D E, Bennett M J. Fatty acid oxidation disorders. A new class of metabolic diseases. J Pediatr 1992; 121: 1–11

617a. Vockley J. The changing face of disorders of fatty acid oxidation. Mayo Clin Proc 1994; 69: 249–257

618. Karpati G, Carpenter S, Engel A G et al. The syndrome of systemic carnitine deficiency. Clinical, morphologic, biochemical and pathophysiologic features. Neurology 1975; 25: 16–24

619. Weber L J, Valle D, Neil C, DiMauro S, Shug A. Carnitine deficiency presenting as familial cardiomyopathy: a treatable defect in carnitine transport. J Pediatr 1982; 101: 700–705

620. Treem W R, Stanley C A, Finegold D N, Hale D E, Coates P M. Primary carnitine deficiency due to failure of carnitine transport in kidney, muscle and fibroblasts. N Engl J Med 1988; 319: 1331–1336

621. Stanley C A, DeLeeuw S, Coates P M et al. Cartinine uptake defect: Chronic myopathy or acute coma in children with a

defect in carnitine uptake. Ann Neurol 1991, 30: 709–716

622. Ericksson B O, Lindstedt S, Mordlin I. Hereditary defect in carnitine membrane transport in expressed in skin fibroblasts. Eur J Pediatr 1988; 147: 662–663

623. Bremmer J. Carnitine metabolism and functions. Physiol Rev 1983; 63: 1420–1480

624. Stanley C A, Hale D E, Berry G T, DeLeeuw S, Boxer J, Bonnefont J-P. Brief report: A deficiency of carnitine-acylcarnitine transferase in the inner mitochondrial membrane. N Engl J Med 1992; 327: 19–23

625. Bougneres P-F, Saudubray J M, Marsac C, Bernard O, Odievre M, Girard J. Fasting hypoglycemia resulting from hepatic carnitine palmitoyl transferase deficiency. J Pediatr 1981; 98: 742–746

626. De Maugre F, Bonnefont J-P, Mitchell G et al. Hepatic and muscular presentations of carnitine palmitoyl transferase deficiency: two distinct entities. Pediatr Res 1988; 24: 308–311

627. Fahk-Borenstein Z C, Jordan S C, Saudubary J-M et al. Brief report: renal tubular acidosis in cartinine palmitoyltransferase type I deficiency. N Engl J Med 1992; 327: 24–27

628. DiMauro S, DiMauro M M. Muscle carnitine palmitoyl transferase deficiency and myoglobinuria. Science 1973; 182: 929–931

629. Hug G, Bove K E, Soukup S. Lethal neonatal multiorgan deficiency of carnitine palmitoyl-transferase II. N Engl J Med 1991; 325: 1862–1864

630. De Maugre F, Bonnefont J-P, Colonna M, Cipahic C, Lerouy J-P, Saudubray J-M. Infantile form of carnitine palmitoyl-transferase II deficiency with hepatomuscular symptoms and sudden death. J Clin Invest 1991; 87: 859–864

631. Finocchiaro G, Taroni F, Rochli M et al. CDNA cloning, sequence analysis and chromosomal localization of the gene for human carnitine palmitoyl-transferase. Proc Natl Acad Sci USA 1991; 88: 661–665

632. Hale D E, Batshaw M L, Coates P M et al. Long-chain acyl coenzyme A dehydrogenase deficiency: an inherited cause of nonketotic hypoglycemia. Pediatr Res 1985; 19: 666–671

633. Treem W R, Witzelben C A, Piccoli D A et al. Medium-chain and long-chain acyl CoA dehydrogenase deficiency: clinical, pathologic and ultrastructural differentiation from Reye syndrome. Hepatology 1986; 6: 1270–1278

634. Stanley C A. New genetic defects in mitochondrial fatty acid oxidation and carnitine deficiency. Adv Pediatr 1987; 34: 59–88

635. Kolvras S, Gregersen N, Christensen E, Holboth N. In vivo fibroblast studies in a patient with C_6-C_{10}-dicarboxylic aciduria: evidence for a defect in general acyl-CoA dehydrogenase. Clin Chim Acta 1982; 126: 53–67

636. Stanley C A, Hale D E, Coates P M et al. Medium chain acyl-CoA dehydrogenase deficiency in children with non-ketotic hypo-glycinemia and low carnitine levels. Pediatr Res 1983; 17: 877–884

637. Roe C R, Coates P M. Acyl-CoA dehydrogenase deficiency. In: Scriver C R, Beaudet A L, Sly W S, Valle D, eds. The metabolic basis of inherited diseases, 6th edn. McGraw-Hill: New York, 1989: pp 889–914

638. Blakemore A I F, Singleton H, Pollitt R J et al. Frequency of the G985 MCAD mutation in the general population. Lancet 1991; 337: 298–299

639. Ikeda Y Y, O'Kamura-Ikeda K, Tanaka K. Purification and characterization of short chain, medium chain, and long chain acyl-CoA dehydrogenase from rat liver mitochondria: isolation of the holo- and apoenzymes and conversion of the apoenzyme to holoenzyme. J Biol Chem 1985; 260: 1311–1325

640. Matsubara Y, Kraus J P, Yang-Feng T L, Franke U, Rosenberg L E, Tanaka K. Molecular cloning of cDNAs encoding rat and human medium chain acyl-CoA dehydrogenase and assignment of the gene to human chromosome 1. Proc Natl Acad Sci 1986; 83: 6543–6547

641. Rinaldo P, O'Shear J J, Coates P M, Hale D E, Stanley C A, Tanaka K. Medium chain acyl-CoA dehydrogenase deficiency: Diagnosis by stable-isotope dilution measurement of urinary n-hexanoylglycine and 3-phenylpropionylglycine. N Engl J Med 1988; 319: 1308–1313

642. Roe C R, Mellington D S, Maltley D A, Kinnebreau P. Recognition of medium chain acyl-CoA dehydrogenase deficiency

in asymptomatic siblings of children dying of sudden infant death or Reyes-like syndromes. J Pediatr 1986; 108: 13–18

643. Amendt B A, Green C, Sweetman L et al. Short-chain acyl-CoA dehydrogenase deficiency: clinical and biochemical studies in 2 patients. J Clin Invest 1987; 79: 1303–1309

644. Coates P M, Hale D E, Finocchioro G, Tanaka K, Winter S C. Genetic deficiency short-chain acyl-coenzyme A dehydrogenase in cultured fibroblasts from a patient with muscle carnitine deficiency and severe skeletal weakness. J Clin Invest 1987; 81: 171–175

645. Barton D E, Yang-Feng T L, Finocchioro G, Ozasa H, Tanaka K, Franke U. Short chain acyl-CoA dehydrogenase (ACADS) maps to chromosome 12(q22-qter) and the electron transfer flavoprotein (ETFA) to 15(q23–q25). Cytogenet Cell Genet 1987; 46: 577–578

646. Natio E, Indo Y, Tanaka K. Short chain acyl-coenzyme A dehydrogenase (SCAD) deficiency. Immunochemical demonstration of molecular heterogeneity due to variant SCAD with differing stability. J Clin Invest 1989; 84: 1671–1674

647. Natio E, Indo Y, Tanaka K. Identification of two variant short chain acyl-coenzyme A dehydrogenase alleles, each containing a different point mutation in a patient with short chain acyl-coenzyme A dehydrogenase deficiency. J Clin Invest 1990; 85: 1575–1582

648. Gregerson N, Wintzensen H, Holorua S et al. C_6-C_{10} decarboxylic aciduria: Investigations of a patient with riboflavin responsive multiple acyl-CoA dehydrogenase defects. Pediatr Res 1982; 16: 861–868

649. Glasgow A M, Engel A G, Bier D M et al. Hypoglycemia, hepatic dysfunction, muscle weakness, cardiomyopathy, free carnitine deficiency and long-chain acyl carnitine excess responsive to medium chain triglyceride diet. Pediatr Res 1983; 17: 319–326

650. Vici C P, Burlima A B, Bertini E et al. Progressive neuropathy and recurrent myoglobinuria in a child with long chain 3 hydroxyacyl-coenzyme A dehydrogenase deficiency. J Pediatr 1992; 118: 744–760

651. Wanders R J A, Duran M, Ijlst L et al. Sudden infant death and long-chain-3-hydroxyacyl-CoA dehydrogenase. Lancet 1989; ii: 52–53

652. Tein I, De Vivo D C, Hale D E et al. Short-chain L-3 hydroxyacyl-CoA dehydrogenase deficiency in muscle: a new cause for recurrent myoglobinuria and encephalopathy. Ann Neurol 1991; 30: 415–419

653. Moser H W, Moser A B, Chen W W, Shram A W. Ceramidase deficiency: Farber lipogranulomatosis. In: Scriver C R, Beaudet A L, Sly W S, Valle D, eds. The metabolic basis of inherited disease, 6th edn. New York: McGraw-Hill, 1989: pp 1645–1654

654. Rutsaert J, Tondeur M, Vamos-Hurwitz E, Dustin P. The cellular lesions of Farber's disease and their experimental reproduction in tissue culture. Lab Invest 1977; 36: 474–480

655. Antonarakis S, Valle D, Moser H W, Moser A, Qualinan S J, Zinkham W H. Phenotypic variability in siblings with Farber disease. J Pediatr 1984; 104: 406–409

656. Abul-Haj S K, Martz D G, Douglas W F, Geppert L J. Farber's disease. Report of a case with observations and notes on the nature of the stored material. J Pediatr 1962; 61; 221–232

657. Crocker A C, Cohen J, Farber S. The "lipogranulomatosis" syndrome: review with report of patient showing milder involvement. In: Aronson S M, Volk B W, eds. Inborn diseases of sphingolipid metabolism. Oxford: Pergamon, 1967: pp 485–503

658. Van Hoof F, Hers H G. Other lysosomal storage disorders. In: Hers H G, Van Hoof F, eds. Lysosomes and storage diseases. New York: Academic Press, 1973: pp 553–573

659. Tanaka T, Takahashi K, Hakozaki H, Kimoto H, Suzuki Y. Farber's disease (disseminated lipogranulomatosis): a pathological histochemical and ultrastructural study. Acta Pathol Jpn 1979; 29: 135–155

660. Burck U, Moser H W, Goebel H H, Gruttner R, Held K R. A case of lipogranulomatosis Farber: some clinical and ultrastructural aspects. Eur J Pediatr 1985; 143: 203–208

661. Koga M, Ishihara T, Uchino F. Farber bodies found in murine phagocytes after injection of ceramides and related sphingolipids. Virchows Arch (B) 1992; 82: 297–302

662. Rauch H J, Aubock L. "Banana bodies" in disseminated lipogranulomatosis (Farber's disease). Am J Dermatopathol 1983; 5: 263–266

663. Lepoutre C. Calcules de voie urinaire chez un infant: infiltration du parenchyme renal par des depots cristallins. J Urol (Paris) 1925; 20: 424

664. Latta K. Die Klinik der Hyperoxalurien, Fallberichte under Literatur. Thesis. Medizinische Hochschule, Hannover, 1990

665. Williams H E, Smith L H. L-glyceric aciduria: a new genetic variant of primary hyperoxaluria. N Engl J Med 1968; 278: 233–239

666. Chalmers R A, Tracey B M, Mistry J, Griffith K D, Green A, Winterborn M H. L-glyceric aciduria (primary hyperoxaluria type 2) in siblings in two unrelated families. J Inherited Metab Dis 1985; 7(Suppl 2): 133–134

667. Seargeant L E, de Grout G W, Dilling L A, Mallory C J, Haworth J C. Primary oxaluria type 2 (L-glycerine aciduria): a rare cause of nephrolithiasis in children. J Pediatr 1991; 118: 912–914

668. Latta K, Brodehl J. Primary hyperoxaluria type 1. Eur J Pediatr 1990; 149: 518–522

669. Hockaday T D R, Clayton J F, Fredrick E W, Smith L H. Primary hyperoxaluria. Medicine 1964; 43: 315–345

670. Scheinman J I, Najarian J S, Mauer S M. Successful strategies for renal transplantation in primary oxalosis. Kidney Int 1984; 25: 804–811

671. Hricik D E, Hussain R. Pancytopenia and hepatomegaly in oxalosis. Arch Intem Med 1984; 144: 167–168

672. Blackburn W E, McRoberts J W, Bhathena D, Vazquez M, Lake R G. Severe vascular complications in oxalosis after bilateral nephrectomy. Ann Intem Med 1975; 82: 44–46

673. Gottlieb K P, Ritter J A. Flecked retina — an association with primary hyperoxaluria. J Pediatr 1977; 90: 939–942

674. Fielder A R, Garner A, Chambers T L. Ophthalmic manifestations of primary oxalosis. Br J Ophthalmol 1980; 64: 782–788

675. Brennan J N, Diwan R V, Makker S P, Cromer B A, Bellon E M C. Ultrasound diagnosis of primary hyperoxaluria in infancy. Radiology 1982; 145: 147–148

676. Day D L, Scheinman J I, Mahan J. Radiological aspects of primary hyperoxaluria. Am J Roentgenol 1986; 146: 395–401

677. Danpure C J, Jennings P R. Enzymatic heterogeneity in primary hyperoxaluria type I (hepatic peroxisomal alanine: Glyoxylate aminotransferase). J Inherited Metab Dis 1988; 11 (Suppl 2): 205–207

678. Wanders R J A, Roermund van C W T, Jurrimans S et al. Diversity in residual alanine glyoxylate aminotransferase activity in primary hyperoxaluria type I: Correlation with pyridoxine responsiveness. J Inherited Metab Dis 1988; 11 (Suppl 2): 208–211

679. Wise P J, Danpure C J, Jennings P R. Immunological heterogeneity of hepatic alanine: Glycooxylate aminotransferase in primary hyperoxaluria. FEBS Lett 1987; 222: 17–20

680. Leumann E R, Matasovic A, Niederwieser A. Primary hyperoxaluria: Oxalate and glycolate unsuitable for prenatal diagnosis. Lancet 1986; ii: 340

681. Iancu T C, Danpure C J. Primary hyperoxaluria type I: ultrastructural observations in liver biopsies. J Inherited Metab Dis 1987; 10: 330–338

682. Burke E C, Baggenstoss A H, Owen C A, Power M H, Lohr O W. Oxalosis. Pediatrics 1955; 15: 383–391

683. Yendt E R, Cohanium M. Response to a physiologic dose of pyridoxine in type I primary hyperoxaluria. N Engl J Med 1985; 312: 953–957

684. Mitwalli A, Oreopoulos D G. Hyperoxaluria and hyperoxalemia: one more concern for the nephrologist. Int J Artif Organs 1985; 8: 571–575

685. Watts R W E, Caine R Y, Williams R et al. Primary hyperoxaluria (type I): Attempted treatment by combined hepatic and renal transplantation. Q J Med 1987; 57: 697–703

686. Raby R A, Tyszka T S, Williams J W. Reversal of cardiac dysfunction secondary to type I primary hyperoxaluria after combined liver–kidney transplantation. Am J Med 1991; 90: 498–504

687. Siemerling E, Creutzfeldt H G. Bronzekrankheit und

sklerorisiende encephalomyelitis (diffuse sklerose). Arch Psychiatry 1923; 68: 217–244

688. Igarashi M, Schaumberg H H, Powers J, Kishimoto V, Kolodny E, Suzuki K. Fatty acid abnormality in adrenoleukodystrophy. J Neurochem 1976; 26: 851–860

689. Moser H W, Moser A B. Adrenoleukodystrophy (X-linked). In: Scriver C R, Beaudet A L, Sly W S, Valle D, eds. The metabolic basis of inherited disease, 6th edn. New York: McGraw-Hill, 1989: pp 1511–1532

690. Whitcomb R W, Linehan W M, Knazek R A: Effects of long-chain, saturated fatty acids on membrane microviscosity and adrenocorticotropin responsiveness in human adrenocortical cell in vitro. J Clin Invest 1988; 81: 185–188

691. Wanders R J A, van Roermund C W T, Schutgens R B H, Tager J M. Disorders of peroxisomal fatty acid ß -oxidation. In: Schaub J, Van Hoof F, Vis H L, eds. Inborn errors of metabolism. New York: Raven Press, 1991: pp 43–53

692. Wanders R J A, van Roermund C W T, Wyland M J A, Schutgens R B H, van der Bosch H, Schram A W, Toger J M. Direct demonstration that the deficient oxidation of very long chain fatty acids in X-linked adrenoleukodystrophy is due to an impaired ability of peroxisomes to activate very long chain fatty acids. Biochem Biophys Res Commun 1988; 153: 618–624

693. Lazo O, Contreras M, Bhusnan A, Stanley W, Singh I. Adrenoleukodystrophy: impaired oxidation of fatty acids due to peroxisomal lignoceroxyl-CoA ligase deficiency. Arch Biochem Biophys 1989; 270: 722–728

694. Poll-The B T, Roels F, Ogier H et al. A new peroxisomal disorder with enlarged peroxisomes and a specific deficiency of acyl-CoA oxidase (pseudoneonatal adrenoleukodystrophy). Am J Hum Genet 1988; 42: 422–434

695. Watkins P A, Chen W W, Harris C J et al. Peroxisomal bifunctional enzyme deficiency. J Clin Invest 1989; 83: 771–777

696. Goldfischer S, Collins H, Rapin I et al. Pseudo-Zellweger syndromes: Deficiencies in several peroxisomal oxidative activities. J Pediatr 1986; 108: 25–32

697. Suzuki Y, Shimozawa N, Orii T et al. Zellweger-like syndrome; Deficiencies in several peroxisomal oxidative activities. J Pediatr 1986; 108: 25–32

698. Poulos A, Sheffield L, Sharp P et al. Rhizomelic chondrodysplasia punctata: Clinical, pathologic, and biochemical findings in two patients. J Pediatr 1988; 113: 685–690

699. Brown P, Lee C S M, Zellweger H, Lindenberg R. A familial syndrome of multiple congenital defects. Bull Johns Hopkins Hosp 1964; 114: 402–414

700. Goldfischer S, Moore C L, Johnson A B et al. Peroxisomal and mitochondrial defects in the cerebro-hepato-renal syndrome. Science 1973; 182: 62–64

701. Martinez R D, Martin-Jimenez R, Matalon R. Zellweger syndrome. Pediatrics 1991; 6: 91–93

702. Moser H W, Moser A B, Chen W W, Watkins P A. Adrenoleukodystrophy and Zellweger syndrome in fatty acid oxidation: clinical, biochemical and molecular aspects. In: Tanaka K, ed. Progress in clinical and biological research. New York: Alan R Liss, 1990: Vol 321, pp 511–535

703. Ulrich J, Herschowitz N, Hertz T, Baerlocher P. Adrenoleukodystrophy: preliminary report of a conatal case. Acta Neuropath 1978; 43: 77–83

704. Vamecq J, Drayl J P, Van Hoof F et al. Multiple peroxisomal enzymatic deficiency disorders: A comparative biochemical, and morphological study of Zellweger cerebro-hepato-renal syndrome and neonatal adrenoleukodystrophy. Am J Pathol 1986; 125: 525–535

705. Scotto J M, Hadchouel L M, Odiever M et al. Infantile phytanic acid storage disease. A possible variant of Refsum's disease. J Inher Metabolic Dis 1982; 5: 83–90

706. Brul S, Westerveld A, Strijland A et al. Genetic heterogeneity in the cerebrohepatorenal (Zellweger) syndrome and other inherited disorders with a generalized impairment of peroxisomal functions. J Clin Invest 1988; 81: 1710–1715

707. Tager J M, Brul S, Weimer A C et al. Genetic relationship between the Zellweger syndrome and other peroxisomal disorders

708. Santos M H, Inanaka T, Shie H, Smale O M, Lazarow P B. Peroxisomal membrane ghosts in Zellweger syndrome — aberrant organelle assembly. Science 1988; 239: 1536–1538

709. Shimozawa N, Tsukamoto T, Suzuki Y et al. A human gene responsible for Zellweger syndrome that affects peroxisome assembly. Science 1992; 255: 1132–1134

710. Patton R G, Christie D L, Smith D W, Beckwith J B. Cerebro-hepatorenal syndrome of Zellweger. Am J Dis Child 1972; 124: 840–844

711. Gilchrist R W, Gilbert E G, Goldfarb S et al. Studies of malformation syndromes of man. IIB. Cerebro-hepato-renal syndrome of Zellweger: comparative pathology. Eur J Pediatr 1976; 122: 99–118

712. Danks D M, Tippett P, Adams C, Campbell P. Cerebro-hepato-renal syndrome of Zellweger: a report of eight cases with comments upon the incidence, the liver lesion, and a fault of pipecolic acid metabolism. J Pediatr 1975; 86: 382–387

713. Jan J E, Hardwick D F, Lowry R B, McCormick A Q. Cerebro-hepatorenal syndrome of Zellweger. Am J Dis Child 1970; 119: 274–277

714. Pfeifer U, Sandhage K. Licht- und Elektron microscopische Leberfunde beim Cerebro-Hepato-Renalen Syndrom nach Zellweger (Peroxisomen-Defizienz). Virchows Arch A Pathol Anat Histol 1979; 384: 269–284

715. Mooi W J, Dingemans K P, Weerman M A V B, Jobsis A C, Heymans H S A, Barth P G. Ultrastructure of the liver in the cerebrohepatorenal syndrome of Zellweger. Ultrastr Pathol 1983; 5: 135–144

716. Goldfischer S L. Peroxisomal disease. In: Arias I M, Jakoby W B, Popper H, Schachter D, eds. The liver. biology and pathobiology, 2nd edn. New York: Raven Press, 1988: pp 255–265

717. Powers J M, Moser H W, Moser A B et al. Fetal cerebrohepatorenal (Zellweger) syndrome. Dysmorphic, radiologic, biochemical, and pathologic findings in four affected fetuses. Hum Pathol 1985; 16: 610–620

718. Smith D W, Opitz J M, Inhorn S L. A syndrome of multiple developmental defects including polycystic kidneys and intrahepatic dysgenesis in two siblings. J Pediatr 1965; 67: 617–624

719. Passarge E, McAdams A J. Cerebro-hepato-renal syndrome. J Pediatr 1967; 71: 691–702

720. Nakamura K, Takenouchi T, Aizawa M et al. Cerebro-hepato-renal syndrome of Zellweger. Clinical and autopsy findings and a review of previous cases in Japan. Acta Pathol Jpn 1986; 36: 1727–1735

721. Hanson R F, Szczepanik-Van Leeuwen P, Williams G C, Grabowski G, Sharp H L. Defects of bile acid synthesis in Zellweger's syndrome. Science 1979; 203: 1107–1108

722. Mathis R K, Watkins J B, Szczepanik-Van Leeuwen P, Lott I T. Liver in the cerebro-hepato-renal syndrome: defective bile acid synthesis and abnormal mitochondria. Gastroenterology 1980; 79: 1311–1317

723. Litwin J Q, Volkl A, Muller-Hocker J, Hashimoto T, Fahimi H D. Immunohistochemical localization of peroxisomal enzymes in human liver biopsies. Am J Pathol 1987; 128: 141–150

724. Haas J E, Johnson E S, Farrell D L. Neonatal-onset adrenoleukodystrophy in a girl. Ann Neurol 1982; 12: 449–457

725. Jaffe R, Crumrine P, Hashida Y, Moser H W. Neonatal adrenoleukodystrophy. Clinical, pathologic, and biochemical delineation of a syndrome affecting both males and females. Am J Pathol 1982; 108: 100–111

726. Dimmick J E. Liver pathology in neonatal adrenoleukodystrophy. Lab Invest 1984; 50: 3P (abstract)

727. Hughes J L, Poulos A, Robertson E et al. Pathology of hepatic peroxisomes and mitochondria in patients with peroxisomal disorders. Virchows Arch (A) 1990; 416: 255–264

728. Budden S S, Kennaway N G, Buist N R M, Poulos A, Weleber R G. Dysmorphic syndrome with phytanic acid oxidase deficiency, abnormal very long chain fatty acids, and pipecolic acidemia: studies in four children. J Pediatr 1986; 108: 33–39

729. Torvik A, Torp S, Kase B F, Skjeldal O, Stokke O. Refsum's

characterized by an impairment in the assembly of peroxisomes host-like structures. Prog Clin Biol Res 1990; 321: 545–558 disease—a generalized peroxisomal disorder. Case with postmortem examination. J Neurol Sci 1988; 85: 39–53

730. Scotto J M, Hadchoul M, Odievre M et al. Infantile phytanic acid storage disease, a possible variant of Refsum's disease. Three cases, including ultrastructural studies of the liver. J Inher Metabol Dis 1982; 5: 83–90

731. Roels F, Cornelis A, Poll-The B T et al. Hepatic peroxisomes are deficient in infantile Refsum disease. A cytochemical study of four cases. Am J Med Genet 1986; 25: 257–271

732. DiMauro S, Bonilla E, Zerani M, Nakagawa M, De Vivo D C. Mitochondrial myopathies. Ann Neurol 1985; 17: 521–538

733. Clarke L A. Mitochondrial disorders in pediatrics. Pediatr Clin N Am 1992; 39: 319–334

734. Boustany R N, Aprille J R, Halperin J, Levy H, DeLong G R. Mitochondrial cytochrome deficiency presenting as a myopathy with hypotonic, external ophthalmoplegia, and lactic acidosis in an infant and as fatal hepatopathy in second cousin. Ann Neurol 1983; 14: 462–470

735. Cormier V, Rustin P, Bonnefont J-P et al. Hepatic failure in disorders of oxidative phosphorylation with neonatal onset. J Pediatr 1991; 119: 951–954

736. Fayon M, Lamireau T, Bioulac-Sage P et al. Fatal neonatal liver failure and mitochondrial cytopathy: an observation with antenatal ascites. Gastroenterology 1992; 103: 1332–1335

736a. Bioulac-Sage P, Parrot-Rouland F, Mazat J P et al. Fatal neonatal liver failure and mitochondrial cytopathy (oxidative phosphorylation deficiency): a light and electron microscopic study of the liver. Hepatology 1993; 18: 839–846

737. Sternlieb I. Perspectives in Wilson's disease. Hepatology 1990; 1234–1239.

738. Frydman M, Bonne-Tamir B, Farrer L A et al. Assignment of the gene for Wilson's disease to chromosome 13: linkage to the esterase D locus. Proc Natl Acad Sci 1985; 82: 1819–1821

739. Bowcock A M, Farrer L A, Herbert J M et al. Eight closely linked loci place the Wilson's disease locus within 13q 14–q21. Am J Hum Genet 1988; 43: 664–674

740. Czaja M J, Weiner F R, Schwarzenberg S J et al. Molecular studies of ceruloplasmin deficiency in Wilson's disease. J Clin Invest 1987; 80: 1200 –1204

741. Barrow L, Tanner M S, Critchley D R. Expression of the ceruloplasmin gene in the adult and neonatal liver. Clin Sci 1989; 77: 259–263

742. Scheinberg I H, Sternlieb I. Wilson's disease. Philadelphia: W B Saunders, 1984

743. McCullough A J, Fleming C R, Thistle J L et al. Diagnosis of Wilson's disease presenting as fulminant hepatic failure. Gastroenterology 1983; 84: 161–167

744. Rector W G, Uchida T, Kanel G C, Redeker A G, Reynolds T B. Fulminant hepatic failure and renal failure complicating Wilson's disease. Liver 1984; 4: 341–347

745. Gur H, Aderrka D, Finkelstein A et al. Fulminant Wilsonian hepatitis: difficulties in diagnosis and treatment. Am J Gastroenterol 1988; 83: 679–681

746. Berman D H, Leventhal R I, Gavaler J S, Cadoff E M, Van Thiel D H. Clinical differentiation of fulminant Wilsonian hepatitis from other causes of hepatic failure. Gastroenterology 1991; 100: 1129–1134

747. Sallie R, Katsiyiannakesh L, Baldwin D et al. Failure of simple biochemical indexes to reliably differentiate fulminant Wilson's disease from other causes of fulminant liver failure. Hepatology 1992; 16: 1206 –1211

748. Schulsky M L, Schienberg I H, Sternlieb Z. Prognosis of Wilsonian chronic active hepatitis. Gastroenterology 1991; 100: 762–767

749. Cheng W S C, Govindarajan S, Redeker A G. Hepatocellular carcinoma in a case of Wilson's disease. Liver 1992; 12: 42–45

750. Rosenfield N, Grand R J, Watkins J B, Ballantine T V N, Leevy R H. Cholelithiasis and Wilson's disease. J Pediatr 1978; 92: 210–213

751. Derue G, Geubel A P, Rahier J, Michaux J L, Reynaert M. Acute Wilson's disease and thalassemia minor. A case report. Am J Gastroenterol 1984; 79: 562–566

752. Sternlieb I. Evolution of the hepatic lesion in Wilson's disease (hepatolenticular degeneration). Prog Liver Dis 1972; 4: 511– 525

753. Levi A J, Sherlock S, Scheuer P J, Cumings J N. Presymptomatic Wilson's disease. Lancet 1967; ii: 575–579

754. Lindahl J M, Sharp H L. Screening asymptomatic family members for Wilson's disease. Minnesota Med 1982; 65: 473–475

755. Farrer L A, Bonne-Tamier B, Frydman M et al. Predicting genotypes at loci for autosomal recessive disorders using linked genetic markers: application to Wilson's disease. Hum Genet 1988; 79: 109–117

756. Figus A, Lampis R, Devoto M et al. Carrier detection and early diagnosis of Wilson's disease by restriction fragment length polymorphism analysis. J Med Genet 1989; 26: 78–82

757. Clossu P, Pirastu M, Mucaro A et al. Prenatal diagnosis of Wilson's disease by analysis of DNA polymorphism. N Engl J Med 1992; 327: 57

758. Stromeyer F W, Ishak K G. Histology of the liver in Wilson's disease: a study of 34 cases. Am J Clin Pathol 1980; 73: 12–24

759. Sternlieb I, Scheinberg I H. Chronic hepatitis as a first manifestation of Wilson's disease. Ann Intern Med 1972; 76: 59–64

760. Archer G J, Morrie R D. Wilson's disease and chronic active hepatitis. Lancet 1977; i: 486–487

761. Scott J, Gollan J L, Samourian S, Sherlock S. Wilson's disease presenting as chronic active hepatitis. Gastroenterology 1978; 74 645–651

762. Goldfischer S, Sternlieb I. Changes in the distribution of hepatic copper in relation to the progression of Wilson's disease (hepatolenticular degeneration). Am J Pathol 1968; 53: 883–901

763. Lindquist R R. Studies on the pathogenesis of hepatolenticular degeneration. II. Cytochemical methods for the localization of copper. Arch Pathol 1969; 87: 370–379

764. Irons R D, Schenk E A, Lee J C K. Cytochemical methods for copper. Arch Pathol Lab Med 1977; 101: 298–301

765. Salaspuro M, Sipponen P. Demonstration of an intracellular copper-binding protein by orcein staining. Gut 1976; 13: 787–790

766. Jain S, Scheuer P J, Archer B B, Newman S P, Sherlock S. Histological demonstration of copper-associated protein in chronic liver diseases. J Clin Pathol 1978; 31: 784–790

767. Sumithran E, Looi L M. Copper-binding protein in liver cells. Hum Pathol 1985; 16: 677–682

768. Graul R S, Epstein O, Sherlock S, Scheuer P J. Immunocytochemical identification of caeruloplasmin in hepatocytes in patients with Wilson's disease. Liver 1982; ii: 207–211

769. Nartey N O, Frei J V, Cherian M G. Hepatic copper and metallothionein distribution in Wilson's disease (hepatolenticular degeneration). Lab Invest 1987; 57: 397–401

770. Davies S E, William S R, Portmann B. Hepatic morphology and histochemistry of Wilson's disease as fulminant hepatic failure: a study of 11 cases. Histopathology 1989; 15: 385–394

771. Sternlieb I. Fraternal concordance of abnormal hepatocellular mitochondria in Wilson's disease. Hepatology 1992; 16: 728–732

772. Hayashi H, Sternlieb I. Lipolysosomes in human hepatocytes. Ultrastructural and cytochemical studies of patients with Wilson's disease. Lab Invest 1975; 33: 1– 7

773. Lough J, Wiglesworth F W. Wilson's disease. Comparative ultrastructure in a sibship of nine. Arch Pathol Lab Med 1976; 100: 659–663

774. Sternlieb I, Feldmann G. Effects of anticopper therapy on hepatocellular mitochondria in patients with Wilson's disease Gastroenterology 1976; 71: 457–461

775. Brewer G J, Terry C A, Aisen A M, Hill G M. Worsening of neurologic syndrome in patients with Wilson's disease with initial penicillamine therapy. Arch Neurol 1987; 44: 490–494

776. Scheinberg I H, Sternlieb I, Schilsky M L, Stockert R J. Penicillamine may detoxify copper in Wilson's disease. Lancet 1987; ii: 95

777. Heilmaier H E, Jiang J L, Green H, Schramel P, Summer K H. D-penicillamine induces rat hepatic metallothionein. Toxicology 1986; 42: 23–31

778. Brewer G J, Hill G M, Prasad A S, Cossack Z T, Rabbani P. Oral zinc therapy for Wilson's disease. Ann Intern Med 1983; 99: 314–320

779. Brewer G J, Hill G M, Dick R D et al. Treatment of Wilson's disease with zinc. II. Prevention of accumulation of hepatic copper. J Lab Clin Med 1987; 109: 526–531

780. Brewer G J, Yuzbasiyan-Gurkan V, Lee D-V. Use of zinc-copper metabolic interaction in treatment of Wilson's disease. J Am Coll Nutr 1990; 9: 487–491

781. Rakela K, Kurtz S B, McCarthy J T et al. Fulminant Wilson's disease treated with hemofiltration and orthotopic liver transplantation. Gastroenterology 1986; 90: 2004–2007

782. Peleman R R, Gavaler J S, Van Thiel D H et al. Orthotopic liver transplantation for acute and subacute hepatic failure in adults. Hepatology 1987; 7: 484–489

783. Paradis K J B, Freese D K, Sharp H L. A pediatric perspective on liver transplantation. Pediatr Clin North Am 1988; 35: 409–433

783a. Rela M, Heaton N D, Vougas V et al. Orthotopic liver transplantation for hepatic complications of Wilson's disease. Br J Surg 1993; 80: 909–911

783b. Schilsky M L, Scheinberg I H, Sternlieb I. Liver transplantation for Wilson's disease: indications and outcome. Hepatology 1994; 19: 583–587

784. Landing B H, Shirkey H S. A syndrome of recurrent infection and infiltration of viscera by pigmented lipid histiocytes. Pediatrics 1957; 20: 431–438

785. Bridges R A, Berendes H, Good R A. A fatal granulomatous disease of childhood. Am J Dis Childh 1959; 97: 387–408

786. Forehand J R, Nausell W B, Johnston R B. Inherited disorders of phagocyte killing. In: Scriver C R, Beaudet A L, Sly W S, Valle D, eds. The metabolic basis of inherited disease, 6th edn. New York: McGraw-Hill, 1989: pp 2779–2801

787. Harris B H, Boles E T. Intestinal lesions in chronic granulomatous disease of childhood. J Pediatr Surg 1973; 8: 955–956

788. Griscom N T, Kirkpatrick J A, Girdany B R, Berdon W E, Grand R J, Mackie G G. Gastric antral narrowing in chronic granulomatous disease of childhood. Pediatrics 1974; 54: 456–460

789. Markowitz J F, Aranow E, Rausen A R, Aiges H, Silverberg M, Daum F. Progressive esophageal dysfunction in chronic granulomatous disease. J Pediatr Gastroenterol Nutr 1982; 1: 146–149

790. Ament M E, Ochs H D. Gastrointestinal manifestations of chronic granulomatosis disease. N Engl J Med 1973; 228: 382–387

791. Yogman M W, Touloukian R J, Gallagher R. Intestinal granulomatosis in chronic granulomatous disease and in Crohn's disease. N Engl J Med 1974; 290: 228

792. Sty J R, Chusid M F J, Babbit D P, Werlin S L. Involvement of the colon in chronic granulomatous disease of childhood. Radiology 1973; 132: 618

793. Werlin S L, Chusid M J, Caya J, Oechler H W. Colitis in chronic granulomatous disease. Gastroenterology 1982; 82: 328–331

794. Lindahl J A, Williams F H, Newman S L. Small bowel obstruction in chronic granulomatous disease. J Pediatr Gastroenterol Nutr 1984; 3: 637–640

795. Quie P G. Pathology of bactericidal power of neutrophils. Semin Hematol 1975; 12: 143–160

796. Shapiro B L, Newburger P E, Dlempner M S, Dinauer M C. Chronic granulomatous disease presenting in a 69 year old man. N Engl J Med 1991; 325: 1786–1790

797. Smith R M, Curnutte J T. Molecular basis of chronic granulomatous disease. Blood 1991; 77: 673–686

798. Chin T W, Stiehm E R, Falloon J, Gallin J I. Corticosteroids in treatment of obstruction lesions of chronic granulomatous disease. J Pediatr 1987; 111: 349–352

799. Kamani N, August C S, Campbell D E, Hassan N F, Douglas S D. Marrow transplantation in chronic granulomatous disease: An update with 6-year-follow-up. J Pediatr 1985; 13: 697–700

800. The International Chronic Granulomatous Disease Cooperative Study Group. Controlled trial of interferon gamma to prevent infection in chronic granulomatous disease. N Engl J Med 1991; 324: 509–516

801. Johnston R B Jr, Newman S L. Chronic granulomatous disease. Pediatr Clin N Am 1977; 24: 365–376

802. Nakhleh R E, Glock M, Snover D C. Hepatic pathology of chronic granulomatous disease of childhood. Arch Pathol Lab Med 1992; 116: 71–75

803. Tauber A I, Borregaard N, Simons E, Wright J. Chronic granulomatous disease. Medicine 1983; 62: 286–309

804. Rodey D E, Landing B H. Chronic granulomatous disease of males. In: Bergsma D, ed. Birth defects atlas and compendium. Baltimore: Williams & Wilkins, 1973: pp 255–256

805. Carson M J, Chadwick D L, Brubaker C A, Cleland R S, Landing B H. Thirteen boys with progressive septic granulomatosis. Pediatrics 1965; 35: 405–412

806. Anderson D H. Cystic fibrosis of the pancreas and its relationship to celiac disease. A clinical and pathologic study. Am J Dis Childhood 1938; 58: 344–399

807. Boat T F, Welsh M J, Beaudet A L. Cystic fibrosis. In: Scriver C R, Beaudet A L, Sly W S, Valle D, eds. The metabolic basis of inherited disease, 6th edn. New York: McGraw-Hill, 1989: pp 2649–2680

808. Rommens J M, Iannuzzi M C, Kerem B-S et al. Identification of the cystic fibrosis gene: chromosome walking and jumping. Science 1989; 242: 1059–1065

809. Riordan J R, Rommens J M, Kerem B S et al. Identification of the cystic fibrosis gene: cloning and characterization of complimentary DNA. Science 1989; 245: 1066–1073

810. Kerem B S, Rommens J M, Buchanan J A et al. Identification of the cystic fibrosis gene: genetic analysis. Science 1989; 245: 1073–1080

811. Rommens J M, Dho S, Bear C E et al. cAMP-inducible chloride conductance in mouse fibroblast lines stably expressing the human cystic fibrosis transmembrane conductance regulator. Proc Natl Acad Sci USA 1991; 88: 7500–7504

812. Kerem B, Corey M, Kerem B-S, Rommens J. The relationship between genotype and phenotype in cystic fibrosis — analysis of the most common mutation (508). N Engl J Med 1990; 323: 1517–1522

813. Sorscher E J, Kirk K L, Weaver M L, Jilling T, Blalock J E, LaBoeuf R D. Antisense oligodeoxy nucleotide to the cystic fibrosis gene inhibits anion transport in normal cultures of sweat duct cells. Proc Natl Acad Sci USA 1991; 88: 7759–7762

814. Shouwaert J N, Brigman K K, Latour A M et al. An animal model for cystic fibrosis made by gene targeting. Science 1992; 257: 1083–1088

815. Park R W, Grand R J. Gastrointestinal manifestations of cystic fibrosis. A review. Gastroenterology 1981; 81: 1143–1161

816. Isenberg J N, Cystic fibrosis. Its influence on the liver, biliary tree, and bile acid metabolism. Semin Liver Dis 1982; 2: 301–313

817. Roy C C, Weber A M, Morin C L, LePage G, Youssef I, LaSalle R. Hepatobiliary disease in cystic fibrosis: a survey of current issues and concepts. J Pediatr Gastroenterol Nutr 1982; 1: 469–478

818. Rodman H M, Matthews L W, Hyperglycemia in cystic fibrosis: A review of the literature and our own patient experience. In: Warwick J W, ed. 1000 Years of cystic fibrosis: collected papers. St Paul: University of Minnesota Press, 1981: pp 67–76

819. Di Sant'Agnese P, Davis P B. Cystic fibrosis in adults: seventy-five cases and a review of 232 cases in the literature. Am J Med 1979; 66: 122–132

820. Finkelstein S M, Wielinski C L, Elliot G R et al. Diabetes mellitus associated with cystic fibrosis. J Pediatr 1988; 112: 373–377

821. Moran A, Diem P, Klein D, Levitt M, Robertson R P. Pancreatic endocrine function in cystic fibrosis. J Pediatr 1991; 118: 715–723

822. Stern R C, Boat T F, Abramowsky C R, Matthews L W, Wodd R E, Doershuk C F. Intermediate-range sweat chloride concentration and pseudomonas bronchitis, a cystic fibrosis variant with preservation of exocrine pancreatic function. JAMA 1978; 239: 2676–2680

823. Gatzemas C D, Javitt R H. Jaundice in mucoviscidosis. Am J Dis Child 1955; 89: 182–186

824. Valman H B, France N E, Wallis P G. Prolonged neonatal jaundice in cystic fibrosis. Arch Dis Childh 1971; 46: 805–809

825. Rosenstein B J, Oppenheimer E H. Prolonged obstructive jaundice and giant cell hepatitis in an infant with cystic fibrosis. J Pediatr 1977; 91: 1022–1023

826. Psacharopoulos H T, Howard E R, Portmann B, Mowat A P, Williams R. Hepatic complications of cystic fibrosis. Lancet 1981; ii: 78–80

827. Strandvik B, Hjelte L, Gabrielsson N, Glaumann H. Sclerosing cholangitis in cystic fibrosis. Scand J Gastroenterol 1988; 23 (Suppl 143): 121–124

828. Nagel R A, Westaby D, Javaid A et al. Liver disease and bile duct abnormalities in adults with cystic fibrosis. Lancet 1989; ii: 1422–1425

829. O'Brien S, Keogan M, Casey M et al. Biliary complications of cystis fibrosis. Gut 1992; 33: 387–391

830. Gaskin K J, Waters D L M, Howman-Giles R et al. Liver disease and common-bile duct stenosis in cystic fibrosis. N Engl J Med 1988; 318: 340–346

831. Isenberg J N, L'Heureux P R, Warwick W J, Sharp H L. Clinical observations on the biliary system in cystic fibrosis. Am J Gastroenterol 1976; 65: 134–141

832. Gorup W, Richalm P P, Delylal P, Schmerling P H. Cholelithiasis als erst manifestation der zystischen pankrease fibrose. Helv Paediatr Acta 1980; 35: 177–184

833. Bass S, Connon J J, Ho C S. Biliary tree in cystic fibrosis: biliary tract abnormalities in cystic fibrosis demonstrated by endoscopic retrograde cholangiography. Gastroenterology 1983; 84: 1592–1596

834. Feigelson J, Pecan Y, Cathelineau L, Navarro J. Additional data on hepatic function tests in cystic fibrosis. Acta Paediatr Scand 1975; 64: 337–344

835. Warwick W J, L'Heureaux P R, Sharp H L, Isenberg J N. Gallstones in cystic fibrosis. Proceedings of the International Cystic Fibrosis Congress, Paris, 1976, pp 100–104

836. Watkins J B, Tercyak A M, Szczpanik P, Klein P D. Bile salt kinetics in cystic fibrosis: influence of pancreatic enzyme replacement. Gastroenterology 1977; 73: 1023–1028

837. Fondaro J D, Heubi J E, Kellogg F W. Intestinal bile acid malabsorption in cystic fibrosis: a primary mucosal defect. Pediatr Res 1982; 16: 494–498

838. Angelico M, Gandin C, Canuzzi P et al. Gallstones in cystic fibrosis: a critical reappraisal. Hepatology 1991; 14: 768–775

839. Vawter G F, Schwachman H. Cystic fibrosis in adults. An autopsy study. Pathol Annu 1979; 14: 357–382

840. Masaryk T J, Achkar E. Pancreatitis as initial presentation of cystic fibrosis in young adults: a report of two cases. Dig Dis Sci 1983; 28: 874–878

841. Lambert J R, Cole M, Crozier D N, Connor J J. Intrapancreatic common bile duct compression causing jaundice in an adult with cystic fibrosis. Gastroenterology 1981; 80: 169–172

842. Lindblad A, Hultcranz R, Strandvik B. Bile-duct destruction and collagen deposition: a prominent ultrastructural feature of the liver in cystic fibrosis. Hepatology 1992; 16: 372–381

843. Abdul-Karim F W, King T A, Dahms B B, Gauderer W L, Boat T F. Carcinoma of the extrahepatic biliary system in an adult with cystic fibrosis. Gastroenterology 1982; 758–762

844. Biberstein M, Wolf P, Pettross B, Fanestil D, Vasquez M. Amyloidosis complicating cystis fibrosis. Am J Clin Pathol 1983; 80: 752–754

845. Castile R, Shwachman H, Travis W, Hadley C A, Warwick W, Missmahl H P. Amyloidosis as a complication of cystic fibrosis. Am J Dis Child 1985; 139: 728–732

846. Travis W D, Castile R, Vawter G et al. Secondary (AA) amyloidosis in cystic fibrosis. Am J Clin Pathol 1986; 85: 419–424

847. Bodian M. Fibrocystic disease of the pancreas. A congenital disorder of mucus production—mucosis. London: William Heinemann Medical, 1952

848. Craig J M, Haddad H, Shwachman H. The pathological changes in the liver in cystic fibrosis of the pancreas. Am J Dis Child 1957; 93: 357–369

849. de Sant' Agnese P A, Blanc W A. A distinctive type of biliary cirrhosis of the liver with cystic fibrosis of the pancreas. Pediatrics 1956; 18: 387–409

850. Oppenheimer E H, Esterly J R. Hepatic changes in young infants with cystic fibrosis: possible relation to focal biliary cirrhosis. J Pediatr 1975; 86: 683–689

851. Oppenheimer E H, Esterly J R. Pathology of cystic fibrosis: review of the literature and comparison with 146 autopsied cases. Persp Pediatr Pathol 1975; 2: 244–278

852. Porta E A, Stein A A, Patterson D. Ultrastructural changes of the pancreas and liver in cystic fibrosis. Am J Clin Pathol 1964; 41: 451–465

853. Park R W, Grand R J. Gastrointestinal manifestations of cystic fibrosis: a review. Gastroenterology 1981: 81: 1143–1163

854. Dominick H C. Cystic fibrosis. In: Bianchi L, Gerok W, Landmann L, Sickinger K, Stalder G A, eds. Liver in metabolic diseases. Lancaster: MTP Press, 1983: pp 283–290

855. Esterly J R, Oppenheimer E H. Observations in cystic fibrosis of the pancreas. I. The gallbladder. Bull Johns Hopkins Hosp 1962; 110: 247–255

856. Arends P, von Bassewitz D B, Dominick H C. Ultrastructure of liver biopsies in cystic fibrosis. Cystic Fibrosis Quarterly Annotated References 1974; 13: 13 (Abstract)

857. Bradford W, Allen D, Sheburne J, Spock A. Hepatic parenchymal cells in cystic fibrosis: ultrastructural evidence for abnormal intracellular transport. Pediatr Pathol 1983; 1: 269–279

858. Hultcrantz R, Mengareli S, Strandvik B. Morphological findings in the liver of children with cystic fibrosis: a light and electron microscopical study. Hepatology 1986; 6: 881–889

859. Gowen C W, Lawson E E, Gingras-Leatherman J, Gatzy J T, Boucher R C, Knowles M R. Increased nasal potential difference and amiloride sensitivity in neonates with cystic fibrosis. J Pediatr 1986; 108: 517–521

860. Sauder R A, Chesrown S E, Loughlin G. Clinical application of transepithelial potential difference measurements in cystic fibrosis. J Pediatr 1987; 111: 353–358

861. Hammond K B, Abman S H, Sokol R J, Aecurso F J. Efficacy of statewide neonatal screening for cystic fibrosis by assay of trypsinogen concentration. N Engl J Med 1991; 325: 769–774

862. Holtzman N A. What drives neonatal screening programs? N Engl J Med 1991; 325: 802–803

863. Thompson G N. Excessive fecal taurine loss predisposes to taurine deficiency in cystic fibrosis. J Pediatr Gastroenterol Nutr 1988; 7: 214–219

864. Colombo C, Roda A, Roda E et al. Bile acid malabsorption in cystic fibrosis with and without pancreatic insufficiency. J Pediatr Gastroent Nutr 1984; 3: 556–562

865. Darling P B, LePage G, Leroy C, Musson P, Roy C C. Effect of taurine supplements on fat absorption in cystic fibrosis. Pediatr Res 1985; 19: 578–582

866. Colombo C, Arlati S, Curceo L et al. Effect of taurine supplementation on fat and bile acid absorption in patients with cystic fibrosis. Scand J Gastroenterol 1988: 23 (Suppl 143): 151–156

867. Robb T A, Davidson G P, Kirubakaran C. Conjugated bile acids in serum and secretions in response to cholecystokinin/secretion stimulation in children with cystic fibrosis. Gut 1985; 26: 1246–1256

868. Colombo C, Setchell K D R, Podda M et al. Effects of ursodeoxycholic acid therapy for liver disease associated with cystic fibrosis. J Pediatr 1990; 117: 982–989

869. Knowles R M, Clark L L, Boucher R C. Activation by extracellular nucleotides of chloride secretion in the airway epithelia of patients with cystic fibrosis. N Engl J Med 1991; 325: 533–538

870. Fiel S B. Heart-lung transplantation for patients with cystic fibrosis. Arch Intern Med 1991; 151: 970–972

871. Cox K L, Ward R E, Furgiuele T L, Cannon R A, Saunders K D, Kurland G. Orthotopic liver transplantations in patients with cystic fibrosis. Pediatrics 1987; 80: 571–574

872. Evans J S, George D E, Mollit D. Biliary infusion therapy of the inspissated bile syndrome of cystic fibrosis. J Pediatr Gastroenterol Nutr 1991; 12: 131–135

873. DiLiberti J H, Whitington P F. Shwachman syndrome. In: Buyse M L, ed. Birth defects encyclopedia. Dover, MA: Center for Birth Defects Information Services, 1990: pp 1535–1536

874. Hill R W, Durie P R, Gaskin K J, Davidson G P, Forstner G G. Steatorrhea and pancreatic insufficiency in Shwachman syndrome. Gastroenterology 1982; 83: 22–27

875. Saunders E F, Gall G, Freedman M H. Granulopoiesis in Shwachman's syndrome (pancreatic insufficiency and bone marrow dysfunction). Pediatrics 1979; 64: 515–519

876. Goldstein R. Congenital lipomatosis of the pancreas. Malabsorption, dwarfism, leukopenia with relative granulocytopenia and thrombocytopenia. Clin Pediatr 1968; 7: 419–422

877. Doe W F. Two brothers with congenital pancreatic exocrine insufficiency, neutropenia and dysgammaglobulinemia. Proc Roy Soc Med 1973; 66: 1125–1126

878. Woods W C, Roloff J S, Lukens J N, Krivit W. The occurrence of leukemia in patients with Shwachmann syndrome. J Pediatr 1981; 99: 424–428

879. Bodian M, Sheldon W, Lightwood R. Congenital hypoplasia of the exocrine pancreas. Acta Paediatr 1964; 53: 582–593

880. Brueton M V, Mavromichalis J, Goodchild M C, Anderson M. Hepatic dysfunction in association with pancreatic insufficiency

and cyclical neutropenia. Shwachman-Diamond syndrome. Arch Dis Childh 1977; 52: 76–78

881. Shmerling D H, Prader A, Hitzig W H, Giedion A, Hadorn B, Kuhni M. The syndrome of exocrine pancreatic insufficiency, neutropenia, metaphysical dysostosis and dwarfism. Helv Paediatr Acta 1968; 24: 547–575

882. Lebenthal E, Shwachman H, The pancreas—development, adaptation and malfunctions in infancy and childhood. Clin Gastroenterol 1977; 6: 404–405

883. Shwachman H, Diamond L K, Oski F A, Khaw K T. The syndrome of pancreatic insufficiency and bone marrow insufficiency. J Pediatr 1964; 65: 645–663

884. Burke V, Colebatach J H, Anderson C M, Simon M J. Association of pancreatic insufficiency and chronic neutropenia in childhood. Arch Dis Childh 1976; 42: 147–157

885. Graham A R, Walson P D, Paplanus S H, Payne C M. Testicular fibrosis and cardiomegaly in Shwachman's syndrome. Arch Pathol Lab Med 1980; 104: 242–244

886. Wefring K W, Kamvik J O. Familial progressive poliodystrophy with cirrhosis of the liver. Acta Paediatr Scand 1967; 56: 295–300

887. Huttenlocher P R, Solitaire G B, Adams G. Infantile diffuse cerebral degeneration with hepatic cirrhosis. Arch Neurol 1975; 33: 186–192

888. Harding B N, Egger J, Portmann B, Erdohaz M. Progressive neuronal degeneration of childhood with liver disease. Brain 1986; 109: 181–206

889. Vedanarayanan V V, Kandt R S. Alpers disease. In: Buyse M L, ed. Birth defects encyclopedia. Dover, M A: Center for Birth Defects Information Services, 1990: p 90

890. Narkewicz M R, Sokol R J, Beckwith B, Sondheimer J, Silverman A. Liver involvement in Alpers disease. J Pediatr 1991; 119: 260–267

891. Aarskog D. A familial syndrome of short stature associated with facial dysplasia and genital anomalies. J Pediatr 1970; 77: 856–861

892. Escobar V, Weaver D D. Aarskog syndrome. New findings and genetic analysis. JAMA 1978; 240: 2638–2644

893. Aarskog D, Aarskog syndrome. In: Buyse M L, ed. Birth defects encyclopedia. Dover, M A: Center for Birth Defects Information Services, 1990: pp 1–2

894. Senior B, Gellis S S. The syndromes of total lipodystrophy and of partial lipodystrophy. Pediatrics 1964; 33: 593–612

895. Ruvalcara R H A, Kelley V C. Lipoatrophic diabetes. II. Metabolic studies concerning the mechanism of lipemia. Am J Dis Child 1965; 109: 287–294

896. Case Records of the Massachusetts General Hospital. Case 1 — 1975. N Engl J Med 1975; 292: 35–41

897. Ipp M M, Howard N J, Tervo R C, Gelfand E W. Sicca syndrome and total lipodystrophy. A case in a fifteen-year-old female patient. Ann Intern Med 1975; 85; 443–446

898. Berge T, Brum A, Hansing B, Kjellman B. Congenital generalized lipodystrophy. Acta Pathol Microbiol Scand Sect A 1976; 84: 47–54

899. Klar A, Livni N, Gross-Kieselstein E, Navon P, Shahin A, Branski D. Ultrastructural abnormalities of the liver in total lipodystrophy. Arch Pathol Lab Med 1987; 111: 197–199

900. Johnson J P, Wilson D E. Lipodystrophy syndrome, Berardinelli type. In: Buyse M L, ed. Birth defects encyclopedia. Dover, M A: Center for Birth Defects Information Services, 1990: pp 1067–1068

901. Harbour J R, Rosenthal P, Smuckler E A, Ultrastructural abnormalities of the liver in total lipodystrophy. Hum Pathol 1981; 12: 856–862

902. Peremans J, Degraef P J, Strubble G, De Block G. Familial metabolic disorder with fatty metamorphosis of the viscera. J Pediatr 1966; 69: 1103–1112

903. Satran L, Sharp H L, Sehenken J R, Krivit W. Fatal neonatal hepatic steatosis. A new familial disorder. J Pediatr 1969; 75: 39–46

904. Rasanen O, Korhonen M, Simila S, Autere T, Hakosalo J. Fatal familial steatosis of the liver and kidney in two siblings. Z Kinderheilk 1971; 110: 267–275

905. Wadlington W B, Riley J D. Familial disease characterized by neonatal jaundice and probable hepatosteatosis and kernicterus. A new syndrome? Pediatrics 1973; 51: 192–198

906. Suprun H, Freundlich E. Fatal familial steatosis of myocardium, liver and kidneys in three siblings. Acta Paediatr

Scand 1981; 70: 247–252

907. Lorenz G, Barenwald G. Histologic and electron-microscopic liver changes in diabetic children. Acta Hepato-Gastroenterol 1979; 26: 435–438

908. Moran J R, Ghishan F K, Halter S A, Greene H L. Steatohepatitis in obese children: a cause of chronic liver dysfunction. Am J Gastroenterol 1983; 78: 374–377

909. Kinugasa A, Tsunamoto K, Furukawa N, Sawada T, Kusunoki T, Shimada N. Fatty liver and its fibrous changes found in simple obesity in children. J Pediatr Gastroenterol Nutr 1984; 3: 408–414

910. Paolucci F, Cinti S, Cangiotti A et al. Steatosis associated with immotile cilia syndrome: an unrecognized relationship. J Hepatol 1992; 14: 317–324

911. Donohue W L, Uchida I. Leprechaunism: a euphemism for a rare familial disorder. J Pediatr 1954; 45: 505–519

912. Evans P R. Leprechaunism. Arch Dis Childh 1955; 30: 479–483

913. Patterson J H, Watkins W L. Leprechaunism in a male infant. J Pediatr 1962; 60: 730–739

914. Dekaban A. Metabolic and chromosomal studies in leprechaunism. Arch Dis Childh 1965; 40: 632–636

915. Kallo I L, Lakatos I, Szijarto L. Leprechaunism (Donohue's syndrome). J Pediatr 1965; 66: 372–379

916. Rogers D R. Leprechaunism (Donohue's syndrome): a possible case, with emphasis on changes in the adrenohypophysis. Am J Clin Pathol 1966; 15: 614–619

917. Summitt R L, Favara B E. Leprechaunism (Donohue's syndrome): a case report. J Pediatr 1960; 74: 601–610

918. Ordway N K, Stout L C. Intrauterine growth retardation, jaundice and hypoglycemia in a neonate. J Pediatr 1973; 83: 867–874

919. Rosenberg A M, Howorth J C, Degroot G W, Trevenen C L, Rechler M M. A case of leprechaunism with severe hyperinsulinemia. Am J Dis Child 1980; 134: 170–175

920. Elsas L J. Leprechaunism. In: Buyse M L, ed. Birth defects encyclopedia. Dover, MA: Center for Birth Defects Information Services, 1990: pp 1044–1045

921. Elsas L J. Leprechaunism: an inherited defect in a high-affinity insulin receptor. Am J Hum Genet 1985; 37: 73–88

922. Reddy S S-K, Lauris V, Kahn C R. Insulin receptor function in fibroblasts from patients with leprechaunism. J Clin Invest 1988; 82: 1359–1365

923. Kadowski T, Bevins C, Cama A et al. Two mutant alleles of the insulin receptor in a patient with extreme insulin resistance. Science 1988; 240: 787–790

924. Klinkhauer M D, Goren N A, Van der Zon B C M. A leucine to proline mutation in the insulin receptor in family with insulin resistance. EMBO J 1989; 8: 2503–2507

925. Hermansky F, Pudlak P. Albinism associated with hemorrhagic diathesis and unusual pigmented reticular cells in the bone marrow: report of two cases with histochemical studies. Blood 1959; 14: 162–169

926. Bednar B, Hermansky F, Lojda Z. Vascular pseudohemophilia associated with ceroid pigmentophagia in albinos. Am J Pathol 1964; 45: 283–294

927. Schinella R A, Greco M A, Garay S M, Lackner H, Wolman S R, Fazzini E P. Hermansky Pudlak syndrome. A clinico-pathologic study. Hum Pathol 1985; 16: 366–376

928. Witkop C J Jr, Quevedo W C Jr, Fitzpatrick T B, King R A. Albinism. In: Scriver C R, Beaudet A L, Sly W S, Valle D, eds. The metabolic basis of inherited disease, 6th edn. New York: McGraw-Hill, 1989: pp 2905–2947

929. Boxer G J, Holmsen H, Robkin L, Bank N O, Boxer L A, Boehner R L. Abnormal platelet function in Chediak-Higashi syndrome. Br J Haematol 1977; 35: 521–533

930. White J G. The Chediak-Higashi syndrome: cytoplasmic sequestration in circulating leukocytes. Blood 1967; 29: 435–451

931. Hug G. Nonbilirubin genetic disorders of the liver. In: Gall E A, Mostofi F K, eds. The liver. Baltimore: Williams & Wilkins, 1973: pp 21–71

932. Valenzuela R, Aikawa M, O'Regan S, Makker S. Chediak-Higashi syndrome in black infant. Am J Clin Pathol 1976; 65: 483–494

933. Bedoya V, Grimley P M, Dugue O. Chediak-Higashi syndrome. Arch Pathol 1969; 88: 340–349

5

Iron storage disease

J. Searle   J. F. R. Kerr   J. W. Halliday   L. W. Powell

NORMAL IRON METABOLISM

INTRODUCTION

Iron is essential to mammalian life and yet, despite extensive study, the pathways of normal iron metabolism in human beings remain tantalizingly elusive. The body of a healthy adult male contains about 5 g of iron; the figure for females is slightly less. Approximately one-third of the total is present as storage iron, which can be drawn upon as needed, and approximately one-third of this storage is in the liver. No physiological mechanism has evolved for the excretion of excess iron, and normal iron balance is maintained by regulation of iron absorption via the duodenum and proximal jejunum. Increase in iron absorption or parenteral administration of iron thus results in an increase in body iron. Much of the excess iron will accumulate in the liver.

Iron is chemically reactive and potentially highly toxic. Stored iron must therefore be sequestered in a non-toxic form, while at the same time being readily available when needed for biosynthesis of essential iron proteins such as haemoglobin, myoglobin and catalase. In mammals, the dual requirements of storage in an innocuous form and continuous bioavailability are catered for by two specific iron-binding proteins, transferrin and ferritin. Transferrin is a single chain polypeptide which maintains iron in a non-toxic form during its transport via the blood whilst ferritin is the major storage protein that sequesters iron in tissues.[1] Both transferrin and ferritin are capable of the necessary tight, but reversible, binding of iron; transferrin has only two binding sites, whereas each molecule of ferritin is capable of holding up to 4000 atoms of iron within its centre.[2] The liver plays a central role in the metabolism of both of these proteins. However, Kupffer cells and hepatocytes have somewhat different properties in relation to the handling of iron. Thus the major function of the Kupffer cell is ingestion of effete red cells and colloidal iron, such as iron dextran, increased

219

synthesis of ferritin being stimulated as a result. The hepatocyte synthesizes and secretes transferrin, takes up transferrin with or without iron, and releases iron to plasma apotransferrin. Secondly, it synthesizes ferritin and takes up ferritin from the plasma, and it is also capable of taking up non-transferrin bound iron from the plasma.[3,4] Lastly, it takes up haemoglobin and haemoglobin bound to haptoglobin, and haem-haemopexin complexes.[5,6]

IRON ABSORPTION

Iron is absorbed both as haem and as non-haem compounds. Haem is taken up by the intestinal mucosal cell, in which iron is released from the porphyrin ring by the action of haem oxygenase. Approximately 12–20% of the haem iron ingested is absorbed, and this absorption is not influenced by dietary composition or luminal factors.[5] Most of the non-haem iron presented to the jejunum (e.g. from vegetable sources) is in a high molecular weight form, which is less well absorbed. Ferrous iron is more readily absorbed than ferric. Normal gastric juice provides an acid pH that assists in the formation of readily absorbable soluble iron complexes. However, the presence of hydrochloric acid is not essential for iron absorption. Natural chelating agents, which include sugars, amino acids, ascorbic acid and glycoproteins, may form complexes with iron, maintaining it in a soluble form and thus promoting absorption. In contrast, phytate, phosphate, carbonate, oxalate, pancreatic bicarbonate, tea and dietary fibre bind iron to form relatively insoluble complexes and thus result in a decrease in absorption.[6] The dietary absorption of iron can also be decreased by drugs such as cholestyramine[7] and tetracyclines.[8]

The most important factor in the physiological regulation of iron absorption is the total body iron content. When this is decreased, iron absorption in normal people is increased, and vice versa. Another factor is the rate of erythropoiesis.[5] The precise means by which the body's needs for iron are communicated to the intestinal mucosal cell are, nevertheless, still poorly understood. Cavill et al[9] proposed the concept of an exchangeable or labile iron pool for each tissue. This pool consisted of iron available for binding to circulating transferrin, and the total exchangeable iron in the body was considered to be directly related to the level of storage iron. They suggested that physiological regulation of iron absorption could be explained by consideration of the kinetics of internal iron exchange, with iron transfer from the intestinal epithelium to plasma varying directly as the product of intestinal exchangeable iron and plasma iron turnover, and inversely as the total exchangeable iron in stores. A possible mechanism whereby erythropoietic activity might influence intestinal absorption has been revealed by experiments

conducted by Finch & Huebers.[10] They produced an increase in iron absorption of 50–130% in normal rats by exchange transfusion with reticulocyte-rich blood, and this was not mediated by a decrease in plasma iron or an increase in unsaturated iron binding capacity of the plasma. Reticulocytes have been shown to possess receptors for the transferrin-iron complex[11] and it is possible that such receptors might influence the rate of plasma iron turnover. Recent evidence, however, indicates that mucosal transferrin receptors do not play a direct role in the absorption of iron and that the increases seen in transferrin receptors on the serosal surfaces of mucosal cells in iron-deficiency states may relate more to the demand for iron within the proliferating epithelial cells in the crypts than to a deficiency in body iron stores.[12] Transferrin receptors are shed into the plasma and the measurement of such receptors can now be used in the detection of iron deficiency states, in which the level is increased.[13,14]

Several newly identified iron-binding proteins have recently been described in the intestine. Peters and his colleagues[15,16] have identified a basolateral iron-binding site on luminal epithelial cell membranes, which shows increased binding in vivo following chronic hypoxia, a condition associated with increased iron absorption. Conrad et al[17] have reported two novel iron-binding proteins in the mucosa, which are distinct from ferritin and transferrin, and which they suggest may play a role in the regulation of iron absorption. Teichmann & Stremmel[18] have reported evidence of a facilitated transport system, which is mediated by a 54 kilodalton iron-binding protein in the microvillous membranes of enterocytes. This protein has also been located by immunofluorescent techniques on the serosal side of the mucosal cells and in the liver. Some recent evidence indicates that it may be up-regulated in genetic haemochromatosis, but further studies are needed to confirm this.

IRON TRANSPORT

Iron bound to transferrin is transported from the basal surface of the intestinal mucosal cell via the plasma to the liver, bone marrow and other tissues. Transferrin in plasma exists in mono- and diferric forms. In normal human plasma, most of the monoferric transferrin contains iron which is bound at the more labile N-terminal binding site. Studies have shown no difference in either the half-life or utilization of iron bound to the N-terminal or the C-terminal site.[19]

Plasma iron shows a diurnal variation in which morning values are approximately 30% higher than those in the evening. The normal plasma iron ranges from 10 to 30 µmol/l, and the total plasma iron-binding capacity from 50 to 70 µmol/l. The iron-binding capacity is normally approximately one-third saturated. It is now known that, in addition to transferrin, small amounts of ferritin also circulate in the plasma in normal individuals[20,21] and ferritin, unlike transferrin, can bind up to 4500 atoms of iron per molecule. The concentration of plasma ferritin in iron overload uncomplicated by tissue necrosis is elevated in proportion to the increase in the tissue iron stores. Where tissue necrosis is present, this relationship does not hold, since ferritin may act like an acute phase protein. Thus, although the origin and function of plasma ferritin are unknown, its concentration has been found to provide a reliable indication of body iron stores in the absence of hepatocellular necrosis, leukaemia or inflammatory disease. The normal values for plasma ferritin have been quoted as $12-250\,\mu g/l$ for males and $10-150\,\mu g/l$ for females. However, some recent studies have suggested that in certain populations where meat consumption is high the reference values may be higher, perhaps as a result of higher body iron stores.[22] The values rise slowly with advancing age, especially in males. Circulating ferritin has a much lower iron concentration than ferritin found in tissues, both in normal subjects and in patients with severe iron overload, and it seems unlikely that ferritin acts as an iron transport protein in the blood in normal subjects. However, ferritin with a high iron content is released following tissue damage, and may be taken up by the liver via the hepatic ferritin receptor (see p. 220).

IRON DELIVERY TO TISSUES

Some of the iron that is absorbed by the intestine and carried by transferrin in the portal blood is deposited within hepatocytes. Transferrin receptors have been described on isolated rat hepatocytes,[23] but the extent to which they are involved in the uptake of iron by the normal liver in vivo is unclear. Much information has been derived from study of haemopoietic tissue.[24] It is known that the interaction between transferrin and erythroid cells involves several steps; the binding of an iron–transferrin complex to specific cell receptors,[11] the shift of the bound complex into the cell, and the subsequent release of iron.[24] The latter occurs in intracellular organelles close to the Golgi apparatus, where an intravesicular acid pH facilitates the removal of iron from transferrin.[25] Little is known of the pathways taken by iron within the cell after its release from transferrin and before incorporation into the ferritin molecule. At least three different pathways of iron uptake by hepatocytes have been described[26,27] and the uptake of transferrin and of iron by hepatocytes occurs by both saturable and non-saturable processes.

Ferritin receptors have now been described in a variety of tissues, including mammalian liver, guinea pig reticulocytes and malignant tumours. Such receptors permit the uptake of ferritin[28,29] and although their role in normal iron metabolism remains to be elucidated, it has been suggested that hepatocyte ferritin receptors may play a role in the redistribution of iron from Kupffer cells to hepatocytes.[30,31]

IRON STORAGE

Under physiological conditions, iron is stored in the liver mainly in the form of ferritin, although some haemosiderin may also be present.

The ferritin molecule comprises a large spherical protein shell of molecular weight approximately 445 kilodaltons with a central hollow core capable of containing up to 4500 atoms of iron. The shell consists of 24 subunits of two distinct types, designated H and L, which differ in molecular weight, immunological properties and amino acid composition.[2] The relative numbers of H and L subunits in the molecule are to some extent responsible for the fact that each tissue exhibits a characteristic isoferritin profile (microheterogeneity) that changes in differing physiological and pathological states, particularly in iron overload, following phlebotomy and in malignancy.[21,32] Much recent work has been devoted to studies of the possible role of these subunits, not only in relation to iron uptake by the molecule, but also with respect to function. It has been proposed that the H subunit may play a regulatory role in the haemopoietic system.[33]

Haemosiderin is a chemically ill-defined, water-insoluble deposit of hydrated iron oxide micelles of indiscriminate size, which are associated with varying amounts of partly denatured protein.[34] This protein appears to be largely derived from ferritin, possibly following polymerization. Both storage forms provide iron that is accessible for haemoglobin production, although iron mobilization from haemosiderin is relatively slow. Iron in haemosiderin is also less accessible than ferritin iron to chelating agents such as desferrioxamine (see Electron microscopy, p. 222).

THE REGULATION OF IRON METABOLISM

Because of its importance in iron uptake into cells, the transferrin receptor (TfR) pathway is an obvious candidate for a mechanism by which iron leaves the mucosal cell of the gut and is transported via transferrin to other organs of the body. However, as pointed out in the section on iron absorption, Anderson et al[12] have shown that, in the neonatal rat, mucosal transferrin receptors are unlikely to be directly related to the regulation of iron absorption. Transferrin receptors have been detected on the serosal surface of mucosal cells[35,36] and are increased in iron deficiency, when the ferritin content of the cells is decreased. Recent studies have revealed a most interesting mechanism for the control of the translation of both ferritin and transferrin messenger RNA (mRNA). It is now known that the iron-mediated control of ferritin translation[37,38] can be explained by the presence of a folded hairpin (a 'stem-loop') structure with conserved unpaired nucleotides, known as the iron-regulatory element (IRE) in the 5' untranslated region of ferritin mRNAs. A 90-kilodalton protein known as the IRE-binding protein (IRE-BP) binds to the IRE and acts as a translation repressor.[37] The IRE-BP exists in a reduced and an oxidized form, each of which can react specifically with the IRE but the affinity for which differs according to the oxidation state. The reduced form has a higher binding affinity. This has been shown to be related to the reversible oxidation of a sulphydril group. The protein also contains a reactive iron-sulphur cluster. The total IRE-BP in the cytosol appears to be unaffected by prior treatment of the cell by iron; rather, the affinity of its binding to the IRE varies with the concentration of iron within the cell. Five similar stem-loop structures have now been demonstrated in the TfR mRNA and at least four of these IREs can simultaneously bind the same cytosolic IRE-BP as does the ferritin IRE.[39,40] Binding of the IRE-BP appears to protect the TfR mRNA from degradation, allowing translation to occur while binding to the ferritin mRNA prevents translation of the ferritin. This reciprocal mechanism thus provides very neatly for the coordinated regulation of ferritin and TfR proteins by iron. The IRE-BP has now been cloned[41] and localized to the human chromosome 9.[42] The haemochromatosis gene on the other hand has been localized to chromosome 6, thus making it unlikely that an abnormality in the IRE-BP is the basic defect in genetic haemochromatosis.

ANATOMICAL LOCALIZATION AND ASSESSMENT OF STORED IRON

ELECTRON MICROSCOPY

From the earliest stages of disorders in which there is excessive iron storage, both ferritin and haemosiderin accumulate in cells.[43–45] Tiny, electron-opaque cores of ferritin are seen dispersed throughout the cell sap (Fig. 5.1), and ferritin and haemosiderin are found together within siderosomes.[43,44] The latter are membrane-delimited bodies derived from secondary lysosomes of various types, including those originating from

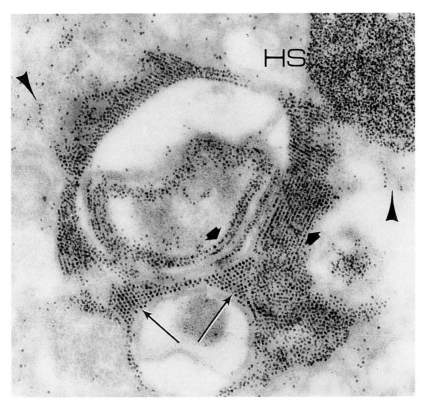

Fig. 5.1 Part of an hepatocyte from a 5-year-old thalassaemic patient. Ferritin particles are randomly dispersed in the cytosol (arrow heads). Larger, more electron-dense particles form arrays (short arrows) and hexagonal arrangements (long arrows) in relationship with membranous material. Such iron-rich ferritin molecules are preferentially located with lysosomes (siderosomes). Aggregates in which individual ferritin particles cannot be resolved are termed haemosiderin (HS). Unstained, × 90 000. Courtesy of Professor T C Iancu.

autophagosomes and heterophagosomes.[45] Inside siderosomes, the ferritin cores may be arranged in parallel arrays (Fig. 5.1) or show hexagonal configurations, and haemosiderin appears as electron-dense aggregates in which individual ferritin particles cannot be resolved (Fig. 5.1). Ferritin cores are conspicuously absent from all other cytoplasmic organelles.

Progressive iron loading results in a plateau being reached in the concentration of free cell-sap ferritin, but the amount of siderosomal iron continues to increase indefinitely.[44] Most of the haemosiderin within siderosomes is derived from ferritin,[34,46] but it includes iron (ferric hydroxide) micelles of various sizes associated with partly denatured protein.[46] Aggregation of parenterally administered iron compounds inside phagosomes may result in a similar ultrastructural appearance.[45] Siderosomes in hepatocytes frequently contain amorphous osmiophilic and membranous masses as well as haemosiderin, and they have been shown to be chemically as well as structurally heterogeneous.[34,35,47] The ultrastructure of Kupffer cell siderosomes suggests that they are more homogeneous.[44] The structure of the iron cores appears to differ in genetic haemochromatosis and thalassaemia major, and to change with the duration of iron loading, becoming more crystalline with time.[47,48] This influences the accessibility of iron to chelating agents. Whether the difference in haemosiderin structure results from the different primary storage cells in the two diseases (i.e. hepatocytes versus Kupffer cells), or whether it represents a more fundamental difference related to the diseases themselves, is unknown.

LIGHT MICROSCOPY

Both ferritin and haemosiderin are ferric compounds, and with acid ferrocyanide solutions they give the Prussian blue reaction. Perls' staining technique is recommended because of its high degree of sensitivity and specificity;[49] acidic tissue fixatives should be avoided and care must be taken to control the acid hydrolysis of iron and possible diffusion of the reaction product.[45] Occasionally, the Tirmann–Schmelzer modification of the reaction has been used,[50] but this is considered too insensitive to demonstrate more than a small proportion of the iron present and it is not recommended.[49] Using Perls' stain, ferritin dispersed through the cell sap produces a diffuse bluish tint to the cytoplasm, whereas intense blue granules correspond to ferritin and haemosiderin stored together within siderosomes.[45] In liver parenchymal cells, siderosomes characteristically tend to be aligned along the bile canaliculi, which is in accord with the localization of most lysosomes to this part of their cytoplasm.[51] All figures illustrating increased iron storage in this chapter represent sections stained by Perls' technique.

In iron storage diseases, haemosiderin-packed siderosomes may be most prominent in either the parenchymal or the sinusoid-lining cells of the liver. The patterns will be described in detail in the section dealing with the pathology of iron overload. However, it is worth pointing out at this stage that genetic haemochromatosis is characterized by preferential loading of parenchymal cells, whilst heavy loading of Kupffer cells and macrophages with relatively less in hepatocytes is a feature of most other types of excessive storage.

HISTOLOGICAL ASSESSMENT OF HEPATIC IRON STORES

Visual assessment of the amount of iron revealed by a Perls' stain on liver sections can rapidly provide valuable information about the level of iron stores in a particular patient, and often also about the manner by which any excessive amounts might have been acquired. There are three elements to be considered in such an assessment — the grade (or amount) of stainable iron present, its distribution in the various cell types of the acinus and portal tract, and the presence or absence of fibrosis or cirrhosis. Several studies using different criteria but with a common 0–4+ grading system for iron storage have been described and these have been reviewed previously.[52] A practical scheme of grading that is suitable for use in routine histological diagnosis is set out in Table 5.1. The advantages of this system are that iron in all cell types in the liver is included in the assessment, no subjective estimation of the percentage of cells containing iron is required, and the magnifications used to make judgments about the amount of iron visible are specified.

It should be emphasized, however, that all such grading methods remain subjective, and in this system grades less than 4+ are assigned according to the magnification at which discrete granules of haemosiderin can be resolved and not according to the lowest magnification at which a positive Prussian blue reaction can be discerned. Problems will arise occasionally, such as the difficulty in grading a diffuse blue staining of the cytosol due to the presence of abundant ferritin (see Miscellaneous conditions, p. 235), but in practice haemosiderin granules will be present also, either in nearby cells or in the cells containing the ferritin.

Table 5.1 Histological grading of iron storage

Grade	Ease of observation and magnification (eyepiece × objective) required
0	Granules absent or barely discernible × 400
1+	Barely discernible × 250
	Easily confirmed × 400
2+	Discrete granules resolved × 100
3+	Discrete granules resolved × 25
4+	Masses visible × 10, or naked eye

Another difficulty may be encountered in grading the iron in a biopsy taken during the course of phlebotomy for removal of excess iron from a patient with genetic haemochromatosis. In this instance, established heavy iron overload is characterized by the presence of large coalescent granular masses of haemosiderin in periportal hepatocytes and some macrophages (see Homozygotes, late changes, p. 226), and while smaller granules are removed from other cells at a comparatively early stage following regular venesections, these larger masses may remain for some time (see Homozygotes, effects of iron removal, p. 228). They are readily resolved at relatively low magnification, and, if assessed out of clinical context, an inappropriately high grading might be assigned in such cases.

Despite these limitations, this grading system has been found to give consistent results when used by different observers, with grades 0 and 1+ being within normal limits (corresponding to chemically estimated tissue iron concentrations of 5–40 µmol/g dry weight) and 3+ and 4+ representing significant increases in hepatic iron concentration (130–850 µmol/g dry weight). A grading of 2+ is suggestive of mild iron overload, particularly if haemosiderin is found almost exclusively in parenchymal cells. Calculation of the hepatic iron index usually allows the clinical significance of grade 2+ parenchymal iron stores to be determined. The grades recorded in the legends to figures in this chapter have been derived using this system.

CALCULATION OF THE HEPATIC IRON INDEX

Chemical determination of tissue iron concentration remains the ultimate criterion by which iron overload is diagnosed, and it has been recommended that a sample of liver tissue for the measurement of its iron concentration be taken at the time of liver biopsy in all patients being investigated for iron storage disorders.[53] Where no sample of the fresh biopsy has been taken, reliable results may be obtained by removing some of the tissue from the paraffin block and de-waxing it. The hepatic iron index is a derived value calculated by dividing the hepatic iron concentration (in µmol/g dry weight) by the age of the patient (in years). It is based on the principle that increasing hepatic iron concentration is found in homozygotes for genetic haemochromatosis with increasing age, whereas the same progressive accumulation of hepatic iron does not occur in patients with alcoholic liver disease or in those who are heterozygotes for genetic haemochromatosis. In a detailed study, the hepatic iron index was found to be greater than 2 in homozygotes, but in heterozygotes and in patients with alcoholic siderosis it was less than 2.[53,53a]

A rapid and reproducible method of measuring hepatic iron concentration in a Perls'-stained tissue section using a microcomputer and image analysis has been devised.[54] This technique permits a morphometric hepatic iron index to be calculated, which similarly may help discriminate between genetic haemochromatosis and other disorders of hepatic iron overload,[54] and which does not require any chemical analysis to be performed. Nevertheless, in the great majority of diagnostic laboratories, initial visual assessment followed by chemical measurement of tissue iron concentration will continue to be the mainstay of investigations into iron storage diseases. Another method of visually estimating tissue iron has been devised in which values are assigned according to the ease with which haemosiderin granules in the various cell types in the liver can be seen.[55] A weighting value for haemosiderin in parenchymal cells is part of this system, and although it is clearly useful in a specialized unit, the method appears too complex for routine use.

MECHANISMS AND CLASSIFICATION OF IRON OVERLOAD

Given that mammals possess no natural pathway for excretion of excess iron, iron overload may occur in one of three ways:

1. Increased absorption of iron from the diet. This is the sole mechanism operating in genetic haemochromatosis, where excess iron is absorbed from a normal diet. It also occurred in the past in the black South African ('Bantu'), in whom increased absorption followed extremely high oral intake of iron in a readily available form.

2. Parenteral administration of excess iron, either as therapeutic iron compounds or as blood transfusions. The latter occurs in the course of management of patients with chronic aplastic or hypoplastic anaemias, where increased intestinal absorption is minimal (see Transfusional overload, p. 230).

3. A combination of 1 and 2 above, where increased absorption of ingested iron coexists with excessive parenteral iron administration. This occurs in chronic anaemias characterized by ineffective erythropoiesis and a hyperplastic bone marrow, such as thalassaemia major and many sideroblastic anaemias.

Depending on the route and mechanism of iron loading, excess iron stored in ferritin and haemosiderin may be found predominantly in hepatocytes and biliary epithelial cells, Kupffer cells and portal tract macrophages, connective tissue cells, or in combinations of these. The excess iron may also be associated with fibrosis that ranges in degree from minimal to advanced, or with cirrhosis. Thus, the histological appearances of hepatic iron overload vary depending on the stage at which the biopsy is taken as well as the cause, so that close clinicopathological consultation is required in order to reach a specific and complete diagnosis in most cases of iron storage disease. Using this combined approach, genetic haemochromatosis emerges as a distinctive disease entity. The other examples of iron overload are best considered in the clinicopathological contexts in which they occur.

Genetic haemochromatosis is an iron storage disorder caused by one or more inherited defects in iron metabolism which result in iron absorption inappropriate to the level of body iron stores. The trait is inherited in an autosomal recessive mode[56] and recent evidence suggests that it is one of the commonest autosomal recessive disorders in certain Caucasian groups. The frequency of the gene in such populations has been estimated to be as high as 4.5%, which corresponds to a disease frequency of 0.2%.[57] The disease-susceptibility gene is located on chromosome 6, close to the locus of the alleles of the major histocompatibility complex (MHC), and significant linkage with the class I antigen HLA-A3 has been demonstrated in many countries. However, linkage with HLA-B14 and HLA-B7 has also been recorded, though less frequently.[58] In homozygous subjects, life-long excessive iron absorption may result in a massive increase in body iron. In such cases, parenchymal cell loading eventually results in functional organ failure as seen in cirrhosis, cardiac failure, diabetes mellitus and gonadal atrophy. The basic metabolic defect that leads to such inappropriate uptake of iron is unknown (for review, see Halliday & Powell).[59]

A classification of iron storage disease is set out in Table 5.2. It avoids the confusion engendered by use of the terms haemosiderosis and haemochromatosis as synonyms for iron loading (and sometimes as different stages in the same process), and it specifically dispenses with the problem of assessing the degree of parenchymal damage in order to classify a particular case. The extent of fibrosis and the presence of cirrhosis are clearly of great importance. However, they must be sharply distinguished from features that provide information about the aetiology and pathogenesis of the excessive iron accumulation. The pattern of organ dysfunction associated with parenchymal iron overload is similar, irrespective of the cause of the excessive iron storage, and it is not entirely dependent on the presence of structural parenchymal damage.[53,60,61]

PATHOLOGY OF IRON OVERLOAD

GENETIC HAEMOCHROMATOSIS

Homozygotes — early changes

Biopsies from young homozygotes, including those from the series of Bassett et al,[62] show that considerable amounts of iron have accumulated by the mid-teens (Fig. 5.2), with young males generally being more affected than females of

Table 5.2 Classification of iron overload

Genetic haemochromatosis
Familial iron overload (non-MHC linked)
Iron overload associated with chronic anaemia:
   Increased absorption (ineffective erythropoiesis with marrow
     hyperplasia)
   Multiple transfusions (marrow hypoplastic)
   Combination of increased absorption and transfusions
Iron overload associated with high dietary intake
Iron overload associated with alcoholic and other types of cirrhosis
Neonatal iron overload
Miscellaneous conditions

the same age.[62a] Haemosiderin is found first in hepatocytes in the vicinity of portal tracts, particularly those in zone 1 of the hepatic acinus (Fig. 5.2), the pattern resembling that seen in some older heterozygotes (compare Fig. 5.2 with Fig. 5.8). This distribution of stored iron may

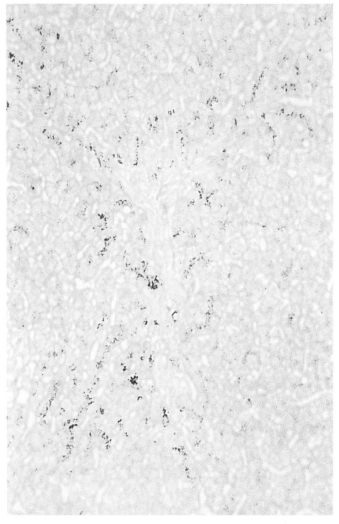

Fig. 5.2 Female aged 14. Mother has genetic haemochromatosis with cirrhosis; father is a probable heterozygote. Plasma ferritin was 160 µg/l and transferrin saturation was 73% at time of liver biopsy. She is almost certainly a homozygote. Haemosiderin (grade 2+) is present in periportal hepatocytes and extends along zone 1 of the hepatic acini. The granules form a cruciate pattern about the portal tract (centre). Perls' stain.

result in haemosiderin-containing hepatocytes forming a cruciate pattern around a portal tract (Fig. 5.2). The liver architecture is normal, Kupffer cells do not show excess iron storage at this stage, and there is no visible fibrosis.

Homozygotes — late changes

With increasing age, the deposition of haemosiderin becomes progressively heavier in parenchymal cells, such that the early periportal cruciate pattern becomes obscured by a more general distribution of larger granules. The increased iron storage remains, however, most marked around portal tracts and in acinar zone 1 (Fig. 5.3), and it attenuates towards the perivenular zones. Some Kupffer cells and occasional portal tract macrophages also become laden with haemosiderin at this stage (Fig. 5.3), although the involvement of both is greatly overshadowed by the large amount in hepatocytes. With the accumulation of still more iron, increasing fibrosis develops around portal tracts, and fine connective tissue septa begin to extend into the adjacent parenchyma (Fig. 5.4). This gradually evolves into a diffuse irregular fibrosis that first causes architectural distortion and later dissection with nodule formation. The combination of heavily iron-laden discrete parenchymal nodules and partially preserved acini (Fig. 5.5) is characteristic of the cirrhosis of untreated genetic haemochromatosis.[63] Further progression of fibrosis at this stage results in a diffuse micronodular pattern that resembles that occurring in secondary biliary cirrhosis,[64] but without the bile ductular proliferation that is typical of this condition.

In the later stages of heavy iron overload occasional

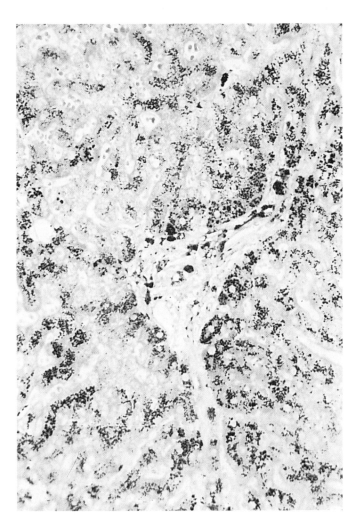

Fig. 5.3 Male aged 23 with genetic haemochromatosis (homozygous subject M-111-3 from Bassett et al).[62] Grade 3+ iron stores (liver iron concentration was 147 μmol/g dry weight). Haemosiderin is predominantly in periportal parenchymal cells with a little in Kupffer cells. There is little fibrosis. Perls' stain.

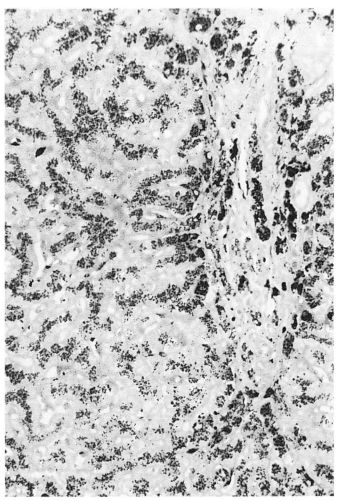

Fig. 5.4 Female aged 63 with genetic haemochromatosis (homozygous subject H-11-1 from Bassett et al).[62] Grade 4+ iron stores (liver iron concentration was 289 μmol/g dry weight). Haemosiderin is still predominantly in parenchymal cells, but some portal tract macrophages are now heavily laden. A connective tissue spur extends from the portal tract. Perls' stain.

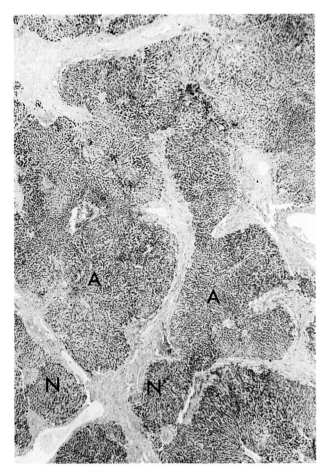

Fig. 5.5 Male aged 70 with untreated genetic haemochromatosis and cirrhosis. Massive iron stores in parenchymal cells outline the pattern of discrete nodules (N) and partially preserved acini (A) that characterizes this condition. Perls' stain. For a series of figures illustrating these features at higher magnification, see Powell & Kerr[63]

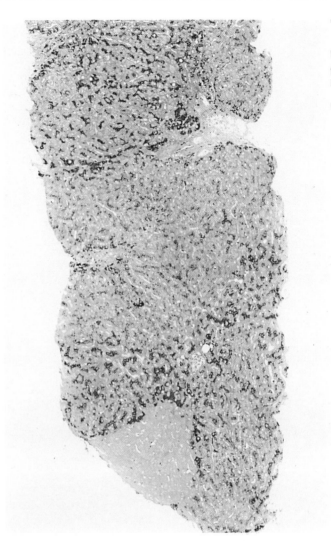

Fig. 5.6 Male aged 58 with untreated genetic haemochromatosis. A parenchymal iron-free focus is present surrounded by liver tissue that shows grade 4+ iron storage. There is no cirrhosis. Perls' stain.

discrete small areas may be found where hepatocytes contain either very little haemosiderin or apparently none at all. However, Kupffer cells lining the sinusoids in these areas invariably contain some iron (Fig. 5.6). Such parenchymal iron-free foci are seen most often in established cirrhosis,[63,64a] but they may also occur in its absence (Fig. 5.6). Similar non-siderotic foci may be seen in secondary (i.e. non-haemochromatotic) iron overload (Fig. 5.7). In both circumstances, their cause and significance are unknown. In general, the more advanced stages of evolution of the liver disease are seen at an earlier age in males than in females, but females in their thirties occasionally present with fully developed cirrhosis. The youngest recorded case with established disease was a male aged 13.[65]

Heterozygotes

Although full clinical, biochemical and pathological expression of genetic haemochromatosis occurs only in homozygotes, up to 25% of heterozygotes will develop partial biochemical expression of the disease associated with a limited increase in hepatic iron concentration.[62,66]

Biopsies from known heterozygotes (from the series of Bassett et al)[62] show architecturally normal liver with histologically graded iron stores in the range of 0–2+. Hepatic iron concentration in the group studied ranged from 10 to 68 μmol/g dry weight (reference range 5–40 μmol/g dry weight). When it is visible, the haemosiderin is contained in hepatocytes close to the portal tracts, often appearing heaviest in zone 1 of the hepatic acinus (Fig. 5.8). There is no fibrosis, and Kupffer cells show no excess of iron. A similar pattern may be found in young homozygotes who are liable to develop massive stores as they grow older, so that an hepatic iron index should be calculated, and clinical details and biochemical investigations should be assessed together with the biopsy appearances when the possibility of progressive primary iron storage disease

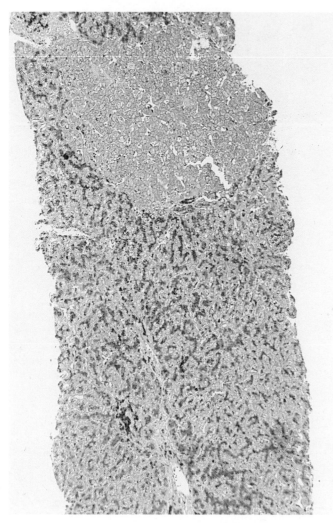

Fig. 5.7 Female, aged 37, given multiple transfusions over many years for chronic haemolytic anaemia. A relatively iron-free parenchymal focus is present, but Kupffer cells in this area show marked iron storage. Perls' stain.

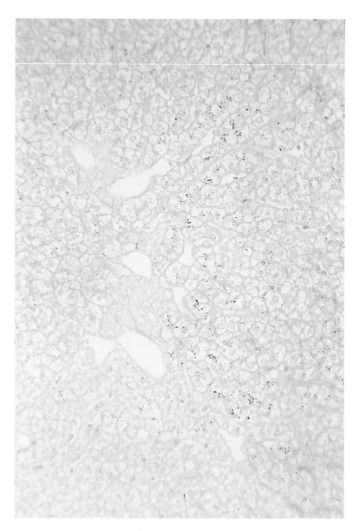

Fig. 5.8 Female aged 32 with genetic haemochromatosis (heterozygous subject J-11-6 in Bassett et al).[62] Grade 2+ iron stores (liver iron concentration was 58 µmol/g dry weight). Haemosiderin is predominantly in periportal hepatocytes and extends along zone 1 of the hepatic acinus. Perls' stain.

is being considered.[53,66a] Heterozygotes show no evidence of progression to massive iron accumulation with increasing age, and excessive alcohol consumption does not appear to result in significant iron overload.[62]

Homozygotes — effects of iron removal

In patients with genetic haemochromatosis and marked iron overload, an adequate course of therapeutic phlebotomies results in the disappearance of stored iron from the tissues. Biopsies taken during such treatment indicate that the pattern of removal of haemosiderin is the reverse of that which occurred during its accumulation, so that the last cells to contain stainable iron (often as relatively large granules) are periportal and scattered acinar zone 1 hepatocytes (Fig. 5.9). Occurring *pari passu* with the removal of iron from the

liver, in patients in whom cirrhosis had developed, there are changes in the pattern of fibrosis and in the parenchymal architecture. Occasional case reports of reversal of cirrhosis after phlebotomy have been published,[67-69] but a subsequent necropsy study of two patients originally thought on biopsy to have shown such reversal revealed that an iron-free macronodular cirrhosis was present in both,[63] and this finding has been repeated on other patients treated since then (Fig. 5.10). The macronodules are partly delineated by fine connective tissue septa, and often contain increased numbers of terminal hepatic veins (Fig. 5.10). Detailed microscopy shows that they also often contain tiny portal tract-like structures.[63] In a series reported by Niederau et al[70] a reduction in fibrosis was noted after phlebotomy but, in particular, complete reversal of cirrhosis was not observed.

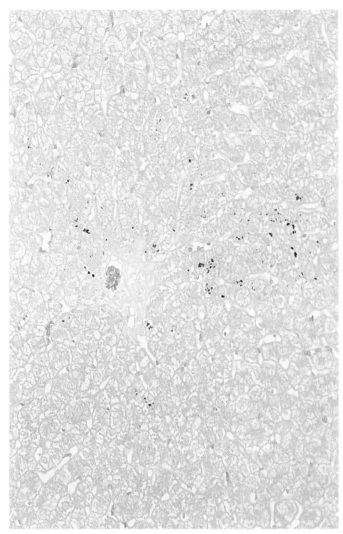

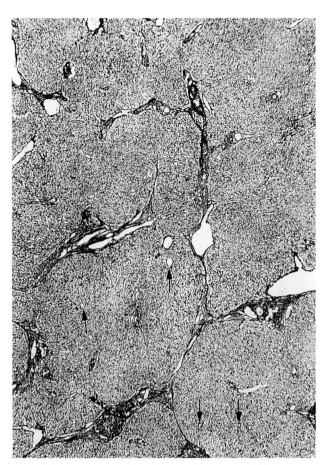

Fig. 5.10 Male aged 71. Macronodular cirrhosis present at necropsy 4 years after completion of treatment by repeated phlebotomies for biopsy-proven haemochromatosis with cirrhosis of classic pattern. Nodules are delineated by fine septa, and contain numerous hepatic vein tributaries. Death was due to a primary hepatocellular carcinoma. Reticulin stain.

Fig. 5.9 Male aged 43 with genetic haemochromatosis one year after beginning regular venesections for the removal of excess iron. Originally grade 3+ parenchymal iron storage was present, but now only a few coalescent granular aggregates of haemosiderin remain in the periportal zone. Perls' stain.

In general, such changes in the degree of fibrosis and architectural pattern have been described between 4 and 8 years after treatment, but in one patient who survived 32 years after iron removal from what was unequivocal haemochromatotic cirrhosis, restoration of liver architecture to almost normal has been recorded.[71]

Homozygotes — occurrence of primary hepatic carcinoma

Primary carcinoma of the liver may supervene in genetic haemochromatosis, as in other forms of cirrhosis, and its frequency appears to be gradually increasing. In 1935, Sheldon[72] recorded in incidence of 6.5%, and by 1951 Warren & Drake[73] found it to be 19%. By the mid-1970s an incidence of approximately 24% was reported.[74,75] In 1985, Niederau et al[70] reported an incidence of approxi-

mately 15%. The rise in incidence of liver carcinoma in haemochromatosis between the mid-1930s and mid-1970s might be related to longer patient survival as other lethal complications were successfully managed.[76] The malignancy develops against a background of established cirrhosis, although two patients with hepatocellular carcinoma have been described who were considered to show hepatic fibrosis rather than cirrhosis.[77] The tumours occur predominantly in males, and are not prevented by removal of iron.[70,75,78] The malignant transformation usually takes the form of hepatocellular carcinoma, but cholangiocarcinomas have been described.[70,79] The apparent decline in the incidence of malignancy complicating haemochromatosis in the decade to the mid-1980s might reflect earlier diagnosis and iron removal before the development of fibrosis or cirrhosis, but this is not yet certain.

Opinions differ concerning the relative risk of developing liver carcinoma in genetic haemochromatosis as compared with other types of cirrhosis. Warren & Drake[73] found a fourfold increase in risk with haemochromatosis over other types of cirrhosis, and Powell et al[80] reported a twofold increase. However, since haemochromatosis with cirrhosis is predominantly a disease of males, MacSween & Scott[74] restricted their comparison to figures for males and found that there was no significant difference in the incidence of primary hepatic cancer between haemochromatotics and cirrhotics generally. None of these studies has been able to take into account the incidence of either hepatitis B or hepatitis C virus infection in all cirrhotics with hepatic carcinoma, so that uncertainty remains about the relative risks and the possible mechanisms of liver carcinogenesis in genetic haemochromatosis. There is no doubt, however, that liver cancer is over 200 times more frequent in patients with genetic haemochromatosis than in the normal population.[70,81,81a] Bomford & Williams[75] observed a significantly higher rate of death from neoplasms in a variety of sites other than the liver in their series of patients treated by venesection; this, however, was not observed in the series of either Niederau et al[70] or Bradbear et al.[81]

FAMILIAL IRON OVERLOAD: NON-MHC LINKED

A large kindred of Melanesians from the Solomon Islands has been described in whom there is a very high incidence of iron overload.[82] The excess iron storage is predominantly in parenchymal cells (Fig. 5.11) and resembles that seen in genetic haemochromatosis in Caucasians. Genetic analysis, however, suggests autosomal dominant inheritance, and a study of a small part of the kindred has shown no linkage to any MHC locus.[82] Definitive diagnosis of this particular iron-loading disorder will depend on a more detailed linkage analysis. (See also Iron overload associated with ingestion of excessive amounts of dietary iron, p. 232)

IRON OVERLOAD ASSOCIATED WITH CHRONIC ANAEMIA

Overload associated with increased iron absorption

In patients with chronic anaemias characterized by a mild increase in erythropoiesis and not requiring transfusion therapy, slightly increased iron absorption might be expected. However, their liver iron stores do not appear to have been systematically investigated. Occasional cases of severe iron overload have been described in hereditary spherocytosis,[83,84] beta thalassaemia minor,[85] mild sideroblastic anaemia[61,86] and congenital pyruvate kinase deficiency.[87,88] In all of these reports, increased dietary absorption alone has been suggested as the cause for the overloading. Hepatic iron storage is predominantly parenchymal and fibrosis, or even cirrhosis, may occur (Fig. 5.12). Some of these patients have been found to have HLA genotypes commonly associated with genetic haemochromatosis[85,86] (Fig. 5.12), but in others no

evidence suggesting such an association has been found.[61] The frequency with which haemochromatosis-associated genotypes occur in chronic anaemias that are complicated by increased iron absorption from the gut remains to be determined.

Transfusional overload

Regular transfusions are the mainstay of therapy for many chronic anaemias, and in aplastic or hypoplastic anaemias, where increased intestinal absorption is minimal,[60,89] transfused blood provides the major source of the excess iron that accumulates.[90] Such iron is stored in Kupffer cells and macrophages of the spleen, liver, bone marrow and lymph nodes,[91] but the capacity of these cells can be exceeded by as little as 10–15 units of blood, after which increasing amounts of iron may be taken up by parenchymal cells as well.[90] Schafer et al[60] have shown

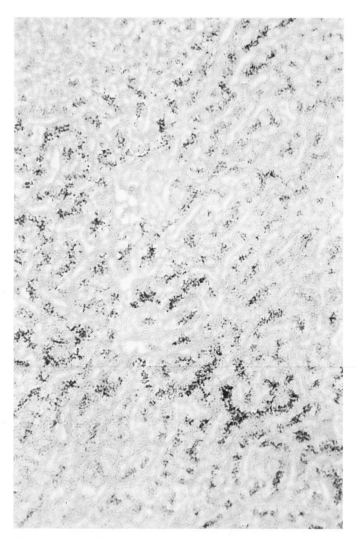

Fig. 5.11 Melanesian male aged 14 with familial iron overload (subject V-5 from Eason et al).[82] Grade 3+ iron stores (liver iron concentration was 190 µmol/g dry weight). Haemosiderin is present almost exclusively in acinar zone 1 hepatocytes. Perls' stain.

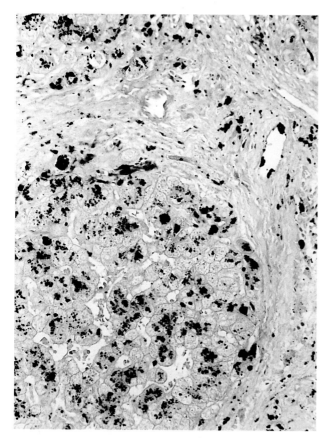

Fig. 5.12 Male aged 48 with congenital pyruvate kinase deficiency. The liver is cirrhotic, with grade 4+ iron stores predominantly in parenchymal cells (liver iron concentration was 388 μmol/g dry weight). Histocompatibility typing revealed both A3 and B14 antigens, suggesting that he might suffer from genetic haemochromatosis as well. Perls' stain.

that widespread, subclinical organ dysfunction resembling that found in genetic haemochromatosis can result from even relatively short-term transfusional iron loading.

It has been claimed that the histological appearances of transfusional overload are similar to those of genetic haemochromatosis.[90] However, in addition to iron being present in periportal and outer acinar parenchymal cells (Fig. 5.13), regular transfusion results in large amounts of iron being stored in Kupffer cells and groups of macrophages both within the liver parenchyma (Fig. 5.13) and in the portal tracts. Moreover, in perivenular (acinar zone 3) regions, sinusoidal lining cells consistently show heavy preferential iron storage (Fig. 5.14). This is unlike the pattern of genetic haemochromatosis, even in its advanced phase. Fibrosis is usually only mild, even with heavy iron stores (Fig. 5.13). Cirrhosis in patients of this type is extremely rare.[5]

Increased iron absorption combined with transfusional overload

Anaemias characterized by severely ineffective erythro-poiesis, a markedly hyperplastic marrow and a high

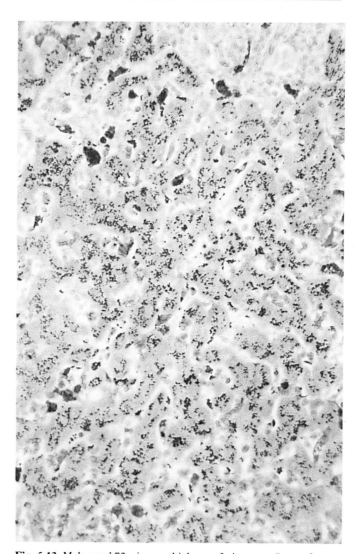

Fig. 5.13 Male, aged 72, given multiple transfusions over 5 years for chronic aplastic anaemia. Both Kupffer cells and hepatocytes are heavily laden with haemosiderin, and some is present in portal tract macrophages (top) as well. There is no fibrosis. Perls' stain.

plasma iron turnover, such as thalassaemia major and most sideroblastic anaemias, are associated with increased iron absorption from a normal diet, and this results in progressive iron overload.[92,93] For many patients with ineffective erythropoiesis, repeated blood transfusions may be the only effective treatment,[92] and this may result in marked acceleration of the rate of iron accumulation.

The most severe consequences of such a combined type of iron overload are typified by the progressive changes seen in children with thalassaemia major, the histological features of which have been described by Iancu et al.[94] In young thalassaemics (up to 3 years old), granular deposits of haemosiderin are present in hepatocytes, Kupffer cells and some portal tract macrophages, with the parenchymal accumulation being more prominent in the periportal zones. By the age of 5 years, iron deposition in these sites

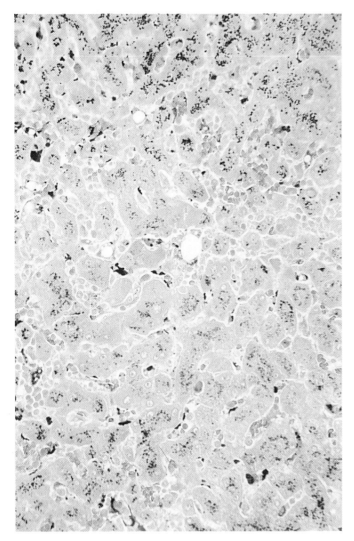

Fig. 5.14 Same case as Fig. 5.13. Acinar zone 3. Kupffer cells and endothelial cells contain abundant haemosiderin, with relatively less in parenchymal cells. Perls' stain.

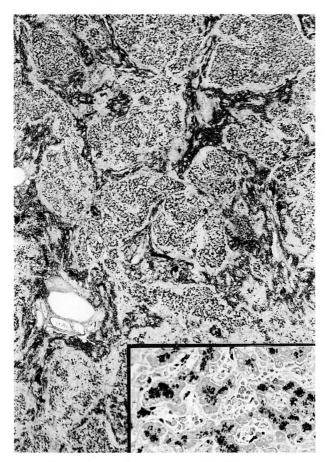

Fig. 5.15 Male aged 16 with thalassaemia major. There is dissection of the parenchyma into irregular nodules of various sizes by connective tissue septa that show heavy ferrocalcinosis. Inset: at higher magnification both parenchymal and Kupffer cells are heavily laden with iron. Perls' stain.

is heavier, and haemosiderin is present in clumps of macrophages in the parenchyma. Subsequently, further iron storage is associated with progressive periportal and septal fibrosis with some nodule formation, and in patients aged 10 years and over, the heavily iron-laden liver is cirrhotic and shows ferrocalcinosis of vessel walls and septal connective tissue (Fig. 5.15). The severity of the fibrosis in thalassaemics is directly related to both the liver iron concentration and the duration of its accumulation,[95] and the general pattern of architectural disturbance that develops often resembles that seen in the cirrhosis of genetic haemochromatosis,[63] though transfusion-related hepatitis C may modify the histological picture. Progressive periportal fibrosis with septum formation also occurs in association with heavy parenchymal iron storage in chronic sideroblastic anaemia (Fig. 5.16). However, in both of these anaemias, clusters of macrophages heavily laden with iron are far more prominent in the fibrotic areas and

in the parenchyma (Fig. 5.16) than they are in genetic haemochromatosis (compare Fig. 5.16 with Fig. 5.4).

There is currently no evidence that the incidence of primary hepatic carcinoma is increased in conditions of iron overload associated with chronic anaemia.[90]

IRON OVERLOAD ASSOCIATED WITH INGESTION OF EXCESSIVE AMOUNTS OF DIETARY IRON

Iron storage disease has been described occasionally in non-anaemic patients who are habituated to self-medication with iron compounds.[76,96] Whether or not such ingestion can result in excessive absorption of iron in the absence of one or both genes for genetic haemochromatosis is unknown at present.

By far the most extensively studied group with dietary iron overload is the black South African, whose source of surplus iron was the containers used for brewing traditional beers.[97] However, even here, it has been suggested that genetic factors may be involved in this form of iron overload.[98] Most of the excessive storage iron is found in

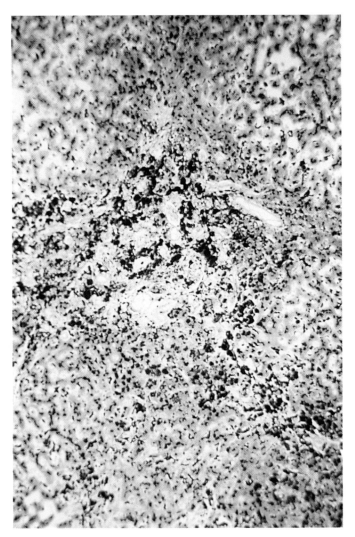

Fig. 5.16 Male aged 67 with idiopathic sideroblastic anaemia treated with numerous transfusions over the previous 4 years. Heavy iron stores are present (grade 4+) with loading of both parenchymal cells and macrophages. Periportal fibrosis with architectural distortion is discernible, but there is no cirrhosis. Perls' stain.

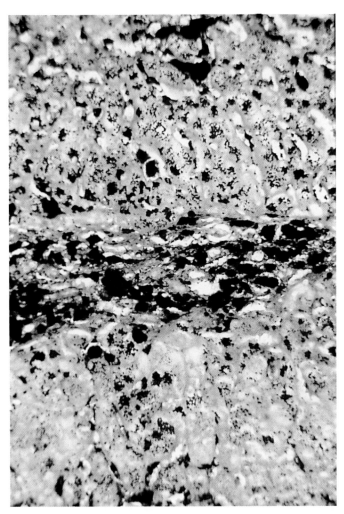

Fig. 5.17 South African black ('Bantu' siderosis). Massive iron storage in macrophages in portal tracts and in Kupffer cells. Considerably less is present in hepatocytes. Perls' stain. Courtesy of Professor T Bothwell

the liver, bone marrow and spleen.[99] In the liver, the major deposits of iron are present in portal tract macrophages and Kupffer cells, with moderately heavy deposits in hepatocytes and only scanty amounts in the biliary epithelium (Fig. 5.17). Fibrosis increases with rising hepatic iron concentration,[100] and the massive accumulation of haemosiderin that develops in the late stages of the disease is predominantly in the portal tracts and fibrous tissue (Fig. 5.18). This results in a pattern of iron storage that is quite unlike the predominantly parenchymal storage of genetic haemochromatosis[101] (compare Fig. 15.8 with Fig. 5.5). It does, however, resemble the pattern reported in experimental animals placed on nutritionally deficient diets with heavy oral iron supplements.[102] In the siderotic South African blacks, parenchymal deposits in tissues such as pancreas, heart and endocrine glands are uncommon, except in a small proportion

with severe iron overload who always gave a long history of excessive alcohol consumption and who were invariably cirrhotic.[101]

IRON OVERLOAD IN ALCOHOLIC AND OTHER TYPES OF CIRRHOSIS

The incidence of excessive alcohol consumption is usually high in groups of patients with genetic haemochromatosis, with figures ranging from 15%[75] to 41%.[78] Dubin[79] was the first to recognise that alcohol-induced injury may have a marked effect on the distribution of iron in the liver in 'idiopathic' (genetic) haemochromatosis. He described a shift of haemosiderin from parenchymal to Kupffer cells and macrophages in the fibrous septa, with much less remaining in the epithelial cells of the nodules (Fig. 5.19). These findings were confirmed by Powell & Kerr,[63] who described similar differences in haemosiderin distribution between two brothers with genetic

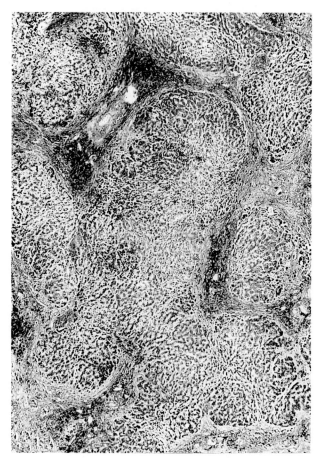

Fig. 5.18 South African black ('Bantu' siderosis). Cirrhosis with heavy iron deposition in cells in connective tissue septa. Iron stores in parenchymal nodules are patchy. Perls' stain. Courtesy of Professor T Bothwell

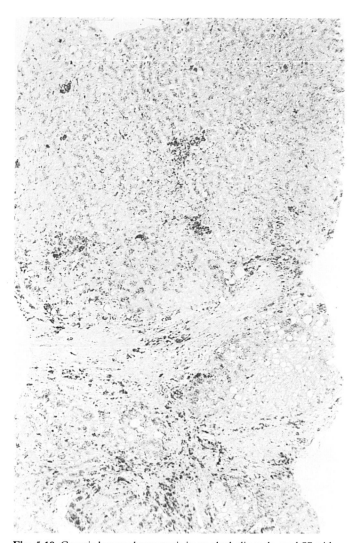

Fig. 5.19 Genetic haemochromatosis in an alcoholic male aged 57 with cirrhosis. Within the parenchymal nodules, hepatocellular iron storage is variable and aggregates of iron-laden macrophages are present at the edges of nodules and in the fibrous septa. Perls' stain.

haemochromatosis, one of whom was a total abstainer and the other a chronic alcoholic. In addition to the change in the pattern of excess iron storage, they observed that the alcoholic patient had a micronodular cirrhosis unlike the variable pattern of nodules and partially preserved acini seen in the uncomplicated genetic disease. More recently, it has been found that the concentration of hepatic iron is lower in alcoholic than non-alcoholic patients with genetic haemochromatosis, despite equal total body iron stores, and it has been suggested that alcohol may have been responsible for altering the distribution of the stored iron.[103]

Some degree of hepatic siderosis is common among cirrhotic patients in general,[104,105] but it is usually only slight[106] and is patchy in distribution (Fig. 5.20). The mechanism for increased iron storage in such patients is unclear.[107] Whether all such patients suffer from genetic haemochromatosis is uncertain, but there is growing evidence that the majority of alcoholics in whom iron accumulation is massive also suffer from genetic haemochromatosis.[103,108]

NEONATAL IRON OVERLOAD

A rare perinatal syndrome termed neonatal haemochromatosis has been defined, in which infants who are stillborn, born prematurely, or show signs of intrauterine growth retardation manifest clinical evidence of liver failure, and pathologically show a characteristic pattern of heavy iron storage.[109,110] The condition may recur in sibs, and signs in live-born infants include hypoglycaemia, hypoalbuminaemia and oedema, a haemorrhagic diathesis, and ultimately hyperbilirubinaemia; these signs are present either at birth or develop shortly thereafter.[111] Pathologically, this process is characterized by severe hepatic parenchymal cell loss, with either patchy or massive confluent acinar collapse (Fig. 5.21). Surviving hepatocytes may show giant cell or pseudoacinar transformation, and foci of nodular regeneration may be present (Fig. 5.21). Liver cell siderosis is usually marked

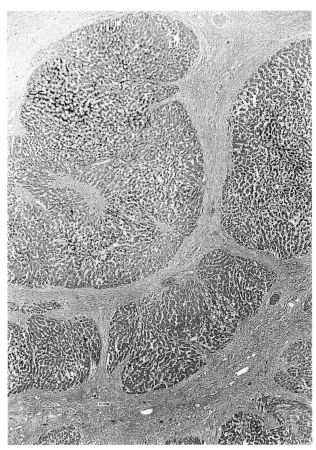

Fig. 5.20 Mild, patchy iron deposition in a cirrhotic alcoholic male aged 56. This was an incidental finding at necropsy; death was caused by pneumonia. Perls' stain.

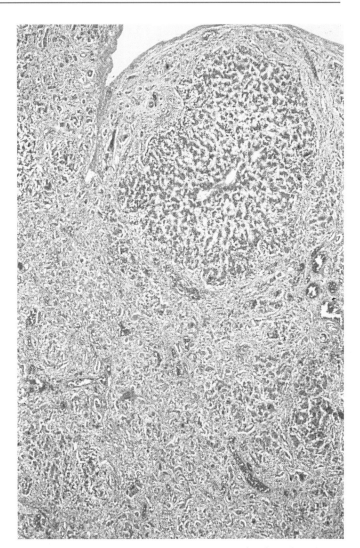

Fig. 5.21 Premature male neonate who died from fulminant hepatic failure. There is confluent panacinar collapse with occasional areas of nodular regeneration. Abundant stainable iron was present in the surviving hepatocytes. H&E.

(Fig. 5.22), and haemosiderin can also be demonstrated in parenchymal cells of the heart, thyroid, pancreas and glands of the upper respiratory and digestive tracts.[111] The aetiology of this condition is unknown, but current evidence favours the view that severe antenatal liver disease leads to abnormal feto-placental iron handling, with subsequent tissue siderosis.[111] There is no evidence that this condition is related to genetic haemochromatosis in adults.[112]

Variable degrees of hepatic parenchymal iron overload may be seen in infants with the cerebro-hepato-renal (Zellweger) syndrome and with tyrosinaemia. Such iron excess does not appear to be part of the primary disorder in these conditions, which are described elsewhere in this book (see ch. 4).

MISCELLANEOUS CONDITIONS

Iron overload associated with chronic renal failure

Intermittent blood transfusions have commonly been used in the past for the treatment of the anaemia that invariably accompanies chronic renal failure, and mildly

increased hepatic iron storage involving both sinusoidal lining cells and hepatocytes occurs in such patients.[113] Increasingly, such transfusion-dependent patients are being treated with erythropoietin, so that the risk of their developing siderosis is being reduced. The use of maintenance haemodialysis in the management of more advanced chronic renal insufficiency has led to a great reduction in the need for transfusions for anaemia, but has introduced the problem of recurrent blood loss that results in significant losses of body iron from patients managed in this way.[114] Although oral iron supplementation has been shown to be effective in replacing these losses,[114] some dialysis units continue to use parenteral iron or blood transfusions[115,116] which can lead to hepatic iron overload (Fig. 5.23). Under these conditions, iron storage is greater the longer the period of haemodialysis but concomitant fibrosis has not yet been described.[113]

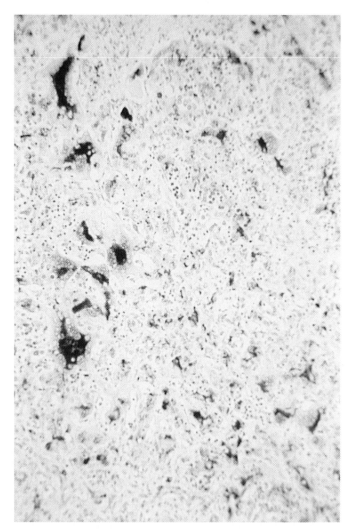

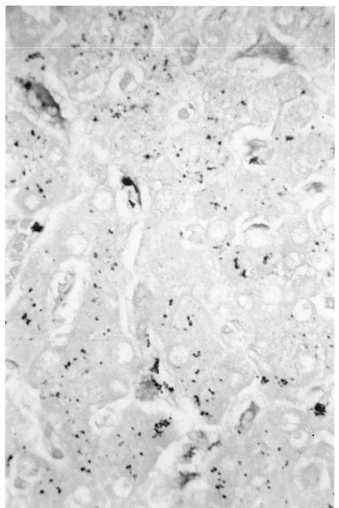

Fig. 5.22 Female sib of the case shown in Fig. 5.21. She also died in the neonatal period of hepatic failure. There is widespread hepatocellular loss with parenchymal collapse, and surviving liver cells, some showing giant cell transformation, show marked siderosis. Perls' stain.

Fig. 5.23 Grade 2+ iron storage in a female aged 20 who died of chronic renal failure. During the 6 months prior to death she had been transfused with 18 units of blood. Granular deposits of haemosiderin are present in hepatocytes and some Kupffer cells. The cytoplasm of other Kupffer cells shows a diffuse staining reaction indicating a marked increase in ferritin in the cell sap. Perls' stain.

Iron overload in porphyria cutanea tarda (PCT)

A common but not universal feature of the liver histology in PCT is iron overload involving periportal hepatocytes and Kupffer cells (Fig. 5.24). This is usually only mild,[117,118] but occasional patients with heavy iron deposition have been described.[119,120] The excessive storage frequently, but not invariably, coexists with alcoholic liver disease,[121] and Felsher & Kushner[122] considered that hepatic siderosis in PCT was the result of an enhanced rate of iron absorption from the diet, although no mechanism of increased absorption was proposed. Increased frequencies of MHC class I antigens A3 and B7 have been described in patients with PCT[123] and evidence has been presented that heterozygosity for MHC-linked (genetic) haemochromatosis could be responsible for the hepatic siderosis associated with sporadic PCT[124] However, no such association was

found by Beaumont et al.[125] Since the study protocols of these latter two investigations were dissimilar, further epidemiological study is needed to resolve this question.[126]

Iron overload after portacaval shunt

Conn[127] reviewed the literature and reported a series of his own patients which indicated that portacaval anastomosis in cirrhotic patients is sometimes accompanied by an accelerated tendency to deposit haemosiderin in the liver. In particular, he described a threefold increase in the degree of iron storage in affected livers.[127] Almost simultaneously, Koff et al[128] reported contrasting experience with a smaller series of cirrhotics in which they were able to demonstrate only minimal changes in both the incidence and the degree of hepatic iron storage

Fig. 5.24 Grade 2+ iron storage in a male aged 55 with sporadic porphyria cutanes tarda. Haemosiderin is present mainly in parenchymal cells around the portal tract, Perls' stain.

after portacaval shunt surgery. It appears that, while post-shunt iron overload can occur and may even be severe,[129,130] it is neither inevitable nor necessarily very heavy. The mechanism by which it occurs is unknown.

Congenital atransferrinaemia

This is an exceptionally rare disorder in which children develop a chronic hypochromic anaemia that is complicated by massive iron overload.[131] Affected children usually have received multiple transfusions, and in some, increased absorption of iron from the gut has been recorded. This suggests that in this condition the mechanism of iron overload is a combination of increased absorption and parenteral administration.

EXPERIMENTAL IRON OVERLOAD

Early experiments in which iron overload was induced in a wide variety of animal species, using many different iron compounds and various parenteral routes of administration, resulted in the production of features of transfusional siderosis without coincident hepatic fibrosis.[132] Subsequently, after more prolonged periods of iron administration were employed, fibrosis and even cirrhosis have been recorded.[133,134,134a] In all of these experiments, large amounts of iron accumulated first in the cells of the monocyte-macrophage system, and only later in hepatocytes. Marked Kupffer cell iron storage together with heavy hepatocellular siderosis was produced in rats by combining excessive oral iron administration with cyclic starvation,[135] but fibrosis did not occur. Parenchymal and Kupffer cell iron overload associated with hepatic fibrosis and cirrhosis have been induced in rats after iron feeding was augmented by the use of hepatotoxins or dietary deficiency,[102,136] and this pattern of excess iron storage and tissue damage simulates that of dietary iron overload in the South African black.

More recently, dietary administration of carbonyl iron[137] to rats for several months has been shown to result in a pattern of hepatocellular iron overload that closely resembles that seen in genetic haemochromatosis[138,139] (Fig. 5.25). In one of these experiments, prolonged feeding with such iron resulted in marked overload in Kupffer cells and portal tract macrophages in addition to parenchymal siderosis, and marked hepatic fibrosis developed, so that the pattern of storage again came to resemble that seen in the South African black.[139] In the other experiment, however, feeding carbonyl iron for up to 15 months failed to induce hepatic fibrosis.[138] This difference might reflect the higher concentration of dietary iron used in the former experiment, or alternatively, some degree of inflammatory activity may have coexisted with the iron loading.

THE GENESIS OF FIBROSIS IN IRON OVERLOAD

Although human organ dysfunction may result from relatively mild iron overload with only slight fibrosis,[60] in tissues where iron deposition is heavy, such as liver and pancreas, progressive fibrosis may develop which results in severe structural disorganization. In untreated, uncomplicated genetic haemochromatosis, hepatic fibrosis develops as iron storage increases with time.[53] In both thalassaemia major[95] and 'Bantu' siderosis[100] fibrosis increases with the duration of storage and the tissue iron concentration, and similar results have been obtained experimentally.[139] Whether this fibrosis is a consequence of hepatocyte injury and necrosis or is a direct effect of iron accumulation is controversial.

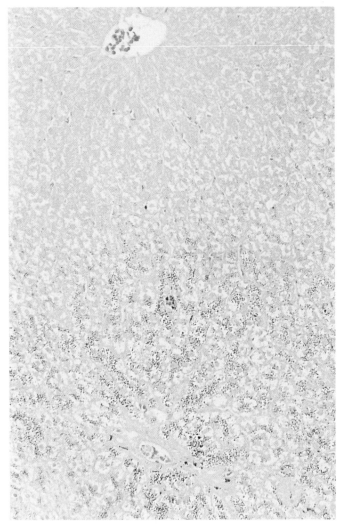

Fig. 5.25 Rat liver 3 months after continuous dietary administration of 2.5% (w/w) carbonyl iron. There is marked hepatocellular iron storage in acinar zones 1 and 2, but no fibrosis. Perls' stain.

Trump et al[43] suggested that iron toxicity might be expressed through membrane lipid peroxidation with the production of a series of free radicals capable of inflicting cell injury. This concept was supported by Bacon et al[137] who demonstrated lipid peroxidation of hepatic organelle membranes in vivo after inducing iron overload, and who obtained similar results from in vitro experiments.[140] Further, membranes of iron-laden lysosomes (siderosomes) have been shown to have increased fragility,[141] and lysosomal disruption has been proposed as a mechanism for tissue damage in conditions of iron storage.[142] However, it has not been demonstrated that the increased lysosomal fragility observed in vitro reflects increased lysosomal permeability in vivo, and organelles in the vicinity of hepatocyte siderosomes show no ultrastructural abnormality in either human beings[44] or experimental animals.[138,139] Moreover, no evidence of lethal cell injury has been found in a number of studies by electron microscopy of either experimental iron over-load[43,138,139,143] or human iron storage disease,[94] although non-specific ultrastructural changes interpreted as evidence of cell damage have been described in heavily iron-laden human livers that also showed established cirrhosis.[144] Nevertheless, in a light microscopic study, Deugnier et al[55] reported the occurrence of 'sideronecrosis' in most liver biopsies from haemochromatotic patients that showed heavy iron overload. They proposed that this was an important precursor to the development of hepatic fibrosis. But 'sideronecrosis' is described by these authors as being both rare and difficult to identify,[55] and review of many biopsies from our series of patients with all levels of iron loading has failed to reveal any such lesions, save for occasional possible foci in some patients with massive iron overload and established fibrosis or cirrhosis. The significance of such lesions in the initiation of the diffuse portal and periportal fibrosis typical of chronic progressive parenchymal iron overload in human beings remains to be determined.

Collagen deposition has been observed ultrastructurally at a very early stage of iron loading in children with thalassaemia major,[44] as well as in experimental iron overload when no fibrosis was visible by light microscopy.[145] In the latter experiment there was also a 50% increase in hepatic hydroxyproline content. All of these observations suggest that excess iron might be a direct stimulus for collagen biosynthesis. In this context, the finding that iron-induced lipid peroxidation of cultured human fibroblasts resulted in increased collagen gene transcription and in collagen production[146] appears significant. A similar process in hepatocytes and sinusoidal cells, both of which are capable of forming collagen,[147] could explain the development of iron-associated hepatic fibrosis without antecedent cell death (for review, see Bacon & Britton).[148]

ACKNOWLEDGEMENT

This work was supported in part by the National Health and Medical Research Council of Australia.

REFERENCES

1. Aisen P, Listowsky I. Iron transport and storage proteins. Annu Rev Biochem 1980; 49: 357–393
2. Harrison P M, Clegg G A, May K. Ferritin structure and function. In: Jacobs A, Worwood M, eds. Iron in biochemistry and medicine II. London: Academic Press, 1980
3. Brissot P, Wright T L, Ma W-L, Weisiger R A. Efficient clearance of non-transferrin-bound iron by rat liver. J Clin Invest 1985; 76: 1463–1470
4. Wright T L, Brissot P, Ma W-L, Weisiger R A. Characterization of non-transferrin-bound iron clearance by rat liver. J Biol Chem 1986; 261:(23) 10909–10914
5. Bothwell T H, Charlton R W, Cook J D, Finch C A. Iron metabolism in man. Oxford: Blackwell, 1979
6. Aisen P. Current concepts in iron metabolism. Clin Haematol 1982; 11: 241–258
7. Thomas F B, Salsburey D, Greenberger N J. Inhibition of iron absorption by cholestyramine. Am J Dig Dis 1972; 17: 263–269

8. Greenberger N J, Ruppert R D, Cuppage F E. Inhibition of intestinal iron transport induced by tetracycline. Gastroenterology 1967; 53: 590–599

9. Cavill I, Worwood M, Jacobs A. Internal regulation of iron absorption. Nature 1975; 256: 328–329

10. Finch C A, Huebers H. The regulation of iron exchange. Clin Res 1989; 29: 570A

11. van Bockxmeer F M, Morgan E H. Identification of transferrin receptors in reticulocytes. Biochim Biophys Acta 1977; 468: 437–450

12. Anderson G J, Walsh M D, Powell L W, Halliday J W. Intestinal transferrin receptors and iron absorption in the neonatal rat. Br J Haematol 1991; 77: 229–236

13. Kohgo Y, Niitsu Y, Kondo H et al. Serum transferrin receptor as a new index of erythropoiesis. Blood 1987; 70: 1955–1958

14. Flowers C H, Skikne B S, Covell A M, Cook J D. The clinical measurement of serum transferrin receptor. J Lab Clin Med 1989; 114: 368–377

15. Osterloh K R S, Simpson R J, Snape S, Peters T J. Intestinal iron absorption and mucosal transferrin in rats subjected to hypoxia. Blut 1987; 55: 421–431

16. Simpson R J, Moore R, Peters T J. Significance of non-esterified fatty acids in iron uptake by intestinal brush-border membrane vesicles. Biochim Biophys Acta 1988; 941: 39–47

17. Conrad M E, Umbreit J N, Moore E G, Peterson R D A, Jones MBA. A newly identified iron binding protein in duodenal mucosa of rat. J Biol Chem 1990; 265: 5273–5279

18. Teichmann R, Stremmel W. Iron uptake by human upper small intestine microvillus membrane vesicles. Indication for a facilitated transport mechanism mediated by a membrane iron-binding protein. J Clin Invest 1990; 86: 2145–2153

19. van der Heul C, Kroos M J, van Noort W L, van Eijk H G. No functional difference of the two iron-binding sites of human transferrin in vitro. Clin Sci 1981; 60: 185–190

20. Jacobs A, Miller F, Worwood M, Beamish M R, Wardrop C A J. Ferritin in the serum of normal subjects and patients with iron deficiency and iron overload. Br Med J 1972; 4: 206–208

21. Halliday J W, Powell L W. Serum ferritins and isoferritins in clinical medicine. Prog Hematol 1979; 11: 229–266

22. Leggett B A, Brown N N, Bryant S J, Duplock L, Powell L W, Halliday J W. Factors affecting the concentrations of ferritin in serum in a healthy Australian population. Clin Chem 1990; 36: 1350–1355

23. Young S P, Aisen P. Transferrin receptors and the uptake and release of iron by isolated hepatocytes. Hepatology 1981; 1: 114–119

24. Morgan E H. Transferrin, biochemistry, physiology and clinical significance. Mol Aspects Med 1981; 4: 1–122

25. Aisen P. Transferrin metabolism and the liver. Semin Liver Dis 1984; 4: 193–206

26. Trinder D, Morgan E, Baker E. The mechanisms of iron uptake by fetal rat hepatocytes in culture. Hepatology 1986; 6: 852–858

27. Trinder D, Batey R G, Morgan E H, Baker E. Effect of cellular iron concentration on iron uptake by hepatocytes. Am J Physiol 1990; 259: G611–G617

28. Mack U, Powell L W, Halliday J W. Detection and isolation of an hepatic receptor for ferritin. J Biol Chem 1983; 258: 4672–4675

29. Adams P C, Powell L W, Halliday J W. Isolation of a human hepatic ferritin receptor. Hepatology 1988; 8: 719–721

30. Kondo H, Saito K, Grasso J P, Aisen P. Iron metabolism in the erythrophagocytosing Kupffer cell. Hepatology 1988; 8: 32–39

31. Sibille J-C, Kondo H, Aisen P. Interactions between isolated hepatocytes and Kupffer cells in iron metabolism: a possible role for ferritin as an iron carrier protein. Hepatology 1988; 8: 296–301

32. Worwood M. Ferritin in human tissues and serum. Clin Haematol 1982; 11: 275–307

33. Broxmeyer H E, Williams D E, Geissler K et al. Suppressive effects in vivo of purified recombinant human H-subunit (acidic) ferritin on murine myelopoiesis. Blood 1989; 73: 74–79

34. Wixom R L, Prutkin L, Munro H N. Hemosiderin: nature, formation, and significance. Int Rev Exp Pathol 1980; 22: 193–225

35. Banerjee D, Flanagan P R, Cluett J, Valberg L S. Transferrin receptors in the human gastrointestinal tract. Relationship to body iron stores. Gastroenterology 1986; 91: 861–869

36. Lombard M, Bomford A B, Polson R J, Bellingham A J, Williams R. Differential expression of transferrin receptor in duodenal mucosa in iron overload. Evidence for a site-specific defect in genetic haemochromatosis. Gastroenterology 1990; 98: 976–984

37. Rouault T A, Hentze M W, Caughman S W, Harford J B, Klausner R D. Binding of a cytosolic protein to the iron-responsive element of human ferritin messenger RNA. Science 1988; 241: 1207–1210

38. Haile D J, Hentze M W, Rouault T A, Harford J B, Klausner R D. Regulation of interaction of the iron-responsive element binding protein with iron-responsive RNA elements. Mol Cell Biol 1989; 9: 5055–5061

39. Koeller D M, Casey J L, Hentze M W et al. A cytosolic protein binds to structural elements within the iron regulating region of the transferrin receptor mRNA. Proc Natl Acad Sci USA 1989; 86: 3574–3578

40. Mullner E W, Neupert B, Kuhn L C. A specific mRNA binding factor regulates the iron-dependent stability of cytoplasmic transferrin receptor mRNA. Cell 1989; 58: 373–382

41. Rouault T A, Tang C K, Kaptain S et al. Cloning of the cDNA encoding an RNA regulatory protein — the human iron-responsive element-binding protein. Proc Natl Acad Sci USA 1990; 87: 7958–7962

42. Hentze M W, Seuanez H N, O'Brien S J, Harford J B, Klausner R D. Chromosomal localisation of nucleic acid-binding proteins by affinity mapping: assignment of the IRE-binding protein gene to human chromosome 9. Nucleic Acids Res 1989; 17: 6103–6108

43. Trump B F, Valigorsky J M, Arstila A U, Mergner W J, Kinney T D. The relationship of intracellular pathways of iron metabolism to cellular iron overload and iron storage diseases. Am J Pathol 1973; 72: 295–336

44. Iancu T C, Neustein H B, Landing B H. The liver in thalassaemia major: ultrastructural observations. In: Porter R, Fitzsimons D W, eds. Iron metabolism. Ciba Foundation Symposium 51. Amsterdam: Elsevier, 1977

45. Richter G W. The iron-loaded cell — the cytopathology of iron storage. Am J Pathol 1978; 91: 362–404

46. O'Connell M J, Ward R, Baum H, Treffry A, Peters T J. Evidence of a biosynthetic link between ferritin and haemosiderin. Biochem Soc Trans 1988; 16: 828–829

47. Ward R J, O'Connell M J, Dickson D P E et al. Biochemical studies of the iron cores and polypeptide shells of haemosiderin isolated from patients with primary or secondary haemochromatosis. Biochim Biophys Acta 1989; 993: 131–133

48. Mann S, Wade V J, Dickson D P E, Reid N M K, Ward R J, O'Connell M, Peters T J. Structural specificity of haemosiderin iron cores in iron-overload diseases. FEBS Lett 1988; 234:69–72

49. Pearse A G E. Histochemistry. Edinburgh: Churchill Livingstone, 1972

50. Brissot P, Bourel M, Herry D et al. Assessment of liver iron content in 271 patients: a reevaluation of direct and indirect methods. Gastroenterology 1981; 80: 557–565

51. Novikoff A B, Essner E. The liver cell. Am J Med 1960; 29: 102–131

52. Searle J W, Kerr J F R, Halliday J W, Powell L W. Iron storage disease. In: MacSween R N M, Anthony P P, Scheuer P J, eds. Pathology of the liver. 2nd ed. Edinburgh: Churchill Livingstone, 1987

53. Bassett M L, Halliday J W, Powell L W. Value of hepatic iron measurements in early hemochromatosis and determination of the critical iron level associated with fibrosis. Hepatology 1986; 6: 24–29

53a. Summers K M, Halliday J W, Powell L W. Identification of homozygous hemochromatosis subjects by measurement of hepatic iron index. Hepatology 1990; 12: 20–25

54. Olynyk J, Hall P, Sallie R, Reed W, Shilkin K, Mackinnon M. Computerised measurement of iron in liver biopsies: a comparison with biochemical iron measurement. Hepatology 1990; 12: 26–30

55. Deugnier Y, Loreal O, Turlin B et al. Liver pathology in genetic hemochromatosis: a review of 135 homozygous cases and their bio-clinical correlations. Gastroenterology 1992; 102: 2050–2059

56. Simon M, Bourel M, Genetet B, Fauchet R. Idiopathic hemochromatosis. Demonstration of recessive transmission and early detection by family HLA typing. N Engl J Med 1977; 297: 1017–1021

57. Edwards C Q, Dadone M M, Skolnick M H, Kushner J P. Hereditary hemochromatosis. Clin Haematol 1982; 11: 411–435

58. Beaumont C, Simon M, Fauchet R et al. Serum ferritin as a possible marker of the hemochromatosis allele. N Engl J Med 1979; 301: 169–174

59. Halliday J W, Powell L W. Hereditary haemochromatosis and other diseases associated with iron overload. In: Lauffer R B, ed. Iron and human disease. Boca Raton: CRC Press, 1992

60. Schafer A I, Cheron R G, Pluhy R et al. Clinical consequences of acquired transfusional iron overload in adults. N Engl J Med 1981; 304: 319–324

61. Peto T E A, Pippard M J, Weatherall D J. Iron overload in mild sideroblastic anaemias. Lancet 1983; 1: 375–378

62. Bassett M L, Halliday J W, Powell L W. HLA typing in idiopathic hemochromatosis: distinction between homozygotes and heterozygotes with biochemical expression. Hepatology 1981; 1: 120–126

62a. Crawford D H G, Halliday J W, Summers K M, Burke M, Powell L W. Concordance of iron storage in siblings with genetic hemochromatosis: evidence for a predominantly genetic effect on iron storage. Hepatology 1993; 17: 833–837

63. Powell L W, Kerr J F R. The pathology of the liver in hemochromatosis. Pathobiol Annu 1975; 317–337

64. Scheuer P J. Liver biopsy interpretation. 4th ed. London: Baillière Tindall, 1988

64a. Deugnier Y M, Charalambous P, Le Quilleuc D et al. Preneoplastic significance of hepatic iron-free foci in genetic hemochromatosis: a study of 185 patients. Hepatology 1993; 18: 1363–1369

65. Perkins K W, McInnes I W S, Blackburn C R B, Beal R W. Idiopathic haemochromatosis in children. Am J Med 1965; 39: 118–126

66. Cartwright G E, Edwards C Q, Kravitz K et al. Hereditary hemochromatosis. N Engl J Med 1979; 301: 175–179

66a. Deugnier Y M, Halliday J W, Summers K M et al. Differentiation between heterozygotes and homozygotes in genetic hemochromatosis by means of a histological hepatic iron index: a study of 192 cases. Hepatology 1993; 17: 30–34

67. Knauer C M, Gamble C N, Monroe L S. The reversal of hemochromatotic cirrhosis by multiple phlebotomies. Gastroenterology 1965; 49: 667–671

68. Weintraub L R, Conrad M E, Crosby W H. The treatment of hemochromatosis by phlebotomy. Med Clin North Am 1966; 50: 1579–1590

69. Powell L W, Kerr J F R. Reversal of 'cirrhosis' in idiopathic haemochromatosis following long-term intensive venesection therapy. Aust Ann Med 1970; 1: 54–57

70. Niederau C, Fischer R, Sonnenberg A, Stremmel W, Trampisch H J, Strohmeyer G. Survival and causes of death in cirrhotic and in noncirrhotic patients with primary hemochromatosis. N Engl J Med 1985; 313: 1256–1262

71. Blumberg R S, Chopra S, Ibrahim R et al. Primary hepatocellular carcinoma in idiopathic hemochromatosis after reversal of cirrhosis. Gastroenterology 1988; 95: 1399–1402

72. Sheldon J H. Haemochromatosis. London: Oxford University Press, 1935

73. Warren S, Drake W L. Primary carcinoma of the liver in hemochromatosis. Am J Pathol 1951; 27: 573–609

74. MacSween R N M, Scott A R. Hepatic cirrhosis: a clinicopathological review of 520 cases. J Clin Pathol 1973; 26: 936–942

75. Bomford A, Williams R. Long term results of venesection therapy in idiopathic haemochromatosis. Q J Med 1976; 45: 611–623

76. Walker R J, Williams R. Haemochromatosis and iron overload. In: Jacobs A, Worwood M, eds. Iron in biochemistry and medicine. London: Academic Press, 1974

77. Fellows I W, Stewart M, Jeffcoat W J, Smith P G, Toghill P J. Hepatocellular carcinoma in primary haemochromatosis in the absence of cirrhosis. Gut 1988; 29; 1603–1606

78. Milder M S, Cook J D, Stray S, Finch C A. Idiopathic hemochromatosis, an interim report. Medicine (Baltimore) 1980; 59: 34–49

79. Dubin I N. Idiopathic hemochromatosis and transfusion siderosis. Am J Clin Pathol 1955; 25: 514–542

80. Powell L W, Mortimer R, Harris O D. Cirrhosis of the liver. Med J Aust 1971; 1: 941–950

81. Bradbear R A, Bain C, Siskind V et al. Cohort study of internal malignancy in genetic hemochromatosis and other chronic nonalcoholic liver diseases. J N C I 1985; 75: 81–84

81a. Deugnier Y M, Guyader D, Crantock L et al. Primary liver cancer in genetic hemochromatosis: a clinical, pathological and pathogenetic study of 54 cases. Gastroenterology 1993; 104: 228–234

82. Eason R J, Adams P C, Aston C E, Searle J. Familial iron overload with possible autosomal dominant inheritance. Aust NZJ Med 1990; 20: 226–230

83. Wilson J D, Scott P J, North J D K. Hemochromatosis in association with hereditary spherocytosis. Arch Intern Med 1967; 120: 701–707

84. Barry M, Scheuer P J, Sherlock S, Ross C F, Williams R. Hereditary spherocytosis with secondary haemochromatosis. Lancet 1968; 2: 481–485

85. Edwards C Q, Skolnick M H, Kushner J P. Coincidental nontransfusional iron overload and thalassaemia minor: association with HLA-linked hemochromatosis. Blood 1981; 58: 844–848

86. Cartwright G E, Edwards C Q, Kravitz K et al. Hereditary hemochromatosis. N Engl J Med 1979; 301: 175–179

87. Salem H H, van der Weyden M B, Firkin B G. Iron overload in congenital erythrocyte pyruvate kinase deficiency. Med J Aust 1980; 1: 531–532

88. Rowbotham B J, Roeser H P. Iron overload associated with pyruvate kinase deficiency and high dose ascorbic acid ingestion. Aust N Z J Med 1984; 14: 667–669

89. Cook J D, Barry W E, Hershko C, Fillett G, Finch C. Iron kinetics with emphasis on iron overload. Am J Pathol 1973; 72: 337–343

90. Ley T J, Griffith P, Nienhuis A W. Transfusion haemosiderosis and chelation therapy. Clin Haematol 1982; 11: 437–464

91. Finch C A, Deubelbeiss K, Cook J D et al. Ferrokinetics in man. Medicine (Baltimore) 1970; 49: 17–54

92. Jacobs A. Iron overload — clinical and pathological aspects. Semin Hematol 1977; 14: 89–113

93. Bottomley S S. Sideroblastic anaemia. Clin Haematol 1982; 11: 389–409

94. Iancu T C, Landing B H, Neustein H B. Pathogenetic mechanisms in hepatic cirrhosis in thalassaemia major: light and electron microscope studies. Pathol Annu 1977; 12: 171–200

95. Risdon R A, Barry M, Flynn D M. Transfusional iron overload: the relationship between tissue iron concentration and hepatic fibrosis in thalassaemia. J Pathol 1975; 116: 83–95

96. Turnberg L A. Excessive oral iron therapy causing haemochromatosis. Br Med J 1965; 1: 1360

97. Bothwell T H, Charlton R W. Dietary iron overload. In: Kief H, ed. Iron metabolism and its disorders. Amsterdam. Excerpta Medica, 1975

98. Gordeuk V, Mukiibi J, Hasstedt S J et al. Iron overload in Africa. Interaction between a gene and dietary iron content. N Engl J Med 1992; 326: 95–100

99. Charlton R W, Bothwell T H, Seftel H C. Dietary iron overload. Clin Haematol 1973; 2: 383–403

100. Bothwell T H, Isaacson C. Siderosis in the Bantu: a comparison of incidence of males and females. Br Med J 1962; 1: 522–524

101. Bothwell T H, Abrahams C, Bradlow B A, Charlton R W. Idiopathic and Bantu hemochromatosis. Arch Pathol 1965; 79: 163–168

102. MacDonald R A, Pechet G S. Experimental hemochromatosis in rats. Am J Pathol 1965; 46: 85–109

103. Le Sage G D, Baldus W P, Fairbanks V F et al. Hemochromatosis: genetic or alcohol-induced? Gastroenterology 1983; 84: 1471–1477

104. Pechet G S, French S W, Levy J, MacDonald R A. Histologic and chemical tissue iron. Arch Pathol 1965; 79: 452–461

105. Williams R, Williams H S, Scheuer P J, Pitcher C S, Loizeau E, Sherlock S. Iron absorption and siderosis in chronic liver disease. Q J Med 1967; 36: 151–166

106. Kent G, Popper H. Liver biopsy in diagnosis of hemochromatosis. Am J Med 1968; 44; 837–841

107. Grace N D. Iron metabolism and hemochromatosis. In: Zakim D, Boyer T D, eds. Hepatology: a textbook of liver diseases. Philadelphia: Saunders, 1982

108. Bassett M L, Halliday J W, Powell L W. Genetic hemochromatosis. Semin Liver Dis 1984; 4: 217–227

109. Goldfischer S, Grotsky H W, Chang C H et al. Idiopathic neonatal iron storage involving the liver, pancreas, heart and endocrine and exocrine glands. Hepatology 1981; 1: 58–64

110. Knisely A S, Magid M S, Dische M R et al. Neonatal hemochromatosis. In: Gilbert E F, Opitz J M, eds. Genetic aspects of developmental pathology. New York: Alan R Liss, 1987

111. Knisely A S. Neonatal hemochromatosis. Adv Pediatr 1992; 39: 383–403

112. Hardy L, Hansen J, Kushner J P et al. Neonatal hemochromatosis: genetic analysis of transferrin-receptor, H-apoferritin, and L-apoferritin loci and of the HLA class 1 region. Am J Pathol 1990; 137: 149–153

113. Kothari T, Swamy A P, Lee J C K, Mangla J C, Cestero R V M. Hepatic hemosiderosis in maintenance hemodialysis (MHD) patients. Dig Dis Sci 1980; 25: 363–368

114. Cook J D, Eschbach J W. Iron absorption and loss in chronic renal disease. In: Kief H, ed. Iron metabolism and its disorders. Amsterdam: Excerpta Medica, 1975

115. Gokal R, Millard P R, Weatherall D J, Callender S T E, Ledingham J G G, Oliver D O. Iron metabolism in haemodialysis patients. Q J Med 1979; 48: 369–391

116. Ali M, Fayemi A O, Rigolosi R, Frascino J, Marsden T, Malcolm D. Hemosiderosis in hemodialysis patients. An autopsy study of 50 cases. J A M A 1980; 244: 343–345

117. Turnbull A, Baker H, Vernon-Roberts B, Magnus I A. Iron metabolism in porphyria cutanea tarda and in erythropoietic protoporphyria. Q J Med 1973; 42: 341–355

118. Cortes J M, Oliva H, Paradinas F J, Hernandez-Guio C. The pathology of the liver in porphyria cutanea tarda. Histopathology 1980; 4: 471–485

119. Sauer G F, Funk D D. Iron overload in cutaneous porphyria. Arch Int Med 1969; 124: 190–196

120. Reizenstein P, Höglund S, Landegren J, Carlmark B, Forsberg K J. Iron metabolism in porphyria cutanea tarda. Acta Med Scand 1975; 198: 95–99

121. Pimstone N R. Porphyria cutanea tarda. Semin Liver Dis 1982; 2: 132–142

122. Felsher B E, Kushner J P. Hepatic siderosis and porphyria cutanea tarda; relation of iron excess to the metabolic defect. Semin Hematol 1977; 14: 243–251

123. Kuntz B M E, Goerz G, Sonneborn H H, Lissner R. HLA-types in porphyria cutanea tarda. Lancet 1981; 1: 155

124. Kushner J P, Edwards C W, Dadone M M, Skolnick M H. Heterozygosity for HLA-linked hemochromatosis as a likely cause of the hepatic siderosis associated with sporadic porphyria cutanea tarda. Gastroenterology 1985; 88: 1232–1238

125. Beaumont C, Fauchet R, Phung L N, De Verneuil H, Gueguen M, Nordmann Y. Porphyria cutanea tarda and HLA-linked hemochromatosis. Evidence against a systematic association. Gastroenterology 1987; 92: 1833–1838

126. Adams P C, Powell L W. Porphyria cutanea tarda and HLA-linked hemochromatosis — all in the family? Gastroenterology 1987; 92: 2033–2035

127. Conn H O. Portacaval anastomosis and hepatic hemosiderin deposition: a prospective, controlled investigation. Gastroenterology 1972; 62: 61–72

128. Koff R S, Go T B, Oliai A. Hepatic hemosiderosis after portacaval shunt surgery in alcoholic cirrhosis: a sometime thing. Gastroenterology 1972; 63: 834–836

129. Tuttle S G, Figueroa W G, Grossman M I. Development of hemochromatosis in a patient with Laennec's cirrhosis. Am J Med 1959; 26: 655–658

130. Lombard C M, Strauchen J A. Postshunt hemochromatosis with cardiomyopathy. Hum Pathology 1981; 12: 1149–1151

131. Fairbanks V F, Beutler E. Congenital atransferrinemia and idiopathic pulmonary hemosiderosis. In: Williams W J, Beutler E, Erslev A J, eds. Hematology, 3rd ed. New York: McGraw-Hill, 1983

132. Brown E B, Dubach R, Smith D E, Reynafarje C, Moore C V. Studies in iron transportation and metabolism. J Lab Clin Med 1957; 50: 862–893

133. Lisboa P E. Experimental hepatic cirrhosis in dogs caused by chronic massive iron overload. Gut 1971; 12: 363–368

134. Brissot P, Campion J P, Guillouzo A et al. Experimental hepatic iron overload in the baboon: results of a two-year study. Evolution of biological and morphologic hepatic parameters of iron overload. Dig Dis Sci 1983; 28: 616–624

134a. Halliday J W, Searle J. Hepatic iron deposition in human disease and animal models. BioMetals 1994 (in press)

135. Richter G W. Effects of cyclic starvation-feeding and of splenectomy on the development of hemosiderosis in rat livers. Am J Pathol 1974; 74: 481–506

136. Golberg L, Smith J P. Iron overloading and hepatic vulnerability. Am J Pathol 1960; 36: 125–149

137. Bacon B R, Tavill A S, Brittenham G M, Park C H, Recknagel R O. Hepatic lipid peroxidation in vivo in rats with chronic iron overload. J Clin Invest 1983; 71: 429–439

138. Iancu T C, Ward R J, Peters T J. Ultrastructural observations in the carbonyl iron-fed rat, an animal model for hemochromatosis. Virchows Arch [B] 1987; 53: 208–217

139. Park C H, Bacon B R, Brittenham G M, Tavill A S. Pathology of dietary carbonyl iron overload in rats. Lab Invest 1987; 57: 555–563

140. Bacon B R, Healey J F, Brittenham G M et al. Hepatic microsomal function in rats with chronic dietary iron overload. Gastroenterology 1986; 90: 1844–1853

141. Seymour C A, Peters T J. Organelle pathology in primary and secondary haemochromatosis with special reference to lysosomal changes. Br J Haematol 1978; 40: 239–253

142. Selden C, Owen M, Hopkins J M P, Peters T J. Studies on the concentration and intracellular localisation of iron proteins in liver biopsy specimens from patients with iron overload with special reference to their role in lysosomal disruption. Br J Haematol 1980; 44: 593–603

143. Hultcrantz R, Arborgh B. Studies on the rat liver following iron overload. Acta Pathol Microbiol Scand [A] 1978; 86: 143–155

144. Stal P, Glaumann H, Hultcrantz R. Liver cell damage and lysosomal iron storage in patients with idiopathic hemochromatosis. A light and electron microscopic study. J Hepatol 1990; 11: 172–180

145. Weintraub L R, Goral A, Grasso J, Granzblau C, Sullivan A, Sullivan S. Pathogenesis of hepatic fibrosis in experimental iron overload. Br J Haematol 1985; 59: 321–331

146. Chojkier M, Houglum K, Solis-Heruzo J, Brenner D A. Stimulation of collagen gene expression by ascorbic acid in cultured human fibroblasts. A role for lipid peroxidation? J Biol Chem 1989; 264: 16957–16962

147. Tseng S C G, Lee P C, Ellis P F, Bissell D M, Smuckler E A, Stern R. Collagen production by rat hepatocytes and sinusoidal cells in primary monolayer culture. Hepatology 1982; 2: 13–18

148. Bacon B R, Britton R S. The pathology of hepatic iron overload: a free radical-mediated process? Hepatology 1990; 11: 127–137

6

Viral hepatitis

P. J. Scheuer

The subject of this chapter is infection with the hepatitis viruses and its acute pathological consequences. Several of the viruses can lead to chronic disease also, and this is described in detail in Chapters 9 and 10. However, acute and chronic hepatitis are closely related to each other, and some discussion of chronicity is therefore necessary in the present chapter.

The hepatitis viruses (Table 6.1) are grouped together not because of any biological relationship but because they are hepatotropic; their main effect is on the liver. Other agents such as cytomegalovirus and Epstein-Barr virus also produce liver lesions, but these are usually part of a systemic infection in which the liver is only one of several organs or systems affected. These agents are therefore not included in the list but are discussed in the next chapter.

Table 6.1 The human hepatitis viruses

Virus	Type	Disease
Hepatitis A (HAV)	RNA; hepatovirus	Sporadic or epidemic; acute only. Faecal–oral spread
Hepatitis B (HBV)	DNA; hepadnavirus	Acute or chronic, including hepatocellular carcinoma (HCC). Parenteral spread
Hepatitis C (HCV)	RNA; flavi- and pestivirus-like	Acute and often chronic, including HCC. Spread typically parenteral, but also sporadic
Hepatitis D (HDV, delta agent)	RNA, defective virus	Needs HBV for pathogenicity and increases severity of type B hepatitis
Hepatitis E	RNA virus	Epidemic or sporadic; probably acute disease only. Faecal–oral spread
Hepatitis F	RNA; toga virus-like	Implicated in fulminant hepatitis
Other	e.g. paramyxovirus	Various

Details of the hepatitis viruses are discussed in a later part of this chapter.

ACUTE VIRAL HEPATITIS IN MAN: CLINICAL FEATURES

Acute hepatitis may be sporadic or epidemic. It may be spread by the faecal–oral route, or parenterally by drug abuse, sexual intercourse or blood transfusion. The mode of spread of each virus is specified later in this chapter, when individual viruses are discussed.

The acute attack is often subclinical. If symptoms are present, they may either be characteristic or non-specific and not readily identifiable as due to hepatitis. Typical symptoms include anorexia and nausea in the early stages, followed in the icteric form by dark urine and jaundice. In the anicteric form, jaundice is absent or unnoticed. The attack varies from a mild illness to fatal, fulminant hepatitis. The latter is almost always associated with a histological picture of multiacinar or severe bridging necrosis (see below). The terms 'subacute hepatitis' and 'subacute hepatic necrosis' are sometimes used to describe a serious and often fatal course over a period of several weeks or months. In fatal cases varying degrees of nodular hyperplasia of the surviving parenchyma are superimposed on extensive hepatocellular necrosis. Death sometimes results from complications such as sepsis rather than from pure hepatocellular failure.

Portal hypertension and ascites, more typically associated with chronic liver disease, develop in some patients with acute hepatitis. These complications are at least partly the result of liver-cell loss and consequent collapse of the sinusoidal network.[1]

Cholestatic hepatitis is characterized by unusually severe and prolonged clinical and biochemical cholestasis, and needs to be distinguished from bile-duct obstruction. The degrees of clinical and histological cholestasis do not necessarily correspond, and the term is best used in a clinical sense rather than as a histological entity.

More commonly, the biochemical changes in acute hepatitis are those associated with hepatocellular damage. Serum aminotransferase activities are characteristically high, their peak sometimes preceding the onset of jaundice. The prothrombin time gives a good indication of the severity of liver-cell injury. Serum bilirubin levels correlate with the degree of clinical jaundice. The rise in serum alkaline phosphatase activity is generally modest.

ACUTE VIRAL HEPATITIS IN MAN: PATHOLOGICAL FEATURES

Acute viral hepatitis is characterized morphologically by a combination of inflammatory-cell infiltration, macrophage activity, hepatocellular damage and regeneration. The proportion and detailed nature of these components vary widely according to the particular virus responsible, the host response and the passage of time. The pathological features are very different from those of classic acute inflammation, because they mainly represent a response of the patient's immune system to viral antigens displayed on cells, rather than a vascular and cellular response to injury. Some features of acute inflammation are nevertheless present to a limited extent; thus, for instance, the liver in acute viral hepatitis is swollen and tender, its capsule is tense, blood vessels are engorged and polymorphonuclear leucocytes may be seen as a secondary response to epithelial injury.

MACROSCOPIC APPEARANCES

Information on the macroscopic appearances of the liver in non-fatal acute hepatitis is mainly derived from laparoscopy.[2] Initially the liver is swollen and red, its capsule oedematous and tense; exuded tissue fluid may be seen on the capsular surface. Focal depressions are the result of localized subcapsular necrosis and collapse. In patients with severe cholestasis, the colour of the liver is bright yellow or green. In fulminant hepatitis the organ shrinks and softens as a result of extensive necrosis, and the capsule becomes wrinkled. The left lobe may be more severely affected than the right. If the patient survives for weeks or months, yellow or green nodules of regenerating parenchyma may be seen protruding from the capsular surface. At autopsy, similar nodules are seen deep within the liver in some patients, separated by red necrotic areas. In others, necrosis is uniform throughout the organ.

In patients dying of fulminant hepatitis, there is often damage to organs other than the liver and this may contribute to, or indeed form, the immediate cause of death.[3] Findings at autopsy include pneumonia, septicaemia, cerebral oedema, gastrointestinal haemorrhage and pancreatitis. Such lesions help to explain death when liver-cell damage is limited in extent or when there has already been substantial regeneration.

LIGHT-MICROSCOPIC APPEARANCES: TYPES OF NECROSIS

The histological classification of acute hepatitis given in this chapter is based on different patterns of hepatocellular necrosis (Table 6.2). These patterns will therefore be briefly discussed before the microscopic changes of acute hepatitis are described in detail. More than one of the patterns of necrosis described below may be seen in

Table 6.2 Morphological patterns of acure hepatitis

- Classic acute hepatitis with spotty (focal) necrosis
- Acute hepatitis with bridging necrosis
- Acute hepatitis with panacinar or multicinar necrosis
- Acute hepatitis with periportal necrosis

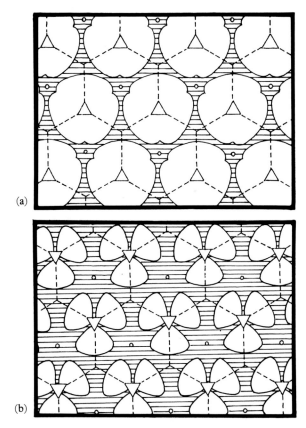

(a)

(b)

Fig. 6.1 Schematic representation of bridging necrosis; necrotic areas are cross-harched. ----= outlines of classic lobules; Δ = portal tracts; ◯ = terminal hepatic venules. (a) Confluent necrosis at the periphery of the complex acinus, linking terminal hepatic venules ('central–central' bridging). (b) Necrosis involves the peripheral parts of simple acini as well as the areas shown in (a); this has led to linking of terminal hepatic venules and portal tracts by bridges of confluent necrosis ('central–portal' bridging). Reproduced from Bianchi et al[5] with permission.

different parts of the same liver, and even within a single biopsy specimen.

Spotty (focal) necrosis. In this form of necrosis, which represents the fundamental lesion of acute viral hepatitis, individual hepatocytes within otherwise intact parenchyma die and are removed. The mode of death of hepatocytes probably includes both lytic necrosis and apoptosis, but the relative contribution of each is uncertain. In the case of apoptosis, or formation of Councilman bodies, it is likely that T-lymphocytes olay a role. The remnants of cells affected by either process are rapidly removed from the site by blood flow or phagocytosis.

Confluent and bridging necrosis. Groups of adjacent hepatocytes die, so that areas of confluent necrosis are formed. These are often perivenular in location. Confluent necrosis linking vascular structures is known as bridging necrosis. The topographical relationships between different kinds of bridging necrosis and Rappaport's acinus[4] are discussed in detail by Bianchi et al[5] and will only be reviewed briefly here. Bridging at the periphery of

complex acini links terminal hepatic venules to each other, but does not involve portal tracts (Fig. 6.1a). This is called 'central–central' bridging in the lobular nomenclature. The more serious and important form of bridging necrosis, and one to which the term bridging is sometimes restricted (p. 249), links terminal hepatic venules to portal tracts ('central–portal' bridging in the lobular nomenclature). This form is best explained as necrosis of zone 3 of the simple acinus (Fig. 6.1b), because this zone touches both terminal hepatic venule and portal tract. Zone 3 bridges are sometimes curved, in keeping with the shape of the zone. When confluent necrosis is more extensive, involving zones 2 and 1 in addition to zone 3 so that entire acini are destroyed, the process is described as panacinar necrosis.

Piecemeal necrosis. Piecemeal necrosis can be defined as death of hepatocytes at the interface of parenchyma and connective tissue, accompanied by a

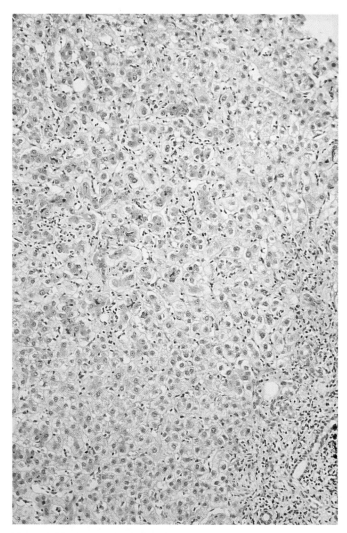

Fig. 6.2 Classic acute hepatitis. Liver-cell swelling, cholestasis and lymphocytic infiltration are seen in the perivenular area (above left). The portal tract (below right) is also inflamed. H & E.

variable degree of inflammation and fibrosis. Interface hepatitis is an alternative term. The sites of piecemeal necrosis are the margins of portal tracts and of connective tissue septa. In the acinar concept, piecemeal necrosis typically involves zone 1, and leads to apparent widening of portal tracts. These are therefore more likely to be cut longitudinally by a microtome knife, and this is seen in two-dimensional sections as linking of adjacent portal tracts, that is to say portal–portal bridging. Because such zone 1 necrosis is thought to be fundamentally different from zone 3 bridging as described above, the author prefers to restrict the term bridging necrosis to the zone 3 type in order to avoid possible confusion, and for reasons discussed on page 250.

Piecemeal necrosis is a defining feature of chronic active hepatitis[6] (for discussion of the applicability of this diagnosis see Ch. 9), but very similar periportal necrosis is found in some cases of acute hepatitis, as described on page 252.

Classic acute hepatitis

Features seen in the acini in this form of acute hepatitis include liver-cell damage, potentially leading to cell death, liver-cell regeneration, cholestasis, infiltration with inflammatory cells, and prominence of sinusoidal cells. There is a variable degree of condensation of the reticulin framework but, in the classic form of hepatitis, this does not amount to substantial alteration of acinar structure and vascular relationships. Portal tracts are inflamed and bile ducts may be damaged.

Little is known about the earliest changes of acute viral hepatitis in man. Available information suggests that Kupffer cells are prominent and may show mitotic activity, and that hepatocellular necrosis occurs early in the course of the disease.[7]

Lesions can be seen in all parts of the acini, but are usually most severe in zone 3, near the terminal hepatic venules (Fig. 6.2). The reason for this zonal distribution has not been established, but possible explanations include metabolic and functional differences between hepatocytes in different zones, and the lower oxygen content of the blood in zone 3. Changes include hepatocyte swelling, shrinkage, fragmentation and death. Bile pigment may accumulate within the damaged cells. Macrovesicular fatty change (steatosis) is relatively uncommon in the fully developed stage of hepatitis.

Hepatocyte swelling is a common feature in acute hepatitis, and results mainly from dilatation of the endoplasmic reticulum (p. 253). The swollen cells are pale-staining as a result of intracellular oedema (Fig. 6.3). Because of the combination of swelling and rounding of the affected cells, the term 'ballooning degeneration' is sometimes applied. It should be noted, however, that such ballooning degeneration is not a diagnostic feature of viral hepatitis, since it may also be seen in other

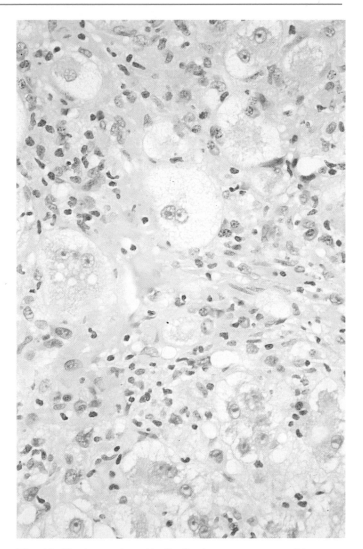

Fig. 6.3 Classic acute hepatitis. Swollen hepatocytes, some of them multinucleated, are seen together with an inflammatory infiltrate in a perivenular area. Loss of hepatocytes has led to disarray of the plate architecture. H & E.

circumstances, for example in alcoholic or drug-induced hepatitis and following liver transplantation. The nuclei of the affected cells are also swollen, because of the accumulation of protein.[8] Nucleoli of hepatocytes may be more prominent than usual, and mitotic figures are occasionally seen. Multinucleation may be increased, and giant cells containing large numbers of nuclei may be present (Fig. 6.4). When this change is widespread the appearances resemble those of neonatal giant-cell hepatitis.

In addition to swollen cells, there are hepatocytes with deeply acidophilic cytoplasm, in which the nucleus is sometimes seen to be undergoing pyknosis. Such acidophilic hepatocytes are small in comparison with ballooned cells, but may nevertheless be larger than normal hepatocytes. This suggests that the two types of cell change could represent stages of cell degeneration rather than fundamentally different responses to injury. Acidophilic

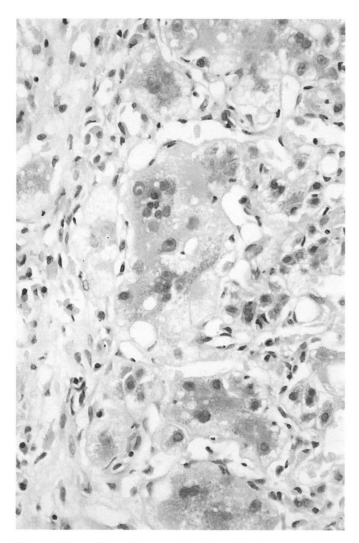

Fig. 6.4 Giant-cell hepatitis in an adult. Many of the hepatocytes in a perivenular area contain large numbers of nuclei. H & E.

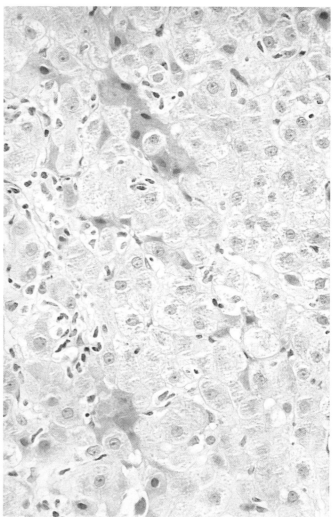

Fig. 6.5 Classic acute hepatitis. Hepatocytes with intensely eosinophilic cytoplasm have irregular outlines because of compression by adjacent cells. Section of non-A, non-B hepatitis kindly provided by Professor L Bianchi, Basel, and photographed with permission; figure previously published as half-tone in *Recent Advances in Histopathology 12*. H & E.

cells have round or irregular outlines, sometimes assuming rhomboid, angular shapes, apparently determined by the pressures of adjacent swollen hepatocytes (Fig. 6.5). The formation of acidophil (Councilman) bodies (Fig. 6.6) is probably a later stage of this process. Affected cells eventually undergo fragmentation, the whole process representing an example of apoptosis.[9–12] Acidophilic bodies may or may not contain nuclear remnants. Some acidophilic bodies appear thick and refractile, and extend beyond the plane of a thin paraffin section. Many acidophil bodies are rounded, although ovoid and irregular forms are also seen. Some acidophil bodies are in close contact with lymphocytes or Kupffer cells, while others appear to lie free within liver-cell plates or sinusoids, with no other cells in close proximity. Like ballooned hepatocytes, acidophil bodies are not specific for acute viral hepatitis, although they often constitute a striking histological feature of the disease.

Loss of individual hepatocytes leads to localized defects in the liver-cell plates, with consequent distortion and condensation of the supporting reticulin framework, especially when the necrosis is confluent. While an overall increase in connective tissue fibres is probably slight in acute hepatitis and therefore difficult to detect by light microscopy (with conventional staining methods), immunocytochemical and ultrastructural evidence indicates synthesis of fibres and associated proteins. This is presumably balanced initially by degradation of these components, so that there is a dynamic balance which determines the degree of fibrosis in an individual case. Type III and type V collagen were found to be increased both in portal tracts and in areas of focal necrosis in hepatitis A.[13] In the parenchyma an increase in transitional

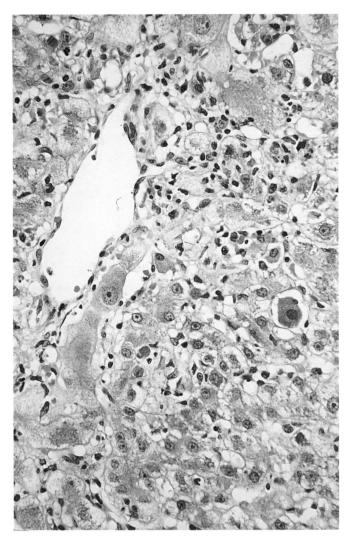

Fig. 6.6 Classic acute hepatitis. There is hepatocyte swelling and inflammation near a terminal venule (above left). A rounded acidophil body with nuclear remnant is seen lying free within a sinusoid (right). H & E.

perisinusoidal cells was seen on electron microscopy, while fibroblasts were prominent within the portal tracts. Increased amounts of type IV collagen and fibronectin were found near areas of focal necrosis.

The distortion of cell plates mentioned above is accentuated by regeneration of hepatocytes. This is recognized by the appearance of mitotic figures, rare in normal liver, and by a change in the structure of the cell plates; these become more than one cell thick, or assume the structure of short cylinders known as liver-cell rosettes. The occurrence of liver-cell regeneration is supported by an increased frequency of interploid DNA values in nuclei.[14] The end result of focal necrosis, reticulin condensation and regeneration is a diagnostically helpful disarray of the liver-cell plates (Fig. 6.3).

Cholestasis is common in acute hepatitis. It varies from the presence of scanty small bile plugs in perivenular

canaliculi to extensive bile plug formation with canalicular dilatation. Intracellular bile is more difficult to recognize because bile is easily confused with lipofuscin pigment. For this reason cholestasis should only rarely be diagnosed on the basis of routine stains in the absence of canalicular bile plugs, an exception being the bile staining of hepatocytes after liver transplantation. Morphological cholestasis may be accompanied by clinical and biochemical features of cholestasis, but this is not invariable.

The inflammatory infiltrate of acute viral hepatitis is mainly composed of lymphocytes, plasma cells and macrophages in varying proportions. Within the acini, the infiltrate is most abundant where liver-cell damage is greatest, usually the perivenular areas. Lymphocytes are often attached to endothelial cells of the terminal hepatic and portal venules.[15] Mononuclear phagocytes, either activated Kupffer cells or circulating phagocytes, are seen as large irregular cells in areas of liver-cell drop-out. They often show brown pigmentation, due to phagocytosis of bile or to the accumulation of lipid-rich ceroid pigment. Iron is also abundant in some cases (Fig. 6.7), particularly in men.[16] The iron-containing phagocytes are sometimes found in the form of small clumps composed of several cells.[17] Whatever the pigment, the PAS reaction after diastase digestion is usually strongly positive (Fig. 6.8).

Most portal tracts in acute viral hepatitis are infiltrated with inflammatory cells to a greater or lesser extent, and, in the classic form, lymphoid cells predominate as in the acini. Plasma cells are common, the majority containing IgG.[18] Perls-positive iron-rich macrophages may be present. Minimal or absent portal inflammation in an acute hepatitis, or an infiltrate rich in segmented leucocytes, should alert the pathologist to the possibility that the hepatitis is not viral but drug-induced (see Ch. 15). Portal infiltration may be diffuse or focal. The formation of lymphoid follicles is discussed later in this chapter under the heading of hepatitis C. Mild bile-duct damage is common, and is seen as minor irregularity of shape, size and arrangement of the epithelial nuclei of the small, interlobular ducts. Less commonly, the duct epithelium becomes vacuolated and disrupted,[19] such lesions being seen most often near or within lymphoid follicles (Fig. 6.9). Absence of granuloma formation and presence of acinar changes of hepatitis help to distinguish such bile-duct lesions from those of primary biliary cirrhosis. Irregular dilatation of ductules has been described in type A hepatitis.[20] In general, however, a finding of dilated, bile-containing ductules or canals of Hering should arouse a suspicion of sepsis, a complication of severe acute hepatitis in some patients. Bile-duct damage in acute hepatitis does not usually correlate with a cholestatic clinical course, probably because there is not the widespread and progressive destruction of the duct system found in disorders such as primary biliary cirrhosis.

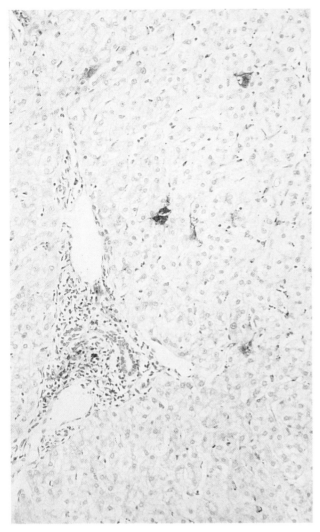

Fig. 6.7 Classic acute hepatitis. Kupffer cells and portal tract macrophages contain iron. Perls' stain.

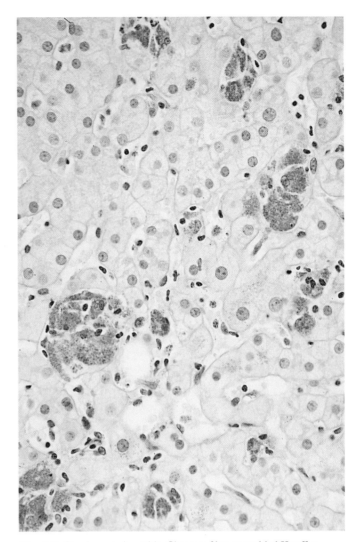

Fig. 6.8 Classic acute hepatitis. Clumps of hypertrophied Kupffer cells in a perivenular area stain strongly with diastase–PAS. DPAS.

The outlines of the portal tracts may remain intact and sharp in classic acute hepatitis with spotty necrosis. More often, infiltration by lymphoid cells and accompanying disruption of the limiting plate of hepatocytes leads to an irregular outline. Severe periportal necrosis and inflammation is described below, under the heading of acute hepatitis with periportal necrosis.

All the above pathological features of classic acute hepatitis with spotty (focal) necrosis vary in extent. There is thus a wide range of appearances, from a mild hepatitis with little cell damage or inflammatory-cell infiltration, to one with widespread changes throughout the acini. In the latter case the diagnosis presents no great difficulty, but in the former the distinction from non-specific reactive changes or from non-hepatitic cholestasis may be difficult or even impossible.

These characteristics of classic acute hepatitis with spotty (focal) necrosis also form the basis of the other three forms of acute hepatitis; the latter may be regarded as exaggerations of one or other component of the classic form described in the above paragraphs.

Acute hepatitis with bridging necrosis

In this form of acute hepatitis, the features described under classic acute hepatitis with spotty (focal) necrosis are seen but there is in addition zone 3 bridging in the form of confluent necrosis linking terminal hepatic venules to portal tracts ('central–portal' bridging in the lobular nomenclature). Bridging necrosis linking terminal hepatic venules to each other but not extending to portal tracts ('central–central' bridging) is not included under hepatitis with bridging necrosis in the present classification, but may be seen in the 'classic' form. It should be noted, however, that authors differ in the use of the term 'bridging', which thus needs careful definition in

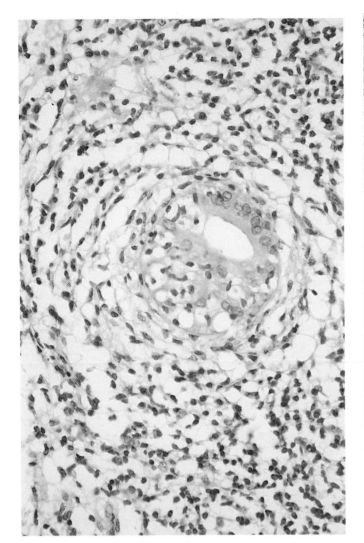

Fig. 6.9 Acute hepatitis. Part of the wall of a bile duct within a portal inflammatory infiltrate is swollen. Bile duct epithelial cells are vacuolated and infiltrated by lymphocytes. H & E.

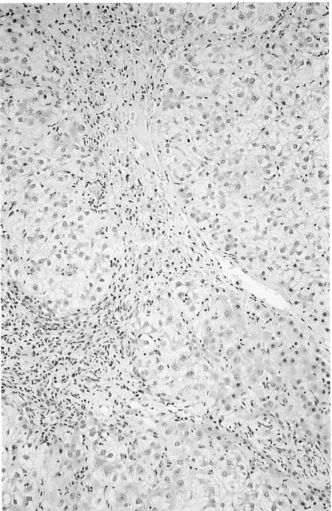

Fig. 6.10 Acute hepatitis with bridging necrosis. Curving bridges formed as a result of confluent necrosis link vascular structures. H & E.

each publication and study. The principal reason for separating zone 3 bridging from the other types is that it forms the anatomical basis for portal–systemic shunting within the liver. Furthermore, in patients who develop chronic liver disease, zone 3 bridging hastens the onset of cirrhosis by creating early disruption of the normal architectural relationships. This is later accentuated by conversion of the bridges into fibrous septa which undergo contraction.

The appearance of the bridges varies according to the stage of the illness. In the early stages of bridge formation, there is death of substantial numbers of hepatocytes. This is followed by disappearance of the affected cells, leaving a loose connective tissue stroma infiltrated with lymphocytes and macrophages (Fig. 6.10). With time, the stroma collapses to form more or less dense 'passive' septa which intersect the liver tissue. The combination of necrosis, collapse and hepatocellular regeneration leads to architec-

tural distortion which can easily be mistaken for that of chronic hepatitis or cirrhosis. Helpful differentiating features include the presence of other lesions of acute viral hepatitis; and staining properties of the septa; recently formed passive septa are virtually devoid of elastic fibres (Fig. 6.11) whereas the older septa of chronic hepatitis and cirrhosis contain increasing numbers of these fibres.[21]

Extensive liver-cell destruction in acute hepatitis with bridging necrosis may lead to a more florid portal inflammatory reaction than is normally found in classic acute hepatitis. Polymorphonuclear leucocytes are more abundant, and there may be bile-duct proliferation, mimicking bile-duct obstruction.

The prognostic significance of bridging necrosis is controversial. Boyer & Klatskin,[22] in their seminal paper, considered that patients with bridging necrosis were more likely to develop chronic hepatitis, a conclusion later supported by another study.[23] However, both groups of

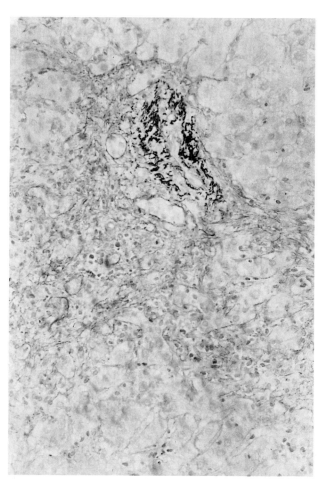

Fig. 6.11 Acute hepatitis with bridging necrosis. Deeply stained elastic fibres are seen in a portal tract. Adjacent areas of collapse are virtually unstained. Orcein.

to multiacinar necrosis involving a substantial part of the whole liver, a situation judged at autopsy rather than on liver biopsy. Massive hepatic necrosis is a morphological counterpart of the clinical condition of fulminant hepatitis, and is often fatal. For reasons as yet unknown, such necrosis may spare large areas of the liver, though these usually show lesser degrees of damage, including bridging necrosis. The cause of panacinar necrosis is also unknown; suggested mechanisms include overwhelming virus infection, superinfection with a second virus[26] and microcirculatory failure.[27] In some instances, mutants of the hepatitis B virus have been implicated.[28,29] Specific, as yet incompletely characterized, hepatitis viruses may be involved in some cases.[30,31] Panacinar necrosis on a smaller scale is not necessarily accompanied by severe disease clinically, and may be seen particularly in a subcapsular location, overlying less severely damaged liver tissue. It is even likely that panacinar necrosis can occur in the entire absence of severe symptoms, because areas of old panacinar necrosis and collapse may be found incidentally in the livers of patients with no history of acute hepatitis. Conversely, some patients have severe clinical hepatitis in the absence of panacinar necrosis, and it must then be assumed that a large proportion of hepatocytes has sustained sublethal damage.

The macroscopic appearances in acute hepatitis with severe necrosis have already been described above. Microscopically, acute hepatitis with panacinar necrosis is characterized by extensive liver-cell loss, proliferation of duct-like structures around portal tracts, inflammatory-cell infiltration and collapse (Fig. 6.12). Inflammation in areas of surviving parenchyma is sometimes surprisingly mild in comparison with classic acute hepatitis.[27] The degree of collapse may be judged by the extent of approximation of adjacent portal tracts, which increases with time, and by the density of the collapsed reticulin framework. As in the case of bridging necrosis, areas of recent collapse contain few if any elastic fibres whereas, later, stains for these fibres become positive.[32] Inflammatory-cell infiltration is mixed and variable in degree, when it is mild, the main infiltrating cells are macrophages. These contain yellow-brown ceroid pigment. The duct-like structures are partly of bile-duct and partly of hepatocellular origin; there is evidence of substantial liver-cell regeneration even in fatal cases.[14] Many of the tubular structures contain both liver-cell and bile-duct elements, and these have been termed neocholangioles.[33] They may reflect proliferation of a hepatic stem cell population analogous to the oval cell of rat liver.[34]

In some patients with clinically fulminant hepatitis, liver biopsies obtained early in the course of the disease show widespread microvesicular change of hepatocytes rather than cell loss. This has been documented in infection with the delta virus in South America,[35] and has also been seen in hepatitis A (unpublished observation).

authors included not only zone 3 bridging as described above, but also bridges linking portal tracts, probably representing periportal necrosis. Others have not considered bridging as a good predictor of chronicity.[24,25] It must nevertheless be regarded as a serious histological feature, for the reasons given in the first part of this section.

Bridging necrosis can develop in the early weeks of acute hepatitis, but its absence from a biopsy does not exclude the possibility that it will develop later. In patients who do not develop chronic hepatitis, bridging inevitably leads to a certain degree of scarring and distortion, sometimes seen in biopsy specimens taken many months after the acute attack.

Acute hepatitis with panacinar necrosis

This form of acute hepatitis represents the most severe degree of necrosis, with complete or near-complete destruction of hepatocytes in entire acini. When several adjacent acini undergo necrosis, the term 'multiacinar' is applicable. Massive (or submassive) hepatic necrosis refers

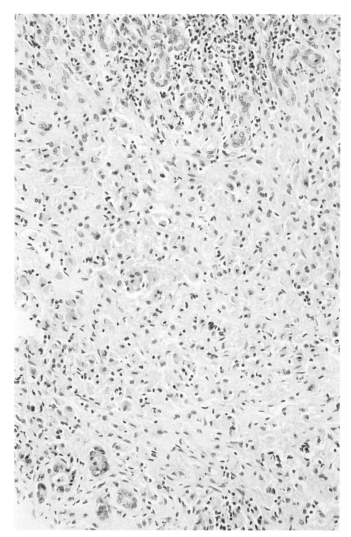

Fig. 6.12 Acute hepatitis with panacinar necrosis. Most of the hepatocytes have been destroyed, leaving debris and pigmented macrophages. Duct-like structures are seen in the portal tracts (above and below) and intervening areas are lightly infiltrated with inflammatory cells. H & E.

Acute hepatitis with periportal necrosis

In this pattern of hepatitis, the usual changes of classic acute hepatitis are seen to a greater or lesser extent, but there is additionally a substantial degree of necrosis in the periportal zones, accompanied by much periportal inflammatory infiltration (Fig. 6.13). The pattern was previously described as 'acute hepatitis with possible transition to chronic aggressive hepatitis'.[36] However, as discussed below in the section on the individual aetiological forms of hepatitis, the prognostic significance of periportal necrosis and inflammation depends on the particular virus responsible, so that a descriptive term is used in this chapter to avoid a possibly misleading prognostic implication.

Lymphocytes and plasma cells usually predominate in the portal and periportal infiltrate. There may be ductular proliferation. In contrast to the periportal (piecemeal) necrosis of chronic active hepatitis, trapped hepatocytes are usually absent from the necrotic periportal zone in acute hepatitis, or scanty. Differences between 'true' piecemeal necrosis and the periportal necrosis of acute hepatitis are further discussed in Chapter 9. There is, nevertheless, a close resemblance between these two kinds of necrosis; biopsies from patients with acute hepatitis may thus be wrongly diagnosed as chronic hepatitis, an error usually avoidable if the patient's history is both unequivocal and available to the pathologist, and if the typical acinar changes of acute hepatitis are looked for. One effect of the periportal necrosis is to cause apparent widening of the portal tracts, and linking of tracts as seen in two-dimensional sections. This portal–portal bridging necrosis should be distinguished from the zone 3 ('central–portal') bridging described above under acute hepatitis with bridging necrosis, as it probably has a different pathogenesis and different prognostic significance.

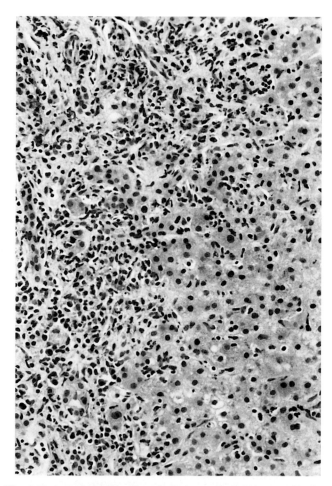

Fig. 6.13 Acute hepatitis with periportal necrosis. In this example of type A hepatitis, extensive inflammation and necrosis are seen at the edge of a portal tract. H & E.

Changes in other parts of the acini may be mild or severe. In some examples of type A hepatitis, for instance, the portal and periportal changes may be accompanied by very little perivenular necrosis. In contrast, there are patients in whom biopsy shows a combination of periportal necrosis with zone 3 bridging.

ULTRASTRUCTURAL CHANGES

These have been extensively reviewed by Phillips and co-workers.[37] The most striking alterations are seen in ballooned hepatocytes, in acidophil bodies and in the sinusoidal cell populations. Hepatocellular changes have been attributed mainly to interference with mechanisms for maintaining normal ion concentrations within the cells.[38] Such interference might result from direct action of a virus on the cell membrane, or from immunological reactions mounted by the host The latter mechanism is likely to be the more important. Changes in hepatic function are attributable mainly to sublethal cell damage and to interference with the nutrition of cells rather than to loss of cells and reduction of the hepatocellular mass.[39]

Ballooned hepatocytes (Fig. 6.14) have dilated, vesicular endoplasmic reticulum.[37,40] Attached ribosomes are reduced in number. There is overall loss of glycogen. Mitochondria are swollen, with matrix of increased density. Paracrystalline inclusions are seen, some of them in giant mitochondria. Autophagic vacuoles are prominent, and there are inclusions of bile within hepatocytes. Bile canaliculi are normal or show changes of cholestasis (p. 439). At the sinusoidal poles there is loss of microvilli and bleb formation. The latter is an important, though relatively non-specific, feature of liver-cell injury, possibly related to disruption of the cortical cytoskeleton immediately beneath the plasma membrane.[41] The plasma membrane may rupture, allowing escape of organelles from the cell. Nuclei have undulating outlines. There is dilatation of the perinuclear space, and both this and the dilated endoplasmic reticulum contain sparse flocculent material. Nuclear inclusions usually consist of glycogen. Nuclear bodies are increased in number, and nucleoli are enlarged or fragmented.[40] Nuclear pseudoinclusions are formed by invagination of adjacent cytoplasm.

Some hepatocytes, corresponding to the acidophilic cells described in the section on classic acute hepatitis, contrast

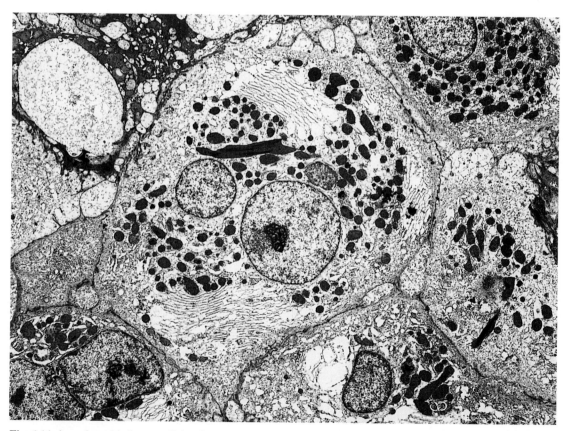

Fig. 6.14 Acute hepatitis: hepatocellular changes. A swollen, binucleated hepatocyte has prominent, dilated endoplasmic reticulum and swollen sinusoidal microvilli (top centre). An elongated mitochondrion is seen. Surrounding hepatocytes show a variety of changes, including acidophilic degeneration (top left). Electron micrograph, × 4100, kindly provided by Dr K A Bardadin.

sharply with the ballooned cells in that they have electron-dense hyaloplasm. Free acidophil bodies (Councilman bodies) have rounded contours, absent microvilli and densely packed organelles.[42] Mitochondria are irregular, with shortened cristae, and glycogen is sparse.

Regenerating hepatocytes have prominent nucleoli, and polyribosomes in the cytoplasm. They may contain glycogen bodies, arrays of smooth endoplasmic reticulum interspersed with glycogen rosettes.[43]

There are extensive changes in sinusoidal cell populations and in the spaces of Disse (Fig 6.15). Kupffer cells are swollen, and contain prominent lysosomal structures. Pinocytosis is increased, and the endoplasmic reticulum is often dilated. Endothelial cells are also increased in size. Their cytoplasm contains large, electron-dense granules corresponding to iron-containing, Perls-positive granules seen by light microscopy.[44] Basement membrane material sometimes develops beneath the endothelium within the space of Disse. A variety of other cells including lymphocytes is seen in the sinusoids and spaces of Disse, some of them in close contact with hepatocytes. These infiltrating cells may obstruct the sinusoidal lumens.

EVOLUTION OF THE LESION

As already noted, little is known about the early stages of acute hepatitis in man. The descriptions given in this chapter refer to the fully developed acute lesion, but the time over which this lesion develops varies widely from patient to patient. In some, the lesion begins to regress after a few weeks, while in others the course is one of many months. There is international agreement that the term 'chronic hepatitis' should be used for inflammation of the liver continuing without improvement for more than six months,[45] but there is overlap between acute and chronic disease: the former may last for more than six months in some instances, regressing slowly thereafter, while the latter possibly becomes established in the first few weeks or months of the disease.[46]

Following the fully developed stage of acute hepatitis, there is a stage of regressing and finally residual hepatitis. During regression, necrosis diminishes or ceases and phagocytic activity predominates. In patients with marked cholestasis, this may continue unabated, often in association with a cholestatic clinical course. Portal inflammation is still seen, and in severe hepatitis there may be ductular

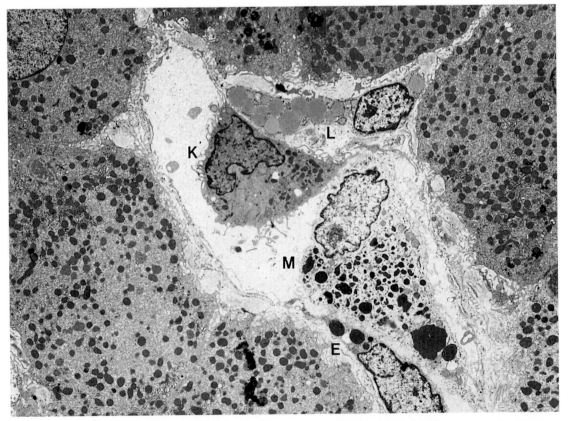

Fig. 6.15 Acute hepatitis: sinusoidal reaction. The sinusoid contains two macrophages, one of them (K) a typical Kupffer cell, the other (M) swollen and filled with lysosomes of various shapes and sizes. Also seen are a perisinusoidal cell or lipocyte (L) containing many lipid droplets, and part of an endothelial cell (E) with four electron-dense granules. Electron micrograph, × 3500, kindly provided by Dr K A Bardadin.

proliferation. Condensation of the reticulin framework marks zones of liver-cell loss, and necrotic bridges undergo collapse to form passive septa. The risk of confusion with chronic liver disease thus increases. In this regressing stage, however, the lesion can still be recognized as acute hepatitis on the basis of hepatocellular changes, acinar inflammation and phagocytic activity.

The stage of regression passes imperceptibly into a residual stage (Fig. 6.16) which is much less characteristic and easily mistaken for a non-specific reaction unconnected with viral hepatitis. Changes include slight alterations of acinar architecture, minor degrees of septum formation, focal liver-cell regeneration as shown by variation in liver-cell size and appearance from one area to another, inflammatory infiltration and Kupffer cell activation. Clumps of ceroid-containing Kupffer cells may still contain iron. Cholestasis, if still present, is mild. Gradually these residual changes fade and the liver returns to normal. Minor degrees of inflammation and phagocytic activity may be seen as long as a year or more after onset.

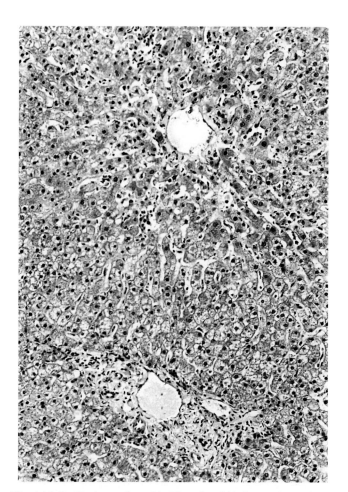

Fig. 6.16 Residual acute hepatitis. There is mild inflammation and expansion of a portal tract (below), and small foci of Kupffer cells and lymphocytes are seen near the terminal hepatic venule (above). H & E.

Persistence of substantial portal or periportal inflammation forms the basis of a diagnosis of chronic hepatitis (see Ch. 9).

DIFFERENTIAL DIAGNOSIS OF ACUTE HEPATITIS IN LIVER BIOPSIES

The lesions of acute hepatitis are sufficiently diffuse within the liver to be diagnosable with confidence in small biopsy specimens.[47] As discussed above, some examples of panacinar necrosis form an exception to this rule, but this rarely presents real diagnostic problems when clinical data are taken into account.

In cholestasis from any cause, secondary changes in hepatocytes and accompanying inflammation may cause confusion with acute hepatitis. In cholestasis the changes are confined to the cholestatic areas, and liver-cell plates show little or no disruption. Portal changes vary according to the cause of the cholestasis, and may help to establish a correct diagnosis.

As discussed in the last sections of this chapter, different causes of acute viral hepatitis are difficult to distinguish morphologically, although there may be histological clues. Hepatitis due to other viruses occasionally mimics that due to the established hepatitis viruses. In infectious mononucleosis (p. 273) liver-cell damage is usually absent or mild, and the atypical lymphocytes are seen in sinusoids and portal tracts.

Drugs should always be suspected as a possible cause of hepatitis. Features that should arouse a greater than average degree of suspicion include a poorly developed or absent portal inflammatory reaction, abundant neutrophil or eosinophil leucocytes, granuloma formation and sharply defined perivenular necrosis with little inflammation. Bile-duct damage may be a prominent feature. In alcoholic hepatitis (see Ch. 8), the typical ballooning of protein-retaining hepatocytes is accompanied by a predominantly neutrophil leucocytic infiltrate and by formation of new collagen fibres around affected hepatocytes; fatty change and Mallory bodies may be present.

The bile-duct lesion of acute hepatitis (Fig. 6.9) can usually be distinguished from that of biliary tract diseases such as primary biliary cirrhosis (see Ch. 12) by the presence of the acinar features of acute hepatitis and by clinical and biochemical findings. Granulomas associated with bile-duct lesions are virtually never seen in hepatitis, although portal granulomas are occasionally found in drug abusers.

Lastly, areas of collapse in acute hepatitis must be distinguished from the fibrous septa of chronic liver disease, as discussed above under 'acute hepatitis with bridging necrosis'.

SEQUELAE OF ACUTE HEPATITIS

The morphological consequences of acute viral hepatitis

Table 6.3   Sequelae of acute hepatitis

- Restitution to normal morphology
- Death from severe liver damage or its complications
- Post-hepatitic scarring
- Viral carrier state
- Chronic hepatitis and cirrhosis
- Hepatocellular carcinoma

are shown in Table 6.3. Restitution to normal liver is described in the preceding section, and fulminant hepatitis under 'acute hepatitis with panacinar necrosis'. The spectrum of lesions of chronic hepatitis is discussed in Chapter 9. A viral carrier state without significant histological changes (other than ground-glass hepatocytes in hepatitis B virus carriers) may develop and has recently been demonstrated in hepatitis C virus infection.[48] Karvountzis et al[49] followed 22 patients surviving acute hepatitis with coma, and concluded that such patients rarely if ever developed chronic hepatitis. On the other hand, Horney & Galambos[27] reported that chronic hepatitis had developed in 3 of 9 patients having follow-up biopsies 6 to 60 months after fulminant hepatitis. It is likely that most cirrhosis following acute hepatitis develops via chronic hepatitis. The idea that cirrhosis can develop directly from massive hepatic necrosis, without the intervention of chronic hepatitis, is expressed in the old term 'post-necrotic cirrhosis'. Certainly, nodular regeneration of surviving parenchyma is seen in patients dying some weeks or months after the acute attack, but this cannot be considered as cirrhosis in that the nodularity is not usually diffuse, and in so far as septa are formed by collapse of pre-existing fibres rather than by true fibrosis. It is possible that in a small number of patients who recover from the acute attack there is sufficient nodularity, portal–systemic shunting, fibrosis and portal hypertension to warrant a diagnosis of inactive cirrhosis even in the absence of chronic hepatitis,[25,50] but this is probably the exception rather than the rule.

There are patients, however, in whom collapse of bridges and regeneration of parenchyma lead to a morphological picture somewhat like that of inactive cirrhosis, and easily mistaken for it in needle biopsy specimens. Macroscopically the liver is irregularly nodular. Portal hypertension and other clinical features of cirrhosis are lacking, and liver function is good. The lesion does not progress. This state is best designated as post-hepatitic or post-necrotic scarring, and corresponds to the 'scar liver' (Narbenleber) or 'potato liver' (Kartoffelleber) of the German literature.[51]

Hepatocellular carcinoma (Ch. 16) is a long-term complication of viral hepatitis, usually but not always on the basis of a hepatitis virus carrier state with cirrhosis.

VIRAL HEPATITIS IN ANIMALS

Many viruses are hepatotropic and cause liver damage. Examples include the canine adenovirus of infectious canine hepatitis, and the mouse hepatitis virus. Rats and mice are susceptible to frog virus 3, which damages Kupffer cells and endothelium. Destruction of sinusoidal lining cells is followed by secondary hepatocellular damage, probably by endotoxins.[52]

The hepadna group of viruses is of special interest to hepatologists. The members of this group share properties of virion size, ultrastructure, DNA size and structure and replication strategy.[53] The best studied hepadna viruses are the hepatitis B virus of man (HBV), the woodchuck hepatitis virus (WHV),[54] the ground squirrel hepatitis virus (GSHV)[55] and the duck hepatitis B virus (DHBV).[56] Similar viruses are found in a variety of rodents, carnivores, marsupials, birds and reptiles.

The woodchuck is infected with WHV in the wild. The presence of a surface antigen in serum and liver is regularly associated with acute or chronic hepatitis as well as hepatocellular carcinoma.[54,57] The disease differs from human type B hepatitis in that hepatocellular carcinoma is seen together with histologically active hepatitis, characterized by abundant plasma cells, in the absence of cirrhosis. Woodchucks chronically infected with WHV can be experimentally superinfected with the human delta virus, HDV.[58]

Duck hepatitis B virus differs from WHV and human HBV in having a larger surface antigen particle, 30–60 nm in diameter. Natural infection is associated with chronic hepatitis, cirrhosis and liver cancer,[56] thus providing a useful model for therapy of human disease. Integrated viral DNA has been demonstrated in hepatocellular carcinoma tissue.[59] Experimental inoculation of ducklings with DHBV was found to lead to chronic inflammation in the liver of some animals, and viral DNA was demonstrable in a number of organs including pancreas, spleen and kidney as well as liver.[60]

INDIVIDUAL TYPES OF VIRAL HEPATITIS IN MAN

There are more histological similarities than differences between the various viral hepatitides. All share the same basic features of liver-cell damage and inflammation, and the four principal histological patterns of acute hepatitis (Table 6.2) may all be found in association with any of the viruses, with the possible exception of panacinar necrosis which is rarely if ever due to HCV infection. It is not currently possible to differentiate reliably between the viruses on histological grounds alone. However, there are different, sometimes characteristic patterns associated with some of the agents, and these will now be described. They represent tendencies rather than definitive differential diagnostic criteria.

TYPE A HEPATITIS

The infective agent (hepatitis A virus, HAV) is a small unenveloped RNA hepatovirus. The genome is a linear, single-stranded plus-sense RNA. Virus particles approximately 27 nm in diameter were first demonstrated in faeces of infected volunteers by Feinstone and co-workers in the early 1970s.[61] A single viral antigen can be demonstrated in the cytoplasm of Kupffer cells and hepatocytes,[62,63] and in situ hybridization has been used to detect viral RNA.[64] In practice, however, diagnosis rests on demonstration of antibody to the virus in serum rather than on tissue methods. Current infection is shown by the presence of the IgM form of the antibody, and past infection by the corresponding IgG antibody.

Spread is by the faecal–oral route, either directly from person to person or via contaminated food or water.[65] Improving hygiene in many countries has led to later and less frequent infection of the population, so that the prevalence of immunity to the virus is falling. This, together with the commonly greater severity of infection in older subjects, has determined a need for the development of vaccines, some of which are now in use.

Type A hepatitis is characteristically mild in the young, although protracted or relapsing hepatitis is not uncommon and a very small number of patients develop fulminant, potentially fatal disease that may require liver transplantation. At the other end of the spectrum, asymptomatic attacks are probably very common. Chronic type A hepatitis, if it occurs at all, is extremely rare. McDonald and colleagues[66] reported a patient in whom chronic disease developed over a period of 4 years, with persistence of IgM anti-HAV for an unusually long period. Of particular interest is the possibility that HAV might be one of several viruses capable of triggering the onset of autoimmune chronic hepatitis. In a prospective study of healthy relatives of patients with autoimmune chronic active hepatitis, 3 out of 58 developed subclinical HAV infection over a period of 4 years, and 2 of these developed autoimmune hepatitis shortly thereafter.[67]

The mechanism whereby HAV produces liver disease has been the subject of several studies. T-lymphocytes of CD8 type derived from the livers of patients with hepatitis A were shown to exhibit specific anti-HAV activity, and killed skin fibroblasts infected with the virus.[68] Immunocytochemical staining of lymphoid cells in liver biopsy sections of 2 patients showed that the portal infiltrate was mainly composed of plasma cells, other lymphocytes of B lineage and helper/inducer T cells, supporting the concept of a humoral immune response. In peripheral blood, the most striking early change is an increase in the number of NK lymphocytes, consistent with the view that non-MHC-restricted cellular cytotoxicity is involved in the control of viral infection.[69] A substantial directly cytopathic effect of the virus on hepatocytes seems unlikely.

The histological features of HAV infection are those of acute hepatitis in general, but two features are especially common. One is a periportal pattern of inflammation and necrosis, with little or no perivenular necrosis.[70] Plasma cells are prominent, and the lesion may be mistaken for that of chronic active hepatitis (Fig. 6.13). The other feature is perivenular cholestasis with little or no associated hepatocellular necrosis (Fig. 6.17). The periportal hepatitis and cholestasis are sometimes found in the same biopsy, and it is possible that the cholestasis is then the result of interruption of bile drainage by the periportal damage.[20] In other patients there is classic perivenular hepatitis with hepatocellular ballooning, multinucleation and necrosis.[71,72] In the rare fulminant form of hepatitis A the histological features are those of panacinar necrosis. Microvesicular change in surviving hepatocytes, similar to that reported in delta hepatitis in Venezuelan Indians,[35] has been observed in a patient with fatal HAV infection

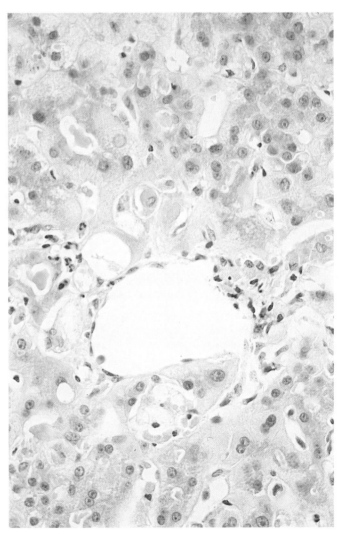

Fig. 6.17 Type A hepatitis. There is severe cholestasis in the form of bile plugs in dilated canaliculi and bile-laden Kupffer cells. Inflammation and liver-cell loss are relatively slight. H & E.

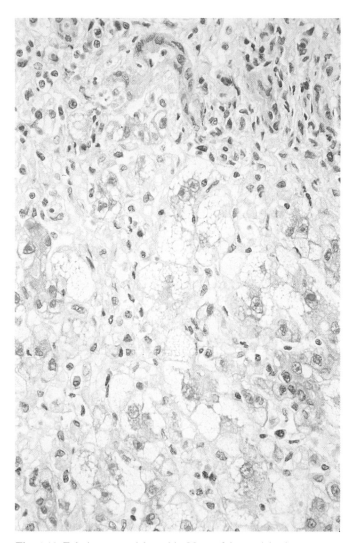

Fig. 6.18 Fulminant type A hepatitis. Many of the surviving hepatocytes are swollen and finely vacuolated. H & E.

(Fig. 6.18). Fibrin-ring granulomas have been reported in hepatitis A.[73,74]

TYPE B HEPATITIS

This major worldwide disease is the result of infection with the hepatitis B virus (HBV), a member of the hepadna virus family. The virus is transmitted by parenteral routes and by close contact, including sexual acitivty. Transmission from infected mothers to neonates commonly takes place at or soon after birth, and is important in countries with a high carrier rate.

The complete virion or Dane particle is composed of a 27 nm core containing circular, incompletely double-stranded DNA, surrounded by an envelope of surface material. The whole particle measures 42 nm in diameter. It is assembled in the endoplasmic reticulum of hepatocytes by the addition of surface material to core particles.

The envelope bears an antigen, HBsAg, which was discovered by Blumberg and colleagues in the early 1960s[75] and first named Australia antigen because of the origin of the infected patient. This discovery opened the floodgates to a rapidly growing stream of research on the hepatitis viruses. Two separate but chemically related antigens, HBcAg and HBeAg, are associated with the viral core particles. Other antigens include pre-SI[76] which is considered important for attachment of the virus to liver-cell membranes, pre-S2, and a gene product designated X. The latter is very common in hepatocytes in chronic type B hepatitis[77] and may be found in the tumour cells of hepatocellular carcinoma in the absence of HBsAg and HBcAg.[78] All these antigens can be demonstrated in tissues by immunocytochemical techniques. HBV-DNA can be identified by means of in situ hybridization,[79] which may be combined with immunocytochemical staining for HBsAg and HBcAg.[80] While infection of the liver by HBV has obviously been the main focus of study, molecular methods have shown that viral DNA is also present in many other organs, notably lymphoid tissue.[81] Its presence in cells of the genital tract may contribute to sexual transmission.[82]

Most of the antigens are demonstrable in serum at one or other time during acute and chronic HBV infection, the exception being HBcAg. Antibodies include anti-HBs, anti-HBc, anti-HBe, anti-pre-S1, anti-pre-S2 and anti-X. In a self-limiting attack of type B hepatitis, HBsAg, HBeAg and a specific DNA polymerase appear in the blood, followed by anti-HBc; antibody of IgM class is characteristic of acute infection, while IgG antibody persists after recovery. Anti-HBe appears soon after disappearance of the corresponding antigen, and finally anti-HBs develops. The sequence of events is different when HBV infection leads to chronic disease: HBsAg and HBeAg then persist in the blood, and appearance of the corresponding antibodies is delayed. Serum HBeAg is associated with viral replication, but more accurate measures are the serum level of HBV-DNA and the presence of HBcAg in hepatocytes.

Demonstration of HBsAg in liver biopsies, either by specific immunocytochemical staining or by non-immunological methods such as the orcein or Victoria blue stain, serves to distinguish the ground-glass hepatocytes (p. 370) of chronic HBV infection from their imitators. It also indicates that infection is chronic, because HBsAg can rarely be demonstrated in acute type B hepatitis, and then only in small amounts in fulminant disease. Staining for HBcAg is more informative, since in chronic hepatitis it is associated with active viral replication. In the replicative phase of HBV infection the antigen is mainly nuclear in location while histological activity and elimination of virus-producing hepatocytes are associated with cytoplasmic positivity in addition to the nuclear staining. The phases of chronic HBV infection are discussed in more detail in Chapter 9.

In recent years, considerable interest has focused on the ability of the hepatitis B virus to undergo mutation.[83–87] This is probably much more frequent than was previously suspected. A genomic variant affecting the pre-core region leads to inability of the virus to express HBeAg, although anti-HBe is found in the serum.[83] Patients with this variant may show active virus replication in the absence of HBeAg. The variant probably emerges spontaneously during infection, and has been particularly associated with severe acute disease. The virus can revert to its original form after transmission to another subject, and the mutant may coexist with wild-type virus. Another mutation induced by vaccination against HBV leads to escape from protection by the vaccine.[84] This so-called 'escape mutant' is characterized by a point mutation leading to substitution of a single amino acid in a highly antigenic region of HBsAg. The mutant is stable, and has been shown to be present five years after its appearance. As already noted, mutant forms of HBV have been implicated in the pathogenesis of fulminant hepatitis.[28,29]

The histological changes of acute type B hepatitis are not substantially different from those of other forms.[16,70,72,88] Differences observed in various studies probably reflect selection of patients rather than the infective agent. Lymphocytes and macrophages are often in close contact with hepatocytes and the lymphocytes may even lie within them (emperipolesis), in keeping with immunological mechanisms of liver damage. Prediction of chronicity is very difficult on histological grounds, and the clinician can obtain more accurate information from study of the various antigens and antibodies in serum. HBs antigenaemia is sometimes associated with glomerulonephritis of secondary membranous type.[89]

The mechanisms whereby HBV infection causes disease have mostly been studied in chronic hepatitis, but some information is available for acute hepatitis. There is general agreement that the virus is not cytotoxic to any substantial degree under ordinary circumstances. One possible exception is liver transplantation, after which reinfection of the graft may be characterized by the rapid accumulation of large amounts of HBsAg and HBcAg without much infiltration by lymphoid cells.[90] Under other circumstances it is assumed that the main mechanisms of liver-cell damage are immunological. Sequential study of cellular immunity in acute infection indicates that the initial response is to pre-S, followed by HBcAg and HBsAg.[91] The main mode of hepatocyte death is probably apoptosis,[10–12] although rupture of ballooned hepatocytes or lysis of smaller cells may also be involved, especially in hepatitis with confluent necrosis. Expression of HLA antigens,[92] adhesion molecules[93,94] and viral antigens on the surface of hepatocytes is considered to be important. This expression may lead to T-cell activity against HBcAg[95] and possibly HBsAg.[96] On the other hand, one

study of 6 patients with acute type B hepatitis revealed a preponderance of non-T-lymphocytes in the inflammatory infiltrate, many of them natural killer (NK) cells.[97] IgM-containing B-lymphocytes were found in the portal tracts. It seems likely, therefore, that liver-cell damage in acute type B hepatitis is usually immunologically mediated, and that it involves both humoral and cellular mechanisms.[97–100]

TYPE C HEPATITIS

In 1989, Choo et al[101] reported the isolation of a cDNA clone from a viral genome derived from a chimpanzee infected with a blood borne non-A, non-B hepatitis virus. This made it possible to construct an assay for antibodies in the serum of infected patients,[102] and to identify what is now universally known as hepatitis C and the hepatitis C virus (HCV).[103–105] It is apparent that this virus is responsible for most post-transfusion non-A, non-B hepatitis, as well as for much sporadic infection.

HCV is a small single-stranded RNA virus with some of the properties of the flaviviruses and pestiviruses. It appears to be present in only small amounts in the blood of infected patients, which helps to explain the paucity of reports on its structure. Virus-like particles in the serum of chimpanzees and humans with non-A, non-B hepatitis[106] may represent HCV.

The putative genome has regions coding for the viral core (c), an envelope (e) and several non-structural components (NS1 to NS5) including enzymes necessary for replication.[107] There is variation in the nucleotide sequence in isolates from different parts of the world[107] and also within the same geographical area.[108,109] The first generation of tests for anti-HCV in serum was based on a non-structural protein, c-100. More recent tests utilize both structural and non-structural proteins coded by different regions of the genome;[110–112] these tests have enabled HCV infection to be identified earlier in the course of the disease.[113] The most direct method of testing is the identification of HCV-RNA in serum and in liver tissue.[114,115] The polymerase chain reaction (PCR) has made this task much easier,[116–117] but because of the above-mentioned genetic variability of the viral genome, primers need to be carefully chosen.[118,119] PCR enables infection to be detected within weeks of onset, earlier than is possible with current antibody tests.[118]

The newer methods for detection of serum antibodies and the application of PCR to serum and tissues have both helped to improve the accuracy of diagnosis of HVC infection. They have therefore clarified the epidemiology of hepatitic C and the role which infection plays in various forms of liver disease. Blood transfusion and treatment with blood products are important modes of transmission,[120–122] well illustrated by the high incidence of infection among patients with haemophilia[123–125] and multiply transfused patients with thalassaemia.[126] A history of intravenous drug abuse is common. This virus can be transmitted by organ transplantation.[127] However, these methods of transmission cannot account for the very large numbers of patients infected, or for all instances of sporadic, non-transfusion-related disease. Sexual transmission has been postulated,[128,129] but is not currently thought to be important. Vertical transmission from infected mothers to newborn babies is described.[130] Health personnel are at risk of contracting HCV infection.[131]

The virus is associated with a wide range of liver diseases. In acute self-limiting hepatitis anti-HCV usually disappears from the serum whereas in chronic infection it persists.[132] Fulminant hepatitis is rarely attributed to HCV. Chronic hepatitis is common in parenterally acquired HCV infection, developing in at least half of the patients. The pathological lesions are often mild, on the borderline of chronic persistent and chronic active hepatitis (see below). In spite of this, cirrhosis appears to develop in a substantial proportion of patients,[120,133–135] probably on the basis of repeated episodes of acinar necrosis. Hepatocellular carcinoma may ensue as in cirrhosis of any cause, and HCV is currently regarded as a major factor in the worldwide incidence of this cancer.[136–142] Loss of serum HCV-RNA has been reported after treatment of chronic hepatitis C with alpha-interferon.[143] Treatment may lead to a reduction in the degree of piecemeal necrosis and lobular injury,[144] and diminution of fibrosis has been reported.[145]

The pathological features of hepatitis C are essentially those already described in previous years for parenterally transmitted and sporadic non-A, non-B hepatitis.[88,146–150] Acute infection is characterized by liver-cell swelling, acidophil body formation, cholestasis and infiltration of sinusoids by lymphocytes.[151] Prediction of a chronic course cannot easily be made on histological grounds; indeed, an often striking lymphocytic portal reaction early in the course of infection, and extensive lobular changes in chronic infection, make the histological distinction between acute and chronic disease difficult (Fig. 6.19). Bile-duct damage[120] and formation of portal lymphoid follicles, the most characteristic feature of chronic hepatitis C, may be seen.[152–154] Once chronic disease is established, the most frequently observed picture is one of mild chronic hepatitis, on the borderline of chronic persistent and chronic active hepatitis, with lymphoid follicles and focal intra-acinar damage in the form of acidophilic change, acidophil body formation and liver-cell drop-out. There may also be mild to moderate fatty change which is principally of macrovesicular type. As already noted, cirrhosis develops in a substantial number of patients in spite of the mildness of this earlier histological pattern, probably on the basis of repeated attacks of bridging and other forms of acinar necrosis, but possibly also to some extent as a result

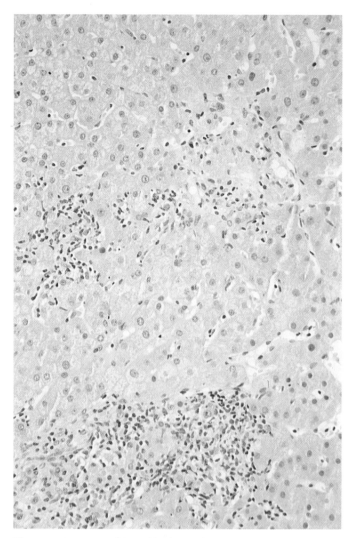

Fig. 6.19 Acute type C hepatitis. A portal tract (below) and sinusoids are infiltrated by lymphocytes. Liver-cell damage is slight in this example. The hepatitis followed a needle-stick injury. H & E.

of piecemeal necrosis.[155] A relationship between histological exacerbations and the typically episodic clinical course is speculative but likely. The histological appearances in cirrhosis due to HCV infection are not specific, although lymphoid aggregates may still be seen. The progression to cirrhosis may take many years or even decades.[120,122] The pathological features of chronic type C hepatitis are further discussed in Chapter 9.

Several groups have demonstrated viral antigens[156–158] and the hepatitis C genome[158,159] in liver biopsy tissue, but the techniques and reagents are not currently suitable for routine use. The pathogenesis of liver damage in HCV infection remains speculative. Demonstration of adhesion molecules in areas of inflammation in non-A, non-B hepatitis[93] and attachment of lymphocytes to the endothelium of portal and terminal hepatic venules[15] support the concept, generally held for most viral hepatitides, that the pathological lesions result mainly from an interaction of the patient's immune system with hepatocytes displaying viral antigens.

There is accumulating evidence to suggest that HCV infection modifies other forms of liver disease. Infection with both HBV and HCV is common among intravenous drug abusers. Superinfection of HBV carriers with HCV was found to be uncommon in a Chinese population, but was associated with a higher prevalence of cirrhosis.[160] On the other hand it has been suggested that HCV might exert a suppressive effect on HBV and trigger both HBeAg/anti-HBe seroconversion and clearance of HBsAg.[161] Infection with the human immunodeficiency virus (HIV) together with HCV can lead to severe liver damage.[162,163] In patients with alcoholic liver disease, HCV infection has been implicated as a pathogenetic factor, responsible for more severe liver-cell damage and progression to cirrhosis.[164–166] The histological lesion of chronic active hepatitis in alcohol abusers may be the result of HCV infection.[167–168]

The relationship between HCV infection and autoimmune hepatitis has been the subject of much debate, particularly because of a high prevalence of anti-HCV seropositivity by first-generation testing in patients with a diagnosis of autoimmune chronic hepatitis. This has been partly explained by false-positive results due to high serum globulin levels,[169] but more sophisticated tests for antibodies and testing of serum and liver by PCR have made it clear that there is a real relationship. Evidence of HCV infection has been demonstrated in patients with different types of autoimmune hepatitis,[170–172] and is associated with an unexpectedly poor response to corticosteroid therapy;[173] such patients may, however, respond to interferon.[172] A high proportion of patients with acute or chronic type C hepatitis have serum antibodies to a nonviral host epitope, GOR.[174] In a study of patients with type 2 autoimmune hepatitis characterized by LKM-1 antibodies, the presence of anti-GOR and anti-HCV identified a subgroup with less severe disease activity and a poor response to immunosuppression.[175] It therefore seems reasonable to assume that HCV infection plays a part in the pathogenesis of some hepatitides previously regarded as autoimmune in origin. The finding of Sjögren's syndrome in many patients with HCV infection[176] suggests that there is also a link with immunologically mediated disease of other organs.

TYPE D (DELTA) HEPATITIS

In 1977 Rizzetto and colleagues described a new antigen–antibody system in the serum of patients with HBV infection.[177] The antigen, delta or HDAg, has since been shown to be a marker for a defective RNA virus. This is capable of surviving in hepatocytes on its own, but requires the surface material of HBV for release from cells and for its pathogenetic effect.[178] HDAg is readily demon-

strable in paraffin sections of formalin-fixed material by immunoperoxidase. It is mainly located in hepatocyte nuclei (Fig. 6.20), with smaller amounts in cytoplasm. Nuclei rich in HDV sometimes have a homogeneous, finely textured 'sanded' appearance previously attributed to HBV core particles.[179] Immunocytochemical localization of HDAg correlates well with in situ hybridization[180] but not with degenerative changes in hepatocytes. The antibody corresponding to HDAg, anti-HD or anti-δ, is found in serum in present and past infection. Because the presence of anti-δ fails to distinguish reliably between active and past infection, immunocytochemical demonstration of HDAg in hepatocytes plays an important part in diagnosis. However, the high molecular weight form of IgM anti-δ (19S) is mainly found in acute infection, while the low molecular weight form (7S) denotes chronic disease.[181] IgA anti-δ is almost exclusively found in chronic infection; its presence correlates with histological severity.[182]

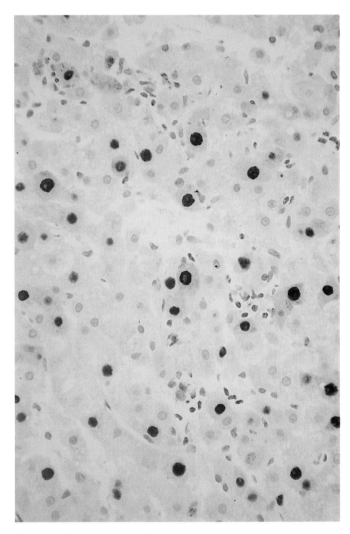

Fig. 6.20 Hepatitis D virus (delta virus) infection. Positive staining is seen in many hepatocyte nuclei and there is weak cytoplasmic positivity. Polyclonal anti-HDV antibody; immunoperoxidase.

HDV infection has a worldwide distribution and is an important factor in modifying both acute and chronic type B hepatitis. It can be acquired simultaneously with HBV (coinfection), in which case the illness is often more severe than simple acute type B hepatitis and is sometimes fulminant.[26] Alternatively an HBV carrier may be secondarily infected with HDV (superinfection), an event which encourages chronic HDV infection but which may also lead to a severe and potentially fatal illness.[26,183]

There are few pathological features of HDV infection that distinguish it from other forms of acute or chronic viral hepatitis, but HDV is usually associated with histologically and biochemically active disease.[184–186] In some series cirrhosis has been shown to develop more rapidly than in hepatitis B without delta,[184] and has been found in younger patients.[185] However, slow progression of the disease to cirrhosis has also been noted.[187]

Acute delta infection in parts of South America and Africa has been associated with a peculiar microvesicular change in hepatocytes.[35] This so-called 'morula cell degeneration' or 'spongiocytic change' is attributed to the accumulation of finely divided fat in damaged hepatocytes. Similar appearances are, however, occasionally found in severe acute hepatitis of other cause. In chronic infection, eosinophilic degeneration of hepatocytes is common.[185] Ultrastructural changes in hepatocytes include dilatation of the endoplasmic reticulum, abnormal density of the matrix of mitochondria and shortened, curled mitochondrial cristae.[188]

The eosinophilic change noted above, and the microvesicular appearance of hepatocytes in acute delta infection in some parts of the world, have led to the suggestion that the virus may have a direct cytopathic effect. Degenerative changes in cultured HeLa and HepG2 cells transfected with a plasmid containing HDAg have been cited in support.[189] On the other hand, there is evidence for immune-mediated damage, including close contact between HDAg-containing hepatocytes and lymphocytes,[188] correlation between portal lymphocytic infiltration and the number of HDAg-containing hepatocytes,[190] and predominance of suppressor/cytotoxic T-lymphocytes in areas of piecemeal and intralobular necrosis.[191] There appears to be no direct correlation between expression of HDAg in hepatocyte nuclei and necro-inflammatory changes in liver biopsies,[186] but in one study hepatocytes with cytoplasmic HDAg were often seen in contact with lymphocytes.[188] The current balance of opinion is therefore that the pathogenetic effects of the virus are usually mediated by the patient's immune system.

TYPE E HEPATITIS

Hepatitis E, formerly classified as one of the forms of non-A, non-B hepatitis,[192] resembles hepatitis A in that it is spread by the faecal-oral route. It is common in Asia, where the virus gives rise to water-borne epidemics[193] as well as to sporadic disease. The infection has also been identified in Africa and Latin America,[194] and occasional cases are reported in the Western world[195] following travel to endemic areas. Infection is reported to be more severe in pregnancy.[196]

The infective agent is an unenveloped, single-stranded RNA virus. Virus particles measure approximately 27–34 nm in diameter, and have a spiky outline. They are found in faeces of infected patients, and were also demonstrated within bile ductules and hepatic sinusoidal cells of a patient with fatal cholestatic hepatitis E.[197] The virus can be transmitted to a number of primates.[198–201] The viral genome has been cloned after isolation from gallbladder bile of infected cynomolgus monkeys.[202] Close contact between lymphocytes and damaged hepatocytes in the latter suggests that immunological mechanisms are involved in the pathogenesis of the disease.[203]

There is relatively little information to date on detailed histological appearances in hepatitis E. The picture has been reported to resemble hepatitis A, with dense portal and periportal inflammatory infiltration and canalicular cholestasis.[204] In the fatal case cited above[197] there was extensive necrosis and collapse. Surviving hepatocytes were swollen and foamy, and sometimes formed cholestatic rosettes. Other features included bile ductular proliferation and phlebitis involving both portal and terminal hepatic venules. Portal inflammation was mild. Cholestasis and transformation of hepatocytes to bile ductule-like structures was reported in a patient who developed the disease during an epidemic in Pakistan.[205]

TYPE F HEPATITIS

This designation has been very provisionally applied[206] to infection with a toga-like virus found in the nuclei of hepatocytes of patients with fulminant hepatitis.[30] Particles typically 60–70 nm in diameter, with a spiked envelope, were seen on electron microscopy in the livers of 9 patients with severe hepatitis requiring liver transplantation.[31] In 7 of these the disease had been attributed to a non-A, non-B virus. In a different study of 15 patients referred for liver transplantation for fulminant non-A, non-B hepatitis or subacute hepatic failure[207] it was shown that none had evidence of HCV infection. It is therefore possible that the toga-like virus described represents an important cause of fulminant hepatitis not attributable to any of the previously known hepatitis viruses. Of the 9 patients with the toga virus-like particles who underwent liver transplantation, 5 developed acute liver failure one week after operation; similar particles were found in all the grafts, and were more abundant than before. Histologically, the native livers of affected patients showed extensive necrosis with broad areas of collapse alternating with map-like areas of surviving, bile-stained parenchyma. There was heavy infiltration by lymphocytes and plasma cells. The grafts examined one week later were red and swollen, and histological examination showed haemorrhagic necrosis.

It should be noted that the designation of hepatitis F has also been used for chronic non-A, non-B hepatitis of unproven cause.

OTHER FORMS OF VIRAL HEPATITIS

In a series of 10 patients with severe acute and chronic hepatitis characterized by formation of syncytial giant hepatocytes, Phillips and co-workers[208] described intracytoplasmic structures with the ultrastructural features of a paramyxovirus. A label of hepatitis G has been very tentatively suggested.[209] In other examples of giant-cell hepatitis no virus-like inclusions were demonstrated, and it is thought that giant-cell hepatitis may have several causes.[210,211]

Because not all episodes of viral hepatitis can currently be proved to be due to one or other of the above agents, it is possible that there are other, as yet undiscovered, hepatitis viruses.

REFERENCES

1. Valla D, Flejou J-F, Lebrec D et al. Portal hypertension and ascites in acute hepatitis: clinical, hemodynamic and histological correlations. Hepatology 1989; 10: 482–487
2. Bruguera M, Bordas J M, Rodés J. Atlas of laparoscopy and biopsy of the liver. Philadelphia: Saunders, 1979: p 49
3. Gazzard B G, Portmann B, Murray-Lyon I M, Williams R. Causes of death in fulminant hepatic failure and relationship to quantitative histological assessment of parenchymal damage. Q J Med 1975; 44: 615–626
4. Rappaport A M. The microcirculatory acinar concept of normal and pathological hepatic structure. Beitr Pathol 1976: 157: 215–243
5. Bianchi L, Zimmerli-Ning M, Gudat F. Viral hepatitis. In: MacSween R N M, Anthony P P, Scheuer P J, eds. Pathology of the liver. Edinburgh: Churchill Livingstone, 1979: p 164
6. De Groote J, Desmet V J, Gedigk P et al. A classification of chronic hepatitis. Lancet 1968; ii: 626–628
7. Thaler H. Die Virushepatitis. In: Thaler H, ed. Leberbiopsie. Berlin: Springer, 1969: p 51
8. Ranek L. Cytophotometric studies of the DNA, nucleic acid and protein content of liver cell nuclei from patients with virus hepatitis. Acta Pathol Microbiol Scand [A] 1976; 84: 1–8
9. Kerr J F R, Wyllie A H, Currie A R. Apoptosis: a basic biological phenomenon with wide-ranging implications in tissue kinetics. Br J Cancer 1972; 26: 239–257
10. Searle J, Harmon B V, Bishop C J, Kerr J F R. The significance of cell death by apoptosis in hepatobiliary disease. J Gastroenterol Hepatol 1987; 2: 77–96
11. Powell L W. The nature of cell death in piecemeal necrosis: is order emerging from chaos? Hepatology 1987; 7: 794–796
12. Wyllie A H. Apoptosis: cell death in tissue regulation. J Pathol 1987; 153: 313–316
13. Inuzuka S, Ueno T, Torimura T, Sata M, Abe H, Tanikawa K. Immunohistochemistry of the hepatic extracellular matrix in acute viral hepatitis. Hepatology 1990; 12: 249–256
14. Milandri M, Gaub J, Ranek L. Evidence for liver cell proliferation during fatal acute liver failure. Gut 1980; 21: 423–427
15. Nomomura A, Mizukami Y, Matsubara F, Kobayashi K. Clinicopathological study of lymphocyte attachment to endothelial cells (endothelialitis) in various liver diseases. Liver 1991; 11: 78–88
16. Kryger P, Christoffersen P. Liver histopathology of the hepatitis A virus infection: a comparison with hepatitis type B and non-A, non-B. J Clin Pathol 1983; 36: 650–654
17. Hengeveld P, Zuyderhoudt F M J, Jöbsis A C, van Gool J. Some aspects of iron metabolism during acute viral hepatitis. Hepato-gastroenterol 1982; 29: 138–141
18. Mietkiewski J M, Scheuer P J, Immunoglobulin-containing plasma cells in acute hepatitis. Liver 1985; 5: 84–88
19. Poulsen H, Christoffersen P. Abnormal bile duct epithelium in liver biopsies with histological signs of viral hepatitis. Acta Pathol Microbiol Scand [A] 1969; 76: 383–390
20. Sciot R, Van Damme B, Desmet V J. Cholestatic features in hepatitis A. J Hepatol 1986; 3: 172–181
21. Scheuer P J, Maggi G. Hepatic fibrosis and collapse: histological distinction by orcein staining. Histopathology 1980; 4: 487–490
22. Boyer J L, Klatskin G. Pattern of necrosis in acute viral hepatitis. Prognostic value of bridging (subacute hepatic necrosis). N Engl J Med 1970; 283: 1063–1071
23. Ware A J, Eigenbrodt E H, Combes B. Prognostic significance of subacute hepatic necrosis in acute hepatitis. Gastroenterology 1975; 68: 519–524
24. Spitz R D, Keren D F, Boitnott J K, Maddrey W C. Bridging hepatic necrosis. Etiology and prognosis. Dig Dis 1978; 23: 1076–1078
25. Nisman R M, Ganderson A P, Vlahcevic R, Gregory D H. Acute viral hepatitis with bridging necrosis. An overview. Arch Intern Med 1979; 139: 1289–1291
26. Smedile A, Farci P, Verme G et al. Influence of delta infection on severity of hepatitis B. Lancet 1982; ii: 945–947
27. Horney J T, Galambos J T. The liver during and after fulminant hepatitis. Gastroenterology 1977; 73: 639–645
28. Omata M, Ehata T, Yokosuka O, Hosoda K, Ohto M. Mutations in the precore region of hepatitis B virus DNA in patients with fulminant and severe hepatitis. N Engl J Med 1991; 324: 1699–1704
29. Liang T J, Hasegawa K, Rimon N, Wands J R, Ben-Porath E. A hepatitis B virus mutant associated with an epidemic of fulminant hepatitis. N Engl J Med 1991; 324: 1705–1709
30. Fagan E A, Ellis D S, Tovey G M et al. Toga-like virus as a cause of fulminant hepatitis attributed to sporadic non-A, non-B. J Med Virol 1989; 28: 150–155
31. Fagan E A, Ellis D S, Tovey G M et al. Toga virus-like particles in acute liver failure attributed to sporadic non-A, non-B hepatitis and recurrence after liver transplantation. J Med Virol 1992; 38: 71–77
32. Thung S N, Gerber M A. The formation of elastic fibers in livers with massive hepatic necrosis. Arch Pathol Lab Med 1982; 106: 468–469
33. Phillips M J, Poucell S. Modern aspects of the morphology of viral hepatitis. Hum Pathol 1981; 12: 1060–1084
34. Roskams T, De Vos R, van den Oord J J, Desmet V. Cells with neuroendocrine features in regenerating human liver. APMIS 1991; Suppl. 23: 32–39
35. Popper H, Thung S N, Gerber M A et al. Histologic studies of severe delta agent infection in Venezuelan Indians. Hepatology 1983; 3: 906–912
36. Bianchi L, De Groote J, Desmet V J et al. Morphological criteria in viral hepatitis. Lancet 1971; i: 333–337
37. Phillips M J, Poucell S, Patterson J, Valencia P. Viral hepatitis. In: Phillips M J, Poucell S, Patterson J, Valencia P, eds. The liver: an atlas and text of ultrastructural pathology. New York: Raven Press, 1987: pp 37–51
38. Trump B F, Kim K M, Iseri O A. Cellular pathophysiology of hepatitis. Am J Clin Pathol 1976; 65: 828–847
39. Schaffner F. The structural basis of altered hepatic function in viral hepatitis. Am J Med 1970; 49: 658–668
40. Schaff Z, Lapis K. Fine structure of hepatocytes during the etiology of several common pathologies. J Electron Microsc Tech 1990; 14: 179–207
41. Gores G J, Herman B, Lemasters J J. Plasma membrane bleb formation and rupture: a common feature of hepatocellular injury. Hepatology 1990; 11: 690–698
42. Klion F M, Schaffner F. The ultrastructure of acidophilic 'Councilman-like' bodies in the liver. Am J Pathol 1966; 48: 755–767

43. Wills E J. Acute infective hepatitis. Fine structural and cytochemical alterations in human liver. Arch Pathol 1968; 86: 184–207

44. Bardadin K A, Scheuer P J. Endothelial cell changes in acute hepatitis. A light and electron microscopic study. J Pathol 1984; 144: 213–220

45. Leevy C M, Popper H, Sherlock S, eds. Diseases of the liver and biliary tract. Standardization of nomenclature, diagnostic criteria, and diagnostic methodology. Washington: US Government Printing Office, 1976: p 9

46. Shikata T, Karasawa T, Abe K. Two distinct types of hepatitis in experimental hepatitis B virus infection. Am J Pathol 1980; 99: 353–368

47. Hölund B, Poulsen H, Schlichting P. Reproducibility of liver biopsy diagnosis in relation to the size of the specimen. Scand J Gastroenterol 1980; 15: 329–335

48. Brillanti S, Foli M, Gaiani S, Masci C, Miglioli M, Barbara L. Persistent hepatitis C viraemia without liver disease. Lancet 1993; 341: 464–465

49. Karvountzis G G, Redeker A G, Peters R L. Long-term follow-up studies of patients surviving fulminant viral hepatitis. Gastroenterology 1974; 67: 870–887

50. Thaler H. Hepatitis und Zirrhose. Dtsch Med Wochenschr 1975; 100: 1018–1025

51. Gedigk P, Bechtelsheimer H. Leber. In: Eder M, Gedigk P, eds. Lehrbuch der allgemeinen Pathologie und der pathologischen Anatomie. Berlin: Springer, 1975: p 513

52. Kirn A, Gut J-P, Bingan A, Steffan A-M. Murine hepatitis induced by frog virus 3: a model for studying the effect of sinusoidal cell damage on the liver. Hepatology 1983; 3: 105–111

53. Robinson W S, Klote L, Aoki N. Hepadnaviruses in cirrhotic liver and hepatocellular carcinoma. J Med Virol 1990; 31: 18–32

54. Paronetto F, Tennant B C. Woodchuck hepatitis virus infection: a model of human hepatic diseases and hepatocellular carcinoma. Prog Liver Dis 1990; 9: 463–483

55. Marion P L, Knight S S, Salazar F H, Popper H, Robinson W S. Ground squirrel hepatitis virus infection. Hepatology 1983; 3: 519–527

56. Omata M, Uchiumi K, Ito Y et al. Duck hepatitis B virus and liver diseases. Gastroenterology 1983; 85: 260–267

57. Popper H, Shih J W-K, Gerin J L et al. Woodchuck hepatitis and hepatocellular carcinoma: correlation of histologic with virologic observations. Hepatology 1981; 1: 91–98

58. Dourakis S, Karayiannis P, Goldin R, Taylor M, Monjardino J, Thomas H C. An in situ hybridization, molecular biological and immunohistochemical study of hepatitis delta virus in woodchucks. Hepatology 1991; 14: 534–539

59. Yokosuka O, Omata M, Zhou Y-Z, Imazeki F, Okuda K. Duck hepatitis B virus DNA in liver and serum of Chinese ducks: integration of viral DNA in a hepatocellular carcinoma. Proc Natl Acad Sci USA 1985; 82: 5180–5184

60. Freiman J S, Jilbert A R, Dixon R J et al. Experimental duck hepatitis B virus infection: pathology and evolution of hepatic and extrahepatic infection. Hepatology 1988; 8: 507–513

61. Feinstone S M, Kapikian A Z, Purcell R H. Hepatitis A: detection by immune electron microscopy of a virus-like antigen associated with acute illness. Science 1973; 182: 1026–1028

62. Mathiesen L R, Fauerholdt L, Moller A M et al. Immunofluorescence studies for hepatitis A virus and hepatitis B surface and core antigen in liver biopsies from patients with acute viral hepatitis. Gastroenterology 1979; 77: 623–628

63. Shimizu Y K, Shikata T, Beninger P R et al. Detection of hepatitis A antigen in human liver. Infect Immun 1982; 36: 320–324

64. Fagan E, Yousef G, Brahm J et al. Persistence of hepatitis A virus in fulminant hepatitis and after liver transplantation. J Med Virol 1990; 30: 131–136

65. Tilzey A J, Banatvala J E, Hepatitis A: changing prevalence and possible vaccines. Br Med J 1991; 302: 1552–1553

66. McDonald G S A, Courtney M G, Shattock A G, Weir D G. Prolonged IgM antibodies and histopathological evidence of chronicity in hepatitis A. Liver 1989; 9: 223–228

67. Vento S, Garofano T, Di Perri G, Dolci L, Concia E, Bassetti D. Identification of hepatitis A virus as a trigger for autoimmune chronic hepatitis type 1 in susceptible individuals. Lancet 1991; 337: 1183–1187

68. Vallbracht A, Maier K, Stierhof Y-D, Wiedmann K H, Flehmig B, Fleischer B. Liver-derived cytotoxic T cells in hepatitis A virus infection. J Infect Dis 1989; 160: 209–217

69. Müller C, Gödl I, Göttlicher J, Wolf H M, Eibl M M. Phenotypes of peripheral blood lymphocytes during acute hepatitis A. Acta Paediatr Scand 1991; 80: 931–937

70. Abe H, Beninger P R, Ikejiri N, Setoyama H, Sata M, Tanikawa K. Light microscopic findings of liver biopsy specimens from patients with hepatitis type A and comparison with type B. Gastroenterology 1982; 82: 938–947

71. Teixeira M R J Jr, Weller I V D, Murray A M et al. The pathology of hepatitis A in man. Liver 1982; 2: 53–60

72. Okuno T, Sano A, Deguchi T et al. Pathology of acute hepatitis A in humans. Comparison with acute hepatitis B. Am J Clin Pathol 1984; 81: 162–169

73. Ponz E, Garcia-Pagan J C, Bruguera M, Bruix J, Rodes J. Hepatic fibrin-ring granulomas in a patient with hepatitis A. Gastroenterology 1991; 100: 268–270

74. Ruel M, Sevestre H, Henry-Biabaud E, Courouce A M, Capron J P, Erlinger S. Fibrin ring granulomas in hepatitis A. Dig Dis Sci 1992: 37: 1915–1917

75. Blumberg B S, Alter H J, Visnich S. A 'new' antigen in leukemia sera. JAMA 1965; 191: 541–546

76. Hadzic N, Alberti A, Portmann B, Vergani D. Detection of hepatitis B virus pre-S1 and pre-S2 determinants in paraffin wax embedded liver tissue: importance of reagents used. J Clin Pathol 1991; 44: 554–557

77. Wang W, London W T, Lega L, Feitelson M A. HBxAg in the liver from carrier patients with chronic hepatitis and cirrhosis. Hepatology 1991; 14: 29–37

78. Wang W, London W T, Feitelson M A, Hepatitis B x antigen in hepatitis B virus carrier patients with liver cancer. Cancer Res 1991; 51: 4971–4977

79. Infantolino D, Pinarello A, Ceccato, R, Barbazza R. HBV-DNA by in situ hybridization. A method to improve sensitivity on formalin-fixed, paraffin-embedded liver biopsies. Liver 1989; 9: 360–366

80. Lau J Y N, Naoumov N V, Alexander G J M, Williams R. Rapid detection of hepatitis B virus DNA in liver tissue by in situ hybridisation and its combination with immunohistochemistry for simultaneous detection of HBV antigens. J Clin Pathol 1991; 44: 905–908

81. Yoffe B, Burns D K, Bhatt H S, Combes B. Extrahepatic hepatitis B virus DNA sequences in patients with acute hepatitis B infection. Hepatology 1990; 12: 187–192

82. Pao C C, Yao D-S, Lin M-Y, Lin C-Y, Hsieh T-T. Hepatitis B virus DNA in cervicovaginal cells. Arch Pathol Lab Med 1991; 115: 607–609

83. Carman W F, Jacyna M R, Hadziyannis S et al. Mutation preventing formation of hepatitis B e antigen in patients with chronic hepatitis B infection. Lancet 1989; ii: 588–591

84. Carman W F, Zanetti A R, Karayiannis P et al. Vaccine-induced escape mutant of hepatitis B virus. Lancet 1990; 336: 325–329

85. Carman W F, Fagan E A, Hadziyannis S et al. Association of a precore genomic variant of hepatitis B virus with fulminant hepatitis. Hepatology 1991; 14: 219–222

86. Liang T J, Hasegawa K, Rimon N, Wands J R, Ben-Porath E. A hepatitis B mutant associated with an epidemic of fulminant hepatitis. N Engl J Med 1991; 324: 1705–1709

87. Omata M, Ehata T, Yokosuka O, Hosoda K, Ohto M, Mutations in the precore region of hepatitis B virus DNA in patients with fulminant and severe hepatitis. N Engl J Med 1991; 324: 1699–1704

88. Rugge M, Vanstapel M-J, Ninfo V et al. Comparative histology of acute hepatitis B and non-A, non-B in Leuven and Padova. Virchows Arch [A] 1983; 401: 275–288

89. Wrzolkowa T, Zurowska A, Uszycka-Karcz M, Picken M M. Hepatitis B virus-associated glomerulonephritis: electron microscopic studies in 98 children. Am J Kidney Dis 1991; 18: 306–312

90. Davies S E, Portmann B C, O'Grady J G et al. Hepatic histological findings after transplantation for chronic hepatitis B

virus infection, including a unique pattern of fibrosing cholestatic hepatitis. Hepatology 1991; 13: 150–157

91. Vento S, Rondanelli E G, Ranieri S, O'Brien C J, Williams R, Eddleston A L W F. Prospective study of cellular immunity to hepatitis-B-virus antigens from the early incubation phase of acute hepatitis B. Lancet 1987; ii: 119–122

92. Nagafuchi Y, Scheuer P J. Expression of β_2-microglobulin on hepatocytes in acute and chronic type B hepatitis. Hepatology 1986; 6: 20–23

93. Volpes R, van den Oord J J, Desmet V J. Immunohistochemical study of adhesion molecules in liver inflammation. Hepatology 1990; 12: 59–65

94. Volpes R, van den Oord J J, Desmet V J. Hepatic expression of intercellular adhesion molecule-1 (ICAM-1) in viral hepatitis B. Hepatology 1990; 12: 148–154

95. Jung M-C, Spengler U, Schraut W et al. Hepatitis B virus antigen-specific T-cell activation in patients with acute and chronic hepatitis B. J Hepatol 1991; 13: 310–317

96. Mohite B J, Rath S, Bal V et al. Mechanisms of liver cell damage in acute hepatitis B. J Med Virol 1987; 22: 199–210

97. Eggink H F, Houthoff H J, Huitema S, Wolters G, Poppema S, Gips C H. Cellular and humoral immune reactions in chronic active liver disease. II. Lymphocyte subsets and viral antigens in liver biopsies of patients with acute and chronic hepatitis B. Clin Exp Immunol 1984; 56: 121–128

98. Thomas H C, Jacyna M, Waters J, Main J. Virus–host interaction in chronic hepatitis B virus infection. Semin Liver Dis 1988; 8: 342–349

99. Desmet V J. Liver lesions in hepatitis B viral infection. Yale J Biol Med 1988; 61: 61–83

100. Desmet V J. Immunopathology of chronic viral hepatitis. Hepato-gastroenterol 1991; 38: 14–21

101. Choo Q-L, Kuo G, Weiner A J, Overby L R, Bradley D W, Houghton M. Isolation of a cDNA clone derived from a blood-borne non-A, non-B viral hepatitis genome. Science 1989; 244: 359–362

102. Kuo G, Choo Q-L, Alter H J et al. An assay for circulating antibodies to a major etiologic virus of human non-A, non-B hepatitis. Science 1989; 244: 362–364

103. Zuckerman A J. The elusive hepatitis C virus. A cause of parenteral non-A, non-B hepatitis. Br Med J 1989; 299: 871–873

104. Anon. Hepatitis C virus upstanding. Lancet 1990; 335: 1431–1432

105. Sherlock S, Dusheiko G. Hepatitis C virus updated. Gut 1991; 32: 965–967

106. Abe K, Kurata T, Shikata T. Non-A, non-B hepatitis: visualization of virus-like particles from chimpanzee and human sera. Arch Virol 1989; 104: 351–355

107. Houghton M, Weiner A, Han J, Kuo G, Choo Q-L. Molecular biology of the hepatitis C viruses: implications for diagnosis, development and control of viral disease. Hepatology 1991; 14: 381–388

108. Chan S-W, Simmonds P, McOmish F et al. Serological responses to infection with three different types of hepatitis C virus. Lancet 1991; 338: 1391

109. Takada N, Takase S, Enomoto N, Takada A, Date T. Clinical backgrounds of the patients having different types of hepatitis C virus genomes. J Hepatol 1991; 14: 35–40

110. Fagan E A. Testing for hepatitis C virus. Br Med J 1991; 303: 535–536

111. Chiba J, Ohba H, Matsuura Y et al. Serodiagnosis of hepatitis C virus (HCV) infection with an HCV core protein molecularly expressed by a recombinant baculovirus. Proc Natl Acad Sci USA 1991; 88: 4641–4645

112. van der Poel C L, Cuypers H T M, Reesink H W et al. Confirmation of hepatitis C virus infection by new four-antigen recombinant immunoblot assay. Lancet 1991; 337: 317–319

113. Alberti A. Diagnosis of hepatitis C. Facts and perspectives. J Hepatol 1991; 12: 279–282

114. Hosoda K, Yokosuka O, Omata M, Kato N, Ohto M. Detection and partial sequencing of hepatitis C virus RNA in the liver. Gastroenterology 1991; 101: 766–771

115. Shieh Y S C, Shim K-S, Lampertico P et al. Detection of hepatitis

C virus sequences in liver tissue by the polymerase chain reaction. Lab Invest 1991; 65: 408–411

116. Garson J A, Tedder R S, Briggs M et al. Detection of hepatitis C viral sequences in blood donations by 'nested' polymerase chain reaction and prediction of infectivity. Lancet 1990; 335: 1419–1422

117. Villa E, Ferretti I, De Palma M et al. HCV RNA in serum of asymptomatic blood donors involved in post-transfusion hepatitis (PTH). J Hepatol 1991; 13: 256–259

118. Farci P, Alter H J, Wong D et al. A long-term study of hepatitis C virus replication in non-A, non-B hepatitis. N Engl J Med 1991; 325: 98–104

119. Inchauspe G, Abe K, Zebedee S, Nasoff M, Prince A M. Use of conserved sequences from hepatitis C virus for the detection of viral RNA in infected sera by polymerase chain reaction. Hepatology 1991; 14: 595–600

120. Di Bisceglie A M, Goodman Z D, Ishak K G, Hoofnagle J H, Melpolder J J, Alter H J. Long-term clinical and histopathological follow-up of chronic posttransfusion hepatitis. Hepatology 1991; 14: 969–974

121. Tremolada F, Casarin C, Tagger A et al. Antibody to hepatitis C virus in post-transfusion hepatitis. Ann Intern Med 1991; 114: 277–281

122. Patel A, Sherlock S, Dusheiko G, Scheuer P, Ellis L A, Ashrafzadeh P. Clinical course and histological correlations in post-transfusion hepatitis C: the Royal Free Hospital experience. Eur J Gastroenterol Hepatol 1991; 3: 491–495

123. Makris M, Preston F E, Triger D R et al. Hepatitis C antibody and chronic liver disease in haemophilia. Lancet 1990; 335: 1117–1119

124. Lim S G, Lee C A, Charman H, Tilsed G, Griffiths P D, Kernoff P B A. Hepatitis C antibody assay in a longitudinal study of haemophiliacs. Br J Haematol 1991; 78: 398–402

125. Tedder R S, Briggs M, Ring C et al. Hepatitis C antibody profile and viraemia prevalence in adults with severe haemophilia. Br J Haematol 1991; 79: 512–515

126. Wonke B, Hoffbrand A V, Brown D, Dusheiko G. Antibody to hepatitis C virus in multiply transfused patients with thalassaemia major. J Clin Pathol 1990; 43: 638–640

127. Pareira B J G, Milford E L, Kirkman R L, Levey A S. Transmission of hepatitis C virus by organ transplantation. N Engl J Med 1991; 325: 454–460

128. Schouler L, Dumas F, Mesnier F et al. Possibilité de transmission du virus de l'hépatite C par voie sexuelle. Presse Med 1991; 20: 1886–1888

129. Tedder R S, Gilson R J C, Briggs M et al. Hepatitis C virus: evidence for sexual transmission. Br Med J 1991; 302: 1299–1302

130. Thaler M M, Park C-K, Landers D V et al. Vertical transmission of hepatitis C virus. Lancet 1991; 338: 17–18

131. Klein R S, Freeman K, Taylor P E, Stevens C E, Occupational risk for hepatitis C virus infection among New York City dentists. Lancet 1991; 338: 1539–1542

132. Dittmann S, Roggendorf M, Dürkop J, Wiese M, Lorbeer B, Deinhardt F. Long-term persistence of hepatitis C virus antibodies in a single source outbreak. J Hepatol 1991; 13: 323–327

133. Mattsson L, Weiland O, Glaumann H. Chronic non-A, non-B hepatitis developed after transfusions, illicit self-injections or sporadically. Outcome during long-term follow-up — a comparison. Liver 1989; 9: 120–127

134. Hopf U, Möller B, Küther D et al. Long-term follow up of posttransfusion and sporadic chronic hepatitis non-A, non-B and frequency of circulating antibodies to hepatitis C virus (HCV). J Hepatol 1990; 10: 69–76

135. Westjål R, Hermodsson S, Norkrans G. Long-term follow-up of chronic hepatitis non-A, non-B — with special reference to hepatitis C. Liver 1991; 11: 143–148

136. Bruix J, Barrera J M, Calvet X et al. Prevalence of antibodies to hepatitis C virus in Spanish patients with hepatocellular carcinoma and hepatic cirrhosis. Lancet 1989; ii: 1004–1006

137. Colombo M, Kuo G, Choo Q L et al. Prevalence of antibodies to hepatitis C virus in Italian patients with hepatocellular carcinoma. Lancet 1989; ii: 1006–1008

138. Hasan F, Jeffers L J, De Medina M et al. Hepatitis C-associated hepatocellular carcinoma. Hepatology 1990; 12: 589–591
139. Kew M C, Houghton M, Choo Q L, Kuo G. Hepatitis C virus antibodies in southern African blacks with hepatocellular carcinoma. Lancet 1990; 335: 873–874
140. Kiyosawa K, Sodeyama T, Tanaka E et al. Interrelationship of blood transfusion, non-A, non-B hepatitis and hepatocellular carcinoma: analysis by detection of antibody to hepatitis C virus. Hepatology 1990; 12: 671–675
141. Caporaso N, Romano M, Marmo R et al. Hepatitis C virus infection is an additive risk factor for development of hepatocellular carcinoma in patients with cirrhosis. J Hepatol 1991; 12: 367–371
142. Tsukuma H, Hiyama T, Tanaka S et al. Risk factors for hepatocellular carcinoma among patients with chronic liver disease. New Eng J Med 1993; 328: 1797–1801
143. Shindo M, Di Bisceglie A M, Cheung L et al. Decrease in serum hepatitis C viral RNA during alpha-interferon therapy for chronic hepatitis C. Ann Intern Med 1991; 115: 700–704
144. Di Bisceglie A M, Martin P, Kassianides C et al. Recombinant interferon alfa therapy for chronic hepatitis C. A randomized, double-blind, placebo-controlled trial. N Engl J Med 1989; 321: 1506–1510
145. Schvarcz R, Glaumann H, Weiland O, Norkrans G, Wejstål R, Frydén A. Histological outcome in interferon alpha-2b treated patients with chronic posttransfusion non-A, non-B hepatitis. Liver 1991; 11: 30–38
146. De Vos R, de Wolf-Peeters C, Vanstapel M J et al. New ultrastructural marker in hepatocytes in non-A, non-B viral hepatitis. Liver 1982; 2: 35–44
147. Dienes H P, Popper H, Arnold W, Lobeck H. Histologic observations in human hepatitis non-A, non-B. Hepatology 1982; 2: 562–571
148. Realdi G, Alberti A, Rugge M et al. Long-term follow-up of acute and chronic non-A, non-B post-transfusion hepatitis: evidence of progression to liver cirrhosis. Gut 1982; 23: 270–275
149. Schmid M, Pirovino M, Altorfer J, Gudat F, Bianchi L. Acute hepatitis non-A, non-B; are there any specific light microscopic features? Liver 1982; 2: 61–67
150. Lefkowitch J H, Apfelbaum T F, Non-A, non-B hepatitis: characterization of liver biopsy pathology. J Clin Gastroenterol 1989; 11: 225–232
151. Bamber M, Murray A, Arborgh B A et al. Short incubation non-A, non-B hepatitis transmitted by factor VIII concentrates in patients with congenital coagulation disorders. Gut 1981; 22: 854–859
152. Bach N, Thung S N, Schaffner F. The histological features of chronic hepatitis C and autoimmune chronic hepatitis: a comparative analysis. Hepatology 1992; 15: 572–577
153. Scheuer P J, Ashrafzadeh P, Sherlock S, Brown D, Dusheiko G M. The pathology of hepatitis C. Hepatology 1992; 15: 567–571
154. Lefkowitch J H, Schiff E R, Davis G L et al. Pathological diagnosis of chronic hepatitis C: a multicenter comparative study with chronic hepatitis B. Gastroenterology 1993; 104: 595–603
155. Mattsson L, Weiland O, Glaumann H. Application of a numerical scoring system for assessment of histological outcome in patients with chronic posttransfusion non-A, non-B hepatitis with or without antibodies to hepatitis C. Liver 1990; 10: 257–263
156. Hiramatsu N, Hayashi N, Haruna Y et al. Immunohistochemical detection of hepatitis C virus-infected hepatocytes in chronic liver disease with monoclonal antibodies to core, envelope and NS3 regions of the hepatitis C virus genome. Hepatology 1992; 16: 306–311
157. Krawczynski K, Beach M J, Bradley D W et al. Hepatitis C virus antigen in hepatocytes: immunomorphologic detection and identification. Gastroenterology 1992; 103: 622–629
158. Yamada G, Nishimoto H, Endou H et al. Localization of hepatitis C viral RNA and capsid protein in human liver. Dig Dis Sci 1993; 38: 882–887
159. Haruna Y, Hayashi N, Hiramatsu N et al. Detection of hepatitis C virus RNA in liver tissues by an in situ hybridization technique. J Hepatol 1993; 18: 96–100
160. Chan C-Y, Lee S-D, Wu J-C, Hwang S-J, Huang Y-S, Lo K-J.

161. Liaw Y F, Lin S M, Sheen I S, Chu C M. Acute hepatitis C virus superinfection followed by spontaneous HBeAg seroconversion and HBsAg elimination. Infection 1991; 19: 250–251
162. Martin P, Di Bisceglie A M, Kassianides C, Lisker-Melman M, Hoofnagle J H. Rapidly progressive non-A, non-B hepatitis in patients with human immunodeficiency virus infection. Gastroenterology 1989; 97: 1559–1561
163. Berk L, Schalm S W, Heijtink R A. Severe chronic active hepatitis (autoimmune type) mimicked by coinfection of hepatitis C and human immunodeficiency viruses. Gut 1991; 32: 1198–1200
164. Halimi C, Dény P, Gotheil C et al. Pathogenesis of liver cirrhosis in alcoholic patients: histological evidence for hepatitis C virus responsibility. Liver 1991; 11: 329–333
165. Nishiguchi S, Kuroki T, Yabusako T et al. Detection of hepatitis C virus antibodies and hepatitis C virus RNA in patients with alcoholic liver disease. Hepatology 1991; 14: 985–989
166. Parés A, Barrera J M, Caballer'a J et al. Hepatitis C virus antibodies in chronic alcoholic patients: association with severity of liver injury. Hepatology 1990; 12: 1295–1299
167. Brillanti F, Masci C, Siringo S, Di Febo G, Miglioli M, Barbara L. Serological and histological aspects of hepatitis C virus infection in alcoholic patients. J Hepatol 1991; 13: 347–350
168. Noguchi O, Yamaoka K, Ikeda T et al. Clinicopathological analysis of alcoholic liver disease complicating chronic type C hepatitis. Liver 1991; 11: 225–230
169. Lenzi M, Johnson P J, McFarlane I G et al. Antibodies to hepatitis C virus in auto-immune liver disease: evidence for geographical heterogeneity. Lancet 1991; 338: 277–280
170. Lenzi M, Ballardini G, Fusconi M et al. Type 2 autoimmune hepatitis and hepatitis C virus infection. Lancet 1990; 335: 258–259
171. Magrin S, Craxi A, Fabiano C et al. Hepatitis C virus replication in 'autoimmune' chronic hepatitis. J Hepatol 1991; 13: 364–367
172. Todros L, Touscoz G, D'Urso N et al. Hepatitis C virus-related chronic liver disease with autoantibodies to liver-kidney microsomes (LKM). Clinical characterization from idiopathic LKM-positive disorders. J Hepatol 1991; 13: 128–131
173. Magrin S, Craxi A, Fiorentino G et al. Is autoimmune chronic active hepatitis a HCV-related disease? J Hepatol 1991; 13: 56–60
174. Mishiro S, Hoshi Y, Takeda K et al. Non-A, non-B hepatitis specific antibodies directed at host-derived epitope: implication for an autoimmune process. Lancet 1990; 336: 1400–1403
175. Michel G, Ritter A, Gerken G, Meyer zum Büschenfelde K H, Decker R, Manns M P. Anti-GOR and hepatitis C virus in autoimmune liver diseases. Lancet 1992; 339: 267–269
176. Haddad J, Deny P, Munz-Gotheil C et al. Lymphocytic sialadenitis of Sjögren's syndrome associated with chronic hepatitis C virus liver disease. Lancet 1992; 339: 321–323
177. Rizzetto M, Canese M G, Aricò S et al. Immunofluorescence detection of a new antigen–antibody system (δ/anti-δ) associated to hepatitis B virus in liver and in serum of HBsAg carriers. Gut 1977; 18: 977–1003
178. Bonino F, Brunetto M R, Negro F, Smedile A, Ponzetto A. Hepatitis delta virus, a model of liver cell pathology. J Hepatol 1991; 13: 260–266
179. Moreno A, Ramón y Cahal S, Marazuela M et al. Sanded nuclei in delta patients. Liver 1989; 9: 367–371
180. Negro F, Bonino F, Di Bisceglie A, Hoofnagle J H, Gerin J L. Intrahepatic markers of hepatitis delta virus infection: a study by in situ hybridization. Hepatology 1989; 10: 916–920
181. Jardi R, Buti M, Rodriquez-Frias F et al. Clinical significance of two forms of IgM antibody to hepatitis delta infection. Hepatology 1991; 14: 25–28
182. McFarlane I G, Chaggar K, Davies S E, Smith H M, Alexander G J M, Williams R. IgA class antibodies to hepatitis delta virus antigen in acute and chronic hepatitis delta virus infections. Hepatology 1991; 14: 980–984
183. Liaw Y-F, Chen T-J, Chu C-M, Lin H-H. Acute hepatitis delta virus superinfection in patients with liver cirrhosis. J Hepatol 1990; 10: 41–45
184. Verme G, Amoroso P, Lettieri G et al. A histological study of hepatitis delta virus liver disease. Hepatology 1986; 6: 1303–1307

Superinfection with hepatitis C virus in patients with symptomatic chronic hepatitis B. Scand J Infect Dis 1991; 23: 421–424

185. Sagnelli E, Felaco F M, Filippini P et al. Influence of HDV infection on clinical, biochemical and histological presentation of HBsAg positive chronic hepatitis. Liver 1989; 9: 229–234

186. Lau J Y N, Hansen L J, Bain V G et al. Expression of intrahepatic hepatitis D viral antigen in chronic hepatitis D virus infection. J Clin Pathol 1991; 44: 549–553

187. Lin H-H, Liaw Y-F, Chen T-J, Chu C-M, Huang M-J. Natural course of patients with chronic type B hepatitis following acute hepatitis delta virus superinfection. Liver 1989; 9: 129–134

188. Kojima T, Callea F, Desmyter J, Sakurai I, Desmet V J. Immuno-light and electron microscopic features of chronic hepatitis D. Liver 1990; 10: 17–27

189. Cole S M, Gowans E J, Macnaughton T B, Hall P de la M, Burrell C J. Direct evidence for cytotoxicity associated with expression of hepatitis delta virus antigen. Hepatology 1991; 13: 845–851

190. Negro F, Baldi M, Bonino F et al. Chronic HDV (hepatitis delta virus) hepatitis. Intrahepatic expression of delta antigen, histologic activity and outcome of liver disease. J Hepatol 1988; 6: 8–14

191. Chu C-M, Liaw Y-F. Studies on the composition of the mononuclear cell infiltrates in liver from patients with chronic active delta hepatitis. Hepatology 1989; 10: 911–915

192. Khuroo M S. Study of an epidemic of non-A, non-B hepatitis. Am J Med 1980; 68: 818–824

193. Ramalingaswami V, Purcell R H. Waterborne non-A, non-B hepatitis. Lancet 1988; i: 571–573

194. Velázquez O, Stetler H C, Avila C et al. Epidemic transmission of enterically transmitted non-A, non-B hepatitis in Mexico, 1986–1987. JAMA 1990; 263: 3281–3285

195. Skidmore S J, Yarbough P O, Gabor K A, Tam A W, Reyes G R, Flower A J E. Imported hepatitis E in UK. Lancet 1991; 337: 1541

196. Khuroo M S, Teli M R, Skidmore S, Sofi M A, Khuroo M I. Incidence and severity of viral hepatitis in pregnancy. Am J Med 1981; 70: 252–255

197. Asher L V S, Innis B L, Shrestha M P, Ticehurst J, Baze W B. Virus-like particles in the liver of a patient with fulminant hepatitis and antibody to hepatitis E virus. J Med Virol 1990; 31: 229–233

198. Inoue O, Nagataki S, Itakura H et al. Liver morphology in marmosets infected with epidemic non-A, non-B hepatitis in India. Liver 1986; 6: 178–183

199. Arankalle V A, Ticehurst J, Sreenivasan M A et al. Aetiological association of a virus-like particle with enterically transmitted non-A, non-B hepatitis. Lancet 1988; i: 550–554

200. Panda S K, Datta R, Kaur J, Zuckerman A J, Nayak N C. Enterically transmitted non-A, non-B hepatitis: recovery of virus-like particles from an epidemic in South Delhi and transmission studies in rhesus monkeys. Hepatology 1989; 10: 466–472

201. Zuckerman A J. Hepatitis E virus. The main cause of enterically transmitted non-A, non-B hepatitis. Br Med J 1990; 300: 1475–1476

202. Reyes G R, Purdy M A, Kim J P et al. Isolation of a cDNA from the virus responsible for enterically transmitted non-A, non-B hepatitis. Science 1990; 247: 1335–1339

203. Soe S, Uchida T, Suzuki K et al. Enterically transmitted non-A, non-B hepatitis in cynomolgus monkeys: morphology and probable mechanism of hepatocellular necrosis. Liver 1989; 9: 135–145

204. Dienes H P, Hütteroth T, Bianchi L, Grün M, Thoenes W. Hepatitis A-like non-A, non-B hepatitis: light and electron microscopic observations of three cases. Virchows Arch [A] 1986; 409: 657–667

205. De Cock K M, Bradley D W, Sandford N L, Govindarajan S, Maynard J E, Redeker A G. Epidemic non-A, non-B hepatitis in patients from Pakistan. Ann Intern Med 1987; 106: 227–230

206. Anon. The A to F of viral hepatitis. Lancet 1990; 336: 1158–1160

207. Wright T L, Hsu H, Donegan E et al. Hepatitis C virus not found in fulminant non-A, non-B hepatitis. Ann Intern Med 1991; 115: 111–112

208. Phillips M J, Blendis L M, Poucell S et al. Syncytial giant-cell hepatitis. Sporadic hepatitis with distinctive pathological features, a severe clinical course, and paramyxoviral features. N Engl J Med 1991; 324: 455–460

209. Anon. Hepatitis G? Lancet 1991; 337: 1070

210. Devaney K, Goodman Z D, Ishak K G, Postinfantile giant-cell transformation in hepatitis. Hepatology 1992; 16: 327–333

211. Lau J Y N, Koukoulis G, Mieli-Vergani G, Portmann B C, Williams R, Syncytial giant-cell hepatitis — a specific disease entity? J Hepatol 1992; 15: 216–219

7

Other viral and infectious diseases and HIV-related liver disease

S. B. Lucas

As a major blood-filtering organ, the liver is affected in many infections — be they systemic or arriving via the portal venous system. The large component of phagocytic Kupffer cells, which engulf blood-borne bacteria, fungi and protozoa, ensures that hepatomegaly is almost as frequent as fever. In addition, several viral infections are solely hepatotropic; the commonest viral hepatitides are described in chapter 6, and the remainder here.

The infections are described in taxonomic groupings. The final section discusses the hepatic manifestations of human immunodeficiency virus (HIV) infection and AIDS. Parasite life cycles are not detailed in this chapter, and the reader is referred to standard texts on parasitology.[1,2] For clinico-pathological aspects of liver disease in the tropics, their description by Cook[3] is useful, as are the earlier but relevant histopathological observations of Hutt.[4] Covering dozens of different infectious agents, this chapter cannot detail all the appearances that aid differential diagnosis. The pathology of protozoal and helminthic diseases of the liver and other organs is illustrated and discussed by Gutierrez,[5] and the AFIP fascicles cover the pathology of most infections.[6] An encyclopaedic description of the clinical and pathogenetic aspects of infectious diseases can be found in the textbook by Mandell et al.[7]

VIRAL INFECTIONS

VIRAL HAEMORRHAGIC FEVERS

This group of viral infections shares several epidemiological and clinico-pathological features, and their liver pathologies are similar. The diseases caused by these agents and their geographical distribution are listed in Table 7.1. Although much attention has been paid to the hepatic pathology of the viral haemorrhagic fevers, and abnormal liver function tests are common, clinically

Table 7.1 The viral haemorrhagic fevers (adapted from Johnson[12])

Disease	Virus group	Geography
Yellow fever	Flaviviridae	Africa, South America
Dengue	Flaviviridae	Africa, Asia, tropical America
Lassa fever	Arenaviridae	West Africa
Argentine haemorrhagic fever (Junin virus)	Arenaviridae	Argentina
Ebola fever	Filoviridae	Central Africa
Marburg fever	Filoviridae	Central and southern Africa
Rift valley fever	Bunyaviridae	Africa
Haemorrhagic fever with renal syndrome (Hantaan virus)	Bunyaviridae	Northern Eurasia
Congo-Crimea haemorrhagic fever	Bunyaviridae	Former Soviet Union, central-west Asia, Africa

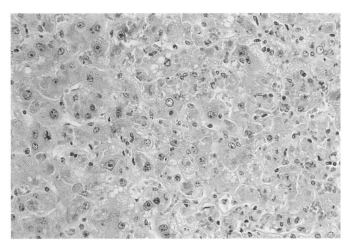

Fig. 7.1 Yellow fever. Mid-zonal liver necrosis with minimal inflammation. Note the acidophilic (Councilman) bodies. H&E.

significant liver disease and death from liver failure are rare except in yellow fever. The viruses cause small vessel damage, in multiple organs, which is often associated with haemorrhage. The clinico-pathological correlations of the viral haemorrhagic fevers were reviewed by Ishak et al.[8]

Yellow fever

Despite the existence of a safe and effective vaccine against yellow fever for over 50 years, the disease is still endemic in Africa and South America. This flavivirus is transmitted by several *Aedes* species of mosquito. Young adult males are predominantly affected. During a recent epidemic in rural West Africa, the clinical attack rate was estimated to be 5% and the mortality was nearly 3% of the local population.[9] The presenting features are an acute illness of sudden onset with fever, myalgia and headache, followed by jaundice after a few days; death occurs in the second week after onset, and is preceded by coma. The diagnosis is usually confirmed by the serological demonstration of specific IgM by an ELISA method, or by virus isolation from blood.

The histopathological appearances depend on the stage of the disease, and the classic features are seen only in the acute stage. At autopsy the liver is yellow and soft. Microscopically, there is confluent focal necrosis with a predominantly mid-zonal distribution. Some hepatocytes undergo acidophilic degeneration and lose their nuclei, forming the classic (but non-specific) Councilman bodies (Fig. 7.1). Rarely, eosinophilic intranuclear inclusions (Torres bodies) are present. Fatty change may be prominent. The surviving liver shows ballooned hepatocytes and regenerative hyperplasia; multinucleate hepatocytes are common. Cholestasis is unusual. Some portal lymphocytic infiltration may be seen. Biopsies taken from survivors up to 2 months after the acute illness show a non-specific intra-acinar hepatitis.[10]

Dengue

Dengue is also transmitted by *Aedes* mosquitoes. The initial disease is influenza-like with a rash. The more important dengue haemorrhagic fever follows from re-infection but with a different serotype of the virus. There is shock, widespread petechial haemorrhages and multiple organ damage; in untreated cases, the mortality approaches 50%. The liver is often enlarged. Microscopically, there are focal necroses or more coalescent perivenular necrosis in acinar zone 3, with little inflammation.

Lassa fever

The natural reservoir of Lassa virus is the multimammate rat *Mastomys natalensis*. Man is infected directly from its urine. Following the alarming emergence of the disease in the early 1970s, serological surveys have shown that the infection is widespread in West Africa, but clinical disease occurs in 5–10% and the case fatality rate is less than 25%. The features include abdominal pain, pharyngitis and fever, but not jaundice.

The liver is mottled in appearance (Fig. 7.2a). Histologically, there is necrosis without inflammation. Individual hepatocytes or groups of cells are acidophilic in all parts of the acinus (Fig. 7.2b). There is no cholestasis, nor fatty change, but lipofuscin deposition is evident.[11] Arenaviruses are present in large numbers under electron microscopy, but there are no light-microscopic viral inclusions.

Lassa virus is readily transmitted by inoculation of infected blood. The pathologist who performed the early autopsies in West Africa died of the disease following an accident during these examinations.

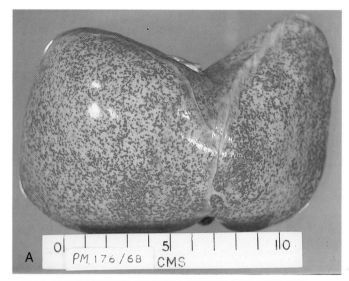

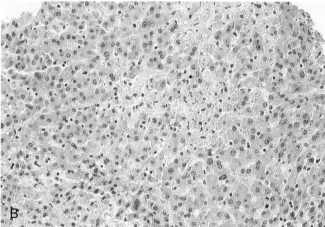

Fig. 7.2 Lassa fever. (a) Autopsy liver showing foci of haemorrhagic necrosis under the capsule. Photograph courtesy of Prof MSR Hutt. (b) Focal liver-cell necrosis without associated inflammation. H&E.

Ebola and Marburg fevers

The natural reservoirs of these viruses are unknown. Between 1976 and 1979, three epidemics of Ebola disease occurred in Zaire and Sudan with a rapid course and 70% mortality. Marburg disease first occurred in 1967 in people who had been in contact with African green monkeys imported from Uganda. The mortality was 25%; subsequently there were isolated cases in Kenya and South Africa up to 1982. Clinically, patients had fever and widespread haemorrhages, shock and disseminated intravascular coagulation.[12] The hepatic pathology is similar to that in Lassa fever: hepatocyte necrosis that ranges from spotty to widespread, no cholestasis, and minimal inflammation.[13]

These infections are still relevant. In 1989, monkeys imported into the United States from the Philippines were found to be dying of Ebola virus infection. Transmissions to some laboratory staff occurred although no clinical disease developed.

HERPES VIRUS GROUP AND OTHER VIRUSES

The four members of this group of DNA viruses that may affect the liver are herpes simplex, herpes zoster, cytomegalovirus, and the Epstein–Barr virus.

Herpes simplex

Primary herpes simplex infection produces oral or genital lesions, and latent infection lasts for life. There are two strains of this virus: type 1 is responsible for generalized infections in older children and adults, and type 2 affects the genital tract in the neonate. In the latter, dissemination may occur, with necrotizing hepatitis. The liver is also involved in the severe fulminant systemic herpes infection that immunocompromised patients may suffer. Organ transplantation and treatment for haematological malignancy are the most frequent underlying predispositions[14] but HIV infection is increasingly important. Fatal herpetic hepatitis also occurs in apparently immunocompetent adults.[15] The clinical features resemble those of septic shock; jaundice is not always present.

At autopsy the liver is enlarged and mottled with yellow or white foci surrounded by congestion (Fig. 7.3a). Microscopically, there is little inflammation but irregular coagulative necrosis of the parenchyma is present. At the margins, hepatocytes show purple nuclear inclusions with a clear surrounding halo, and some hepatocytes are multinucleate (Fig. 7.3b).

Herpes zoster

Herpes zoster causes chicken pox and — as a reactivation of latent infection — shingles. After infection, there is a primary viraemia with viral replication in the epithelium of the gut, respiratory tract, liver, pancreas and adrenal. A secondary viraemia leads to skin infection with the usual rash. Liver disease is restricted to those patients who are immunocompromised, most often from cancer treated with chemotherapy. Rarely, steroid therapy given during the phases of viral dissemination may precipitate severe zoster.[16] In these severe infections there is focal or massive liver necrosis without much inflammation, similar to the lesions of herpes simplex infection. Intranuclear inclusions may be plentiful or scanty.

In herpetic lesions, electron microscopy shows abundant herpes virions. Immunocytochemistry is useful for confirming the presence of a herpes virus although, depending on the specificity of the antibodies used, it may not identify which one is present. Polymerase chain reaction

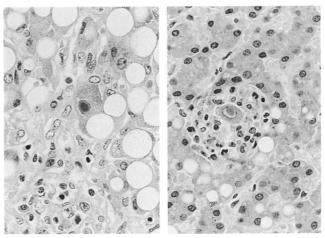

Fig. 7.4 Cytomegalovirus infection. Two cytomegalovirus lesions with intranuclear inclusions, and no or little associated inflammation. The basophilic material within the cytoplasm is also viral. H&E. See also Fig. 7.48

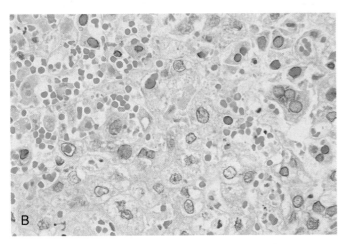

Fig. 7.3 Herpes simplex. (a) Autopsy liver (fixed) of an HIV-positive child with disseminated herpes. The extensive, paler areas are necrotic, with adjacent congested liver. (b) At the edge of a necrotic zone, some hepatocytes are multinucleate and many nuclei contain eosinophilic viral inclusions. H&E.

analysis, even of formalin-fixed paraffin-embedded material, is highly sensitive and specific

Cytomegalovirus

Most adult populations have a prevalence of latent, asymptomatic cytomegalovirus infection greater than 50%, as judged by serological surveys. Primary infection with clinical disease does occur in immunocompetent adults, but most significant cytomegalovirus disease occurs in the newborn or in the immunocompromised host. In renal transplant recipients, it is the commonest specific cause of hepatitis and, in liver transplant recipients, cytomegalovirus hepatitis needs to be distinguished from graft rejection (see Ch. 17).

In immunocompetent individuals, cytomegalovirus produces an infectious mononucleosis-like syndrome. Liver biopsy shows focal hepatocyte and bile duct damage with lymphocytic infiltration of sinusoids. In some cases, there are non-caseating epithelioid cell granulomas, but neither viral inclusions nor immunocytochemically demonstrable antigen are seen.[17,18]

Cytomegalovirus is a cause of neonatal hepatitis with giant cell transformation, cholestasis, inflammation and viral inclusions. The characteristic finding is an enlarged cell (endothelial, hepatocyte, or bile-duct epithelium) that contains basophilic granules in the cytoplasm and a swollen nucleus. An amphophilic intranuclear inclusion is surrounded by a clear halo, so that it resembles an owl's eye. Both the nuclear and cytoplasmic inclusions represent closely packed virions[19] (Fig 7.4). Immunocytochemical staining for cytomegalovirus will highlight evident and ambiguous inclusions, but usually does not provide a positive signal if inclusions are absent on ordinary stains.

In immunocompromised hosts, cytomegalovirus inclusions are often seen without necrosis or inflammation — a 'passenger infection', but when tissue damage is evident, then the virus is presumed to be pathogenic. In the fetal liver, cytomegalovirus disease has been associated with obliteration of bile ducts.[20] The commonest predisposition to cytomegalovirus hepatitis at present is HIV infection.

Epstein-Barr virus

In the tropics, Epstein-Barr virus is transmitted early in childhood and is aetiologically associated with Burkitt's lymphoma. In industrialized countries, infection usually occurs in adolescence and causes infectious mono-nucleosis. Abnormal liver function tests indicate frequent hepatic involvement, but jaundice is rare.

The usual liver histopathology in infectious mononucle-osis is of a diffuse lymphocytic infiltrate in the sinusoids.[21] When this is marked, focal apoptotic hepatocytes are seen.[22] The infiltrate—which is composed of infected B-lymphocytes, activated T-lymphocytes and natural killer cells—can be atypical and suggest leukaemia/lymphoma. Any part of the liver acinus is affected. Fatty change may occur and cholestasis is not a feature. Non-necrotic tuber-culoid granulomas are occasionally found in infectious mononucleosis.[23] Patients with the X-linked lymphopro-liferative syndrome are especially vulnerable to Epstein–Barr virus infection[24] and may suffer severe liver necrosis (Fig. 7.5). In a fatal case, herpes-like viral intranuclear in-clusions were seen.[25]

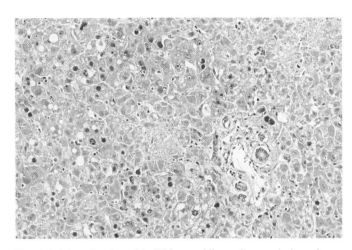

Fig. 7.6 Adenovirus hepatitis. Widespread liver cell necrosis; irregular dark viral inclusions are seen in the nuclei of some surviving hepatocytes. H&E

THE ADENOVIRUS GROUP

These DNA viruses usually affect the respiratory tract and conjunctiva. In children and in adults immunosuppressed because of HIV infection, severe combined immuno-deficiency, haematological malignancy or organ trans-plantation, adenovirus may cause a severe hepatitis and liver failure.[26–28] The pathology is similar to that seen in herpes simplex infection. There are extensive areas of liver cell necrosis with little inflammation; intranuclear inclu-sions may be frequent (Fig. 7.6).

ENTEROVIRUSES

Group B Coxsackie virus infections can produce multi-system disease in neonates, including liver involvement, but in adults they are a rare cause of hepatitis.[29] The histopathology in neonates is of haemorrhagic necrosis. In adults, there is perivenular bile stasis and hydropic swelling of hepatocytes, accompanied by infiltration of mononuclear cells and polymorphs in sinusoids and portal tracts.

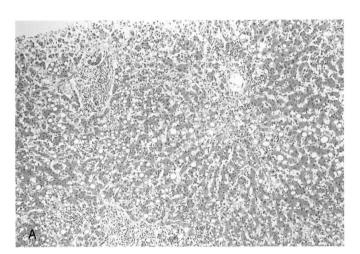

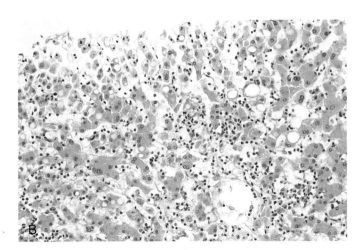

Fig. 7.5 Epstein–Barr virus infection. (a) There is a diffuse portal tract and intra-acinar mononuclear cell infiltrate of the fatty liver; at a higher power (b) there is perivenular focal liver-cell necrosis and an intense intra-sinusoidal mononuclear cell infiltrate. H&E.

MEASLES (RUBEOLA)

In children dying of measles, the liver usually shows non-specific features. There is frequently fatty change, especially when associated with malnutrition in the tropics, portal inflammation and focal necroses.[30] Viral inclusions and giant cells are rarely seen, but have been reported in a patient with immunoglobulin deficiency.[31] Inclusions are not present in the liver when measles is associated with HIV infection. Measles can also cause an acute hepatitis syndrome in adults.[32]

RUBELLA

Childhood rubella is not associated with liver disease. However, this virus can be associated with giant cell transformation in neonatal hepatitis. In mild cases, focal necroses, cholestasis and a lymphocytic infiltrate occur.[33] Rarely, there is massive necrosis.

PARVOVIRUS

Human parvovirus (B19 virus) is the cause of erythema infectiosum in childhood. If a pregnant woman acquires the infection, it can be transmitted to the fetus and cause hydrops fetalis. Many fetal organs, including the liver, are damaged. There is excessive erythropoietic activity; erythroblasts and hepatocytes have eosinophilic nuclear inclusions as well as swollen hydropic nuclei.[34]

RICKETTSIAL AND CHLAMYDIAL INFECTIONS

Rickettsiae are obligate intracellular parasites that contain both DNA and RNA. They are coccobacilli, $1 \times 0.3\,\mu m$ in size, and in human infection they are found in endothelial cells. Although mild derangement of liver function tests may occur in any of the rickettsial fevers, including typhus, clinical liver disease is seen only in Q fever, Boutonneuse fever, and bacillary angiomatosis.

Q fever

Q fever, caused by *Coxiella burnettii*, exists as a zoonosis in domestic and other animals. Transmission to man is probably via inhalation, with a resulting rickettsaemia. Clinical presentations include pneumonia, hepatitis and fever of unknown origin. Liver function tests are usually abnormal. The typical microscopic hepatic lesions are intra-acinar granulomas.[35] These have a central fat vacuole, an intermediate ring of fibrin, and a peripheral rim of activated macrophages (Fig. 7.7). Non-vacuolated granulomas and tuberculoid granulomas with giant cells and central necrosis may also occur. Thus, the differential diagnosis on histology includes brucellosis and tuberculosis.

The fibrin-ring granuloma itself is not a lesion specific for Q fever. It is also been in patients with lymphoma, staphylococcal bacteriaemia, Epstein–Barr virus infection, cytomegalovirus infection, leishmaniasis, and allopurinol hypersensitivity.[36,37]

Boutonneuse fever

The tick-borne infection, *Rickettsia conorii*, occurs around

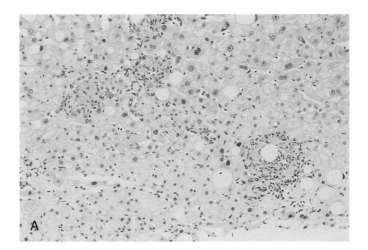

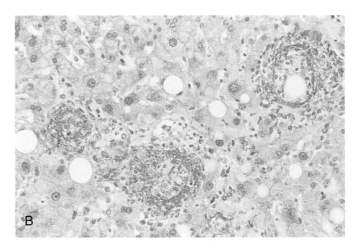

Fig. 7.7 Liver biopsy from a patient with proven Q fever. (a) The granulomas have a central fatty vacuole and the surrounding macrophages are trapped in a mesh of fibrin, H&E; this is better seen on an MSB stain (b).

the Mediterranean, in East and South Africa, and in India. Although it usually takes the form of a mild febrile disease, there is a fatality rate of up to 5%. The liver lesions have been described as granulomatous.[38] However, a series of biopsies taken from Boutonneuse fever patients without clinical hepatitis showed focal hepatocyte necrosis without granulomas, and a local lymphocytic infiltrate; the portal tracts were normal.[39] Immunocytochemical staining may reveal rickettsial antigen in endothelial cells lining the sinusoids.

The newly identified rickettsial pathogen *Rochalimaea henselae* is the agent of bacillary angiomatosis, which occurs only in HIV-infected individuals (see p. 303).

Chlamydia infection

Chlamydiae are obligate intracellular parasites that contain both RNA and DNA and have a characteristic life cycle with inclusion bodies. The liver is involved in two chlamydial diseases — psittacosis and genital infection.

Infection with *Chlamydia psittaci* causes pneumonia and systemic illness with hepatomegaly and sometimes jaundice. Focal hepatocyte necrosis and Kupffer cell hypertrophy have been described in autopsy material.[6] The intracellular inclusion bodies are difficult to identify even with a Giemsa stain. Genital tract infection with *Chlamydia trachomatis* causes salpingitis and may produce the Fitz-Hugh–Curtis syndrome of perihepatitis.[40]

BACTERIAL INFECTIONS

SEPTICAEMIA AND PYOGENIC LIVER ABSCESS

Hepatomegaly and jaundice are commonly associated with septicaemia, i.e. bacteriaemia with clinical shock.[41] Various histological features may be seen depending on the aetiology and severity of the condition. Canalicular cholestasis is frequent, sometimes with inspissated bile in cholangioles. Fatty change and perivenular ischaemic necrosis are non-specific but common. Microabscesses may occur in the parenchyma and contain visible bacteria.

Bacterial infection may reach the liver via the portal vein, the hepatic artery and the biliary tree. The first route is less common now in industrialized countries; the sources of sepsis are the appendix, colon and pancreas. This results in septic portal thrombophlebitis and hepatic abscesses. In some developing countries, a significant proportion of idiopathic splenomegaly has been attributed to a late complication of neonatal portal pyaemia and secondary splenic vein occlusion that originated from umbilical sepsis.[42]

Hepatic arterial spread of infection is common, but patients often succumb before visible abscesses can develop. One of the more frequent identifiable lesions is seen in staphylococcal sepsis: clusters of Gram-positive cocci are surrounded by necrosis and polymorphs. In chronic granulomatous disease (see Ch. 4), disseminated bacterial infection (commonly staphylococcal) also involves the liver;[43] portal macrophages with lipofuscin pigment, parenchymal necrotizing granulomas, and portal fibrosis are seen. In septicaemia due to *Neisseria gonorrhoeae* jaundice is a common complication with focal necrosis and neutrophil infiltration in the liver. Liver tenderness described as perihepatitis can complicate pelvic infection by gonococci and *Chlamydia trachomatis* (the Fitz-Hugh–Curtis syndrome); it may simulate acute cholecystitis.[44,45] The liver parenchyma is normal in this condition, but the organisms can be isolated from the capsule.

Septicaemic plague, caused by *Yersinia pestis*, is occasionally encountered at autopsy in developing countries; it is a highly virulent infection and stringent safety measures must be employed to ensure that material is not inhaled or inoculated accidentally into skin. The liver shows multiple necrotic foci with little inflammatory response, but they are packed with short Gram-negative rods.[46]

Spread via the biliary tree follows an acute ascending cholangitis (see Fig. 7.57a). This often complicates large duct obstruction due to stones, but may follow suppurative cholecystitis, postoperative biliary strictures, acute or chronic pancreatitis, and tumours in the biliary tree or pancreas.

In many cases of pyogenic abscess, the origin of the infection is not obvious. Underlying causes include diabetes mellitus, perforated duodenal ulcer or diverticular disease. The commonest aetiological agents are *E. coli* and other coliforms, but anaerobes are reported with increasing frequency.[7,47] *Streptococcus milleri* is also common. The differential diagnosis of pyogenic liver abscess includes amoebiasis and several worm infections of the biliary tree that predispose to bacterial cholangitis (ascariasis, clonorchiasis and fascioliasis).

TYPHOID FEVER, BRUCELLOSIS, MELIOIDOSIS AND LISTERIOSIS

This group of infections has common clinicopathological features. They are intracellular parasites of macrophages, and all may cause granulomatous hepatitis.

Typhoid fever

Salmonella typhi is a Gram-negative bacillus. The classic clinicopathological phases of typhoid disease are incubation, active invasion (dissemination throughout the lymphoreticular system), fastigium, and lysis. During the phase of invasion, the liver shows a range of non-specific histological lesions: sinusoidal and portal lymphocytosis, focal parenchymal necrosis, and Kupffer cell hypertrophy, sometimes with erythrophagocytosis. Small macrophage clusters, which evolve into non-necrotizing epithelioid cell granulomas, are often seen. Microvesicular fatty change in hepatocytes is common. In the symptomatic phase of fastigium, there is hepatomegaly and sometimes jaundice. The granulomas in the liver enlarge and become necrotic, as they do in the lymph nodes of the bowel and mesentery (Fig. 7.8). There are no Langhans' giant cells, and bacilli are very hard to detect with standard methods such as Gram stains. Although typhoid bacilli multiply readily in the bile and gallbladder, ascending cholangitis is rare.

Brucellosis

Brucellosis is a zoonosis of ruminants. Man may be infected by the Gram-negative bacilli *Brucella melitensis*, *B. abortus*, or *B. suis*, and infection comes through occupational exposure or ingestion of milk products. The clinical manifestations are protean — brucellosis is a great mimic.

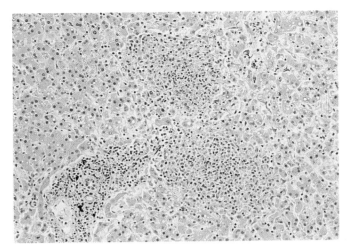

Fig. 7.8 Typhoid fever. Autopsy liver showing portal and parenchymal granulomas. H&E.

Three main patterns occur, all including fever and weakness: acute, recurrent, and chronic. In all, there is haematogenous dissemination of bacteria to all lymphoreticular organs, including the liver. Hepatomegaly and altered liver function tests are common. Histological examination shows a non-specific reactive hepatitis, microgranulomas, or epithelioid cell granulomas (Fig. 7.9). The latter may have giant cells and, in the chronic pattern of brucellosis, there may be fibrinoid necrosis, rendering the histological appearances indistinguishable from tuberculosis or histoplasmosis. Patients with large caseous granulomas (coin lesions) in the liver have been reported.[48] When granulomatous hepatitis without evident cause is encountered in biopsy material, brucellosis should always be considered. Serology is the means of establishing the diagnosis.

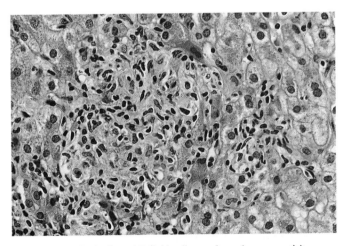

Fig. 7.9 Brucellosis. An epithelioid cell granuloma (non-necrotic) within the liver parenchyma. In addition to tuberculosis and sarcoidosis, the presence of such granulomas should also prompt a suspicion of brucellosis. H&E.

Melioidosis

Disease due to the Gram-negative bacillus *Pseudomonas pseudomallei* is endemic in South-East Asia, and sporadic cases occur in other parts of the tropics. The organism is a saprophyte of soil and water. Clinically, it presents as acute pulmonary, septicaemic, or chronic suppurative disease. Hepatomegaly and jaundice are complications. The histopathology of the liver in acute melioidosis includes small and large abscesses, in which the rods may be seen on a Gram or Giemsa stain. In the chronic form of the disease, there are necrotic granulomas. These may mimic tuberculosis, or be stellate in form, resembling cat-scratch disease. Bacteria are rarely seen.[49]

Listeriosis

Listeria monocytogenes is a Gram-positive bacillus that is saprophytic in soil and water. It may be transmitted to man through soft cheeses. Disease occurs in pregnant women and their infants via the transplacental route, in immunosuppressed patients and, less commonly, in immunocompetent individuals. HIV infection does not play a predisposing role. The clinical disease in neonates is septicaemia with multiple organ lesions. The liver shows miliary microabscesses that contain abundant Gram-positive rods (Fig. 7.10). In routine sections, this may resemble acute neonatal syphilis. In adults with listeriosis, the clinical picture can mimic viral hepatitis, though microabscesses with bacilli are common and some patients have a granulomatous hepatitis.[50]

CAT-SCRATCH DISEASE

Although most cases of cat-scratch disease manifest only as a skin lesion and local lymphadenopathy, dissemination to the viscera, including the liver, occurs in a small proportion.[51] Occasionally this can occur without lymphadenopathy.[52] Clinically, disseminated cat-scratch disease is an illness presenting in children as fever with tender hepatosplenomegaly. The liver lesions have the same histological features as the typical lymph node: stellate microabscesses with a granulomatous border. With a Warthin–Starry stain, extracellular clumps of short Gram-negative bacilli may be demonstrated at the edges of the necrosis. The taxonomy of the cat-scratch bacillus has recently been determined as *Afipia felis*.[53]

ACTINOMYCETE INFECTIONS

Most cases of actinomycosis in man are caused by *Actinomyces israelii*, a globally distributed soil organism. Actinomycosis of the liver is usually secondary to intra-abdominal or thoracic infection, the bacilli reaching the liver by direct extension or via the portal vein.[54] The latter

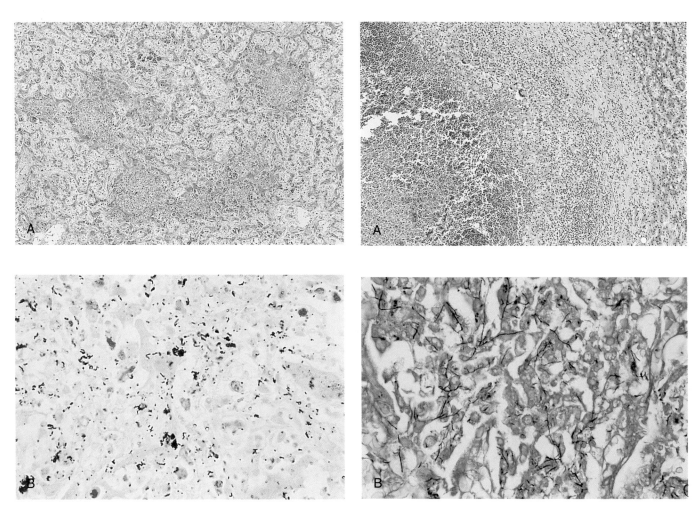

Fig. 7.10 Listeriosis. (a) Necrotic granulomas in the parenchyma. H&E. (b) Gram stain shows abundant Gram-positive bacilli.

Fig. 7.11 Nocardiosis. (a) Edge of a liver abscess with a purulent centre and a granulomatous border. Note the giant cell. H&E. (b) Clusters of thin branching filaments of *N. asteroides* within the abscess. Grocott stain.

follows caecal or appendiceal infection. Occasionally an apparently primary hepatic lesion is seen,[55] which presents clinically as other liver abscesses. Grossly, there is usually a honeycomb of confluent small abscesses, containing greenish pus. Microscopically, amidst the acute inflammation there are grains (colonies) of *Actinomyces*, which are basophilic in H&E-stained sections. These are composed of closely packed, radiating, Gram-positive bacilli, 1 μm across, which can be impregnated with silver by the Grocott method. There is often a fibrinoid Hoeppli–Splendore reaction at the perimeter. These abscesses may rupture, forming sinuses into the retroperitoneum.

A related infection, *Nocardia brasiliensis* or *asteroides*, may also spread to the liver as part of haematogenous dissemination. *N. asteroides* is usually an opportunistic infection in immunosuppressed individuals (due to transplantation or HIV infection). The bacilli within the abscess may form grain-like colonies or be more diffusely

spread (Fig. 7.11). They are also Gram-positive and beaded, and are silver-positive on Grocott stains but, unlike *Actinomyces*, they are weakly acid-fast, staining well with a Wade–Fite method.[56]

SPIROCHAETE INFECTIONS

Syphilis

Congenital syphilis often manifests early as intra-uterine death or infantile disease, both with hepatosplenomegaly. In the earlier phases there may be miliary necroses, portal inflammation and a hepatocyte giant cell response. In neonatal deaths, the degree of persistent haemopoiesis is excessive for gestational age. The Warthin–Starry stain demonstrates large numbers of spirochaetes, particularly when there is necrosis. Later, the liver shows a characteristic progressive pericellular fibrosis with apparent withering of the liver-cell plates (Fig. 7.12).[57]

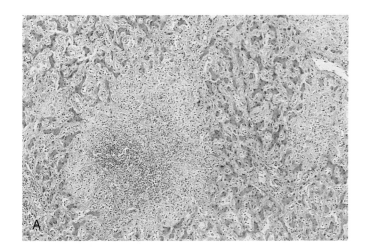

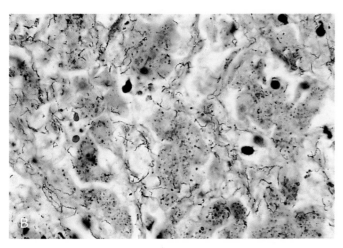

Fig. 7.12 Congenital syphilis. (a) Liver showing both a focal necrotic and inflammatory lesion, and the typical diffuse sinusoidal fibrosis with attenuation of the liver plates. H&E. (b) The focal lesion contains abundant silver-positive spirochaetes. Warthin–Starry stain.

Primary syphilis has no notable liver histology, but in the secondary phase there is focal hepatocyte necrosis, portal inflammation with numerous polymorphs around bile ductules, and sometimes granulomas. The portal vessels may show vasculitis.[58,59] Spirochaetes are less often seen compared with congenital lesions. The lesion of tertiary disease is the gumma. In the liver these are single or multiple, ranging in size from millimetres to centimetres. They are tuberculoid giant cell granulomas with amorphous pale necrotic centres, mimicking caseation, although the classic description emphasizes the preservation of cellular architecture within the necrotic zone. Accompanying this are plasma cells and endarteritis obliterans. Healing is by fibrosis and broad bands of scarring which may distort the liver to produce 'hepar lobatum'.

Relapsing fever (borreliosis)

Relapsing fever may be louse- or tick-borne and is caused by many *Borrelia* spp. The louse-borne infection is due to *B. recurrentis*. Most infections occur in East Africa. As the name suggests, it presents as periodic fever lasting a week and recurring another week or so later. The diagnosis is made by finding the spirochaetes in peripheral blood smears.

In severe infections, jaundice and hepatosplenomegaly occur. In fatal cases an enlarged, congested liver is seen. There are foci of hepatocyte necrosis with surrounding haemorrhage in acinar zones 2 and 3. The sinusoids are infiltrated by lymphocytes and polymorphs, which are associated with Kupffer cell hypertrophy and erythrophagocytosis.[60] Warthin–Starry or Dieterle stains may reveal the 10–20 μm long spirochaetes lying free in the sinusoids.

Leptospirosis (Weil's disease)

Leptospirosis is a zoonosis of rats, dogs and pigs. The agent, *Leptospira icterohaemorrhagica*, is ubiquitous in wet environments, and man acquires the infection via water contaminated with animal urine. The clinical features are fever with jaundice and renal failure, and bleeding into conjunctiva, skin and viscera. Hepatomegaly is often present. The haemorrhagic phenomena are not due to liver failure, but to direct damage to small vessels by leptospirae. With appropriate therapy, mortality is now low.

At autopsy the liver may be normal or enlarged and icteric. The major histological features are individual hepatocyte damage, regeneration, canalicular cholestasis, and only slight portal or sinusoidal lymphocytosis. Ballooning and hydropic change of hepatocytes is less marked than that seen in viral hepatitis; apoptotic bodies are the more prominent evidence of liver damage. Many liver-cells are binucleate and show mitoses; variation in size is a further indication of regenerative activity. Autopsy material shows dissociation and separation of liver-cell plates, but biopsy samples have intact plates, so the separation is probably a post-mortem artefact (Fig. 7.13). Kupffer cells are hypertrophied and contain erythrocytes. In a proportion of cases, a Warthin–Starry stain shows the spirochaetes, which are 10–20 μm long. Immunocytochemical staining with specific polyclonal antibodies can demonstrate leptospiral antigen in Kupffer cells, portal tracts and endothelium.[61]

Lyme disease

Lyme disease is a multisystem infection caused by *Borrelia burgdorferi*. It is tick borne and occurs throughout the world. It has acute and chronic clinical patterns, and the liver may be involved in both. Hepatomegaly and

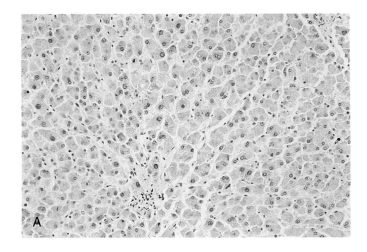

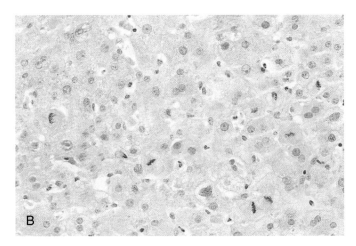

Fig. 7.13 Leptospirosis. (a) Autopsy liver: the liver cells appear dissociated and there is cholestasis. H&E. Slide courtesy of Dr C Corbett, Brazil. (b) Liver biopsy: no dissociation of liver cells is seen but there are numerous mitoses. H&E.

abnormal liver function tests, associated with portal tract inflammation on biopsy, are noted in the acute disease. Recurrent Lyme disease may cause a more marked hepatitis, with ballooned hepatocytes, mitotic activity, microvesicular fatty change, Kupffer cell hyperplasia, and sinusoidal infiltration by lymphocytes and polymorphs. On Warthin–Starry or Dieterle silver stains, the spirochaetes can be seen in the sinusoids and in liver cells.[62,63]

MYCOBACTERIAL INFECTIONS

Of the 50-odd mycobacterial species, *M. tuberculosis* and *M. leprae* are the most frequent causes of disease in man. However, the advent of the HIV pandemic has highlighted the predisposition of immunosuppressed people to develop other mycobacterioses, particularly of the *M. avium* complex.

Tuberculosis

Some 20% of the global population are infected with *M. tuberculosis*, generating more than 8 million cases per annum.[64] Since this organism is a parasite of macrophages, the liver is frequently involved. There are broadly three patterns of hepatic tuberculosis:

Primary tuberculosis. During the primary infection, whether it be in lung or intestine, the liver is involved if there is haematogenous dissemination leading to miliary tuberculosis. Hepatomegaly is common but jaundice is unusual. In rare cases of congenital tuberculosis, the infection is transmitted via the umbilical vein and the liver is the most severely affected organ. At autopsy or on liver biopsy, there is a range of histological appearances. The classic pattern is of miliary portal and parenchymal tubercles composed of epithelioid cells and a Langhans' giant cell. There may or may not be central fibrinoid necrosis, and acid-fast bacilli are often scanty or absent on Ziehl–Neelsen stain. In severe cases (including congenital tuberculosis), the tubercles are of the 'soft' type. These are immature granulomas with much central fibrinoid necrosis, no giant cells and numerous acid-fast bacilli.[65] Rarely, a tuberculoma may form; this is a solitary caseating mass measuring up to several centimetres in size. Microscopy shows the classic giant cell granuloma pattern at the border, with scanty acid-fast bacilli.

Post-primary tuberculosis. This, the commonest manifestation of tuberculosis, is a pulmonary disease and is usually considered to arise from reactivation of previous infection. Bacilli (or antigen) are shed into the blood stream, and in many organs including the liver, granulomas are found. These are usually of the 'hard' non-necrotic type, with epithelioid and giant cells. Acid-fast bacilli are demonstrated infrequently.[65]

Anergic (immunosuppressed, non-reactive) tuberculosis. Patients with primary or reactivated tuberculosis who are immunocompromised often manifest a non-specific disease with wasting, termed 'cryptic tuberculosis'.[66] The underlying causes range from old age and immunosuppressive chemotherapy to leukaemia and HIV infection. Multiple organs, including the liver, show miliary necrotic lesions 1 mm–2 cm in diameter (see Fig. 7.49). Histological examination shows a rim of unactivated macrophages with clear cytoplasm (hydropic swelling) surrounding a necrotic centre with much haematoxyphilic debris. Enormous numbers of acid-fast bacilli are characteristic in these lesions (Fig. 7.14).

Leprosy (Hansen's disease)

Leprosy as a clinical disease affects some 10 million people, mainly in the tropics and subtropics. However, significant involvement of the liver is uncommon and is mainly due to drug reactions and amyloidosis.

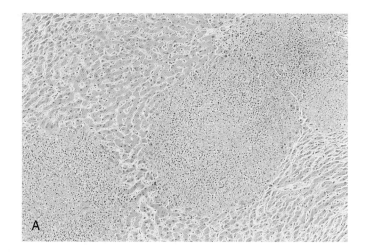

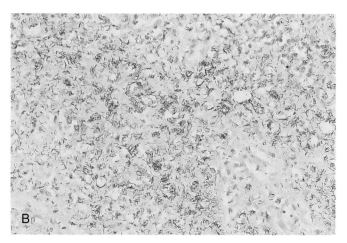

Fig. 7.14 Tuberculosis (anergic). (a) Multiple necrotic lesions within the parenchyma; these are not true granulomas, being composed of 'non-activated' hydropic and dead macrophages. H&E. (b) Ziehl–Neelsen stain of same liver, showing vast numbers of extra cellular acid-fast bacilli. See also Fig. 7.49, and contrast with *M. avium* complex infection illustrated in Fig. 7.50

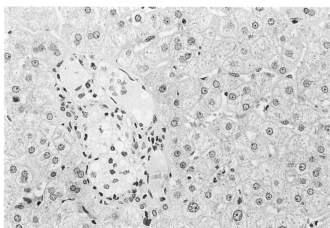

Fig. 7.15 Lepromatous leprosy. Biopsy showing a cluster of foamy macrophages. On Wade–Fite stain, these contained degenerate acid-fast bacilli. H&E.

Systematic studies of large numbers of leprosy patients show that about 20% of those with paucibacillary (tuberculoid) disease have liver lesions, rising to about 60% of those with multibacillary (lepromatous) disease.[67] Abnormalities of liver function tests are mild. Histological examination reveals good correlation between the patterns of skin and liver lesions. In the liver of paucibacillary leprosy patients, there are tuberculoid granulomas with few or no acid-fast bacilli. Conversely, lepromatous patients have foamy macrophage aggregates (Virchow cells) with acid-fast bacilli, distributed randomly within the acinus or near the portal tracts (Fig. 7.15). Such patients may also have acid-fast bacilli in Kupffer cells: this is a result of mycobacteraemia that may reach 10^5 bacilli per ml of blood.[68] It is possible that the liver is a source of bacilli in cases of relapse.

Occasionally, multibacillary patients undergoing the leprosy reaction of erythema nodosum leprosum are jaundiced and have hepatomegaly. These lepromatous hepatic lesions are accompanied by neutrophil polymorph infiltrates, as in the skin lesions of such patients.[69]

The incidence of systemic amyloidosis in leprosy varies widely, depending on geography, and thus host factors.[70] The liver is usually affected.[71] Concerning drug reactions, these are due to dapsone, rifampicin, ethionamide and prothionamide, the main hepatotoxic drugs that patients with leprosy receive.

Other mycobacterioses

Many other mycobacteria cause disease in man, especially when the subject is immunocompromised: the predispositions include congenital immunodeficiency states, chronic granulomatous disease, HIV infection, myeloid and hairy cell leukaemias, pancytopenia, steroid and cytotoxic therapy, alcoholism and old age.[70] Systemic infection often involves the liver as a lymphoreticular organ, and unexplained hepatomegaly may be a presenting feature. The mycobacteria known to cause hepatic lesions are listed in Table 7.2.

Table 7.2 Liver disease caused by non-tuberculosis, non-leprosy mycobacterial infections

Species	Reference
BCG	72
M. avium complex	73,74
M. bovis	75
M. chelonei	76
M. fortuitum	77–79
M. gordonae	80
M. kansasii	81–83
M. scrofulaceum	82, 84
M. simiae	85
M. terrae	86
M. xenopi	87,88

The pathologies of these mycobacterioses vary widely according to the species of infection and the underlying state of the host. At one end of a spectrum, immunological responses result in epithelioid cell granulomas with or without giant cells, with few or no acid-fast bacilli evident on Ziehl–Neelsen stains, and necrosis (caseating or often admixed with a neutrophil infiltrate). At the anergic end of the spectrum, the more virulent mycobacteria (e.g. *M. kansasii*) produce parenchymal necrosis with no granulomatous reaction and numerous acid-fast bacilli, whilst the less virulent infections (e.g. *M. avium* and BCG) result in nodules of histiocytic cells in the sinusoids and parenchyma. Here, the macrophages are stuffed with acid-fast bacilli (see Fig. 7.50).

MYCOTIC INFECTIONS

The liver is involved in many fungal infections as part of haematogenous dissemination. With the exception of candidiasis and zygomycosis, these organisms enter the body by inhalation. They produce a primary lesion in the lung, with contemporary or later spread to other organs: the sequence is similar to that of tuberculosis. Significant visceral disease, including liver involvement, is often precipitated by immunosuppression.

Identification of the fungus on histological examination alone is usually possible from the size and morphology of the yeasts or the hyphae.[89] Some fungi — the commonest of which is Candida — manifest both forms within a lesion. The special stains of Grocott or PAS are helpful in clarifying the morphology of fungi in tissues. Sometimes (particularly with yeast forms), this is misleadingly atypical in size or shape. Culture of tissue or blood, serological techniques and, more recently, detection of specific fungal antigenaemia are aids to speciation. Immunocytochemical techniques using antibodies and lectins can identify fungi in sections, but are of limited availability.[90,91] A comprehensive atlas of the clinical pathology of mycoses has been produced by Chandler et al.[56]

Aspergillosis

Aspergilli are abundant in the environment and cause a wide range of diseases. Disseminated infection that involves the liver is opportunistic and the host is debilitated by malignancy (typically leukaemia), immunosuppressive therapy, steroids and antibiotics. Hepatic failure is also a predisposing cause.[92] The commonest agents are *Aspergillus fumigatus* and *flavus*. The liver is affected in about one-fifth of such cases. Macroscopically, there are multiple foci of haemorrhagic necrosis. Microscopically, the hyphae are seen to penetrate blood vessel walls and produce thrombosis and infarction. The hyphae are basophilic, 3–6 μm in diameter, septate, and branch regularly at a 45° angle.

Candidiasis

Candida infection is global. *C. albicans* is the most frequent species, being a commensal organism in the mouth and intestine of most healthy individuals. Liver infection is usually encountered in neonates and in the immunocompromised host, such as leukaemic patients with low blood neutrophil counts. Occasionally it occurs in pregnant women and as a result of hyperalimentation. Multiple portal and periportal chronic abscesses form, sometimes with granulomas. The yeasts and hyphae may be plentiful or scanty (Fig. 7.16). This infection is very hard to eliminate, and persistent lesions can induce considerable scarring.

Cryptococcosis

Cryptococcus neoformans is also distributed globally. Clinical disease is usually a meningo-encephalitis or pneumonia, and the liver is involved during dissemination in an immunosuppressed host. The usual association was

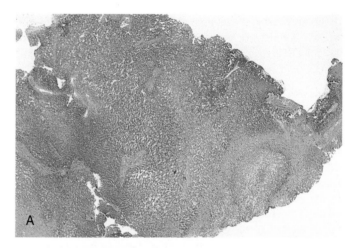

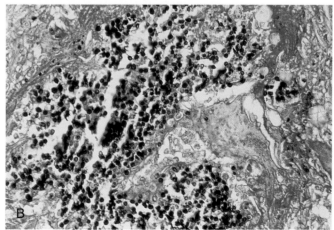

Fig. 7.16 Candidiasis associated with leukaemia. (a) Low-power view of liver with a focal inflammatory lesion surrounded by fibrosis. H&E. (b) Multiple small budding yeasts within the inflammation. Grocott stain.

chemotherapy for lymphoma, but HIV-associated opportunism is now more important. Macroscopically, liver cryptococcosis is usually unremarkable. Rarely, there are multiple foci of necrosis,[93] and occasionally the extrahepatic biliary tree is involved, mimicking sclerosing cholangitis.[94] The fungal yeasts have a wide range of size, from 5 to 20 μm, relatively thin walls, and are usually encapsulated. This characteristic thick mucoid capsule appears as an empty space on H&E, PAS and Grocott stains, and is best shown with a mucicarmine stain (or by dark-ground illumination in cerebrospinal fluid). Sometimes the yeasts are small and non-encapsulated, in which case the distinction from histoplasmosis can be made only on culture or by specific immunostaining. The usual host reaction is single or multiple budding yeasts engulfed by Kupffer cells in the sinusoids or by portal macrophages, with minimal accompanying lymphocytic inflammation (Fig. 7.17). Sometimes, epithelioid cell granulomas develop and large multinucleate giant cells may be seen containing many yeasts.

Histoplasmosis

There are two organisms causing histoplasmosis. *Histoplasma capsulatum* is found in most parts of the world; *H. duboisii* is restricted to Africa. In some zones endemic for *H. capsulatum*, such as the southern United States, infection is almost universal. The various clinico-pathological patterns of histoplasmosis (analogous to tuberculosis) have been described in Goodwin et al.[95] Disseminated infection is usually associated with deficient cell-mediated immunity, of which the commonest cause is now HIV infection, or with age over 50 years.[96] Histoplasmosis is a classic example of an infection that may lie latent in the body for decades after primary infection, becoming manifest if host defences decline, and causing diagnostic

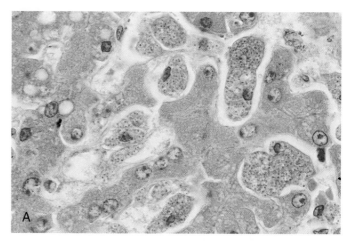

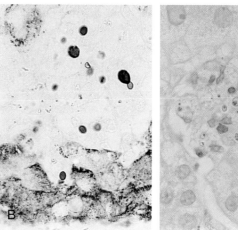
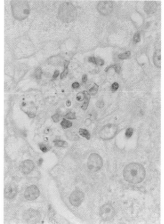

Fig. 7.18 Histoplasmosis capsulatum. (a) Kupffer cells contain abundant yeasts, with purple nuclei. The yeasts are about the same size as *Leishmania* amastigotes, but the latter have a smaller nucleus. H&E. (b) In a case with granulomas and fewer organisms, special stains highlight the *H. capsulatum*: right — PAS stain emphasizes the cell membrane and the nucleus; left — Grocott silver stain shows a budding yeast (same case as Fig. 7.52).

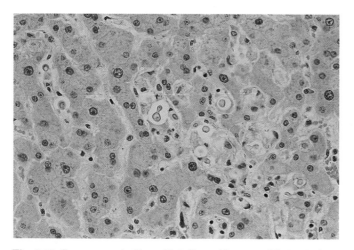

Fig. 7.17 Cryptococcosis. Sinusoids infiltrated by yeasts. The central one is budding. They have thick walls and all show an apparently empty rim which is the mucoid capsule. H&E.

confusion in non-endemic countries if a travel history is not sought.

The liver in histoplasmosis is usually enlarged. The yeast forms are 3–4 μm across and parasitize Kupffer cells and portal macrophages (Figs 7.18 and 7.52). They may be seen budding and in chains, and are best visualized with a Grocott silver stain. Various histological patterns are seen: diffuse or focal parasitization of sinusoidal Kupffer cells or the formation of small tuberculoid granulomas with fewer yeasts. Rarely, a large 'histoplasmoma' forms, consisting of a central fibronecrotic mass, often calcified and containing variable numbers of yeasts, which is surrounded by a granulomatous rim. The yeasts are refractile and have an amphophilic central nucleus, yet can resemble amastigotes of leishmaniasis on H&E stains. However, the latter possess a kinetoplast and are negative with fungal special stains. On Grocott silver stains, the fungi may also resemble cysts of *Pneumocystis carinii* but these appear as an extracellular honeycomb agglomeration, the cysts do not bud, and they often appear bent over.

H. duboisii rarely involves the liver. The yeasts are larger, 10 to 15 μm in diameter, and similar to *Blastomyces*. They are usually contained within macrophages of giant cell granulomas.

Blastomycosis (North American)

Blastomyces dermatitidis infection occurs in the Americas, Africa and Israel. Liver lesions are incidental to widespread dissemination and take the form of miliary nodules. The histological reaction shows a range from purulent abscesses to chronic granulomas, or a mixture of the two. Yeasts may be seen surrounded by polymorphs; in the granulomatous pattern they may be inside or outside epithelioid cells and giant cells. The fungi are 6–15 μm diameter yeasts with a thick refractile cell wall (Fig. 7.19). They bud with a distinctively broad base, but in histological sections they may resemble *Cryptococcus* or *H. duboisii*.

Paracoccidioidomycosis (South American blastomycosis)

In rural areas of South America, infection with *Paracoccidioides brasiliensis* is endemic. Systemic infection follows from pulmonary disease. In the liver there are miliary nodules related to portal tracts.[97] The host cell reaction is similar to that of blastomycosis. A variable amount of portal fibrosis is seen. The morphology is characteristic: the round to oval amphophilic yeasts are 5–60 μm in diameter and show small peripheral buds that resemble a ship's steering wheel.

Coccidioidomycosis

The agent *Coccidioides immitis* is restricted to the southern United States and Central and South America. Pulmonary disease is the commonest manifestation but, like tuberculosis, it may disseminate to viscera, including the liver. The pleomorphic host reaction is like that in blastomycosis. The fungi are large spherules ranging in size from 20 to 200 μm in diameter and contain endospores.[56]

Penicilliosis

Infection with *Penicillium marneffei* is endemic in South-East Asia. Clinically it presents much like disseminated tuberculosis. All parts of the lymphoreticular system are involved, including the liver and spleen.[98] The host inflammatory reaction varies from tuberculoid granulomas, with or without suppuration, to a diffuse histiocytosis. Like *H. capsulatum*, which it closely resembles, *P. marneffei* is

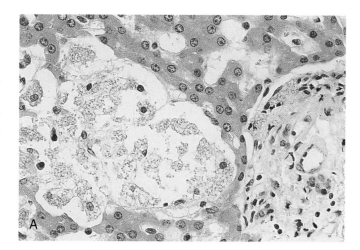

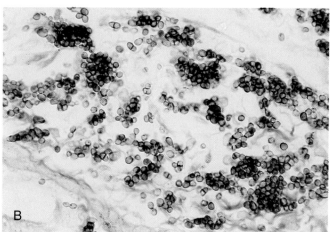

Fig. 7.20 Penicilliosis. (a) Small yeasts filling the Kupffer cells and expanding the sinusoids. H&E. (b) Grocott silver stain shows the yeasts: they are similar in size to *H. capsulatum*, but some show characteristic transverse septae. Slides courtesy of Dr W Tsui, Hong Kong

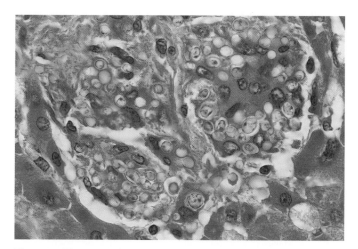

Fig. 7.19 Blastomycosis. A giant cell granuloma containing abundant large yeasts with prominent nuclear material. H&E.

an intracellular macrophage infection. The yeasts are ovoid, 5 × 2 μm in size, do not bud but multiply by schizogony, and have a prominent septum which distinguishes them from histoplasmosis. Tubular forms are also seen (Fig. 7.20).

Zygomycosis

This group of diseases, which includes mucormycosis and phycomycosis, is caused by several fungal genera such as *Rhizopus*, *Mucor* and *Absidia*. They share a characteristic morphology: broad, branching hyphae, 6–25 μm in diameter with few or no septae. The fungi are ubiquitous and cause opportunistic, disseminated disease when the host is immunocompromised, usually from haematological malignancy or transplantation.[99] Liver involvement, as seen at autopsy, may show multiple, necrotic, 1 cm diameter nodules. Histologically, there is coagulative necrosis infiltrated by hyphae.[90] This pattern of widespread vascular invasion with ischaemic necrosis is similar to that seen in aspergillosis, but the hyphae in the latter infection are narrower and septate.

PROTOZOAL INFECTIONS

Malaria

Clinical and epidemiological features

The *P. falciparum* parasite — clinically the most important malarial species — continues to infect more than 1 billion people in Africa, Asia and South America, and in many African countries it is a major cause of childhood mortality. Chronologically, there are three phases to malaria in endemic areas:

1. Up to three months of age, children are protected by maternal antibodies.
2. Thereafter, repeated attacks of acute malaria occur, which may be fatal, until immunity is acquired in survivors by late childhood.
3. Adults maintain immunity by repeated clinically silent infections. This immunity may be broken in women by pregnancy, and in anyone who leaves and endemic zone. A few adults go on to develop the 'tropical splenomegaly syndrome'.

Thus, clinical malaria is encountered in children and pregnant women; in adults who have lost acquired immunity by emigration and have been reinfected; and in non-immune travellers to endemic malarial areas. HIV infection does not influence the prevalence or severity of falciparum malaria.[100] In malaria, death from hepatic failure that is directly due to plasmodial infection does not occur. None the less, many liver-related phenomena may develop: jaundice, hepatomegaly, hypoglycaemia, low serum albumin, prolonged prothrombin time, and mildly elevated transaminases.[101]

Pathology

The initial phase of infection after a mosquito bite requires multiplication in the liver. Schizonts develop within hepatocytes and then seed into the blood. There are no clinical sequelae until the erythrocytic part of the life cycle with consequent haemolysis commences.

The gross appearance of the liver at autopsy in severe malaria is of an enlarged, congested dark brown or grey organ, the colour being due to pigment deposition (Fig. 7.21). This colour may be mimicked by severe a cute schistosomiasis and by dissemination of gas-producing Gram-negative bacilli after death.

Microscopically, in the liver as in other organs of the mononuclear phagocyte system, the striking feature is the accumulation of malarial pigment, *haemozoin*. It is seen as small dark-brown dots in parasitized erythrocytes and as larger lumps within macrophages. In acute attacks, the pigment accumulates in Kupffer cells, which are increased in number and size. When parasitaemia subsides, the pigment shifts to portal tract macrophages and is eventually cleared. The sinusoids are usually distended by erythrocytes. Parasites are visible in them as faint, clear rings with a haematoxyphilic dot, the nucleus (Fig. 7.22), but they are often obscured by the pigment. The hepatocytes may show steatosis (a non-specific product of

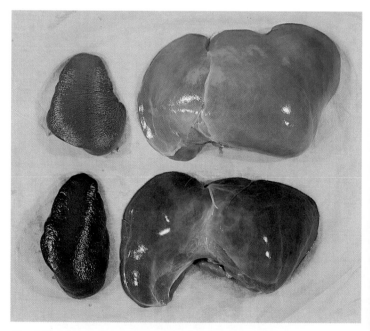

Fig. 7.21 Malaria. Pairs of liver and spleen from autopsied young children, one of whom died of malaria. The lower set is dark brown owing to the haemozoin pigment of malaria

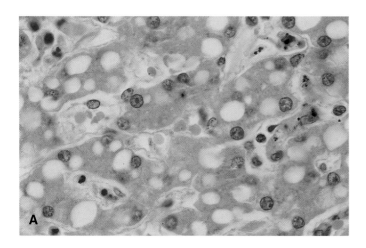

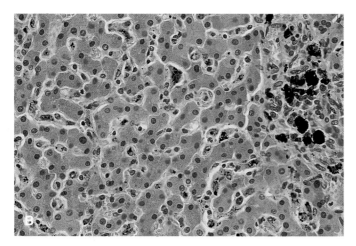

Fig. 7.22 Malaria. (a) Acute falciparum malaria with some fatty change; haemozoin pigment is in Kupffer cells, and two erythrocytes (centre, top) contain falciparum ring forms. H&E. (b) Acute falciparum malaria showing large clumps of haemozoin in portal tract macrophages and Kupffer cells. H&E.

anaemia and infection) but in most cases are otherwise unaffected. A mild portal lymphocytosis and plasmacytosis are often present.[102]

The old-fashioned clinical entity 'malarial hepatitis' does not exist. Significant clinico-biochemical liver damage is associated with shock in severe malaria; histopathologically there is perivenular ischaemic necrosis and sometimes cholestasis.[103] The hypoglycaemic state — mainly seen in African children and adult pregnant women[101] — has its histological counterpart in a complete absence of glycogen in hepatocytes. Electron microscopic studies of the liver in malaria have shown mitochondrial damage, and swelling and loss of microvilli: these are secondary non-specific effects of shock.[104]

Pathogenesis

Haemozoin is an iron porphyrin proteinoid complex

formed by the parasite from the breakdown of haemoglobin. It does not react with Prussian blue stain and can be removed from tissue sections by a saturated alcoholic solution of picric acid. Haemozoin is birefringent under polarized light in a red-yellow colour. It is to be distinguished from porphyria pigment, which is darker red in polarized light and is seen in hepatocytes and ductules. It is ordinarily indistinguishable from schistosomal haemozoin pigment, but differences are revealed by electron microscopy and biochemical methods.[105] There is evidence that the haemozoin in macrophages compromises their functions of phagocytosis and cell-mediated immunity.[106]

The jaundice of malaria is mainly haemolytic, as erythrocytes rupture and the merozoites are released. The mechanisms causing the shock state of severe malaria and the uncommon hepatic necrosis and cholestasis are uncertain.[101] They include sequestration of parasitized erythrocytes in the splanchnic vasculature with subsequent hypoperfusion, endotoxaemia, and elevated production of tumour necrosis factor.

'Tropical splenomegaly syndrome'

In malarial areas, chronic splenomegaly has many causes, but a syndrome of 'big spleen disease' in adults, without evident cause, has long been recognized. In such cases the spleen may weigh 2–4 kg. The splenic morphology is a non-specific hyperplasia, whilst the liver, which is only slightly enlarged, shows a characteristic lymphocytic infiltrate — 'hepatic sinusoidal lymphocytosis' — morphologically resembling that seen in Felty's syndrome (Fig. 7.23). The lymphocytes are T-cells, and may form fairly dense clusters. The Kupffer cells are hypertrophied and contain phagocytosed immune complexes; there is no haemozoin pigment.

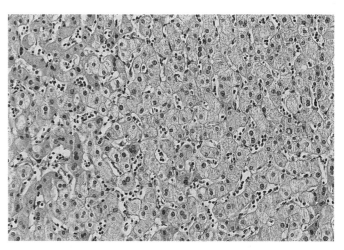

Fig. 7.23 'Tropical splenomegaly syndrome'. Liver sinusoids contain numerous reactive T-lymphocytes. Note the absence of haemozoin pigment. H&E.

The evidence that the underlying pathogenesis of tropical splenomegaly syndrome is an idiosyncratic immune response to *P. falciparum* infection comes from several sources. The geographical epidemiology, its rarity in people with sickle-cell trait, the good response to antimalarial chemotherapy, and serological abnormalities with raised IgM levels all implicate a low-grade chronic *P. falciparum* infection. The entity has recently been renamed 'hyper-reactive malarial splenomegaly'.[107]

Other malaria infections

The clinically mild *P. vivax*, *P. ovale* and *P. malariae* infections cause less haemolysis than *P. falciparum*, and jaundice is rare. Grossly the liver may be grey, but as death seldom occurs, it is rarely encountered at autopsy. The histological findings are similar to those in falciparum malaria though less marked.

Babesiosis

Babesia species are transmitted by ticks, and the disease is a zoonotic infection. In Europe, people who have had splenectomy may occasionally become infected by the cattle babesia parasite *B. divergens*. The clinical course is similar to falciparum malaria with fever, renal failure and haemolysis, but jaundice is more severe.[108] Mortality is high. At autopsy, the liver is enlarged and congested. Microscopically, there is focal ischaemic necrosis, hypertrophied Kupffer cells, and erythrocytes containing parasites morphologically similar to *P. falciparum*. However, there is no production of haemozoin pigment.

Visceral leishmaniasis

Clinical and epidemiological features

Visceral leishmaniasis (kala azar) is endemic in southern Europe, the Middle East, Asia, China, South America and Africa. In recent years, epidemics have occurred in Italy, India and Sudan. *Leishmania donovani* is the agent except in Europe, where its variant, *L. infantum*, is responsible, and in South America where it is the related *L. donovani chagasi*. Infection follows the bite of an infected sandfly. Apart from India, where leishmaniasis is an anthroponotic infection, visceral leishmaniasis is a zoonosis and canines are the reservoir.

The ratio of those infected to those who develop disease is between 10 and 30 to one[109] The clinical spectrum of manifestations is protean. It ranges from mild malaise, through growth retardation in children, to the classic picture of hepatosplenomegaly, lymphadenopathy, fever, pancytopenia and hypergammaglobulinaemia.[110] Liver function tests are little altered, apart from a low albumin,

and jaundice is uncommon. Untreated clinical visceral leishmaniasis is usually fatal; treated leishmaniasis has a mortality range of 2–17%. Children suffer a more acute form of the disease than adults, with a higher mortality.

Pathology

The liver is enlarged, sometimes massively, up to 4 kg, with no specific macroscopic appearance. Accounts of the histopathology are confusing. Liver biopsies taken during an epidemic in Italy showed that infected but asymptomatic patients (with positive anti-leishmanial serology) had epithelioid cell granulomas scattered throughout the parenchyma. These only rarely contained the parasite.[111]

In patients with acute overt leishmaniasis, the liver generally shows two overlapping histopathological patterns. The classic type consists of Kupffer cell hypertrophy and hyperplasia, portal inflammation and a diffuse sinusoidal chronic inflammatory infiltrate with conspicuous plasma cells. The parasites are present in Kupffer cells and portal macrophages, but the numbers vary widely (Fig. 7.24). They are seen as 2–3 µm diameter, ovoid or round, clear blobs of cytoplasm with a basophilic nucleus (the amastigote form); the characteristic paranuclear rod-shaped kinetoplast is not always evident in sections. Rarely, parasites are seen in hepatocytes also.[112] In the second pattern, the macrophages are seen within the acinus as small nodules with scanty parasites.[113] Sometimes epithelioid cell granulomas are found. Fatty change is common, but non-specific, and cholestasis is seen in some fatal cases. Occasionally, fibrin-ring granulomas form within the nodules, similar to those seen in Q fever.[114]

Necrosis is not normally a feature of the liver in leishmaniasis but it occurs in some acute fatal cases. The granulomas may show central necrosis and resemble those of tuberculosis and brucellosis, but amastigotes are usually visible. Hepatic necrosis around granulomas with bile-duct proliferation has been described and sometimes haemorrhagic necrosis is seen.[115,116] The extent to which terminal shock or other processes contribute to these more severe lesions is unclear.

In chronic adult cases of visceral leishmaniasis, a diffuse panacinar fibrosis may develop, similar to that seen in congenital syphilis. Amastigotes are scanty in this phase.[117] A denser form of fibrosis, leaving the portal structures intact but dividing the parenchyma into small groups of hepatocytes, was described as 'Rogers' cirrhosis'[118] It is not a true cirrhosis and is now uncommon (Fig. 7.25).

Liver biopsy is not the most sensitive diagnostic technique for leishmaniasis, but a liver aspirate can demonstrate parasites in 75% or more of cases.[119] The main treatment for visceral leishmaniasis is pentavalent antimo-

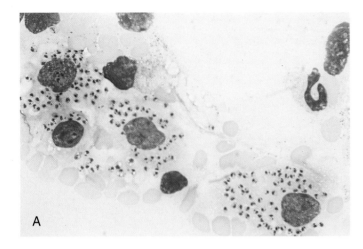

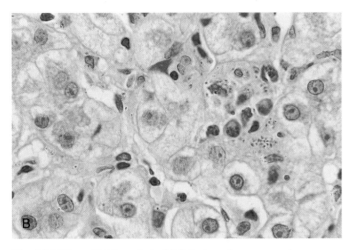

Fig. 7.24 Visceral leishmaniasis. (a) Splenic aspirate: macrophages contain amastigotes that have a nucleus and an eccentric bar of DNA, the kinetoplast. Giemsa. (b) Liver biopsy showing Kupffer cells with amastigotes and associated plasma cells. H&E.

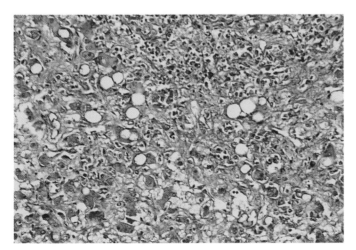

Fig. 7.25 Chronic leishmaniasis: 'Rogers' cirrhosis'. Progressive sinusoidal fibrosis separating the liver plates. Trichrome stain. Photograph courtesy of Dr C Corbett, Brazil.

nial chemotherapy, and these agents are occasionally hepatotoxic.[109]

Many cases of leishmaniasis in HIV-1-positive patients are now reported although it is not an AIDS-defining disease.

Pathogenesis

Resistance to leishmaniasis depends on cell-mediated immunity. In the mouse, a single autosomal gene controls the persistence or elimination of the infection.[120] In patients with clinical leishmaniasis, interleukin-2 and γ-interferon production are poor, resulting in a lack of macrophage activation to eliminate the parasites. Macrophages throughout the body are also parasitized. A major contribution to the morbidity and mortality is the immune paralysis consequent upon macrophage malfunction, and secondary bacterial infections are common. Conversely, the granulomatous lesions in asymptomatic, infected cases reflect parasite elimination.

Amoebiasis

Epidemiology and clinical features

Entamoeba histolytica infection is globally distributed, with about 10% of the world's population being infected. Whilst most of these reside in tropical and subtropical areas, no country is exempt. However, only 10% overall of people infected develop amoebiasis — either colorectal or extra-intestinal. The remaining 90% are asymptomatic carriers of amoebic trophozoites in the gut. Infection is via the faecal–oral route and results from ingestion of cysts. An invasive lesion in the large bowel is a prerequisite for the parasite to pass into the portal vein circulation, but only one-third of patients with amoebic liver abscess have a history of bowel symptoms.

Amoebic liver abscess presents with an enlarged, tender liver, fever and leucocytosis. Ultrasound is now the usual mode of diagnosis in hospital practice, supported by serology which is positive in nearly all cases. Aspiration of an abscess is usually performed as a therapeutic measure to prevent rupture rather than as a diagnostic procedure, but amoebae may be identified in the aspirate.

The major differential diagnoses are hepatocellular carcinoma and pyogenic abscess. Jaundice is more common in pyogenic than in amoebic liver abscess. However, in a large series studied in India, cholestasis was present in nearly 30% of patients. This was associated with large, inferior abscesses and compression of the hepatic ducts. The mortality is increased (up to 43%, despite treatment) in such patients.[121]

Pathology

Most amoebic abscesses are in the right lobe, reflecting

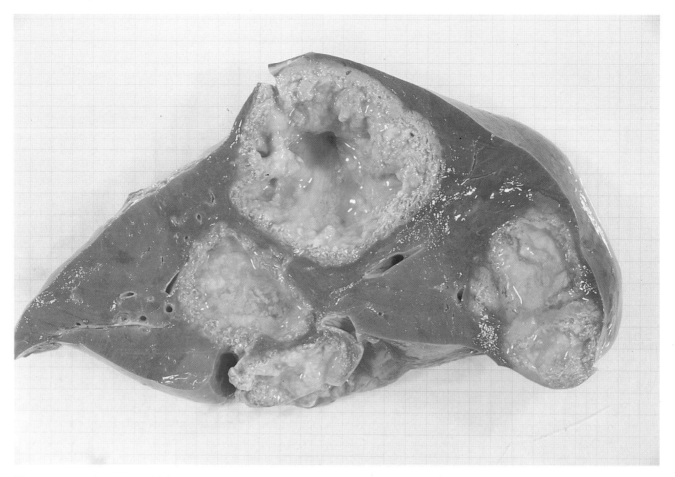

Fig. 7.26 Amoebiasis. Liver with four large amoebic abscesses. Photograph courtesy of Prof MSR Hutt and the late Dr F MacDonald

its greater portal venous drainage compared with the left lobe, and are often multiple (Fig. 7.26). The earliest macroscopic lesion, which is rarely encountered, is one or more small nodules of pale necrotic liver tissue. Fully developed abscesses have a ragged margin without a fibrous rim, and liquid contents. These have been likened to anchovy sauce, being brown-red and often paste-like in consistency. The size of an abscess varies greatly, but most are between 5 and 20 cm in diameter. Old lesions can develop a fibrotic capsule up to a centimetre thick.

The earliest histological finding is the presence of amoebic trophozoites in the sinusoids, associated with coagulative necrosis between the portal tract and terminal venule of an acinus.[122] There is a mild polymorph reaction with oedema. Trophozoites are 20–50 μm in diameter. They have a cytoplasm that ranges from nearly clear to purple and granular, depending on fixation and quality of staining. Phagocytosed erythrocytes are often present. The round nucleus is the size of a red cell with a sharp nuclear membrane and a prominent central karyosome. The usual confusion is with macrophages; the latter are smaller, have more basophilic nuclei and less granular cytoplasm.

Amoebae are intensely PAS positive due to glycogen in the cytoplasm. Immunocytochemical stains (human anti-amoeba serum works well) also highlight amoebae (Fig. 7.27), even in tissues stored for over a century.

As the lesion enlarges, amoebae cluster at the advancing edge of the abscess, leaving behind haemorrhagic granular necrotic material with much nuclear debris. Oedema is prominent around the abscess, associated with lymphocytes and plasma cells, but polymorphs are scanty — hence it is technically not a true 'abscess'. Older lesions generate peripheral granulation tissue and, eventually, dense fibrosis.

Amoebic abscesses may rupture through the liver capsule. Sub-diaphragmatic lesions may penetrate into the pleural cavity and the lung tissue. A sinus may drain through the abdominal wall and progressively digest away the surrounding skin. Rupture into the peritoneal cavity has a particularly high mortality from the resulting amoebic peritonitis.

Pathogenesis

The majority of people with *E. histolytica* in the bowel

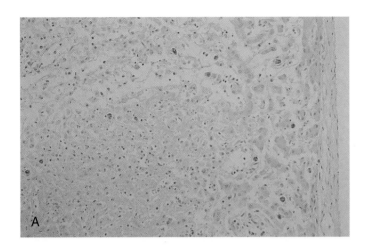

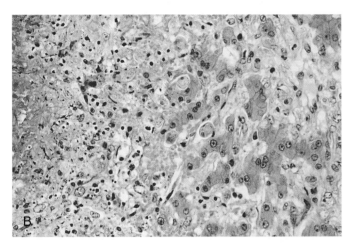

Fig. 7.27 Amoebiasis. (a) Early stage of invasive amoebiasis in liver: single trophozoites visible in sinusoids and around a focus of necrosis. Anti-*Entamoeba* immunoperoxidase stain. (b) Edge of an established amoebic abscess: necrotic liver on left; several purple-staining trophozoites in the centre and between hepatocytes. H&E.

by lethal leak of ions.[124] Tissue dissolution may be mediated by secretion of collagenase and cysteine proteinase by trophozoites. The amoeba phagocytoses the injured cell, and continues its motion through the tissue by pseudopodial action.

Balantidiasis

Balantidium coli, a rare cause of enteritis, may occasionally pass via the portal vein and produce a liver abscess.[5] This parasite is the largest protozoon that infects man, the trophozoites measuring 50–100 μm.

Toxoplasmosis

Infection with *Toxoplasma gondii*, whose definitive host phase is in the enterocytes of cats, is ubiquitous. Man is infected from cat faeces or, more usually, from consuming undercooked meat. Most infections in adults are asymptomatic and toxoplasmosis is a latent, lifelong infection. The prevalence depends on climate, contact with pets, and culinary habits. In France and West Africa, adult seroprevalence rates are over 80%, but in dry, hot countries only 10% of adults may have serological evidence of infection.

A giant cell hepatitis may occur in congenital toxoplasmosis, but more frequently there are focal necroses associated with parasitized sinusoidal cells. Toxoplasmosis acquired after birth is only rarely associated with liver problems in normal hosts. Immunocompromised individuals, however, can have a marked toxoplasmic hepatitis with focal necroses and cholestasis.[125] The parasites are seen as cysts containing many zoites or as free tachyzoites (Fig. 7.28). The commonest clinical association is now HIV infection. Toxoplasmosis is also a cause of granulo-

harbour strains that are non-pathogenic but morphologically identical to the potentially invasive and disease-associated virulent strains. It is now established that the pathogenic and non-pathogenic strains (zymodemes), originally described by enzyme electrophoresis, are distinct genotypic entities.[123]

The pathogenicity of *E. histolytica* depends on direct contact with the target cell. The process has five stages: binding, cytolysis of target cells, dissolution of tissue, phagocytosis, and spread of amoebae. Binding involves a 170 kD galactose/*N*-acetyl galactosamine-inhibitable lectin which is expressed on the surface of the parasite. The mechanisms of amoebic cytotoxicity are still unclear. Under investigation are contact-dependent calcium influx into the target cell, a phospholipase associated with the plasma membrane, and an ionophore secreted by the amoeba. This 'amoebapore' is a 14 000 MW dimer which produces large pores in the target cell membrane, followed

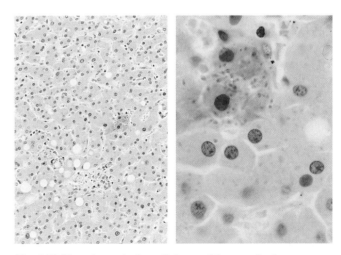

Fig. 7.28 Toxoplasmosis. A small cluster of degenerating hepatocytes containing small haematoxyphilic zoites of *T.gondii*. H&E.

matous hepatitis with non-necrotic epithelioid and giant cell lesions.[126]

HELMINTH INFECTIONS

NEMATODES

Ascariasis

In the tropics and subtropics, more than one billion people are infected with *Ascaris lumbricoides* — it is the commonest helminth infection of man. These 25 cm long roundworms inhabit the small bowel, but the liver is involved as a phase in the life cycle and by adult worms causing biliary obstruction. Infection occurs via the faecal–oral route by ingesting eggs and, when heavy, it may cause hepatomegaly during larval migration. If the liver is biopsied, an eosinophilic granulomatous reaction may be seen around degenerate small larvae. Ascaris worms migrate, and as they move into and out of the biliary tree and pancreatic duct, complications may arise. These include acalculous cholecystitis, biliary colic, acute bacterial cholangitis and hepatic abscess.[127] The diagnosis may be made by ERCP and ultrasound, in addition to finding the ova in the faeces. The organisms causing secondary cholangitis are usually *E.coli*, *Klebsiella* spp., and *Pseudomonas aeruginosa*. These complications usually resolve with appropriate chemotherapy and removal or spontaneous migration of the worms. Once a hepatic abscess has developed it may perforate the liver capsule or lead to septicaemia.

The worms may be seen obstructing and distending the bile ducts (Fig. 7.29). If they are trapped and die within the biliary tree, the remnants can form nidi for biliary calculi to form. Such remnants may adhere to the biliary epithelium, and cause glandular proliferation and intestinal metaplasia.[128] Eggs deposited by adult worms may also be seen within necrotic peribiliary foci, where they induce a mixed suppurative and granulomatous reaction around the characteristic brown-shelled and mamillated eggs.

Enterobiasis

Enterobius (Oxyuris) vermicularis, or the pinworm, is endemic in temperate zones, but less so in the tropics. Normally the only clinical sequel is pruritus from the eggs that the gravid female worm deposits around the anus. Occasionally the worm migrates up the female genital tract and into the peritoneal cavity. There, a florid inflammatory reaction occurs around the adult worm and eggs to produce a mass which causes abdominal pain and is associated with blood eosinophilia. Several cases of such nodules in the liver ('enterobioma') have been reported.[129,130] These join the list of non-neoplastic lesions that

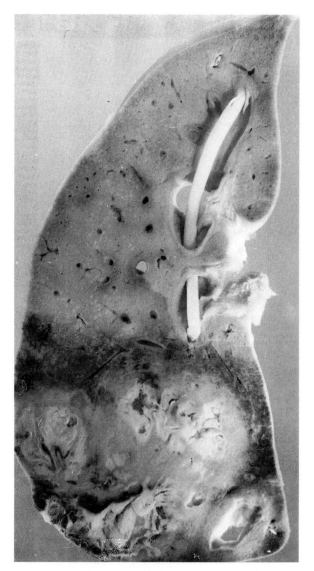

Fig. 7.29 Ascariasis. Ascarid worm within a dilated bile duct, associated with several cholangitic abscesses in the lower half. Photograph courtesy of the Wellcome Museum of Medical Science

can mimic a benign tumour or a deposit of metastatic carcinoma in the liver.

Macroscopically, the lesions are about 1 cm in diameter and white or greenish in colour. Histologically, there is usually a fibrous and granulomatous rim surrounding a bland eosinophilic necrotic centre. This contains the degenerate worm, which may be seen to have characteristic triangular, pointed alae along the cuticle. The eggs are 25×50 μm in size, and one lateral aspect is flattened; they are seen within and outside the worm (Fig. 7.30).

Strongyloidiasis

Strongyloides stercoralis is endemic in tropical and

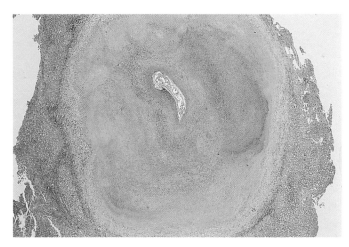

Fig. 7.30 Enterobiasis. Necrotic nodule with a central female *E. vermicularis* worm. The extensive surrounding eosinophilic necrosis is typical. H&E.

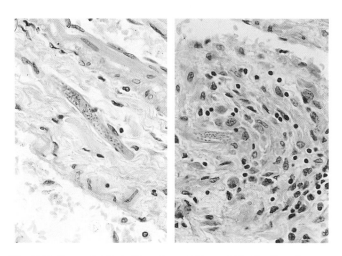

Fig. 7.31 Strongyloidiasis. Two views of *Strongyloides* filariform larvae invading a portal tract; they contain many small nuclei. On the right, the larva has evoked a granulomatous reaction with eosinophils. H&E.

subtropical areas around the world, including the southern United States. It is almost unique in that, once a person is infected, the autoinfection cycle perpetuates the infection indefinitely in many instances. Thus, decades after leaving an endemic zone, an infected but previously asymptomatic patient may present with unsuspected strongyloidiasis.

The liver is involved, like other visceral organs, when immunosuppression precipitates a hyperinfection syndrome. In this situation, the autoinfection process is accelerated and the infection load in the intestine augments rapidly. Predisposing events include malnutrition, high-dose steroid therapy and cytotoxic drugs for organ transplantation and cancer.[131] Human T-cell leukaemia virus type 1 (HTLV-1) infection has a particularly high risk of promoting the hyperinfection syndrome. This may occur before or after the HTLV-1-associated adult T-cell leukaemia/lymphoma has developed, and may be a presenting feature of leukaemia.[132] HIV infection, however, is not epidemiologically associated with strongyloidiasis.

The filariform larvae disseminate haematogenously and there is often an associated Gram-negative septicaemia. The larvae are 600 × 16 µm, but they are rarely seen in a complete longitudinal section. In the liver, they are present in small portal vessels and sinusoids without any inflammation; or they may be surrounded by a chronic inflammatory infiltrate, often with giant cells but usually not many eosinophils (Fig. 7.31).[133]

Capillariasis

Infection with *Capillaria hepatica* is a worldwide zoonosis of small mammals, and human disease is rare. Man is infected by ingesting eggs in foodstuffs contaminated with soil. Clinically, there is fever, hepatomegaly and eosinophilia, and mortality is high.[134] Macroscopically, the liver

is enlarged, sometimes fibrotic, and shows numerous small white foci of necrosis. Histologically, there are many eosinophils and a granulomatous reaction to adult worms (20×0.1 mm) and abundant eggs (60×30 µm). The eggs have characteristic striated shells and bipolar plugs (Fig. 7.32).

Visceral larva migrans (toxocariasis)

Certain ascarid intestinal worms of dogs (*Toxocara canis*) and cats (*T. cati*) are able to parasitize virtually any host paratenically: that is, larvae migrate through the body for years but they do not develop or mature. The term 'visceral larva migrans', when used unqualified, is taken to indicate infection with *T. canis* larvae.

Visceral larva migrans is a disease of children, who ingest the larvae from faeces of infected dogs. Seroprevalence surveys have shown that many infections are

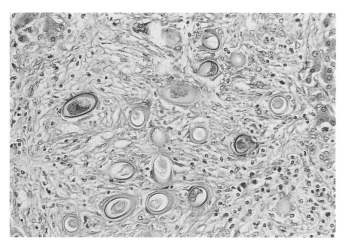

Fig. 7.32 Capillariasis. Intrahepatic granuloma around numerous eggs. H&E.

asymptomatic. Hepatomegaly and blood eosinophilia are part of the syndromes of both mild ('covert') and overt visceral larva migrans disease.[135,136] Histologically, the liver may show small foci of necrosis, many degranulating eosinophils and some giant cells. This is the track lesion of a migrating larva. Rarely, part of a larva, which is 300 × 20 µm in size, is seen within the granuloma.

Other hepatic larval helminthic diseases

The life cycles of many anthroponotic worm infections involve the liver, so larvae and an attendant inflammatory reaction may occasionally be encountered in liver biopsy or autopsy material as an incidental finding. These infections include not only *Ascaris lumbricoides*, the hookworms, and *Strongyloides stercoralis*, but also certain zoonotic infections. These include *Baylisascaris*, *Gnathostoma*, and *Sparganum*.[5]

CESTODES

Hydatid disease is caused by the larval forms of *Echinococcus* tapeworms. *E. granulosus* is the most frequent parasite, the adults being found in dogs and jackals in all continents including Europe. Many mammals can serve as intermediate hosts, but sheep are the most frequent. *E. multilocularis* is less common but causes a more aggressive clinical disease. The definitive host is the fox and the infection occurs in eastern Europe, Turkey, the southern Russian states and the northern states of the United States and Canada. Intermediate hosts are usually rodents.

Unilocular hydatidosis

This is the classic hydatid cyst, caused by *E. granulosus*. After ingestion, the eggs hatch and the larval oncospheres pass to the liver by the portal vein. About 75% of infected individuals develop one or more cysts in the liver. These grow slowly, about 1 cm a year. The right lobe of the liver is affected more often than the left. Many hepatic hydatid cysts are asymptomatic and are discovered incidentally on X-ray. Clinical symptoms arise from large cysts as space-occupying lesions, when they compress the biliary tree, become bacterially infected or, rarely, press on the portal vein and produce portal hypertension. A small proportion of liver cysts rupture into the peritoneal cavity, resulting in secondary dissemination of infection there. *E. granulosus* cysts may also develop in the lung, kidneys, spleen, brain and musculo-skeletal system.

The typical hydatid cyst is spherical, up to 30 cm or more in diameter, and has a fibrous rim. It may be single and unilocular or, more frequently, contain several daughter cysts which have developed by growth and invagination of the germinal membrane (Fig. 7.33). The wall has three structural components: (i) an outer acellular laminated

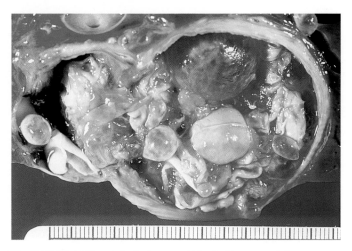

Fig. 7.33 Hydatid cyst. A single cyst within the liver, containing numerous daughter cysts. The white laminated membranes are seen and also the thin fibrous rim around the cyst.

membrane, which is 1 mm thick, ivory white, friable, and rather slippery to touch; (ii) the germinal membrane, a transparent nucleated lining; and (iii) the protoscolices, which are attached to the membrane and budding from it. These are about 100 µm across, ovoid in shape, and contain two circles of hooklets, and a sucker (Figs 7.34 and 7.35). Many cysts are partly or wholly degenerate. Collapsed daughter cysts have closely rolled laminated membranes. Histologically, these are anucleate and devoid of viable protoscolices. They may contain many shed hooklets, which have a characteristic scimitar shape, and small calcareous bodies.

The host reaction to unilocular hydatid cyst is slight: there is some granulation tissue and a relatively thin fibrous wall. Eosinophils are not conspicuous but if a cyst has died or ruptured, they may be more evident, along with giant cell granulomas.

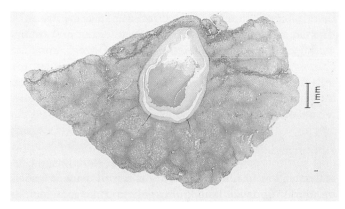

Fig. 7.34 Hydatid cyst. A liver resection containing a small apparently dead cyst. There is a fibrous rim, a detached laminated membrane, and granular or fluid contents. H&E.

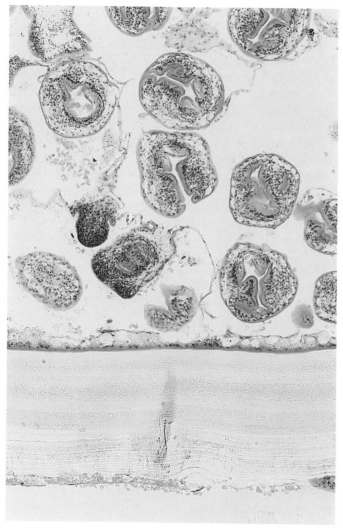

Fig. 7.35 Hydatid cyst. From bottom to top: non-staining laminated membrane, the thin nucleated germinal membrane, and several protoscolices with sucker and refractile hooklets. H&E.

The diagnosis is usually made by ultrasound or CT scan, supported by positive hydatid serology. Leakage of antigen-laden hydatid cyst fluid into the circulation may result in anaphylactic shock, which can be fatal. Thus, liver biopsy is not encouraged if a hydatid cyst is suspected. Fine needle aspiration, however, is a safe diagnostic procedure.[137] The fluid obtained should be spun down and searched for protoscolices or hooklets. The latter are acid-fast on Ziehl–Neelsen stain and also stain well with trichrome methods.

Modern surgical treatment avoids hepatectomy if possible: the laminated membrane and contents are sucked out, taking care not to disseminate germinal membrane or protoscolices. Current chemotherapy is with albendazole. The histopathologist is often asked whether resected or aspirated cysts are sterile, searching for an end-point to therapy. This is impossible to answer. The presence of germinal membrane with nuclei or of protoscolices indicates that the cyst is potentially viable;

however, retained remnants of hydatid cysts, even in the absence of apparent nucleated membrane or protoscolices, are capable of continued growth and dissemination.

Alveolar (multilocular) hydatidosis

The liver is also the primary site of infection with *E. multilocularis*. Patients present with hepatomegaly, jaundice and ascites.[138] Untreated, this infection is fatal, for spontaneous resolution rarely occurs. Surgery and chemotherapy have improved this dismal outlook.

The liver lesions appear as multilocular, necrotic, cystic cavities, containing thick pasty material. A fibrous rim is absent (Fig. 7.36). Rupture into the abdominal cavity or biliary tree and distant spread to other organs may occur. Histologically, the irregular cysts have a laminated membrane, but no nucleated germinal membrane or protoscolices are seen. The laminated membrane is often fragmented and is highlighted by PAS stain. These structures invade necrotic liver tissue much like a malignant tumour. The host response is variable. There may be a granulomatous reaction with polymorphs and eosinophils, or an extensive peripheral rim of necrosis, fibrosis and focal calcification (Fig. 7.37).

TREMATODES

The four major genera of trematode flatworms or flukes that affect man are *Schistosoma*, *Clonorchis*, *Opisthorchis* and *Fasciola*, and all cause liver damage. Trematodes require specific aquatic snail intermediate hosts for their life cycles.

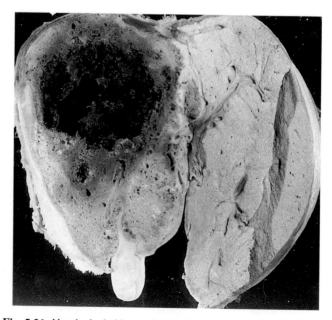

Fig. 7.36 Alveolar hydatid cyst. Autopsy liver with a large irregular necrotic and invasive mass on the left. Photograph courtesy of the Wellcome Museum of Medical Science

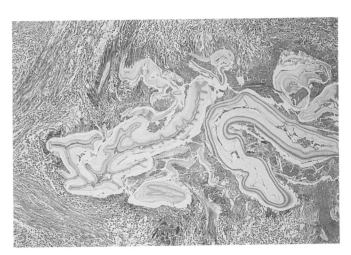

Fig. 7.37 Alveolar hydatid cyst. Necrotic and fibrotic liver tissue infiltrated by irregular membranes that have no apparent nuclei. Protoscolices are not seen in human infection. H&E.

Schistosomiasis

Epidemiology and clinical features

Schistosomiasis (bilharzia) is one of the great tropical diseases, with more than 200 million people infected. However, only 10% of those infected have clinically evident disease. Hepatosplenic schistosomiasis is the commonest cause of portal hypertension in the world. It results from infection with *Schistosoma mansoni*, *S. japonicum* and *S. mekongi*. *S. mansoni* is endemic in Africa, the Caribbean and South America; *S. japonicum* is prevalent in several countries in South-East Asia including the Philippines, China, Indonesia and Thailand; *S. mekongi* occurs in Laos and Cambodia.[139,140] Of the other species, *S. haematobium* and *S. intercalatum* mainly involve the bladder or bowel respectively, and cause minor non-symptomatic hepatic lesions.[141,142]

After infection by schistosome cercariae, there is a latent period before the worms settle in the veins of their preferred visceral sites. For *S. mansoni*, *S. japonicum* and *S. mekongi* these are the mesenteric and portal veins. Adult worms are 10–20 mm long and up to 1 mm in diameter. About 4 weeks after infection, female worms commence egg-laying. Eggs not retained in the intestinal wall or excreted in the faeces are carried to the liver; about 50% of all eggs laid are retained in the body. An acute infection syndrome called 'Katayama fever' may occur at this time, with fever, systemic upset, eosinophilia and transient hepatosplenomegaly.[143] No histopathological studies of Katayama fever are available, but one might expect in the liver an infiltrate of eosinophils and, in some cases, young schistosome eggs in the portal tracts.

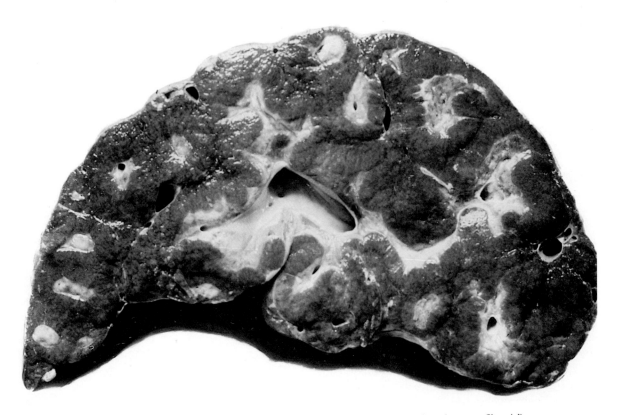

Fig. 7.38 Schistosomiasis. Autopsy liver showing the thick periportal fibrosis ('Symmers' clay-pipe stem fibrosis')

Clinical hepatosplenic schistosomiasis presents with splenomegaly and gastrointestinal bleeding from oesophageal varices. Young adults are the main age group affected. Liver metabolic function is generally well preserved, and encephalopathy is rare after variceal haemorrhage. Ascites is found in up to one-third of patients presenting with haemorrhage,[144] but is more frequent in advanced decompensated cases.[145]

Pathology

The typical macroscopic features of advanced hepatosplenic schistosomiasis are a firm, enlarged liver with a bosselated thickened capsule, and a characteristic portal fibrosis termed Symmers' clay-pipe stem fibrosis.[146] On cut section, there are thick, white tracts of collagen around major portal tracts, in rounded or stellate shapes (Fig. 7.38). Liver acinar architecture is preserved and there is no cirrhosis.

The microscopic features depend on duration of infection.[147] Eggs arriving in the liver are trapped in portal vein radicles of about 50 µm diameter. In early lesions the live eggs are surrounded by eosinophils and an eosinophil abscess may form with fibrinoid material surrounding the egg, a Hoeppli–Splendore reaction. Later an epithelioid granuloma with or without giant cells develops around the egg, the eosinophils being distributed round the periphery (Fig. 7.39). Schistosomal haemozoin pigment, which is indistinguishable from malarial pigment on light microscopy, is phagocytosed by macrophages in granulomas and in the portal tracts and sinusoids. This pigment is a product of haemoglobin catabolism by adult worms. Fibrous scar tissue forms around the granulomas and it eventually replaces them. The eggs live for about 3 weeks then gradually degenerate into empty shells which may be seen in longstanding lesions (Fig. 7.40). Within the thick clay-pipe stem fibrous lesions, one sees variable numbers

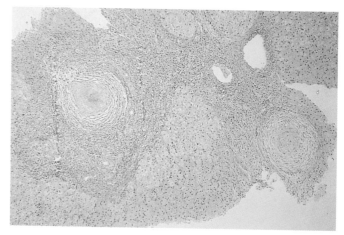

Fig. 7.40 Schistosomiasis. Portal fibrosis associated with two peri-oval granulomas, each with concentric fibrosis. Van Gieson.

of dead eggs, healing granulomas, fibroblasts, myofibroblasts, dense collagen, hypertrophied elastic fibres, tortuous arterioles and venules, and entrapped bile ducts.[148] Electron microscopic studies reveal deposition of collagen in the space of Disse, resulting in obstruction of sinusoidal fenestrations.[149]

S. mansoni eggs are 60×140 µm in size and bear a lateral spine; *S. japonicum* eggs measure 60×85 µm, *S. mekongi* eggs are 50×60 µm and both have a small lateral knob. The shells of these eggs are characteristically brown in colour, and they are acid-fast with Ziehl–Neelsen stain. Occasionally in biopsy material and more often at autopsy, a pair of adult worms, eliciting no inflammatory reaction, may be seen within a portal vein (Fig. 7.41).

Where schistosomiasis is common so is cirrhosis, thus a proportion of patients will have incidental schistosome eggs in a liver biopsy showing cirrhosis. The distinction between cirrhosis and schistosomal fibrosis is usually

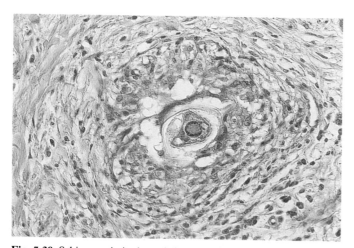

Fig. 7.39 Schistosomiasis. Acute infection: within the granuloma is a live egg with brown shell and spine, and the circular ring of nuclei. H&E.

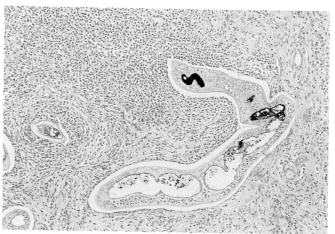

Fig. 7.41 Schistosomiasis. Wedge liver biopsy: the adult worm within a portal vein has haemozoin pigment within its intestine, and is causing no host inflammatory reaction; the egg (left) is surrounded by eosinophils. H&E.

straightforward on wedge biopsies, but there may be problems with needle biopsies. If schistosome eggs are seen in a fibrotic liver, features in favour of cirrhosis as the main disease are small liver nodules, hyperplastic liver-cell plates, piecemeal necrosis, fibrotic bands of uniform thickness around the nodules, and the absence of granulomas and eosinophilia. If a biopsy of liver from a patient in an endemic area shows a portal lymphocytic infiltrate, non-necrotic tuberculoid granulomas and eosinophils, this is evidence that the process is due to schistosomiasis even in the absence of eggs.

Pathogenesis

The portal hypertension of hepatosplenic schistosomiasis is pre-sinusoidal in type. It results from fibrosis due to the host's cell-mediated granulomatous reaction to secreted egg antigens.[150–152] The major determinants of liver disease are the intensity and duration of infection. Autopsy studies of *S. mansoni* show that clinically significant hepatic fibrosis does not usually develop until there has been chronic infection from more than 160 worms.[153] However, the degree of fibrosis does not correlate closely with infection load. Individuals vary in their fibrogenic potential to given stimuli. Hepatosplenic schistosomiasis is associated with various HLA types which may influence the degree of fibrosis. Linkage disequilibrium has been demonstrated with HLA-A1, -A2, -B5 and -B12, according to the population studied. T-lymphocyte responses to schistosomal antigens show a correlation with the degree of fibrosis. Blood mononuclear cells from patients with hepatic fibrosis show a higher blastogenic response to antigen than from schistosomiasis patients without fibrosis; the latter also have a lower blood CD4:CD8 T-cell ratio than fibrotic patients and uninfected controls.[154,155] *S. japonicum* is considered to cause more severe liver disease than *S. mansoni* since adult females lay more than 1000 eggs/day, in comparison with 300/day from *S. mansoni* females. It is also possible that, within species, different strains of the parasite vary in their propensity to cause fibrosis.

It is not clear why the typical localized clay-pipe stem pattern develops rather than a more diffuse peri-acinar portal fibrosis. Morphological and haemodynamic studies of portal veins and hepatic arteries in schistosomiasis are conflicting. In schistosomal fibrosis, total hepatic blood flow is normal. Impregnation of vessels in autopsy material suggests an augmented arterial network and arterio-portal venous shunting.[156] However, radiographic studies during life indicate amputation of the large portal veins, proliferation of smaller vein branches around them, diminished hepatic arterial diameters, and shunting of hepatic arterial blood towards the spleen.[145] It is possible that once portal fibrosis has developed, with the accompanying distortion of vascular architecture, incoming eggs are swept into the smaller veins proliferating around the large portal veins, and via the granuloma/fibrosis sequence this results in progressively expanding tracts of collagen that characterize the clay-pipe stem pattern.

The mechanisms of pre-sinusoidal portal hypertension in hepatosplenic schistosomiasis are thus multifactorial. In addition, since schistosomiasis is an intravascular infection, reactive lymphoid hyperplasia contributes to splenomegaly.

Clinically decompensated hepatosplenic schistosomiasis is characterized by wasting, low serum albumin, prolonged prothrombin time, ascites and hepatic encephalopathy. Its pathogenesis is disputed but the factors proposed include malnutrition, severe deposition of collagen in the space of Disse, ischaemic damage from repeated variceal bleeding, and severely distorted arterio-venous relationships in the portal tracts. Alcohol abuse and viral hepatitis types B and C will produce additional effects.[157]

Hepatitis B virus (HBV) infection is common in areas where schistosomiasis is endemic. However, there is no epidemiological association between the prevalences of HBV and *S. mansoni* or *S. japonicum* infections. HBV coinfection may be important in determining the prognosis of individual patients with hepatosplenic schistosomiasis. Thus, mortality from acute viral hepatitis is increased, and splenomegaly and HBsAg carriage are prolonged after acute B viral hepatitis in patients with schistosomiasis. Cross-sectional studies have also indicated that the chronic sequelae of HBV infection — chronic active hepatitis and cirrhosis — are more likely to develop.[158] An explanation for these associations may lie in the interactions of cytokines, T-lymphocytes and macrophage responses to both infections. Epidemiological studies have not shown that schistosomiasis per se is a risk factor for hepatocellular carcinoma.

Ultrasound studies

Most clinicopathological studies of hepatosplenic schistosomiasis have relied on hospitalized patients studied clinically, parasitologically, and histopathologically by biopsy and autopsy. Ultrasonography has changed this perspective. It provides a non-invasive means of assessing hepatic fibrosis and can be correlated with morphological studies.[159] The technology is suitable for epidemiological studies of schistosomal liver disease in the community (Fig. 7.42). In rural Zimbabwe, ultrasonography showed that an overall 10% of the population studied had schistosomiasis-related portal fibrosis, rising to 19% in those over 50 years of age, but severe fibrosis was rare.[160] Ultrasound studies in Egypt also suggest that a mild degree of fine portal fibrosis accompanies mild hepatosplenomegaly in children infected only with *S. haematobium*.[142]

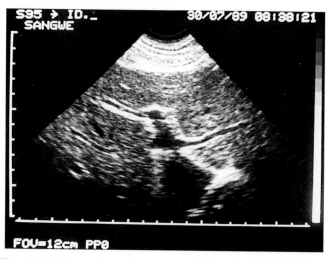

Fig. 7.42 Schistosomiasis. Liver ultrasound shows thick white bands of fibrous tissue around major portal tracts. Photograph courtesy of Dr S Houston, Canada

Therapy

The fibrosis of advanced hepatosplenic schistosomiasis is not reversible on anti-schistosomal therapy with praziquantel. Biochemical studies of patients treated before variceal haemorrhage has occurred show a reduction in fibrogenesis and a diminution of the obstruction to portal vein blood flow.[161] Ultrasound evaluation of patients with *S. japonicum* has indicated that moderate but not severe hepatic fibrosis diminishes on praziquantel with a reduction in spleen size, and that serum total bile acid levels can predict which patients are more likely to improve with chemotherapy.[162]

Comprehensive, recent reviews of the clinical pathology of the schistosomiases have been provided by Chen & Mott.[151,152,163,164].

Clonorchiasis and opisthorchiasis

Epidemiology and clinical features

Infection with the human liver flukes *Clonorchis* and *Opisthorchis* mainly occurs in the Far East. *C. sinensis* is prevalent in China, Taiwan, Hong Kong, Korea, and Vietnam. *O. viverrini* is frequent in the adult population of north-east Thailand. There are foci of *O. felineus* infection in eastern Europe, and apparently many cases in the former Soviet Union. The infection is acquired by ingesting cercariae in uncooked freshwater fish. Immature worms ascend and settle in the biliary tract, and occasionally the pancreatic duct.

Clonorchiasis and opisthorchiasis are clinically and pathologically similar and will be described together. Adult *C. sinensis* flukes are 8–25 mm long, 2–5 mm wide and 1 mm thick; *O. viverrini* is smaller, 11–20 mm long

and 3 mm wide. They usually live less than 10 but occasionally up to 25 years. They excrete their eggs into the bile. The diagnosis is usually made by identifying eggs in the faeces, but ultrasonography is increasingly important.

One-third of chronically infected people are asymptomatic. Surveys in Thailand found a prevalence of 5–10% of symptomatic cases in the population. Symptoms and pathology broadly correlate with the intensity of infection. The clinical disease is usually insidious. Blood eosinophilia is usual. Patients may present with abdominal pain, hepatomegaly and, less commonly, jaundice.[165] Portal hypertension and splenomegaly do not develop. Specific complications of the infection include biliary obstruction from the worms themselves, stricture and calculus formation, secondary ascending cholangitis and liver abscess, and occasionally cholecystitis. An important sequel in adults is cholangiocarcinoma. In endemic areas clonorchiasis and opisthorchiasis increase the incidence of this carcinoma by a factor of 20–40.[166] In some areas, the incidence reaches 87 per 100 000 per annum, approaching the frequency of hepatocellular carcinoma. One large hospital-based autopsy study in Thailand found that 55% of cadavers with opisthorchiasis had liver cancer, of which 44% were cholangiocarcinoma.[167]

Pathology

In light infections, worms are mainly found in the distal bile ducts, but with heavier loads the proximal ducts and the gallbladder are parasitized (Fig. 7.43). Worms in the gallbladder are usually dead. The left lobe of the liver is more commonly affected than the right because the left intrahepatic bile duct is straighter and wider, allowing more ready access to worms. The largest number of *Clonorchis* worms found in a liver was 27 000.

The pathology of heavy *Clonorchis* infection is detailed in the classic description by Hou.[168] The liver is enlarged

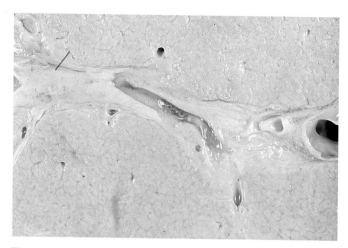

Fig. 7.43 Clonorchiasis. Fluke within a bile duct.

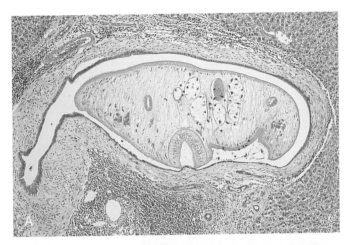

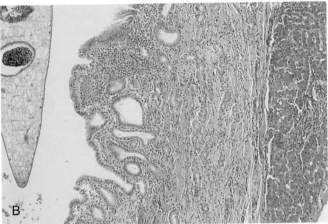

Fig. 7.44 Opisthorchiasis. (a) Fluke in bile duct, attached to the epithelium via its sucker. H&E. (b) Biliary epithelial proliferation associated with a fluke. H&E.

but not cirrhotic. The commonest macroscopic feature is focal dilatation of segments of smaller bile ducts to a diameter of 3–6 mm. The walls are thickened and worms are visible in the lumen (Fig. 7.44). Generalized bile-duct dilatation is uncommon and signifies a proximal stricture, stone or tumour.

Histologically, the bile-duct lining adjacent to the worms is hyperplastic, with infoldings of the epithelium ('adenomatous hyperplasia'). There is fibrosis and variable eosinophilia. Eggs are not seen in the tissues. Ascending cholangitis, usually due to *E. coli* infection, produces a purulent exudate in the dilated ducts and sometimes liver abscesses may form. Stones in the ducts often have dead worms as their nidus.

The cholangiocarcinoma associated with clonorchiasis is usually intrahepatic, multicentric and mucin-secreting. The pathogenesis is not certain. Malnutrition, and carcinogens, either ingested or formed in the bile, are factors proposed. The fluke itself may be only weakly carcinogenic, but constant irritation of biliary epithelium by the worms could act as a promoting agent.[169] This subject is discussed further in chapter 16.

For a comprehensive review of the recent literature on the clinical pathology of clonorchiasis, see Chen et al.[170]

Fascioliasis

Fasciola hepatica is a common zoonotic infection of sheep, goats and cattle. Man is only occasionally affected although many infections may be subclinical. Human infections are distributed globally but most cases occur in Europe. Eating watercress contaminated by metacercariae is the mode of infection. The immature fluke penetrates the liver capsule and migrates through the parenchyma to reside in the large bile ducts and the gallbladder. The leaf-like worm is up to 30 mm long and 13 mm wide, and lives for about 9 years. It adheres to and irritates the biliary epithelium via its suckers.

The clinical features are fever, upper abdominal pain and hepatomegaly during the phase of invasion and, in the chronic phase, ascending bacterial cholangitis with obstructive jaundice. Severe bleeding may occur from the biliary tract. A marked blood eosinophilia, reaching 30% or more of total white cell count, is typical. The diagnosis is made at laparotomy, ERCP, or by finding eggs in the faeces. Fatalities due to fascioliasis are uncommon.

Because the parasite migrates through the parenchyma, the liver may show yellow surface nodules 5–20 mm across. As in enterobiasis, these may be mistaken for metastatic carcinoma. Histologically, tracks are seen with much necrosis and eosinophilia around the worm. Subsequently, scars develop under the capsule.

Up to 40 worms may be found in an infected liver. Focal bile-duct dilatation is associated with a worm and there may be an acute cholangitis. Histologically, the bile epithelium is eroded, inflamed, and hyperplastic, and the surrounding portal tract is thickened and fibrotic (Fig. 7.45). Large necrotic granulomas can develop around trapped eggs. Tissue eosinophilia is typical in all these

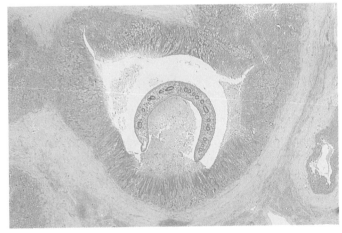

Fig. 7.45 Fascioliasis. Cross-section of a bile duct with a fluke exciting florid epithelial proliferation. H&E.

lesions. Adult flukes are often seen, along with gallstones, in the gallbladder which shows a hypertrophied muscle coat and hyperplastic inflamed mucosal epithelium.[171]

Fascioliasis is not associated with cholangiocarcinoma. A comprehensive, recent review of the clinical pathology of this infection has been provided by Chen & Mott.[172]

PENTASTOMIASIS

Pentastomes are worm-like organisms that share morphological features of helminths and arthropods. In Africa, most cases of visceral infection are caused by *Armillifer (Porocephalus) armillatus*. In Asia, other species are prevalent. Occasional cases of pentastomiasis with hepatic lesions have been reported in the United States.[173] The adult pentastomes live in snakes, and man is infected from ingesting either eggs in contaminated drinking water or larvae in raw snake meat. The larval nymphs migrate within the abdominal organs, including the liver; they do not mature to adults but die and degenerate. Most hepatic pentastomiasis is encountered as calcified nodules enclosing dead parasites. Autopsy and radiological surveys have produced remarkably high prevalences of healed pentastomiasis, such as 25% in West Africans[174] and 45% among certain groups of Malaysians.[175] In Africa, it is said to be the commonest cause of calcification in the liver.

The calcified lesions are 5–10 mm in diameter and histologically are often non-specific; there is old necrotic tissue and surrounding fibrosis. Earlier lesions show an identifiable or even viable parasite. It is folded in a C shape, has a thick crenellated cuticle, and contains an intestinal canal and striated muscle (Fig. 7.46).

HIV INFECTION AND AIDS

Infection by the human immunodeficiency viruses type 1 (HIV-1) and type 2 (HIV-2) causes the acquired im-

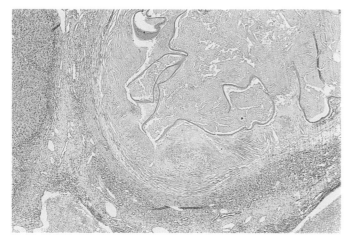

Fig. 7.46 Pentastomiasis. Typical appearance of a dead pentastome in liver. The irregular cuticle is surrounded by fibrous and granulomatous reaction. H&E.

munodeficiency syndrome, AIDS. First observed in the United States in the early 1980s, the epidemic of HIV-1 infection is now global and some 13 million people are currently infected. The worldwide prevalence of HIV infection varies greatly. Current predictions for HIV infections among adults by 1995 are 1.5 million in North America, 1.4 million in South America, 1.2 million in Western Europe, 1.2 million in Asia, and 11.5 million in sub-Saharan Africa.[176] In certain capital cities of Africa, HIV-1 seroprevalence rates in sentinel groups such as women of child-bearing age may reach 32%.[177] HIV-2 infection is mainly restricted to West Africa, although cases are occasionally seen elsewhere in immigrants or their sexual partners. It is a depressing fact that, within a decade, HIV-related disease has come totally to dominate hospital medicine and pathology in many countries in Africa.

Transmission of the HIVs is through sexual intercourse (vaginal and anal), transfusion of blood and blood products, needle sharing among intravenous drug users, and from mother to fetus. Among HIV-positive people in European countries, homosexual males and intravenous drug users predominate. However, heterosexual transmission is the dominant mode in developing countries, and the prevalence of infection is similar among males and females.[178]

Pathogenesis

The essential pathogenesis of the disease is the initial HIV infection and immune response, followed by the progressive destruction of CD4+ T-lymphocytes (T-helper cells) by the virus and, ultimately, AIDS.[179] The course runs from the time of infection, when there may be a seroconversion illness, through the latent asymptomatic phase, to the development of certain diseases that constitute AIDS. The latter are indicative of severely compromised cellular immunity, the most commonly used marker of which is the blood CD4+ T-lymphocyte count. These diseases include, according to the surveillance criteria for cases of AIDS: (i) specific opportunistic infections and tumours, (ii) clinically defined states such as wasting and dementia and, recently, (iii) the documentation of a blood CD4+ T-lymphocyte count less than 200/mm³ (normal range 500 – 2000 in adults) irrespective of symptoms.[180,181] Once AIDS has developed, death is inevitable. The survival period with HIV infection and disease varies widely according to geographical location and the availability of medical treatment; in industrialized countries, 10 or more years is now typical (Fig. 7.47).

GENERAL PATHOLOGICAL FEATURES IN THE LIVER

The liver and biliary tree are commonly affected by HIV-associated opportunistic infections and tumours, and liver

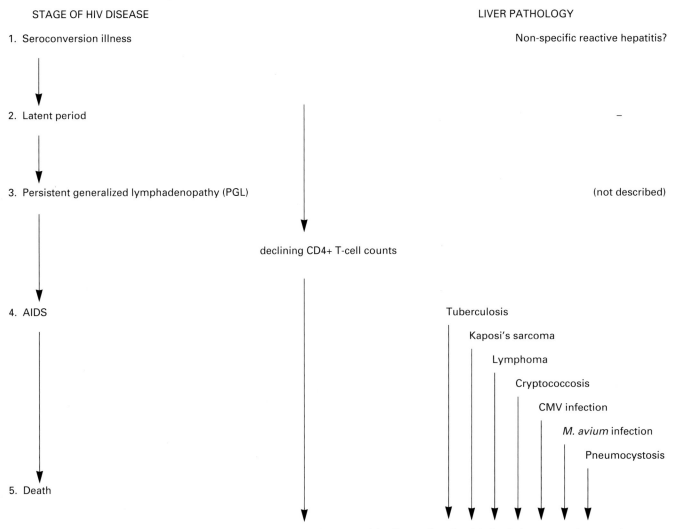

Fig. 7.47 The time course of HIV disease and liver pathology, indicating some of the diseases found and their relative presentation over time.

biopsy is a means of establishing such diagnoses (Table 7.3). However, HIV infection rarely produces liver failure. There is no evidence of a direct 'HIV-hepatitis' although other viral hepatitides are modified by HIV infection. HIV-positive people consume numerous drugs as prophylaxis and therapy, some of which are hepatotoxic. As the pandemic spreads and seroprevalence rates augment, any disease may be encountered in the liver of an HIV-infected person by chance. The HIV-associated diseases are those whose prevalences are significantly increased in HIV-positive people compared with the HIV-negative population, and/or whose clinico-pathological features are distinctly worsened by HIV infection.

The following account is primarily of HIV-1 disease, the major infection (see below for HIV-2 infection). There are several autopsy and biopsy series documenting the hepatic pathology in HIV disease,[182–185] and recent reviews of same.[83,186–188] All emanate from industrialized countries. However, the patterns of infections and tu-

mours in AIDS depend both on the mode of HIV transmission and where the infected person lives. For example, Kaposi's sarcoma is common in HIV-positive homosexuals but rare in HIV-positive haemophiliacs. Many of

Table 7.3 The main HIV-associated opportunistic diseases found in the liver of HIV-infected patients. Those marked* are AIDS-defining conditions for surveillance purposes

1. Non-specific: peliosis hepatis; sclerosing cholangitis (some cases are pathogen negative).
2. Specific infections:
   a. viral: cytomegalovirus*, herpes simplex virus*, Epstein–Barr virus, adenovirus, hepatitis B and C viruses.
   b. bacterial: *Mycobacterium tuberculosis**, *M. avium* complex and other mycobacteria*; *Rochalimaea henselae* (bacillary angiomatosis); Gram-negative bacillus sepsis*.
   c. fungal: *Candida**, *Cryptococcus neoformans**, *Histoplasma capsulatum**, *Penicillium marneffei*, *Pneumocystis carinii**, *Coccidioides immitis.**
   d. protozoal: *Toxoplasma gondii**, *Cryptosporidium parvum**, microsporidia, *Leishmania* spp.
3. Tumours: Kaposi's sarcoma*, high-grade B-cell lymphoma*.

the most significant opportunistic infections in AIDS are reactivations of latent asymptomatic infections acquired since birth, and these are often regionally restricted. Thus the hepatic pathology is not uniform around the world.

HIV seroconversion illness

Some 50% of HIV-infected people experience a seroconversion illness resembling infectious mononucleosis between 3 weeks and 6 months after infection. A small proportion of these develop an acute hepatitis syndrome with vomiting, upper abdominal pain and hepatomegaly. The serum transaminases are raised but there is no jaundice nor elevated serum alkaline phosphatase.[189,190] Serological evidence is against co-infection by other hepatitis viruses in these patients, and the liver disease resolves. No histopathological reports of liver biopsies are available, and the pathogenesis of this 'HIV-associated hepatitis' is uncertain.

Other general features

At some time during HIV disease, hepatomegaly is seen in 60% of patients in industrialized countries, and at autopsy the liver weight is more than 1800 g in 72% of cases.[188] This may not be universal: in a West African autopsy study, the mean liver weight (approximately 1550 g) was no different in HIV-negative and HIV-positive patients, nor different between those dying with or without an AIDS-defining condition (personal observations).

Mild to moderate degrees of macrovesicular fatty change are common in liver biopsy and autopsy material in HIV-positive patients, particularly those with AIDS. Moderate chronic lymphocytic inflammation of portal tracts is common as a non-specific reactive hepatitis. These are regarded as the non-specific consequences of a chronic wasting disease. Haemosiderin deposits in Kupffer cells are common in those to whom blood transfusions have been given to maintain haemoglobin levels. If there is bone marrow failure, haemopoiesis may be seen in the sinusoids. Rarely, massive and sometimes fatal macrovesicular fatty change occurs, with the liver at autopsy weighing 5 kg or more.[191] In the cases reported, such patients have not had terminal AIDS (their CD4 counts were more than 100/mm³). Anti-retroviral therapy with azidothymidine has been implicated as the cause.

Granulomas are found in liver biopsy and autopsy material in up to one-third of HIV-positive patients.[184,192] The main causes are *M. avium* complex infection, tuberculosis, and mycoses. In patients with AIDS, HIV-1 can usually be demonstrated in the liver by in-situ hybridization probes and by immunocytochemistry against p24 antigen.[193,194] Kupffer cells and endothelial cells contain more virus than hepatocytes, and the liver is probably a site of active replication of the virus.

Peliosis hepatis

The term refers to the presence of multiple blood-filled cystic spaces in the liver, previously associated with tuberculosis, cancer cachexia and androgen therapy. It is infrequently seen in patients with AIDS.[195] The lesions are visible as red spots beneath the capsule of the liver, which may be greatly enlarged. Histologically, they appear as 1–4 mm cysts within the parenchyma, containing blood. A partial endothelial lining may be present and adjacent sinusoids are ectatic. The aetiology is unclear; degeneration of hepatocytes is indicated by residual reticulin fibres in the lesions.

Amyloidosis

Amyloidosis is reported in HIV patients without other predisposing conditions, and the liver may be affected.[196,197] In Africa, despite the high frequency of tuberculosis associated with HIV infection, amyloidosis is only occasionally seen.

INFECTIONS OF THE LIVER

Viral infections

Cytomegalovirus

Reactivation of cytomegalovirus (CMV) is frequent in HIV disease but significant pathology is unusual until CD4+ T-lymphocyte counts are very low (less than 50/mm³). Hepatic disease due to parenchymal cytomegalovirus infection is minor.[186] In up to 10% of patients, microscopic examination shows scanty cytomegalovirus inclusions in hepatocytes, Kupffer cells and endothelial cells. This is usually associated with only a small zone of necrosis and inflammation. However, cytomegalovirus infection can occasionally be a cause of severe bile-duct necrosis (Fig. 7.48), and it is also associated with sclerosing cholangitis.

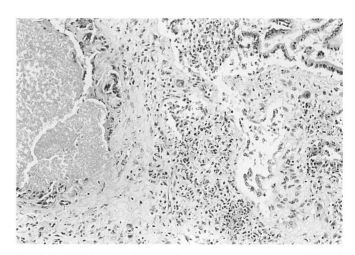

Fig. 7.48 CMV infection. Large, inflamed portal tract with two CMV inclusions and necrotic bile duct (at left). H&E. See also Fig. 7.4

Herpes simplex virus

Disseminated Herpes simplex virus infection is uncommon in HIV disease. However, it can present with liver failure. At autopsy, the enlarged liver shows hepatic necrosis affecting zones 2 and 3 of the acini, multinucleate hepatocytes, ground-glass nuclear inclusions, and minimal inflammation[198] (Fig. 7.3).

Epstein-Barr virus

An Epstein–Barr-virus-associated lymphoproliferative disorder affecting many lymphoreticular organs is associated with HIV infection. Histologically, the liver shows an infiltrate of immunoblasts in sinusoids but no necrosis.[199]

Adenovirus

Adenovirus hepatitis in HIV-positive patients appears to be restricted to children and, occasionally, to young adults.[27,28] As well as fever and hepatomegaly, it presents with a bleeding diathesis. Histologically, there is extensive zone 3 hepatocyte necrosis, little inflammation, and abundant intranuclear viral inclusions.

Viral hepatitides—HAV, HBV, HCV, HDV

Risk factors that greatly increase the likelihood of hepatotropic virus infections are intravenous drug use (HBV, HCV and HDV), homosexual activity (HBV), and being African (HBV). There is no evidence of an association between HIV and hepatitis A virus infections.

Hepatitis B. HIV-positive men infected with HBV are at an increased risk of becoming chronic carriers as CD4+ T-lymphocyte counts fall.[200] Moreover, HIV infection seems to permit the reactivation of, or reinfection by, HBV infection in those who had earlier become HBsAg-seronegative.[201] In terms of clinical manifestations, HIV-positive patients are less likely to be icteric following HBV infection than HIV-negative individuals.[200] Liver biopsy studies have also demonstrated that HIV-positive patients have less active chronic HBV disease and less scarring, and HBV-associated cirrhosis is less frequent. Further, expression of HBeAg and HBV-DNA polymerase is greater, indicating that HBV viral replication is more active in HIV-positives.[202] Within HIV-positive cohorts, acute hepatitis (HBV, and 'non-A, non-B') and chronic active hepatitis are found more often in those who have not developed AIDS, and therefore have better cell-mediated immunity than those with AIDS.[203]

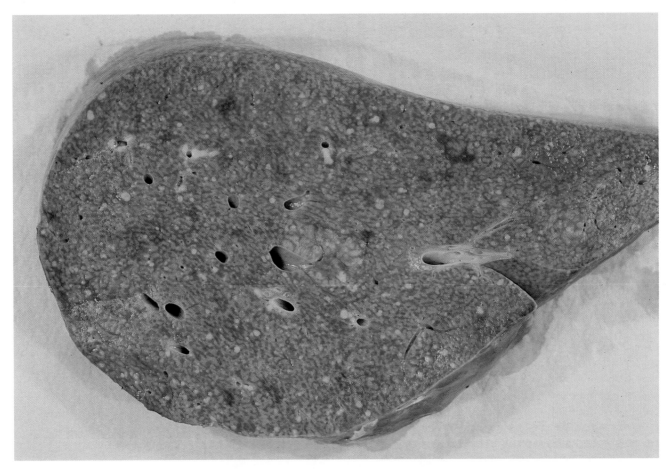

Fig. 7.49 Miliary tuberculosis of the liver in an HIV-positive adult. Slice of liver with numerous small white spots of necrosis. See also Fig. 7.14

Concerning the effect of HBV infection on the biology of HIV disease, one European study has suggested that, among HIV-positive men, those who are HBcAg-sero-positive progress to AIDS faster than those without evidence of active HBV infection,[204] but this association may be spurious, confounded by other behaviour and infection co-factors.

Hepatitis C. The biological sequelae of co-infection with HCV and HIV are still unclear, although it appears that the cadence of HCV disease is unchanged or milder in HIV-positive patients.[205]

Hepatitis D. Although HDV is dependent on HBV infection, it is not known whether its pathogenicity is modified by HIV co-infection.[186]

Bacterial infections

Tuberculosis

From being rare initially, the prevalence of tuberculosis in HIV-positive patients in industrialized countries is increasing, and it is high in Africa and India.[206] An autopsy study in West Africa found that 50% of adults dying of AIDS had active tuberculosis and in 85% of them the liver was involved (Fig. 7.49). Tuberculosis was, in fact, the commonest specific hepatic HIV-associated lesion.[207]

The macroscopic features include single or multiple mass lesions, and miliary tuberculosis which is the commonest pattern in AIDS patients. Depending on the cellular immune status of the patient, the pathology of the lesions varies. Granulomas with Langhans' giant cells and caseation may be seen, or non-giant cell epithelioid cell granulomas. Acid-fast bacilli are usually scanty in these cases. However, at the extreme of immune deficiency commonly seen in terminal AIDS patients with tuberculosis, the histological pattern is that of non-reactive (anergic) tuberculosis. Foci of granular necrosis are surrounded by degenerate swollen macrophages, and large numbers of acid-fast bacilli are present[208] (Fig. 7.14).

Other mycobacterioses

The prevalence of *M. avium* complex infection in HIV-positive patients depends on geography, being rare in developing countries, and on survival. Some 25% of those with *M. avium* bacillaemia have liver infection on biopsy or at autopsy.[209] However, the prevalence is inversely correlated with CD4+ T-lymphocyte count, rising to 40% when it is less than 10/mm³. *M. avium* may eventually infect most patients who do not die earlier from another HIV-related event.[210]

M. avium complex infection is frequently associated with raised serum alkaline phosphatase as enlarged lymph nodes compress the bile duct, or intrahepatic *M. avium* granulomas obstruct terminal ductules. Abscesses may

develop and contain numerous bacilli on Ziehl–Neelsen stain.[74] More frequently, there are miliary nodules of non-necrotic epithelioid cell granulomas throughout the parenchyma. When immune deficiency is extreme, clusters of histiocytes are seen with bluish and even striated cytoplasm due to the vast numbers of acid-fast bacilli (Fig. 7.50).[73]

Disseminated infections with many other species of mycobacteria are recorded in HIV-positive patients and often involve the liver. The histopathological appearances are not distinct from tuberculosis and culture is required to identify them. Against expectations, leprosy is not more frequent or more severe in HIV-positive people.[211]

Bacillary angiomatosis and cat-scratch disease

In the livers of some patients with HIV-associated peliosis hepatis, lesions resembling bacillary angiomatosis of the skin are also found. Macroscopically these are greyish or haemorrhagic nodules, and microscopically show fibrovascular and vascular proliferation accompanied by neutro-

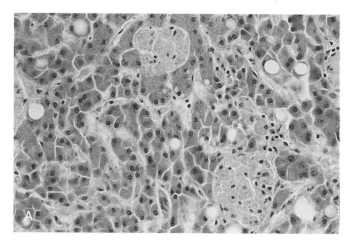

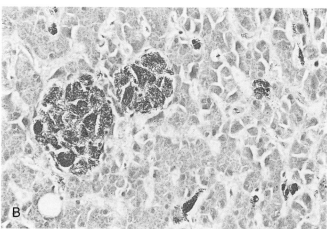

Fig. 7.50 *M. avium* complex infection. (a) Discrete, non-necrotic aggregates of unactivated macrophages in the sinusoids. The blue haematoxyphilic cytoplasm results from the tightly packed mycobacteria. H&E. (b) Ziehl–Neelsen stain of same liver, showing large numbers of intracellular acid-fast bacilli.

phils.[212,213] Between liver-cell plates and the blood vessels, there is a myxoid stroma that contains clumps of granular material.[214] On Warthin-Starry stain (Fig. 7.51), these are masses of bacilli that are morphologically similar to those seen in the lesions of cutaneous bacillary angio-

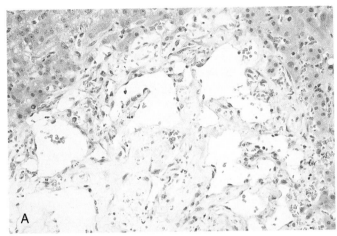

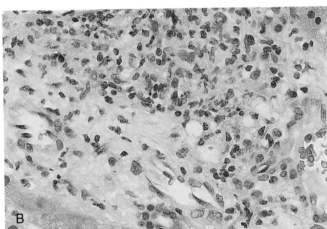

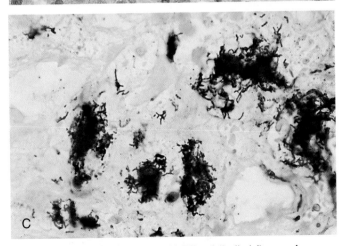

Fig. 7.51 Bacillary angiomatosis. (a) Dilated ('peliotic') avascular components with surrounding myxoid stroma. (b) Portal tract with chronic inflammatory cells around blood vessels, and granular greyish stroma which contains abundant bacteria. (c) Warthin–Starry stain of the same liver showing clumps of silver-positive bacilli. Slides courtesy of Dr T J Stephenson, Sheffield

matosis. This agent is now characterized as the rickettsial organism *Rochalimaea henselae*.[215] It is possible that it secretes an angiogenic factor that leads to bacillary angiomatosis and/or peliosis.

Rarely, cat-scratch disease also affects the liver in HIV-positive patients, with pathology similar to that in non-HIV-infected individuals.[216]

Q fever

Recent serological evidence suggests that infection with *Coxiella burnetii* is 3 times more frequent among HIV-positive individuals than in HIV-negative controls, and cases of disease are 12 times more frequent. However, the course of the disease with treatment is unaffected by HIV status. There is fever and sometimes hepatomegaly. Liver biopsy shows a granulomatous hepatitis.[217]

Gram-positive and Gram-negative sepsis

Septicaemia due to Gram-positive cocci (staphylococci and streptococci) and Gram-negative bacilli (particularly non-typhoid salmonellae) is strongly associated with HIV infection.[218,219] These infections may produce hepatic abscesses.

Fungal infections

Many disseminated fungal infections involving the liver have been reported.[184] The most important infections are by *Candida albicans*, *Cryptococcus neoformans*, *Histoplasma capsulatum*, *Penicillium marneffei*, *Coccidioides immitis*, and *Pneumocystis carinii*. *Histoplasmosis duboisii*, blastomycosis and aspergillosis have also been encountered occasionally.[220-223] Liver biopsy may detect these diseases, but the most sensitive techniques for identifying them (except pneumocystosis) are blood culture or blood antigenaemia tests.[188]

Candidiasis and cryptococcosis

Candidiasis and cryptococcosis are ubiquitous infections and are documented in the liver in 2–14% of HIV-positive patients in industrialized countries.[192] Candidiasis often presents as small purulent abscesses containing the yeasts and hyphae. Cryptococcosis may cause hepatomegaly. It is a diffuse intracellular infection of Kupffer cells and portal macrophages (Fig. 7.17). Foreign-body-type giant cells may also be seen containing many yeasts.

Histoplasmosis

The prevalence of histoplasmosis in HIV disease depends on geography since the infection is rare in Europe or Australasia. A 1–4% prevalence of hepatic histoplasmosis

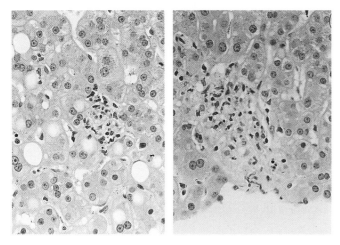

Fig. 7.52 Histoplasmosis. Liver biopsy of an HIV-positive man with fever revealed small non-necrotic granulomas. The yeasts are difficult to see, but can be highlighted by special stains. H&E. See also Fig. 7.18b

in the United States has been quoted.[188,192] Histologically, small non-giant cell granulomas may be seen throughout the parenchyma or portal tracts, containing budding yeasts 3–5 μm in diameter (Figs 7.18 and 7.52). In heavy infections, Kupffer cells may be filled with yeasts.

Penicilliosis

Although infection with *Penicillium marneffei* is not currently an AIDS-defining condition, it is strikingly frequent in patients with HIV infection in Thailand and Hong Kong. Histologically, a diffuse infiltrate of yeast-laden macrophages replaces the liver parenchyma (Fig. 7.20).[224] The 3–4 μm diameter yeasts closely resemble *H. capsulatum* in size, but also show the characteristic features of forming tubes and elongated, septate spores.

Coccidioidomycosis

This mycosis is endemic in the Americas only, and is found in the liver as part of disseminated disease in AIDS patients. Histologically there are multiple granulomas containing the characteristic 20–200 μm diameter spherules.[183,225]

Nocardiosis

Nocardiosis (mainly *N. asteroides*) is uncommon but appears to be associated with HIV infection.[226] Hepatic lesions occur as part of disseminated disease. Macroscopically, they resemble miliary tuberculosis. Histologically the lesions are small or large purulent abscesses, sometimes with a granulomatous edge, containing branching and beaded bacilli. These are invisible in H&E-stained sections but are clearly demonstrated by Grocott silver stain; they are also Gram-positive and are weakly acid-fast by the Wade–Fite method (Fig. 7.11).

Pneumocystis carinii

P.carinii is an enigmatic organism. Previously it was considered to be a protozoon but now — on the basis of studies of ribosomal RNA homology — it is classed as a fungus. It is probably ubiquitous in soil or air, and, globally, most children manifest a subclinical antibody response to infection before the age of 10 years.[227] Immunodepression from malnutrition, steroid therapy and HIV infection predisposes to pneumocystis pneumonia. Before systematic anti-pneumocystis prophylaxis was instituted, more than 85% of patients with AIDS in industrialized countries developed pneumocystis pneumonia some time before death. Spread of the infection outside the lungs is common in HIV-positive patients with CD4+ T-lymphocyte counts less than 50/mm³, often associated with use of nebulized (inhaled) pentamidine therapy for pneumocystosis. The liver may then be involved in up to 40% of such cases.[184,228,229] Extra-pulmonary pneumocystosis has not yet been seen in HIV disease in Africa.

There is no notable macroscopic appearance. Microscopically there are focal areas where the sinuses are widened and the liver cells are necrotic, being replaced by extracellular frothy pink material on H&E stain. On high power, pale cysts containing a haematoxyphilic dot are seen amongst the eosinophilic material (Fig. 7.53). With a Grocott stain, the characteristic cysts are more evident, their membranes often folded over and bearing a solid dark spot.

Protozoal infections

The protozoa that are more frequent in the liver in HIV-positive patients are *Toxoplasma gondii*, *Leishmania* spp., *Cryptosporidium parvum*, and microsporidia. The last two primarily affect the biliary tree and are considered below.

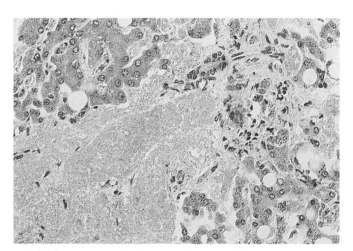

Fig. 7.53 *Pneumocystis carinii* infection. Post-mortem liver: eosinophilic granular material composed of cysts has infiltrated the sinusoids and replaced the liver cells. H&E. Slide courtesy of Dr R Goldin, London

Toxoplasmosis

Disseminated toxoplasmosis (i.e. outside the usual location of the brain) is uncommon in AIDS patients. Hepatic lesions are occasionally encountered in autopsy material, with microscopic lesions composed of one or more parasitized parenchymal cells which contain zoites and are surrounded by a few lymphocytes or polymorphs (Fig. 7.28).

Leishmaniasis

The prevalence of leishmaniasis in the liver in HIV-positive patients depends on geography, since the species and strains of *Leishmania* that cause visceral infection are restricted to southern Europe, South America and Africa. Like *H. capsulatum* and *M. tuberculosis*, leishmanial parasites can remain latent in the body for years, only to reactivate as immune competence declines.

The majority of HIV-positive patients with visceral leishmaniasis are intravenous drug users in Europe, and the agent is *L. infantum*. Three-quarters present with leishmaniasis when they already have AIDS and the CD4+ T-lymphocyte counts are about 150/mm³. This infection is not currently an AIDS-defining condition for surveillance purposes, although it seems that HIV-positive people are more likely to develop disease than HIV-negative individuals.[230] The potential magnitude of this co-infection is illustrated by a 17% prevalence of leishmanial infection in one Spanish series of HIV-positive people with a fever of unknown origin.[231]

The presentation in HIV-positive people may be atypical, a smaller proportion having hepatosplenomegaly or positive anti-leishmanial serology. The response to chemotherapy is more variable and there is a greater likelihood of relapse.[232] However, the liver pathology is the same as in non-HIV-infected people: numerous amastigotes within Kupffer cells and portal macrophages (Fig. 7.24).[184,233]

Amoebiasis

Amoebiasis (infection with *Entamoeba histolytica*) was expected to be an opportunistic infection in HIV-infected patients, but there is no epidemiological evidence for this association.[234] In regions where amoebiasis is common, incidental co-infection may occur.

Helminthic infections

Helminthic infections are not more virulent in immunocompromised patients since few of them proliferate in the host. Common infections (e.g. schistosomiasis) and rarities (e.g. dicrocoeliasis) have been reported in the livers of HIV-positive patients, but their effects are not modified by HIV infection.[235,236] Disseminated infection by *Strongyloides stercoralis* — a worm which does multiply in the host — was initially expected to occur with increased frequency in HIV-positive patients and to be an AIDS-defining disease.[234] Although a few cases have been reported with hepatic involvement,[237] epidemiological studies have not found a significant association between strongyloidiasis and HIV infection.

TUMOURS

The established HIV-associated tumours are Kaposi's sarcoma and non-Hodgkin's lymphoma.

Kaposi's sarcoma

The notable increase in the incidence of Kaposi's sarcoma in the United States was one of the first indications of the HIV pandemic. It involves the liver in up to one fifth of autopsied AIDS patients in industrialized countries, though its prevalence elsewhere is less. Only rarely is hepatic Kaposi's sarcoma the first presentation of AIDS since the liver is usually involved as part of cutaneous and visceral disseminated disease.[238] Macroscopically, there may be capsular deposits of tumour, 5–10 mm in diameter, appearing as dark-red blebs. On cut section, Kaposi's sarcoma radiates out from the portal tracts and follows the bile ducts.[239] It also causes multiple dark-red spots in the parenchyma (Fig. 7.54). Histologically, the typical lesion is a bland spindle-cell tumour arising around bile ducts and forming a mesh that contains erythrocytes (Fig. 7.55). Early lesions may be difficult to diagnose. They consist of irregular thin-walled dilated vessels which separate the collagen fibres of capsular and portal connective tissue. Clues to the diagnosis of Kaposi's sarcoma include the diffuse presence of plasma cells, infrequent and normal mitoses, and clusters of intracytoplasmic eosinophilic

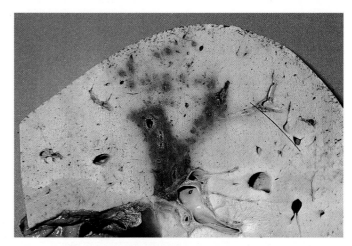

Fig. 7.54 Kaposi's sarcoma. Purplish lesions infiltrating the portal tracts and spreading into the parenchyma. Fixed liver

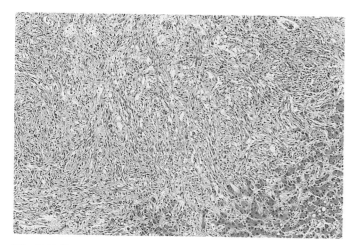

Fig. 7.55 Kaposi's sarcoma. Interlacing bands of Kaposi spindle cells infiltrating a portal tract and extending into the parenchyma. H&E.

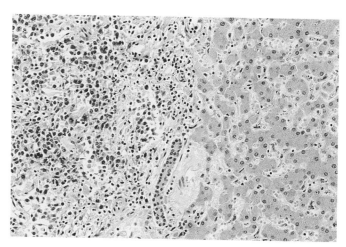

Fig. 7.56 HIV-associated non-Hodgkin's lymphoma. Autopsy liver showing malignant lymphoid cells infiltrating a portal tract. H&E.

inclusions which resemble erythrocytes but are smaller. Although it is called a sarcoma, it is likely that Kaposi's 'disease' is probably a benign reactive vascular hyperplasia.[240]

Lymphomas

HIV-infected people are at high risk of developing non-Hodgkin's lymphoma. It is nearly always a high-grade B-cell lymphoma and the proportion having extra-nodal disease is greater than among HIV-negative patients. Typically, B-cell lymphoma develops when the CD4+ T-lymphocyte counts are below 100/mm³. As treatment of complications prolongs the survival of HIV-infected patients, it is expected that the proportion with lymphoma will increase, perhaps to one-third or more of those who survive more than 3 years with AIDS.[241]

The liver is involved in over a quarter of HIV-positive patients with lymphoma and it may be primary there.[242] Infiltration is often diffuse but mass lesions also occur, with multifocal pale tumours several centimetres in diameter. These are often necrotic and can mimic tuberculosis or *M. avium* complex infection. Primary bile-duct lymphoma, clinically and radiologically mimicking sclerosing cholangitis, has also been reported.[243] Histologically, the lymphoma cells are centroblastic or immunoblastic, often with bizarre polylobated nuclei (Fig. 7.56).

Although Hodgkin's disease has been reported in AIDS patients, it is not clear whether it is aetiologically associated with HIV infection.[244] However, it tends to pursue a more rapidly progressive clinical course.

Other tumours

There is no evidence for an increased frequency of visceral carcinomas but there is an impression that such tumours

are more aggressive in HIV-positive patients. Whilst earlier studies in the United States suggested that hepatocellular carcinoma was associated with HIV infection, more recent larger series have not confirmed this.[245] None the less, the more frequent persistence of HBV envelope protein in HIV-positive people suggests the potential for an association.

CHOLANGITIS

Two types of cholangitis are seen in HIV-positive patients: ascending bacterial cholangitis and HIV-associated sclerosing cholangitis. The frequency of bacterial cholangitis is not known; the organisms are usually Gram-negative bacilli. The disease resembles that seen in non-HIV-infected people, with dilated biliary tracts and parenchymal abscesses (Fig. 7.57).

Sclerosing cholangitis

HIV-associated sclerosing cholangitis is increasingly recognized as a complication of advanced immune depression: the median CD4+ T-lymphocyte count of patients at diagnosis was 24/mm³.[246] It is characterized by chronic abdominal pain, fever, and cholestasis with dilatation and irregularities of the bile ducts, both intra- and extrahepatic. The diagnosis is usually made by ERCP; some cases are virtually identical to primary sclerosing cholangitis (see Ch. 12).

The role of infectious agents

Cryptosporidiosis. Cryptosporidiosis (*C. parvum*) and cytomegalovirus infections are the most frequently documented. Two-thirds of patients with cholangitis are infected with one or both agents.[246] In a study of HIV-positive men with cryptosporidial diarrhoea, 26% had

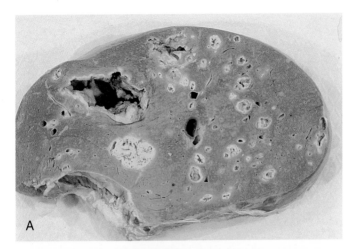

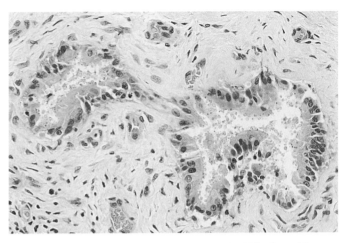

Fig. 7.58 Cryptosporidial cholangitis. Medium-sized bile duct with numerous *Cryptosporidium* bodies at the luminal surface of epithelial cells. With electron microscopy, these are seen to reside just within the plasma membrane. H&E.

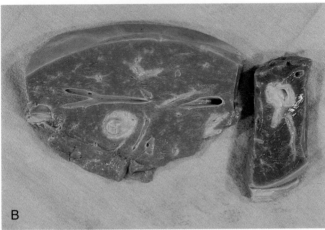

Fig. 7.57 Cholangitis in HIV-positive patients. (a) Slice of liver with bacterial ascending cholangitis and several associated hepatic abscesses. (b) Sclerosing cholangitis with fibrotic portal tracts.

sclerosing cholangitis.[247] The extrahepatic biliary mucosa is inflamed, often fibrotic, and the epithelium is hyperplastic. The cryptosporidia are seen adhering to the surface of biliary epithelial cells (Fig. 7.58), although electron microscopy shows them to be intracellular, covered by brush-border membrane. Intrahepatic portal tracts are frequently normal but may show mild inflammation, periductal fibrosis or ductal obliteration. Uncommonly, one sees the cryptosporidia attached to small intrahepatic bile ducts in liver biopsies. Similarly, cytomegalovirus inclusions are more often seen in the extrahepatic than in the intrahepatic ducts. Currently, it is thought that *C. parvum* is the major aetiological agent in HIV-associated sclerosing cholangitis, and that cytomegalovirus is usually a passenger infection (Fig. 7.48).

Analysis of MHC class I and II antigens in the liver in HIV disease has shown that HLA-DR II expression is only found in biliary epithelium, but this does not correlate with biliary pathology.[248] Whether HIV itself causes cholangitis is not clear. Since a similar association with cryptosporidiosis is seen in congenitally immunodeficient children without HIV infection,[249] it is considered that *C. parvum* is a sufficient cause of sclerosing cholangitis. However, the pathogenetic mechanisms are unknown.

Microsporidiosis. Microsporidiosis is being diagnosed in an increasing number of the 'pathogen-negative' cases of HIV-associated sclerosing cholangitis. Microsporidia are small oval obligate intracellular protozoan parasites that live and multiply in the cytoplasm of host cells. In man, two genera are important, *Enterocytozoon* and *Encephalitozoon*.[250] They are recognizable with some difficulty on H&E-stained sections in the supranuclear cytoplasm as clusters of pale refractile spores with a tiny haematoxyphilic nucleus. More sensitive is toluidine blue stain on semi-thin resin sections, or electron microscopy, which is needed to determine the genus and species (Fig. 7.59). A characteristic feature of microsporidia is an electron-dense coiled polar tube.

Enterocytozoon bieneusi is a parasite of small bowel enterocytes found in a proportion of HIV-positive patients with diarrhoea. It has also been observed in the bile of patients with HIV-associated sclerosing cholangitis, and within the cytoplasm of biliary epithelial cells of liver, extrahepatic ducts and gallbladder. There is usually an associated mild mononuclear inflammation of the lamina propria. Cases of co-infection of the biliary tree involving microsporidia, cytomegalovirus, *Cryptosporidium* and *M. avium* infection are being reported.[251–254]

Encephalitozoon has been noted within hepatocytes in a patient with a necrotizing granulomatous and suppurative hepatitis.[255] The same organism has also been seen in sinusoidal lining cells and lying free in clusters in the portal vein.[251]

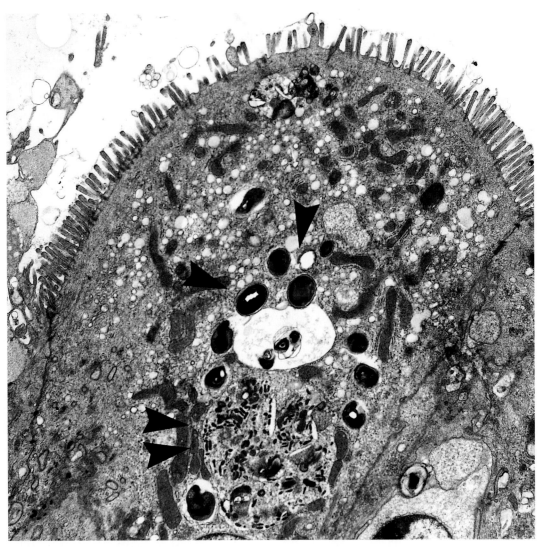

Fig. 7.59 Microsporidiosis. Electron micrograph of *Enterocytozoon bieneusi* forms within an epithelial cell: spores (single arrowheads); proliferating plasmodia (double arrowheads). x 5000. Photograph courtesy of Mr G Tovey, London

PAEDIATRIC HIV-ASSOCIATED LIVER DISEASE

By 1995, the WHO estimates that there will be 2.3 million HIV-infected children, 90% of them residing in sub-Saharan Africa.[176] An increasing majority are infected by their mothers. The course of HIV disease in children is bimodal: a proportion, perhaps mainly those infected in utero, become ill and die within 1–2 years of birth; those infected perinatally, or by transfusion later, present when some years older.[256]

The liver is often enlarged and shows non-specific features of fatty change and mild portal chronic inflammation. Whilst cytomegalovirus and *M. avium* complex infections, tuberculosis, Kaposi's sarcoma and lymphoma occur in HIV-positive children, they are less frequent than in adults. Hepatic granulomas are uncommon, and hepatic pneumocystosis has not been reported; neither has HIV-associated cholangitis, despite the fact that intestinal cryptosporidiosis is common in children.

Conversely, two hepatic lesions are restricted to children: *giant cell transformation* and a *nodular lymphoplasmacytic portal infiltrate*. It has been suggested that these changes represent abnormal responses to Epstein–Barr virus.[257,258] Some children with hepatomegaly have chronic active hepatitis and bile-duct damage.[259] Unlike in hepatitis B virus infection and autoimmune liver disease, these HIV-positive children have predominantly CD8+ T-lymphocytes in the portal tracts. Adenovirus hepatitis is also usually confined to children.

In African children dying with HIV infection, specific hepatic lesions are uncommon although cytomegalovirus, necrotizing herpes simplex, miliary tuberculosis and toxoplasmosis have all been noted. Severe malaria infection is not more prevalent in HIV-positive children than in controls.[100]

DRUG TOXICITY IN HIV DISEASE

The polypharmacy of HIV-positive patients in industrialized countries is such that drug reactions are an important concern. The prevalence of raised liver enzymes and of clinical hepatitis varies widely. The major potential hepatotoxic drugs are listed in Table 7.4. The widely used anti-retroviral agent, azidothymidine, is only rarely associated with hepatotoxicity though it has been implicated in fatal macrovesicular steatosis.[191,260] Dideoxyinosine may induce microvesicular damage in hepatocytes and fulminant liver failure.[261] The other drugs can cause acute hepatitis, to be distinguished from infective hepatitis.

HIV-2 AND LIVER DISEASE

HIV-2 infection is mainly confined to West Africa, although patients with this infection, with or without HIV-1 co-infection, are also encountered in Europe. HIV-2 causes AIDS, although the progression of disease may be slower than with HIV-1. The same range of pathological manifestations is seen in the liver of such patients, including tuberculosis, sclerosing cholangitis and leishmaniasis.[262,263]

THE ROLE OF LIVER BIOPSY IN HIV DISEASE

Many studies of HIV-positive patients with fever, hepatomegaly and abnormal liver function tests of unknown aetiology have been published, and diagnostic strategies involving liver biopsy proposed.[183,186,188,264] Diagnostic yields of up to 50% are quoted, higher than in the investigation of fever of unknown origin in non-HIV patients.[265] The common histological findings include specific infective conditions and tumours, and non-specific features such as lymphocytic infiltrate of the portal tracts, haemosiderosis, and macrovesicular steatosis which reflect systemic illness and repeated blood transfusions.

The diagnostic sensitivity of liver histology for disseminated infections such as mycobacterioses and mycoses is lower than other techniques such as blood culture, marrow and lymph node examination, and the detection of fungal antigenaemia. Liver biopsy is most useful in evaluation of liver masses, drug hepatotoxicity versus infections, biliary tree abnormalities, and undiagnosed fever and hepatosplenomegaly.

It is essential to examine liver biopsies from all HIV-positive patients with Grocott silver stain for fungi and nocardiosis, Ziehl–Neelsen for mycobacteria and, if bacillary angiomatosis is suspected, a Warthin–Starry stain.

Table 7.4 Potentially hepatotoxic drugs commonly used in HIV-positive people (see also Ch. 16)

Drug	Indication
Azidothymidine	anti-retroviral
Dideoxyinosine	anti-retroviral
Co-trimoxazole	*Pneumocystis carinii* infection
Pentamidine	*Pneumocystis* and *Toxoplasma* infections
Ketoconazole	anti-fungal
Fluconazole	anti-fungal
Rifampicin	anti-mycobacterial
Isoniazid	anti-mycobacterial
Ganciclovir	anti-cytomegalovirus

REFERENCES

1. Beaver P C, Jung R C, Cupp E W. Clinical parasitology. Philadelphia: Lea & Febiger, 1984
2. Lucas S B. Pathology of tropical infections. In: McGee J O, Isaacson P G, Wright N A, eds. Oxford textbook of pathology. Oxford: Oxford University Press, 1992: pp 2187–2266
3. Cook G C. Tropical gastroenterology. Oxford: Oxford University Press, 1980
4. Hutt M S R. Some aspects of liver disease in Ugandan Africans. Trans R Soc Trop Med Hyg 1971; 65: 273–285
5. Gutierrez Y. Diagnostic pathology of parasitic infections with clinical correlations. Philadelphia: Lea & Febiger, 1990
6. AFIP. Pathology of tropical and extraordinary diseases. Washington, D C: Armed Forces Institute of Pathology, 1976
7. Mandell G L, Douglas R G, Bennett J E. Principles and practice of infectious diseases. New York: Churchill Livingstone, 1990
8. Ishak K G, Walker D H, Coetzer J A W, Gardner J J, Gorelkin L. Viral hemorrhagic fevers with hepatic involvement: pathologic aspects with clinical correlations. In: Popper H, Schaffner F, eds. Progress in liver diseases, vol VII. New York: Grune & Stratton, 1982: pp 495–515
9. De Cock K M, Nasidi A, Enriquez J et al. Epidemic yellow fever in Eastern Nigeria, 1986. Lancet 1989; i: 630–633
10. Francis T I, Moore D L, Edington G M, Smith J A. A clinicopathological study of human yellow fever. Bull WHO 1972; 46: 659–667
11. Edington G M, White H A. The pathology of Lassa fever. Trans R Soc Trop Med Hyg 1972; 66: 381–389
12. Johnson K M. Marburg and Ebola viruses. In: Mandell G L, Douglas R G, Bennett J E, eds. Principles and practice of infectious diseases, 3rd edn. New York: Churchill Livingstone, 1990: pp 1303–1305
13. Rippey J J, Schepers N J, Gear J H S. The pathology of Marburg virus disease. S Afr Med J 1984; 66: 50–54
14. Walker D P, Longson M, Lawler W, Mallick N P, Davies J S, Johnson R W G. Disseminated herpes simplex virus infection with hepatitis in an adult renal transplant recipient. J Clin Pathol 1981; 34: 1044–1046
15. Goodman Z D, Ishak K G, Sesterhenn I A. Herpes simplex hepatitis in apparently immunocompetent adults. Am J Clin Pathol 1986; 85: 694–699
16. Kasper W J, Howe P M. Fatal varicella after a single course of corticosteroids. Pediatr Infect Dis J 1990; 9: 729–732
17. Clarke J, Craig R M, Saffro R, Murphy P, Yokoo H. Cytomegalovirus granulomatous hepatitis. Am J Med 1979; 66: 264–269
18. Snover D C, Horwitz C A. Liver disease in cytomegalovirus mononucleosis: a light microscopical and immunoperoxidase study of six cases. Hepatology 1984; 4: 408–412
19. Vanstapel M-J, Desmet V J. Cytomegalovirus hepatitis: a histological and immunohistochemical study. Appl Pathol 1983; 1: 41–49
20. Finegold M J, Carpenter R J. Obliterative cholangitis due to cytomegalovirus: a possible precursor of paucity of intrahepatic bile ducts. Hum Pathol 1982; 13: 662–665

21. Purtilo D T, Sakamoto K. Epstein–Barr virus and human disease: immune response determines the clinical and pathologic expression. Hum Pathol 1981; 12: 677–679

22. Kilpatrick Z M. Structural and functional abnormalities of liver in infectious mononucleosis. Arch Intern Med 1966; 117: 47–53

23. Ishak K G. Granulomas of the liver. In: Ioachim H L, ed. Pathology of granulomas. New York: Raven Press, 1983: pp 309–369

24. Purtilo D T, DeFlorio D, Hutt L M et al. Variable phenotypic expression of an X-linked recessive lymphoproliferative syndrome. N Engl J Med 1977; 297: 1077–1080.

25. Chang M Y, Campbell W G. Fatal infectious mononucleosis. Association with liver necrosis and herpes-like virus particles. Arch Pathol Lab Med 1975; 99: 185–191

26. Carmichael G P, Zahradnik J M, Moyer G H, Porter D D. Adenovirus hepatitis in an immunosuppressed adult patient. Am J Clin Pathol 1979; 71: 352–355

27. Janner D, Petru A M, Belchis D, Azimi P H. Fatal adenovirus infection in a child with acquired immunodeficiency syndrome. Pediatr Infect Dis J 1990; 9: 434–436

28. Krilov L R, Rubin L G, Frogel M et al. Disseminated adenovirus infection with hepatic necrosis in patients with human immunodeficiency virus infection and other immunodeficiency states. Rev Infect Dis 1990; 12: 303–307

29. Sun N C, Smith V C. Hepatitis associated with myocarditis: unusual manifestations of infection with coxsackie Group B, type 3. N Engl J Med 1966; 274: 190–193

30. Williams A O. Autopsy study of measles in Ibadan, Nigeria. Ghana Med J 1970; 9: 23–27

31. Scully R E, Mark E J, McNeely W F, McNeely B U. Case records of the Massachusetts General Hospital [measles hepatitis]. N Engl J Med 1988; 319: 495–509

32. McLellan R K, Gleiner J A. Acute hepatitis in an adult with rubeola. JAMA 1982; 247: 2000–2001

33. Heathcote J, Deodhar K P, Scheuer P J, Sherlock S. Intrahepatic cholestasis in childhood. N Engl J Med 1976; 295: 801–805

34. Anand A, Gray E S, Brown T, Clewley J P, Cohen B J. Human parvovirus infection in pregnancy and hydrops fetalis. N Engl J Med 1987; 316: 183–186

35. Pellegrin M, Delsol G, Auvergant J C et al. Granulomatous hepatitis in Q fever. Hum Pathol 1980; 11: 51–57

36. Lobdell D H. 'Ring' granulomas in cytomegaloviral hepatitis. Arch Pathol Lab Med 1987; 111: 88–882

37. Murphy E, Griffiths M R, Hunter J A, Burt A D. Fibrin-ring granulomas: a non-specific reaction to liver injury? Histopathology 1991; 19: 91–93

38. Guardia J, Martinez-Vazquez J M, Moragas A. The liver in boutonneuse fever. Gut 1974; 15: 549–551

39. Walker D H, Staiti A, Mansueto G, Tringali G. Frequent occurrence of hepatic lesions in boutonneuse fever. Acta Trop 1986; 43: 175–181

40. Wollner-Hanssen P, Weström L, Mårdh P-A. Perihepatitis and chlamydial salpingitis. Lancet 1980; i: 901–904

41. Rackow E C, Astiz M E. Pathophysiology and treatment of septic shock. JAMA 1991; 266: 548–554

42. Bagshawe A, Miller J R M. The aetiology of portal hypertension associated with gross haemorrhage in Kenya. East Afr Med J 1970; 47: 185–187

43. Nakhleh R E, Glock M, Snover D C. Hepatic pathology of chronic granulomatous disease in childhood. Arch Pathol Lab Med 1992; 116: 71–75

44. Kimball M W, Knee S. Gonococcal perihepatitis in a male. N Engl J Med 1970; 282: 1082–1083

45. Lopez-Zeno J A, Keith L G, Berger G S. The Fitz-Hugh–Curtis syndrome revisited: changing perspectives after half a century. J Reprod Med 1985; 30: 567–582

46. Butler T. Plague and other *Yersinia* infections. New York: Plenum, 1983

47. Greenstein A J, Lowenthal B A, Hammer G F S, Schaffner F, Aufses A H. Continuing patterns of disease in pyogenic liver abscess: a study of 38 cases. Am J Gastroenterol 1984; 79: 217–226

48. Cervantes F, Carbonell J, Bruguera M, Force L, Webb S. Liver disease in brucellosis. A clinical and pathologic study of 40 cases. Postgrad Med J 1982; 58: 346–350

49. Piggot J A, Hochholzer L. Human melioidosis. A histopathologic study of acute and chronic melioidosis. Arch Pathol Lab Med 1970; 90: 101–111

50. Yu V L, Miller W P, Wing E J, Romano J M, Ruiz C A, Bruns F J. Disseminated listeriosis presenting as acute hepatitis. Am J Med 1982; 73: 773–777

51. Rizkallah M F, Meyer L, Ayoub E M. Hepatic and splenic abscesses in cat-scratch disease. Pediatr Infect Dis J 1988; 7: 191–195

52. Delbeke D, Sandler M P, Shaff M I, Miller S F. Cat-scratch disease: report of a case with liver lesions and no lymphadenopathy. J Nucl Med 1988; 29: 1454–1456

53. Brenner D J, Hollis D G, Moss C W et al. Proposal of *Afipia* gen. nov. with *Afipia felis* sp. nov. (formerly the cat scratch bacillus), *Afipia clevelandensis* sp. nov. (formerly the Cleveland Clinic Foundation strain), *Afipia broomeae* sp. nov., and three unnamed genospecies. J Clin Microbiol 1991; 29: 2450–2460

54. Putman H C, Dockerty M B, Waugh J M. Abdominal actinomycosis: an analysis of 122 cases. Surgery 1993; 28: 781–790

55. Kazmi K A, Rab S M. Primary hepatic actinomycosis: a diagnostic problem. Am J Trop Med Hyg 1989; 40: 310–311

56. Chandler F W, Kaplan W, Ajello L. A color atlas and text of the histopathology of mycotic diseases. London: Wolfe Medical Publications, 1980

57. Brooks S E H, Audretsch J J. Hepatic ultrastructure in congenital syphilis. Arch Pathol Lab Med 1978; 102: 502–505

58. Sobel H J, Wolf E H. Liver involvement in early syphilis. Arch Pathol Lab Med 1972; 93: 565–568

59. Romeu J, Rybak B, Dave P, Coven R. Spirochetal vasculitis and bile ductular damage in early hepatic syphilis. Am J Gastroenterol 1980; 74: 352–354

60. Judge D M, Samuel I, Perine P L, Vukotic D. Louse-born relapsing fever in man. Arch Pathol Lab Med 1974; 97: 136–140

61. Ferreira V A, Vianna M R, Yasuda P H, de Brito T. Detection of leptospiral antigen in the human liver and kidney using an immunoperoxidase staining procedure. J Pathol 1987; 151: 125–131

62. Duray P H. Clinical pathologic correlations of Lyme disease. Rev Infect Dis 1989; 11 (suppl 6): S1487–S1493

63. Goellner M H, Agger W A, Burgess J H, Duray P H. Hepatitis due to recurrent Lyme disease. Ann Intern Med 1988; 108: 707–708

64. Snider D E. Introduction [to symposium on tuberculosis]. Rev Infect Dis 1989; 11: S336–S338

65. Rich A R. The pathogenesis of tuberculosis. Springfield: C C Thomas, 1951

66. O'Brien J R. Non-reactive tuberculosis. J Clin Pathol 1954; 7: 216–225

67. Karat A B A, Job C K, Rao P S S. Liver in leprosy: histological and biochemical findings. Br Med J 1971; i: 307–310

68. Chen T S N, Drutz D J, Whelan G E. Hepatic granulomas in leprosy. Arch Pathol Lab Med 1976; 100: 182–185

69. Kramarsky B, Edmondson H A, Peters R L, Reynolds T B. Lepromatous leprosy in reaction. Arch Pathol Lab Med 1968; 85: 516–531

70. Lucas S B. Mycobacteria and the tissues of man. In: Ratledge C, Stanford J, eds. The biology of the mycobacteria, vol 3. London: Academic Press, 1988: pp 107–176

71. Desikan K V, Job C K. A review of post mortem findings in 37 cases of leprosy. Int J Lepr 1968; 36: 32–44

72. MacKay A, Alcorn M J, MacLeod I M et al. Fatal disseminated BCG infection in a 16-year old boy. Lancet 1980; ii: 1332–1334

73. Sohn C C, Schroff R W, Kliewer K E, Lebel D M, Fligiel S. Disseminated *Mycobacterium avium-intracellulare* infection in homosexual men with acquired cell-mediated immunodeficiency: a histological and immunologic study of two cases. Am J Clin Pathol 1983; 79: 247–252

74. Maasenkeil G, Opravil M, Salfinger M, Von Graevenitz A, Lüthy R. Disseminated coinfection with *Mycobacterium avium* complex

and *Mycobacterium kansasii* in a patient with AIDS and liver abscess. Clin Infect Dis 1992; 14: 618–619

75. Simor A E, Patterson C. Disseminated *Mycobacterium bovis* infection in an elderly patient. Diagn Microbiol Infect Dis 1987; 7: 149–153

76. Ausina V, Gurgui M, Verger G, Prats G. Iatrogenic disseminated *Mycobacterium chelonei* infection. Tubercle 1984; 65: 53–57

77. Dreisin R B, Scoggin C, Davidson P T. The pathogenicity of *Mycobacterium fortuitum* and *Mycobacterium chelonei* in man: a report of seven cases. Tubercle 1976; 57: 49–57

78. Bültmann B D, Flad H D, Kaiserling E et al. Disseminated mycobacterial histiocytosis due to *M. fortuitum* associated with helper T-lymphocyte immune deficiency. Virchows Arch [A] 1982; 395: 217–225

79. Razon-Veronesi S, Visconti A, Boeri R, Casiraghi G, Canova G. Linfogranulomatosi disseminata da *Mycobacterium fortuitum* in eta pediatrica. Minerva Pediatr 1983; 35: 775–783

80. Kurnik P B, Padmanabh U, Bonatsos C, Cynamon M H. *Mycobacterium gordonae* as a human hepato-peritoneal pathogen, with a review of the literature. Am J Med Sci 1983; 285: 45–48

81. Stewart C, Jackson L. Spleno-hepatic tuberculosis due to *Mycobacterium kansasii*. Med J Aust 1976; 2: 99–101

82. Zamorano J, Tompsett R. Disseminated atypical mycobacterial infection and pancytopenia. Arch Intern Med 1968; 121: 424–427

83. Bach N, Thung S N, Berk P D. The liver in acquired immunodeficiency syndrome (AIDS). In: Bianchi L, Gerok W, Maier K P, Deinhardt F J, eds. Infectious diseases of the liver. Dordrecht: Kluwer Academic, 1990: pp 333–351

84. Patel K M. Granulomatous hepatitis due to *Mycobacterium scrofulaceum*: report of a case. Gastroenterology 1981; 81: 156–158

85. Torres R A, Nord J, Feldman R, LaBombardi V, Barr M. Disseminated mixed *Mycobacterium simiae–Mycobacterium avium* complex infection in acquired immunodeficiency syndrome. J Infect Dis 1991; 164: 432–433

86. Cianculli F D. The radish bacillus (*Mycobacterium terrae*): saprophyte or pathogen?. Am Rev Respir Dis 1974; 109: 138–141

87. Weinberg J R, Gertner D, Dootson G, Chambers S T, Smith H. Disseminated *Mycobacterium xenopi* infection. Lancet 1985; 1: 1033–1034

88. Tecson-Tumang F T, Bright J L. Mycobacterium xenopi and the acquired immunodeficiency syndrome. Ann Intern Med 1984; 100: 461–462

89. Anthony P P. A guide to the histological identification of fungi in tissues. J Clin Pathol 1973; 26: 828–831

90. Benbow E W, Delamore I W, Stoddart R W, Reid H. Disseminated zygomycosis associated with erythroleukaemia: confirmation by lectin stains. J Clin Pathol 1985; 38: 1039–1044

91. Moskowitz L B, Ganjei P, Ziegels-Weissman J, Clergy TJ, Penneys N S, Nadji M. Immunohistologic identification of fungi in systemic and cutaneous mycoses. Arch Pathol Lab Med 1986; 110: 433–436

92. Walsh T J, Hamilton S R. Disseminated aspergillosis complicating hepatic failure. Arch Intern Med 1983; 143: 1189–1191

93. Sabesin S M, Fallon H J, Andriole VT. Hepatic failure as a manifestation of cryptococcosis. Arch Intern Med 1963; 111: 661–669

94. Buculvalas J C, Bove K E, Kaufman R A, Gilchrist M J R, Oldham K T, Balistreri W F. Cholangitis associated with *Cryptococcus neoformans*. Gastroenterology 1985; 88: 1055–1059

95. Goodwin R A, Shapiro J L, Thurman G H, Thurman S S, Des Prez R M. Disseminated histoplasmosis: clinical and pathologic correlations. Medicine 1980; 59: 1–33

96. Wheat L J, Slama T G, Norton J A et al. Risk factors for disseminated or fatal histoplasmosis. Ann Intern Med 1982; 96: 159–163

97. Teixeira F, Gayotto L C D C, de Brito T. Morphological patterns of the liver in South American blastomycosis. Histopathology 1978; 2: 231–237

98. Jayanetra P, Nitiyanant P, Ajello L et al. Penicilliosis marneffei in Thailand: report of five human cases. Am J Trop Med Hyg 1984; 33: 637–644

99. Meyer R D, Rosen P, Armstrong D. Phycomycosis complicating leukaemia and lymphoma. Ann Intern Med 1972; 77: 871–879

100. Butcher G A. HIV and malaria: a lesson in immunology. Parasitology Today 1992; 8: 307–311

101. Warrell D A, Molyneux M E, Beales P F. Severe and complicated malaria. Trans R Soc Trop Med Hyg 1990; 84 (suppl 2): S1–S65

102. Deller J J, Cifarelli P S, Berque S, Buchanan R. Malaria hepatitis. Milit Med 1967; 132: 614–620

103. Joshi Y K, Tandon S K, Acharya S K, Babu S, Tandon M. Acute hepatic failure due to *Plasmodium falciparum* liver injury. Liver 1986; 6: 357–360

104. de Brito T, Barone A A, Faria R M. Human liver biopsy in *P. falciparum* and *P. vivax* malaria: a light and electron microscopy study. Virchows Arch [A] 1969; 348: 220–229

105. Moore G, Homewood C A, Gilles H M. A comparison of pigment from *S. mansoni* and *P. berghei*. Ann Trop Med Parasitol 1975; 69: 373–374

106. Turrini F, Schwarzer E, Arese P. The involvement of hemozoin toxicity in depression of cellular immunity. Parasitology Today 1993; 9: 297–300

107. Crane G G. Hyperreactive malarious splenomegaly (tropical splenomegaly syndrome). Parasitology Today 1986; 2: 4–9

108. Entrican J H, Williams H, Cook I A et al. Babesiosis in man: report of a case from Scotland with observations on the infecting strain. J Infect 1979; 1: 227–234

109. Bryceson A D M. The liver in leishmaniasis. In: Bianchi L, Maier K-P, Gerok W, Deinhardt F, eds. Infectious diseases of the liver. Dordrecht: Kluwer Academic Press, 1989: pp 215–223

110. Badaró R, Jones T C, Carvalho E M et al. New perspectives on a subclinical form of visceral leishmaniasis. J Infect Dis 1986; 154: 1003–1011

111. Pampiglione S, Manson-Bahr P E C, Giungi F, Giunti G, Parenti A, Trotti G C. Studies in Mediterranean leishmaniasis 2. Asymptomatic cases of visceral leishmaniasis. Trans R Soc Trop Med Hyg 1974; 68: 447–453

112. Duarte M I S, Mariano O N, Corbett C E P. Liver parenchymal cell parasitism in human visceral leishmaniasis. Virchows Arch [A] 1989; 415: 1–6

113. Khaldi F, Bennaceur B, Othman H B, Achouri E, Ayachi R, Regaieg R. Les formes sévères d'atteinte hépatique au cours de la leishmaniose viscérale. A propos de 7 cas. Arch Fr Pediatr 1990; 47: 257–260

114. Moreno A, Marazuela M, Yerba M et al. Hepatic fibrin ring granulomas in visceral leishmaniasis. Gastroenterology 1988; 95: 1123–1126

115. Daneshbod K. Visceral leishmaniasis (kala azar) in Iran: a pathologic and electron microscopic study. Am J Clin Pathol 1972; 57: 156–166

116. Pampiglione S, La Placa M, Schlick G. Studies on Mediterranean leishmaniasis. 1. An outbreak of visceral leishmaniasis in Northern Italy. Trans R Soc Trop Med Hyg 1974; 68: 349–359

117. Duarte M I S, Corbett C E P. Histopathological patterns of the liver involvement in visceral leishmaniasis. Rev Inst Med Trop Sao Paulo 1987; 29: 131–136

118. Rogers L. A peculiar intralobular cirrhosis of the liver produced by the protozoal parasite of kala-azar. Ann Trop Med Parasitol 1908; 2: 147–152

119. Ho E A, Suong T-H, Li Y. Comparative merits of sternum, spleen and liver puncture in the study of human visceral leishmaniasis. Trans R Soc Trop Med Hyg 1948; 41: 315–320

120. Bradley D J, Taylor B A, Blackwell J A et al. Regulation of *Leishmania* populations within the host: III. Mapping of the locus controlling susceptibility to visceral leishmaniasis in the mouse. Clin Exp Immunol 1979; 37: 7–14

121. Nigam P, Gupta A K, Kapoor K K, Sharan G R, Goyal B M, Joshi L D. Cholestasis in amoebic liver abscess. Gut 1985; 26: 140–145

122. Palmer R B. Changes in the liver in amebic dysentery. With special reference to the origin of amebic abscess. Arch Pathol Lab Med 1938; 25: 327–335

123. Spice W M, Cruz-Reyes J A, Ackers J P. *Entamoeba histolytica*. In: Myint S, Cann A, eds. Molecular and cell biology of opportunistic infections in AIDS. London: Chapman & Hall, 1993: pp 95–137

124. Young J D, Young T M, Lu L P, Unkless J C, Cohn Z A. Characterization of a membrane pore-forming protein from *Entamoeba histolytica*. J Exp Med 1982; 156: 1677–1690

125. Tiwari I, Rolland C F, Popple A W. Cholestatic jaundice due to toxoplasma hepatitis. Postgrad Med J 1982; 58: 299–300

126. Weitberg A B, Alper J C, Diamond I, Fligiel Z. Acute granulomatous hepatitis in the course of acquired toxoplasmosis. N Engl J Med 1979; 300: 1093–1096

127. Khuroo M, Zargar SA, Mahajan R. Hepatobiliary and pancreatic ascariasis in India. Lancet 1990; i: 1503–1506

128. Gayotto L C D C, Muszkat R M L, Souza I V. Hepatobiliary alterations in massive biliary ascariasis. Histopathological aspects of an autopsy case. Rev Inst Med Trop Sao Paulo 1990; 32: 91–95

129. Daly J J, Baker G F. Pinworm granuloma of the liver. Am J Trop Med Hyg 1984; 33: 62–64

130. Mondou E N, Gnepp D R. Hepatic granuloma resulting from *Enterobius vermicularis*. Am J Clin Pathol 1989; 91: 97–100

131. Genta R M. Global prevalence of strongyloidiasis: critical review and epidemiologic insights into the prevention of disseminated disease. Rev Infect Dis 1989; 11: 755–767

132. Nakada K, Yamaguchi K, Furgen S et al. Monoclonal integration of HTLV-1 proviral DNA in patients with strongyloidiasis. Int J Canc 1987; 40: 145–148

133. Poltera A A, Katsimbura N. Granulomatous hepatitis due to *Strongyloides stercoralis*. J Pathol 1974; 113: 241–246

134. Choe G, Lee H S, Seo J K et al. Hepatic capillariasis: first case report in the Republic of Korea. Am J Trop Med Hyg 1993; 48: 610–625

135. Taylor M R H, Keane C T, O'Connor P, Mulvihill E, Holland C. The expanded spectrum of toxocaral disease. Lancet 1988; i: 692–695

136. Schantz P M. *Toxocara* larva migrans now. Am J Trop Med Hyg 1989; 41 (suppl): 21–34

137. Hira P R, Lindberg L G, Francis I et al. Diagnosis of cystic hydatid disease: role of aspiration cytology. Lancet 1988; ii: 655–657

138. Akinoglu A, Demiryurek H, Guzel C. Alveolar hydatid disease of the liver: a report on thirty-nine surgical cases in eastern Anatolia. Am J Trop Med Hyg 1991; 45: 182–189

139. WHO. The control of schistosomiasis. Second report of the WHO expert committee. Geneva: WHO, 1993

140. Wittes R, MacLean J D, Law C, Lough J O. Three cases of schistosomiasis mekongi from northern Laos. Am J Trop Med Hyg 1984; 33: 1159–1163

141. Van Wijk H B, Elias E A. Hepatic and rectal pathology in *Schistosoma intercalatum* infection. Trop Geogr Med 1975; 27: 237–248

142. Nafeh M A, Medhat A, Swifae Y et al. Ultrasonographic changes of the liver in *Schistosoma haematobium* infection. Am J Trop Med Hyg 1992; 47: 225–230

143. Hiatt R A, Sotomayor Z R, Sanchez G, Zambrana M, Knight W B. Factors in the pathogenesis of acute schistosomiasis mansoni. J Infect Dis 1979; 139: 659–666

144. De Cock K M, Awadh S, Raja R S, Wankya B M, Lucas S B. Eosophageal varices in Nairobi, Kenya: a study of 68 cases. Am J Trop Med Hyg 1982; 31: 579–588

145. Da Silva L C, Carrilho F J. Hepatosplenic schistosomiasis. Pathophysiology and treatment. Gastroenterol Clin N Am 1992; 21: 163–177

146. Symmers W S C. Note on a new form of liver cirrhosis due to the presence of the ova of *Bilharzia haematobia*. J Path Bact 1903; 9: 237–239

147. Bhagwandeen S B. The histopathology of early hepatic schistosomiasis. Afr J Med Sci 1976; 5: 125–130

148. Andrade Z A, Peixoto E, Guerret S, Grimaud J-E. Hepatic connective tissue changes in hepatosplenic schistosomiasis. Hum Pathol 1992; 23: 566–573

149. Grimaud J A, Borojevic R. Chronic human schistosomiasis mansoni: pathology of the Disse's space. Lab Invest 1977; 36: 268–273

150. Dunn M A, Kamel R. Hepatic schistosomiasis. Hepatology 1981; 1: 653–661

151. Chen M G, Mott K E. Progress in assessment of morbidity due to *Schistosoma japonicum* infection. A review of recent literature. Trop Dis Bull 1988; 85 (6): R1–R45

152. Chen M G, Mott K E. Progress in assessment of morbidity due to *Schistosoma mansoni* infection. A review of recent literature. Trop Dis Bull 1988; 85 (10): R1–R56

153. Cheever A W. A quantitative post-mortem study of schistosomiasis mansoni in man. Am J Trop Med Hyg 1968; 17: 38–64

154. Colley D G, Garcia A A. Lambertucci J R et al. Immune responses during human schistosomiasis. XII. Differential responsiveness in patients with hepatosplenic disease. Am J Trop Med Hyg 1986; 35: 793–802

155. Hafez M, Hassan S A, El-Tahan H et al. Immunogenetic susceptibility for post-schistosomal hepatic fibrosis. Am J Trop Med Hyg 1991; 44: 424–433

156. Andrade Z A, Cheever A W. Alterations of the intrahepatic vasculature in hepatosplenic schistosomiasis mansoni. Am J Trop Med Hyg 1971; 20: 425–432

157. Watt G, Padre L, Tuazon M, Wotherspoon A, Adapon B. Hepatic parenchymal dysfunction in *Schistosoma japonicum* infection. J Infect Dis 1991; 164: 186–192

158. Ghaffar Y A, Fatah S A, Kamel M, Badr R M, Mahomed F F, Strickland G T. The impact of endemic schistosomiasis on acute viral hepatitis. Am J Trop Med Hyg 1991; 45: 743–750

159. Homeida M, Abdel-Gadir A F, Cheever A W, Bennett J L. Diagnosis of pathologically confirmed Symmers' periportal fibrosis by ultrasonography: a prospective blinded study. Am J Trop Med Hyg 1988; 38: 86–91

160. Houston S, Munjoma M, Kanyimo K, Davidson RN, Flowerdew G. Use of ultrasound in a study of schistosomal periportal fibrosis in rural Zimbabwe. Acta Trop 1993; 53: 51–58

161. Zwingenberger K, Richter J, Vergetti J G S, Feldmeier H. Praziquantel in the treatment of hepatosplenic schistosomiasis: biochemical disease markers indicate deceleration of fibrogenesis and diminution of portal flow obstruction. Trans Roy Soc Trop Med Hyg 1990; 84: 252–256

162. Ohmae H, Tanaka M, Hayashi M et al. Improvement of ultrasonographic and serologic changes in *Schistosoma japonicum*-infected patients after treatment with praziquantel. Am J Trop Med Hyg 1992; 46: 99–104

163. Chen M G, Mott K E. Progress in assessment of morbidity due to *Schistosoma intercalatum* infection: a review of recent literature. Trop Dis Bull 1989; 86 (8): R1–R18

164. Chen M G, Mott K E. Progress in assessment of morbidity due to *Schistosoma haematobium* infection. A review of recent literature. Trop Dis Bull 1989; 86 (4): R1–R36

165. Upatham E S, Viyanant V, Kurathong S et al. Relationship between prevalence and intensity of *Opisthorchis viverrini* infection, and clinical symptoms and signs in a rural community in north-east Thailand. Bull WHO 1984; 62: 451–461

166. Vatanasapt V, Uttaravichien T, Mairiang E-O, Pairojkul C, Chartbanchachai W, Haswell E M. Cholangiocarcinoma in north-east Thailand. Lancet 1990; i: 117–118

167. Koompirochana C, Sonakul D, Chinda K et al. Opisthorchis: a clinicopathologic study of 154 autopsy cases. Southeast Asian J Trop Med Public Health 1978; 9: 60–64

168. Hou P C. The pathology of *Clonorchis sinensis* infestation of the liver. J Pathol 1955; 70: 53–64

169. Flavell D J. Liver-fluke infection as an aetiological factor in bile-duct carcinoma of man. Trans Roy Soc Trop Med Hyg 1981; 75: 814–824

170. Chen M G, Lu W P, Hua X J, Mott K E. Progress in assessment of morbidity due to *Clonorchis sinensis* infection: a review of recent literature. Trop Dis Bull 1994; in press

171. Acosta-Ferreira W, Vercelli-Hetta J, Falconi L M. *Fasciola hepatica* human infection. Histopathological study of 16 cases. Virchows Arch [A] 1979; 383: 319–327

172. Chen M G, Mott K E. Progress in assessment of morbidity due to *Fasciola hepatica* infection: a review of recent literature. Trop Dis Bull 1990; 87 (4): R1–R37

173. Gardiner C H, Dyke J W, Shirley S F. Hepatic granuloma due to a nymph of *Linguatula serrata* in a woman from Michigan. A case

report and review of the literature. Am J Trop Med Hyg 1984; 33: 187–189

174. Self J T, Hopps H C, Williams A O. Pentastomiasis in Africans. Trop Geogr Med 1975; 27: 1–13

175. Prathap K, Lau K S, Bolton J M. Pentastomiasis: a common finding at autopsy in Malaysian aborigines. Am J Trop Med Hyg 1969; 18: 20–27

176. Mann J M, Tarantola D J M, Netter T W. AIDS in the world. Cambridge, Mass: Harvard University Press, 1992

177. Allen S, Lindan C P, Serufilira A et al. Human immunodeficiency virus infection in urban Rwanda. JAMA 1991; 266: 1657–1663

178. Quinn T C, Mann J M, Curran J W, Piot P. AIDS in Africa: an epidemiologic paradigm. Science 1986; 234: 955–963

179. Pantaleo G, Graziosi C, Fauci A S. The immunopathogenesis of human immunodeficiency virus infection. N Engl J Med 1993; 328: 327–335

180. Centers for Disease Control and Prevention. Revision of the CDC surveillance case definition for AIDS. MMWR 1987; 36: 1S–15S

181. Buehler J W, Ward J W. A new case definition for AIDS surveillance. Ann Intern Med 1993; 118: 390–392

182. Nakanuma Y, Liew C I, Peters RL, Govindarajan S. Pathologic features of the liver in AIDS. Liver 1986; 6: 158–166

183. Schneiderman D J, Arenson D M, Cello JP, Margaretten W, Weber T E. Hepatic disease in patients with the acquired immunodeficiency syndrome (AIDS). Hepatology 1987; 7: 925–930

184. Wilkins M J, Lindley R, Doukaris S P, Goldin R D. Surgical pathology of the liver in HIV infection. Histopathology 1991; 18: 459–464

185. Cello J P. Acquired immunodeficiency syndrome cholangiopathy: spectrum of disease. Am J Med 1989; 86: 539–546

186. Palmer M, Braly L F, Schaffner F. The liver in AIDS disease. Semin Liver Dis 1987; 7: 192–202

187. Dowsett J F, Miller R, Davidson R et al. Sclerosing cholangitis in acquired immunodeficiency syndrome. Case reports and a review of the literature. Scand J Gastroenterol 1988; 23: 1267–1274

188. Bonacini M. Hepatobiliary complications in patients with human immunodeficiency virus infection. Am J Med 1992; 92: 404–411

189. Boag F C, Dean R, Hawkins D A, Lawrence A G, Gazzard B G. Abnormalities of liver function during HIV seroconversion illness. Int J STD AIDS 1992; 3: 46–48

190. Molina J M, Welker Y, Ferchal F, Decazes J M, Shenmetzler C, Modaï J. Hepatitis associated with primary HIV infection. Gastroenterology 1992; 102: 739

191. Freiman J P, Helfert K E, Hamrell M R, Stein D S. Hepatomegaly with severe steatosis in HIV-seropositive patients. AIDS 1993; 7: 379–385

192. Klatt E C. Practical AIDS pathology. Chicago: ASCP Press, 1992

193. Housset C, Bouchier O, Girard PM et al. Immunohistochemical evidence for human immunodeficiency virus-1 infection of liver Kupffer cells. Hum Pathol 1990; 21: 404–408

194. Cao Y, Dieterich D, Thomas P A, Huang Y, Mirabile M, Ho DD. Identification and quantification of HIV-1 in the liver of patients with AIDS. AIDS 1992; 6: 65–70.

195. Czapar C A, Weldon-Linne C M, Moore D M, Rhone DP. Peliosis hepatis in acquired immunodeficiency syndrome. Arch Pathol Lab Med 1986; 110: 611–613

196. Welch K, Finkbeiner W, Alpers C E et al. Autopsy findings in the acquired immune deficiency syndrome. JAMA 1984; 252: 1152–1159

197. Cozzi P J, Abu-Jawdeh G M, Green R M, Green D. Amyloidosis in association with human immunodeficiency virus infection. Clin Infect Dis 1992; 14: 189–191

198. Zimmerli W, Bianchi L, Gudat F et al. Disseminated herpes simplex type 2 and systemic Candida infection in a patient with previous asymptomatic HIV infection. J Infect Dis 1988; 157: 597–598

199. Beissner R S, Rappaport E S, Diaz J A. Fatal case of Epstein–Barr virus-induced lymphoproliferative disorder associated with a human immunodeficiency virus infection. Arch Pathol Lab Med 1987; 111: 250–253

200. Bodsworth N J, Cooper D A, Donovan B. The influence of human immunodeficiency virus type 1 infection on the development of hepatitis B virus carrier state. J Infect Dis 1991; 163: 1138–1140

201. Waite J, Gilson R J C, Weller I V D et al. Hepatitis B virus reactivation or reinfection associated with HIV-1 infection. AIDS 1988; 2: 443–448

202. Goldin R D, Fish D E, Hay A et al. Histological and immunohistochemical study of hepatitis B virus in human immunodeficiency virus infection. J Clin Pathol 1990; 43: 203–205

203. Prufer-Kramer L, Kramer A, Weigel R et al. Hepatic involvement in patients with human immunodeficiency virus infection: discrepancies between AIDS patients and those with earlier stages of infection. J Infect Dis 1991; 163: 866–869

204. Eskild A, Magnus P, Petersen G et al. Hepatitis B antibodies in HIV-infected homosexual men are associated with more rapid progression to AIDS. AIDS 1992; 6: 571–574

205. Vento S, Cruciani M, Di Perri G et al. Hepatitis C virus with normal liver histology in symptomless HIV-1 infection. Lancet 1992; 340: 1161

206. De Cock K M, Soro B, Coulibaly I-M, Lucas S B. Tuberculosis and HIV infection in sub-Saharan Africa. JAMA 1992; 268: 1581–1587

207. Lucas S B, Hounnou A, Peacock C et al. The mortality and pathology of HIV infection in a West African city. AIDS 1993; 7: 1569–1579

208. Nambuya A, Sewankambo N, Mugerwa J, Goodgame R W, Lucas S B. Tuberculous lymphadenitis associated with human immunodeficiency virus (HIV) in Uganda. J Clin Pathol 1988; 41: 93–96

209. Wallace J M, Hannah J B. Mycobacterium avium complex infection in patients with the acquired immunodeficiency syndrome. A clinicopathologic study. Chest 1988; 93: 926–932

210. Nightingale S D, Byrd L T, Southern P M, Jockusch J D, Cal SX, Wynne B A. Incidence of Mycobacterium avium-intracellulare complex bacteremia in human immunodeficiency virus-positive patients. J Infect Dis 1992; 165: 1082–1085

211. Lucas S B. HIV and leprosy (editorial). Lepr Rev 1993; 64: 97–103

212. Slater L N, Welch D F, Min K W. Rochalimaea henselae causes bacillary angiomatosis and peliosis hepatis. Arch Intern Med 1992; 152: 602–606

213. Steeper T A, Rosenstein H, Weiser J, Inampudi S, Snover D C. Bacillary epithelioid angiomatosis involving the liver, spleen, and skin in an AIDS patient with concurrent Kaposi's sarcoma. Am J Clin Pathol 1992; 97: 713–718

214. Perkocha L A, Geaghan S M, Yen T S B et al. Clinical and pathological features of bacillary peliosis hepatitis in association with human immunodeficiency virus infection. N Engl J Med 1990; 323: 1581–1586

215. Reed J A, Brigati D J, Flynn S D et al. Immunocytochemical identification of Rochalimaea henselae in bacillary (epithelioid) angiomatosis, parenchymal bacillary peliosis, and persistent fever with bacteremia. Am J Surg Pathol 1992; 16: 650–657

216. Schlossberg D, Morad Y, Krouse T B, Wear D J, English C K. Culture-proven disseminated cat-scratch disease in acquired immunodeficiency syndrome. Arch Intern Med 1989; 149: 1437–1439

217. Raoult D, Levy P-Y, Dupont H T et al. Q fever and HIV infection. AIDS 1993; 7: 81–86

218. Nichols L, Balogh K, Silverman M. Bacterial infections in the acquired immunodeficiency syndrome. Clinicopathologic correlations in a series of autopsy cases. Am J Clin Pathol 1989; 92: 787–790

219. Gilks C F, Ojoo S A, Brindle R J. Non-opportunistic bacterial infections in HIV-seropositive adults in Nairobi, Kenya. AIDS 1991; 5 (suppl 1): S113–S116

220. Carme B, Ngaporo A I, Ngolet A, Ibara J R, Ebikili B. Disseminated African histoplasmosis in a Congolese patient with AIDS. J Med Vet Mycol 1992; 30: 245–248

221. Harding C V. Blastomycosis and opportunistic infections in patients with acquired immunodeficiency syndrome. An autopsy study. Arch Pathol Lab Med 1992; 115: 1133–1136

222. Pursell K J, Telzak E E, Armstrong D. Aspergillus species colonization and invasive disease in patients with AIDS. Clin Infect Dis 1992; 14: 141–148

223. Filce C, Brunetti E, Carnevale G, Dughetti S, Pirola F, Rondanelli E G. Ultrasonographic and microbiological diagnosis of mycolic liver abscess in patients with AIDS. Microbiologica 1989; 12: 101–104

224. Tsui W M S, Ma K F, Tsang D N C. Disseminated *Penicillium marneffei* infection in HIV-infected subject. Histopathology 1992; 20: 287–291

225. Bronnimann D A, Adam R D, Galgiani J N et al. Coccidioidomycosis in the acquired immunodeficiency syndrome. Ann Intern Med 1987; 106: 372–379

226. Kim J, Minamoto G Y, Grieco M H. Nocardial infection as a complication of AIDS: report of six cases and review. Rev Infect Dis 1991; 13: 624–629

227. Wakefield A E, Stewart T J, Moxon E R, Marsh K, Hopkin J M. Infection with *Pneumocystis carinii* is prevalent in healthy Gambian children. Trans Roy Soc Trop Med Hyg 1990; 84: 800–802.

228. Telzak E E, Cote R J, Gold J W M, Campbell S W, Armstrong D. Extrapulmonary *Pneumocystis carinii* infection. Rev Infect Dis 1990; 12: 380–386

229. Coker R J, Clark D, Claydon E L et al. Disseminated *Pneumocystis carinii* infection in AIDS. J Clin Pathol 1991; 44: 820–823

230. Altes J, Salas A, Riera M et al. Visceral leishmaniasis: another HIV-associated opportunistic infection? Report of eight cases and review of the literature. AIDS 1991; 5: 201–207

231. Alvar J, Gutierrez-Solar B, Molina R, et al. Prevalence of *Leishmania* infection among AIDS patients. Lancet 1992; 339: 1427

232. Peters B S, Fish D, Goldin R, Evans D A, Bryceson A D M, Pinching A J. Visceral leishmaniasis in HIV infection and AIDS: clinical features and response to therapy. Q J Med 1990; 77: 1101–1111

233. Falk S, Helm E B, Hübner K, Stutte H J. Disseminated visceral leishmaniasis (kala azar) in acquired immunodeficiency syndrome (AIDS). Pathol Res Pract 1989; 183: 253–255

234. Lucas S B. Missing infections in AIDS. Trans Roy Soc Trop Med Hyg 1990; 84 Suppl 1: 34–38

235. Tuur S M, Macher A M, De Vinatea M L et al. Case for diagnosis. Milit Med 1987; 152: M10–M16

236. Drabick J J, Egan J E, Brown S L, Vick R G, Sandman B M, Neafie R C. Dicroceliasis (lancet fluke disease) in an HIV seropositive man. JAMA 1988; 259: 567–568

237. Harcourt-Webster J N, Scaravilli F, Darwish A H. *Strongyloides stercoralis* hyperinfection in an HIV positive patient. J Clin Pathol 1991; 44: 346–348

238. Hasan F A, Jeffers L J, Welsh S W, Reddy K R, Schiff E R. Hepatic involvement as the primary manifestation of Kaposi's sarcoma in the acquired immune deficiency syndrome. Am J Gastroenterol 1989; 84: 1449–1451

239. Glasgow B J, Anders K, Layfield L J, Steinsapir K D, Gitnick G L, Lewin K J. Clinical and pathologic findings of the liver in acquired immune deficiency syndrome (AIDS). Am J Clin Pathol 1985; 83: 582–588

240. Bayley A C, Lucas S B. Kaposi's sarcoma or Kaposi's disease? A personal reappraisal. In: Fletcher C D M, McKee P M, eds. Pathobiology of soft tissue tumours. Edinburgh: Churchill Livingstone, 1990: pp 141–164

241. Pluda J M, Yarchoan R, Jaffe E S et al. Development of non-Hodgkin lymphoma in a cohort of patients with severe human immunodeficiency virus (HIV) infection on long-term antiretroviral therapy. Ann Intern Med 1990; 113: 276–282

242. Caccamo D, Pervez N K, Marchevsky A. Primary lymphoma of the liver in the acquired immunodeficiency syndrome. Arch Pathol Lab Med 1986; 110: 553–555

243. Kaplan L D, Kahn J, Jacobson M, Bottles K, Cello J. Primary bile duct lymphoma in the acquired immunodeficiency syndrome (AIDS). Ann Intern Med 1989; 110: 161–162

244. Ioachim H L, Dorsett B, Cronin W, Maya M, Wahl S. Acquired immunodeficiency syndrome-associated lymphomas: clinical, pathologic, immunologic, and viral characteristics of 111 cases. Hum Pathol 1991; 22: 659–673

245. Rabkin C S, Blattner W A. HIV infection and cancers other than non-Hodgkin lymphoma and Kaposi's sarcoma. In: Beral V, Jaffe H W, Weiss R A, eds. Cancer, HIV and AIDS. New York: Cold Spring Harbor Laboratory Press, 1991: pp 151–160

246. Forbes A, Blanshard C, Gazzard B G. Natural history of AIDS sclerosing cholangitis: a study of 20 cases. Gut 1993; 34: 116–121

247. McGowan I, Hawkins A S, Weller I V D. The natural history of cryptosporidial diarrhoea in HIV-infected patients. AIDS 1993; 7: 349–354

248. Sieratzki J, Thung S N, Gerber M A, Ferrone S, Schaffner F. Major histocompatibility antigen expression in the liver in acquired immunodeficiency syndrome. Arch Pathol Lab Med 1987; 111: 1045–1049

249. David J J, Heyman M B, Ferrell L, Kerner J, Kerlan R, Tahler M M. Sclerosing cholangitis associated with chronic cryptosporidiosis in a child with a congenital immunodeficiency disorder. Am J Gastroenterol 1987; 82: 1196–1202

250. Shadduck J A. Human microsporidiosis and AIDS. Rev Infect Dis 1989; 11: 203–207

251. Orenstein J M, Dieterich D T, Kotler D P. Systemic dissemination by a newly recognised intestinal microsporidia species in AIDS. AIDS 1992; 6: 1143–1150

252. Beaugerie L, Teilhac M F, Deluol A-M et al. Cholangiopathy associated with *Microsporidia* infection of the common bile duct mucosa in a patient with HIV infection. Ann Intern Med 1992; 117: 401–402

253. Pol S, Romana C, Richard S et al. *Enterocytozoon bieneusi* infection in acquired immunodeficiency syndrome-related sclerosing cholangitis. Gastroenterology 1992; 102: 1778–1781

254. Pol S, Romana C, Richard S et al. Microsporidia infection in patients with the human immunodeficiency virus and unexplained cholangitis. N Engl J Med 1993; 328: 95–99

255. Terada S, Reddy K R, Jeffers L J, Cali A, Schiff E R. Microsporidian hepatitis in the acquired immunodeficiency syndrome. Ann Intern Med 1987; 107: 61–62

256. Blanche S, Tardieu M, Duliege A-M et al. Longitudinal study of 94 symptomatic infants with perinatally acquired human immunodeficiency virus infection. Am J Dis Child 1990; 144: 1210–1215

257. Kahn E, Greco M A, Daum F et al. Hepatic pathology in pediatric acquired immunodeficiency syndrome. Hum Pathol 1991; 22: 1111–1119

258. Jonas M M, Roldan E O, Lyons H J, Fojaco R M, Reddy R K. Histopathologic features of the liver in pediatric acquired immunodeficiency syndrome. J Pediatr Gastroenterol Nutr 1989; 9: 73–81

259. Duffy L F, Daum F, Kahn E et al. Hepatitis in children with acquired immune deficiency syndrome. Gastroenterology 1986; 90: 173–181

260. Chen S C A, Barker S M, Mitchell D H, Stevens S M B, O'Neill P, Cunningham A L. Concurrent zidovudine-induced myopathy and hepatotoxicity in patients treated for human immunodeficiency virus (HIV) infection. Pathology 1992; 24: 109–111

261. Lai K K, Gang D L, Zawacki J K, Cooley T P. Fulminant hepatic failure associated with 2',3'-dideoxyinosine (ddI). Ann Intern Med 1991; 115: 283–284

262. Roulot D, Valla D, Brun-Vezinet F, et al. Cholangitis in the acquired immunodeficiency syndrome: report of two cases and review of the literature. Gut 1987; 28: 1653–1660

263. Sabbatani S, Isulerdo Calzado A, Ferro A et al. Atypical leishmaniasis in an HIV-2 seropositive patient from Guinea-Bissau. AIDS 1991; 5: 899–901

264. Taillan B, Garnier G, Fuzibet J-G et al. Liver biopsy in patients with serum antibodies to HIV. Am J Med 1990; 89: 694

265. Mitchell D P, Hanes T E, Hoyumpa A M, Schenker S. Fever of unknown origin: assessment of the value of percutaneous liver biopsy. Arch Intern Med 1977; 137: 1001–1004

8

Alcoholic liver disease

P. de la M. Hall

Archaeological records of the earliest civilizations show that the history of alcohol dates back over 50 000 years.[1] Alcohol-related diseases are recorded in Ayurveda, an ancient text of medicine from India, written about 567 BC.[2] Many reviews of the epidemiology of alcoholic liver disease document a direct relationship between alcohol consumption per capita and the mortality from alcoholic cirrhosis; both are increasing inexorably.[3-7] After heart disease and cancer, alcoholism and alcohol-related diseases constitute the third largest health problem in the USA, affecting over 10 million people, causing about 200 000 deaths each year and costing in the region of 60 billion dollars annually.[8]

The spectrum of alcoholic liver disease includes fatty change (steatosis), perivenular fibrosis, alcoholic foamy degeneration, alcoholic hepatitis, occlusive venous lesions, cirrhosis and hepatocellular carcinoma. Numerous reviews on the pathology and pathogenesis of alcohol-associated liver injury have appeared in the last few years.[9-18] While there is no doubt that alcohol is a direct hepatotoxin there is now a growing realization that both genetic and environmental factors influence the susceptibility of the individual to alcohol-associated liver injury.[19-22] The increased susceptibility of women to alcoholic injury can now be explained, at least in part, by differences in the first-pass metabolism of alcohol[23] while racial differences in susceptibility are associated with genetic polymorphisms of alcohol dehydrogenase and acetaldehyde dehydrogenase.[24]

THE METABOLISM OF ALCOHOL

Alcohol metabolism, and the associated metabolic disturbances, are comprehensively reviewed elsewhere[25-30] and will be discussed only briefly.

Alcohol is readily absorbed from the gastrointestinal tract and is distributed throughout the body in proportion to the amount of fluid in the tissues. Less than 10% is

317

eliminated through the lungs and kidneys and the remainder is oxidized in the body, predominantly in the liver; this probably explains the marked metabolic disturbances that occur in that organ. In addition, the liver has a limited capacity for safe disposal of large amounts of alcohol.

There are three pathways for alcohol metabolism in the liver.

1. Alcohol dehydrogenase (ADH) pathway. ADH catalyses the oxidative metabolism of alcohol to acetaldehyde

$$CH_3CH_2OH \;+\; NAD^+$$
Ethanol

$$\downarrow ADH$$

$$CH_3CHO \;+\; NADH \;+\; H^+$$
Acetaldehyde

Hydrogen is transferred from alcohol to the cofactor nicotinamide adenine dinucleotide (NAD), converting it to the reduced form NADH, and acetaldehyde is produced. The generation of excess reducing equivalents (NADH) in the cytosol results in a marked shift in the redox potential, as indicated by the increased lactate : pyruvate ratio. Some of the hydrogen equivalents are transferred from the cytosol, via several shuttle systems, to the mitochondria.

The major rate-limiting factor in the ADH pathway is the ability of the liver to reoxidize NADH; the regeneration of NAD from NADH ultimately requires oxygen. Chronic alcohol consumption accelerates ADH-related alcohol metabolism to a limited extent. ADH activity, however, does not increase and a hypermetabolic state has been proposed as a possible mechanism for this acceleration.[31]

2. The microsomal ethanol-oxidizing system (MEOS). This is a cytochrome P-450-dependent pathway.

$$CH_3CH_2OH \;+\; NADPH \;+\; H^+ + O_2$$
Ethanol

$$\downarrow MEOS$$

$$CH_3CHO \;+\; NADP^+ \;+\; 2H_2O$$
Acetaldehyde

Increased MEOS activity following chronic alcohol consumption is probably the major mechanism for the increased rates of clearance of alcohol from the blood, and

for the metabolic tolerance that develops in regular drinkers.[32] Increased MEOS activity is associated with the appearance of an 'ethanol specific' form of cytochrome P-450[33] which has been designated P-450 2E1.[34] The P-450 2E1 gene has been isolated, characterized and localized to chromosome 10 in humans.[35] Animal studies have shown that the activity of this isoenzyme increases after relatively short-term alcohol consumption in doses that do not cause fatty change.[36] The increased xenobiotic toxicity and carcinogenicity seen in association with chronic alcohol consumption, in both humans and a variety of animal models, can be explained largely by the enhanced metabolism of a wide variety of agents that are also metabolized by cytochrome P-450 2E1.[28,37–39]

3. Catalase pathway. Catalase, located in peroxisomes, plays only a minor role in alcohol metabolism.

$$CH_3CH_2OH + H_2O_2 \xrightarrow{\text{catalase}} CH_3CHO + 2H_2O$$
Ethanol   Acetaldehyde

THE METABOLISM OF ACETALDEHYDE

Acetaldehyde is oxidized to acetate; again, this occurs predominantly in the liver. Some of the acetaldehyde and most of the acetate are excreted by the liver into the blood stream and are metabolized peripherally. Chronic alcoholics have accelerated alcohol metabolism and higher levels of blood acetaldehyde than non-drinkers.[40] Chronic alcohol consumption impairs mitochondrial oxidation of acetaldehyde, which can lead to a relative imbalance between the production and disposition of this metabolite; increased levels of acetaldehyde further impair mitochondrial functions.

METABOLIC DISTURBANCES ASSOCIATED WITH ALCOHOL METABOLISM (Fig. 8.1)

The increased NADH : NAD ratio which results from the oxidation of ethanol causes:

1. An increase in the lactate : pyruvate ratio, because of both decreased utilization and increased lactate production by the liver. There is lactic acidosis with a reduced renal capacity for uric acid excretion and a secondary hyperuricaemia.

2. Impaired carbohydrate metabolism with reduced gluconeogenesis from amino acids; this may produce hypoglycaemia.

3. Impaired fat metabolism:[41] H^+ ions replace two-carbon fragments derived from fatty acids as the main energy source of hepatocyte mitochondria and also depress the citric acid cycle. There is decreased fatty acid oxidation. There is also an increase in α-glycerophosphate, a consequent increase in trapping of fatty acids and an accompanying increased synthesis of triglycerides. In

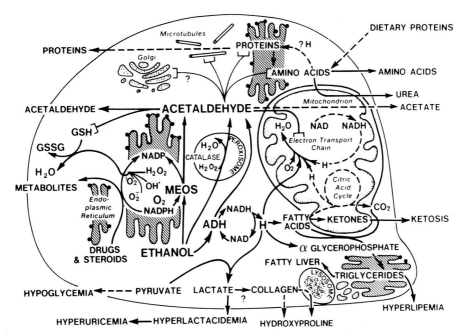

Fig. 8.1 Metabolism of ethanol. Oxidation of ethanol in the hepatocyte and link of the two products (acetaldehyde and H$^+$ ions) to disturbances in intermediary metabolism, including abnormalities of lipid, carbohydrate and protein metabolism. The broken lines indicate pathways that are depressed by ethanol. The symbol –[denotes interference or binding. NAD = nicotinamide adenine dinucleotide; NADH = reduced NAD; NADP = nicotinamide adenine dinucleotide phosphate; NADPH = reduced NADP; MEOS = microsomal ethanol oxidizing system; ADH = alcohol dehydrogenase. Reproduced with permission from Lieber[25].

long-standing alcohol abuse protein synthesis is depressed and this, together with impaired liver-cell secretory function, causes retention of lipoproteins and contributes to the accumulation of fat in hepatocytes.

4. Impaired metabolism of galactose, serotonin and other amines.

5. Alterations in steroid metabolism; this may explain some of the hormonal disturbances in chronic alcoholism.

PATHOLOGY OF ALCOHOLIC LIVER DISEASE

ALCOHOLIC STEATOSIS (FATTY CHANGE)

Steatosis is the earliest and the most common manifestation of alcoholic liver injury. It was seen in up to 90% of patients presenting for treatment of chronic alcoholism.[42] The clinical spectrum of manifestations ranges from asymptomatic hepatomegaly, through non-specific digestive symptoms, to life-threatening hepatic failure.[7] Sudden death may occur in alcoholics whose liver shows severe fatty change at autopsy. Blood alcohol levels in such cases have been reported as low, generally less than 50 mg/100 ml, and it has been suggested that death is due to alcohol withdrawal.[43]

Fatty change occurs predominantly in zone 3 of the liver acinus and is seen initially in hepatocytes adjacent to the terminal hepatic venule. It spreads from there to involve hepatocytes in all zones. However, the zonal distribution of fat may vary and is not helpful in indicating the aetiology of fatty change. Fat disappears from the hepatocytes in 2–4 weeks following abstinence from alcohol but may persist in macrophages in the portal tracts.

Initially fat droplets are membrane-bound, presumably by endoplasmic reticulum. As the droplets become larger they fuse, forming non-membrane-bound droplets. Fat droplets are seen as clear, intracytoplasmic vacuoles in haematoxylin and eosin stained sections after paraffin embedding (Fig. 8.2a). Formalin-fixed liver biopsies can be post-fixed in osmium tetroxide to demonstrate fat; the fat, seen as black osmicated droplets, can be readily measured and routine stains can still be performed (Fig. 8.2b).[44,45] Fat is seen predominantly as single, large vacuoles which displace the nuclei of the hepatocytes, so-called macrovesicular fatty change.

Liver-cell necrosis and inflammation are not usually seen at the fatty liver stage other than in association with lipogranuloma formation. Rupture of distended hepatocytes leads to the release of fat and an inflammatory response comprising lymphocytes, macrophages and occasionally eosinophils (Fig. 8.3).[46,47] Rarely, true epithelioid granulomas are seen, serial sectioning being required in order to demonstrate the presence of fat droplets.[48] Lipogranulomas usually occur in the region of the terminal hepatic venules,

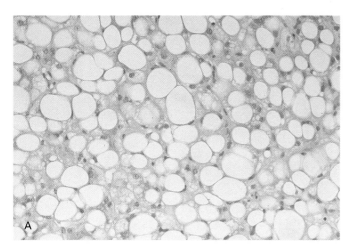

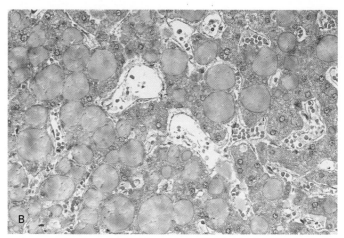

Fig. 8.2 Macrovesicular fatty change. (a) Most of the hepatocytes are distended by single, large fat droplets. The liver-cell nuclei are situated peripherally. H & E. (b) Liver tissue which has been 'post-fixed' in osmium tetroxide. The osmicated fat is seen as brown droplets of varying sizes. H & E.

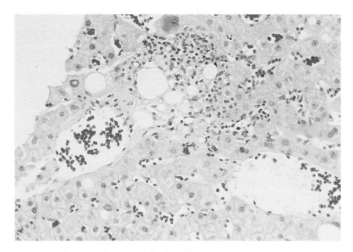

Fig. 8.3 Lipogranuloma. Mildly fatty liver with a lipogranuloma in the region of a terminal hepatic venule. H & E.

are usually present in association with marked elevations of serum transaminases, alkaline phosphatase and bilirubin. The clinical and biochemical features are highly suggestive of extrahepatic biliary obstruction. The liver shows striking microvesicular fatty change which is maximal in acinar zone 3, may extend into zone 2 but usually spares zone 1 (Fig. 8.4). Some macrovesicular fat droplets may also be present. Bile is frequently seen in perivenular hepatocytes and canaliculi, while Mallory bodies and a neutrophil polymorph infiltrate are usually minimal or absent. Perivenular fibrosis is usually present as is a small amount of perisinusoidal fibrosis. Enzyme histochemical studies revealed marked functional impairment of hepatocytes in the perivenular regions. Electron microscopy showed widespread damage or loss of organelles, particularly mitochondria and endoplasmic reticulum.[51]

and are seen most frequently in severe fatty change. Small amounts of fibrous tissue may be present. However, lipogranulomas usually disappear without sequelae.

Alcoholic foamy degeneration (microvesicular fatty change)

Microvesicular fatty change has been previously described in alcohol-induced liver injury.[49,50] The term alcoholic foamy degeneration has been used to describe severe liver injury occurring at the fatty liver stage, in the absence of alcoholic hepatitis.[51] Uchida and co-workers[51] described 20 patients with alcoholic foamy degeneration, all of whom recovered rapidly once alcohol was withdrawn. They considered alcoholic foamy degeneration to be a purely degenerative process since it occurred in the absence of inflammation. Jaundice and hepatomegaly

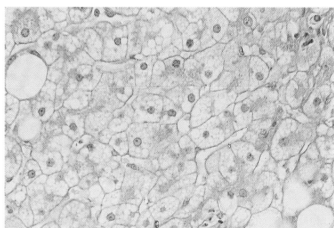

Fig. 8.4 Microvesicular fatty change. Most of the liver cells are distended by large numbers of small fat droplets. The cells have centrally situated nuclei. Chromotrope aniline blue.

PERIVENULAR FIBROSIS

Baboons fed alcohol chronically have been observed to progress from the fatty liver stage to cirrhosis, without an intermediate stage of alcoholic hepatitis.[52,53] Perivenular fibrosis was present in the baboons' livers in association with alcoholic steatosis. A similar lesion occurs in humans[52,54] and it is now accepted as a probable intermediate stage in the development of alcoholic cirrhosis and distinct from alcoholic hepatitis.

Perivenular fibrosis has been defined as fibrosis extending around at least two-thirds of the perimeter of the terminal hepatic venule, the fibrous rim measuring over 4 μm in thickness (Fig. 8.5).[54] Serial liver biopsy studies have shown that patients with perivenular fibrosis at the fatty liver stage are likely to have progressive liver injury if drinking continues.[52,55] In the study of Worner & Lieber,[55] 13 of 15 patients with perivenular fibrosis in the first biopsy developed more severe disease within 4 years; 9 had more extensive fibrosis, 1 incomplete cirrhosis and 3 established cirrhosis.[55] However, several recent quantitative studies of 'early alcoholic liver disease' failed to demonstrate fibrous thickening of the walls of the terminal hepatic venules.[56,57]

Ultrastructural studies have shown myofibroblast proliferation around the terminal hepatic venule, occurring in association with perivenular fibrosis.[54] Perivenular fibrosis is thought to be the first lesion in a sequence of events which leads ultimately to the development of cirrhosis. The recognition of perivenular fibrosis at the fatty liver stage may permit the identification of patients who are likely to have progressive liver injury if they continue to drink.

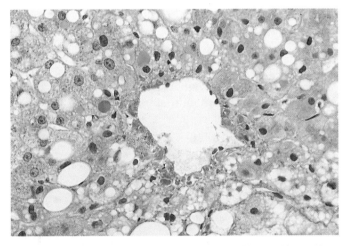

Fig. 8.5 Perivenular fibrosis. Alcoholic fatty liver without evidence of alcoholic hepatitis. The terminal hepatic venule is surrounded by an abnormally thick rim of fibrous tissue; fibrous tissue also extends focally into the surrounding liver in a pericellular pattern. Several hepatocytes contain large mitochondria (discrete, pink globular masses). Chromotrope-aniline blue.

ALCOHOLIC HEPATITIS

Beckett et al[58] used the term 'acute alcoholic hepatitis' to describe a clinicopathological syndrome. Many subsequent studies have shown that a wide variety of clinical features and biochemical abnormalities may accompany the same morphological pattern of liver injury.[59-61] The term 'steatonecrosis', used by some authors, is synonymous with alcoholic hepatitis.[62,63] Alcoholic hepatitis can only be reliably diagnosed morphologically, and histological severity cannot be reliably predicted from the clinical features. A liver biopsy study of patients presenting for treatment of alcoholism revealed alcoholic hepatitis in 17%.[64] Alcoholic hepatitis may be asymptomatic[65] but it is usually associated with non-specific digestive symptoms, hepatomegaly and raised liver enzymes.[59,61] About 25% of patients with severe liver injury show evidence of liver failure or hepatic encephalopathy.[59,61] Since alcoholic hepatitis may be asymptomatic, and up to 39% of patients have established cirrhosis at the time of first presentation,[66] the true incidence of alcoholic hepatitis remains to be determined. Alcoholic hepatitis is reported to occur less commonly in Japan than in other parts of the world.[67] Several recent reviews discuss the prognosis and treatment of alcoholic hepatitis as well as the clinical and pathological features of the condition.[14,17,68]

The liver injury is characterized by fatty change, liver-cell necrosis and a neutrophil polymorph infiltrate.[11,69] Mallory bodies, which are irregularly shaped masses of deeply eosinophilic intracytoplasmic material, are usually seen but their presence is not obligatory for the diagnosis. Unlike fat droplets, Mallory bodies persist in liver cells for some months after alcohol consumption ceases. Giant mitochondria may be seen on light microscopy (Fig. 8.5) as eosinophilic, globular and occasionally needle-shaped cytoplasmic inclusions;[70,71] the presence of giant mitochondria, where the liver injury is very mild, may be a 'diagnostic hint' of chronic alcohol consumption.[72]

When the liver injury is mild, only occasional foci of liver-cell necrosis are seen in the perivenular region accompanied by a light neutrophil polymorph infiltrate; occasional enlarged hepatocytes may contain Mallory bodies, and minimal pericellular fibrosis may be present. In fully developed alcoholic hepatitis liver-cell necrosis is extensive; liver-cell enlargement is a prominent feature and ballooned hepatocytes frequently contain Mallory bodies (Fig. 8.6a). The neutrophil infiltrate is often concentrated around hepatocytes containing Mallory bodies (Fig. 8.6b). Monoclonal antibodies to hepatocyte cytokeratins, K8 and K18, can be used to confirm the presence of Mallory bodies (Fig. 8. 6c) and to detect small Mallory bodies that are not readily apparent in routinely stained sections. Fatty change is usually present but is variable in severity. Other features that may be seen include lipogranulomas, acidophilic necrosis of hepato-

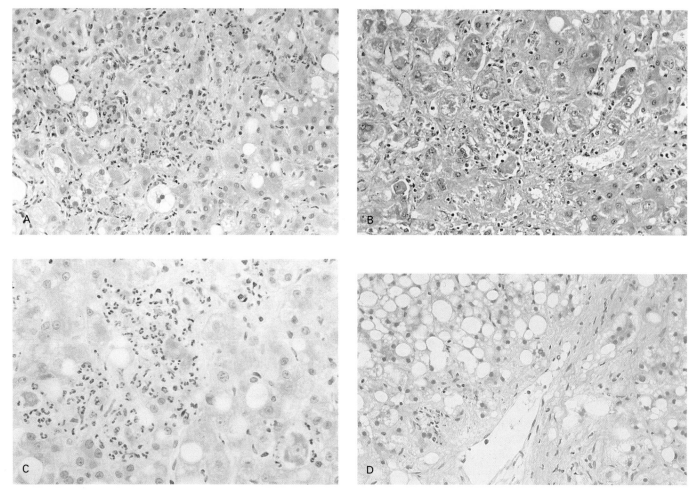

Fig. 8.6 Alcoholic hepatitis. (a) The acinar architecture is disturbed and there is a considerable liver-cell necrosis with an associated neutrophil polymorph infiltrate. Macrovesicular fat droplets are present in some hepatocytes. The patient, a woman aged 30 years, had a 12-year history of heavy drinking. H & E. (b) Several enlarged hepatocytes contain Mallory bodies and a heavy neutrophil polymorph infiltrate is seen in proximity to these cells. A marked degree of liver-cell necrosis is apparent and a few large fat droplets are seen. H & E. (c) Mallory bodies. A monoclonal antibody to cytokeratins K8, K18 (CAM 5.2, Becton Dickinson, Santa Barbara, CA) reacts strongly with Mallory bodies while the hepatocytes show a weaker staining reaction. PAP. (d) Sclerosing hyaline necrosis. Alcoholic hepatitis is apparent in the region of a terminal hepatic venule. Increased amounts of fibrous tissue surround the venule. Mild fatty change is seen and some of the hepatocytes contain Mallory bodies. H & E.

cytes (apoptotic bodies), induced (i.e. 'ground-glass') hepatocytes, oncocytic hepatocytes, ductal metaplasia of hepatocytes, bile stasis, Kupffer cell proliferation, bile-duct proliferation, 'microscopic cholangitis', a lympho-cytic infiltrate, and variable degrees of perivenular and pericellular fibrosis.

Sclerosing hyaline necrosis, described by Edmondson et al,[73] forms part of the morphological spectrum of alcoholic hepatitis,[69] representing a more extensive degree of perivenular liver-cell necrosis associated with the deposition of fibrous tissue (Fig. 8.6d). The terminal hepatic venules may become occluded and portal hyper-tension can occur in the absence of cirrhosis.[74]

Initially, fibrosis is seen only in the perivenular region and in association with foci of necrosis. With progression, widespread pericellular fibrosis is seen (Fig. 8.7). More severe bridging necrosis between adjacent terminal hepatic venules or between terminal hepatic venules and portal tracts results in condensation of pericellular fibrosis tissue and the formation of septa.[75] Elastic fibres, which stain with orcein, can be seen in active fibrous septa, but not in areas of passive collapse of the reticulin framework.[76]

The histopathologist is frequently asked on the basis of the liver biopsy to assess prognosis and the likelihood of the liver injury being reversible. The features which indicate a risk of progression to cirrhosis are:

(i) The extent and degree of liver-cell necrosis and fibrosis; active liver-cell necrosis and pericellular fibrosis are bad prognostic indicators;[77] the formation of fibrous septa with elastic fibre deposition[76] and architectural disturbance are also bad features.

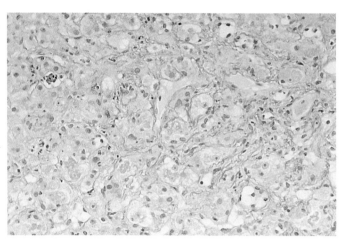

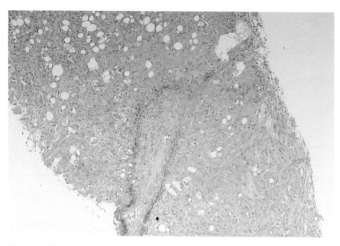

Fig. 8.7 Pericellular fibrosis. The liver shows the features of severe alcoholic hepatitis and prominent fibrosis. Thin bands of pericellular collagen, situated in the perisinusoidal space of Disse, surround cords of hepatocytes and hepatocytes showing ductal metaplasia. Mallory bodies are seen in several hepatocytes. Sirius red.

Fig. 8.8 Veno-occlusive lesion in alcoholic liver disease: note the intimal proliferation producing considerable narrowing of the hepatic vein branch. van Gieson–Verhoef

(ii) Diffuse parenchymal disease; this may per se have a poor outlook and result in an acute fulminant course.

(iii) Widespread obliteration of hepatic venules (see below).

(iv) Widespread Mallory body formation. The significance of Mallory bodies in relation to the severity of liver injury has been reviewed by Harinasuta & Zimmerman,[62] Christoffersen et al,[78] and by Boitnott & Maddrey;[76] in non-cirrhotic livers parenchymal fibrosis appears to be more marked when Mallory bodies are present.

Bouchier et. al[80] reported a prospective study of 510 patients with a liver biopsy diagnosis of alcoholic liver disease who were followed for a 10-year period; 72% of those with simple fatty liver were alive at 10 years while only 37% of patients in whom alcoholic hepatitis was the predominant histological lesion survived. The highest mortality rate for patients with alcoholic hepatitis, both with and without cirrhosis, is in the first year after diagnosis.[81] Patients with alcoholic hepatitis are likely to have progressive injury leading to cirrhosis;[82] in one study 50% of patients with alcoholic hepatitis, who continued drinking, developed cirrhosis in 10–13 years.[83] Pares et al[84] documented three variables that independently increase the risk of progression to cirrhosis: the severity of the initial histological injury, continuation of drinking, and female sex.

Occlusive venous lesions in alcoholic liver disease

Goodman & Ishak[85] reviewed 200 autopsy cases of alcoholic liver disease, and described three types of venous lesions:

1. lymphocytic phlebitis;
2. phlebosclerosis, due to perivenular fibrosis gradually obliterating vein lumens;
3. veno-occlusive lesions characterized by intimal proliferation, fibrosis of the vein wall and varying degrees of luminal obliteration.

Lymphocytic phlebitis was noted in 16% of patients with alcoholic hepatitis and in 4% of those with cirrhosis. Phlebosclerosis was found in all cases of alcoholic hepatitis and cirrhosis. Veno-occlusive lesions (Fig. 8.8) were found in 52% of cases of alcoholic hepatitis with portal hypertension, totally occluded veins were found in 47%, and partial occlusion of varying severity was found in 74% of cirrhotics. Portal hypertension correlated significantly with the degree of phlebosclerosis and veno-occlusive change. In biopsy material Burt & MacSween[86] confirmed that phlebosclerosis was a universal finding in alcoholic hepatitis and cirrhosis but they found veno-occlusive lesions in only 10% of 256 biopsies and lymphocytic phlebitis in 4%. These occlusive venous lesions may contribute to the atrophy of hepatic parenchyma and functional impairment. Atrophy of the left lobe of the liver has been reported in association with endophlebitis of the left hepatic vein.[87]

ALCOHOLIC CIRRHOSIS

Alcohol is the most common cause of cirrhosis in Western countries.[3,4] In the USA, in the 35–54 age group, cirrhosis, predominantly alcoholic, is the fourth commonest cause of death in men and the fifth commonest cause in women.[6]

A WHO group[88] has defined cirrhosis as 'a diffuse process characterized by fibrosis and the conversion of the normal liver architecture into structurally abnormal nodules'. Micronodular cirrhosis is the most common type of cirrhosis seen in association with alcohol.[89] This is characterized by remarkably uniform-sized regenerative nodules, most of which are less than 3 mm in diameter (Fig. 8.9). Bands of fibrous tissue completely surround the regenerative nodules; the terminal hepatic venules are not recognizable, but new vessel formation is apparent within the fibrous tissue (Fig. 8.9).

Cirrhotic livers may also show the features of alcoholic hepatitis; liver-cell necrosis occurs predominantly at the periphery of the regenerative nodules. A variable mixture of neutrophils, lymphocytes, plasma cells and macrophages is seen in the fibrous tissue. The presence of alcoholic hepatitis usually means continued drinking, even though there may be little or no fatty change.

Superimposed hepatitis C virus infection explains some of the reported cases of chronic active hepatitis in alcoholic patients[90–95] (Fig. 8.10). However, cases of chronic active hepatitis that are serologically negative for both hepatitis B and C virus are still being described[96] and the role of alcohol per se as a cause of a chronic active hepatitis-like injury remains controversial.

Bile ductular proliferation is commonly seen in alcoholic liver disease; ultrastructural studies have demonstrated a transition of cords of hepatocytes to bile ductules, while special stains and enzyme histochemical studies have demonstrated glycogen, α_1-antitrypsin and glucose-6-phosphatase in the ductular cells.[97] Immunohistochemical studies using a variety of monoclonal and polyclonal antibodies to cytokeratins have demonstrated the presence of the bile-duct cytokeratins K7 and K19 in these ductular cells[98] (Fig. 8.11). The proliferating ductules seen in the periportal regions have been considered to be regenerating hepatocytes showing 'ductal metaplasia'.[98]

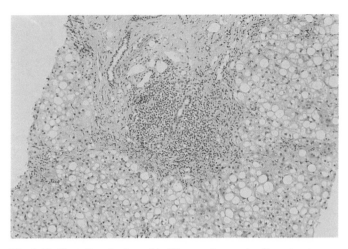

Fig. 8.10 Chronic active hepatitis. Piecemeal necrosis of hepatocytes and a focal lymphocytic infiltrate are present at the periphery of several regenerative nodules. Lymphoid aggregates are prominent in the portal areas. The liver also showed evidence of mild alcoholic hepatitis superimposed on established micronodular cirrhosis; the hepatitis C serology was positive. H & E.

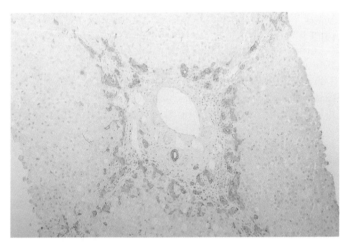

Fig. 8.11 'Ductal metaplasia' of hepatocytes. Hepatocytes at the periphery of several regenerative nodules show ductal features and contained bile-duct cytokeratin; a small bile duct also shows positive staining with a polyclonal *anti*-cytokeratin antibody. PAP.

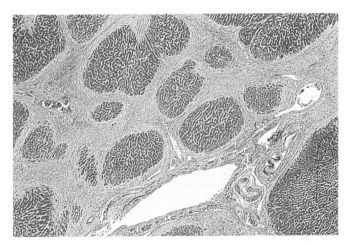

Fig. 8.9 Alcoholic cirrhosis. Broad bands of fibrous tissue surround a number of small regenerative nodules. Masson's trichrome.

Cirrhosis may become macronodular, particularly if drinking ceases.[89,99,100] The regenerative nodules then vary greatly in size, and many measure up to several centimetres in diameter; many such nodules contain portal tracts and terminal hepatic venules which are abnormally related to each other (Fig. 8.12). A mixed micro- and macronodular cirrhosis, with equal proportions of micro- and macronodules, is not an uncommon finding at autopsy. Large regenerative nodules may, on occasion, have clinical and radiological features suggestive of hepatocellular carcinoma. Nagasue et al[101] reported several such cases and proposed the term 'hepatocellular pseudotumour in the cirrhotic liver' to describe these nodules.

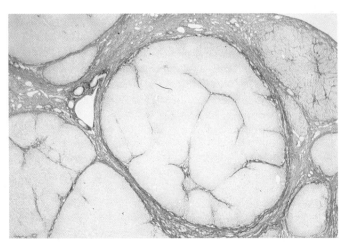

Fig. 8.12 Macronodular cirrhosis. Portions of several macroregenerative nodules are apparent; there is no evidence of active liver injury. The patient, a man aged 61 with a long history of heavy drinking, had abstained for several years. An open, wedge biopsy of liver was performed in conjunction with a cholecystectomy. Sirius red.

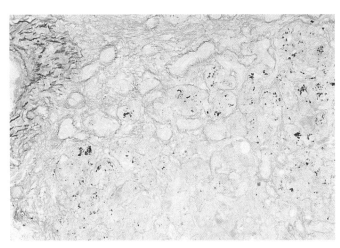

Fig. 8.13 Copper accumulation in alcoholic cirrhosis. Some of the hepatocytes in a regenerative nodule contain red-brown granules of copper. Elastic fibres are apparent in the fibrous tissue seen at the periphery of the nodule. Shikata's orcein stain.

Steatosis and alcoholic hepatitis are reliably diagnosed by needle biopsy of the liver, but cirrhosis may be under-diagnosed because of sampling difficulty, particularly when an aspiration Menghini type of needle is used.[102] Macronodular cirrhosis may be suspected, but cannot be confidently diagnosed by needle biopsy, because of the large size of the nodules. Helpful criteria for needle biopsy diagnosis have been described[88,103] and are discussed in Chapters 10 and 19.

Globules of α_1-antitrypsin are frequently seen in hepatocytes at the periphery of regenerative nodules, the accumulation being considered to be a consequence of impaired protein secretion.[104] Copper may also accumulate in hepatocytes in alcoholic liver disease. Copper bound to protein is seen as PAS-positive, diastase-resistant globules which stain positively with orcein[105] (Fig. 8.13).

Oxyphilic granular hepatocytes, which have been termed 'hepatic oncocytes', are frequently seen at the periphery of regenerative nodules in alcoholic cirrhosis.[106,107] Oncocytes and induced hepatocytes can be differentiated from classic 'ground-glass' hepatocytes which contain HBsAg, by orcein staining or immunohistochemistry.[108]

Prognosis and reversibility of cirrhosis

A Veterans Administration Cooperative Study Group followed 281 alcoholic patients prospectively for 4 years to assess prognosis;[109] the worst prognosis, 35% survival at 48 months, was seen in patients with alcoholic hepatitis superimposed on cirrhosis. The most significant predictors of survival included age, grams of alcohol consumed, the ratio of serum aminotransferases (AST : ALT), and the histological and clinical severity of the disease.

Numerous studies have shown that abstinence can prolong survival in alcoholic cirrhosis.[59,110,111] In Powell & Klatskin's series,[110] 68% of cirrhotics who abstained survived 5 years, compared with 41% of those who continued to drink. Traditionally, cirrhosis has been thought to be an irreversible process; this concept is now being challenged. Cirrhosis in animal models is reversible, provided that the aetiological agent, e.g. carbon tetrachloride, is removed, and that sufficient time is allowed for the liver to return to its normal structure.[112] Reversal of established cirrhosis in the human is rare, however, and reported instances are open to some doubt.[112,113]

Colchicine, an anti-inflammatory drug which is an inhibitor of collagen synthesis, has been studied in a randomized, double-blind, placebo-controlled trial in which 100 cirrhotic patients (45 of whom had alcoholic cirrhosis) were followed for 14 years;[114] the overall survival was considerably better in the colchicine group than in the placebo group (median survival 11 and 3.5 years, respectively). Histological improvement was seen only in the colchicine group, with an apparent decrease in hepatic fibrosis. These are preliminary results and this important study is continuing.

OTHER MORPHOLOGICAL FEATURES OF ALCOHOLIC LIVER INJURY

Cholestatic syndromes

Alcoholic liver disease may present with clinical and biochemical features that are strongly suggestive of extrahepatic biliary obstruction.[49,115-117] The features include jaundice, right upper quadrant pain and tenderness, hepatomegaly, and marked elevation of serum

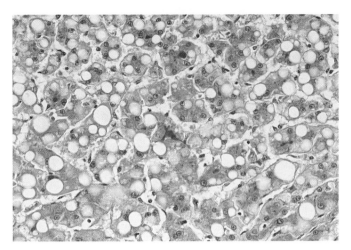

Fig. 8.14 Fatty liver and cholestasis. The hepatocytes show fatty change and bile is present in some canaliculi. H & E.

bilirubin, serum alkaline phosphatase and serum cholesterol. Biliary obstruction due to gallstones or alcoholic pancreatitis[118] can be excluded by ultrasound, transhepatic cholangiography or endoscopic retrograde cholangiopancreatography (ERCP).

A high index of clinical suspicion of intrahepatic cholestasis is required in order to avoid unnecessary surgery in patients with alcoholic liver disease, as the risk of postoperative hepatic and/or renal failure is considerable. Severe cholestasis has been described in association with: (i) fatty liver (Fig. 8.14);[49,50,119] (ii) alcoholic foamy degeneration (Fig. 8.4);[51] (iii) alcoholic hepatitis;[59,62,63,119] (iv) decompensated alcoholic cirrhosis; and (v) Zieve's syndrome which comprises alcoholic steatosis, jaundice, hyperlipidaemia and haemolytic anaemia.[120] A recent Veterans Administration Cooperative Study[121] has shown a significant correlation between tissue cholestasis and mortality in alcoholic liver disease. The possibility that jaundice occurring in patients with a history of excess alcohol consumption may be due to non-alcoholic liver disease, such as viral hepatitis or drug-induced cholestasis, must also be considered.[122]

In patients with a severe fatty liver who develop a cholestatic syndrome, the liver biopsy may show portal tract changes with oedema, increased prominence of marginal bile ducts and a mild to moderate cholangitis with a neutrophil polymorph infiltrate ('microscopic cholangitis').[123]

Portal tract changes

Portal fibrosis is said not to occur as a result of alcohol injury per se. However, it may sometimes be a feature; Morgan et al[124] found that the presence of portal fibrosis correlated with a previous history of viral hepatitis or episodes of acute pancreatitis. Increased numbers of

portal tract macrophages are seen frequently in alcoholic liver disease. A recent study describes this feature at virtually all stages and has shown that the macrophages have markedly enhanced lysosomal enzymal release, compared with the resident macrophages in normal livers, suggesting that cytotoxic mediators released by these activated cells may be contributing to liver injury.[125]

Hepatic siderosis (see Ch. 5)

Excess stainable iron is found in both hepatocytes and Kupffer cells in many patients with alcoholic liver disease. In one study 57% of patients had mild siderosis while 7% had grade 3+/4+ siderosis.[126] The excessive iron accumulation has been attributed to the high iron content of alcoholic beverages[127,128] and to a direct effect of alcohol, enhancing iron absorption,[129] and possibly a promotion of desialylation of transferrin by endothelial cells in the liver, followed by deposition of iron in hepatic lysosomes.[130]

It is now generally accepted that only mild siderosis, grade 1+/2+, is alcohol-related; patients with alcoholic liver disease in whom iron accumulation is massive (grade 3+/4+) are also suffering from genetic haemochromatosis (Fig. 8.15).[131] Biochemical measurement of the hepatic iron concentration is used to differentiate the two conditions;[131,132] an hepatic iron index (hepatic iron concentration divided by the patient's age) of greater than 2 is virtually diagnostic of genetic haemochromatosis.[132,133] In cases where marked iron overload is an unexpected finding in a biopsy specimen from an alcoholic patient the hepatic iron, demonstrated by the Perls' method, can be measured by computerized image analysis[134] or the remainder of the liver tissue can be removed from the

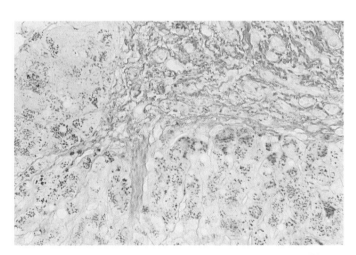

Fig. 8.15 Genetic haemochromatosis and alcoholic liver disease. The liver shows the features of established micronodular cirrhosis, mild fatty change and grade 4+ siderosis with blue granules of iron being seen in 100% of hepatocytes and also in bile-duct epithelium. The patient, a man aged 54 years, had a history of heavy alcohol consumption for many years. Perls'/Sirius red.

paraffin block for biochemical measurement of the iron concentration (manuscript in preparation). In patients with genetic haemochromatosis, alcohol-associated liver injury may alter the distribution of liver iron, with haemosiderin appearing in Kupffer cells and portal tract macrophages as well as in hepatocytes (see Ch 5).

Porphyria cutanea tarda

Alcohol is thought to hasten the onset of the hepatic and cutaneous manifestations of porphyria cutanea tarda; alcohol withdrawal is followed by a dramatic clinical and biochemical improvement.[128] The hepatocytes contain birefringent acicular cytoplasmic inclusions which are specific for porphyria cutanea tarda.[135] Other features include red autofluorescence in hepatocytes under ultraviolet light, and usually some degree of siderosis; in addition there may be evidence of alcoholic liver disease.

Hepatocellular carcinoma (see Ch. 16)

Primary liver carcinoma develops in 5–15% of patients with alcoholic cirrhosis, usually in association with macronodular cirrhosis[89,136] (Fig. 8.16). There is some evidence that alcohol may play a specific role in hepatic carcinogenesis, particularly since liver-cell carcinoma may rarely occur in the alcoholic in the absence of cirrhosis.[137,138] While there is no evidence that alcohol is a direct hepatic carcinogen it could certainly act as a promoter or co-carcinogen because of its ability to induce the hepatic microsomal P-450-dependent biotransformation system, in particular the ethanol-inducible isoenzyme cytochrome P-450 2E1.

The role of the hepatitis B virus (HBV) in the pathogenesis of hepatocellular carcinomas associated with alcoholic

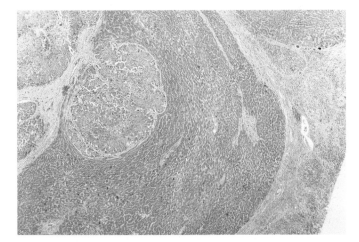

Fig. 8.16 Hepatocellular carcinoma arising in a liver showing macronodular cirrhosis. The patient, a man aged 58 years, had a past history of heavy drinking but had abstained for several years. H & E.

cirrhosis remains controversial; clinical studies by Ohnishi et al[139] and molecular biological studies by Brechot et al[140] support a role for the virus, while a recent study by Walter et al[141] failed to demonstrate integrated HBV in the livers of alcoholic cirrhotic patients with hepatocellular carcinomas. Preliminary studies suggest that the hepatitis C virus (HCV) may play a role in the pathogenesis of hepatocellular carcinomas in alcoholics.[142,143]

Several autopsy studies have suggested that dysplastic nodules, which develop within large (greater than 5 mm diameter) regenerative nodules in cirrhotic livers, may be the precursor lesion to hepatocellular carcinoma.[144,145] Cells within the dysplastic nodules exhibit increased cytoplasmic basophilia and enlarged nuclei and nucleoli; nuclear crowding with thickening of the liver cell plates is often seen and sometimes microacinar formation is apparent. Wada et al[145] suggest that the morphology of the dysplastic nodule is that of a lesion intermediate between that of the large regenerative nodule (sometimes referred to as adenomatous hyperplasia) and small nodules of hepatocellular carcinoma.

THE ROLE OF LIVER BIOPSY IN ALCOHOLIC LIVER DISEASE

In a study by Levin et al[122] only 80% of patients with a heavy alcohol intake were found to have alcohol-associated liver injury. The other 20% had various types of non-alcoholic liver disease including cholangitis, viral hepatitis, granulomatous hepatitis, passive venous congestion and non-specific changes; however, a more recent study[146] showed that a clinical diagnosis of alcoholic liver disease was significantly associated with a histological diagnosis of alcoholic liver disease, with a 98% specificity and a 79% sensitivity. Nevertheless, a liver biopsy is recommended in patients suspected of having alcoholic liver disease since it not only allows the clinical diagnosis of alcoholic liver disease to be confirmed or refuted but it also permits assessment of the severity and stage and thus the prognosis of the liver injury. This information will sometimes be used in counselling patients to obtain from alcohol. In addition, the liver biopsy may reveal coexisting and sometimes treatable liver disease such as infections or genetic haemochromatosis (Fig. 8.15). The role of liver biopsy will become increasingly important in monitoring the effects of anti-inflammatory and anti-fibrinogenic drugs used in the treatment of alcoholic hepatitis[17] and as part of the work-up of patients being considered for orthotopic liver transplantation.[147]

DIFFERENTIAL DIAGNOSIS

The entire histopathological spectrum of alcohol-associated liver injury is non-specific — for example, macrovesicular fatty change is seen frequently in association with diabetes mellitus, obesity and drugs, e.g. corticosteroids; microvesicular fatty change is the lesion seen characteristically in Reye's syndrome, fatty liver of pregnancy and in association with a variety of drugs,[148] e.g. sodium valproate, tetracycline, amiodarone.

Non-alcoholic steatohepatitis

The term 'non-alcoholic steatohepatitis' (NASH) was introduced by Ludwig et al[149] to describe an alcoholic hepatitis-like injury occurring in the livers of non-drinkers. Synonyms for NASH include fatty liver hepatitis, diabetic hepatitis and non-alcoholic Laennec's cirrhosis. Table 8.1 lists a variety of conditions in which NASH has been described and Table 8.2 lists drugs that have been associated with a similar pattern of liver injury.

The pathogenesis of non-alcoholic steatohepatitis is uncertain but may eventually provide insight into alcohol-associated hepatitis. Risk factors for non-alcoholic steatohepatitis include female gender, obesity, rapid weight loss and type II diabetes mellitus.[149,152,176] The histological features mimic those of alcoholic hepatitis (Fig. 8.17) although the injury tends to be less severe and Mallory bodies may be sparse or absent.[177] The diagnosis of non-alcoholic steatohepatitis is best restricted to cases in which there is a complete absence of alcohol abuse, particularly since some women can sustain alcoholic liver injury in association with low doses of alcohol ('social' drinking). The non-alcoholic injury tends to have a more indolent course than the alcohol-associated liver injury; nevertheless, progressive hepatic fibrosis and cirrhosis have been described.[177–180] In contrast, drugs such as perhexiline maleate[166] (Fig. 8.18) and amiodarone,[167–169] can cause severe, and sometimes fatal, alcoholic hepatitis-like injury;

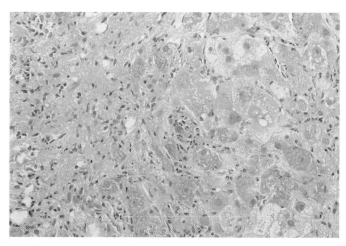

Fig. 8.18 Perhexiline maleate-induced hepatitis. The liver shows a moderately severe alcoholic hepatitis-like injury with numerous enlarged hepatocytes containing Mallory bodies, and widespread focal necrosis of liver cells with a prominent infiltrate of neutrophils. Pronounced pericellular fibrosis was also apparent. H&E.

progression to cirrhosis is well described with both drugs.[165,170]

Viral and drug hepatitis

Both acute and chronic viral hepatitis occur in patients with a history of excess alcohol consumption; the liver biopsy may show only viral hepatitis[122] or may show viral hepatitis superimposed on alcoholic liver disease[181] (Fig. 8.10). Chronic alcohol ingestion also increases the risk of acute drug-induced liver injury due to the induction of the isoenzyme cytochrome P-450 2E1 by alcohol.[37,38] The pattern of liver injury may be purely that of drug-associated injury but may also be superimposed on the various stages of alcoholic injury.

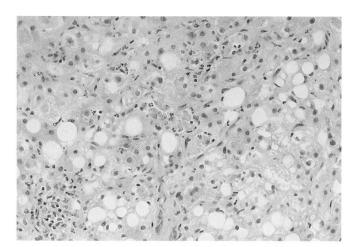

Fig. 8.17 Non-alcoholic steatohepatitis. The liver shows prominent fatty change, several enlarged hepatocytes containing Mallory bodies, focal liver-cell necrosis with drop-out of cells and a mild infiltrate of neutrophil polymorphs. The patient, a woman aged 48, a non-drinker, was mildly overweight. H&E.

Table 8.1 Conditions associated with non-alcoholic steatohepatitis

Obesity[149,150,152]
Diabetes mellitus[149,152–155]
Jejuno-ileal bypass surgery for obesity[156]
Gastroplasty for obesity[157]
Massive small intestinal resection[158]
Pancreato-duodenectomy for pancreatic carcinoma[159]
Limb lipodystrophy[160]
Small intestinal diverticulosis with bacterial overgrowth[161]
Abetalipoproteinaemia[162]
Weber–Christian disease[163]

Table 8.2 Drugs causing an alcoholic hepatitis-like injury

Perhexiline maleate[164–166]
Amiodarone[167–170]
Glucocorticoids[171]
Synthetic oestrogens[172]
Nifedipine[173]
4,4'-diethylaminoethoxyhexestrol[174]
Insulin[175]

Genetic haemochromatosis

As discussed earlier in this chapter and in chapter 5, alcoholic siderosis (grade 1+/2+ siderosis) must be differentiated from genetic haemochromatosis (grade 3+/4+ siderosis) that may occur in people with a history of excess alcohol consumption. The liver biopsy may show only the features of haemochromatosis or may show evidence of both alcoholic liver disease and genetic haemochromatosis (Fig. 8.15).

PATHOGENESIS OF ALCOHOLIC LIVER DISEASE

ULTRASTRUCTURAL CHANGES

The direct hepatotoxic effect of alcohol has been clearly demonstrated in numerous human[182–184] and animal studies.[185–187] Various forms of dietary manipulation failed to prevent the hepatotoxic effects of alcohol.[184,188] Non-intoxicating doses of alcohol given to healthy non-alcoholic volunteers caused liver injury in only 2–4 days;[184] the ultrastructural changes included the accumulation of fat droplets, proliferation of smooth endoplasmic reticulum (SER) and mitochondrial damage.

The mitochondria are enlarged and distorted in shape, with disrupted cristae and sometimes crystalline inclusions. Alterations in mitochondrial structure and function are due to the effects of alcohol metabolism, particularly acetaldehyde accumulation and the shift in redox potential.[25–28,189] Mitochondrial damage is always present at the fatty liver stage and persists as liver disease progresses. The presence of giant mitochondria, although non-specific, is highly suggestive of alcoholic liver disease (Fig. 8.19).[72] Giant mitochondria may be seen at all stages of alcoholic injury but are seen most frequently in association with alcoholic hepatitis.[190] They are often easily recognized in hepatocytes showing microvesicular steatosis. Chronic ethanol consumption results in a generalized depression in hepatic mitochondrial energy metabolism,[191] but the extent to which mitochondrial structure and functional damage contributes to the progression of alcoholic liver disease remains controversial.[192,193]

Proliferation of SER (Fig. 8.20) has been confirmed by the isolation and chemical measurement of microsomes.[182,194] The proliferation of SER is an adaptive response that accelerates alcohol metabolism and increases acetaldehyde production.[32,195] The associated enhancement of vitamin metabolism can lead to a reduction in hepatic vitamin A and the appearance of multivesicular lysosomes in hepatocytes and macrophages (Fig. 8.21).[196] Enhanced metabolism of drugs, e.g. paracetamol (acetaminophen),[197,198] exogenous vitamin A[199] and environmental chemicals, e.g. xylene[200] and carbon tetrachloride,[201] potentiates their hepatotoxic effects.

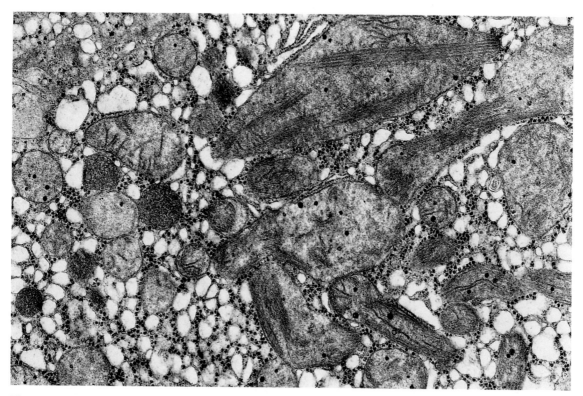

Fig. 8.19 Electron microscopy: giant mitochondria containing crystalline inclusions; a number of normal-sized mitochondria are also seen, some with inclusions. × 17 500.

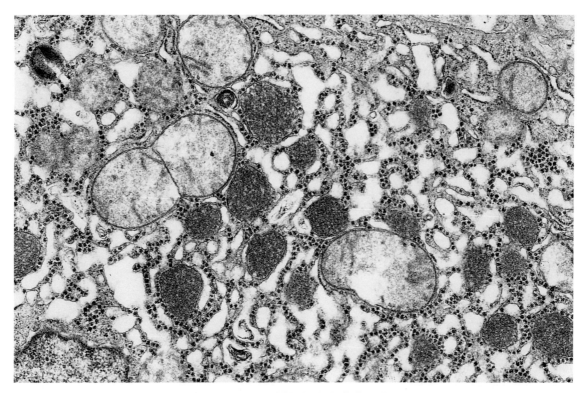

Fig. 8.20 Proliferation of smooth endoplasmic reticulum (SER) in alcoholic liver disease: note the prominent, vesiculated SER, a number of mitochondria, and also a few dense bodies. × 24 000.

Mitochondrial and plasma membranes exhibit increased fluidity after acute ethanol ingestion but become more rigid following chronic alcohol consumption.[189,202-204] The increased rigidity is thought to be due to changes in the lipid composition of the membranes.[205,206] Episodes of acute liver-cell injury may occur in association with chronic alcohol consumption, because liver cells with membranes altered by alcohol are more susceptible to other membrane toxins such as products of intestinal bacteria, viruses and drugs. Influx of calcium ions across damaged liver-cell membranes has been proposed as a final common pathway for acute liver-cell necrosis.[207,208] Hoek et al[209] have reviewed recent studies on the interaction of ethanol with biological membranes, in particular the actions of ethanol on hormonal signal transduction systems.

There is growing interest in the role of peroxidative decomposition of membrane lipids (lipid peroxidation) initiated by oxygen free radicals as a mechanism for alcohol-associated liver injury.[210-212] Oxygen radicals are formed during the metabolism of alcohol;[213] naturally occurring antioxidant and free radical-scavenging enzymes offer some protection but human and animal studies have shown that chronic alcohol consumption decreases the hepatic glutathione content, possibly making the liver more susceptible to oxidative stress and radical-related hepatic injury.[214] Lipid peroxidation results in the formation of more free radicals which can further damage cell and organelle membranes causing more liver-cell

injury. Recent studies suggest that antioxidant free radical scavengers are hepatoprotective;[215] the use of such agents in alcoholic liver disease merits further investigation.

PERIVENULAR HYPOXIA AND ENHANCED OXYGEN REQUIREMENTS

Alcohol-induced liver injury selectively affects the perivenular region in its early stages, and it has been postulated that a relatively lower oxygen tension in this zone may exaggerate the shift in redox potential that accompanies alcohol metabolism.[216] Hypoxia has been shown to induce perivenular liver-cell necrosis in chronic ethanol-fed rats.[217] However, Lieber et al[218] have studied the role of oxygenation in the pathogenesis of alcoholic liver injury in the baboon model and suggest that impaired oxygen utilization rather than lack of oxygen supply is a factor in alcohol-associated liver injury. Zone 3 hepatocytes contain the most SER and cytochrome P-450;[219] consequently, enzyme induction by alcohol and alcohol metabolism are thought to occur maximally in the perivenular region of the liver acini. Israel et al[31] have likened the acceleration of alcohol metabolism with an associated enhancement of oxygen requirement to 'a hypermetabolic state' and this has been the basis for animal and human studies of propylthiouracil;[220,221] for more details see a recent review by Orrego & Carmichael.[222]

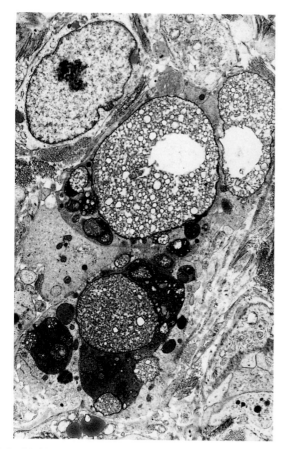

Fig. 8.21 Multivesicular lysosomes. Portion of a cell containing several multivesicular lysosomes of the type also seen in vitamin A deficiency. × 4570.

HEPATOCYTE ENLARGEMENT

Hepatomegaly, seen in association with chronic alcohol consumption, is due to the accumulation of both lipid and protein in hepatocytes (Fig. 8.6a,b).[223] Acetaldehyde and acetate are thought to impair microtubule-mediated protein secretion by hepatocytes.[224] Water is retained in proportion to protein, leading to liver-cell enlargement which may progress through ballooning degeneration to necrosis. Microtubules have a role in the maintenance of the liver-cell shape, and a decrease in the number of microtubules may thus also contribute to the ballooning of hepatocytes.[225]

Some studies report a strong positive correlation between hepatocyte enlargement and intrahepatic pressure;[226–228] however, other studies in baboons[229] and humans[230] failed to demonstrate this relationship. Okanoue et al[231] performed liver biopsies and measured the intrahepatic portal vein pressure in 12 patients immediately after abstinence from alcohol and repeated both investigations after the biochemistry improved; the reduction in intrahepatic pressure correlated with the reduction in size of swollen hepatocytes in patients with mild

fibrosis but in those with severe fibrosis the intrahepatic portal pressure remained high despite the reduction in hepatocyte size. It would seem that hepatocyte enlargement is only one of the mechanisms responsible for portal hypertension in pre-cirrhotic, alcoholic liver disease.

MALLORY BODIES (MALLORY'S HYALIN, ALCOHOLIC HYALIN)

Mallory,[232] in 1911, described amorphous, eosinophilic material in hepatocytes in alcoholic liver disease. The term 'Mallory body' is favoured since the same material is seen in a wide variety of non-alcoholic liver diseases. They are seen in all forms of NASH outlined in Tables 8.1 and 8.2. Mallory bodies are also seen in prolonged cholestasis[233] including primary biliary cirrhosis,[234] in Wilson's disease,[235] Indian childhood cirrhosis,[236] focal nodular hyperplasia,[237] and hepatocellular carcinoma.[238] Mallory bodies have been seen in the lung in asbestosis,[239] in radiation damage and interstitial fibrosis,[240] and have been produced experimentally using griseofulvin,[241] diethylnitrosamine,[242] and dieldrin.[243]

Three ultrastructurally distinct forms of Mallory bodies have been described:[244]

Type I — bundles of filaments in parallel arrays;
Type II — clusters of randomly oriented fibrils;
Type III — granular or amorphous substance containing only scattered fibrils.

The filament thickness varies from 5 to 20 nm, depending on the method of measurement. Type II Mallory bodies (Fig. 8.22) are the type seen most frequently in alcoholic liver disease.

Isolation of Mallory bodies in a purified fraction has made chemical analysis possible.[245] Human Mallory bodies are composed predominantly of protein; five polypeptide bands have been detected by electrophoretic analysis, with molecular weights ranging from 32 kD to 56 kD.[246] Small amounts of carbohydrate have also been detected.[246–248] The polypeptides resemble, but are not identical, to those of the keratin intermediate filaments in the cytoskeleton of the hepatocyte.[249,250] Mallory body formation is thought to result from derangement of the intermediate filament component of the cytoskeleton of the hepatocyte,[251–254] but they are not composed only of intermediate filament proteins. Antibodies to Mallory bodies react with the cytoplasmic filament system of normal hepatocytes.[255,256] However, Mallory bodies also contain a number of unique antigenic determinants.[256,257] Mallory bodies from alcoholic and non-alcoholic liver disease have been shown to share a common antigenic determinant.[258]

Currently there are three main hypotheses concerning the pathogenesis of Mallory bodies — see Denk et al,[248] French,[252–254] French et al[259] and Worman:[260]

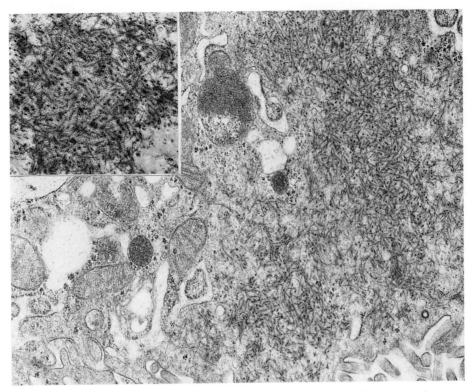

Fig. 8.22 Mallory body, type II. It consists of a mass of randomly orientated filaments, seen in greater detail in the inset. × 23 000 and 27 500

1. Microtubular failure. This theory is based on the observation that agents such as colchicine and alcohol cause microtubular disassembly and an increase of perinuclear intermediate filaments, which are thought to favour the development of Mallory bodies. However, several morphometrical studies have failed to show a relationship between microtubular abnormalities and Mallory body formation.

2. Preneoplasia with a structural phenotypic change. Hepatic carcinogens, such as griseofulvin[249] and diethylnitrosamine,[242] induce Mallory body formation and also the appearance of oncofetal markers in the same benign and malignant cells. It has therefore been postulated that Mallory body formation is part of the disorganization of the cytoskeleton caused by oncogenic transformation. This hypothesis obviously does not explain the presence of Mallory bodies in non-neoplastic liver disease but would be consonant with the presence of Mallory bodies in hepatocellular carcinoma.[261]

3. Vitamin A deficiency. Mallory body formation is considered to be a pathological and a predominantly hepatocytic form of keratinization. This is based on the observation that vitamin A deficiency can induce Mallory body formation in mice[262] and that serum vitamin A levels show a significant inverse correlation with the number of hepatocytes containing Mallory bodies.[263]

Irrespective of the mechanism of formation, all current data suggest that Mallory bodies form as a consequence of disruption of the normal intermediate filament network in the hepatocyte and that they are composed, at least in part, of the pre-existing intermediate filaments. A variety of cytokeratin antibodies have been developed and are useful not only for confirming the presence of Mallory bodies but also in the detection of small, not readily apparent, Mallory bodies.[264,265] Another reagent that can be used in the detection of Mallory bodies is monoclonal anti-ubiquitin antibody (ubiquitin, a polypeptide, is present on keratin intermediate filaments in a variety of cells and on Mallory bodies).[266] The use of sensitive immunohistochemical techniques has confirmed the presence of Mallory bodies in a wide variety of non-alcoholic liver diseases; nevertheless Mallory bodies are seen most frequently in alcoholic (71%) compared with non-alcoholic liver disease (40%).[264] Mallory bodies may also contain bile-duct cytokeratins K7 and K19; Van Eyken et al[98] have suggested that hepatocytes that exhibit 'ductal metaplasia' and express K7 and K19 (Fig. 8.11) may be showing pre-Mallory body changes. A recent electron microscopic study by De Vos & Desmet[267] describes previously unrecognized undifferentiated small cells, possibly a progenitor cell or stem cell population; the relationship of these to cells showing pre-Mallory body changes remains to be elucidated.

LIVER REGENERATION

Hepatic regeneration is controlled by a complex interaction between a wide variety of hormones and growth factors; the responsiveness of hepatocytes is strongly influenced by their prior metabolic state — see recent reviews by Fausto[268] and Bucher[269] and Chapter 10. Chronic alcohol consumption has been shown to significantly impair rat liver regeneration after partial hepatectomy; regenerative activity returned to normal after abstinence for one week.[270] Impaired liver regeneration associated with chronic alcohol ingestion could be an additional factor contributing to the severity and outcome of liver injury in humans.

Epidermal growth factor may be one of the hepatotrophic factors with an important role in maintaining hepatocellular function and aiding cellular repair and regeneration.[271] Studies on isolated rat hepatocytes suggest that chronic alcohol administration impairs endocytosis of epidermal growth factor which may in turn contribute to the alcohol-associated impairment of liver regeneration.[272]

HEPATIC FIBROGENESIS

A recent issue of *Seminars in Liver Disease* was devoted to 'Connective Tissue Metabolism and Hepatic Fibrosis' with an introductory overview by Bissell[273] and a series of excellent review articles.[274–278] Alcohol produces several highly characteristic; although not entirely specific, patterns of fibrosis. The early lesion may be that of perivenular fibrosis[52,54] (Fig. 8.5); while a 'chicken-wire' pattern of pericellular fibrosis may be seen in association with both perivenular fibrosis and alcoholic hepatitis (Fig. 8.7). Progressive alcoholic fibrosis apparently unrelated to alcoholic hepatitis is seen frequently in the livers of heavy drinkers in Japan;[279–281] the role of the hepatitis C virus in this progressive injury remains to be elucidated.

In the normal liver the perisinusoidal extracellular matrix consists predominantly of type III collagen and fibronectin, with small amounts of type IV collagen, laminin and proteoglycans,[282] while in alcoholic fibrosis and cirrhosis, as in cirrhosis of other aetiologies, fibrillar collagens, particularly type I with lesser amounts of type V and type III collagen, are deposited in the space of Disse.[283]

Cells involved in collagen synthesis in the liver

Perisinusoidal cells (lipocytes, fat-storing cells, stellate cells, Ito cells; see Ch. 1) are situated in the perisinusoidal space of Disse and are characterized by the presence of numerous vitamin A-containing fat droplets[284,285] (Fig. 8.23a). Perisinusoidal cells also contain bundles of microfilaments, intermediate filaments, dense bodies, pinocytotic vesicles, small amounts of RER and a few mitochondria. The cytoplasmic processes of these cells extend between adjacent hepatocytes. The ratio of perisinusoidal cells to hepatocytes in the normal human liver is approximately 1:20.[286] Perisinusoidal cells in culture have been shown to divide and to produce collagen type I, collagen type III, and laminin.[287] Anti-desmin antibodies can be used to demonstrate the presence of increased numbers of perisinusoidal cells in areas of necrosis in experimental models of injury,[288] but human perisinusoidal cells do not appear to express this protein.

Transitional cells. The term 'transitional cell' is used to describe 'activated' perisinusoidal cells which show a morphological transition towards fibroblastic differentiation[289–294] (Fig. 8.23b). Studies in the chronic alcohol-fed baboon model and in humans[290–293] suggest that this 'activation' is associated with alcohol or, more likely, its metabolite acetaldehyde. Less than 20% of the volume of transitional cells is composed of lipid droplets. The cells contain prominent RER, microfilaments, dense bodies, pinocytotic vesicles and an oval or slightly irregular nucleus. Following chronic alcohol consumption, over 50% of perisinusoidal cells are seen to have the features of transitional cells,[289] and they are thought to increase in number. Perisinusoidal cells and transitional cells are closely related to collagen fibres in the space of Disse (Fig. 8.23a,b).[290] There is a significant correlation between the percentage of transitional cells, the area of their RER and the amount of collagen in the space of Disse, suggesting that alcohol, or its metabolites, has a direct effect on collagen synthesis by perisinusoidal cells.[289,292]

Myofibroblasts were first described in human livers in association with cirrhosis.[295] They are seen in the perivenular region in normal baboon liver; their number increases following alcohol ingestion and shows a correlation with the thickness of the rim of fibrous tissue around the terminal hepatic venules.[54,296] Myofibroblasts are characterized by prominent bundles of actin microfilaments which usually run parallel to the long axis of the cell. Microtubules are closely related to the microfilaments. The cell also contains numerous dense bodies, sub-plasmalemmal densities, prominent RER, a Golgi apparatus and a few mitochondria; the nucleus is folded or indented. Immunohistochemical studies have shown both desmin and vimentin intermediate filaments as well as contractile protein, actin, within myofibroblasts.[297] Myofibroblasts in the liver are probably activated perisinusoidal cells and are thought to be responsible for the fibrosis that occurs in the perivenular region.[54,296] Both acetaldehyde and lactate have been shown to stimulate collagen production by baboon myofibroblasts in culture.[298] The contractile properties of myofibroblasts may contribute to scar contraction in cirrhosis and, by occluding hepatic venules, to the development of portal hypertension.[295,299]

Fibroblasts contain large amounts of RER, which has

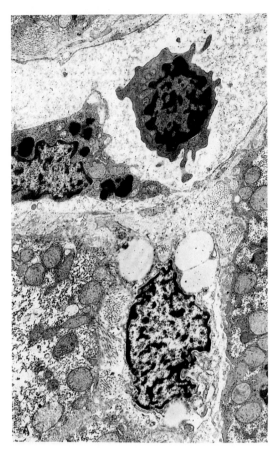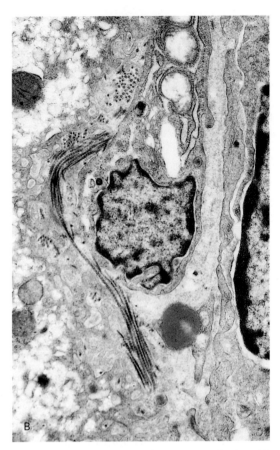

Fig. 8.23 (a) A lipid-containing perisinusoidal cell is situated in the space of Disse, between two hepatocytes and a sinusoid; some collagen fibres are seen cut in cross-section. A lymphocyte and portion of a Kupffer cell are present in the lumen of the sinusoid. (b) Transitional cell. The cell is situated in the space of Disse, bundles of collagen are closely apposed to the outer surface of the cell; note the prominent rough endoplasmic reticulum and the absence of lipid. (a) × 6160. (b) × 12 700

dilated cisternae filled with fluffy material thought to be procollagen. They have a crenated nucleus and contain intermediate filaments of the vimentin type. The number of fibroblasts in the perivenular region and the perisinus-oidal space increases as fibrosis progresses.[54] Fibroblasts predominantly produce type I collagen and lesser amounts of type III, and also collagenase, fibronectin and glycos-aminoglycans;[299] acetaldehyde has been shown to stimu-late the production of both collagen and non-collagenous proteins by human fibroblasts.[300]

It is now generally accepted that perisinusoidal cells, transitional cells, myofibroblasts and fibroblasts belong to the same lineage and that these are the principal collagen-producing cells in the liver. Cultured perisinusoidal cells produce mainly type I collagen[301] and are now thought to be responsible for much of the collagen production in hepatocyte cultures.[302]

The pathogenesis of hepatic fibrosis is complex and largely unresolved. Inflammatory/immune mechanisms certainly contribute. A recent study by Moshage et al[303] suggests that acetaldehyde is directly fibrogenic. The role

of this metabolite in alcoholic fibrogenesis is reviewed by Friedman.[304]

Regulation of collagen synthesis in the liver

Current evidence suggests that a complex interplay of cytokines with one another and with the extracellular matrix of the liver modulates collagen synthesis in vivo; Friedman[275] has proposed a model for perisinusoidal cell activation in hepatic fibrosis in which: (i) the quiescent perisinusoidal cell is firstly activated by Kupffer cell-derived cytokines, e.g. transforming growth factor (TGF) β; and (ii) perpetuation of activation results in a switch from type III to type I collagen production, expression of receptors for platelet-derived growth factor (PDGF) and possibly other cytokines, and increased secretion of type IV collagenase.

Collagenization of the space of Disse ('capillarization of sinusoids')

In 1963 Schaffner & Popper introduced the term 'capillarization of hepatic sinusoids';[305] today this phenomenon is recognized as being due to disruption of the normal extracellular matrix in the space of Disse and replacement by type I collagen and basal lamina-like material containing laminin and type IV collagen produced by activated perisinusoidal cells. This process occurs in early alcoholic liver injury and is seen first in zone 3;[306] capillarization occurs independently of parenchymal necrosis, alcoholic hepatitis or Mallory bodies in alcohol-fed baboons[297] and humans.[306]

The presence of extracellular matrix proteins in the space of Disse can be demonstrated by immunogold techniques,[307] and immunohistochemical techniques can demonstrate alterations in sinusoidal endothelial cells by *Ulex europaeus* 1 lectin binding.[308] Capillarization of the sinusoids results in a significant barrier between the blood and the hepatocyte which may provoke further activation of perisinusoidal cells and may also be a factor in hepatocyte dysfunction and injury.

Defenestration of hepatic sinusoids

Recent review articles, such as that of Brouwer et al,[309] and Chapter 1 discuss in detail the structure and function of the sinusoidal lining cells. The unique endothelial cells have flattened processes perforated by small fanestrae about 0.1 μm in diameter; the fenestrae are arranged in groups termed the 'sieve plate'. Since the normal sinusoidal lining does not have a basement membrane, the presence of the fenestrae permits a full exchange of fluid, solutes and particles between the blood and the space of Disse. Alcohol has been shown to increase the diameter but decrease the number of fenestrae in the alcohol-fed baboon.[310] The term 'defenestration' is used to describe changes in the fenestrae which lessen the 'porosity' of the sinusoidal lining. Scanning electron micrographic studies of needle biopsies from non-cirrhotic alcoholic patients have shown evidence of defenestration in zone 3, occurring both in the presence and absence of collagenization of the space of Disse.[311] A morphometric study of the 'sinusoidal barrier' in alcoholic fatty liver without fibrosis showed no difference in the volume and surface density of endothelial cells and perisinusoidal cells in control livers and alcoholic fatty livers.[312] The authors of this study suggested that alteration of the sinusoidal barrier leading to impaired blood–hepatocyte exchange may be a necessary step in the development of hepatic fibrosis. Horn et al[313] demonstrated a positive correlation between defenestration and the occurrence and localization of subendothelial basal laminas, and between the presence of a basal lamina and the occurrence of collagen in the space of Disse, again suggesting that the phenomenon of defenestration is involved in the pathogenesis of hepatic fibrosis. The process of defenestration has been shown to be associated with increased vascular resistance in the sinusoidal bed, which suggests that alterations in the hepatic sinusoidal lining may be involved in the pathogenesis of portal hypertension.[314]

Clark et al[315] made the interesting suggestion that defenestration of the hepatic sinusoids could be a cause of hyperlipoproteinaemia in alcoholics while Fraser et al[316] suggested that defenestration could also contribute to hepatic steatosis.

The sinusoidal endothelial cells are thought to contribute to the production of non-collagenous matrix proteins and may play a small but important role in the process of capillarization of the sinusoids.[317]

Serum markers of hepatic fibrosis

Liver biopsy provides the only reliable means for assessing the presence, distribution and severity of hepatic fibrosis. Nevertheless, the use of serial biochemical tests may provide a useful non-invasive method for objective assessment of progression of hepatic fibrosis and for monitoring antifibrotic therapy, perhaps using a panel of tests consisting of the aminoterminal peptide of type III procollagen, laminin and hyaluronate as discussed by Plebani & Burlino.[318]

IMMUNE MECHANISMS

This topic has been comprehensively reviewed by MacSween & Anthony,[319] Isreal et al,[320] and Zetterman.[321] Many immunological disturbances occur as a consequence of alcoholic liver injury and may be considered secondary events. Nevertheless, some of the morphological features, the progression of liver disease despite abstinence and the possible association of certain histocompatibility haplotypes with progression to cirrhosis, raise the possibility that immunological mechanisms play a primary role in the liver injury.

Morphological pointers

The neutrophil infiltrate seen in and around hepatocytes which contain Mallory bodies could indicate a local Arthus reaction with humoral sensitization to Mallory bodies. Antibody to Mallory body antigen has been reported in alcoholic hepatitis, but could not be demonstrated in patients with fatty liver or inactive cirrhosis.[322] These workers also demonstrated the presence of Mallory body antigen in IgA- and IgG-containing complexes eluted from livers showing alcoholic hepatitis or active cirrhosis. In vitro evidence of sensitization to Mallory body antigens has been reported with production of migration inhibition factor,[323] blastogenic factor,[324] fibrogenic factor[325] and lymphocytotoxins.[326] Neutrophil polymorphs frequently surround hepatocytes which contain Mallory bodies (Fig. 8.6b); Mallory bodies per se do not appear to be chemotactic but peripheral mononuclear cells incubated with Mallory bodies secrete a chemotactic factor which may explain the accumulation of neutrophils seen around Mallory bodies in alcoholic hepatitis.[327]

A chronic active hepatitis-like injury is sometimes seen in association with chronic alcohol consumption and negative hepatitis B serology;[90-93,96] in some cases this pattern of injury has been shown to be associated with chronic hepatitis C virus infection (Fig. 8.10).[94,95] The suggestion that alcohol per se can cause chronic active hepatitis remains controversial.[96] The presence of serum antibodies to liver-specific protein (LSP) correlates with morphological piecemeal necrosis.[328,329] Antibody to LSP was not found in 'uncomplicated' alcoholic hepatitis, i.e. hepatitis without chronic active-like features, suggesting that sensitization to LSP may be causal in piecemeal necrosis.[330]

Other immunological features

Humoral immunity. Hypergammaglobulinaemia in alcoholic liver disease is characterized by a polyclonal increase in all classes of immunoglobulins, but with serum IgA levels being particularly increased and correlating closely with the severity of liver damage.[331-333] Perisinusoidal deposition of IgA has been reported in all forms of alcoholic liver disease, but it is not clear whether the antibody is present in immune complexes.[334] Van de Wiel et al[335] suggest that the linear deposition of IgA along the sinusoids in alcoholic liver disease has such a high prevalence and specificity that this feature can be used as a reliable marker for the alcoholic aetiology of the liver disease.

Some studies have reported an increased prevalence of antinuclear and anti-smooth muscle autoantibodies;[331,333] these antibodies have sometimes been present in high titre.[336] IgG and IgA antibodies to liver-cell membrane antigens have been demonstrated in all forms of alcoholic liver injury[337] and the same group reported that IgG class antibodies reacting with ethanol-altered rabbit hepatocytes were detected in 74% of patients with biopsy-proven alcoholic liver disease.[338] Recent studies have suggested that antibodies to liver membrane antigens may be directed against acetaldehyde–protein adducts that are formed during the metabolism of alcohol.[339] Several different proteins have been detected in these adducts in hepatocytes; these include a 37kD protein in the cytosol,[340] and cytochrome P-450 2E1 in microsomes.[341] Immunohistochemical studies have demonstrated the presence of protein–acetaldehyde adducts in zone 3 hepatocytes at an early stage of alcoholic injury.[342]

Laskin et al[343] have drawn attention to the high prevalence of autoantibodies in patients with alcoholic liver disease and suggest that, in at least some patients, autoimmune mechanisms play a role in the pathogenesis of the liver injury. They found serum antibodies to single- or double-stranded DNA in 60% of patients with advanced alcoholic liver disease while antinuclear antibodies were found in 22% of patients. Israel et al[320] suggest that the protein–acetaldehyde adducts may be involved in cytotoxic T-cell recognition and stimulation of lymphocytes, in addition to stimulating a humoral response, and that these mechanisms lead to inflammation and necrosis in the liver.

Cell-mediated immunity. Impaired delayed hypersensitivity is described in patients with alcoholic liver disease; this appears to be due to both nutritional deficiencies and a reduction in the number of circulating T-cells.[344] Circulating lymphocytes cytotoxic for autologous liver cells have been described in alcoholic hepatitis and active cirrhosis;[345,346] there is some evidence that these are antibody-dependent K-cells directed at LSP in hepatocyte membranes.[347]

Several studies have demonstrated an increased production of the cytokine tumour necrosis factor α in alcoholic liver disease;[348-351] increased production of interleukin-1α[351] and interleukin-6[351,352] has also been observed. Tumour necrosis factor α is a mediator of many of the biological actions of endotoxin, and the raised levels of this cytokine that have been observed in alcoholic hepatitis and cirrhosis may be related to endotoxaemia that complicates chronic alcohol consumption. As discussed above, disturbances of IgA metabolism, with elevated total serum IgA and a characteristic linear deposition of IgA in the hepatic sinusoids, are well described in alcoholic liver disease;[334,335] IgA has also been shown to trigger the secretion of tumour necrosis factor α by monocytes and to enhance synergistically the endotoxin-induced secretion of this cytokine.[353] These observations suggest that both endotoxaemia and IgA could contribute to cell-mediated immunological disturbances that may be involved in the pathogenesis of alcoholic liver injury.

Kupffer cells. Studies of human liver biopsies[354] and animal studies[355] suggest that chronic alcohol consumption impairs Kupffer cell activity, particularly phagocytosis, which is reflected in increased levels of endotoxin and of antibodies to intestinal microorganisms.[356] Kupffer cells, isolated from a rat model of alcoholic fibrosis, have been shown to be an important source of the cytokine transforming growth factor β that stimulates collagen formation by perisinusoidal cells.[357]

Histocompatibility antigens. Membrane expression of MHC class I antigens, which are not detected normally on hepatocytes, was observed in all patients with alcoholic hepatitis;[358] continuing liver injury could therefore be mediated by sensitized cytotoxic T-lymphocytes which bind to these antigens.

In summary, the presence of alcohol-induced neoantigens and autoantigens could result in an immunological response directed against liver cells. Alternatively, liver injury may occur only in a genetically predisposed subgroup (see below) who demonstrate abnormal immunological reactivity.

NUTRITIONAL DEFICIENCIES

The role of nutritional factors in liver disease has been reviewed recently by Mezey[359] and Marsano & McClain.[360] Primary malnutrition, due to poor diet, is well recognized in the alcoholic. Moreover, secondary malnutrition is now being increasingly recognized in alcoholics in whom the diet is adequate. A complete nutritional assessment of 284 patients with alcoholic hepatitis showed that none was completely free from malnutrition.[361] Secondary malnutrition may be due to: (i) malabsorption with alcohol-related impairment of enterocyte function;[362] (ii) disturbed carbohydrate metabolism; (iii) impaired protein secretion by hepatocytes; (iv) impaired hepatic metabolism of vitamins; and (v) increased catabolic loss of zinc, magnesium and calcium.[363] Vitamin A supplementation together with chronic alcohol administration has been shown to cause hepatic fibrosis in the rat;[364] it is consequently difficult to determine a safe dose of vitamin A supplementation for chronic alcoholics who are often deficient in vitamin A.[365]

As discussed earlier, the recognition that nutritional factors contribute to the pathogenesis of 'non-alcoholic steatohepatitis'[149-159] has stimulated a renewal of interest in the role of nutritional factors in the pathogenesis of alcoholic liver disease. The liver injury of alcoholic hepatitis may well have the same pathogenesis as the histologically similar non-alcoholic steatohepatitis. Predisposing factors for both conditions appear to include nutritional deficiencies, metabolic disturbances and gut-derived endotoxins which stimulate cytokine production.

Several trials of parenteral nutrition have shown that nutritional supplementation results in more rapid recovery from moderately severe, biopsy-proven alcoholic hepatitis.[336,367] Hepatocellular necrosis and inflammation in the initial and follow-up liver biopsies were highly correlated with the nitrogen balance on admission.[366]

FACTORS AFFECTING INDIVIDUAL SUSCEPTIBILITY TO ALCOHOLIC LIVER DISEASE

Numerous studies since the 1960s[182-188] have established alcohol as a direct hepatotoxin and until recently alcoholic liver injury was thought to be purely dose related.[3] The possibility of genetic and acquired factors playing a role in the susceptibility of the individual to alcohol-associated liver disease is a relatively new concept.[19-22]

DOSE AND DURATION OF ALCOHOL CONSUMPTION

Lelbach[3] has clearly demonstrated a relationship between the risk of developing cirrhosis and the dose and duration of alcohol consumption. Nevertheless, even with an intake as high as 226 g for a mean duration of 11.4 years, only 25% of drinkers develop cirrhosis. On the other hand, an intake as low as 20 g for women and 40 g for men has been claimed to be associated with the development of cirrhosis.[368,369] Indeed, a recent Australian case–control study has shown that the risk of both women and men developing cirrhosis increases significantly above the baseline when alcohol intake is greater than 40 g per day.[370] Sorensen et al[83] performed serial liver biopsies over a 10–13-year period in 258 males, none of whom were cirrhotic at the beginning of the study; the average daily consumption of alcohol was over 50 g per day. Cirrhosis developed in 38, an overall risk of about 15%, and similar to that documented in other series.[3,64]

Analysis of the quantitative relationship between alcohol consumption and the occurrence of cirrhosis has led Sorensen to ask if 'alcohol abuse has a permissive rather than a dose-related effect'.[21] Sorensen suggests that the risk of cirrhosis at a given level of alcohol consumption is higher or lower, dependent on the action of other factors. Such factors could change the threshold for alcohol-associated liver injury as well as changing the level of risk with higher alcohol consumption. The group studied by Sorensen et al[83] developed cirrhosis at a constant rate of 2% per year. This observation led the authors to suggest that other contributing factors affect approximately one in every 50 drinkers every year.

GENETIC AND ETHNIC FACTORS

Female gender. As increasing numbers of women have started to consume alcohol, some of them excessively, alcohol-related disorders have ceased to be an almost exclusively male affliction. A study of cirrhosis mortality in the USA, 1961–1985, has shown a trend amongst an older age group (over 55 years) towards a convergence of cirrhosis mortality in men and women which is largely attributed to the changing patterns of alcohol consumption by women.[371] The greater susceptibility of women to alcohol-associated liver injury is no doubt also contributing to this phenomenon. A critical analysis of four liver biopsy studies of alcoholics from England,[61] France[369] and Australia[372,373] showed that women are more susceptible to the hepatotoxic effects of alcohol than men. This has also been confirmed by Gavaler.[374] The increased susceptibility of women to alcoholic liver disease has a number of manifestations: (i) women tend to present with more severe disease, often associated with a lower daily intake of alcohol for a shorter duration;[370,375-378] (ii) women, particularly those under 45 years, have a higher incidence of alcoholic hepatitis, and a worse long-term prognosis even if they abstain;[60,84] (iii) American Negro women appear to be even more susceptible than Caucasian women to alcoholic hepatitis, and have a poor prognosis;[6] and (iv) women with alcoholic cirrhosis have a higher mortality.[379]

A recent study by Frezza et al[23] has provided new insights into the pathogenesis of the increased susceptibility of women. In non-alcoholic women 'first-pass' metabolism of alcohol (i.e. oxidation in the stomach) and gastric alcohol dehydrogenase were considerably less, 23% and 59% respectively, than those in non-alcoholic men. These differences were even more pronounced in drinkers, where 'first-pass' metabolism was virtually absent in women. The authors concluded that 'increased bioavailability of ethanol resulting from decreased gastric oxidation of ethanol may contribute to the enhanced vulnerability of women to acute and chronic complications of alcohol'. First-pass metabolism occurs in the stomach but not the duodenum; the extent of metabolism is reduced by fasting,[380] does not occur after subtotal gastrectomy[381] and can be significantly decreased by cimetidine.[382]

Genetic polymorphisms of alcohol-metabolizing enzymes. A number of studies during the last few years have demonstrated racial differences in alcohol-metabolizing enzymes and have suggested that polymorphisms at the alcohol and aldehyde dehydrogenase loci play a role in genetic predisposition to alcoholic liver injury;[24,383–387] see also recent reviews by Day & Bassendine[388] and Agarwal & Goedde.[389] An atypical $ALDH_2$ isoenzyme is widely prevalent among Japanese, Chinese and other Orientals of Mongoloid origin and is mainly responsible for their 'sensitivity' to alcohol which manifests as facial flushing, sweating, headache and increased pulse rate. This sensitivity to alcohol acts as a deterrent against drinking which no doubt accounts for the lower incidence of alcoholism and alcohol-related diseases in Oriental races.[383,386] Enomoto et al[390] investigated the relationship between the presence of one mutant $ALDH_2$ gene and the severity of liver injury and found that patients who were homozygous for the normal gene had a lower incidence of alcoholic hepatitis/cirrhosis than those who were heterozygous for this gene. Day et al[24] have demonstrated differences in ADH_2, ADH_3 and $ALDH_2$ allele frequencies in alcoholic cirrhotics compared with controls, giving support for a genetic predisposition for alcohol-related organ damage.

Genetic predisposition to alcohol addiction. A number of epidemiological studies of adoptees, siblings and twins have provided convincing evidence of a genetic component to alcohol addition — see recent reviews.[22,391,392] Blum et al[393] suggest that the dopamine D_2 receptor gene on chromosome 11 may confer susceptibility to at least one form of alcoholism. However, alcohol addiction is not necessarily associated with organ damage; for example, Wodak et al[394] found alcoholic liver disease in only 18% of patients with severe alcohol dependence — an observation which is in keeping with Sorensen's hypothesis of the 'permissive' rather than 'dose-related' role of alcohol in the pathogenesis of liver injury.[21]

Histocompatibility antigens (HLA). MacSween & Anthony[319] reviewed the relationship between MHC antigens and alcoholic liver disease. No strong association between any haplotype and liver injury has been demonstrated. Saunders et al[395] have suggested that genetic determinants linked to the MHC class I antigen B8 are associated with an enhanced rate of development of alcoholic cirrhosis. However, there are conflicting results in other studies; Monteiro et al,[396] for example, found that the presence of HLA-Bw35 and A28 appeared to indicate susceptibility to alcoholic liver injury, particularly cirrhosis, while on the other hand Mills et al[397] failed to demonstrate an HLA-A or B locus genetic susceptibility to alcoholic liver disease.

CHRONIC VIRAL INFECTIONS

Hepatitis B virus infection. A number of studies have shown an increased incidence of serological markers for hepatitis B in patients with alcoholic liver disease, raising the possibility of increased susceptibility to infection,[398–406] although other studies have failed to show this association.[407,408] Consequently, the role of hepatitis B in the pathogenesis of alcoholic liver disease remains controversial. Nevertheless, a number of studies do suggest an HBV-alcohol interaction.[139,402,405,409,410] For example, Villa et al[402] studied 296 HBsAg carriers prospectively for 3.5 years; one-third of the carriers developed raised liver enzymes while drinking less than 60 g alcohol per day. These researchers found that, for a given dose of alcohol, the risk of hepatic injury was much higher in the HBsAg carriers than in the age-and sex-matched HBsAg-negative controls. Similarly, a Japanese study showed that HBsAg-positive men with a 'drinking habit' for more than 10 years developed cirrhosis at an average age of 38.8 — 10.5 years younger than those without a drinking habit.[139] A study by Novick et al[409] of alcoholic cirrhotics under 35 years of age also incriminates the HBV in the development of cirrhosis at a relatively young age — 98% had a history of heroin abuse, serological markers were detected in almost 94%, and 9.4% were carriers.

Hepatitis C virus infection. Although tests for HCV infection have become available only recently, a number of studies have already described an increased prevalence of this viral infection in patients with alcoholic liver disease.[94,95,142,406,411–414] The liver injury appears to be more severe in drinkers who are HCV positive;[143,406,411–414] in addition, the virus may be involved in the pathogenesis of hepatocellular carcinomas that occur in alcohol-related liver disease.[142,143,414] The case for an alcohol–virus interaction already appears stronger for HCV than for HBV but further prospective epidemiological studies are obviously required.

DRUGS AND TOXINS

The potentiation of acute drug-associated liver injury is well recognized,[37–39,148,197–200,415–417] but the idea of an alcohol–drug interaction causing chronic liver disease is a more recent concept. Leo & Lieber[364] observed hepatic fibrosis in the rat following long-term administration of ethanol and a moderate dose of vitamin A, while Hall et al[201] produced hepatic fibrosis and cirrhosis in rats by feeding ethanol in the Lieber–DeCarli diet together with exposure to 'low-dose' carbon tetrachloride vapour for 10 weeks. As discussed earlier, chronic alcohol ingestion has been shown to induce the isoenzyme cytochrome P-450 2E1; this effect is seen maximally in zone 3 hepatocytes[418] (Fig. 8.24). This enzyme induction, in turn, enhances the metabolism of a wide variety of drugs and toxins.[28,37–39] Relatively low doses of alcohol may well potentiate insidious liver injury by therapeutic doses of prescription drugs, non-prescription agents such as vitamin A, and environmental toxins.[201] This type of interaction may explain some cases of chronic liver injury seen in association with relatively low doses of alcohol and account for some cases of cryptogenic cirrhosis.

Chronic alcohol consumption appears to be a risk factor in methotrexate-associated fibrosis and cirrhosis in patients with psoriatic arthropathy[419–421] and also appears to increase the risk of liver injury in rheumatoid patients receiving low doses of oral methotrexate.[422] The mechanism for this interaction has yet to be elucidated.

CONCLUSION

Moderate alcohol consumption, up to 50 g per day, is associated with hyperlipaemia and a lower incidence of coronary artery disease;[423,424] high density lipoprotein HDL_3 is elevated rather than HDL_2. However, since relatively small doses of alcohol have been associated with liver disease,[368] the concept of a risk-free and possibly even beneficial daily dose of alcohol should probably be abandoned.

As knowledge of the pathogenesis of alcohol-associated liver disease has increased, so has the range of therapeutic options for treatment of the various stages of the disease. Orthotopic liver transplantation is now considered, by some, to have a place in the treatment of end-stage alcoholic liver disease;[147,425–427] growing acceptance of the permissive role of alcohol in the pathogenesis of liver injury is helping to overcome some of the resistance to the use of transplantation as a therapeutic option.

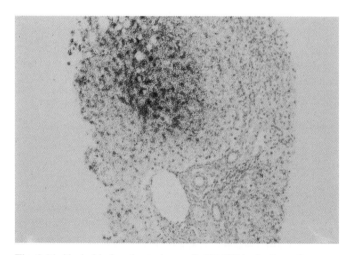

Fig. 8.24 Alcohol-induced cytochrome P-450 2E1 in the liver of a 50-year-old man who had a history of heavy drinking for some years. Increased amounts of the cytochrome P-450 2E1 are seen in zone 3 hepatocytes that surround a terminal hepatic venule. More normal amounts of enzyme are seen in the more peripheral zone 2 hepatocytes. In situ hybridization with a probe for P-450 2E1.

REFERENCES

1. Keller M. A historical overview of alcohol and alcoholism. Cancer Res 1979; 39: 2822–2829
2. Ravi Varma L A. Alcoholism in Ayurveda. Q J Stud Alcohol 1950; 11: 484–491
3. Lelbach W K. Cirrhosis in the alcoholic and its relation to the volume of alcohol abuse. Ann NY Acad Sci 1975; 252: 85–105
4. Lelbach W K. The epidemiology of alcoholic liver disease in continental Europe. In: Hall P de la M, ed. Alcoholic liver disease. London: Edward Arnold, 1985: pp 130–166
5. Saunders J B, Walters J R F, Davies P, Paton A. A 20-year prospective study of cirrhosis. Br Med J 1981; i: 263–266
6. Galambos J T. Epidemiology of alcoholic liver disease in the United States of America. In: Hall P de la M, ed. Alcoholic Liver Disease. London: Edward Arnold 1985: pp 230–249
7. Morgan M Y. Epidemiology of alcoholic liver disease in the United Kingdom. In: Hall P de la M ed. Alcoholic liver disease. London: Edward Arnold, 1985: pp 193–229
8. West L M (moderator). Alcoholism (UCLA Conference). Ann Intern Med 1984; 100: 405–416
9. Orrego H, Israel Y, Blendis L M. Alcoholic liver disease: information in search of knowledge. Hepatology 1981; 1: 267–283
10. Popper H, Thung S N, Gerber M A. Pathology of alcoholic liver diseases. Semin Liver Dis 1981; 1: 203–216
11. MacSween R N M, Burt A D. Histologic spectrum of alcoholic liver disease. Semin Liver Dis 1986; 6: 221–232
12. Hall P de la M. Pathology of pathogenesis of alcoholic liver disease. In: Hall P de la M, ed. Alcoholic liver disease. London: Edward Arnold, 1985: pp 41–68
13. Hall P de la M. Pathologic features of alcohol liver disease. In: Okuda K, Benhamou J-P, eds. Portal hypertension: clinical and physiological aspects. Tokyo: Springer-Verlag, 1991: pp 41–68
14. Maddrey W C. Alcoholic hepatitis: clinicopathologic features and therapy. Sem Liver Dis 1988; 8: 91–102
15. Diehl A M. Alcoholic liver disease. Med Clin North Am 1989; 73: 815–830
16. Rabin L. The morphological spectrum of alcoholic liver disease. In: Seeff L B, Lewis J H, eds. Current perspectives in hepatology. New York: Plenum, 1989: pp 123–139
17. Maddrey W C. Alcoholic hepatitis: pathogenesis and approaches

to treatment. Scand J Gastroenterol 1990; 25 (suppl 175): 118–130

18. Ishak K G, Zimmerman H J, Ray M B. Alcoholic liver disease: pathologic, pathogenic and clinical aspects. Alcoholism: Clin Exp Res 1991; 15: 45–66

19. Saunders J B, Wodak A D, Williams R. What determines susceptibility to liver damage from alcohol? Discussion paper. J R Soc Med 1984; 77: 204–216

20. Johnson R D, Williams R. Genetic and environmental factors in individual susceptibility to the development of alcoholic liver disease. Alcohol Alcoholism 1985; 20: 137–160

21. Sorensen T I A. Alcohol and liver injury: dose-related or permissive effect? Liver 1989; 9: 189–197

22. Hall P de la M. Genetic and acquired factors that influence individual susceptibility to alcohol-associated liver disease. J Gastroenterol Hepatol 1992; 7: 417–426

23. Frezza M, Di Padova C, Pozatto G, Terpin M, Baraona E, Lieber C S. High blood alcohol levels in women: the role of decreased gastric alcohol dehydrogenase activity and first-pass metabolism. N Eng J Med 1990; 322: 95–99

24. Day C P, Bashir R, James O F W et al. Investigation of the role of polymorphisms at the alcohol and aldehyde dehydrogenase loci in genetic predisposition to alcohol-related end-organ damage. Hepatology 1991; 14: 768–801

25. Lieber C S. Metabolism of alcohol. In: Medical disorders of alcoholism: pathogenesis and treatment. Philadelphia: WB Saunders, 1982: pp 1–42

26. Lieber C S. Alcohol metabolism. In: Hall P de la M, ed. Alcoholic liver disease. London: Edward Arnold, 1985: ch 1, pp 3–40

27. Lieber C S. Mechanism of ethanol induced hepatic injury. Pharmacol Ther 1990; 46: 1–41

28. Lieber C S. Metabolism of ethanol and associated hepatotoxicity. Drug Alcohol Rev 1991; 10: 175–202

29. Mezey E. Metabolic effect of alcohol. Fed Proc 1985; 44: 134–138

30. French S W. Biochemical basis for alcohol-induced liver injury. Clin Biochem 1989; 22: 41–49

31. Israel Y, Videla L, Fernandes-Videla V, Bernstein J. Effects of chronic ethanol treatment and thyroxine administration on ethanol metabolism and liver oxidative capacity. J Pharmacol Exp Ther 1975; 192: 565–574

32. Lieber C S, DeCarli L M. Hepatic microsomal ethanol oxidizing system: *in vitro* characteristics and adapative properties *in vivo*. J Biol Chem 1970; 245: 2505–2512

33. Koop D R, Morgan E T, Tarr G E, Coon M J. Purification and characterization of a unique isozyme of cytochrome P-450 from liver microsomes of ethanol-treated rabbits. J Biol Chem 1982; 257: 8472–8480

34. Nebert D W, Adesnick M, Coon M J et al. The P-450-gene superfamily: recommended nomenclature. DNA 1987; 6: 1–11

35. Umeno M, McBride O W, Yang C S, Gelboin H V, Gonzalez F J. Human ethanol-inducible P450IIE1: Complete gene sequence, promoter characterization, chromosome mapping and DNA-directed expression. Biochemistry 1988; 27: 9006–9013

36. Lieber C S, Lasker J M, DeCarli L M, Saeli J, Wojtowicz T. Role of acetone, dietary fat, and total energy intake in the induction of the hepatic microsomal ethanol oxidizing system. J Pharmacol Exp Ther 1988; 247: 791–795

37. Lieber C S, Lasker J M, Alderman J, Leo M A. The microsomal ethanol oxidizing system and its interaction with other drugs, carcinogens, and vitamins. Ann NY Acad Sci 1987; 492: 11–23

38. Lieber C S. Metabolic effects of ethanol and its interaction with other drugs, hepatotoxic agents, vitamins and carcinogens: a 1988 update. Semin Liver Dis 1988; 8: 47–68

39. Watkins P B. Role of cytochromes in drug metabolism and hepatotoxicity. Semin Liver Dis 1990; 10: 235–250

40. Lindros K O, Stowell A, Pikkarainen P, Salaspuro M. Elevated blood acetaldehyde in alcoholics with accelerated ethanol elimination. Pharm Biochem Behav 1980; 13: 119–124

41. Lieber C S, Savolainen M. Ethanol and lipids. Alcoholism: Clin Exp Res 1984; 8: 409–423

42. Edmondson H A, Peters R L, Frankel H H, Borowsky S. The early stage of liver injury in the alcoholic. Medicine 1967; 46: 119–129

43. Randall B. Sudden death and hepatic fatty metamorphosis. JAMA 1980; 243: 1723–1725

44. Hall P, Gormley B M, Jarvis L R, Smith R D. A staining method for the detection and measurement of fat droplets in hepatic tissue. Pathology 1980; 12: 605–608

45. Hall P, Smith R D, Gormley B M. 'Routine' stains on osmicated resin embedded hepatic tissue. Pathology 1982; 14: 73–74

46. Christoffersen P, Braendstrup O, Juhl E, Poulsen H. Lipogranulomas in human liver biopsies with fatty change. A morphological, biochemical and clinical investigation. Acta Pathol Microbiol Scand (A) 1971; 79: 150–158

47. Petersen P, Christoffersen P. Ultrastructure of lipogranulomas in human liver. Acta Pathol Microbiol Scand (A) 1979; 87: 45–49

48. Iversen K, Christoffersen P, Poulsen H. Epithelioid granulomas in liver biopsies. Scand J Gastroenterol 1970; 7 (Suppl): 61–67

49. Ballard H, Bernstein M, Farrar J T. Fatty liver presenting as obstructive jaundice. Am J Med 1961; 30: 196–201

50. Morgan M Y, Sherlock S, Scheuer P J. Acute cholestasis, hepatic failure, and fatty liver in the alcoholic. Scand J Gastroenterol 1978; 13: 299–303

51. Uchida T, Kao H, Quispe-Sjøgren M, Peters R L. Alcoholic foamy degeneration — a pattern of acute alcoholic injury of the liver. Gastroenterology 1983; 84: 683–692

52. Van Waes L, Lieber C S. Early perivenular sclerosis in alcoholic fatty liver: an index of progressive liver injury. Gastroenterology 1977; 73: 646–650

53. Popper H, Lieber C S. Histogenesis of alcoholic fibrosis and cirrhosis in the baboon. Am J Pathol 1980; 98: 695–716

54. Nakano M, Worner T M, Lieber C S. Perivenular fibrosis in alcoholic liver injury: ultrastructure and histologic progression. Gastroenterology 1982; 83: 777–785

55. Worner T M, Lieber C S. Perivenular fibrosis as precursor lesion of cirrhosis. JAMA 1985; 253: 627–630

56. Caulet S, Fabre M, Schoevaert D, Lesty C, Meduri G, Martin E. Quantitative study of centrolobular hepatic fibrosis in alcoholic disease before cirrhosis. Virchows Archiv (A) 1989; 416: 11–17

57. Junge J, Horn T, Vyberg M, Christoffersen P, Svendsen L B. The pattern of fibrosis in the acinar zone 3 areas in early alcoholic liver disease. J Hepatol 1991; 12: 83–86

58. Beckett A G, Livingstone A V, Hill K R. Acute alcoholic hepatitis. Br Med J 1961; ii: 1113–1119

59. Brunt P W, Kew M C, Scheuer P J, Sherlock S. Studies in alcoholic liver disease in Britain. I. Clinical and pathological patterns related to natural history. Gut 1974; 15: 52–58

60. Krasner N, Davis M, Portmann B, Williams R. Changing patterns of alcoholic liver disease in Great Britain: relation to sex and signs of autoimmunity. Br Med J 1977; i: 1497–1500

61. Morgan M Y, Sherlock S. Sex-related differences among 100 patients with alcoholic liver disease. Br Med J 1977; i: 939–941

62. Harinasuta U, Zimmerman H J. Alcoholic steatonecrosis. I. Relationship between severity of hepatic disease and presence of Mallory bodies in the liver. Gastroenterology 1971; 60: 1036–1046

63. Birschbach H R, Harinasuta U, Zimmerman H J. Alcoholic steatonecrosis. Gastroenterology 1974; 66: 1195–1202

64. Bhathal P S, Wilkinson P, Clifton S, Rankin J G, Santamaria J N. The spectrum of liver diseases in alcoholism. Aust NZ J Med 1975; 5: 49–57

65. French S W, Burbridge E J. Alcoholic hepatitis: clinical, morphological and therapeutic aspects. In: Popper P, Schaffner F, eds. Progress in liver diseases. Vol VI. New York: Grune & Stratton, 1979: pp 557–580

66. Hislop W S, Bouchier I A D, Allan J G et al. Alcoholic liver disease in Scotland and Northeastern England: presenting features in 510 patients. Q J Med 1983; 206: 232–243

67. Karasawa T, Kushida T, Shikata T, Kaneda H. Morphologic spectrum of liver disease among chronic alcoholics. A comparison between Tokyo, Japan and Cincinnati, U.S.A. Acta Pathol Jpn 1980; 30: 505–514

68. Sherlock S. Alcoholic hepatitis. Alcohol Alcoholism 1990; 25: 189–196

69. Baptista A, Bianchi L, de Groote et al. Alcoholic liver disease:

morphological manifestations. Review by an international group. Lancet 1981; i: 707–711

70. Yokoo H, Singh K S, Hawasli A H. Giant mitochondria in alcoholic liver disease. Arch Pathol Lab Med 1978; 102: 213–214

71. Uchida T, Kronberg I, Peters R L. Giant mitochondria in alcoholic liver disease; their identification, frequency and pathological significance. Liver 1984; 4: 29–38

72. Bruguera M, Bertran A, Bombi J A, Rodes J. Giant mitochondria in hepatocytes: a diagnostic hint for alcoholic liver disease. Gastroenterology 1977; 73: 1383–1387

73. Edmondson H A, Peters R L, Reynolds T B, Kuzuma O T. Sclerosing hyaline necrosis of the liver in the chronic alcoholic. Ann Intern Med 1963; 59: 646–673

74. Reynolds T B, Hidemura R, Michel H, Peters R L. Portal hypertension without cirrhosis in alcoholic liver disease. Ann Intern Med 1969; 70: 497–506

75. Gerber M A, Popper H. Relation between central canals and portal tracts in alcoholic hepatitis. A contribution to the pathogenesis of cirrhosis in alcoholics. Human Pathol 1972; 3: 199–207

76. Scheuer P J, Maggi G. Hepatic fibrosis and collapse: histological distinction by orcein staining. Histopathology 1980; 4: 487–490

77. Nasrallah S M, Nassar V H, Galambos J T. Importance of terminal hepatic venule thickening. Arch Pathol Lab Med 1980; 104: 84–86

78. Christoffersen P, Eghoje K, Juhl E. Mallory bodies in liver biopsies from chronic alcoholics: a comparative morphological, biochemical and clinical study of two groups of chronic alcoholics with and without Mallory bodies. Scand J Gastroenterol 1973; 8: 341–346

79. Boitnott J K, Maddrey W C. Alcoholic liver disease. I. Interrelationships among histologic features and the histologic effects of prednisolone therapy. Hepatology 1981; 1: 599–612

80. Bouchier I A D, Hislop W S, Prescott R J. A prospective study of alcoholic liver disease and mortality. J Hepatol 1992; 16: 290–297

81. Orrego H, Blake J E, Blendis L M, Medline A. Prognosis of alcoholic cirrhosis in the presence and absence of alcoholic hepatitis. Gastroenterology 1987; 92: 208–214

82. Galambos J T. Natural history of alcoholic hepatitis. III. Histological changes. Gastroenterology 1972; 63: 1026–1035

83. Sorensen T I A, Orholm M, Bentsen K D, Hoybye G, Eghoje K, Christoffersen P. Prospective evaluation of alcohol abuse and alcoholic liver injury in men as predictors of development of cirrhosis. Lancet 1984; ii: 241–244

84. Pares A, Caballeria J, Bruguera M, Torres M, Rodes J. Histological course of alcoholic hepatitis. Influence of abstinence, sex and extent of hepatic damage. J Hepatol 1986; 2: 33–42

85. Goodman Z D, Ishak K G. Occlusive venous lesions in alcoholic liver disease. A study of 200 cases. Gastroenterology 1982; 83: 786–796

86. Burt A D, MacSween R N M. Hepatic vein lesions in alcoholic liver disease: retrospective biopsy and necropsy study. J Clin Pathol 1986; 39: 63–67

87. Lehmann H, Kaiserling E, Schlaak M. Left hepatic lobe atrophy and partial Budd–Chiari syndrome in a patient with alcoholic liver cirrhosis. Hepatogastroenterology 1982; 29: 3–5

88. Anthony P P, Ishak K G, Nayak N C, Poulsen H E, Scheuer P J, Sobin L H. The morphology of cirrhosis. J Clin Pathol 1978; 31: 395–414

89. Lee F I. Cirrhosis and hepatoma in alcoholics. Gut 1966; 7: 77–85

90. Goldberg S J, Mendenhall C L, Connell A M, Chedid A. 'Non-alcoholic' chronic hepatitis in the alcoholic. Gastroenterology 1977; 72: 598–604

91. Hodges J R, Millward-Sadler G H, Wright R. Chronic active hepatitis: the spectrum of disease. Lancet 1982; i: 550–552

92. Crapper R M, Bhathal P S, Mackay I R. Chronic active hepatitis in alcoholic patients. Liver 1983; 3: 327–337

93. Nei J, Matsuda Y, Takada A. Chronic hepatitis induced by alcohol. Dig Dis Sci 1983; 28: 207–215

94. Brillanti S, Barbara L, Miglioli M, Bonino F. Hepatitis C virus: a possible cause of chronic hepatitis in alcoholics. Lancet 1989; ii: 1390–1391

95. Lampertico P, Colombo M, Rumi M G et al. Hepatitis C virus (HCV)-related chronic hepatitis in Italian alcoholic patients. Hepatology 1991; 14: 654 (abstr)

96. Takase S, Takada N, Enomoto N, Yasuhara M, Takada A. Different types of chronic hepatitis in alcoholic patients: does chronic hepatitis induced by alcohol exist? Hepatology 1991; 13: 876–881

97. Uchida T, Peters R L. The nature and origin of proliferated bile ductules in alcoholic liver disease. Am J Clin Pathol 1983; 79: 326–333

98. Van Eyken P, Sciot R, Desmet V J. A cytokeratin immunohistochemical study of alcoholic liver disease: evidence that hepatocytes can express 'bile duct-type' cytokeratins. Histopathology 1988; 13: 605–617

99. Rubin E, Krus S, Popper H. Pathogenesis of postnecrotic cirrhosis in alcoholics. Arch Pathol 1962; 73: 288–299

100. Fauerholdt L, Schlichting P, Christensen E, Poulsen H, Tygstrup N, Jahl E and the Copenhagen Study Group for Liver Diseases. Conversion of micronodular cirrhosis into macronodular cirrhosis. Hepatology 1983; 3: 928–931

101. Nagasue N, Akamizu H, Yukaya H, Yuuki I. Hepatocellular pseudotumour in the cirrhotic liver. Cancer 1984; 54: 2487–2494

102. Abdi W, Millan J C, Mezey E. Sampling variability on percutaneous liver biopsy. Arch Intern Med 1979; 139: 667–669

103. Scheuer P J, Jefkowitch J H. Liver biopsy interpretation, 5th edn. Philadelphia: WB Saunders London: Baillière Tindall, 1994

104. Pariente E-A, Degott C, Martin J-P, Feldmann G, Potet F, Benhamou J-P. Hepatocyte PAS-positive-diastase-resistant inclusions in the absence of alpha-1-antitrypsin deficiency — high prevalence in alcoholic cirrhosis. Am J Clin Pathol 1981; 76: 299–302

105. Berresford P A, Sunter J P, Harrison V, Lesna M. Histological demonstration and frequency of intrahepatic copper in patients suffering from alcoholic liver disease. Histopathology 1980; 4: 637–643

106. Lefkowitch J H, Arborgh B A M, Scheuer P J. Oxyphilic granular hepatocytes. Mitochondrion-rich liver cells in hepatic disease. Am J Clin Pathol 1980; 74: 432–441

107. Gerber M A, Thung S N. Hepatic oncocytes. Incidence, staining characteristics, and ultrastructural features. Am J Clin Pathol 1981; 75: 498–503

108. Hadziyannis S, Gerber M A, Vissoulis C, Popper H. Cytoplasmic hepatitis B antigen in 'ground-glass' hepatocytes of carriers. Arch Pathol 1973; 96: 327–330

109. Chedid A, Mendenhall C L, Gartside P et al. Prognostic factors in alcoholic liver disease. Am J Gastroenterol 1991; 86: 210–304

110. Powell W J Jr, Klatskin G. Duration of survival in patients with Laennec's cirrhosis. Am J Med 1968; 44: 406–420

111. Borowsky S A, Strome S, Lott E. Continued heavy drinking and survival in alcoholic cirrhosis. Gastroenterology 1981; 80: 1405–1409

112. Pérez-Tamayo R. Cirrhosis of the liver: a reversible disease? In: Sommers C, Rosen P P, eds. Pathology Annual 14 (Part 2). New York: Appleton-Century-Crofts, 1979: pp 183–213

113. Baker A L, Elson C O, Jaspan J, Boyer J L. Liver failure with steatonecrosis after jejunoileal bypass: recovery with parenteral nutrition and re-anastomosis. Arch Intern Med 1979; 139:289–292

114. Kershenobich D, Vargos S F, Garcia-Tsao G, Pérez-Tamayo R, Gent M, Rojkind M. Colchicine in the treatment of cirrhosis of the liver. N Engl J Med 1988; 318: 1709–1713

115. Phillips G B, Davidson C S. Liver disease of the chronic alcoholic simulating extrahepatic biliary obstruction. Gastroenterology 1957; 33: 236–244

116. Popper H, Szanto P B. Fatty liver with hepatic failure in alcoholics. J Mt Sinai Hosp 1957; 24: 1121–1131

117. Perrillo R P, Griffin R, DeSchryver-Kecskemeti K, Lander J J, Zuckerman G R. Alcoholic liver disease presenting with marked elevation of serum alkaline phosphatase. Am J Dig Dis 1978; 23: 1061–1066

118. Afroudakis A, Kaplowitz N. Liver histopathology in chronic common bile duct stenosis due to chronic alcoholic pancreatitis. Hepatology 1981; 1: 65–72

119. Glover S C, McPhie J L, Brunt P W. Cholestasis in acute alcoholic liver disease. Lancet 1977; ii: 1305–1307

120. Zieve L. Jaundice, hyperlipaemia and haemolytic anaemia: a heretofore unrecognized syndrome associated with alcoholic fatty liver and cirrhosis. Ann Intern Med 1958; 48: 471–496

121. Nissenbaum M, Chedid A, Mendenhall C, Gartside P and the VA Cooperative Study Group #119. Prognostic significance of cholestatic alcoholic hepatitis. Dig Dis Sci 1990; 35: 891–896

122. Levin D M, Baker A L, Riddell R H, Rochman H, Boyer J L. Non-alcoholic liver disease. Overlooked causes of liver injury in patients with heavy alcohol consumption. Am J Med 1979; 66: 429–434

123. Afshani P, Littenberg G D, Wollman J, Kaplowitz N. Significance of microscopic cholangitis in alcoholic liver disease. Gastroenterology 1978; 75: 1045–1050

124. Morgan M Y, Sherlock S, Scheuer P J. Portal fibrosis in the livers of alcoholic patients. Gut 1978; 19: 1015–1021

125. Karakucuk I, Dilly S A, Maxwell J D. Portal tract macrophages are increased in alcoholic liver injury. Histopathology 1989; 14: 245–253

126. Jakobovits A W, Morgan M Y, Sherlock S. Hepatic siderosis in alcoholics. Dig Dis Sci 1979; 24: 305–310

127. MacDonald R A. Wine and iron in haemochromatosis. Lancet 1963; i: 727

128. Kirsch R E. Epidemiology of alcoholic liver disease in South Africa. In: Hall P de la M, ed. Alcoholic liver disease. London: Edward Arnold, 1985: pp 184–192

129. Jacobs A. Iron-overload — clinical and pathological aspects. Semin Haematol 1977; 14: 89–113

130. Mihas A A, Tavassoli M. The effect of ethanol on the uptake, binding and desialylation of transferrin by rat liver endothelium: implications in the pathogenesis of alcohol-associated hepatic siderosis. Am J Med Sci 1991; 30: 299–304

131. Le Sage G D, Baldus W P, Fairbanks V F et al. Hemochromatosis: genetic or alcohol-induced? Gastroenterology 1983; 84: 1471–1477

132. Bassett M L, Halliday J W, Powell L W. Value of hepatic iron measurements in early haemochromatosis and determination of the critical iron level associated with fibrosis. Hepatology 1986; 6: 24–29

133. Sallie R W, Reed W D, Shilkin K B. Confirmation of the efficacy of hepatic tissue iron index in differentiating genetic haemochromatosis from alcoholic liver disease complicated by alcoholic haemosiderosis. Gut 1991; 32: 207–210

134. Olynyk J, Hall P, Reed W, Sallie R, Mackinnon M. Computerised measurement of iron in liver biopsies: a comparison with biochemical iron measurement. Hepatology 1990; 12: 26–30

135. Cortes J M, Oliva H, Paradinas F J, Hernandez-Guio C. The pathology of the liver in porphyria cutanea tarda. Histopathology 1980; 4: 471–485

136. Hislop W S, Masterton N, Bouchier I A D, Hopwood D. Cirrhosis and primary liver cell carcinoma in Tayside: a five year study. Scot Med J 1982; 27: 29–36

137. Lieber C S, Seitz H K, Garro A J, Worner T M. Alcohol as a co-carcinogen. In: Berk P D, Chalmers T C, eds. Frontiers in liver disease. New York: Thieme-Stratton, 1981: pp 320–335

138. MacSween R N M. Alcohol and cancer. Br Med Bull 1981; 38: 31–33

139. Ohnishi K, Iida S, Iwama S et al. The effect of chronic habitual alcohol intake on the development of liver cirrhosis and hepatocellular carcinoma. Cancer 1982; 49: 672–677

140. Brechot C, Nalpas B, Courouce A-M et al. Evidence that hepatitis B virus has a role in liver-cell carcinoma in alcoholic liver disease. N Engl J Med 1982; 306: 1384–1387

141. Walter E, Blum H E, Meir P et al. Hepatocellular carcinoma in alcoholic liver disease: no evidence for a pathogenic role of hepatitis B virus infection. Hepatology 1988; 8: 745–748

142. Bruix J, Barrera J M, Calvet X et al. Prevalence of antibodies to hepatitis C virus in Spanish patients with hepatocellular carcinoma and hepatic cirrhosis. Lancet 1989; ii: 1004–1006

143. Nalpas B, Driss F, Pol S et al. Association between HCV and HBV infection in hepatocellular carcinoma and alcoholic liver disease. J Hepatol 1991; 12: 70–74

144. Arakawa M, Kage M, Sugihara S, Nakashima T, Suenaga M, Okuda K. Emergence of malignant lesions within an adenomatous hyperplasia nodule in a cirrhotic liver. Gastroenterology 1986; 91: 198–208

145. Wada K, Kondo F, Kondo Y. Large regenerative nodules and dysplastic nodules in cirrhotic livers: a histopathologic study. Hepatology 1988; 6: 1684–1688

146. Talley N J, Roth A, Woods J, Hench V. Diagnostic value of liver biopsy in alcoholic liver disease. J Clin Gastroenterol 1988; 10: 647–650

147. Kumar S, Stauber R E, Gavaler J S et al. Orthotopic liver transplantation for alcoholic liver disease. Hepatology 1990; 11: 159–164

148. Hall P de la M. Histopathological spectrum of drug-induced liver injury. In: Farrell G C, ed. Drug-induced liver disease. Edinburgh: Churchill Livingstone, 1994: pp 115–151

149. Ludwig J, Viggiano T R, McGill D B, Ott B J. Nonalcoholic steatohepatitis. Mayo Clin Proc 1980; 55: 434–438

150. Adler M, Schaffner F. Fatty liver hepatitis and cirrhosis in obese patients. Am J Med 1979; 67: 811–816

151. Capron J-P, Delamarre J, Dupas J-L, Braillon A, Degott C, Quenum C. Fasting in obesity. Another cause of liver injury with alcoholic hyaline? Dig Dis Sci 1982; 27: 265–268

152. Silverman J F, O'Brien K F, Long S et al. Liver pathology in morbidly obese patients with and without diabetes. Am J Gastroenterol 1990; 85: 1349–1355

153. Thaler H. Relation of steatosis to cirrhosis. Clin Gastroenterol 1975; 4: 273–280

154. Falchuk K R, Fiske S C, Haggitt R C, Federman M, Trey C. Pericentral hepatic fibrosis and intracellular hyalin in diabetes mellitus. Gastroenterology 1980; 78: 535–541

155. Batman P A, Scheuer P J. Diabetic hepatitis preceding the onset of glucose intolerance. Histopathology 1985; 9: 237–243

156. Peters R L, Thomas G, Reynolds T B. Post-jejunoileal-bypass hepatic disease. Its similarity to alcoholic hepatic disease. J Clin Pathol 1975; 63: 318–331

157. Hamilton D L, Vest T K Brown B S, Shah A N, Menguy R B, Chey W Y. Liver injury with alcoholic-like hyalin after gastroplasty for morbid obesity. Gastroenterology 1983; 85: 722–726

158. Peura D A, Stromeyer F W, Johnson L F. Liver injury with alcoholic hyaline after intestinal resection. Gastroenterology 1980; 79: 128–130

159. Nakanuma Y, Ohta G, Konishi I, Shima Y. Liver injury with perivenular fibrosis and alcoholic hyalin after pancreatoduodenectomy for pancreatic carcinoma. Acta Pathol Jpn 1987; 37: 1953–1960

160. Powell E E, Searle J, Mortimer R. Steatohepatitis associated with limb lipodystrophy. Gastroenterology 1989; 97: 1022–1024

161. Nazim M, Stamp G, Hodgson H J. Non-alcoholic steatohepatitis associated with small intestinal diverticulosis and bacterial overgrowth. Hepatogastroenterology 1989; 36: 349–351

162. Partin J S, Partin J C, Schubert W K, McAdams A J. Liver ultrastructure in abetalipoproteinemia: evolution of micronodular cirrhosis. Gastroenterology 1974; 67: 107–118

163. Kimura H, Kako M, Yo K, Oda T. Alcoholic hyalins (Mallory bodies) in a case of Weber–Christian disease: electron microscopic observations of liver involvement. Gastroenterology 1980; 78: 807–812

164. Paliard P, Vitrey D, Fournier G, Belhadjali J, Patricot L, Berger F. Perhexilene maleate-induced hepatitis. Digestion 1978; 17: 419–427

165. Pessayre D, Bichara M, Feldman G, Degott C, Potet F, Benhamou J-P. Perhexiline maleate induced cirrhosis. Gastroenterology 1979; 76: 170–177

166. Poupon R, Rosensztaj L, De Saint-Maur P P, Lageron H, Gombeau T, Darnis F. Perhexiline maleate-associated hepatic injury: prevalence and characteristics. Digestion 1980; 20: 145–150

167. Poucell S, Ireton J, Valencia-Mayoral P et al. Amiodarone-associated phospholipidosis and fibrosis of the liver. Gastroenterology 1984; 86: 926–936

168. Gilinksy N H, Briscoe G W, Kuo C-S. Fatal amiodarone hepatotoxicity. Am J Gastroenterol 1988; 83: 161–163

169. Lewis J H, Ranard R C, Caruso A et al. Amiodarone hepatotoxicity: prevalence and clinicopathologic correlation among 104 patients. Hepatology 1989; 9: 679–685

170. Bach N, Schultz B L, Cohen L B et al. Amiodarone hepatotoxicity: progression from steatosis to cirrhosis. Mt Sinai J Med 1989; 56: 293–296

171. Itoh S, Igarashi M, Tsukada Y, Ichinoe A. Nonalcoholic fatty liver with alcoholic hyalin after long-term glucocorticoid therapy. Acta Hepatogastroenterol 1977; 24: 415–418

172. Seki K, Minami Y, Nishikawa M et al. 'Nonalcoholic steatohepatitis' induced by massive doses of synthetic estrogens. Gastroenterol Jpn 1983; 18: 197–203

173. Babany G, Uzzan F, Larrey D et al. Alcoholic-like liver lesions induced by nifedipine. J Hepatol 1989; 9: 252–255

174. Itoh S, Tsukada Y. Clinico-pathological and electron microscopical studies on a coronary dilating agent: 4,4'-diethylaminoethoxyhexestrol-induced liver injuries. Acta Hepatogastroenterol 1973; 20: 204–215

175. Wanless I R, Bargman J M, Oreopoulos D G, Vas S I. Subcapsular steatonecrosis in response to peritoneal insulin delivery: a clue to the pathogenesis of steatonecrosis in obesity. Mod Pathol 1989; 2: 69–74

176. Wanless I R, Lentz J S. Fatty liver hepatitis (steatohepatitis) and obesity: an autopsy study with analysis of risk factors. Hepatology 1990; 12: 1106–1110

177. Diehl A M, Goodman Z, Ishak K G. Alcohol-like liver disease in non-alcoholics. A clinical and histological comparison with alcohol-induced liver injury. Gastroenterology 1988; 95: 1056–1062

178. Lee R G. Nonalcoholic steatohepatitis: a study of 49 patients. Hum Pathol 1989; 20: 594–598

179. Powell E E, Cooksley G E, Hanson R et al. The natural history of nonalcoholic steatohepatitis. A follow-up study of forty-two patients for up to 21 years. Hepatology 1990; 11: 74–80

180. Vyberg M, Ravin V, Andersen B. Pattern of progression in liver injury following jejunoileal bypass for morbid obesity. Liver 1987; 7: 271–276

181. Feller A, Uchida T, Rakela J. Acute viral hepatitis superimposed on alcoholic liver cirrhosis. Liver 1985; 5: 239–246

182. Lane B P, Lieber C S. Ultrastructural alterations in human hepatocytes following ingestion of ethanol with adequate diets. Am J Pathol 1966; 49: 593–603

183. Rubin E, Lieber C S. Early fine structural changes in the human liver induced by alcohol. Gastroenterology 1967; 52: 1–13

184. Rubin E, Lieber C S. Alcohol-induced hepatic injury in nonalcoholic volunteers. N Engl J Med 1968; 278: 869–876

185. Lieber C S, DeCarli L M. An experimental model of alcohol feeding and liver injury in the baboon. J Med Primatol 1974; 3: 153–163

186. Rubin E, Lieber C S. Fatty liver, alcoholic hepatitis and cirrhosis produced by alcohol in primates. N Engl J Med 1974; 290: 128–135

187. Lieber C S, DeCarli L M, Rubin E. Sequential production of fatty liver, hepatitis, and cirrhosis in sub-human primates fed ethanol with adequate diets. Proc Natl Acad Sci USA 1975; 72: 437–441

188. Lieber C S, Leo M A, Mak K M, DeCarli L M, Sato S. Choline fails to prevent liver fibrosis in ethanol-fed baboons but causes toxicity. Hepatology 1985; 5: 561–572

189. Rubin E, Beattie D S, Lieber C S. Effects of ethanol on the biogenesis of mitochondrial membranes and associated mitochondrial functions. Lab Invest 1970; 23: 620–627

190. Inagaki T, Koike M, Ikuta K et al. Ultrastructural identification and clinical significance of light microscopic giant mitochondria and alcoholic liver injuries. Gastroenterol Jpn 1989; 24: 46–53

191. Cunningham C C, Coleman W B, Spach P I. The effects of chronic ethanol consumption on hepatic mitochondrial energy metabolism. Alcohol Alcoholism 1990; 25: 127–136

192. French S W, Ruebner B H, Mezey E, Tamura T, Halstead C H. Effect of chronic ethanol feeding on hepatic mitochondria in the monkey. Hepatology 1983; 3: 34–40

193. Arai M, Leo M A, Nakano M, Gordon E R, Lieber C S. Biochemical and morphological alterations of baboon hepatic mitochondria after chronic alcohol consumption. Hepatology 1984; 4: 165–174

194. Iseri O A, Lieber C S, Gottlieb L S. The ultrastructure of fatty liver induced by prolonged ethanol ingestion. Am J Pathol 1966; 48: 535–555

195. Lieber C S, DeCarli L M. Ethanol oxidation by hepatic microsomes: adaptive increase after ethanol feeding. Science 1968; 162: 917–918

196. Leo M A, Sato M, Lieber C S. Effect of hepatic vitamin A depletion on the liver in humans and rats. Gastroenterology 1983; 84: 562–572

197. McClain C J, Kromhout J P, Peterson F J, Holtzman J L. Potentiation of acetaminophen hepatotoxicity by alcohol. JAMA 1980; 244: 251–253

198. Sato C, Matsuda Y, Lieber C S. Increased hepatotoxicity of acetaminophen after chronic ethanol consumption in the rat. Gastroenterology 1981; 80: 140–148

199. Leo M A, Arai M, Sato M, Lieber C S. Hepatotoxicity of vitamin A and ethanol in the rat. Gastroenterology 1982; 82: 194–205

200. Riihimaki V, Savolainen K, Pfaffli P, Pekari K, Sippel H W, Laine A. Metabolic interaction between m-xylene and ethanol. Arch Toxicol 1982; 49: 253–263

201. Hall P de la M, Plummer J L, Ilsley A H, Cousins M J. Hepatic fibrosis and cirrhosis after chronic administration of alcohol and 'low-dose' carbon tetrachloride vapour in the rat. Hepatology 1991; 13: 815–819

202. Waring A J, Rottenberg H, Ohnishi T, Rubin E. Membranes and phospholipids of liver mitochondria from chronic alcoholic rats are resistant to membrane disordering by alcohol. Proc Natl Acad Sci USA 1981; 78: 2582–2586

203. Rubin E, Rottenberg H. Ethanol-induced injury and adaptation in biological membranes. Fed Proc 1982; 41: 2465–2471

204. Sun G Y, Sun A Y. Ethanol and membrane lipids. Alcohol: Clin Exp Res 1985; 9: 164–180

205. Yamada S, Lieber C S. Decrease in microviscosity and cholesterol content of rat liver plasma membranes after chronic ethanol feeding. J Clin Invest 1984; 74: 2285–2289

206. Taraschi T F, Rubin E. Effects of ethanol on the chemical and structural properties of biologic membrane. Lab Invest 1985; 52: 120–131

207. Schanne F A, Kane A B, Young E E, Farber J L. Calcium dependence of toxic cell death: a final common pathway. Science 1979; 206: 700–702

208. Farber J L. Calcium and mechanisms of liver necrosis. In: Popper H, Schaffner F, eds. Progress in liver diseases, Vol VII. New York: Grune & Stratton, 1982: pp 347–360

209. Hoek J B, Taraschi T F, Rubin E. Functional implications of the interaction of ethanol with biological membranes: actions of ethanol on hormone signal transduction systems. Semin Liver Dis 1988; 8: 36–46

210. Tribble D L, Aw T Y, Jones D P. The pathophysiological significance of lipid peroxidation in oxidative cell injury. Hepatology 1987; 7: 377–387

211. Shaw S, Rubin K P, Lieber C S. Depressed hepatic glutathione and increased diene conjugates in alcoholic liver disease: evidence of lipid peroxidation. Dig Dis Sci 1983; 28: 585–589

212. Younes M, Strubelt O. Alcohol-induced hepatotoxicity: a role for oxygen free radicals. Free Radic Res Commun 1987; 3: 19–26

213. Shigesawa T, Sato C, Marumo F. Significance of plasma glutathione determination in patients with alcoholic and non-alcoholic liver disease. J Gastroenterol Hepatol 1992; 7: 7–11

214. Strubelt O, Younes M, Pentz R. Enhancement by glutathione depletion of ethanol-induced acute hepatotoxicity in vitro and in vivo. Toxicology 1987; 45: 213–223

215. Varga M. How can free radicals cause damage to hepatic cells? A multidisciplinary approach. Drug Alcohol Depend 1991; 27: 117–119

216. Jauhonen P, Baraona E, Miyakawa H, Lieber C S. Mechanisms for selective perivenular hepatotoxicity of ethanol. Alcoholism: Clin Exp Res 1982; 6: 350–361

217. French S W, Benson N C, Sun P S. Centrilobular liver necrosis induced by hypoxia in chronic ethanol-fed rats. Hepatology 1984; 4; 912–917

218. Lieber C S, Baraona E, Hernández-Manoz R et al. Impaired oxygen utilization. A new mechanism for hepatotoxicity of ethanol in sub-human primates. J Clin Invest 1989; 83:1682–1690

219. Gumucio J J, Miller D L. Functional implications of liver cell heterogeneity. Gastroenterology 1981; 80: 393–403

220. Yuki T, Israel Y, Thurman R G. The swift increase in alcohol metabolism: inhibition of propylthiouracil. Biochem Pharmacol 1982; 31: 2403–2407

221. Orrego H, Blake J E, Blendis L M, Compton K V, Israel Y. Longterm treatment of alcoholic liver disease with propylthiouracil. N Engl J Med 1987; 317: 1421–1427

222. Orrego H, Carmichael F J. Effects of alcohol on liver haemodynamics in the presence and absence of liver disease. J Gastroenterol Hepatol 1992; 7: 70–89

223. Israel Y, Orrego H, Coleman J C, Britton R S. Alcohol-induced hepatomegaly: pathogenesis and role in the production of portal hypertension. Fed Proc 1982; 41: 2472–2477

224. Matsuda Y, Takada A, Kanayama R, Takase S. Changes in hepatic microtubules and secretory proteins in human alcoholic liver disease. Pharmacol Biochem Behav 1983; 18: (suppl 1): 479–482

225. Berman W J, Gil J, Jennett R B, Tuma D, Sorrell M F, Rubin E. Ethanol, hepatocellular organelles, and microtubules. A morphometric study in vivo and in vitro. Lab Invest 1983; 48: 760–767

226. Orrego H, Blendis L M, Crossley I R et al. Correlation of intrahepatic pressure with collagen in the Disse space and hepatomegaly in humans and in the rat. Gastroenterology 1981; 80: 546–556

227. Blendis L M, Orrego H, Crossley I R, Blake J E, Medline A, Israel Y. The role of hepatocyte enlargement in hepatic pressure in cirrhotic and noncirrhotic alcoholic liver disease. Hepatology 1982; 2: 539–546

228. Vidins E I, Britton R S, Medline A, Blendis L M, Israel Y, Orrego H. Sinusoidal calibre in alcoholic and nonalcoholic liver disease: diagnostic and pathogenic implications. Hepatology 1985; 5: 408–414

229. Miyakawa H, Iida S, Leo M A, Greenstein R J, Zimmon D S, Lieber C S. Pathogenesis of precirrhotic portal hypertension in alcohol-fed baboons. Gastroenterology 1985; 88: 143–150

230. Krogsgaard K, Gluud C, Henriksen J H, Christoffersen P. Correlation between liver morphology and portal pressure in alcoholic liver disease. Hepatology 1984; 4: 699–703

231. Okanoue T, Sawa Y, Kanaoka H et al. Clinical and experimental studies of the pathophysiology of portal hypertension. Hepatology 1988; 8: 677 (Abstr)

232. Mallory F B. Cirrhosis of the liver. Five different types of lesions from which it may arise. Bull John Hopkins Hosp 1911; 22: 69–75

233. Gerber M A, Orr W, Denk H, Schaffner F, Popper H. Hepatocellular hyalin in cholestasis and cirrhosis: its diagnostic significance. Gastroenterology 1973; 64: 89–98

234. MacSween R N M. Mallory's (alcoholic) hyaline in primary biliary cirrhosis. J Clin Pathol 1973; 26: 340–342

235. Sternlieb I. Evolution of hepatic lesion in Wilson's disease (hepatolenticular degeneration). In: Popper H, Schaffner F, eds. Progress in liver diseases, Vol IV. New York: Grune & Stratton, 1972: pp 511–525

236. Nayak N C, Sagreiya K, Ramalingaswami V. Indian childhood cirrhosis. The nature and significance of cytoplasmic hyaline of hepatocytes. Arch Pathol 1969; 88: 631–637

237. Wetzel W J, Alexander R W. Focal nodular hyperplasia of the liver with alcoholic hyaline bodies and cytologic atypia. Cancer 1979; 44: 1322–1326

238. Keeley A F, Iseri O A, Gottlieb L S. Ultrastructure of hyaline cytoplasmic inclusions in a human hepatoma: relationship to Mallory's alcoholic hyalin. Gastroenterology 1972; 62: 280–293

239. Kuhn C Kuo T-T. Cytoplasmic hyalin in asbestosis. A reaction to injured alveolar epithelium. Arch Pathol 1973; 95: 190–194

240. Warnock M L, Press M, Churg A. Further observations on cytoplasmic hyaline in the lung. Hum Pathol 1980; 11: 59–65

241. Denk H, Gschnait F, Wolff K. Hepatocellular hyalin (Mallory bodies) in long term griseofulvin-treated mice: a new experimental model for the study of hyalin formation. Lab Invest 1975; 32: 773–776

242. Borenfreund E, Bendich A. In vitro demonstration of Mallory body formation in liver cells from rats fed diethylnitrosamine. Lab Invest 1978; 38: 295–303

243. Meierhenry E F, Ruebner B H, Gershwin M E, Hsieh L S, French S W. Mallory body formation in hepatic nodules of mice ingesting dieldrin. Lab Invest 1981; 44: 392–396

244. Yokoo H, Minick O T, Batti F, Kent G. Morphologic variants of alcoholic hyalin. Am J Pathol 1972; 69: 25–40

245. French S W, Ihrig T J, Norum M L. A method of isolation of Mallory bodies in a purified fraction. Lab Invest 1972; 26: 240–244

246. Tinberg H M, Regan R J, Geier E A, Peterson G E, French S W. Mallory bodies: isolation of hepatocellular hyalin and electrophoretic resolution of polypeptide components. Lab Invest 1978; 39: 483–490

247. Luisada-Opper A V, Kanagasundaram N, Leevy C M. Chemical nature of alcoholic hyalin. Gastroenterology 1977; 73: 1374–1376

248. Denk H, Franke W W, Kerjaschi D. Mallory bodies: new facts and findings. In: Berk P D, Chalmers T C, eds. Frontiers in liver disease. New York: Thieme-Stratton, 1981: pp 93–105

249. Franke W F, Denk H, Schmid E, Osborn M, Weber K. Ultrastructural, biochemical and immunologic characterization of Mallory bodies in livers of griseofulvin-treated mice. Fimbriated rods of filaments containing prekeratin-like polypeptides. Lab Invest 1979; 40: 207–220

250. Kimoff R J, Haung S. Immunocytochemical and immunoelectron microscopic studies on Mallory bodies. Lab Invest 1981; 45: 491–503

251. Denk H, Franke W W, Eckerstorfer R, Schmid E, Kerjaschki D. Formation and involution of Mallory bodies ('alcoholic hyalin') in murine and human liver revealed by immunofluorescence microscopy with antibodies to prekeratin. Proc Natl Acad Sci USA 1979; 76: 4112–4116

252. French S W. The Mallory body: structure, composition and pathogenesis. Hepatology 1981; 1: 76–83

253. French S W. Nature, pathogenesis and significance of the Mallory body. Semin Liver Dis 1981; 1: 217–231

254. French S W. Present understanding of the development of Mallory body. Arch Pathol Lab Med 1983; 107: 445–450

255. Denk H, Franke W W, Dragosics B, Zeiler I. Pathology of cytoskeleton of liver cells: demonstration of Mallory bodies (alcoholic hyalin) in murine and human hepatocytes by immunofluorescence microscopy using antibodies to cytokeratin polypeptides from hepatocytes. Hepatology 1981; 1: 9–20

256. Morton J A, Bastin J, Fleming K A, McMichael A, Burns J, McGee JO'D. Mallory bodies in alcoholic liver disease: identification of cytoplasmic filament/cell membrane and unique antigenic determinants by monoclonal antibodies. Gut 1981; 22: 1–7

257. Morton J A, Fleming K A, Trowell J M, McGee JO'D. Mallory bodies — immunohistochemical detection by antisera to unique non-prekeratin components. Gut 1980; 21: 727–733

258. Fleming K A, Morton J A, Barbatis C, Burns J, Canning S, McGee J O'D. Mallory bodies in alcoholic and non-alcoholic liver disease contain a common antigenic determinant. Gut 1981; 22: 341–344

259. French S W, Katsuma Y, Ray M B, Swierenga S H H. Cytoskeletal pathology induced by ethanol. Ann NY Acad Sci 1987; 492: 262–276

260. Worman H J. Cellular intermediate filament networks and their derangement in alcoholic hepatitis. Alcoholism: Clin Exp Res 1990; 14: 789–804

261. Nakanuma Y, Ohta G. Is Mallory body formation a preneoplastic change? A study of 181 cases of liver bearing hepatocellular carcinoma and 82 cases of cirrhosis. Cancer 1985; 55: 2400–2404

262. Akeda S, Fujita K, Kosaka Y et al. Mallory body formation and amyloid deposition in the liver of aged mice fed a vitamin A deficient diet for a prolonged period. Lab Invest 1986; 54: 228–233

263. Ray M B, Mendenhall C L, French S W, Gartside P S and the Veterans Administrative Cooperative Study Group. Serum Vitamin A deficiency and increased intrahepatic expression of cytokeratin antigen in alcoholic liver disease. Hepatology 1988; 8: 1019–1026

264. Ray M B. Distribution patterns of cytokeratin antigen determinants in alcoholic and nonalcoholic liver diseases. Hum Pathol 1987; 18: 61–66

265. Yoshioka K, Kakumu S, Tahara H. Occurrence of immunohistochemically detected small Mallory bodies in liver disease. Am J Gastroenterol 1989; 84: 535–539

266. Ohata M, Marceau N, Perry G et al. Ubiquitin is present on the cytokeratin intermediate filaments and Mallory bodies of hepatocytes. Lab Invest 1988; 59: 848–856

267. De Vos R, Desmet V J. Ultrastructural characteristics of novel epithelial cell types in human pathologic liver specimens with chronic ductular reaction. Am J Pathol 1992; 140: 1441–1450

268. Fausto N. Hepatic regeneration. In: Zakim D, Boyer T D, eds. Hepatology: a text book of liver disease. London: Saunders, 1990: pp 49–65

269. Bucher N L R. Liver regeneration: an overview. J Gastroenterol Hepatol 1991; 6: 615–624

270. Duguay L, Coutu D, Hetu C, Joly J-G. Inhibition of liver regeneration by chronic alcohol administration. Gut 1982; 23:8–13

271. Marti U, Burwen S J, Jones A L. Biological effects of epidermal growth factor, with emphasis on the gastrointestinal tract and liver: an update. Hepatology 1989; 9: 126–138

272. Dalke D D, Sorrell M F, Casey C A, Tuma D J. Chronic ethanol administration impairs receptor-mediated endocytosis of epidermal growth factor by rat hepatocytes. Hepatology 1990; 12: 1085–1091

273. Bissell D M. Connective tissue metabolism and hepatic fibrosis: an overview. Semin Liver Dis 1990; 10: iii–iv

274. Maher J J. Hepatic fibrosis caused by alcohol. Semin Liver Dis 1990; 10: 60–74

275. Friedman S L. Cellular sources of collagen and regulation of collagen production in liver. Semin Liver Dis 1990; 10: 20–29

276. Schuppan D. Structure of the extracellular matrix in normal and fibrotic liver: collagens and glycoproteins. Semin Liver Dis 1990; 10: 1–10

277. Gressner A M, Bachem M G. Cellular sources of noncollagenous matrix proteins: role of fat-storing cells in fibrogenesis. Semin Liver Dis 1990; 10: 30–46

278. Arthur M J P. Matrix degradation in the liver. Semin Liver Dis 1990; 10: 47–55

279. Karasawa T, Chedid A. Sclerosing hyaline necrosis in noncirrhotic chronic alcoholic hepatitis. Am J Clin Pathol 1976; 66: 802–809

280. Takada A, Nei J, Matsuda Y, Kanayama R. Clinicopathological study of alcoholic fibrosis. Am J Gastroenterol 1982; 77: 660–666

281. Ohnishi K, Okuda K. Epidemiology of alcoholic liver disease in Japan. In: Hall P de la M, ed. Alcoholic liver disease. London: Edward Arnold, 1985: pp 167–183

282. Hahn E, Wick G, Pencev D, Timpl R. Distribution of basement membrane proteins in normal and fibrotic human liver: collagen type IV, laminin and fibronectin. Gut 1980; 21: 63–71

283. Rojkind M. Collagen metabolism in the liver. In: Hall P de la M, ed. Alcoholic liver disease. London: Edward Arnold, 1985: pp 90–112

284. Bioulac-Sage P, Lafon M E, Le Bail B, Balabaud C. Perisinusoidal and pit cells in liver sinusoids. In: Bioulac-Sage P, Balabaud C, eds. Sinusoids in human liver: health and disease. Rijswijk: Kupffer Cell Foundation, 1988: pp 39–62

285. Brouwer A, Wisse E, Knook D L. Sinusoidal endothelial cells and perisinusoidal fat-storing cells. In: Arias I M, Jakoby W B, Popper H, Schachter D, Shafritz D A, eds. The liver: biology and pathobiology, 2nd edn. New York: Raven, 1988: pp 665–682

286. Bronfenmajer S, Schaffner F, Popper H. Fat storing cells (lipocytes) in human liver. Arch Pathol 1966; 82: 447–453

287. De Leeuw A M, McCarthy S P, Geerts A, Knook D L. Purified rat liver fat storing cells in culture divide and contain collagen. Hepatology 1984; 4: 392–403

288. Burt A D, Robertson J L, Heir J, MacSween R N M. Desmin-containing stellate cells in rat liver; distribution in normal animals and response to experimental acute liver injury. J Pathol 1986; 150: 29–35

289. Mak K M, Leo M A, Lieber C S. Alcoholic liver injury in baboons: transformation of lipocytes to transitional cells. Gastroenterology 1984; 87: 188–200

290. Minato Y, Hasumura Y, Takeuchi J. The role of fat-storing cells in Disse space fibrogenesis in alcoholic liver disease. Hepatology 1983; 3: 559–566

291. Okanoue T, Burbrige E J, French S W. The role of the Ito cell in perivenular and intralobular fibrosis in alcoholic hepatitis. Arch Pathol Lab Med 1983; 107: 459–463

292. Horn T, Junge J, Christoffersen P. Early alcoholic liver injury. Activation of lipocytes in acinar zone 3 and correlation to degree of collagen formation in the Disse space. J Hepatol 1986; 3: 333–340

293. Mak K M, Lieber C S. Lipocytes and transitional cells in alcoholic liver disease. A morphometric study. Hepatology 1988; 8: 1027–1033

294. Kent G, Gay S, Inouye T, Bahu R, Minick O T, Popper H. Vitamin A-containing lipocytes and formation of type III collagen in liver injury. Proc Natl Acad Sci USA 1976; 73: 3719–3722

295. Bhathal P S. Presence of modified fibroblasts in cirrhotic livers in man. Pathology 1972; 4: 139–144

296. Nakano M, Lieber C S. Ultrastructure of initial stages of perivenular fibrosis in alcohol-fed baboons. Am J Pathol 1982; 106: 145–155

297. Skalli O, Schurch W, Seemayer T et al. Myofibroblasts from diverse pathological settings are heterogeneous in their content of actin isoforms and intermediate filament proteins. Lab Invest 1989; 60: 275–285

298. Savolainen E R, Leo M A, Timpl R, Lieber C S. Acetaldehyde and lactate stimulate collagen synthesis of cultured baboon liver myofibroblasts. Gastroenterology 1984; 87: 777–787

299. Rudolph R, McClure W J, Woodward M. Contractile fibroblasts in chronic alcoholic cirrhosis. Gastroenterology 1979; 76: 704–709

300. Holt K, Bennett M, Chojkier M. Acetaldehyde stimulates collagen and non-collagen protein production by human fibroblasts. Hepatology 1984; 4: 843–848

301. Friedman S L, Roll F J, Boyles J, Bissell D M. Hepatic lipocytes: the principal collagen-producing cells of normal rat liver. Proc Natl Acad Sci USA 1985; 82: 8681–8685

302. Maher J J, Bissell D M, Friedman S L, Roll F J. Collagen measured in primary cultures of normal rat hepatocytes derives from lipocytes within the monolayer. J Clin Invest 1988; 82: 450–459

303. Moshage H, Casini A, Lieber C S. Acetaldehyde selectively stimulates collagen production in cultured rat liver fat-storing cells but not in hepatocytes. Hepatology 1990; 12: 511–518

304. Friedman S L, Acetaldehyde and alcoholic fibrogenesis: fuel to the fire but not the spark. Hepatology 1990; 12: 609–612

305. Schaffner F, Popper H. Capillarization of hepatic sinusoids in man. Gastroenterology 1963; 44: 239–242

306. Horn T, Junge J, Christoffersen P. Early alcoholic liver injury: changes of the Disse space in acinar zone 3. Liver 1985; 5: 301–305

307. Burt A D, Griffiths M R, Schuppan D, Voss B, MacSween R N M. Ultrastructural localization of extracellular matrix proteins in human liver biopsies using ultracryomicrotomy and immunogold labelling. Histopathology 1990; 16: 53–58

308. Petrovic L M, Burroughs A, Scheuer P J. Hepatic sinusoidal endothelium: Ulex lectin binding. Histopathology 1989; 14: 233–234

309. Brouwer A, Wisse E, Knook D L, Sinusoidal endothelial cells and perisinusoidal fat-storing cells. In: Arias I M, Jakoby W B, Popper H, Schachter D, Shafritz D A, eds. The liver: biology and pathobiology, 2nd edn. New York: Raven, 1988: pp 665–682

310. Mak K M, Lieber C S. Alterations in endothelial fenestrations in liver sinusoids of baboons fed alcohol: a scanning electron microscopic study. Hepatology 1984; 4: 389–391

311. Horn T, Christoffersen P, Henriksen J H. Alcoholic liver injury: defenestration in non-cirrhotic livers. A scanning electron microscopic study. Hepatology 1987; 7: 77–82

312. Sztark F, Latry P, Quinton A, Balabaud C, Bioulac-Sage P. The sinusoidal barrier in alcoholic patients without fibrosis. A morphometric study. Virchows Archiv (A) 1986; 409: 385–393

313. Horn T, Lyon H, Christoffersen P. The 'blood–hepatocyte barrier'. A light microscopical transmission and scanning electron microscopic study. Liver 1986; 6: 233–245

314. Oda M, Azuma T, Nishizaki Y et al. Alterations of hepatic sinusoids in liver cirrhosis: their involvement in the pathogenesis of portal hypertension. J Gastroenterol Hepatol 1989; 4 (suppl 1): 111–113

315. Clark S A, Angus H B, Cook H B, George P M, Oxner R B G, Fraser R. Defenestration of hepatic sinusoids as a cause of hyperlipoproteinaemia in alcoholics. Lancet 1988; ii: 1225–1227

316. Fraser R, Bowler L M, Day W A. Damage of rat liver sinusoidal endothelium by ethanol. Pathology 1980; 12: 371–376

317. Clement B, Grimaud J-A, Campion J-P, Deugnier Y, Guillouzo A. Cell types involved in collagen and fibronection production in normal and fibrotic human liver. Hepatology 1986; 6: 225–234

318. Plebani M, Burlino A. Biochemical markers of hepatic fibrosis. Clin Biochem 1991; 24: 219–239

319. MacSween R N M, Anthony R A. Immune mechanisms of alcoholic liver disease. In: Hall P de la M, ed. Alcoholic liver disease. London: Edward Arnold, 1985: pp 69–89

320. Israel Y, Orrego H, Niemelä O. Immune responses to alcohol metabolites: pathogenic and diagnostic implications. Semin Liver Dis 1988; 8: 81–90

321. Zetterman R K. Autoimmune manifestations of alcoholic liver disease. In: Krawitt E L, Wiesner R H, eds. New York: Raven, 1991: pp 247–260

322. Kanagasundaram N, Kakumu S, Chen T, Leevy C M. Alcoholic hyalin antigen (AH Ag) and antibody (AH Ab) in alcoholic hepatitis. Gastroenterology 1977; 73: 1368–1373

323. Triggs S M, Mills P R, MacSween R N M. Sensitisation to Mallory bodies (alcoholic hyalin) in alcoholic hepatitis. J Clin Pathol 1981; 34: 21–24

324. Zetterman R K, Sorrell M F. Immunologic aspects of alcoholic liver disease. Gastroenterology 1981; 81: 616–624

325. Samato A, Chen T, Leevy C M. On the mechanism of progressive liver injury: altered DNA and collagen synthesis induced by Mallory bodies. Gastroenterology 1985; 88: 1692

326. Leevy C M, Chen T, Luisada-Opper A, Kanagasundaram N, Zetterman R. Liver disease in the alcoholic: role of immunological abnormalities in pathogenesis, recognition and treatment. In: Popper H, Schaffner F, eds. Progress in liver diseases, Vol V. New York: Grune & Stratton, 1976: pp 516–530

327. Peters M, Liebman H A, Tong M J, Tinberg H M. Alcoholic hepatitis: granulocyte chemotactic factor from Mallory body-stimulated human peripheral blood mononuclear cells. Clin Immunol Immunopathol 1983; 28: 418–430

328. Manns M, Meyer Zum Buschenfelde K H, Hess G. Autoantibodies against liver-specific membrane lipoprotein in acute and chronic liver diseases; studies on organ-, species-, and disease-specificity. Gut 1980; 21: 955–961

329. Perperas A, Tsantoulas D, Portmann B, Eddleston A L W F, Williams R. Autoimmunity to a liver membrane lipoprotein and liver damage in alcoholic liver disease. Gut 1981; 22: 149–152

330. Meliconi R, Perperas A, Jensen D et al. Anti-LSP antibodies in acute liver disease. Gut 1982; 23: 603–607

331. Bailey R J, Krasner N, Eddleston A L W F et al. Histocompatibility antigens, autoantibodies and immunoglobulins in alcoholic liver disease. Br Med J 1976; 2: 727–729

332. Iturriaga H, Pereda T, Estevez A, Ugarte G. Serum immunoglobulin and changes in alcoholic patients. Ann Clin Res 1977; 9: 39–43

333. Morgan M Y, Ross M G R, Ng C M, Thomas H C, Sherlock S. HLA B8, immunoglobulins, and antibody responses in alcohol-related liver disease. J Clin Pathol 1980; 33: 488–492

334. Swerdlow M A, Chowdhury L N. IgA deposition in liver in alcoholic liver disease. An index of progressive injury. Arch Pathol Lab Med 1984; 108: 416–419

335. Van De Wiel A, Delacroix D L, Van Hattum J. Characteristics of serum IgA and liver IgA deposits in alcoholic liver disease. Hepatology 1987; 7: 95–99

336. Gluud C, Tage-Jensen U, Bahnsen M, Dietrichson O, Svejgaard A. Autoantibodies, histocompatability antigens and testosterone in males with alcoholic liver cirrhosis. Clin Exp Immunol 1981; 44: 31–37

337. Burt A D, Anthony R S, Hislop W S, Bouchier I A D, MacSween R N M. Liver membrane antibodies in alcoholic liver disease: I. Prevalence and immunoglobulin class. Gut 1982; 23: 221–225

338. Anthony R S, Farquharson M, MacSween R N M. Liver membrane antibodies in alcoholic liver disease II. Antibodies to ethanol altered hepatocytes. J Clin Pathol 1983; 36: 1302–1308

339. Niemelä O, Klajner F, Orrego H, Videns E, Blendis L, Israel Y. Antibodies against acetaldehyde-modified protein epitopes in human alcoholics. Hepatology 1987; 7: 1210–1214

340. Lin R C, Smith R S, Lumeng L. Detection of a protein–acetaldehyde adduct in the liver of rats fed alcohol chronically. J Clin Invest 1988; 81: 615–619

341. Behrens V J, Hoerner M, Lasker J M, Lieber C S. Formation of acetaldehyde adducts with ethanol-inducible P450IIE1 in vivo. Biochem Biophys Res Commun 1988; 154: 584–590

342. Niemelä O, Juvonen T, Parkkila S. Immunohistochemical demonstration of acetaldehyde-modified epitopes in human liver after alcohol consumption. J Clin Invest 1990; 87: 1367–1374

343. Laskin C A, Vidins E, Blendis L M, Soloninka C A. Autoantibodies in alcoholic liver disease. Am J Med 1990; 89: 129–133

344. Müller C, Wolf H, Göttlicher J, Eibl M M. Helper-inducer and suppression-inducer lymphocyte subsets in alcoholic cirrhosis. Scand J Gastroenterol 1991; 26: 295–301

345. Actis G, Mieli-Vergani G, Portmann B, Eddleston A L, Davis M, Williams R. Lymphocyte cytotoxicity to autologous hepatocytes in alcoholic liver disease. Liver 1983; 3: 8–12

346. Izumi N, Hasumura Y, Takeuchi J. Lymphocyte cytotoxicity for autologous human hepatocytes in alcoholic liver disease. Clin Exp Immunol 1983; 54: 219–224

347. Cochrane A M G, Moussouros A, Portmann B et al. Lymphocyte cytotoxicity for isolated hepatocytes in alcoholic liver disease. Gastroenterology 1977; 72: 918–923

348. McClain C J, Cohen D A. Increased tumour necrosis factor production by monocytes in alcoholic hepatitis. Hepatology 1989; 9: 349–351

349. Bird G L A, Sheron N, Goka A K J, Alexander G J, Williams R S. Increased tumour necrosis factor in severe alcoholic hepatitis. Ann Intern Med 1990; 112: 917–920

350. Felver M E, Mezey E, McGuire M et al. Plasma tumour necrosis factor a predicts decreased long-term survival in severe alcoholic hepatitis. Alcoholism: Clin Exp Res 1990; 14: 255–259

351. Khoruts A, Stahnke L, McClain C J, Logan G, Allen J I. Circulating tumour necrosis factor, interleukin-1 and interleukin-6 concentrations in chronic alcoholic patients. Hepatology 1991; 13: 267–276

352. Sheron N, Bird G, Goka G, Alexander G, Williams R, Elevated plasma interleukin-6 and increased severity and mortality in alcoholic hepatitis. Clin Exp Immunol 1991; 84: 449–453

353. Devière J, Vaerman J-P, Content J et al. IgA triggers tumour necrosis factor a secretion by monocytes: a study in normal subjects and patients with alcoholic cirrhosis. Hepatology 1991; 13: 670–675

354. Mills L R, Scheuer P J. Hepatic sinusoidal macrophages in alcoholic liver disease. J Pathol 1985; 147: 127–132

355. Shiratori Y, Teraoka H, Matano S, Matsumoto K, Kamii K, Tanaka M. Kupffer cell function in chronic ethanol-fed rats. Liver 1989; 9: 351–359

356. Turunen U, Malkamaki M, Valtonen V et al. Endotoxin and liver diseases: high titres of enterobacterial common antigen antibodies in patients with alcoholic cirrhosis. Gut 1981; 22: 849–853

357. Matsuoka M, Tsukamota H. Stimulation of hepatic lipocyte collagen production by Kupffer cell-derived transforming growth factor β: implication for a pathogenic role in alcoholic liver fibrogenesis. Hepatology 1990; 11: 599–605

358. Barbatis C, Wood J, Morton J A, Fleming K A, McMichael A, McGee JO'D. Immunohistochemical analysis of HLA (A,B,C) antigens in liver disease using a monoclonal antibody. Gut 1981; 22: 985–991

359. Mezey E. Interaction between alcohol and nutrition in the pathogenesis of alcoholic liver disease. Semin Liver Dis 1991; 11: 340–347

360. Marsano L, McClain C J. Nutrition and liver disease. JPEN 1991; 15: 337–344

361. Mendenhall C L, Anderson S, Weesner R E, Goldberg S J, Crolic K A. Protein calorie malnutrition associated with alcoholic hepatitis. Am J Med 1984; 76: 211–222

362. Krasner N, Cochran K M, Russell R I, Carmichael H A, Thompson G G. Alcohol and absorption from the small intestine 1. Impairment of absorption from the small intestine in alcoholics. Gut 1976; 17: 245–248

363. Patek A J. Alcohol, malnutrition and alcoholic cirrhosis. Am J Clin Nutr 1979; 32: 1304–1312

364. Leo M A, Lieber C S. Hepatic fibrosis after long-term administration of ethanol and moderate vitamin A supplementation in the rat. Hepatology 1983; 3: 1–11

365. Leo M A, Lieber C S. Hypervitaminosis A: a liver lover's lament. Hepatology 1988; 8: 412–417

366. Diehl A M, Boitnott J K, Herlong H F et al. Effect of parenteral amino acid supplementation on alcoholic hepatitis. Hepatology 1985; 5: 57–63

367. Bonkovsky H L, Fiellin D A, Smith G S, Slaker D P, Simon D, Galambos J T. A randomized, controlled trial of treatment of alcoholic hepatitis with parenteral nutrition and oxandrolone. I. Short term effects on liver function. Am J Gastroenterol 1991; 86: 1200–1208

368. Péquignot G, Tuyns A J, Berta J L. Ascitic cirrhosis in relation to alcohol consumption. Int J Epidemiol 1978; 7: 113–120

369. Tuyns A J, Péquignot G. Greater risk of ascitic cirrhosis in females in relation to alcohol consumption. Int J Epidemiol 1984; 13: 53–57

370. Batey R G, Burns T, Berson R J, Byth K. Alcohol consumption and the risk of cirrhosis. Med J Aust 1992; 156: 413–416

371. Hasin D S, Grant B, Harford T C. Male and female differences in liver cirrhosis mortality in the United States, 1961–1985. J Stud Alcohol 1990; 51: 123–129

372. Wilkinson P, Santamaria J N, Rankin J A. Epidemiology of alcoholic cirrhosis. Aust Ann Med 1969; 18: 222–226

373. Wilkinson P, Kornaczewski A, Rankin J G, Santamaria J N. Physical disease in alcoholism. Initial survey of 1000 patients. Med J Aust 1971; 1: 1217–1223

374. Gavaler J S. Sex-related differences in ethanol-induced liver disease: artifactual or real? Alcoholism: Clin Exp Res 1982; 6: 186–196

375. Saunders J B, Davis M, Williams R. Do women develop alcoholic liver disease more readily than men? Br Med J 1981; i: 1140–1143

376. Coates R A, Halliday M L, Rankin J G, Feinman S, Fisher M M. Risk of fatty infiltration or cirrhosis of the liver in relation to ethanol consumption: a case–control study. Clin Invest Med 1986; 9: 26–32

377. Norton R, Batey R, Dwyer T, MacMahon S. Alcohol consumption and the risk of alcohol related cirrhosis in women. Br Med J 1987; ii: 80–82

378. Loft S, Olesen K-L, Dossing M. Increased susceptibility to liver disease in relation to alcohol consumption in women. Scand J Gastroenterol 1987; 10: 1251–1256

379. Berglund M. Mortality in alcoholics related to clinical state at first admission. A study of 537 deaths. Acta Psychiatr Scand 1984; 70: 407–416

380. Di Padova C, Worner T M, Julkunen R J, Lieber C S. Effects of fasting and chronic alcohol consumption on the first pass metabolism of ethanol. Gastroenterology 1987; 92: 1169–1173

381. Caballeria J, Frezza M, Hernandez-Munoz R et al. Gastric origin of the first-pass metabolism of ethanol in humans: effect of gastrectomy. Gastroenterology 1989; 97: 1205–1209

382. Caballeria J, Baraona E, Rodamilans M, Lieber C S. Effects of cimetidine on gastric alcohol dehydrogenase activity and blood ethanol levels. Gastroenterology 1989; 96: 388–392

383. Ricciardi B R, Saunders J B, Williams R, Hopkins D A. Hepatic ADH and ALDH isoenzymes in different racial groups and in chronic alcoholism. Pharmacol Biochem Behav 1983; 18 (suppl 1): 61–65

384. Bosron W F, Li T-K. Genetic polymorphism of human liver alcohol and acetaldehyde dehydrogenases, and their relationship to alcohol metabolism and alcoholism. Hepatology 1986; 6: 502–510

385. Bosron W F, Lumeng L, Li T-K. Genetic polymorphism of enzymes of alcohol metabolism and susceptibility to alcoholic liver disease. Mol Aspects Med 1988; 10: 147–158

386. Shibuya A, Yoshida A. Genotypes of alcohol-metabolizing enzymes in Japanese with alcoholic liver diseases: a strong association of the usual Caucasian-type aldehyde dehydrogenase gene (ALDH[2']) with the disease. Am J Hum Genet 1988; 43: 744–748

387. Couzigou P, Fleury B, Groppi A et al. Role of alcohol dehydrogenase polymorphisms in ethanol metabolism and alcohol-related diseases. In: Weiner E, Wermuth B, Crabb D W, eds. Enzymology and molecular biology of carbonyl metabolism 3. New York : Plenum, 1990; pp 263–270

388. Day C P, Bassendine M F. Genetic predisposition to alcoholic liver disease. Gut 1992; 33: 1444–1447

389. Agarwal D P, Goedde W H. Human aldehyde dehydrogenases: their role in alcoholism. Alcohol 1989; 6: 517–523

390. Enomoto N, Takase S, Takada N, Takada A. Alcoholic liver disease in heterozygotes of mutant and normal aldehyde dehydrogenase-2 genes. Hepatology 1991; 13: 1071–1075

391. Goodwin D W. Studies of familial alcoholism: a growth industry. In: Goodwin D W, Van Usen K T, Mednick S A, eds. Longitudinal research in alcoholism. Boston, Kluwer-Nijhoff, 1984: pp 97–105

392. Devor E J, Reich T, Cloninger C R, Genetics of alcoholism and related end-organ damage. Semin Liver Dis 1988; 8: 1–11

393. Blum K, Noble E P, Sheridan P J et al. Allelic association of human dopamine D_2 receptor gene in alcoholism. JAMA 1990; 263: 2055–2060

394. Wodak A D, Saunders J B, Ewusi-Mensah I, Davis M, Williams R. Severity of alcohol dependence in patients with alcoholic liver disease. Br Med J 1983; i: 1420–1421

395. Saunders J B, Wodak A D, Haines A et al. Accelerated development of alcoholic cirrhosis in patients with HLA-B8. Lancet 1982; i: 1381–1384

396. Monteiro E, Alves M P, Santos M L et al. Histocompatibility antigens: markers of susceptibility to and protection from alcoholic liver disease in a Portuguese population. Hepatology 1988; 8: 455–458

397. Mills P R, MacSween R N M, Dick H M, Hislop W S. Histocompatibility antigens in patients with alcoholic liver disease in Scotland and Northeastern England: failure to show an association. Gut 1888; 29: 146–148

398. Mills P R, Pennington T H, Kay P, MacSween R N M, Watkinson G. Hepatitis Bs antibody in alcoholic cirrhosis. J Clin Pathol 1979; 32: 778–782

399. Mills P R, Follett E A C, Urquhart G E D, Watkinson G, MacSween R N M. Evidence for previous hepatitis B virus infection in alcoholic cirrhosis. Br Med J 1981; i: 437–438

400. Hislop W S, Follett E A C, Bouchier I A D, MacSween R N M. Serological markers of hepatitis B in patients with alcoholic liver disease: a multi-centre survey. J Clin Pathol 1981; 34: 1017–1019

401. Orholm M, Aldershvile J, Tage-Jensen U et al. Prevalence of hepatitis B virus infection among alcoholic patients with liver disease. J Clin Pathol 1981; 34: 1378–1380

402. Villa E, Rubbiani L, Barchi T et al. Susceptibility of chronic symptomless HBsAg carriers to ethanol-induced hepatic damage. Lancet 1982; ii: 1243–1244

403. Saunders J B, Wodak A D, Morgan-Capner P et al. Importance of markers of hepatitis B virus in alcoholic liver disease. Br Med J 1983; i: 1851–1854

404. Inoue K, Kojima T, Koyata H et al. Hepatitis B virus antigen and antibodies in alcoholics. Etiological role of HBV in liver diseases in alcoholic patients. Liver 1985; 5: 247–252

405. Nonomura A, Hayashi M, Takayanagi N, Watanabe K, Ohta G. Correlation of morphological subtypes of liver cirrhosis with excess alcohol intake, HBV infections, age at death, and hepatocellular carcinoma. Acta Pathol Jpn 1986; 36: 631–640

406. Mendenhall C L, Seeff L, Diehl A M et al. Antibodies to hepatitis B virus and hepatitis C virus in alcoholic hepatitis and cirrhosis: their prevalence and clinical relevance. Hepatology 1991; 14: 581–589

407. Fong T-L, Govindarijan S A, Valinluck B, Redeker A G, Status of hepatitis B virus DNA in alcoholic liver disease: a study of a large urban population in the United States. Hepatology 1988; 8: 1602–1604

408. Horüke N, Michitaka K, Onji M, Murota T, Ohta Y. HBV-DNA

hybridization in hepatocellular carcinoma associated with alcohol in Japan. J Med Virol 1989; 28: 189–192

409. Novick D M, Enlow R W, Gelb A M et al. Hepatic cirrhosis in young adults: association with adolescent onset of alcohol and parenteral heroin abuse. Gut 1985; 26: 8–13

410. Chung H T, Lai C L, Wu P C, Lok A S. Synergism of chronic alcoholism and hepatitis B infection in liver disease. J Gastroenterol Hepatol 1989; 4: 11–16

411. Pares A, Barrera J M, Caballeria J et al. Hepatitis C virus antibodies in chronic alcoholic patients: association with severity of liver injury. Hepatology 1990; 12: 1295–1299

412 Caldwell S H, Jeffers L J, Ditomaso A et al. Antibody to hepatitis C is common among patients with alcoholic liver disease with and without risk factors. Am J Gastroenterol 1991; 86: 1219–1223

413. Nishiguchi S, Kuroki T, Yabusako T et al. Detection of hepatitis C virus antibodies and hepatitis C virus RNA in patients with alcoholic liver disease. Hepatology 1991; 14: 985–989

414. Shimizu S, Kiyosawa K, Sodeyama T, Tanaka E, Nakano M. High prevalence of antibody to hepatitis C virus in heavy drinkers with chronic liver diseases in Japan. J Gastroenterol Hepatol 1992; 7: 30–35

415. Strubelt O. Interactions between ethanol and other hepatotoxic agents. Biochem Pharmacol 1980; 29: 1445–1449

416. Zimmerman H J. Effects of alcohol on other hepatotoxins. Alcoholism: Clin Exp Res 1986; 10: 3–15

417. Seeff L B, Cucherini B A, Zimmerman H J, Adler E, Benjamin S B. Acetaminophen hepatoxicity in alcoholics: a therapeutic misadventure. Ann Intern Med 1986; 104: 399–404

418. McKinnon R A, Hall P de la M, Gonzalez F J, McManus M E.

Localization of human cytochrome P-450 2E1 mRNA in alcoholic liver disease by in situ hybridisation. In preparation

419. Weinstein G, Roenigh H, Maiback H et al. Psoriasis–liver–methotrexate interactions: Co-operative Study. Arch Dermatol 1973; 108: 36–42

420. Nyfors A. Liver biopsies from psoriatics related to methotrexate therapy. III: findings in postmethotrexate liver biopsies from 160 psoriatics. Acta Pathol Microbiol Immunol Scand [A] 1977, 85: 511–518

421. Zachariae H, Kragballe K, Sogaard H. Methotrexate induced liver cirrhosis. Br J Dermatol 1980; 102: 407–512

422. O'Keefe Q E, Fye K F, Sack K D. Methotrexate and histologic hepatic abnormalities: a meta-analysis. Am J Med 1991; 90: 711–716

423. Devenyi P, Robinson G M, Roncari D A K. Alcohol and high density lipoproteins. Can Med Assoc J 1980; 123: 981–984

424. Duhamel G, Nalpas B, Goldstein S, Laplaud P M, Berthelot P, Chapman M J. Plasma lipoprotein and apolipoprotein profile in alcoholic patients with and without liver disease: on the relative roles of alcohol and liver injury. Hepatology 1984; 4: 577–585

425. Van Thiel D H, Gavaler J S, Tarter R E et al. Liver transplantation for alcoholic liver disease: a consideration of reasons for and against. Alcoholism: Clin Exp Res 1989; 13: 181–184

426. Schenker S, Perkins H S, Sorrell M F. Should patients with end-stage alcoholic liver disease have a new liver? Hepatology 1990; 11: 314–319

427. Lucey M R, Merion R M, Henley K S et al. Selection for and outcome of liver transplantation in alcoholic liver disease. Gastroenterology 1992; 102: 1736–1741

9

Chronic hepatitis

L. Bianchi   F. Gudat

DEFINITIONS AND CAUSES

Chronic hepatitis has been defined as inflammation of the liver continuing without improvement for at least 6 months.[1] This definition is obviously too broad and merely describes a reaction pattern of the liver with a wide spectrum of different clinical, biochemical and histological features due to a variety of causes. Moreover, it is a matter of debate whether cirrhosis should be included in the definition. In this chapter, the term chronic hepatitis is used in a restricted sense, for a chronic necro-inflammatory, primarily hepatocytic lesion with or without cirrhosis, in which the lymphocyte clearly dominates the inflammation. Abbreviations and vocabulary used are listed in Table 9.1, and main aetiological categories in Table 9.2.

Some chronic liver diseases, listed in Table 9.3, are usually not included under the heading of chronic hepatitis although they may have histological features of chronic hepatitis at some stage of their evolution, notably piecemeal necrosis, the hallmark of chronic active hepatitis (CAH). Diseases of intra- or extrahepatic bile ducts, for instance, may show piecemeal necrosis. In our files, 13% of biopsies of histologically typical chronic alcoholic liver disease exhibit, in addition, histological features of chronic active hepatitis, with less than half of the cases being seropositive for antibodies to the hepatitis C virus (HCV) by first generation testing (unpublished own data).

NOMENCLATURE AND CLASSIFICATION

GENERAL CONSIDERATIONS

The current histological classification of chronic hepatitis dates back to 1968.[2] Its major contribution was the distinction of chronic persistent hepatitis (CPH), thought to have a favourable prognosis, from chronic active hepatitis (CAH) which was considered to be progressive and the leading cause of cirrhosis. At this time and for many years

Table 9.1 Abbreviations and vocabulary (for abbreviations and explanations of hepatitis B viral antigens, see Table 9.11)

Active septum	Newly formed sheet of connective tissue rich in inflammatory cells, associated with piecemeal necrosis, giving rise to portal–portal bridging.
AI-CH	Autoimmune chronic hepatitis
Anti-ASGP-R	Antibody against the asialoglycoprotein receptor
Bridging hepatic necrosis	Extensive form of confluent necrosis, connecting different vascular structures. Central–central bridging (i.e. peri-complex acinar necrosis) is distinguished from prognostically more significant central–portal bridging (peri-simple acinar necrosis) (p. 358).
CAH	Chronic active hepatitis: chronic, mainly portal/periportal and predominantly lymphocytic inflammation with the hallmark of piecemeal necrosis and a variable degree of fibrosis. CAH may occur in the absence or presence of cirrhosis (p. 358).
CAH-min	Minimally active chronic hepatitis: mildest form of chronic hepatitis in which only some tongues of piecemeal necrosis are found in few portal tracts (p. 359)
CAH mild	Chronic active hepatitis of mild activity (p. 359)
CAH-mod	Chronic active hepatitis of moderate activity (p. 359)
CAH-sev, very sev	Chronic active hepatitis of severe, or very severe activity (p. 359)
CH	Chronic hepatitis: inflammation of the liver continuing without improvement for at least 6 months (p. 349)
Chronic septal hepatitis	A non-aggressive chronic hepatitis with predominantly lymphocytic infiltration restricted to portal tracts and newly formed fibrous septa. Chronic septal hepatitis represents a regressive stage of CAH[18]
CLH	Chronic lobular hepatitis: chronic hepatitis with pronounced lobular necro-inflammatory changes reminiscent of acute hepatitis but persisting for more than 6 months[5]
Confluent necrosis	Substantial groups of adjacent liver cells affected by necrosis, usually of the lytic type. As a rule, CN affects zone 3, but it may involve whole acini (panacinar necrosis)
CPH	Chronic persistent hepatitis: chronic hepatitis with predominantly lymphocytic inflammation restricted to portal tracts and without piecemeal necrosis, formerly regarded as a separate histological type of CH. For discussion, see p. 351.
LKM	Liver/kidney microsomal antibody
LMA	Liver membrane antibody
Minimal hepatitis	Minimal hepatitis: some small, scattered lobular (and portal) predominantly lymphocytic foci, associated with HBsAg and/or HBcAg expression in tissue. Such features correspond to the permissive and non-permissive HBV carrier state (see pp 351, 377).
Non-specific reactive hepatitis	A usually mild portal and lobular inflammation characterized by mixed histiocytic and neutrophilic infiltrates, and pleomorphism of liver cells and nuclei. NRH is a response of the liver to a variety of primarily extrahepatic diseases.
pANCA	Perinuclear antineutrophil cytoplasmic antibody
Passive septum	Newly formed paucicellular septum reflecting collapse after confluent necrosis, giving rise to central–portal bridging
PBC	Primary biliary cirrhosis
Piecemeal necrosis	Chronic, gradual inflammatory destruction of liver cells at a mesenchymal/parenchymal interface, associated with predominantly lymphocytic infiltration (p. 355)
PSC	Primary sclerosing cholangitis
SLA	Soluble liver antigen
Sleeve necrosis	Extensive periportal piecemeal necrosis forming a contiguous band surrounding the whole perimeter of the portal tract in a sleeve-like manner

Table 9.2 Established aetiological categories of chronic hepatitis

Viral (HBV, HDV, HCV)
Autoimmune (classic 'lupoid' type and subtypes)
Autoimmune overlap syndromes
Drug-induced (e.g. nitrofurantoin, alpha-methyldopa, isoniazid etc.)
'Cryptogenic'

Table 9.3 Chronic liver diseases other than chronic active hepatitis with piecemeal necrosis

Primary biliary cirrhosis
Sclerosing cholangitis
Wilson's disease
α_1-Antitrypsin deficiency
Alcoholic liver disease

thereafter, the underlying aetiology and clinical correlations were ill-defined and histology was a key parameter for prognosis and therapy. The discovery of the hepatitis virus B (HBV) in the late 1960s, of the hepatitis A virus (HAV) some years later and, finally, the identification of several viruses causing non-A, non-B hepatitis, have completely changed the clinical approach to viral hepatitis. It became apparent that CPH and CAH were not separate entities but could merge into each other. Furthermore, chronic lobular hepatitis (CLH), an entity introduced by Popper in 1971,[3–5] is also enigmatic. Although morphologically well-defined, CPH has different prognostic and therapeutic implications, depending on aetiology and the replicative state of infection. This is well-known for CPH due to HBV[6] but has become a renewed issue for HCV since differential diagnosis against CAH is difficult but fundamental because of conceptual and practical consequences. Therefore, in two recent editorials,[7,8] a need for reassessment of the current nomenclature has been duly expressed. In particular, the dualistic concept of CPH and CAH has been challenged. A classification is now envisaged which covers chronic hepatitis as a spectrum of a common inflammatory reaction, the histological presentation of which oscillates in grade, may be modified by structural alterations such as fibrosis or cirrhosis, and may have different prognostic and therapeutic implications according to aetiology.

The reader should be prepared for three possible developments in the classification of chronic hepatitis:[7]

1. Current classification, with specification of aetiology, serology and immunohistochemistry; scoring optional;
2. Entirely new classification, to be defined, and incorporating aetiology, necro-inflammatory activity, serology and immunohistochemistry;
3. Aetiological classification, supplemented with additional qualitative or quantitative information.

Pending a generally accepted revision, option 1 is actually adopted in this chapter. A slight modification of current classification is used and it is postulated that aetiology and replicative state are added. However, it should be realized that the histological types labelled here with old terms are used in a very restrictive way and actually stand for graded inflammatory phenotypes (Table 9.9). This should allow the reader to translate these entities into other systems of concurrent or future classification. For instance, the eight phenotypes listed in Table 9.9 may be communicated to the clinician in terms of defined gradings, scores, histological terms or all together. The state of replication should be determined as far as possible by serology, molecular biology or immunohistology as outlined on page 377. For instance, in an HBsAg-seropositive patient, a lymphocytic inflammation strictly limited to portal tracts may be diagnosed as hepatitis B–CPH, likewise as chronic hepatitis of mild activity (with inflammatory score 3 or 4; fibrosis/cirrhosis score 0); HBc-free type of generalized HBc-type (depending on relevant blood or tissue markers).

These histological phenotypes are:

MINIMAL HEPATITIS

In the context of proven viral aetiology (hepatitis B or C) we use the term minimal hepatitis to replace the formerly used designation 'non-specific reactive hepatitis'.[9] The latter term then is reserved for inflammatory reactions of the liver in primarily extrahepatic disease or for reactions to a focal intrahepatic space-occupying process. In hepatitis B, minimal hepatitis may be associated either with high

viral replication or, more often, with the non-replicative HBV carrier state. In the same way as for CPH the prognosis, infectivity and treatment of these two types of HBV-related carrier state will be entirely different.

The histological features (Table 9.4) comprise discrete inflammatory infiltrates of a degree between almost no inflammation and CPH. Some, but certainly not all, portal tracts contain scattered lymphocytic infiltrates, and the same holds true for the hepatic acini (Fig. 9.1a). Late and residual stages of acute (self-limited) viral hepatitis (e.g. hepatitis A) may show similar features. In minimal hepatitis inflammatory foci are as a rule predominantly lymphocytic while in non-specific reactive hepatitis they are usually intermingled with macrophages and neutrophils.

These histological alterations may be graded with score values not higher than 1 (Tables 9.9 and 9.10).

CHRONIC PERSISTENT HEPATITIS (CPH)

The histology of CPH (Table 9.5 and Fig. 9.1b) is precisely defined by a lymphocytic inflammation entirely restricted to widened portal tracts, leaving the parenchymal limiting plate preserved.[10] Acinar architecture remains intact. Portal tracts contain a diffuse infiltrate, predominantly lymphocytic, intermixed with few plasma

Table 9.4 Histological features in minimal hepatitis (MH)

Constant findings:
    Discrete lymphocytic infiltrate in some portal tracts
    Scanty intra-acinar lymphocytic foci

Exclusion criteria:
    Piecemeal necrosis
    All portal tracts densely infiltrated

Inconstant findings:
    HBs-containing ground-glass hepatocytes
    HBc-containing sanded nuclei (rare)
    Fibrosis/inactive cirrhosis

Table 9.5 Histological features in chronic persistent hepatitis (CPH)

Constant findings:
    Acinar architecture preserved
    Chronic inflammation of portal tracts with lymphocytic predominance
    Limiting plate intact
    Slight focal intra-acinar inflammation
    Absence of substantial fibrosis

Exclusion criteria:
    Piecemeal necrosis

Inconstant findings:
    Slight portal fibrosis (and/or septum formation)
    Portal lymphoid follicle formation★
    Bile-duct lesions of the hepatic type★
    HBs-containing ground-glass cells
    HBc-containing sanded nuclei (rare)
    Signs of superimposed acute hepatitis (rare)
    Fatty infiltration★
    Cirrhosis

★mainly in hepatitis C

Table 9.6 Prognosis of (untreated) chronic persistent hepatitis

Viral type	Abbrev.	State of virus	Prognosis
HBV	HB-CPH	Replicative	Transition into CAH associated with HBeAg/anti-HBe seroconversion within ~ 6 years in most cases;[16] annual HBeAg seroconversion rate 15–30%[307,308]
		Non-replicative	Stable, if not superinfected by other virus (e.g. HDV)
		Pre-core mutant	Ill-defined as yet
HCV	HC-CPH		Not specifically investigated: supposedly unstable. Risk of sampling error. Progression to cirrhosis after many years documented.[17]

HB = hepatitis B; HC = hepatitis C

cells (Fig. 9.1b).[11] There may be slight portal fibrosis.[2] Occasionally, lymphoid follicles with germinal centres may be recognized, especially in chronic hepatitis of viral type C.[12] As a rule, intra-acinar changes are minimal and consist of small foci of liver-cell necrosis with modest, predominantly lymphocytic reaction. The histological alterations may be expressed as score values 3–4 (Tables 9.9 and 9.10).

Contrary to the original definition,[2] slight piecemeal necrosis should not be tolerated in the diagnosis of CPH but should rather lead to a diagnosis of minimally active CAH (CAH-min) because of its uncertain prognosis. Follow-up biopsies have shown progression to CAH in many patients with only slight piecemeal necrosis.[13] The morphological peculiarities of hepatitis C are discussed in chapter 6 and on page 381.

Evolution of CPH

In general, CPH is considered to have a good prognosis.[2] Indeed, in many cases the histological features persist for years without progression to CAH. In chronic hepatitis B, 5-year survival of patients with CPH is 97% as compared to 86% in patients with CAH.[14] Transition to CAH and cirrhosis has, however, been reported to occur in about 10% of cases.[15] As discussed on page 377, two biologically and prognostically different types of CPH are recognized for wild-type hepatitis B (Table 9.6 and Fig. 9.15):

(i) A highly replicative phase with extensive HBcAg expression in the liver which is unstable and, as a rule, progresses to CAH (or CLH) after a course of 4–6 years.[16] In this setting, CPH definitely does not indicate the favourable prognosis suggested in the original publication from 1968[2] and also constitutes an active virus reservoir.

In some therapeutic trials, a histological diagnosis of CPH has been used as a criterion for exclusion from interferon treatment regardless of viral replicative state. This of course is not acceptable, since highly replicative phases of chronic HBV infection, associated with CPH but more often with minimally active CAH, tend to respond particularly favourably to interferon.

(ii) A non-replicative form without core expression or other signs of active replication which remains stable in the absence of superinfection by another virus. Spontaneous fluctuations back to aggressive hepatitis with focal core expression are rare (Fig. 9.15).

In chronic hepatitis C, one of the major characteristics is an inflammatory reaction on the borderline between CPH and CAH[12] with piecemeal necrosis, the main histological distinguishing feature, being mild and focal. Such borderline cases should be classified as minimally active CAH which implies a propensity for cirrhotic transformation in the long run. Indeed, development of cirrhosis has been reported in a substantial proportion of patients with chronic HCV infection.[17]

It follows from this discussion that for prognostic and therapeutic reasons the histological diagnosis should be supplemented by the aetiology, and in the case of hepatitis B by the state of viral replication. For monitoring the effect of treatment semiquantitative scoring is advisable.

Morphological variants of CPH

Chronic septal hepatitis[18] is characterized by the formation of septa with conspicuous inflammatory activity but without piecemeal necrosis (Fig. 9.1c). This form may represent a regressive stage of CAH, as seen spontaneously or after immunosuppressive therapy,[19] and is reported to have a poor prognosis.[18] Other terms have been proposed for non-aggressive variants of chronic hepatitis but are not as widely used. These include 'persistent viral hepatitis' and 'unresolved hepatitis'. They are

Fig. 9.1 The four main non-aggressive types of chronic hepatitis. (a) Minimal hepatitis. Minor lymphocytic inflammatory infiltrate in portal tract and parenchyma. Note the many HBsAg-containing ground glass cells in this non-replicative HBV carrier. H&E. (b) Chronic persistent hepatitis (patient anti-HBs-positive, possibly HCV infection). Dense lymphocytic inflammation restricted to enlarged portal tract. Limiting plate preserved. No piecemeal necrosis. Some scattered lymphocytic foci within the acini. H&E. (c) Chronic septal hepatitis (post-transfusion hepatitis, virus type unknown). Septum formation with dense lymphocytic inflammation but without periseptal piecemeal necrosis. Cobblestone pattern of parenchyma. This type of CPH may represent a regressive form of CAH. H&E. (d) Chronic lobular hepatitis. Portal (P) and acinar changes similar to acute hepatitis. Patient anti-HCV positive. HV = Hepatic vein. H&E.

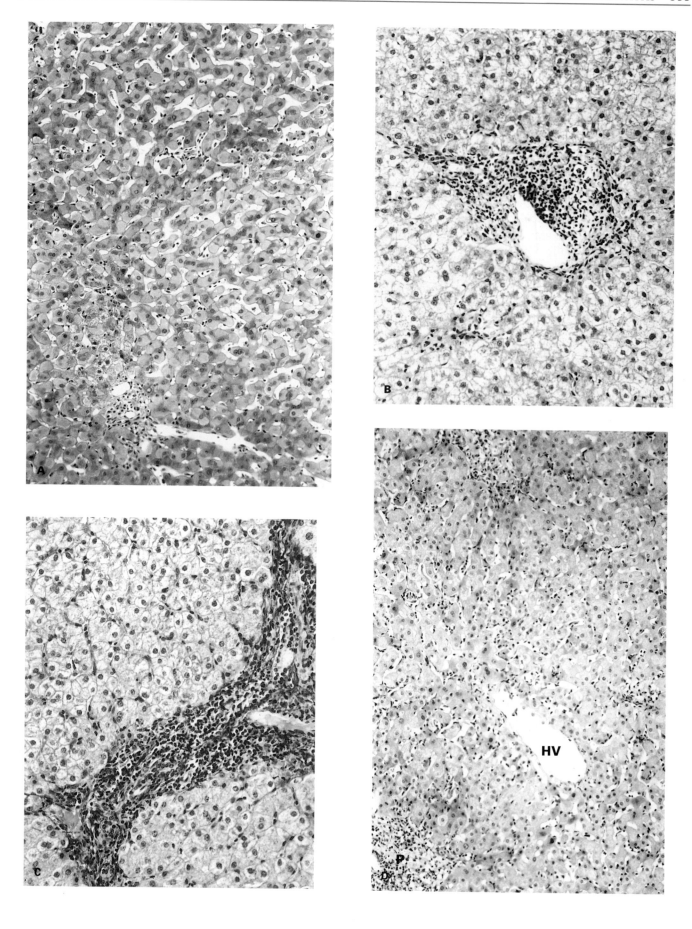

used for cases histologically similar to CPH in which a viral aetiology is established and in which, in contrast to chronic lobular hepatitis, histological features of late and residual stages of acute viral hepatitis persist.[20] As a distinguishing feature from 'non-specific lymphoid hyperplasia', Peters[21] stressed a cobblestone appearance of liver cells.

CHRONIC LOBULAR HEPATITIS (CLH)

In some cases, acute lobular (acinar) features of the degree seen in acute spotty necrotic hepatitis may be present over periods of more than 6 months (Fig. 9.1d). For this the term chronic lobular hepatitis has been coined.[3,4] Most of the cases subside without progression to cirrhosis.[5,22,23] There is no convincing evidence that CLH per se (i.e. without piecemeal necrosis or confluent necrosis) represents an immediate precursor lesion of cirrhosis. CLH may be caused by HCV and other hepatitis viruses.[22] HBV antigen patterns and delta expression have not been investigated systematically in these cases. Histological features of CLH are listed in Table 9.7.

Table 9.7 Histological features in chronic lobular hepatitis

Constant findings:
  Slight, predominantly lymphocytic portal inflammation
  Pronounced spotty necrotic hepatitis, similar to acute viral hepatitis
  Acinar architecture ± preserved

Exclusion criteria:
  Piecemeal necrosis
  Limiting plate eroded

Inconstant findings:
  Abundance of naked acidophilic (apoptotic) bodies*
  Marked sinusoidal infiltration by lymphoid cells in Indian file*
  Minor degrees of fibrosis

*mainly in hepatitis C

While CPH and 'chronic septal hepatitis' describe a phase of activity in chronic hepatitis, the biological meaning and nosological position of chronic lobular hepatitis are not well understood. Although in the evolution of wild-type chronic hepatitis B the histological counterpart of HBeAg/anti-HBe seroconversion is most often CAH, it may alternatively be CLH[16,22] (see also p. 380). Chronic hepatitis C often presents with particularly severe acinar accentuation, the mechanism of which remains to be established. Chronic lobular hepatitis may be taken as a pronounced and prolonged acinar inflammatory component as part of chronic hepatitis, which perhaps may be better assessed by a scoring system than by classifying it as a separate entity. In our scoring system CLH is expressed by values between 4 and 6. It should be appreciated, however, that these score values are based mainly on acinar necro-inflammatory changes (item 3 in Table 9.10).

CHRONIC ACTIVE (AGGRESSIVE) HEPATITIS

The main histological features are summarized in Table 9.8. Histological alterations involve all hepatic territories, comprising portal, periportal, and acinar areas.

Table 9.8 Histological key features in chronic active hepatitis

Constant findings:
  Portal and periportal, mainly lymphocytic inflammation
  Periportal piecemeal necrosis
  Focal intra-acinar inflammation
  Portal tracts with a maple-leaf configuration (Fig. 9.24)

Inconstant findings:
  Signs of acute spotty necrotic hepatitis
  Confluent (bridging) hepatic necrosis
  Active and passive septa
  Periseptal piecemeal necrosis
  Portal lymphoid follicle formation*
  Variable degree of fatty change*
  Sinusoidal lymphoid infiltration in Indian file manner*
  Liver-cell rosetting at parenchymal/mesenchymal interface
  Some derangement of liver architecture
  Minor degrees of ductular proliferation
  Bile-duct lesions of the hepatitic type*
  HBs-containing ground-glass cells†, sanded nuclei†
  Cirrhosis

*mainly in hepatitis C
†only in hepatitis B of HBc-positive types or in hepatitis D

Portal changes

Portal tracts are widened, with a predominantly lymphocytic infiltrate intermixed with plasma cells in varying numbers. In cases of CAH presenting with bridging hepatic necrosis the portal infiltrate may contain a substantial number of neutrophils which accompany ductular proliferation (see below). Although the density of the lymphoid infiltrate may vary from one portal tract to another, the presence of unaffected portal tracts favours HCV infection. Some pigment-laden macrophages may be seen, but less often than in acute forms. Portal lymphoid follicles appear to be far more frequent in hepatitis C than in CAH of other origin.[12] Some portal fibrosis is common, except in very early cases, but the pattern of fibrosis in the periportal area is of greater diagnostic importance.

The bile ducts may show changes morphologically different from those in primary biliary cirrhosis (see Ch. 12): the bile-duct epithelium appears multilayered and swollen, often vacuolated and infiltrated with lymphocytes (Fig. 9.2); the basement membrane remains intact.[24] This duct lesion is reminiscent of salivary duct changes in Sjögren's disease.[25] Such bile-duct changes imply that (i) cirrhosis develops more frequently and more quickly,[26] and (ii) chronic non-A, non-B infection is more likely than hepatitis B.[27] These portal changes are expressed in item 1 of Table 9.10 by score values 3 or 4.

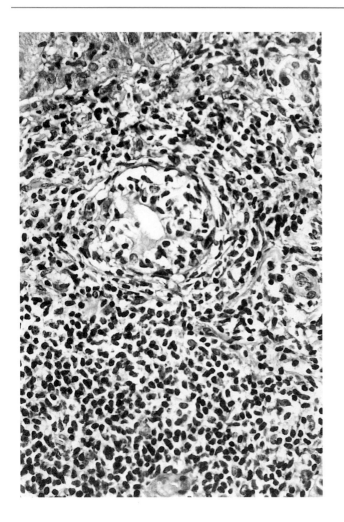

Periportal changes

Periportal hepatitis with progressive erosion of the limiting plate by piecemeal necrosis represents the key feature of CAH. The phenomenon of piecemeal necrosis was originally described as a presumed immunological type of liver-cell necrosis by Popper et al.[28] It may be defined as a chronic, gradual inflammatory destruction of single or small groups of hepatocytes at a mesenchymal/parenchymal interface (periportal, periseptal or at the margin of parenchymal nodules in cirrhosis), associated with lympho-histiocytic inflammatory cells.[29] Close contact between the membranes of clustered lymphocytes/macrophages and hepatocytes (peripolesis; Fig. 9.3)[30] is the hallmark of piecemeal necrosis. The term emperipolesis has been adopted in cases where lymphocytes have invaginated the hepatocyte (Fig. 9.3a). Thus, lymphocytes invade the

Fig. 9.2 Bile-duct lesion in a 77-year-old male with post-transfusional non-A, non-B CAH. Note multilayered, 'reticulated' biliary epithelium with vacuolization. H&E. Courtesy of Prof H Poulsen.

Fig. 9.3 Key features of piecemeal necrosis.
(a) Schematic representation of peripolesis, emperipolesis and apoptosis. LM = light microscopy; EM = electron microscopy; H = hepatocyte; L = lymphocyte; ABs = apoptotic bodies. (b) CAH with severe activity in a 50-year-old female. Piecemeal necrosis with marked lymphocytic peripolesis. Note absence of substantial ductular proliferation. Van Gieson.

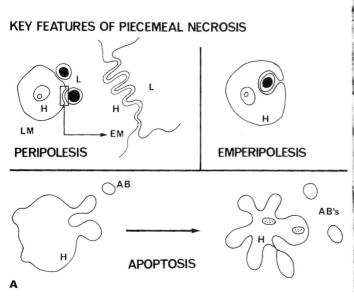

KEY FEATURES OF PIECEMEAL NECROSIS

PERIPOLESIS

EMPERIPOLESIS

APOPTOSIS

A

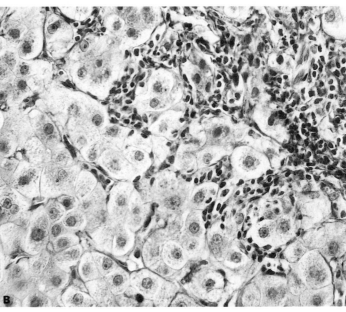

B

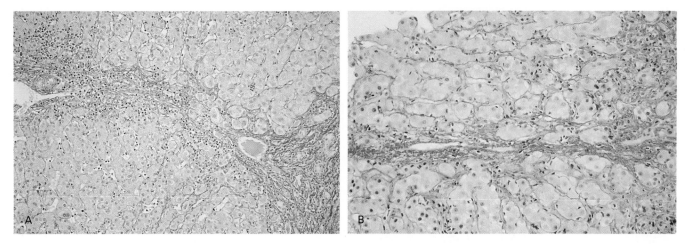

Fig. 9.4 The two types of septum formation in CAH. (a) Active curved portal–portal septum, flanked by piecemeal necrosis. Inflammatory cells are also seen within the septum. Sirius red. (b) Passive straight central–portal septum, paucicellular, produced by collapse of pre-existing reticulin fibres. Sirius red.

periportal parenchyma and destroy and replace periportal hepatocytes. Liver cells in piecemeal necrosis undergo apoptosis, i.e. gradual disintegration by sequential fragmentation of cytoplasm and nuclei.[31] The term apoptosis implies a 'falling-off' as the leaves fall from trees in the autumn[32] due to programmed death induced by cellular immune attack (Fig. 9.3). The result of this liver-cell death is the formation of tiny, darkly acidophilic apoptotic bodies (Fig. 9.16)[33] which are not easily recognizable by light microscopy.[34] Usually they do not markedly attract inflammatory cells but are eventually taken up by sinusoidal macrophages. Larger apoptotic bodies may present as acidophilic (Councilman) bodies.[31] Other hepatocytes within piecemeal necrosis may survive, become hyperplastic, grow in a tubular fashion and become surrounded by a rim of newly formed fibres. Ductular proliferation[3] in piecemeal necrosis is not obligatory and is often overemphasized in textbooks.

Active septa are the result of piecemeal necrosis. The limiting plate is broken, and the periportal parenchyma is progressively destroyed and replaced by newly-formed connective tissue including capillaries (Fig. 9.4a). Unlike passive septa, early active septa are rich in inflammatory cells and are curved.[3,25] The tongue-like extensions give the portal tracts a maple-leaf-like configuration (Fig. 9.24, p. 386), especially in chronic hepatitis B. The advancing edges of piecemeal necrosis may join extensions from neighbouring portal tracts to form portal–portal bridging in zone 1. Unlike central–portal bridges resulting from confluent necrosis, portal–portal bridging in chronic hepatitis is thus piecemeal in nature. More importantly, advancing edges of piecemeal necrosis may connect with confluent necrosis extending from zone 3 to form portal–central bridges, the scaffold for cirrhotic transformation.[29]

Total destruction of a band of periportal hepatocytes by piecemeal necrosis with subsequent ingrowth of granula-tion tissue, including newly formed blood vessels and fibres, may mimic expansion of the portal tract itself — sleeve necrosis.[35] Special staining methods will delineate the original portal tract within the affected zone for a long time. It contains coarse birefringent fibres of type I collagen[35] which stain strongly with collagen stains and are golden brown in untoned silver impregnations,[25] while the newly formed sleeve of type III collagen (reticulin) appears black (Fig. 9.5). Trapped viable liver cells within the enlarged fibrosed portal tract may indicate earlier piecemeal necrosis and are suspected of providing a nidus for perpetuation of disease activity.[29]

This lymphocytic piecemeal necrosis is a major characteristic of CAH, with or without cirrhosis, of any aetiology (Table 9.2). Cases of acute hepatitis may show lymphocytic piecemeal necrosis in addition to the features of acute spotty necrosis. This is particularly seen in drug

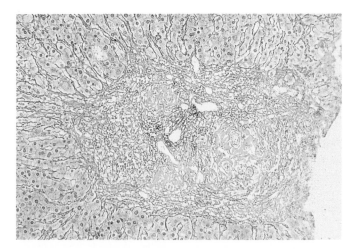

Fig. 9.5 Sleeve necrosis in hepatitis B-CAH. Note a sleeve of black type III collagen fibres surrounding a central core of golden-yellow type I collagen, representing the original portal tract. Untoned silver stain.

addicts and in the elderly and may be taken as an indicator of impending chronicity. However, piecemeal necrosis lacking tubular transformation, ductular proliferation and new fibre formation, particularly if combined with features of acute hepatitis, may regress in some cases. If associated with rosetting of liver-cells, marked liver-cell regeneration and fibre formation, the lesion is considered definitive and progressive.

Organization of inflammatory cells in piecemeal necrosis
(Fig. 9.6)

Piecemeal necrosis may be regarded as an interface hepatitis, i.e. an inflammation at the epithelial/mesenchymal border. There are striking analogies in the inflammatory organization between CAH and the skin lesion in lichen ruber planus.[36-38]

Monoclonal antibodies have identified CD8+ suppressor/cytotoxic T-lymphocytes as the predominant inflammatory cell in the invading front of piecemeal necrosis, whereas CD4+ helper/inducer T cells prevail in the central area of the portal connective tissue[31,38-44] (Fig. 9.6). Some of the portal/periportal mononuclear cells are accessory cells.[38] By electron microscopy, two cell types have been discerned:[45,46]

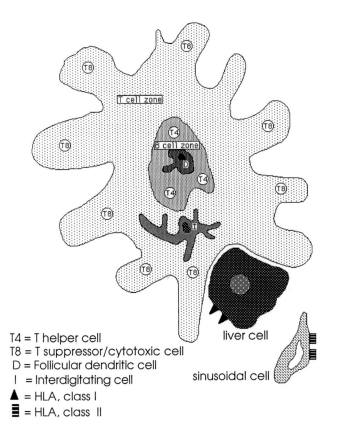

T4 = T helper cell
T8 = T suppressor/cytotoxic cell
D = Follicular dendritic cell
I = Interdigitating cell
▲ = HLA, class I
☰ = HLA, class II

liver cell

sinusoidal cell

Fig. 9.6 Immune architecture of piecemeal necrosis in hepatitis B-CAH. Compiled from literature[31,38-48]

1. Cells with the ultrastructural characteristics of dendritic reticulum cells of lymphoid follicles in B-cell areas of lymph nodes and spleen. Such dendritic reticulum cells were preferentially observed in central parts of the inflamed portal tract.

2. A second cell type, localized mainly in the peripheral parts of piecemeal necrosis, corresponding to interdigitating reticulum cells as they characteristically occur in the paracortical T-cell zones of lymph nodes.

Both dendritic and interdigitating cells are considered to function as antigen-presenting cells for B- and T-lymphocytes respectively.[46]

Based on the topographical distribution of T-cell subsets and of antigen-presenting cells, Desmet[38] considered the central core of the portal inflammation in chronic hepatitis B to represent a B-cell zone and the peripheral invading front of the piecemeal necrosis to correspond to a T-cell zone, as in lymph nodes (Fig. 9.6). Indeed, lymphoid follicle formation is seen quite often at the centre of the portal and periportal infiltrate with piecemeal necrosis.[11]

The participation of endothelial cells in the formation of piecemeal necrosis has been documented in the interesting ultrastructural study of Bardadin & Desmet.[45] Sinusoidal-lining endothelial cells in piecemeal necrosis lose their characteristics and assume the phenotype of the so-called high endothelial venules in the paracortical zones of lymph nodes, where an intense migration of lymphocytes from blood into tissues takes place. This may explain migration and homing of so many lymphocytes in areas of piecemeal necrosis. Bardadin & Desmet[45] have postulated that such transformed endothelial cells may further transform into so-called fibroblastic reticulum cells, thought to be involved in collagen production. This may explain the intimate link between lympho-histiocytic inflammation and fibre formation in CAH.

Unlike normal hepatocytes,[47,48] liver cells in areas of piecemeal necrosis display HLA-I molecules on their surface.[48] Sinusoidal-lining cells surrounding these hepatocytes are hyperplastic and give a strongly positive reaction for HLA class II antigens[48] (Fig. 9.6). Periportal changes are expressed by score values 1, 3, 4-6 in item 2 of Table 9.10.

Differential diagnosis of piecemeal necrosis

Piecemeal necrosis is often overdiagnosed. Attention has to be drawn to the fact that not every example of periportal inflammation with necrosis of liver cells is piecemeal necrosis. The predominance of lymphocytes and the cytological hallmarks of peripolesis and apoptosis have to be looked for carefully. Main confusions include:

1. Simple spillover of inflammatory cells from portal

tracts into the periportal parenchyma as seen in acute hepatitis (see Ch. 6). This lesion may closely resemble the advancing edge of piecemeal necrosis.[29] However, it lacks the diagnostis element of peripolesis as well as substantial liver-cell loss and fibrosis, and readily heals. Oedema, neutrophils and lytic necrosis may be present in addition and help to distinguish the alteration from true piecemeal necrosis.

2. A degenerative and inflammatory alteration in the periportal area seen in chronic cholestatic liver disease has been called 'biliary piecemeal necrosis'.[49] This may be recognized by several details: (i) the cholestatic erosion of periportal parenchyma is mainly characterized by feathery degeneration of liver cells often containing copper;[25] (ii) oedema and neutrophils may be seen in addition to fibre formation; (iii) fibres are more densely packed than in the hepatitic type of piecemeal necrosis and sometimes have a lamellar appearance. There may be considerable ductular proliferation of the elongation type.[25] These features give the periportal region a characteristic halo ('periportal biliary halo effect').

3. Acute hepatitis A (see Ch. 6) may mimic the piecemeal necrosis of CAH when a lympho-plasmocytic periportal inflammation is prominent. A considerable number of plasma cells accompanied by oedema and marked lytic necrosis are features in favour of hepatitis A.[50,51] Essential features of piecemeal necrosis (peripolesis, apoptosis, rosetting and fibre formation) are, however, absent. Complete healing without histological sequelae is the rule. In some cases of early, florid CAH the distinction from acute hepatitis A cannot confidently be made by histology without knowledge of the respective serology.

Acinar (lobular) changes

Basically, all acinar alterations observed in acute viral hepatitis (see Ch. 6) may be seen in chronic hepatitis as a reflection of superimposed acute episodes. The changes may be unevenly distributed and vary from acinus to acinus, especially in chronic hepatitis with advanced architectural disturbances.

Acute exacerbations may present as classic acute hepatitis with spotty necrosis, confluent (bridging) hepatic necrosis or even pan- and multiacinar necrosis. While spotty necrosis and confluent (bridging) hepatic necrosis connecting terminal hepatic venules, i.e. central–central bridging — if not accompanied by piecemeal necrosis — may subside without serious functional implications, central–portal bridging (along zone 3) may create the anatomical basis for intrahepatic porto-caval shunting. The prognostic significance of such bridging hepatic necrosis is discussed on page 359.

A third type of bridging necrosis, on the other hand, is created by extensive piecemeal necrosis, when the advancing edges of piecemeal necrosis from two neighbouring portal tracts connect to form portal–portal bridges ('perilobular', i.e. zone 1 bridging). Such portal–portal bridging alone does not disturb the acinar architecture. These acinar changes are expressed in score values 0, 1, 3, 5, 6, 8, or 10 in item 3 of Table 9.10.

Fibrosis

Except in the very early stages, CAH is accompanied by some degree of acinar fibrosis and a variable degree of portal fibrosis, not interfering with the functional acinar unit. However, intra-acinar formation of active septa as a result of piecemeal necrosis extending from the periportal limiting membrane into the acinar parenchyma dissects the acinus. Active septa are curved and rich in inflammatory cells. Because of capillarization such septa may give rise to intrahepatic shunting. Passive septa originate from perivenular regions as the result of collapse and condensation of the reticulin framework after confluent necrosis (Fig. 9.4b). They are paucicellular and straight, or run in a vaulted fashion along the periphery of zone 3.[25] Ultimately, passive and active septa may link to form fibrous rings, usually along the acinar periphery. In septum formation, type III collagen (reticulin) is the first type to be formed, easily recognizable as black reticulin fibres in untoned silver impregnations (Fig. 9.5). This is followed by deposition of collagen I, staining golden-brown in untoned silver sections. Septa containing elastic fibres (demonstrable with orcein or Victoria blue staining) are considered definite while septa without elastic fibres may be reversible. In livers with massive necrosis, formation of elastic fibres has been shown to appear about 3–4 weeks after onset of necrosis.[52]

Pericellular fibrosis encases hepatocellular rosettes with formation of a new basement membrane, thereby dissecting these structures from vascular supply. Deposition of laminin and collagen IV along sinusoids (perisinusoidal fibrosis) leads to capillarization with functional disturbances.

Regeneration

Portal and periportal fibrosis is almost always accompanied by regeneration, reflected in the formation of twin- or multi-layered liver-cell plates and/or rosetting. Incomplete periportal nodular transformation is thus a frequent feature.

Nodular transformation and cirrhosis (see Ch. 10)

Development of established hepatic cirrhosis within a few months to 4–5 years from the diagnosis of CAH has been observed in 18% of moderately active, and in 45% of severely active CAH with bridging hepatic necrosis.[53] The process of nodular transformation is gradual, so that in

Table 9.9 Phenotypes of chronic hepatitis B*

Category	Old classification	Hallmark	Inflammatory score (portal, periportal, lobular)* (0–20)	Score for fibrosis and cirrhosis* (0 – 6)	Architecture (descriptive)
Minimal hepatitis	Non-specific reactive hepatitis	Sparse focal lymphocytic infiltrate in some portal tracts and within acini	0–1	0	Preserved
CPH	CPH	Moderate to marked lymphocytic portal inflammation without piecemeal necrosis	3–4	0 (–1)	Preserved
CLH		Mild to moderate portal infiltration; widespread and pronounced spotty necrotic hepatitis	4–6	0	Preserved
CAH-min	CPH	Few tongues of PMN in some portal tracts	4–7	0 (–1)	Preserved
CAH-mild	CAH activity (a)	PMN <50% of portal perimeter	6–9	2	+/– disturbed (focally)
CAH-mod		PMN >50% of portal perimeter	10–13	3	Disturbed
CAH-sev	CAH activity (b)	Marked PMN including periseptal PMN and/or perivenular confluent or central–central bridging necrosis	14–15	4–5	Severely disturbed
CAH-very sev		Severe PMN with active septa and bridging and/or pan/multiacinar necrosis	16–20	6	Severely disturbed

*Note that the scores for fibrosis/cirrhosis are correlated with inflammatory scores as indicated in the table but may dissociate from each other during evolution, since inflammation is reversible but cirrhosis is not. Therefore, scoring for both should be done independently for a given biopsy. For details of scores see Table 9.10

sequential biopsies one may be faced for a long time with precirrhotic architectural disturbances, starting with focal incomplete nodular transformation, followed by diffuse incomplete and ultimately diffuse complete nodular transformation. The latter usually reflects established cirrhosis. Repeat liver biopsies may therefore be indicated to assess progression of fibrosis and cirrhotic transformation. This gradually increasing nodular transformation associated with fibrosis may be graded separately as an architectural score. In chronic hepatitis B this process is enhanced by hepatitis D co- or superinfection[54] or HBe- mutant infection (p. 367). Fibrosis/cirrhosis is expressed in score values 0–6 in item 4 of Table 9.10.

Activity and progression

Originally, piecemeal necrosis was regarded as the only mechanism responsible for progression of CAH to cirrhosis.[28] Accordingly, the 1968 classification of CAH by an International Group[2] proposed two degrees of activity based uniquely on extent and severity of piecemeal necrosis. Indeed, in a series of moderately active CAH (i.e. without bridging hepatic necrosis) transition to cirrhosis

was observed in 71% of HBV-positive and in 31% of HBV-negative cases, respectively.[55]

The pivotal publication of Boyer & Klatskin,[56] on the other hand, stressed acinar changes and notably bridging hepatic necrosis as the main pacemaker for cirrhosis. This publication, however, included portal–portal bridging which is piecemeal in nature. A more recent publication from Taiwan,[57] considering only portal–central bridging as an indicator (as proposed in this chapter), calculated for chronic hepatitis B with bridging hepatic necrosis a four times higher relative risk for cirrhosis within 3 years than for CAH without.

This controversy, together with growing experience, triggered a revision and extension of the original classification[2] by the same International Group.[29] Obviously both piecemeal and confluent bridging necrosis are prognostically important. It now appears that piecemeal necrosis alone may, in a moderate number of cases, lead to cirrhosis, but that episodes of bridging hepatic necrosis may accelerate the progression.[58,59] Thus, cases presenting with both piecemeal and bridging hepatic necrosis carry the worst prognosis. A more subtle grading of both extent of piecemeal necrosis and presence of bridging hepatic necrosis is mandatory for a more accurate assessment of activity and severity of chronic hepatitis.

Grading

Depending on the severity of the key histological lesions, the following subtypes of chronic active hepatitis have proved useful in daily practice. Activity may vary from location to location in one biopsy. The most severely affected area will determine the degree of activity reported.

Chronic hepatitis of minimal activity (CAH-min) (Table 9.9 and Fig. 9.7a).

This describes cases in which some but not all portal tracts may exhibit one or few tongues of piecemeal necrosis. Spotty acinar changes are absent or minimal. These cases are often mistaken for CPH; their unstable course with a high incidence of deterioration towards more aggressive forms justifies their classification into CAH.[19] In hepatitis B, they may be recognized as such by their focal HBcAg expression in tissue (Table 9.13, p. 377).

Chronic hepatitis of mild activity (CAH-mild) (Table 9.9 and Fig. 9.7b)

This is characterized by dense inflammatory portal infiltration with piecemeal necrosis involving less than 50% of the perimeter of almost every portal tract. Mild to moderate acinar spotty necrosis may be present.

Chronic hepatitis of moderate activity (CAH-mod) (Table 9.9 and Fig. 9.7c)

This includes piecemeal necrosis involving more than 50% of the portal perimeter and often extending along the

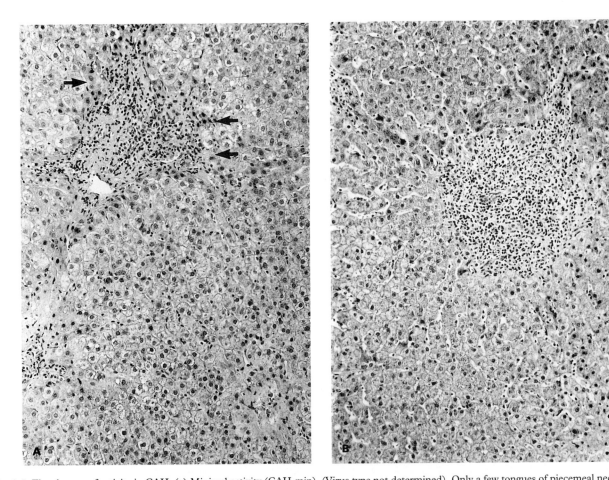

Fig. 9.7 Five degrees of activity in CAH. (a) Minimal activity (CAH-min). (Virus type not determined). Only a few tongues of piecemeal necrosis are seen (arrow). The greater part of the portal tract shows a preserved limiting plate. H&E. (b) Mild activity (CAH mild). (hepatitis C.) Piecemeal necrosis restricted to periportal area, involving less than 50% of portal tract perimeter. Acinar architecture preserved. H&E. (c) Moderate activity (CAH-mod). (Virus type not determined.) Piecemeal necrosis restricted to portal area, involving more than 50% of portal tract perimeter. H&E. (d) Severe activity (CAH-sev). (Virus type unknown). Piecemeal necrosis along fibrous septum extending far into the parenchyma (centre) and along portal–portal bridge. P = portal tract. Van Gieson. (e) Very severe activity (CAH very sev) (hepatitis B). Confluent hepatic necrosis, bridging terminal hepatic venule (central vein, C) with portal tract (P) and flanked by piecemeal necrosis. An additional portal–portal bridge is piecemeal in nature. H&E.

whole portal tract periphery. Spotty necrosis is variable but may be widespread.

Chronic hepatitis of severe activity (CAH-sev) (Table 9.9 and Fig. 9.7d)

This category includes biopsies with piecemeal necrosis in the periportal region and along fibrous septa (periseptal piecemeal necrosis). Alternatively, perivenular non-bridging confluent or central–central bridging necrosis may accompany periportal piecemeal necrosis. There is often a substantial degree or architectural derangement.

Chronic hepatitis of very severe activity (CAH very sev) (Table 9.9 and Fig. 9.7e)

In addition to severe piecemeal necrosis there is confluent porto–central bridging necrosis and/or pan-/multiacinar necrosis. Such porto–central bridging may create the scaffold for cirrhosis even more than does pan- and multilobular necrosis. Acinar derangement is conspicuous and widespread.

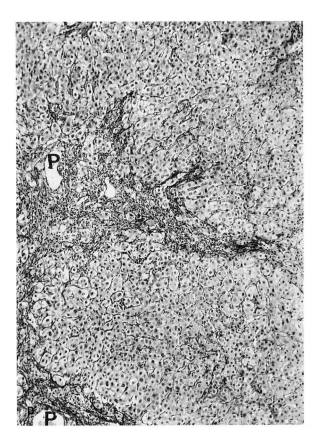

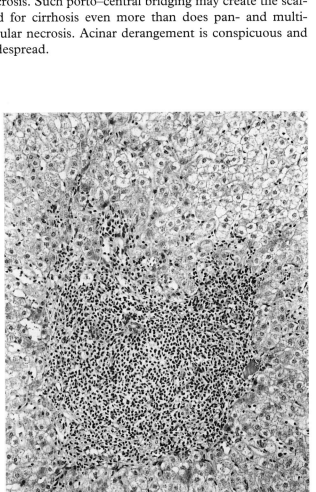

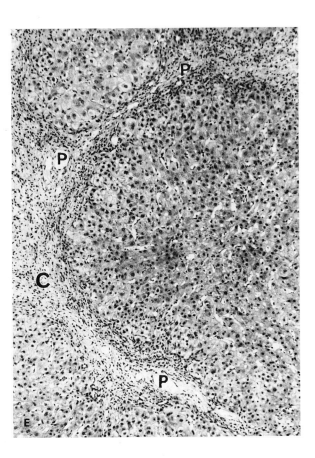

SCORING OF ACTIVITY

Since liver biopsy is an important means of monitoring the effect of therapy (e.g. with interferon) in trials, a reproducible semiquantitative scoring system is desirable. Several attempts have been made to assess disease activity reproducibly:

(i) Knodell et al[60] have presented a scoring system which generates a histological activity index by grading inflammation, necrosis, fibrosis and nodular transformation. This system has the disadvantage of combining active necro-inflammatory changes and fibrotic/cirrhotic alterations which are sequelae of the former and do not indicate activity of inflammation but rather the degree of acinar distortion. Thus, the dynamic evolution of the disease may not become apparent.

(ii) Scheuer[7] proposes a simple grading of 0–4 for necro-inflammatory changes, with separate scores for portal/periportal and acinar components, and a 0–4 grading for fibrosis and architectural disturbances.

(iii) Table 9.10 depicts the form for scoring which we have used for more than 3 years to follow patients with chronic hepatitis B (and C) enrolled in interferon trials and which has proved satisfactory, at least for hepatitis B. It represents a modification of the Knodell score but generates separate scores for both inflammatory (portal, periportal and acinar changes with a maximum of 20 points), and architectural lesions (fibrosis and cirrhotic transformation with a maximum of 6 points). In general terms, this grading system allows the observer to recognize, differentially, whether a particular treatment has had an effect on intra-acinar or periportal necro-inflammatory changes and to analyse its relation to fibrosis. The sum of portal inflammation, piecemeal necrosis, intra-acinar inflammation and fibrosis/cirrhosis, on the other hand, should give an idea about the severity of the disease as a whole.

It should be appreciated that this scheme has primarily been designed for the study of chronic hepatitis B. For hepatitis C, characteristic features (see Ch. 6) such as in-

Table 9.10 Form for scoring biopsies in chronic hepatitis B

SEVERITY INDEX OF CHRONIC HEPATITIS B

Name: _____   First Name: _____   Date of birth: _____

Date of Biopsy: _____   Journal: _____   Pathologist: _____

		SCORE
1. PORTAL INFLAMMATION		
A.	None	0
B.	Mild: Sprinkling of inflammatory cells in < 1/3 of PT	1
C.	Moderate: Numerous inflammatory cells in 1/3–2/3 of PT	3
D.	Marked: Dense inflammatory infiltrate in > 2/3 of PT and/or lymphoid follicles	4
2. PERIPORTAL PIECEMEAL NECROSIS (PMN)		
A.	None	0
B.	Minimal: One or few tongues in single PT	1
C.	Moderate: PMN involving < 50% of circumference of most PT	3
D.	Marked: PMN involving > 50% of circumference of most PT	4
E.	Severe: As in D plus septal PMN	5
F.	Very severe: Portal–portal bridges produced by PMN	6
3. INTRA-ACINAR SPOTTY/CONFLUENT NECROSIS AND INFLAMMATION (SN/I)		
A.	None	0
B.	Mild: SN/I in < 1/3 of acini or nodules	1
C.	Moderate: SN/I in 1/3–2/3 of acini or nodules	3
D.	Marked: SN/I in > 2/3 of acini/nodules and/or bridging confluent necrosis	5
E.	Severe: D plus central–central confluent necrosis	6
F.	Very severe: D plus central–portal confluent necrosis	8
G.	Very severe: Pan- or multiacinar confluent necrosis	10
4. FIBROSIS/CIRRHOSIS		
A.	None	0
B.	Mild: Only portal fibrosis	1
C.	Portal fibrosis plus incomplete septa	2
D.	Septa bridging portal–portal	3
E.	Septa bridging portal–central and/or focal incomplete cirrhosis	4
F.	Diffuse incomplete and/or focal complete cirrhosis	5
G.	Diffuse complete cirrhosis	6
5. BILE-DUCT LESION		ABSENT/PRESENT
TOTAL SCORE		

PT = Portal tracts

flammatory bile-duct lesions should not only be registered but included in the scoring. Lymphoid follicles, in Table 9.10 actually calling for the label 'Portal inflammation — D', might be given an additional point. It seems reasonable to adapt a new staging and grading system to the aetiology of disease and also to combine it with serological and immunological data.

Activity indexes, however, should be interpreted with caution. Although they might provide reproducible values, these score values are arbitrarily chosen and cannot reflect adequately the biological impact of a given histological change.[9]

CHRONIC HEPATITIS B AND INFECTION WITH HEPATITIS D VIRUS (THE DELTA AGENT)

VIRAL REPLICATION AND IMMUNOPATHOLOGY

The early hypothesis that the immune response determines the morphological presentation and course of the non-cytopathic hepatitis B virus infection[6,61,62] has gained general acceptance. Recognized key events are the following:[63]

1. Presentation of endosomally processed viral antigens in association with HLA class II molecules by antigen-

Table 9.11 Virological terms used in this chapter (for detailed description see reference 66)

Designation	Explanation	Immuno-localization
HBV	Complete hepatitis B virus (=Dane particle): 42 nm double-stranded DNA virus (Hepadna virus), composed of a 27 nm core particle and envelope, 7 nm in thickness.	Within endoplasmic reticulum of liver cell (Fig. 9.12b.) In blood by negative staining after immune agglutination (Fig. 9.8).
HBsAg	Glycosylated surface protein of HB virus, composed of 3 gene products: the small, middle and large HBs-protein, governed by the S-, preS2- and preS1 domain, respectively.	
SHBs (gene S)	Small HBs: backbone of HBsAg, coded by gene S (226 amino acids) and representing the main constituent of the virus surface as well as of the tubular and spherical particles in blood	*Liver cell:* Cytoplasmic (immune EM: smooth endoplasmic reticulum)
MHBs (preS2)	Middle HBs: Middle piece of 281 amino acids, coded by additional 55 codons preceding the gene S. Suspected to bind polymerized human serum albumin (pHSA) which, in turn, could mediate attachment to liver cells via pHSA-receptors although there appears to be another receptor on hepatocytes for the glycosylated preS2.[66] Also involved in triggering protective immunity.	Cytoplasmic/membranous membranous *Blood:* Surface of Dane particle Tubular and spherical particles
LHBs (preS1)	Large HBs: protein of 409 amino acids, coded by additional 128 codons preceding the preS2 gene. Also capable of binding to hepatocytes and white blood cells and involved in triggering protective immunity.	
HBcAg	HB core protein of 183 amino acids, which is encoded by the gene C. It is self-assembling and has binding sites for HBV-RNA which is encapsulated together with viral polymerase.	*Liver cell:* Cytoplasmic. Cytoplasmic/membranous. Nuclear
HBeAg	Gene product corresponding to the pre-core region and occurring in 3 molecular forms: 1. 25 kD protein (p25e): full length, probably short-lived transcript of the pre-C/C region. The pre-core transcript acts as a signal sequence for transport through the membrane of the ER. 2. 23 kD cleavage product (p23e). This can be truncated to soluble and secretable HBeAg (see below) and self-asssembling p22c or move back to cytoplasm, nucleus or into cell membrane. 3. 15–18 kD (p15–18e) soluble, non-particulate cleavage product which is released into the blood, probably via smooth ER and Golgi apparatus.	*Liver cell:* Cytoplasmic Nuclear Membranous?
HBxAg	Trans-activating gene product of the X-gene region	*Liver cell:* Cytoplasmic (diffuse, [sub]membranous) ± nuclear[185]
HBV polymerase	Viral polymerase coded by gene P	
HDV	Hepatitis D virus (formerly delta agent): 37 nm particle without internal core particle, enveloped with HBsAg and containing a circular, single-stranded RNA of 1.7 kb and HDAg (delta antigen)	*Blood:* Immune-EM after agglutination with anti-HBs
HDAg	22 kD protein, the only known viral RNA product	*Liver cell:* Diffuse nuclear and/or nucleolar; occasionally cytoplasmic, rarely membrane-associated

presenting cells to CD4+ T-helper lymphocytes (afferent limb of the immune system)

2. Expression of viral epitopes associated with HLA class I antigen for cytolysis by CD8+ T-cytotoxic lymphocytes and/or associated with HLA class II antigen for cytolysis by CD4+/CD56+ cytotoxic T-helper cells (efferent limb)

3. Competent auxiliary mechanism such as proper cytokine production (involved in afferent and efferent limb).

This interplay may be disturbed by viral and host factors as outlined in the following.

Viral factors

The 3.2 kb genome of HBV has been completely sequenced[64] and there are accumulating data on genetic heterogeneity.[65] The viral genome has four open reading frames for two non-structural proteins (gene P for viral polymerase and gene X for the transactivating HBx-protein) and two genes for structural proteins (the genes S and C) (Table 9.11 and Fig. 9.8). The latter have, in addition, different initiation sites allowing for three surface proteins and two core proteins of different length and of different biological functions.[64–66] All can be translated independently. Essentially, this allows two modes of infec-

tion in chronic hepatitis B: a replicative (permissive) and a non-replicative (non-permissive) infection. In its typical presentation, the former produces complete virions (Dane particles) (Fig. 9.9), and expresses associated markers, such as HBV-DNA, DNA-polymerase and HBeAg in liver and blood. The non-replicative infection releases 20 nm spherical and tubular HBs particles only lacks replication markers, has anti-HBe in blood and hence is of low or no infectivity. Neither form has a relevant cytopathic effect on the liver cell, and this is compatible with its ability to produce persistent infections, even without tissue damage or inflammation.

Steps of viral replication are as follows:[66,67]

1. Adsorption to the liver cell and penetration, mediated by binding sites on preS and S proteins
2. Uncoating and transport of viral DNA to the nucleus
3. Completion of the short (+) strand by host polymerase
4. Viral(−) strand DNA is copied into a 3.5 kb strand of RNA which migrates into the cytoplasm and serves as the pregenome for further replication and as matrix for translation of the different proteins
5. The pregenome is packaged into a self-assembling nucleocapsid together with viral DNA polymerase which does a reverse transcription. The newly formed (−) strand DNA is then used by DNA polymerases as a template for a new (+) strand. The RNA-pregenome disintegrates during this process.
6. There are two pathways for core particles, one internal and one for export:
a. Internal pathway: nucleocapsids formed by the shorter, self-assembling gene C product are carried back to the nucleus where they can enter a new round of pregenome transcription.
b. Secretory pathway: nucleocapsid proteins (p25e) read from the pre-C/C gene are primarily stretched and able to pass the membrane of the endoplasmic reticulum by virtue of the leading pre-core protein. When this is cleaved off to become secretable HBeAg, the remaining p22 core protein can self-assemble and be enveloped with the outer coat of pre-S1, pre-S2 and the major HBsAg (i.e. Dane particle formation within the endoplasmic reticulum). Again, reverse transcription, disintegration of the pregenome and reconstitution of the (+) strand goes on simultaneously. The latter, however, is incomplete as elongation is stopped when the completed particle leaves the cells.

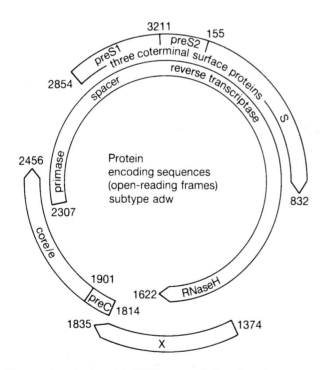

Fig. 9.8 Organization of the HBV genome: indicated are the four functional open reading frames (for C, reverse transcriptase, S and X) and their domains coding for different viral proetins (preC, core/e, preS1, preS2 and S; respectively). From Gerlich & Thomssen[66] with permission

Recently, it has become evident that viral mutants can alter the histological and clinical picture by changing the cytotoxicity of the viral variant and/or by-passing the immune response against the wild-type HBV (see below). The HBe⁻ mutant has particularly pointed to an

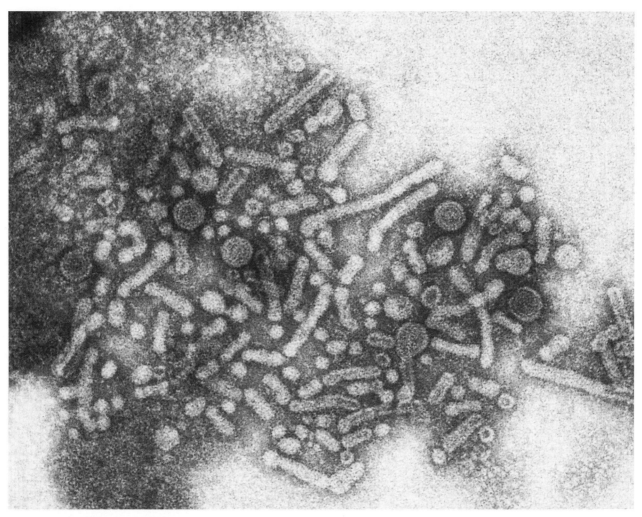

Fig. 9.9 Immune electron microscopy of HBsAg in serum after agglutination with anti-HBs. It consists of small spherical, tubular and double-shelled Dane particles (42 nm) with an internal core particle (27 nm). Negative staining with phosphotungstic acid, × 207 000

immunoregulatory role of secreted HBeAg involved in immune clearance by T-lymphocytes.[68–70]

Molecular hybridization techniques for the demonstration of HBV-DNA in liver extracts and in situ hybridization have added new insights into the natural history of HBV infection. Two different forms of HBV-DNA have been shown: episomal (free, 3.2 kb, single-stranded, circular), and HBV-DNA integrated into the host genome by random non-homologous recombination. Integrated HBV-DNA was first described in cells of a human hepatocellular carcinoma cell line[71,72] and later also in human hepatocellular carcinoma and chronic hepatitis B of variable histology.[73–76] A striking correlation was noted with serum markers: in chronic cases (longer than 6–8 years) positive for anti-HBe and lacking replication markers, the intrahepatic HBV-DNA was mainly in the integrated form, whereas chronic cases with a short history but positive for HBeAg and other markers of active replication exhibited mostly episomal DNA.[74,77] These findings, based on DNA extracts from liver, were supported by in situ hybridization assays.[78–80] Livers with features of active viral replication exhibited large amounts of mainly single-stranded intracytoplasmic HBV-DNA, whereas livers with predominantly non-permissive infection showed low numbers of double-stranded HBV nucleotide sequences in liver nuclei. Moreover, cases of chronic HBV carriage with both episomal and integrated HBV-DNA have been detected.[81] Loriot and co-workers have shown that seroconversion from HBeAg to anti-HBe positive chronic hepatitis is related to a reduction of replication but not disappearance of HBV-DNA from the liver.[82] The latter is less likely to happen after HBsAg to anti-HBs seroconversion, although persistence of HBV-DNA in such patients has been proved by Southern blot analysis.[83]

By combining in situ hybridization and immunohistochemistry it can be shown that HBV-DNA is present in a large proportion of HB-antigen negative cells but it co-localizes mainly with cytoplasmic and less with nuclear HBcAg[84–86] (Fig. 9.14c), indicating that cytoplasmic localization is a marker of active replication. In contrast, cells with nuclear HBcAg are mostly free from label for HBV-DNA, suggesting that this is an accumulation of empty or non-replicating core particles. By analogy, cells with cytoplasmic HBsAg accumulation are not replicative (Fig. 9.14d). Most recently, the highly sensitive polymerase chain reaction for HBV-DNA has revealed a 'carrier' state in which the viral genome can be shown without other detectable HBV markers in blood.[87-90]

Host factors

The armoury of the host includes non-specific (interferon, natural killer cells) and immune mechanisms (cell-mediated immunity [CMI] by T-lymphocytes, antibody-dependent cellular cytotoxicity [ADCC] by Fc-bearing killer cells and antibody/complement-mediated cytotoxicity). Cell-mediated immunity in particular appears to be decisive for clearance of HBV, and this may be impaired by genetic (HLA type, inherited immunodeficiency) or acquired factors, such as congenital tolerance induction,[68] therapeutic immunosuppression[6] or HIV infection.[91] Modulators of the host system may be non-cytotoxic antiviral antibodies which block target antigens and inappropriate production of cytokines and corresponding receptors.[92] Non-lymphoid inflammatory cells also take part in chronic HBV infection.[93] However, their contribution to killing of virus-infected liver cells has not been analysed.

Viral/host interactions

Chronic infection results if non-specific and virus antigen-specific mechanisms fail to eliminate infected liver cells during the acute phase. The relative inefficiency of the clearing mechanism determines the mode and extent of viral antigen expression which is full-blown in complete anergy. Those antigens on the cell surface which normally serve as a target for removal of the cell become visible, and intracellular antigens are allowed to accumulate. Thus, the phenotype of a chronic infection is a selection of cells which escaped immune elimination.

Activated cytotoxic CD8+ T-lymphocytes and natural killer cells have been identified as the main intrahepatic cell population responsible for necro-inflammation.[94,95] CD8+ T-lymphocytes prevail within the invading front of piecemeal necrosis while T4-lymphocytes are the dominant cell type within the core of portal tracts, together with some B-cells. The close contact between CD8+ lymphocytes and HBcAg-positive hepatocytes (Fig. 9.13e,f) is in line with the general assumption that HLA-restricted T-cell cytotoxicity is the main killing mechanism in piecemeal necrosis and probably also in spotty necrosis.[96-99] This is confirmed also by in vitro cytotoxicity

studies.[100-102] Recent studies on the pathogenesis of the hepatocellular injury in transgenic mice[103] have further substantiated the suspected role of immunologically mediated cytotoxicity. Expression of T-dependent surface antigens with proper expression of MHC II molecules on the cell surface was found to be instrumental in the hepatitic lesion.

It is generally accepted that spotty necrosis in hepatitis B results from HLA-restricted cytotoxicity directed against viral antigens (HBcAg and/or HBeAg) expressed on the liver-cell surface.[96-99,104] This assumption comes from a number of in vitro and in situ findings.[105] The pathogenesis of confluent necrosis is not established. Complement activation due to Kupffer cell failure[106,107] and unrestrained activation of cytokines such as interleukins and tumour necrosis factors[92,108,109] are possibilities but definitive proof is lacking.

Almost all viral proteins, HBsAg, HBcAg, HBeAg and HBxAg have been found exposed on the liver-cell membrane and have been shown to contain epitopes suited for the afferent and efferent limb of the B and T system.[110-113] HBsAg is frequently demonstrable in a membranous pattern in tissue sections (Fig. 9.11b) and has also been demonstrated by immuno-electron microscopy in this location.[114] In experimental acute woodchuck hepatitis, HBsAg has been shown in cell membranes but a role of anti-HBs could not be verified.[115] However, in transgenic mice expressing pre-S1 and pre-S2, an HLA class I restricted cytotoxic reaction of CD8+ T-lymphocytes could be proved in addition to an antibody-mediated cell destruction.[103] In man, the convincing demonstration of HBs-specific, cytotoxic T-cells in acute hepatitis B is still lacking. The main role appears to be linked to the humoral immune response via HLA class II restricted T helper cells and generation of protective immunity.[116]

The pre-core/core-associated antigens, HBcAg and HBeAg, appear to play a key role for elimination of the infection because viral replication can be controlled by the immune system via these antigens. There is ample evidence of a T-cell response against HBcAg in acute and chronic infection,[111] including generation of cytotoxic T-cells.[115,117] Anti-HBc is obviously not relevant for elimination since it co-exists in highest titres with cellular HBcAg expression but also in the HBcAg-free state of infection. It is, however, a sensitive marker for an active and post-hepatitic phase of hepatitis B. Likewise, HBeAg epitopes have been localized to the cell membrane as a possible target antigen;[118,119] in the woodchuck model these are separate from membranous HBc.[115]

The notion that there is a shared epitope on HBcAg and m-HBeAg may be important for the action of the T-cell system,[110] since T-cells may be sensitized by HBcAg, a potent T-cell stimulator, and may kill via both targets, HBcAg and HBeAg in the cell membrane. An immunoregulatory role for HBeAg could be that it blocks T-cells from the HBcAg target.

Despite a large body of evidence for the leading role of cellular immunity and replication-associated viral antigens, the interplay between target antigens, cytolytic and helper T-cells, HLA expression, cytokines, circulating viral antigens and antibodies is still poorly understood. Immuno-histochemistry can be used as a functional measure of the net eliminating efficiency which is reflected by the differential expression of hepatitis B antigens.[6]

HBV MUTANTS

Hepadna viruses are prone to single or even multiple genomic mutations ($<2 \times 10^{-4}$ base substitutions/site/year),[120] adding substantially to the complexity of hepatitis B. Such mutations may change viral replication, the expression and quality of involved viral antigens or the ability of the host to respond to the mutant infection.[121] Each alone or in conjunction can change the pathogenicity of hepatitis B, mostly giving rise to a chronic, aggravated course with unusual antigen and antibody presentation. Tests involving conventional antibodies may even miss a mutant infection.

HBsAg mutants

Mutants of the pre-S region have been detected in patients with chronic hepatitis B with or without hepatocellular carcinoma by several groups.[122–124] It has also been documented that such variants can escape vaccine-induced anti-HBs protection.[125] There are, furthermore, observations that phenotypically HBsAg–/HBV–DNA+ infections result from mutations not recognized by current tests.[126]

HBe negative mutant

The best studied mutation is the replacement of guanosine by adenosine at nucleotide 1896 of the pre-core region resulting in a translational stop codon and preventing the formation of HBeAg.[127–130] Despite unaffected replication

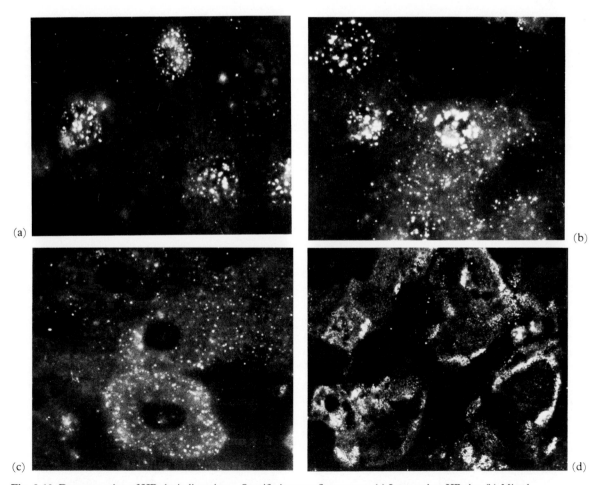

Fig. 9.10 Demonstration of HBcAg in liver tissue. Specific immunofluorescene. (a) Intranuclear HBcAg. (b) Mixed nuclear/cytoplasmic pattern of HBcAg in addition to pure nuclear HBcAg. (c) Pure diffuse cytoplasmic pattern of HBcAg. (d) Submembranous accumulation of HBcAg.

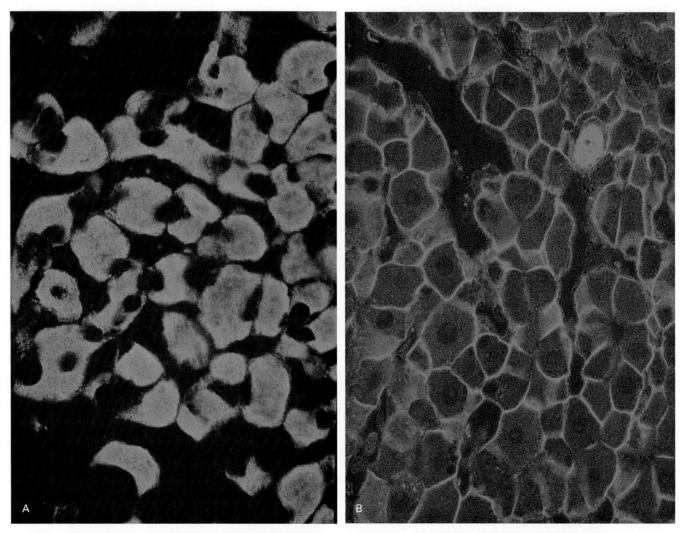

Fig. 9.11 Demonstration of HBsAg in liver tissue. (a) Specific immunofluorescence of purely cytoplasmic HBsAg in an HBcAg-free HBsAg carrier. (b) Honeycomb-like membrane-associated pattern and focal cytoplasmic fluorescence in a kidney transplant recipient. (c) Appearance of cytoplasmic and membranous HBsAg in a case of CAH stained by the avidin–biotin complex method. (d) HBsAg-positive liver cells. Shikata's orcein. (e) HBsAg excess in ground-glass cells. H&E. (f) HBcAg excess in liver-cell nuclei ('sanded nuclei') in an immunosuppressed kidney transplant recipient with CPH. H&E.

of the virus[131] the patients have anti-HBe in serum and usually a fulminant or aggressive type of inflammation which is characterized by progression to cirrhosis and poor responsiveness to interferon therapy.[69,132] Cytoplasmic HBcAg is characteristic for this type of infection.[133] A superimposed HDV infection is better tolerated than in wild-type infection.[134]

Subsequent studies have shown that this point mutation is the most frequent, but a considerable heterogeneity of pre-core mutants is becoming evident.[135] Mixtures of wild-type HBV and mutants can be observed in both HBeAg-positive and anti-HBe-positive patients[127,136,137] with changing ratios during an individual course of infection.[138] Further epidemiological studies are needed to show whether the group of replicative anti-HBe-positive chronic hepatitis is due to co- or superinfection with

mixed inocula or whether the underlying point mutation can spontaneously occur in a pure wild-type infection. The Torino group[138] has forwarded the attractive hypothesis that in these patients the mutant infection will become the prevailing one because of improper immune elimination of cells infected by the mutant strain. This group of patients lacking HBeAg expression also hints at a central pathogenetic role for HBeAg, which is apparently involved in elimination of wild-type virus infection.

HBx mutants

Chronic infections with HBx mutants and low level replication evolving into HBsAg+ wild-type infections have been identified in renal dialysis patients.[139] The fact that such mutations can escape immune elimination indicates

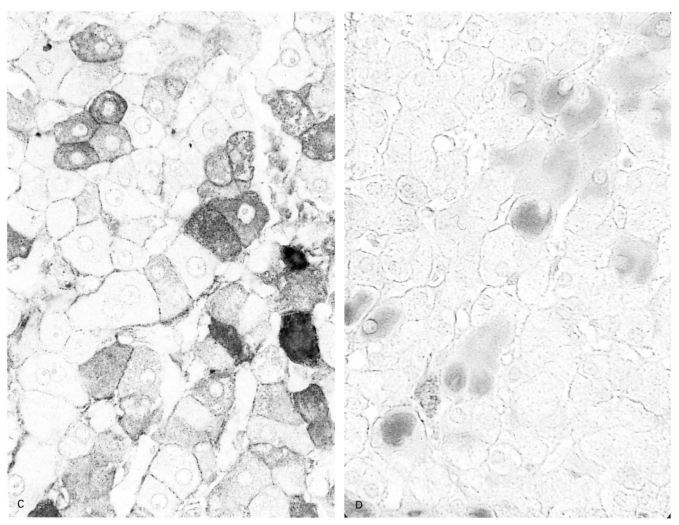

Fig. 9.11 c & d

that HBxAg may be a critical target antigen for eradication of the infection.

MODULATION BY CO-INFECTION WITH OTHER VIRUSES

The effects of HCV superinfection will become more apparent with the detection of viral sequences directly within the liver tissue.[140] The current picture comes largely from anti-HCV antibody determinations. In a group of HBsAg- and HBeAg-positive patients, Fong et al found that HCV co-infection tended to suppress HBV replication and to induce more frequent cirrhosis or decompensated liver disease.[141] Ruiz and colleagues found co-infection in 14% of 70 patients with hepatocellular carcinoma and these were serologically negative for HBsAg but otherwise not conspicuous clinically.[142] In a study of anti-HBe positive chronic carriers, about 10% were anti-HCV-positive without apparent influence on the HBV infection.[143] Among Japanese haemodialysis patients, a co-infection rate of 18% has been reported.[144] It can be concluded that hepatitis C and chronic hepatitis B may co-exist without apparent interference, and termination of a pre-existing chronic hepatitis B[145] appears to be a rare event.

MODULATION BY THERAPY

Both stimulation and suppression of the immune responsiveness have been used as a rationale for therapy.

Immune stimulation is intended to stop the infection by improving the clearance of circulating virus and infected cells. Therefore, viral markers in blood and liver can be expected to drop, but, at the price of increased necro-inflammation which may still be insufficient and even life-threatening. This also holds true for the relative situation when immunosuppression is withdrawn (shift to the right in Fig. 9.15).

Immunosuppression aims at ameliorating the clinical presentation to a healthy carrier state. However, the price is persistence of a highly replicative infection (shift to the

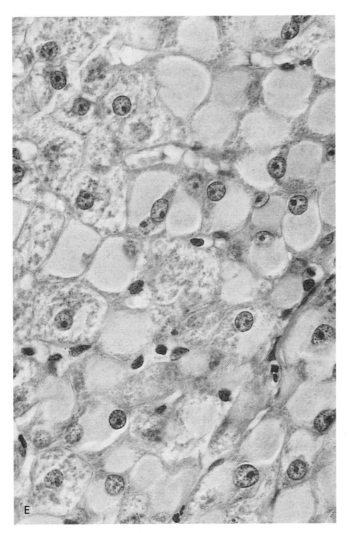

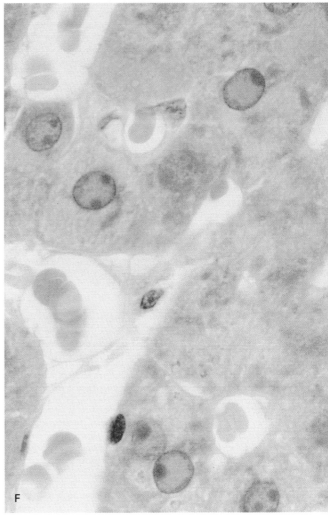

Fig. 9.11 e & f

left in Fig. 9.15). Interferon therapy combines immuno-suppression and direct antiviral activity. Several clinical studies have now shown that α-interferon but not γ-interferon may be efficacious in HBeAg-positive chronic active hepatitis B. However, the long-term effect is not predictable. Loss of HBV replication is seen in 30–50% of patients with HBeAg positive hepatitis. This goes with reduction of intra-acinar and periportal inflammation, including piecemeal necrosis, and reduction of HBcAg in the liver, while HBsAg expression tends to increase[146–153] (shift to the right in Fig. 9.15).

IMMUNOHISTOCHEMISTRY

Specific antibodies can be used to visualize the viral proteins listed in Table 9.11, if their accumulation is permitted because of inadequate clearance of infected cells[6,76,154–161] (Figs 9.10–9.14).

HBcAg is localized preferentially in the liver-cell nucleus and to a lesser extent in the cytoplasm and/or in close association with the cell membrane (Fig. 9.10a–d). The choice of antibody may influence the sensitivity for cytoplasmic HBcAg which is now considered to represent active replication.[162] In very actively replicating infections, cells with cytoplasmic reactivity may outnumber those with nuclear labelling. It appears that the cytoplasmic core expression is mainly responsible for acinar inflammation. Under the electron microscope core particles appear as non-coated spherical structures 24–27 nm in diameter in the nucleoplasm, close to both sides of nuclear pores and between the cisternae of the endoplasmic reticulum — ER (Fig. 9.12c). Encapsulation of core particles within the ER (Dane particle formation, Fig. 9.12c) has been documented repeatedly.[163,164]

Immunohistochemically, HBcAg is best resolved by immunofluorescence which gives a finely granular pattern with monospecific anti-HBc antiserum (Fig. 9.10a–d). Excess accumulation of core particles can be recognized in an H & E stain in rare cases as 'sanded' nuclei (Fig. 9.11f).[165]

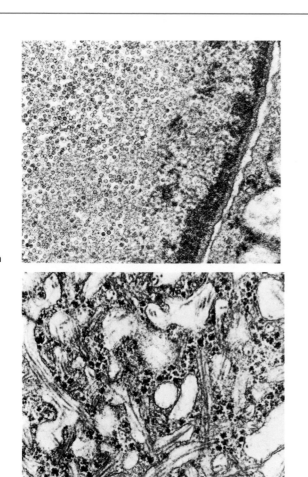

The presence of HBcAg on immunohistochemistry is usually correlated with complete viral synthesis as proved by positivity for viral DNA, DNA polymerase and HBeAg in both liver and blood, as well as by circulating Dane particles in blood.[166,167] Demonstration of HBc in liver cells, therefore, reflects failure to eliminate cells with active (permissive) viral replication. Nuclear HBcAg probably represents accumulation of empty nucleocapsids whereas cytoplasmic HBcAg is now considered to reflect active replication, since cytoplasmic viral DNA can be demonstrated by in situ hybridization in such liver cells (Fig. 9.14c). This is often associated with signs of active disease, characteristically piecemeal necrosis or chronic lobular hepatitis (Fig. 9.14a–b), and with a membrane-associated pattern of HBsAg. It is assumed that viral DNA active in HBcAg production is episomal and not integrated into the host genome.[81,168]

HBsAg (Fig. 9.11). The small, middle and large forms of HBsAg are usually expressed simultaneously in the same location but often in descending order with respect of staining intensity and percentage of stained liver cells. HBsAg in human liver biopsies has two expression patterns with apparently different biological implications:

Fig. 9.12 Electron microscopy of cellular HBAg. (a) Ultrastructure of intranuclear non-coated HBcAg particles (24–27 nm). × 43 500. (b) Ultrastructure of filamentous intracisternal HBsAg within proliferated and distorted smooth endoplasmic reticulum. × 30 600. (c) Uncoated core particles around a cisterna of the endoplasmic reticulum which contains two core particles in the process of encapsulation (arrows). × 104 000

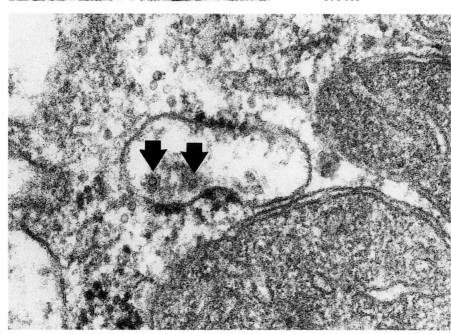

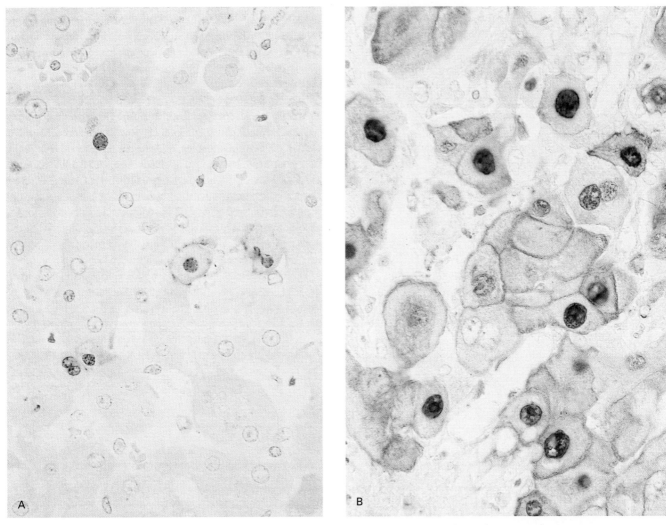

Fig. 9.13 Pathogenetic aspects of viral antigen expression and immune attack. (a) Demonstration of delta antigen in nuclei and cytoplasm of some liver cells. Note conspicuous membranous decoration of the cell in the centre. (b) Extensive HBcAg load in a liver graft, showing pronounced membranous staining in addition to nuclear and cytoplasmic labelling. Note double-nucleated cell below centre, negative for nuclear HBcAg. Same case as Fig. 9.17. (c and d) Specific double-labelling fluorescence of identical area showing expression of HBcAg (c; green) and HBeAg (d; red) in identical cells and comparable distribution pattern. (e and f) Specific double-labelling fluorescence of an HBcAg-harbouring hepatocyte (e; green) attacked by closely attached CD8+ T-lymphocyte in upper portion (f; red); two other HBcAg-positive hepatocytes without contact.

(i) A liver-cell membrane-associated honeycomb-like pattern (Fig. 9.11b), referred to as membranous HBsAg, which may also stain for the middle and less for the large protein. Immune electron microscopic studies showed that it is on or between liver cells in a non-particulate form. Membranous HBsAg is strongly associated with HBc expression and is an indirect indication of replicative HBV infection.[169]

(ii) Intracytoplasmic HBsAg as stained by specific immunohistology and special dyes (orcein, aldehyde thionine, aldehyde fuchsin, Victoria blue) is seen in gradations from a faint localized perinuclear positivity to widespread cytoplasmic involvement (Fig. 9.11) and margination along the cell membrane. Excess cytoplasmic deposition of HBsAg is visible by conventional H & E staining as a homogeneous ground-glass appearance of the cytoplasm (Fig. 9.11e)[170] and stains intensely brown with orcein (Fig. 9.11d). Under the electron microscope, ground-glass cells exhibit a marked proliferation of the smooth endoplasmic reticulum with dislocation of the cytoplasmic organelles to the periphery of the cell. Within the cisternae there are typical filaments (Fig. 9.12b) giving a positive reaction for HBsAg and pre-S by immune electron microscopy.[171,172]

Intracisternal cytoplasmic HBsAg is believed to represent accumulation of surface material which the cell cannot secrete. This may or may not co-exist with active core formation. Hence intracytoplasmic HBsAg is an indicator of chronic elimination insufficiency for this antigen but is an unreliable marker of active replication. If

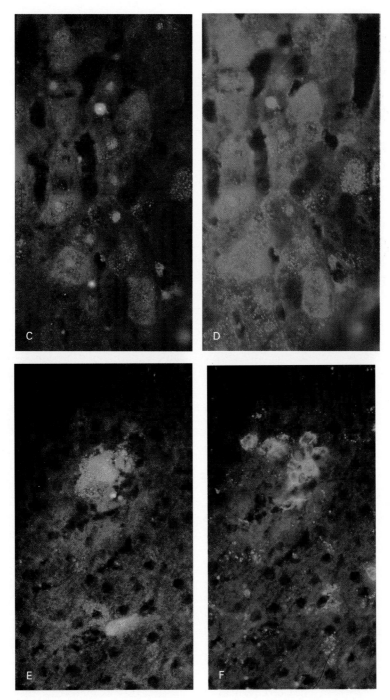

Figure 9.13 *contd*

large aggregates of HBsAg-containing cells are seen, as in the anti-HBe-positive asymptomatic carrier of Western countries, active replication is probably extremely low or absent. In contrast membrane-associated HBsAg should always raise suspicion of active viral replication.

HBeAg. HBeAg, a soluble low-molecular weight component of the nucleocapsid, primarily detected as a non-particulate HBV-associated antigen in serum,[173] has been identified as an HBV core-associated antigen which is coded by the pre-core region,[174,175] and is thus a marker of viral replication. In keeping with this, Arnold and co-workers found HBeAg in liver-cell nuclei, mostly together with HBcAg,[176] but it has also been shown in the cytoplasm.[177-179] Using well-defined monoclonal antibodies, Chu & Liaw[159] could show that cellular HBeAg expression is similar to that of HBcAg, particularly with respect to cytoplasmic localization (Fig. 9.13c,d). The association of HBeAg with the cell membrane has been shown by immune electron microscopy[180] and in transfected hepatoblastoma cells.[181] If HBeAg is a potential target antigen on the liver-cell surface, free HBeAg may have a regulatory role because it could tolerize the T-cell system in the situation of vertical transmission and/or block cytotoxic T-cells in adult infection.[182] The latter mechanism could explain the pronounced necro-inflammation in HBe– mutant infection.

HBxAg. This is the gene product of the X-region and has been characterized as a ubiquitous transcriptional transactivating protein.[183] Its enhancing effect on viral replication[184] and its possible involvement in tumour development are of particular interest. Specific antibodies have been successfully used as additional markers of HBV in chronic hepatitis B and hepatocellular carcinoma.[185–188] In the study of Wang and co-workers[185] HBxAg was visualized in the cytoplasm (diffuse, submembranous ± membranous) and in nuclei of liver cells. Nuclear localization correlated with the presence of dysplastic cells. The expression was sparse, localized or diffuse in most cases of chronic hepatitis B with a preferential labelling of dysplastic cells, particularly in severe CAH and cirrhosis. Clearly, this marker system may become an important diagnostic tool because it may provide the only visible immunohistochemical marker of HBV infection, particularly in hepatocellular carcinoma. Despite cogent circumstantial evidence,[189,190] however, the role of the X gene in the pathogenesis of hepatitis B and hepatocellular carcinoma remains to be clarified.[191,192]

HEPATITIS D INFECTION (Table 9.12)

Hepatitis D is caused by co- or superinfection with a defective RNA virus[193–195] which was detected by its specific delta antigen (HDAg) and extensively characterized as the delta agent by Rizzetto and co-workers.[193–195] The hepatitis D virus (HDV) co-exists with and depends on replicating HBV infection. The viral RNA codes for a short (p24, 195 AA), nucleolar associated[196,197] and an elongated form of HDAg (p27, 214 AA) which is the result of a regularly occurring point mutation at the stop codon of p24.[198,199] HDAg, as a strongly RNA-binding phosphoprotein,[200] is supposedly involved in the replication and assembly of HDV.[195,201–203] The defectiveness of the HDV lies in the fact that the surface of HBV is needed for envelopment and that the release of the latter in a replicating HBV infection is probably necessary for release and propagation of the HDV,[204] whereas replication of HDV can proceed in the absence of HBV.[205]

Immunohistochemically, HDAg is found mainly in liver-cell nuclei (Fig. 9.13a). Using immunofluorescence, Negro and co-workers[206] could define three nuclear patterns: nucleolar with weakly fluorescent nucleoplasm; nucleoplasmic, with negative nucleoli; and intense, homogeneous fluorescence involving the whole nucleus. Excess HDAg may cause 'sanded' nuclei in H&E stains[207] similar to those found in HBcAg excess.[165] Also, similar to HScAg, a cytoplasmic localization[208] and membrane-associated HDAg (Fig. 9.13a) can be observed.

Immunohistochemical double staining shows mostly separate expression of HDAg versus HBsAg or HBcAg (if present at all) but co-expression in the same cell does occur with HBsAg and rarely with HBcAg.[209,210] In situ hybridization always localizes HDV-RNA in nuclei, usually together with HDAg, but RNA may occasionally be present alone.[211]

By transmission and immune electron microscopy HDAg is non-particulate. This is consistent with the lack of a nucleocapsid of the circulating 37 nm delta particle. In the nucleus, it localizes in a granular fashion in the chromatin area and in the cytoplasm on free ribosomes and the cytoplasmic matrix.[209] Yamada & Tsuji[212] described aggregates of an HDAg-positive amorphous substance associated with intranuclear microtubular structures.

The pathogenesis of hepatitis D is still unclear despite considerable progress in the understanding of the molecular biology of this unusual virus and despite several available experimental models.[213] Any explanation must take into account the observation that, in certain settings, HDV infection does not cause disease while, in others, it induces aggravated and accelerated disease.[214] Factors to be considered are the recently recognized molecular heterogeneity of HDV-RNA,[215] a direct toxic effect of HDAg, HDAg as an immunological target, and autoimmune mechanisms. It has been proposed that a replicative and secretorily active HBV infection provides the prerequisite for a toxic effect on the liver cell.[204] In line with this hypothesis are the double-labelling studies of Kojima and co-workers[209] which revealed inflammatory cells preferentially around cells positive for both HDAg and HBsAg but not around those positive for HBsAg alone. Phenotypically, the portal, periportal and intra-acinar infiltrates were dominated by T-lymphocytes in a similar fashion in hepatitis B and D.

With these open questions in mind, a given case of hepatitis D may be assessed in the light of the following considerations:

(i) HDV is cytotoxic, in contrast to HBV, producing direct cellular damage in addition to immunologically mediated cellular cytotoxicity. This explains the fact that inflammation is usually more severe and aggressive, leading to cirrhosis more frequently and in a shorter time[193,216–218] (p. 359). Epidemiological studies indicate, however, that this is mainly valid for populations with rapid circulation of HDV, e.g. in drug addicts or in hyperendemic regions.[219] In several areas a carrier state with low grade HDV replication and lack of tissue damage has been found.[220] Most importantly, the experience with liver transplantation for end-stage hepatitis D has clearly shown that, under immunosuppressive therapy, HDV in-

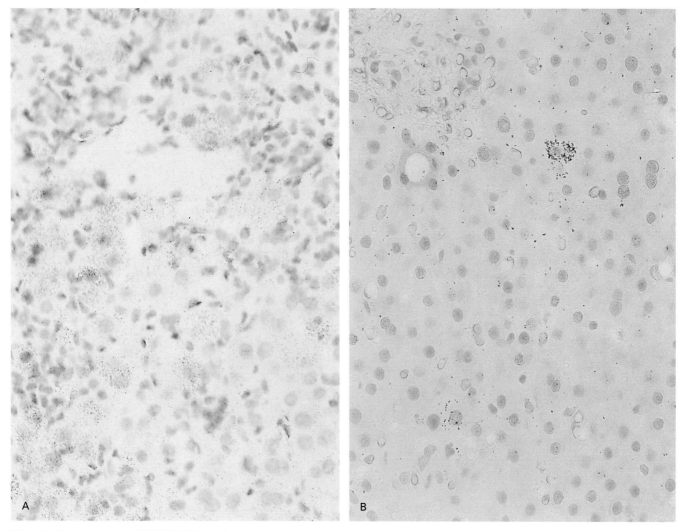

Fig. 9.14 Demonstration of HBV-DNA by in situ hybridization using a ³H-labelled probe (kind gift of Prof R Thomssen, Göttingen, Germany). (a) Replicating cells with cytoplasmic HBV-DNA in an area of piecemeal necrosis in CAH, showing most replicating liver cells without HBcAg accumulation. Autoradiography of frozen section counterstained with H&E. (b) Scattered intra-acinar replicating cells in a case of CLH; same method as in (a).

fection recurred in about 80% of cases but was cytotoxic and symptomatic only when hepatitis B was reactivated.[221] Histological examination in such cases showed the picture of typical acute viral hepatitis. When HBcAg in liver and/or HBV-DNA in serum was negative, HDAg was seen within 17 days as a silent HDV infection with low levels of HDAg expression. This indicates that HDV may replicate as a non-cytotoxic virus in the absence of replicating HBV, at least under the very special conditions of liver transplantation.

(ii) HDV rather selectively suppresses HBcAg and HBeAg[222] and not HBsAg or pre-S,[208,223-226] although it supposedly depends on minimal HBV multiplication and release.[204] This may lead to HBV expression patterns in liver and blood which deviate from those of uncomplicated chronic hepatitis B as outlined above. Conversely,

paradoxical constellations of HBV expression, serology and/or histology should raise a suspicion of HDV co- or superinfection.

(iii) The outcome of the double infection is largely determined by the immunocompetence of the host against the HBV infection. Immunity against HBV protects against hepatitis D. Immuno-insufficiency against HBV results in chronic HBV infection and promotes chronic hepatitis D, whereas efficient elimination of HBV also ends HDV infection.

In acute co-infection, after simultaneous inoculation with both viruses, the disease may resemble acute hepatitis B but may run a fulminant course (see Table 9.12 for details). Usually, this does not allow detectable accumulation of hepatitis B antigens in the liver tissue, and the presence of

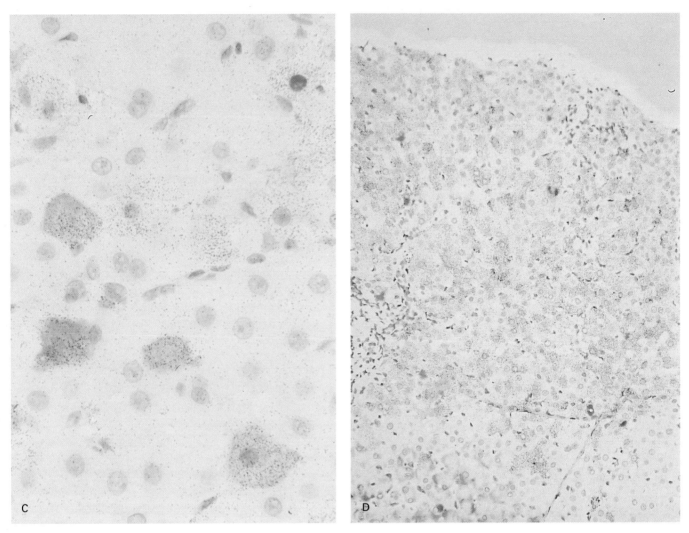

Fig. 9.14 (c) In situ hybridization for HBV-DNA and immunostaining for HBcAg showing differing patterns of co-expression but also negative hepatocytes and others with only one marker in nucleus or cytoplasm. Paraffin sections, autoradiography followed by ABC method. (d) Same procedure as for (c) for HBV-DNA and HBsAg. Note heavy labelling of HBsAg-negative cells and weak or no signs of replication in cells with cytoplasmic HBsAg.

Table 9.12 Types of HDV Infections in Relation to HBV State

Type	HBV infection/host	Clinical presentation	Light microscopy	Immunohistochemistry	Course
Co-infection	Acute/normergic	Acute hepatitis (mono- or bi-phasic)	Acute hepatitis with spotty necrosis	HBcAg – HDAg ±	Limited HBV and HDV infection
	Acute/hyperergic?	Fulminant	Confluent/massive necrosis	HBcAg – HDAg ±	Liver failure or limited hepatitis ± scarring
	Acute/hypoergic	Acute hepatitis with transition into chronicity	Acute hepatitis with piecemeal necrosis → CAH	Co-expression of HBcAg and HDAg → mostly HDAg only	Chronic course with high probability of cirrhosis
	Chronic/hypoergic	Chronic symptomatic hepatitis	Mostly CAH	Mostly HDAg only	
Super-infection	Chronic/hypoergic	Acute episodes in chronic hepatitis	Mostly CAH with lobular hepatitis	HDAg + HBcAg ±	Mostly chronic hepatitis D; rarely limited hepatitis D; extremely seldom limitation of both

HDAg in single liver-cell nuclei (and/or IgM-anti-HDAg and/or HDV-RNA in serum) may be the only clue to the aetiology of fulminant hepatitis.

Superinfection of an existing chronic hepatitis B, including asymptomatic carriers, with an HDV-containing inoculum usually produces an acute inflammatory episode with subsequent undulations of activity (see Table 9.12 for details). Since, during active cytotoxic HDV infection the replication of the HBV becomes suppressed, unusual expression patterns of hepatitis B markers in liver and/or blood may be present. In such a case the prognosis can be overridden by the HDV infection with resulting aggressive inflammation and rapid development of cirrhosis.

THE BASIC REACTION TYPES OF HEPATITIS B
(Table 9.13 and Fig. 9.15)

Infections with mutant strains of HBV have shown that only pure infections with the wild type are comparable with respect to viral expression and host reactions. Therefore, the basic reaction types discussed in the following paragraphs are mainly valid for uncomplicated wild-type infections. For these, we have suggested that viral antigen expression arbitrarily reflects the degree of elimination insufficiency of the host.[227] This hypothesis has gained acceptance, which justifies its adoption with some modifications. The proposed immunopathological classification is primarily derived from viral expression patterns related to complete or incomplete virus replication. HBcAg, Dane particles and associated markers (HBV-DNA, HBeAg) rather than the HBsAg system are taken as the basic discriminating features. Four basic expression patterns with transitional forms are recognized (Fig. 9.15): an acute or elimination type and three chronic forms. This biological classification correlates well with conventional histological findings, indicating an intrinsic

Table 9.14 HBV carrier

Constant findings:
    Chronic HBV infection: replicative or non-replicative
    No or non-aggressive inflammation

Exclusion criteria:
    Chronic active hepatitis
    Chronic lobular hepatitis

association between type and degree of inflammation and the state of viral infection. Whereas an acute limited infection lacks viral over-expression after the establishment of normergic eliminating inflammation, there may be overt and persistent viral expression in chronic hepatitis of any histological type, either with or without active core and Dane particle formation.

Therefore, the identification of a histological diagnosis with one of the basic expression types bears on the evaluation of prognosis, therapy and infectivity. It should be stressed that classification of chronic hepatitis on immunohistological grounds alone is not justified because the borders are not sharp and are also influenced by the sensitivity and set-up of the immunohistochemical methods.

Elimination type: acute self-limited viral hepatitis (Fig. 9.15/I). One of the possible reactions to the infection is the immunocompetent elimination of cells carrying viral antigens by means of spotty necrosis, the hallmark of classic acute viral hepatitis (see Ch. 6). This normergic reaction accomplishes a self-limited course and only transient infectivity of the patient's blood (Fig. 9.15/I). Elimination of the virus associated with liver-cell necrosis may be regarded as an inevitable but beneficial event; immunosuppression might prevent eradication of virus-producing liver cells and be responsible for chronicity. At the height of classic acute viral hepatitis no viral components are found in liver tissue, despite sero-positivity and heavy parenchymal inflammation, except for a very little

Table 9.13 Immunohistopathological types of uncomplicated chronic hepatitis B

	Minimal requirements for definition	Associated histology	Implications	Relation to carrier state (non-aggressive inflammation)
Generalized HBc type (replicative phase, immune tolerant state)	More than 60% of liver cells with nuclear HBcAg and with variable cytoplasmic HBcAg	No inflammation Minimal hepatitis CPH	Course dependent on stability of tolerance; infective focus	High replicative carrier (Table 9.14)
Focal HBc type (replicative phase with inefficient immune elimination)	Less than 60% of liver cells with nuclear core and variable cytoplasmic HBcAg *or* No demonstrable cellular HBcAg but presence of HBeAg, Dane particles or HBV-DNA in serum	CPH CAH minimal CAH severe or CLH	Unstable; imminent cirrhosis; infective focus	High (HBe+) to low (anti-HBe+) replicative carrier
HBcAg-free HBs type (non-replicative phase with viral integration)	Lack of nuclear and cytoplasmic core antigen expression in liver *and* of Dane particles, HBeAg and HBV-DNA in serum.	No inflammation, minimal hepatitis or CPH	Stable, favourable course; imminent HCC; no or low infectivity	Non-replicative carrier (Table 9.14)

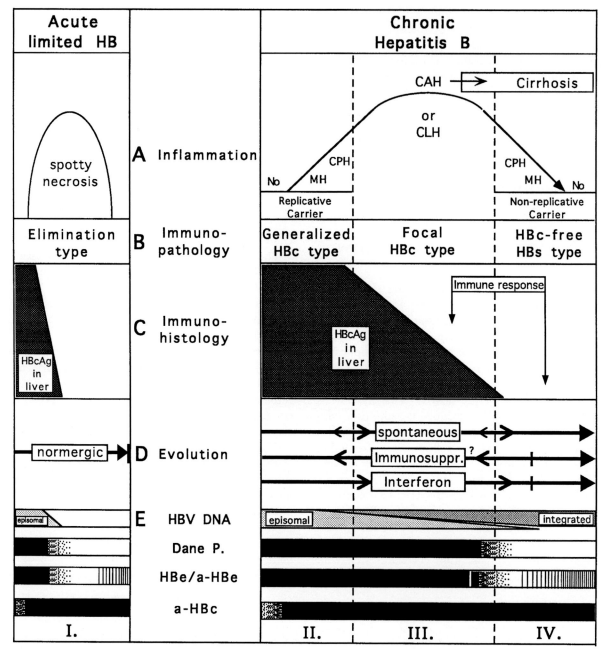

Fig. 9.15 An integrated view of the four basic reaction types of hepatitis B. Correlation between:
A — Inflammatory reaction;
B — Immunopathological expression types (I–IV);
C — Immunohistological expression in the liver tissue;
D — Natural and therapeutically-induced evolution; and
E — Serological markers.
Dark areas indicate presence of respective marker. The indices I-IV correspond to the main expression types described in the text.
Type-associated findings are read vertically and may shift as indicated by the arrows in D (evolution).

HBcAg and membranous HBsAg in the early, immuno-incompetent stages. In the pre-clinical, pre-necrotic stage of infection, however, HBcAg and HBsAg have been shown in chimpanzee[228] and human liver.[229,230] This represents a phase of the infection with permissive replication before elicitation of the immune response. As the normal immune response is mounted, virus-containing cells are eliminated and the infection is terminated. Detection of viral antigens in a biopsy from a patient with acute hepatitis beyond the early stage of infection may therefore be regarded as a sensitive indicator of impending chronicity.

Generalized HBcAg type (Fig. 9.15/II). In effectively immunosuppressed patients (e.g. kidney transplant recipients[6]), in some patients without detectable immune deficiency and in cases of vertically transmitted hepatitis, the response to the infection is not classic acute hepatitis. A subclinical infection with little or no biochemical abnormality and without demonstrable liver-cell damage is accompanied by mild, chronic non-aggressive inflammation (CPH or minimal hepatitis) or no inflammation at all. However, there is marked HBcAg expression (Fig. 9.15/II), accompanied by mostly generalized, honeycomb-like membranous HBs. Cytoplasmic HBsAg is usually sparse and focal and does not discriminate the type. In serum, markers of active viral replication are regularly found (Fig. 9.15/II). Anti-HBc of the IgM and IgG fraction is usually present in spontaneous forms but may be undetectable in immunosuppressed patients, despite active core formation. The generalized HBc type thus represents the prototype of an unrestricted chronic active (permissive) viral replication with high infectivity. Recent findings indicate that most of the viral DNA is episomal (p. 365).

An extreme burden of HBsAg and HBcAg accumulates within weeks in recurrent post-transplant hepatitis B,[231–235] which is probably facilitated not only by the immunosuppression but also by the unusually high infectious dose with which the graft is confronted. In this extreme situation, HBcAg is easily demonstrable as a possible target antigen, in this instance at the level of the cell membrane (Fig. 9.13b).

Focal HBc type (Fig. 9.15/III). Aggressive forms of hepatitis, such as CAH and acute hepatitis with periportal piecemeal necrosis (see Ch. 6), are most often associated with focal expression of HBcAg together with membranous HBsAg in a focal or diffuse display.[155,169] Cytoplasmic HBsAg is usually spotty and again is not type-specific. Concomitant with HBc expression in tissue, markers of active replication (Fig. 9.15/III) appear in blood, implying high infectivity. Inflammatory activity and the amount of HBc expression in tissue are inversely related: the more active the inflammation, the less the tissue expression of HBc and vice versa (shift to right in Fig. 9.15).

Immunosuppressive therapy of CAH usually results in clinical improvement with decrease of the inflammatory reaction (e.g. shift from CAH to CPH), while at the same time HBc synthesis is better tolerated and HBc-expressing cells increase (shift to the generalized Hbc type: Fig. 9.15/II). The hepatic and serological expressions thus represent a whole spectrum, resulting from the interplay of viral and host factors. A finely graded, partial immune insufficiency allows elimination of some but not all infected hepatocytes, facilitating viral propagation. Effective elimination cannot, however, be accomplished, even by confluent necrosis. Persistence of hepatocytes with viral integration and superimposed autoimmunity, possibly related to piecemeal necrosis, may play an additional role.

Cases in which replication and core synthesis are below the detection level of immunohistochemistry present a problem of classification. Such cases might either belong to the HBcAg-free HBs type (type IV in Fig. 9.15) or even the elimination type (type I in Fig. 9.15). Therefore, cases are now included in the focal type in which core replication has been proven by other means, such as demonstration of HBeAg, DNA polymerase or HBV-DNA in serum (Table 9.13).

HBcAg-free HBs type (Fig. 9.15/IV). A further variant with a chronic non-aggressive hepatitis identical to the generalized HBc type, or more often without inflammation, is associated with extensive expression of cytoplasmic HBsAg (Fig. 9.11a), while HBcAg and membranous HBsAg are largely absent. There is again no liver-cell damage, and no biochemical abnormalities are found. In accordance with the lack of HBc formation, the serum lacks Dane particles, HBeAg and anti-HBs but characteristically contains anti-HBe (Fig. 9.15/IV). This type of carrier is regarded as being of low-grade infectivity. It represents the prototype of an incomplete (non-permissive) viral replication, producing exclusively HBsAg. This type probably has viral DNA integrated into the host genome, promoting the development of hepatocellular carcinoma.[74,236] The HBcAg-free HBs type may be seen as a special case in which elimination of liver cells exposing HBcAg-related antigens is normergic and efficient but immune destruction of HBsAg-producing cells is deficient.

The four basic reaction types in a dynamic model of hepatitis B (Fig. 9.15)

When HBV-DNA and HBeAg/anti-HBe in serum are related to the type of hepatitis and age of patients with chronic hepatitis B,[16,167] an evolution becomes apparent which mimics the course of acute, self-limited hepatitis B but which is extended over years. Because the individual phases are of much longer duration, the histological and immune histological expression patterns are more distinct than in acute hepatitis B.

The infection sets in with a highly replicative phase and extensive cellular expression of viral proteins, notably HBcAg. In the pre-clinical, pre-necrotic stage a very discrete lymphocytic reaction may present as minimal hepatitis. With progressive accumulation of lymphoid cells within portal tracts the histological features evolve into CPH while the patient still is asymptomatic.

Within about six years[16] an increasing immune response results in eradication of some but not all HBcAg-bearing liver cells. This is reflected in a reduction of HBAg-expressing cells and, histologically, in increased activity of the disease process, usually CAH with variable degrees of acinar necro-inflammatory changes. This causes architectural disturbances with fibrosis and sometimes development of cirrhosis. It should be appreciated that this attempt at virus elimination is not a continuum, as it may appear from Figure 9.15, but rather proceeds by repeated episodes.

Hand in hand with partial elimination of replicating cells and HBe/anti-HBe seroconversion, the inflammatory response after some further 4–6 years[16] declines and shifts towards non-replicative phases of activity, again CPH, minimal hepatitis or no inflammation, and often in the presence of inactive cirrhosis. During this evolution viral DNA will become integrated into an expanding liver-cell population and this is reflected in lack of HBcAg but purely intracytoplasmic HBsAg expression.

Alternatively (Fig. 9.15), eradication of virus-replicating cells and HBe seroconversion may be accomplished in some patients without piecemeal necrosis. Instead, the liver goes through a prolonged stage of acinar necro-inflammatory changes of the (acute) spotty necrosis type, by definition fulfilling the criteria of CLH. Unlike piecemeal necrosis, the spotty necrosis of CLH does not entail substantial fibrosis or cirrhosis. The declining phase in these cases will show the histological features of a non-replicative carrier such as CPH, minimal hepatitis or even no inflammation. Viral protein expression in the evolution shown in Figure 9.15 is intracytoplasmic HBsAg without HBcAg. Why the immunological attempt to eradicate the virus leads to CAH in one instance and CLH in another is not yet clear.

Another unsolved problem concerns HBc-free HBsAg-positive cells. Their elimination appears to be critical, because release and probably presentation on the liver cell as a target antigen is linked to active core synthesis.[237] Inablity to overcome this second elimination step favours persistence and accumulation of such cells, integration into the host genome and malignant transformation. However, there are also documented patients who accomplish spontaneous HBs-/anti-HBs seroconversion after having lost HBeAg.[238]

This natural evolution of chronic hepatitis B, in comparison to normergic hepatitis B, has been incorporated in a modification of our old scheme (Fig. 9.15) dating back to 1975.[6] Taking the amount of detectable HBc in tissue as a measure of the postulated chronic immune insufficiency, the three types of chronic hepatitis B divide into two extremes that have in common non-aggressive inflammation but differ fundamentally in complete virus (Dane) particle formation and associated markers. Chronic active hepatitis, representing the most active inflammatory attempt to clear the hepatocellular infection, lies between these non-aggressive, inflammatory reactions. The three chronic reaction patterns, however, are not sharply delineated disease entities but rather characteristic types that merge imperceptibly into each other. Transitions may occur in any direction,[239] even as reactivation of a HBeAg-positive hepatitis B.[240] Application and withdrawal of immunosuppressive and antiviral agents result

in simultaneous transition both of histological findings and viral expression pattern.

The term 'carrier' should be used with caution. The clinical attribute 'asymptomatic' or 'healthy' is misleading, since there may be severe inflammation without clinical manifestations. The histological features should therefore be included in the definition, and the term 'carrier' restricted to patients with mild non-aggressive inflammation at most. In addition, the replicative state (non-replicative vs. high or low replicative) should be incorporated, since this has different biological and prognostic implications. The correlation with immunohistological expression is shown in Tables 9.13 and 9.14.

MORPHOLOGY OF CHRONIC HEPATITIS B

Besides the viral expression patterns described above, chronic hepatitis B shows some characteristic, albeit not diagnostic features. In contrast to hepatitis C there is often marked polymorphism and enlargement of hyperbasophilic hepatocellular nuclei together with eosinophilic swelling of the cytoplasm of perivenular hepatocytes (Fig. 9.16). Such cells are reminiscent of hepatocytes described as dysplastic.[241] Fatty change is unusual. Portal lymphoid follicle formation and inflammatory bile-duct lesions may occasionally be seen but are far less common than in hepatitis C. If present, these features are suggestive of HCV or HDV superinfection. Single cell necrosis surrounded by inflammatory cells (satellitosis) is more frequent in hepatitis B, whereas naked acidophilic bodies prevail in hepatitis C. Acute episodes, unlike exacerbations in hepatitis C, are more clearly located in zone III and hepatocyte degeneration is more often of a ballooning or lytic type. The relation of mesenchymal:parenchymal changes is balanced in hepatitis B,

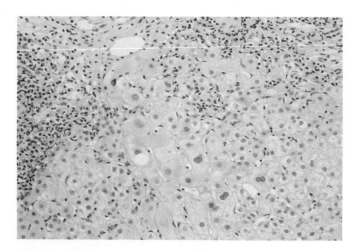

Fig. 9.16 CAH (very severe) in hepatitis B and delta co-infection. Note polymorphism of liver-cell nuclei characteristic for HBV infection. Apoptotic bodies are seen within periportal piecemeal necrosis (top right). H&E.

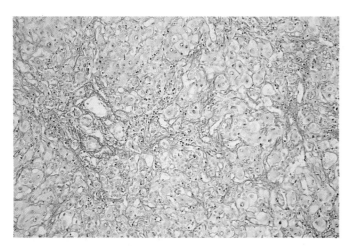

Fig. 9.17 Fibrosing cholestatic hepatitis after liver transplantation for hepatitis B (same case as Fig 9.13b). Note severe pericellular fibrosis, encasing groups of liver cells throughout the acinus. Portal tract at left, perivenular zone at right. Sirius red. Material kindly provided by Dr B Portmann.

whereas in hepatitis C mesenchymal alterations often prevail. Uncomplicated chronic hepatitis B is often of moderate activity.

Fibrosing cholestatic hepatitis

A particular morphological pattern of hepatitis B has been observed in recurrent HBV infection after liver transplantation.[242] It is characterized by impressively high-level expression of intracytoplasmic HBsAg and HBcAg[235] in combination with only mild necrosis and inflammation. In addition, there is severe intrahepatic cholestasis and a marked and characteristic perisinusoidal fibrosis, encasing groups of liver-cells or entire liver-cell plates (Fig. 9.17), possibly related to immunosuppressive therapy. The

disease may be suspected as early as 3 months after transplantation by slight intra-acinar hepatitic changes in the presence of extensive expression of intracytoplasmic HBsAg and HBcAg (Fig. 9.13b)[234,242] and ends in a so-called steatoviral or fibroviral variant.[234]

Chronic hepatitis D

Superinfection of chronic hepatitis B with HDV is usually characterized by severe activity with extensive piecemeal necrosis and rapid progression to cirrhosis.[217,243] Severe panacinar inflammation with a morphology similar to hepatitis C is typical (Fig. 9.18). Chronic hepatitis D may be accompanied by portal lymphoid follicle formation and bile-duct involvement. Fine droplet fatty change has been found in outbreaks of severe hepatitis D in Venezuelan Indians[244] with hepatic failure or rapidly progressing to cirrhosis. For further details, see earlier section on HDAg.

CHRONIC HEPATITIS C

The histological characteristics of both acute and chronic hepatitis C have already been discussed in detail in chapter 6. The main features include portal infiltration by lymphocytes (Fig. 9.7b), often with formation of follicles with or without germinal centres (Fig. 9.19), associated bile-duct damage, and acinar necrosis and inflammation.[12] Piecemeal necrosis varies in degree and the lesion is often on the borderline of CPH and CAH (i.e. low or minimal activity CAH). The intra-acinar activity is characterized by prominent acidophil body formation. Fatty change is common though not usually severe. In spite of the frequently mild histological picture, many patients develop cirrhosis over a period of years. The exact pathogenetic mechanisms of this evolution remain uncertain,

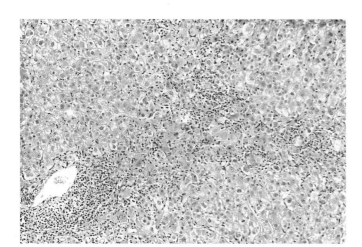

Fig. 9.18 CAH with delta superinfection. Note pronounced acinar necro-inflammatory alterations. Portal tract below left, hepatic vein at centre right. H&E.

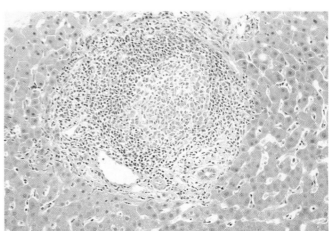

Fig. 9.19 Chronic hepatitis C. The portal tract is expanded by a lymphoid follicle with germinal centre. A small bile duct (below) shows mild epithelial irregularity and its wall contains an infiltrating lymphocyte. Piecemeal necrosis is slight. H&E.

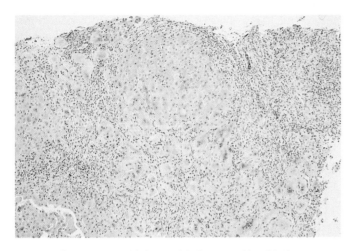

Fig. 9.20 Giant cell hepatitis in an adult (17-year-old male). Severe CAH with extensive nodular transformation. Note many multinucleated syncytial giant cells. (Case published — reference 247). H&E.

but it seems likely that episodes of bridging necrosis play a part in the progression of the lesion.

CHRONIC GIANT CELL HEPATITIS IN THE ADULT

Some forms of CAH are characterized by a varying number of multinucleated syncytial (or plasmodial) giant cells with up to 40 nuclei[245,246] (Fig. 9.20). The course of the disease is often markedly cholestatic and many cases show rapid progression to cirrhosis. About half the cases exhibit serological features of autoimmunity, notably positive antinuclear antibodies.[245] The aetiology is not definitely established. By electron microscopy tubular inclusions (Fig. 9.21) have been observed[245,247] which resemble paramyxovirus, and Phillips et al[245] have presented additional evidence for paramyxovirus infection. If histological cholestasis is pronounced and if giant cells are few, the diagnosis may easily be missed in a needle biopsy.

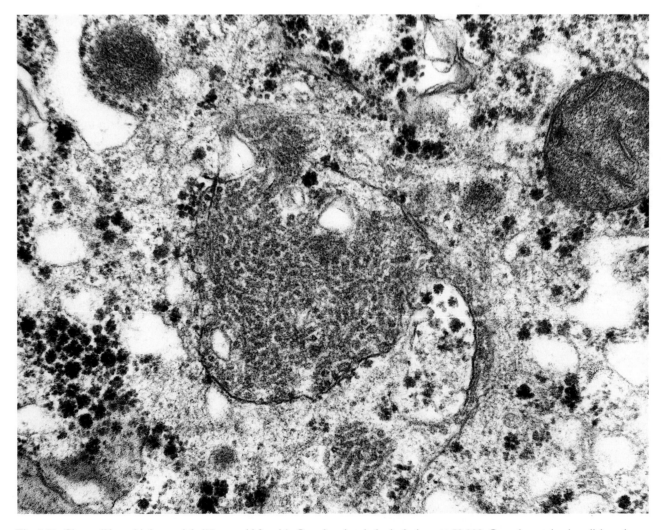

Fig. 9.21 Giant cell hepatitis in an adult (39-year-old female). Cytoplasmic tubular inclusions. × 58 000. Case observation in collaboration with H P Dienes, Mainz and M L Terracciano, Naples

AUTOIMMUNE CHRONIC HEPATITIS (AI-CH)

The recognition of autoimmune chronic (active) hepatitis and its subtypes is important because the patients benefit from immunosuppressive therapy. The main diagnostic features are given in Table 9.15. Although the disease was originally described in young females, it is now well recognized that it affects males as well and may present at any age.[248] Also, the previous apparent association of AI-CH with a North European caucasoid back-ground was based largely on the fact that there were few studies from other areas; there is, however, increasing evidence that the disease also occurs in Japanese and other ethnic groups, making this no longer tenable as a diagnostic criterion.

Based on the serological profiles of autoantibodies, five subtypes may currently be recognized, all but type 2b responding favourably to immunosuppressive therapy.[249]

Type 1 represents classic 'lupoid' hepatitis as described by Mackay;[250] 80% of all AI-CH belongs to this type. Hypergammaglobulinaemia is marked and there is a frequent association with HLA-B8 or HLA-DRw3.[248]

Type 2a is characterized by positivity for LKM-1 (liver kidney microsomal antibody) and negativity for anti-HCV. About 10% of all cases of AI-CH and about two-thirds of cases in children are of this type.[251] There may be an association with other autoimmune phenomena or autoimmune disorders in family members. Without treatment these cases tend to run a rapidly progressive course.

In type 2b, LKM-1 antibodies are positive in the presence of positive anti-HCV antibodies. It differs from all other forms of AI-CH in that anti-GOR is often detectable.[252,253] (GOR 47-1 is a fusion protein expressed by a cDNA clone derived from a chimpanzee infected with non-A, non-B hepatitis). Immunosuppressive treatment of this variant is controversial.

LKM antibodies react with members of the family of drug-metabolizing P-450 enzymes. They are heterogeneous and differ in their immunofluorescent pattern. LKM-1 reacts with P-450 2D6; LKM-2 antibodies, reacting with P-450 2C9, have been observed in drug-induced CAH, e.g. with tienilic acid.[251,255] Liver microsomal antibodies (LM) reacting with P-450 1A2 have been described in patients with dihydralazine hepatitis.[256] In 10% of Italian HDV-positive patients LKM-3 antibodies were described;[257] the latter have not yet been further characterized.

Type 3 is characterized by antibodies against SLA,[258] claimed to be specific for cytokeratins 8 and 18. This pattern is often missed because anti-SLA cannot be detected by immunofluorescence but only by enzyme immunoassay or radioimmunoassay. Clinical presentation is similar to type 1, with conspicuous hypergammaglobulinaemia, and progression is rapid.

Type 4, the form positive for SMA,[259] has high titres of antibodies against F-actin[260] in the absence of any other antibodies, except for liver membrane antibody in some cases.[261] Since low titres of SMA are often present in viral hepatitis differential diagnosis may become a problem.

Histological diagnosis

A diagnosis of AI-CH cannot be made from morphological features in a liver biopsy alone. Suggestive of but not diagnostic for autoimmune CH are high activity of CAH including extensive piecemeal necrosis, often confluent necrosis,[262] notably with bridging, marked liver-cell rosetting (Fig. 9.22) and abundance of plasma cells in the inflammatory exudate.[11] This latter finding, however, is not unequivocally accepted.[263]

Syndromes predominantly producing bile-duct damage but with lymphocytic piecemeal necrosis (e.g. PBC, PSC) should not be regarded as subtypes of classic AI-CH but rather as separate autoimmune entities.

Pathogenesis and aetiology

Despite progress in our knowledge of the immunobiology of AI-CH in the last few years, its pathogenesis is far from understood. Most authors agree, however, that while the large panel of detectable autoantibodies in serum is of diagnostic value, most of these antibodies are not pathogenic, with the possible exceptions of anti-ASGP-R (see below) and anti-LKM-1.[249,264–266]

Cytotoxic T-cells probably play a role in the pathogenesis of the disease.[263] T-lymphocytes constitute the major component of the inflammatory infiltrate in areas of piecemeal necrosis.[39,41,267] Autschbach et al[268] have demonstrated a CD4:CD8 ratio of 1:1 in AI-CAH which differs from viral CAH (ratio 0.37). This may reflect a relatively

Table 9.15 Diagnostic criteria in autoimmune chronic hepatitis (AI-CH). Modified from Johnson and McFarlane.[254]

- Symptoms or signs (including abnormal biochemical liver tests) indicating chronic liver disease of longer than six months duration
- Histological features of CAH
- Elevated serum globulin or gammaglobulin concentrations with specific elevation of IgG
- Circulating ANA and/or SMA and/or LKM-1 autoantibodies at titres of 1:40 or greater
- Seropositivity for other autoantibodies, particularly those apparently more related to the liver such as LMA, anti-SLA, anti ASGP-R, and certain subtypes of AMA
- Multisystem features and/or association with other autoimmune disorders or immunological abnormalities in patients or their first-degree relatives
- Presence of HLA A1-B8-DR3 or B8-DW3 haplotypes
- Exclusion of all other causes of chronic hepatitis (but alcohol abuse does not exclude AI-CH)
- Response to corticosteroid therapy

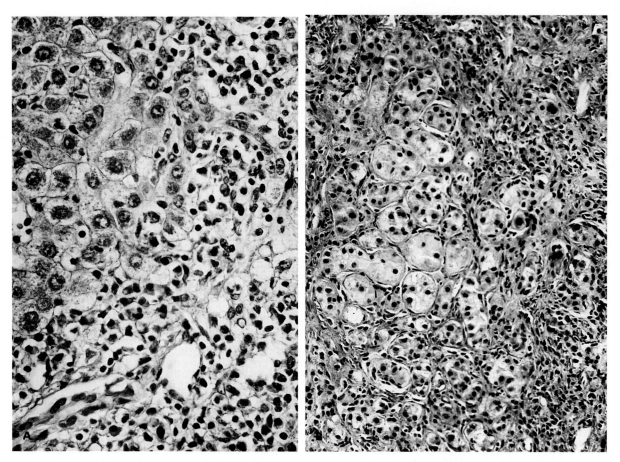

Fig. 9.22 Histology of autoimmune CAH, severe activity, in a 55-year-old female. (a) Note abundance of plasma cells within periportal piecemeal necrosis. Ductular proliferation is absent. H&E. (b) Severe CAH in a 21 year-old female. Piecemeal necrosis with marked tubular transformation of liver cells (rosetting), surrounded by newly formed basement membranes and fibres. H&E.

large number of helper cells and/or a relative diminution of suppressor T-cells. Mori et al[269–271] have shown in a mouse model of CAH which involves immunization with liver proteins that artificial depletion of suppressor T-cell function is essential for development of autoimmune liver damage. It should be appreciated, however, that a certain proportion of the CD4+ subset may have cytotoxic properties.[272]

Further evidence indirectly favouring T-cell cytotoxicity in AI-CH are an increased expression of HLA-I (A,B,C) on liver-cell membranes as well as the demonstration of other components of the effector/target-cell binding complex (CD2, LFA-3, LFA-1 and ICAM-1).[273] Among the infiltrating T-cells, however, there appear to be more activated CD4-positive than CD8-positive T-cells.[272,274–276]

These findings do not exclude additional antibody-dependent cellular cytotoxicity. Various types of AI-CH are characterized by the presence of diagnostic marker autoantibodies in serum, such as ANA, SMA, LKM and SLA.[258,277–278] However, their corresponding antigens have not so far been shown to be expressed on the cell surface and lack organ specificity.[258,278,279] The occurrence of anti-human asialoglycoprotein receptor (ASGP-

R) in 50% of patients with AI-CH has been reported.[264,265] The anti-human ASGP-Rs were predominantly found (88%) in patients with histologically severe inflammatory activity.[264,265] Indeed, a number of investigations, mostly in in-vitro studies, favour antibody-dependent cellular cytotoxicity.[98–100,104,280–283] This would imply that an antibody directed against liver-cell membrane constituents (e.g. anti-ASGP-R[284]) might bind to a cell which then becomes the target for an Fc-receptor-bearing killer cell (K cell). On the other hand, ASGP-R has been found to be preferentially expressed on periportal hepatocytes,[285] the location of piecemeal necrosis. Also, based on in-vitro testing of T-cell clones isolated from biopsy samples of patients with AI-CH, the human hepatic ASGP-R has been identified as a major target antigen not only for humoral but also for T-cell-mediated immune reactions.[284] Therefore, T-cell-mediated cytotoxicity is a realistic pathogenetic alternative for piecemeal necrosis in AI-CH.

LKM-positive AI-CH may provide new insights into pathogenetic mechanisms of autoantibody formation and possibly also into pathogenesis of tissue damage. LKM-2 autoantibodies, reacting with P-450IIC9, have been detected in cases of autoimmune chronic hepatitis induced by tienilic acid.[252] Beaune et al[255] suggested that the drug is metabolized by cytochrome P-450IIC9 and that a reactive metabolite then binds to the P-450 protein which becomes antigenic. A similar mechanism has been proposed for dihydralazine-induced hepatitis.[256] It is premature to speculate on mechanisms mediating tissue destruction in these cases. Löhr et al[286] isolated 189 liver tissue-derived T-cell clones from patients with LKM-1-positive CH. Five of these specifically proliferated in the presence of human recombinant LKM-1 antigen.

Pathogenetic mechanisms of LKM-3 autoantibodies in chronic hepatitis D are not established and the relation of certain forms of hepatitis C to LKM-1 autoantibodies remains to be clarified.

The aetiology of AI-CH is unresolved. Drugs and viruses deserve consideration: LKM-2-positive forms have been observed after tienilic acid or dihydralazine medication. Candidate viruses suspected but not proven so far include paramyxovirus, HDV, HCV, HAV, and herpes simplex virus. There are several lines of evidence in favour of a viral aetiology:

1. There are cases positive for anti-HCV, LKM-1 and anti-GOR but their relation to anti-HCV-negative, LKM-1-positive and anti-GOR-negative cases remains to be investigated further.[249]

2. Measles virus DNA sequences have been detected in lymphocytes from patients with autoimmune hepatitis.[287]

3. The association of herpes simplex virus with autoimmunity is especially intriguing, since there appears to be molecular mimicry between LKM-1 and herpes simplex virus-1.[288]

AUTOIMMUNE OVERLAP SYNDROMES

'Overlap' syndromes have been described for autoimmune CH and primary biliary cirrhosis,[289-294] primary biliary cirrhosis and primary sclerosing cholangitis,[295] as well as for primary biliary cirrhosis and sarcoidosis.[296-298] Recently, we have observed cases of AI-CH overlapping with primary sclerosing cholangitis (Fig. 9.23).[299]

The diagnosis of an overlap syndrome requires both criteria to be fulfilled: a characteristic serological pattern as well as a combination of histological features of CAH and primary biliary cirrhosis of primary sclerosing cholangitis respectively. It has to be borne in mind that piecemeal necrosis per se is an intrinsic phenomenon of both CAH and primary biliary cirrhosis/primary sclerosing cholangitis. The mere presence of piecemeal necrosis in primary biliary cirrhosis or primary sclerosing cholangitis therefore does not establish the diagnosis of an overlap syndrome; the full pattern of CAH, including intra-acinar hepatitis, should be demonstrable in addition to histological criteria for primary biliary cirrhosis or primary sclerosing cholangitis.

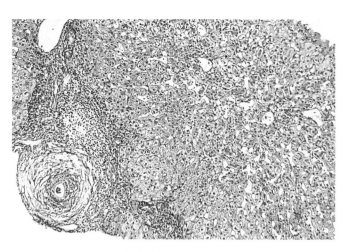

Fig. 9.23 Autoimmune CAH/PSC overlap syndrome in a 28-year-old female. ANA and pANCA strongly positive. Cholangiogram compatible with PSC. Case observation together with Prof P Berg. Tübingen, and Prof. D. Wurbs, Hamburg. There is onion-skin-like periductal fibrosis (lower left) and marked perivenular intra-acinar inflammation in addition to piecemeal necrosis. Chromotrope aniline blue.

The recognition of such overlap syndromes is important because at least some patients will respond favourably to immunosuppressive treatment. Autoimmune overlap syndromes need to be more clearly defined. It is not established whether they represent a coincidence of two diseases[274] or a hybrid of two diseases considered to be autoimmune in nature.[300]

DRUG-INDUCED CHRONIC HEPATITIS

Some drugs (p. 581) have been implicated in the production of a lesion which closely resembles other forms of CAH (e.g. alphamethyldopa, nitrofurantoin, oxyphenisatin, isoniazid).[301-303] In a number of these, autoimmune phenomena such as autoantibodies or the lupus erythematosus cell phenomenon are found:[302] LKM-2 antibodies have been associated with intake of tienilic acid[252,255] and dihydralazine.[256] No definite histological criteria are known but most cases show histological features of the autoimmune type of chronic hepatitis and some additional criteria suggesting a drug-induced reaction.[11] A major characteristic of drug-induced chronic hepatitis is clinical and histological improvement after withdrawal in most cases and relapse after rechallenge.[301]

HISTOLOGICAL DIFFERENTIAL DIAGNOSIS OF CHRONIC HEPATITIS

In the histological diagnosis of chronic hepatitis a wide range of condition has to be considered,[11] including certain forms and stages of acute viral hepatitis, primary biliary cirrhosis and sclerosing cholangitis, secondary biliary lesions, Wilson's disease and α_1-antitrypsin deficiency, certain forms of chronic alcoholic liver disease, and infections with other viruses. Portal tract configuration in a low power view represents a useful diagnostic marker (Fig. 9.24). In general, there is a tendency to over-diagnose CAH, mainly due to misinterpretation of histological features mimicking piecemeal necrosis (p. 357).

Late stages of acute hepatitis

The passage from acute into chronic hepatitis may be gradual and therefore transitional stages may be difficult to classify. Repeat biopsies may be needed. As a rule of thumb, portal and periportal lesions dominate in chronic hepatitis over parenchymal changes, with densely packed portal lymphocytes as the prevailing inflammatory cells. In acute hepatitis, parenchymal changes are prominent. Late stages of acute hepatitis are characterized by predominance of pigment-laden macrophages. In hepatitis C a distinction may be impossible because of the frequent co-existence of acinar and portal lesion.[12] Differentiation becomes difficult also in superimposed acute episodes in chronic hepatitis and, conversely, in acute hepatitis with periportal piecemeal necrosis. It should be recalled that, in the view of some hepatologists, the diagnosis of chronic hepatitis requires two biopsies with an interval of 6 months and pertinent features in both. An exception to this rule is seropositive hepatitis B with demonstrable viral antigens in the liver.

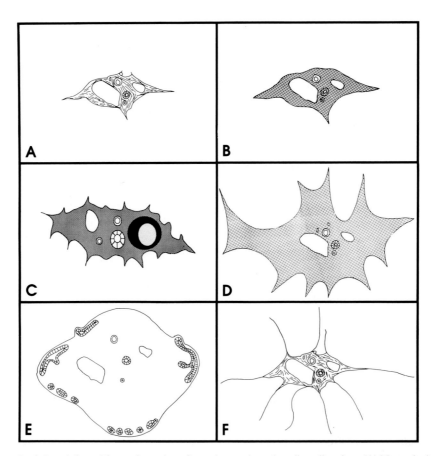

Fig. 9.24 Differential diagnosis of chronic hepatitis: configuration of portal tracts in various liver disorders. (A) Normal triangular preterminal portal tract (terminal portal tracts are round or ovoid).
(B) CPH. Portal tract highly cellular (lymphocytes), increased in size, outline somewhat smooth compared to (A), but not laciniform as in CAH (D).
(C) Typical portal tract of hepatitis C-CAH. Note moderate activity and lymphoid follicle formation.
(D) CAH. Portal tract highly cellular (lymphocytes), expanded in a maple-leaf configuration. Fibrosis mainly at original portal tract borders including active septa giving laciniform aspect.
(E) 'Biliary' portal tract as seen for example in intra- or extrahepatic mechanical bile-duct obstruction. Ballooning and rounding-off due to oedema. Marked marginal ductular proliferation. Interlobular bile duct (near artery) may be normal.
(F) Chronic alcoholic liver disease. Portal tract spider-shaped, paucicellular, with long, slender septa extending into acini. Within portal tract no or little increase in fibres.

Primary biliary cirrhosis (see Ch.12)

Primary biliary cirrhosis may pass through a stage with extensive lymphocytic piecemeal necrosis. In needle biopsies the diagnostic features, bile-duct lesions of primary biliary cirrhosis type[24] and granuloma formation, are often missed. A key observation in later stages is loss of bile ducts, a feature not characteristic of chronic viral hepatitis. Further features helpful in recognizing primary biliary cirrhosis are:

(i)   in addition to lymphocytic piecemeal necrosis, presence of 'biliary piecemeal necrosis' with cholate stasis including periportal/periseptal feathery degeneration and hepatocytic copper accumulation;[11,25]
(ii) marked ductular proliferation;
(iii) variability of the appearance of portal tracts in that some may look unchanged, others present features of non-specific reactive hepatitis or chronic active hepatitis, while in others signs of mechanical bile-duct obstruction may be seen;
(iv) the type of fibrosis with heavily condensed fibres of type I collagen in portal tracts, along marginal ductular proliferation and as septa running in a lamellar fashion parallel to the limiting plate.

Discriminating histological features are summarized in Table 9.16.

Primary sclerosing cholangitis (see Ch. 12)

This may be accompanied by piecemeal necrosis and give rise to confusion with CAH. The characteristic fibro-lamellar, onion-skin-like bile-duct lesion may be missed

Table 9.16 Differential diagnosis of chronic active hepatitis (CAH) and primary biliary cirrhosis (PBC).

	PBC	CAH
Bile-duct lesion	PBC type, ducts >50 mm	Hepatitic type, ducts < 50 μm
Granulomas	+	0 (+ in drug lesions)
Piecemeal necrosis	Broad-based, shallow	Focal, deep
'Biliary piecemeal necrosis'	+++	0 (+ in drug lesions)
Intra-acinar inflammation	Hypertrophy of sinusoidal cells	Hepatitic
Hepatocytolysis	0–+	++
Cholestatic phenomena:	++, late	0–+
Copper accumulation	Periportal ++	0–+
Mallory bodies	Periportal ++	0–+
Configuration of portal tract	Variable, often rounded (Fig. 9.24)	'Hepatitic', maple-leaf-shaped (Fig. 9.24)
Fibrosis	Dense, hypocellular, running parallel to limiting plate	Loose, active and passive septa
Cirrhosis	Biliary type	Hepatitic type

on biopsy.[304] Signs of periportal cholate stasis including copper accumulation and the special type of fibrosis as in primary biliary cirrhosis may be helpful in diagnosis. As in primary biliary cirrhosis, loss of bile ducts in characteristic.

Drug-induced chronic hepatitis (see Ch. 15)

Diagnosis is guided by some additional features reflecting a possible hypersensitivity reaction. These include:

(i)   granuloma formation;
(ii) bile-duct lesions, usually distinct from the primary biliary cirrhosis and hepatitic type and involving the smallest portal ducts and ductules;[304,305]
(iii) portal inflammation varying in density from one portal tract to another and usually less pronounced than in virus-induced forms;
(iv) punched-out perivenular confluent necrosis with or without bridging and which may resemble the effect of toxins such as paracetamol;
(v)   eosinophils may be an indicator but are often missing.

Chronic liver disease in alcoholics (see Ch. 8)

The recognition of pure chronic alcoholic liver disease usually creates no diagnostic problems. The lymphocyte is not the dominant inflammatory cell. There are, however, cases, mostly advanced, with superimposed features of CAH including piecemeal necrosis. It is not established whether this represents induction of secondary autoimmunity or whether there is a coincidence of chronic alcoholic liver disease and independent HCV infection. Prevalence of anti-HBc positivity in alcoholics is recorded as 25–50%, which is about 10 times the prevalence in the normal population.[306,307] Histological diagnosis in these cases should mention both components.

Wilson's disease and α_1-antitrypsin deficiency (see Ch. 4)

Piecemeal necrosis may be seen in some stages of the evolution of both. Wilson's disease is likely to be misinterpreted as CAH and therefore nearly curative treatment may be delayed. A diagnosis of 'cryptogenic CAH' should always arouse suspicion as to the possibility of Wilson's disease. Features favouring Wilson's disease are copper distribution of a type different from secondary ('precholestatic') accumulation as in primary biliary cirrhosis or 'cholestatic' CAH, fatty change, nuclear vacuolation, cytoplasmic swelling, marked lipofuscinosis, Mallory bodies in a periportal location and a more pronounced ductular proliferation and fibrosis than in CAH of other origin. It should be kept in mind that in some phases of Wilson's disease there may be no hepatic copper accumulation.

Despite the presence of piecemeal necrosis, homozygous α_1-antitrypsin deficiency is easily recognized in a PAS stain after diastase digestion by the typical PAS-positive intracytoplasmic globules restricted to periportal hepatocytes.

Malignant lymphoma

Some forms of malignant lymphoma may be mistaken for CAH. The absence of an inflammatory reaction in portal tracts and particularly within acini, together with the presence of an extremely densely packed, monotonous lymphoid portal infiltration, may establish the correct diagnosis, especially if the infiltrating cells can be shown to be monoclonal.

REFERENCES

1. Fogarty International Center Criteria Committee. Diseases of the liver and biliary tract. Standardization of nomenclature, diagnostic criteria, and diagnostic methodology. Washington: US Government Printing Office, 1976: pp 9–11
2. De Groote J, Desmet V, Gedigk P et al. A classification of chronic hepatitis. Lancet 1968; ii: 626–628
3. Popper H, Schaffner F. Chronic hepatitis: taxonomic, etiologic and therapeutic problems. In: Popper H, Schaffner F, eds. Progress in liver diseases, vol V. New York: Grune & Stratton, 1976: pp 531–558
4. Popper H, Schaffner F. The vocabulary of chronic hepatitis. New Engl J Med 1971; 284: 1154–1156
5. Popper H. Changing concepts of the evolution of chronic hepatitis and the role of piecemeal necrosis. Hepatology 1983; 3: 758–762
6. Gudat F, Bianchi L, Sonnabend W, Thiel G, Aenishänslin W, Stalder G. Pattern of core and surface expression in liver tissue reflects state of specific immune response in hepatitis B. Lab Invest 1975; 32: 1–9
7. Scheuer P J. Classification of chronic viral hepatitis: a need for reassessment. J Hepatol 1991; 13: 372–374
8. Gerber M. Chronic hepatitis C: the beginning of the end of a time-honored nomenclature? Hepatology 1992; 15: 733–734
9. Desmet V J. Histopathology of chronic viral hepatitis. In: Callea F, Zorzi M, Desmet V J, eds. Viral hepatitis. Berlin: Springer, 1986: pp 32–40
10. Bianchi L, De Groote J, Desmet V et al. Morphological criteria in viral hepatitis. Lancet 1971; i: 914–919
11. Bianchi L. Liver biopsy interpretation in hepatitis. Part II: Histopathology and classification of acute and chronic hepatitis/ differential diagnosis. Path Res Pract 1983; 178: 180–213
12. Scheuer P J, Ashrafzadeh P, Sherlock S, Brown D, Dusheiko G. The pathology of hepatitis C. Hepatology 1922; 15: 567–571
13. De Groote J, Fevery J, Verbrugghe J, Desmet V, Vandenbroucke J. Less active chronic hepatitis. A follow up of 59 patients. 5th World Congress of Gastroenterology. Mexico: 1974
14. Weissberg J, Andres L, Smith C et al. Survival in chronic hepatitis B: an analysis of 379 patients. Ann Int Med 1984; 101: 613–616
15. Vido I, Selmair H, Wildhirt E, Ortmans H. Zur Prognose der chronischen Hepatitis. I. Formen und Entwicklungsstadien. Dtsch Med Wschr 1969; 94: 2215–2218
16. Chu C M, Karayiannis P, Fowler M J F, Monjardino J, Liaw Y F, Thomas H C. Natural history of chronic hepatitis B virus infection in Taiwan: studies of hepatitis B virus DNA in serum. Hepatology 1985; 5: 431–434
17. Hopf U, Möller B, Küther D et al. Long-term follow-up of posttransfusion and sporadic chronic hepatitis non-A, non-B and frequency of circulating antibodies to hepatitis-C virus (HCV). J Hepatol 1990; 10: 69–76
18. Gerber M, Vernace S. Chronic septal hepatitis. Virchows Arch (A) 1974; 363: 303–309
19. Czaja A, Ludwig J, Baggenstoss A, Wolf A. Corticosteroid-treated chronic active hepatitis in remission: uncertain prognosis of chronic persistent hepatitis. N Engl J Med 1981; 304: 5–9
20. Edmondson H, Peters R. Liver. In: Anderson W, Kissane J, eds. Pathology, 7th edn. St Louis: Mosby, 1977: pp 1321–1438
21. Peters R L. Viral hepatitis: a pathologic spectrum. Am J Med Sci 1975; 270: 17–31
22. Liaw Y F, Chu C M, Chen T J, Lin D Y, Chang-Chien C S, Wu C S. Chronic lobular hepatitis: a clinicopathological and prognostic study. Hepatology 1982; 2: 258–262
23. Wilkinson S P, Portmann B, Cochrane A M G et al. Clinical course of chronic lobular hepatitis. J Med 1978; 188: 421–429
24. Poulsen H, Christoffersen P. Atlas of liver biopsies. Copenhagen: Munksgaard, 1979
25. Bianchi L. Liver biopsy interpretation in hepatitis. Part I: Presentation of critical morphologic features used in diagnosis (Glossary). Path Res Pract 1983; 178: 2–19
26. Christoffersen P, Dietrichson O, Faber V, Poulsen H. The occurrence and significance of abnormal bile duct epithelium in chronic aggressive hepatitis. Acta Path Microbiol Scand A 1972; 80: 294–302
27. Schmid M, Pirovino M, Altorfer J, Gudat F, Bianchi L. Acute hepatitis non-A, non-B; are there any specific light mircoscopic features? Liver 1982; 2: 61–67
28. Popper H, Paronetto F, Schaffner F. Immune processes in the pathogenesis of liver disease. Ann N Y Acad Sci 1965; 124: 781–799
29. Bianchi L, De Groote J, Desmet V et al. Acute and chronic hepatitis revisited. Lancet 1977; ii: 714–719
30. Kerr J F R, Cooksley W G E, Searle J et al. The nature of piecemeal necrosis in chronic active hepatitis. Lancet 1979; ii: 827–828
31. Desmet V. New aspects of piecemeal necrosis. In: Bianchi L, Gerok W, Popper H, eds. Trends in hepatology. Lancaster: MTP Press, 1985: pp 183–200
32. Bianchi L. Necroinflammatory liver diseases. Sem Liver Dis 1986; 6: 185–198
33. Wyllie A, Kerr J, Currie A. Cell death — the significance of apoptosis. Internat Rev Cytol 1980; 68: 251–305
34. Popper H. Hepatocellular degeneration and death. In: Arias I, Jakoby W, Popper H, Schachter D, Shafritz D, eds. The Liver: biology and pathobiology, 2nd edn. New York: Raven Press, 1988: pp 1087–1103
35. Popper H. Pathologic aspects of cirrhosis. A review. Am J Path 1977; 87: 227–264
36. Rebora A, Rongioletti F. Lichen planus and chronic active hepatitis. A retrospective study. Acta Derm Venereol 1984; 64: 52
37. Rebora A. Lichen planus and the liver. Lancet 1981; ii: 805
38. Desmet V J. Liver lesions in hepatitis B viral infection. Yale J Biol Med 1988; 61: 61–83
39. Eggink H F, Houthoff H J, Huitema S, Gips C H, Poppema S. Cellular and humoral immune reactions in chronic active liver disease. I. Lymphocyte subsets in liver biopsies of patients with untreated idiopathic autoimmune hepatitis, chronic active hepatitis B and primary biliary cirrhosis. Clin Exp Immunol 1982; 50: 17–24
40. Eggink H F, Hofstee N, Gips C H, Krom R A F, Houthoff H J. Histopathology of serial graft biopsies from liver transplant recipients. Am J Path 1984; 114: 18–31
41. Montano L, Aranguibel F, Boffill M, Goodall A H, Janossy G, Thomas H C. An analysis of the composition of the inflammatory infiltrate in autoimmune and hepatitis B virus-induced chronic liver disease. Hepatology 1983; 3: 292–296
42. Si L, Whiteside T L. Tissue distribution of human NK cells studied with anti-Leu-7 monoclonal antibody. J Immunol 1983; 130: 2149–2155
43. Si L, Whiteside T L, Van Thiel D, Rabin B S. Lymphocyte subpopulations at the site of "piecemeal" necrosis in end stage chronic liver diseases and rejecting liver allografts in cyclosporine-treated patients. Lab Invest 1984; 50: 341–347
44. Colucci G, Colombo M, Del Ninno E, Paronetto F. In situ characterization by monoclonal antibodies of the mononuclear cell infiltrate in chronic active hepatitis. Gastroenterology 1983; 85: 1138–1145

45. Bardadin K, Desmet V. Ultrastructural observations on sinusoidal endothelial cells in chronic active hepatitis. Histopathology 1985; 9: 171–181

46. Bardadin K A, Desmet V J. Interdigitating and dendritic reticulum cells in chronic active hepatitis. Histopathology 1984; 8: 657–668

47. Thomas H, Shipton U, Montano L. The HLA system: Its relevance to the pathogenesis of liver disease. In: Popper H, Schaffner F, eds. Progress in liver diseases, vol VII. Orlando: Grune & Stratton, 1982: pp 517–527

48. Van den Oord J J, Desmet V J. Verteilungsmuster der Histokompatibilitäts-Hauptantigene im normalen und pathologischen Lebergewebe. Leber Magen Darm 1984; 14: 244–254

49. Popper H. The problem of histologic evaluation of primary biliary cirrhosis. Virchows Arch A 1978; 379: 99–102

50. Abe H, Beninger P, Ikejiri N, Setoyama H, Sata M, Tanikawa K. Light microscopic findings of liver biopsy specimens from patients with hepatitis type A and comparison with type B. Gastroenterology 1982; 82: 938–947

51. Teixeira M R, Weller I V D, Murray A et al. The pathology of hepatitis A in man. Liver 1982; 2: 53–60

52. Thung S, Gerber M. The formation of elastic fibers in livers with massive hepatic necrosis. Arch Path Lab Med 1982; 106: 468–469

53. Thaler H. Leberkrankheiten. Klinisch-morphologische Diagnostik und ihre Grundlagen. Berlin: Springer, 1987

54. Rizzetto M, Verme G. Delta hepatitis — present status. J Hepatol 1985; 1: 187–193

55. De Groote J, Fevery J, Lepoutre L. Long-term follow-up of chronic active hepatitis of moderate severity. Gut 1978; 19: 510–513

56. Boyer J, Klatskin G. Patterns of necrosis in acute viral hepatitis. Prognostic value of bridging (subacute hepatic necrosis). N Engl J Med 1970; 283: 1063–1071

57. Chen T, Liaw Y. The prognostic significance of bridging hepatic necrosis in chronic type B hepatitis: a histopathologic study. Liver 1988; 8: 10–17

58. Cooksley W, Bradbear R, Robinson W et al. The prognosis of chronic active hepatitis without cirrhosis in relation to bridging necrosis. Hepatology 1986; 6: 345–348

59. Combes B. The initial morphologic lesion in chronic hepatitis, important or unimportant? Hepatology 1986; 6: 518–522

60. Knodell R G, Ishak K G, Black W C et al. Formulation and application of a numerical scoring system for assessing histological activity in asymptomatic chronic active hepatitis. Hepatology 1981; 1: 431–435

61. Dudley F J, Fox R A, Sherlock S. Cellular immunity and hepatitis-associated, Australia antigen liver disease. Lancet 1972; i: 723–726

62. Eddleston A L W F, Williams R. Inadequate antibody response to HB Ag or suppressor T-cell defect in development of active chronic hepatitis. Lancet 1974; ii: 1543–1545

63. Barnaba V, Balsano F. Immunologic and molecular basis of viral persistence. The hepatitis B virus model. J Hepatol 1992; 14: 391–400

64. Tiollais P, Pourcel C, Dejean A. The hepatitis B virus. Nature 1985; 317: 489–495

65. Carman W F, Thomas H C. Genetic variation in hepatitis B virus. Gastroenterology 1992; 102: 711–719

66. Gerlich W H, Thomssen R. Terminology, structure, and laboratory diagnosis of hepatitis viruses. In: McIntyre N, Benhamou J-P, Bircher J, Rizzetto M, Rodes J, eds. Oxford textbook of clinical hepatology. Oxford: Oxford University Press, 1991: pp 537–565

67. Tiollais P, Buendia M-A. Hepatitis B virus, Scientific American 1991; 264/4: 48–54

68. Milich D R, Jones J E, Hughes J L, Price J, Raney A K, McLachlan A. Is a function of the secreted hepatitis B e antigen to induce immunologic tolerance in utero? Proc Natl Acad Sci USA 1990; 87: 6599–6603

69. Bonino F, Rizzetto M, Will H. Hepatitis B virus unable to secrete e antigen. Gastroenterology 1991; 100: 1138–1141

70. Thomas H, Carman W. The host immune response may be responsible for selection of envelope and precore/core variants of HBV. J Hepatol 1991; 13, suppl 4: S108–S113

71. Marion P L, Salazar F H, Alexander J J, Robinson W S. State of hepatitis B viral DNA in a human hepatoma cell line. J Virol 1980; 33: 795–806

72. Chakraborty P R, Ruiz-Opazo N, Shouval D, Shafritz D A. Identification of integrated hepatitis B virus DNA and expression of viral RNA in a HBsAg-producing human hepatocellular carcinoma cell line. Nature 1980; 286: 531–533

73. Brechot C, Pourcel C, Louise A, Rain B, Tiollais P. Presence of integrated hepatitis B virus DNA sequences in cellular DNA of human hepatocellular carcinoma. Nature 1980; 286: 533–535

74. Shafritz D, Shouval D, Sherman H et al. Integration of hepatitis B virus DNA into the genome of the liver cells in chronic liver disease and hepatocellular carcinoma. N Engl J Med 1981; 305: 1067–1073

75. Hino O, Kitagawa T, Koike K et al. Detection of hepatitis B virus DNA in hepatocellular carcinomas in Japan. Hepatology 1984; 4: 90–95

76. Hadziyannis S J, Lieberman H M, Karvountzis G G, Shafritz D A. Analysis of liver disease, nuclear HBcAg, viral replication, and hepatitis B virus DNA in liver and serum of HBeAg vs. anti-Hbe positive carriers of hepatitis B virus. Hepatology 1983; 3: 656–662

77. Tozuka S, Uchida T, Suzuki K, Esumi M, Shikata T. State of hepatitis B virus DNA in hepatocytes of patients with noncarcinomatous liver disease. Arch Pathol Lab Med 1989; 113: 20–25

78. Burrell C J, Gowans E J, Jilbert A R, Lake J R, Marmion B P. HBV DNA by in situ cytohybridization; implications for viral replication strategy and pathogenesis of chronic hepatitis. Hepatology 1982; 2: 85S–91S

79. Burrell C J, Gowans E J, Rowland R, Hall P, Jilbert A R, Marmion B P. Correlation between liver histology and markers of hepatitis B virus replication in infected patients: A study by in situ hybridization. Hepatology 1984; 4: 20–24

80. Gowans E, Burrell C J, Jilbert A R, Marmion B P. Patterns of single- and double-stranded hepatitis B virus DNA and viral antigen accumulation in infected liver cells. J General Virol 1983; 64: 1229–1239

81. Brechot C. State of HBV DNA in liver diseases. Hepatology 1982; 2: 278

82. Loriot M A, Marcellin P, Bismuth E et al. Demonstration of hepatitis B virus DNA by polymerase chain reaction in the serum and the liver after spontaneous or therapeutically induced HBeAg to anit-HBe or HBsAg to anti-HBs seroconversion in patients with chronic hepatitis B. Hepatology 1992; 15: 32–36

83. Tanaka Y, Esumi M, Shikata T. Persistence of hepatitis B virus DNA after serological clearance of hepatitis B virus. Liver 1990; 10: 6–10

84. Blum H E, Haase A T, Vyas G N. Molecular pathogenesis of the infection with the hepatitis B virus: simultaneous demonstration of DNA and viral antigens in paraffin-embedded liver sections. Lancet 1984; ii: 771–775

85. Infantolino D, Pinarello A, Ceccato R, Barbazza R. HBV-DNA by in situ hybridization. A method to improve sensitivity on formalin-fixed, paraffin-embedded liver biopsies. Liver 1989; 9: 360–366

86. Lau J Y N, Naoumov N V, Alexander G J M, Williams R. Rapid detection of hepatitis B virus DNA in liver tissue by in situ hybridisation and its combination with immunohistochemistry for simultaneous detection of HBV antigens. J Clin Pathol 1991; 44: 905–908

87. Brechot C, Hadchouel M, Scotto J et al. State of hepatitis B virus DNA in hepatocytes of patients with hepatitis B surface antigen-positive and -negative liver diseases. Proc Nat Acad Sci USA 1981; 78: 3906–3910

88. Diamantis I, McGandy C, Pult I et al. Polymerase chain reaction detects hepatitis B virus DNA in paraffin-embedded liver tissue from patients sero- and histo-negative for active hepatitis B. Virchows Arch (A) 1992; 420: 11–15

89. Lampertico P, Malter J, Colombo M, Gerber M. Detection of hepatitis B virus DNA in formalin-fixed, paraffin-embedded liver tissue by the polymerase chain reaction. Am J Path 1990; 137: 253–258

90. Brechot C, Kremsdorf D, Paterlini P, Thiers V. Hepatitis B virus DNA in HBsAg-negative patients. Molecular characterization and clinical implications. J Hepatol 1991; 13(suppl 4): S49–S55

91. Goldin R D, Fish D E, Hay A et al. Histological and immunohistochemical study of hepatitis B virus in human immunodeficiency virus infection. J Clin Pathol 1990; 43: 203–205

92. Volpes R, van den Oord J J, De Vos R, Desmet V J. Hepatic expression of type A and type B receptors for tumour necrosis factor. J Hepatol 1992; 14: 361–369

93. Van den Oord J J, De Vos R, Facchetti F, Delabie J, De Wolf-Peters C, Desmet V J. Distribution of non-lymphoid, inflammatory cells in chronic HBV infection. J Pathol 1990; 160: 223–230

94. Hata K, Van Thiel D H, Herberman R B, Whiteside T L. Phenotypic and functional characteristics of lymphocytes isolated from liver biopsy specimens from patients with active liver disease. Hepatology 1992; 15: 816–823

95. Garcia-Monzon C, Moreno-Otero R, Pajares J M et al. Expression of a novel activation antigen on intrahepatic CD8+ T lymphocytes in viral chronic active hepatitis. Gastroenterology 1990; 98: 1029–1035

96. Alberti A, Trevisan A, Fattovich G et al. The role of hepatitis B virus replication and hepatocyte membrane expression in the pathogenesis of HBV-related hepatic damage. In: Chisari F V, ed. Advances in hepatitis research. New York: Masson, 1984: pp 134–143

97. Thomas H C, Lok A S F. The immunopathology of autoimmune and hepatitis B virus-induced chronic hepatitis. Sem Liver Dis 1984; 4: 36–46

98. Mondelli M, Eddleston A. Mechanisms of liver cell injury in acute and chronic hepatitis B. Sem Liver Dis 1984; 4: 47–58

99. Gerber M, Immunopathology of chronic hepatitis. In: Farber E, Phillips M, Kaufman N, eds. Pathogenesis of liver diseases. IAP Monographs, no. 28. Baltimore: Williams & Wilkins, 1987: pp 54–64

100. Eddleston A L W F, Mondelli M, Mieli-Vergani G, Williams R. Lymphocyte cytotoxicity to autologous hepatocytes in chronic hepatitis B virus infection. Hepatology 1982; 2: 122S–127S

101. Mieli-Vergani G, Vergani D, Portmann B et al. Lymphocyte cytotoxicity to autologous hepatocytes in HBsAg positive chronic liver disease. Gut 1982; 23: 1029–1036

102. Poralla T, Hütteroth T, Staritz M, Meyer zum Büschenfelde K. Cellular cytotoxicity against autologous hepatocytes in chronic hepatitis B — its relationship to the HBeAg/anti-HBe status. Z Gastroenterol 1985; 23: 183–187

103. Moriyama T, Guilhot S, Klopchin K et al. Immunobiology and pathogenesis of hepatocellular injury in hepatitis B virus transgenic mice. Science 1990; 248: 361–364

104. Thomas H C, Montano L, Goodall A, De Koning R, Oladapo J, Wiedmann K H. Immunologic mechanisms in chronic hepatitis B virus infection. Hepatology 1982; 2: 116S–121S

105. Ferrari C, Penna A, DegliAntoni A, Fiaccadori F. Cellular immune response to hepatitis B virus antigens. J Hepatol 1988; 7: 21–33

106. Liehr H, Grün M. Endotoxins in liver disease. In: Popper H, Schaffner F, eds. Progress in liver diseases, vol VI. New York: Grune & Stratton, 1979: pp 313–326

107. Mori W, Shiga J, Irie H. Shwartzman reaction as a pathogenetic mechanism in fulminant hepatitis. Sem Liver Dis 1986; 6: 267–276

108. Sheron N, Lau J, Daniels H et al. Increased production of tumour necrosis factor alpha in chronic hepatitis B virus infection. J Hepatol 1991; 12: 241–245

109. Lau J, Sheron N, Nouri-Aria K, Alexander G, Williams R. Increased tumour necrosis factor 1α receptor number in chronic hepatitis B virus infection. Hepatology 1991; 14: 44–50

110. Milich D R, McLachlan A, Moriarty A, Thornton G B. Immune response to hepatitis B virus core antigen (HBcAg): localization of T cell recognition sites within HBcAg/HBeAg. J Immunol 1987; 139: 1223–1231

111. Jung M-C, Spengler U, Schraut W et al. Hepatitis B virus antigen-specific T-cell activation in patients with acute and chronic hepatitis B. J Hepatol 1991; 13: 310–317

112. Celis E, Ou D, Otvos Jr L. Recognition of hepatitis B surface antigen by human T lymphocytes. Proliferative and cytotoxic responses to a major antigenic determinant defined by synthetic peptides. J Immunol 1988; 140: 1808–1815

113. Sällberg M, Ruden U, Wahren B, Noah M, Magnius L O. Human and murine B-cells recognize the HBeAg/beta (or HBe2) epitope as a linear determinant. Molecular Immunol 1991; 28: 719–726

114. Sasaki H, Kojima T, Matsui S, Aoyama K, Inoue K. Interaction of lymphocytes with hepatocytes containing hepatitis B antigen: ultrastructural demonstration of target antigen and T-cell subsets by the peroxidase antibody technique. Virchows Arch (A) 1987; 411: 489–498

115. Michalak T I, Lin B, Churchill N D, Dzwonkowski P, Desousa J R B. Hepadna virus nucleocapsid and surface antigens and the antigen-specific antibodies associated with hepatocyte plasma membranes in experimental woodchuck acute hepatitis. Lab Invest 1990; 62: 680–689

116. Ferrari C, Cavalli A, Penna A et al. Fine specificity of the human T-cell response to the hepatitis B virus preS1 antigen. Gastroenterology 1992; 103: 255–263

117. Mondelli M U, Bortolotti F, Pontisso P et al. Definitions of hepatitis B virus (HBV)-specific target antigens recognized by cytotoxic T cells in acute HBV infection. Clin Exp Immunol 1987; 68: 242–250

118. Mondelli M, Mieli-Vergani G, Alberti A et al. T-lymphocyte cytotoxicity to autologous hepatocytes in chronic hepatitis B virus infection: Evidence that T cells are directed against HB core antigen on hepatocytes. J Immunol 1982; 129: 2773–2778

119. Yamada G, Takaguchi K, Matsueda K et al. Immunoelectron microscopic observation of intrahepatic HBeAg in patients with chronic hepatitis B. Hepatology 1990; 12: 133–140

120. Girones R, Miller R H. Mutation rate of the hepadnavirus genome. Virology 1989; 170: 595–597

121. Terre S, Rodmorduc O, Kremsdorf D, Petit M-A, Brechot C. Reverse transcription and packaging of hepatitis B virus (HBV)-RNA generates in vivo defective serum HBV particles. J Hepatol 1991; 13 (suppl 4): S42–S48

122. Gerken G, Kremsdorf D, Petit M A, Manns M, Meyer zum Büschenfelde K-H, Brechot C. Hepatitis B defective virus with rearrangements in the preS gene during HBV chronic infection. J Hepatol 1991; 13 (suppl 4): S93–S96

123. Okamoto H, Imai M, Tsuda F et al. Point mutation in the S gene of hepatitis B virus for a d/y or w/r subtypic change in two blood donors carrying a surface compound subtype adyr or adwr. J Virol 1987; 61: 3030–3034

124. Raimondo G, Campo S, Smedile V et al. Hepatitis B virus variant, with a deletion in the preS2 and two translational stop codons in the precore regions, in a patient with hepatocellular carcinoma. J Hepatol 1991; 13 (suppl 4): S74–S77

125. Carman W F, Zanetti A R, Karayiannis P et al. Vaccine-induced escape mutant of hepatitis B virus. Lancet 1990; 336: 325–329

126. Lee H-S, Ulrich P P, Vyas G N. Mutations in the S-gene affecting the immunologic determinants of the envelope protein of hepatitis B virus. J Hepatol 1991; 13 (suppl 4): S97–S101

127. Brunetto R M, Stemler M, Schödel F et al. Identification of HBV variants which cannot produce precore derived HBeAg and may be responsible for severe hepatitis. Ital J Gastroenterol 1989; 21: 151–154

128. Ulrich P P, Bhat R A, Kelly I, Brunetto M R, Bonino F, Vyas G N. A precore-defective mutant of hepatitis B virus associated with e antigen-negative chronic liver disease. J Med Virol 1990; 32: 109–118

129. Peters M G. Second-generation hepatitis C antibody testing. Am J Clin Pathol 1992; 98: 4

130. Petersen E E, Clemens R, Bock H L, Friese K, Hess G. Hepatitis B and C in heterosexual patients with various sexually transmitted diseases. Infection 1992; 20: 128–131

131. Tong S, Brotman B, Li J et al. In vitro and in vivo replication capacity of the precore region defective hepatitis B virus variants. J Hepatol 1991; 13, (suppl 4): S68–S73

132. Kosaka Y, Takase K, Kojima M et al. Fulminant hepatitis B: induction by hepatitis B virus mutants defective in the precore region and incapable of encoding e antigen. Gastroenterology 1991; 100: 1087–1094

133. Naoumov N V, Schneider R, Grötzinger T et al. Precore mutant hepatitis B virus infection and liver disease. Gastroenterology 1992; 102: 538–543

134. Brunetto M R, Stemler M, Bonino F et al. A new hepatitis B virus strain in patients with severe anti-HBe positive chronic hepatitis B. J Hepatol 1990; 10: 258–261

135. Santantonio T, Jung M, Miska S et al. High prevalence and heterogeneity of HBV preC mutants in anti-HBe-positive carriers with chronic liver disease in Southern Italy. J Hepatol 1991; 13 (suppl 4): S78–S81

136. Carman W F, Jacyna M R, Hadziyannis S et al. Mutation preventing formation of hepatitis B e antigen in patients with chronic hepatitis B infection. Lancet 1989; ii: 588–591

137. Okamoto H, Yotsumoto S, Akahane Y et al. Hepatitis B viruses with precore region defects prevail in persistently infected hosts along with seroconversion to the antibody against e antigen. J Virol 1990; 64: 1298–1303

138. Brunetto M R, Giarin M M, Oliveri F et al. Wild-type and e antigen-minus hepatitis B viruses and course of chronic hepatitis. Proc Natl Acad Sci USA 1991; 88: 4186–4190

139. Feitelson M, Duan L, Horiike N, Clayton M. Hepatitis B X open reading frame deletion mutants isolated from atypical hepatitis B virus infections. J Hepatol 1991; 13 (suppl 4): S58–S60

140. Weiner A J, Kuo G, Bradley D W et al. Detection of hepatitis C viral sequences in non-A, non-B hepatitis. Lancet 1990; 335: 1–3

141. Fong T, Di Bisceglie A, Waggoner J, Banks S, Hoofnagle J. The significance of antibody to hepatitis C virus in patients with chronic hepatitis B. Hepatology 1991; 14: 64–67

142. Ruiz J, Sangro B, Cuende J I et al. Hepatitis B and C viral infections in patients with hepatocellular carcinoma. Hepatology 1992; 16: 637–641

143. Moraleda G, Bartolome J, Molina J, Castillo I, Carreno V. Analysis of hepatitis B virus DNA, liver disease and influence of antibody to hepatitis C virus in anti-HBe chronic carriers. Liver 1991; 11: 352–357

144. Oguchi H, Miyasaka M, Tokunaga S et al. Hepatitis virus infection (HBV and HCV) in eleven Japanese hemodialysis units. Clin Nephrol 1992; 38: 36–43

145. Liaw A F, Lin S M, Sheen I S, Chu D M. Acute hepatitis C virus superinfection followed by spontaneous HBeAg seroconversion and HBsAg elimination. Infection 1991; 19: 250–251

146. Wu P C, Lok A S F, Lau J Y N, Lauder I J, Lai C L. Histological changes in Chinese patients with chronic hepatitis B virus infection after interferon-α therapy. Am J Clin Pathol 1992; 98: 402–407

147. Hoofnagle J H, Peters M, Mullen K D et al. Randomized, controlled trial of recombinant human alpha-interferon in patients with chronic hepatitis B. Gastroenterology 1988; 95: 1318–1325

148. Fevery J, Elewaut A, Michielsen P et al. Efficacy of interferon alpha-2b with or without prednisone withdrawal in the treatment of chronic viral hepatitis B. A prospective double-blind Belgian-Dutch study. J Hepatol 1990; 323: 295–301

149. Hess G, Gerlich W, Slusarczyk J, Hütteroth T H, Meyer zum Büschenfelde K H. Treatment of hepatitis B surface antigen (HBsAg)-positive chronic hepatitis with recombinant leucocyte alpha-A interferon. J Hepatol 1986; 3: S245–S251

150. De Man R A, Schalm S W, Heijtink R A et al. Long-term follow-up of antiviral combination therapy in chronic hepatitis B. Am J Med 1988; 85: 150–154

151. Perez V, Tanno H, Villamil F, Fay O. Recombinant interferon-alpha-2b following prednisone withdrawal in the treatment of chronic type B hepatitis. J Hepatol 1990; 11: S113–S117

152. Liaw Y F, Lin S M, Sheen I S, Chen T J, Chu C M. Treatment of chronic type B hepatitis in Southeast Asia. Am J Med 1988; 85: 147–149.

153. Lok A S, Lai C L, Wu P C, Leung E K. Long-term follow-up in a randomized controlled trial of recombinant alpha 2-interferon in Chinese patients with chronic hepatitis B infection. Lancet 1988; ii: 298–302

154. Huang S N, Neurath A R. Immunohistologic demonstration of hepatitis B viral antigens in liver with reference to its significance in liver injury. Lab Invest 1979; 40: 1–17

155. Rugge M, Guido M, Bortolotti F, Cassaro M, Cadrobbi P, Noventa F, Realdi G. Histology and virus expression in the liver: a prognostic puzzle in chronic hepatitis B. Virchows Arch (A) 1991; 419: 93–97

156. Mondelli M, Tedder R S, Ferns B, Pontisso P, Realdi G, Alberti A. Differential distribution of hepatitis B core and E antigens in hepatocytes: analysis by monoclonal antibodies. Hepatology 1986; 6: 199–204

157. Chu C M, Liaw Y F. Intrahepatic distribution of hepatitis B surface and core antigens in chronic hepatitis B virus infection. Gastroenterology 1987; 92: 220–225

158. Gowans E J, Burrell C J. Widespread presence of cytoplasmic HBcAg in hepatitis B infected liver detected by improved immunochemical methods. J Clin Pathol 1985; 38: 393–398

159. Chu C M, Liaw Y F. Immunohistological study of intrahepatic expression of hepatitis B core and E antigens in chronic type B hepatitis. J Clin Pathol 1992; 45: 791–795

160. Ray M B, Desmet V J, Bradburne A F, Desmyter J, Fevery J, De Groote J. Differential distribution of hepatitis B surface antigen and hepatitis B core antigen in the liver of hepatitis B patients. Gastroenterology 1976; 71: 462–469

161. Nowoslawski A, Brzosko W J, Madalinski K, Krawczynski K. Cellular localization of Australia antigen in the liver of patients with lymphoproliferative disorders. Lancet 1970; i: 494–498

162. Kakumu S, Arao M, Yoshioka K, Tsutsumi Y, Inoue M. Distribution of HBcAg in hepatitis B detected by immunoperoxidase staining with three different preparations of anti-HBc antibodies. J Clin Pathol 1989; 42: 284–288

163. Kamimura T, Yoshiike F, Ichida F et al. Electron microscopic studies of Dane particles in hepatocytes with special reference to intracellular development of Dane particles and their relation with HBeAg in serum. Hepatology 1981; 1: 392–397

164. Yamada G, Sakamoto M, Mizuno T et al. Electron and immuno-electron microscopic study of Dane particle formation in chronic hepatitis B virus infection. Gastroenterology 1982; 83: 348–356

165. Bianchi L, Gudat F. Sanded nuclei in hepatitis B. Lab Invest 1976; 35: 1–5

166. Ballare M, Lavarini C, Brunetto M R et al. Relationship between the intrahepatic expression of e and c epitopes of the nucleocapsid protein of hepatitis B virus and viraemia. Clin Exp Immunol 1989; 75: 64–69

167. Chu C M, Liaw Y F. Intrahepatic expression of HBcAg in chronic HBV hepatitis: lessons from molecular biology. Hepatology 1990; 12: 1443–1445

168. Robinson W S. Hepatitis B virus. In: Deinhardt F, Deinhardt J, eds. Viral hepatitis: laboratory and clinical science. New York: M. Dekker, 1983: pp 57–116

169. Gudat F, Bianchi L. HBsAg: A target antigen on the liver cell? In: Popper H, Bianchi L, Reutter W, eds. Membrane alterations as basis of liver injury. Lancaster: MTP Press, 1977: pp 171–178

170. Hadziyannis S, Gerber M A, Vissoulis C, Popper H. Cytoplasmic hepatitis B antigen in "ground glass" hepatocytes of carriers. Arch Pathol 1973; 96: 327–330

171. Gerber M A, Hadziyannis S, Vissoulis C, Schaffner F, Paronetto F, Popper H. Electron microscopy and immunoelectronmicroscopy of cytoplasmic hepatitis B antigen in hepatocytes. Am J Pathol 1974; 75: 489–502

172. Yamada G, Nakane P K. Hepatitis B core and surface antigens in liver tissue. Light and electron microscopic localization by the peroxidase-labelled antibody method. Lab Invest 1977; 36: 649–659

173. Magnius L O, Espmark J A. New specificities in Australia antigen positive sera distinct from the Le Bouvier determinants. J Immunol 1972; 109: 1017–1021

174. Takahashi K, Akahane Y, Gotanda T et al. Demonstration of hepatitis B-e antigen in the core of Dane particles. J Immunol 1979; 122: 275–279

175. Miyakawa Y, Mayumi M, HBeAg-anti-HBe system in hepatitis B virus infection. In: Szmuness W, Alter H J, Maynard J E, eds. Viral hepatitis. 1981 International Symposium. Philadelphia: The Franklin Institute Press, 1982: pp 183–194

176. Arnold W, Neilsen J O, Hardt F, Meyer zum Büschenfelde K H. Localization of e-antigen in nuclei of hepatocytes in HBsAg-positive liver diseases. Gut 1977; 18: 994–996

177. Mondelli M, Tedder R S, Ferns B, Pontisso P, Realdi G, Albert A. Differential distribution of hepatitis B core and e antigens in hepatocytes: analysis by monoclonal antibodies. Hepatology 1988; 6: 199–204

178. Alberti A, Mondelli M, Pontisso P, Tedder R S, Busachi C A, Realdi G. Hepatitis B core (HBcAg) and e (HBeAg) antigens in the liver detected by immunofluorescence with monoclonal antibodies. European Association for the Study of the Liver. Southampton, 1983: poster abstract

179. Trepo C, Vitvitski L, Neurath R et al. Detection of e antigen by immunofluorescence in cytoplasm of hepatocytes of HBsAg carriers. Lancet 1976; i: 486

180. Yamada G, Takaguchi K, Matsueda K et al. Immunoelectron microscopic observation of intrahepatic HBeAg in patients with chronic hepatitis B. Hepatology 1990; 12: 133–140

181. Gerber M, Sells M, Chen M et al. Morphologic, immunohistochemical, and ultrastructural studies of the production of hepatitis B virus in vitro. Lab Invest 1988; 59: 173–180

182. Thomas H C, Jacyna M, Waters J, Main J. Virus-host interaction in chronic hepatitis B virus infection. Sem Liver Dis 1988; 8: 342–349

183. Twu J S, Schloemer R H. Tanscriptional trans-activating function of hepatitis B virus. J Virol 1987; 61: 3448–3453

184. Haruna Y, Hayashi N, Katayama K et al. Expression of X protein and hepatitis B virus replication in chronic hepatitis. Hepatology 1991; 13: 417–421

185. Wang W, London W, Lega L, Feitelson M. HBxAg in the liver from carrier patients with chronic hepatitis and cirrhosis. Hepatology 1991; 14: 29–37

186. Katayama K, Hayashi N, Sasaki Y et al. Detection of hepatitis B virus X gene protein and antibody in type B chronic liver disease. Gastroenterology 1989; 97: 990–998

187. Zentgraf H, Herrmann G, Klein R et al. Mouse monoclonal antibody directed against hepatitis B virus X protein synthesized in Escherichia coli: Detection of reactive antigen in liver cell carcinoma and chronic hepatitis. Oncology 1990; 47: 143–148

188. Wang W, London W T, Feitelson M A. Hepatitis B x antigen in hepatitis B virus carrier patients with liver cancer. Cancer Res 1991; 51: 4971–4977

189. Kim C M, Koike K, Saito I, Miyamura T, Jay G. HBx gene of hepatitis B virus induces liver cancer in transgenic mice. Nature 1991; 351: 317–320

190. Seifer M, Höhne M, Schaefer S, Gerlich W. In vitro tumorigenicity of hepatitis B virus DNA and HBx protein. J Hepatol 1991; 13 (suppl 4): S61–S65

191. Will H. The X-protein of hepatitis B virus. Facts and fiction. J Hepatol 1991; 13 (suppl 4): S56–S57

192. Koff R S. Hepatocellular carcinoma in transgenic mice: A consequence of continued expression of the HBx gene? Gastroenterology 1992; 102: 1081–1082

193. Rizzetto M, Canese M G, Aricò S et al. Immunofluorescence detection of new antigen-antibody system (δ/anti-δ) associated to hepatitis B virus in liver and serum of HBsAg carriers. Gut 1977; 18: 997–1003

194. Rizzetto M, Bonino F, Verme G. Hepatitis delta virus infection of the liver: Progress in virology, pathobiology, and diagnosis. Sem Liver Dis 1989; 8: 350–356

195. Taylor J. Hepatitis delta virus: cis and trans functions required for replication. Cell 1990; 61: 371–373

196. Kuo M Y P, Chao M, Taylor J. Initiation of replication of the human hepatitis delta virus genome from cloned DNA: role of the delta antigen. J Virol 1989; 63: 1945–1950

197. MacNaughton T B, Gowans E J, Jilbert A R, Burrell C J. Hepatitis delta virus RNA, protein synthesis and associated cytotoxicity in a stably transfected cell line. Virology 1990; 177: 692–698

198. Xia Y-P, Chang M-F, Wei D et al. Heterogeneity of hepatitis delta antigen. Virology 1990; 177: 331–336

199. Luo G, Chao M, Hsieh S-Y et al. A specific base transition occurs on replicating hepatitis delta virus RNA. J Virol 1990; 64: 1021–1027

200. Chang M F, Baker S C, Soe L H et al. Human hepatitis delta antigen is a nuclear phosphoprotein with RNA-binding activity. J Virol 1988; 62: 2403–2410

201. Chao M, Hsieh S Y, Taylor J. Role of two forms of hepatitis delta virus antigen: evidence for a mechanism of self-limiting genome replication. J Virol 1990; 64: 5066–5069

202. Taylor J, Chao M, Hsieh S-Y, Ryu W-S. The roles of the delta antigen in the structure and replication of hepatitis delta virus. J Hepatol 1991; 13 (suppl 4): S119–S120

203. Glenn J S, Watson J A, Havel C M, White J M. Identification of a prenylation site in delta virus large antigen. Science 1992; 256: 1331–1333

204. Smedile A, Rosina F, Saracco G et al. Hepatitis B virus replication modulates pathogenesis of hepatitis D virus in chronic hepatitis D. Hepatology 1991; 13: 413–416

205. Sureau C, Jacob J R, Eichberg J W, Lanford R E. Tissue culture system for infection with human hepatitis delta virus. J Virol 1991; 65: 3443–3450

206. Negro F, Pacchioni D, Bussolati G, Bonino F. Hepatitis delta virus heterogeneity: a study by immunofluorescence. J Hepatol 1991; 13 (suppl 4): S125–S129

207. Moreno A, Ramon Y, Cajal S, Marazuela M et al. Sanded nuclei in delta patients. Liver 1989; 9: 367–371

208. Stöcklin E, Gudat F, Spichtin H P et al. Die Delta-Koinfektion der Hepatitis B in der Schweiz: Histologie und Serologie von 28 Patienten. Schweiz Med Wschr 1984; 114: 1047–1052

209. Kojima T, Callea F, Desmyter J, Sakurai I, Desmet V J. Immuno-light and electron microscopic features of chronic hepatitis D. Liver 1990; 10: 17–27

210. Negro F, Baldi M, Bonino F et al. Chronic HDV (hepatitis delta virus) hepatitis: intrahepatic expression of delta antigen, histologic activity and outcome of liver disease. J Hepatol 1988; 6: 8–14

211. Pacchioni D, Negro F, Chiaberge E, Rizzetto M, Bonino F, Bussolati G. Detection of hepatitis Delta virus RNA by a nonradioactive in situ hybridization procedure. Hum Path 1992; 23: 557–561

212. Yamada G, Tsuji T. Intranuclear inclusion bodies in liver of chronic hepatitis B with delta infection. Acta Pathol Jpn 1988; 38: 759–768

213. Bonino F, Brunetto M, Negro F, Smedile A, Ponzetto A. Hepatitis delta virus, a model of liver cell pathology. J Hepatol 1991; 13: 260–266

214. Ackerman Z, Valinluck B, McHutchison J G, Redeker A G, Govindarajan S. Spontaneous exacerbation of disease activity in patients with chronic delta hepatitis infection: The role of hepatitis B, C or D. Hepatology 1992; 16: 625–629

215. Lai M M C, Lee C-M, Bih F-Y, Govindarajan S. The molecular basis of heterogeneity of hepatitis delta virus. J Hepatol 1991; 13(suppl. 4): S121–S124

216. Lin H-H, Liaw Y-F, Chen T-J, Chu C-M, Huang M-J. Natural course of patients with chronic type B hepatitis following acute hepatitis delta virus superinfection. Liver 1989; 9: 129–134

217. Rizzetto M, Verme G, Gerin J, Purcell R. Hepatitis delta virus disease. In: Popper H, Schaffner F, eds. Progress in liver diseases, vol VIII. New York: Grune & Stratton, 1986: pp 417–431

218. Govindarajan S, De C K M, Redeker A G. Natural course of delta superinfection in chronic hepatitis B virus-infected patients: histopathologic study with multiple liver biopsies. Hepatology 1986; 6: 640–644

219. Saracco G, Macagno S, Rosina F, Rizzetto M. Serologic markers with fulminant hepatitis in persons positive for hepatitis B surface antigen. A worldwide epidemiologic and clinical survey. Ann Intern Med 1988; 108: 380–383

220. Rizzetto M, Durazzo M. Hepatitis delta virus (HDV) infections. Epidemiological and clinical heterogeneity. J Hepatol 1991; 13 (suppl 4): S116–S118

221. Ottobrelli A, Marzano A, Smedile A et al. Patterns of hepatitis delta virus reinfection and disease in liver transplantation. Gastroenterology 1991; 101: 1649–1655

222. Raimondo G, Rodino G, Brancatelli S et al. HBe antibody unrelated to "e minus" hepatitis B virus variant infection in patients with chronic type D hepatitis. J Hepatol 1991; 13(suppl 4): S87–S89

223. Lau J Y N, Portmann B C, Alexander G J M, Williams R. Differential effect of chronic hepatitis D virus infection on intrahepatic expression of hepatitis B viral antigen. J Clin Path 1992; 45: 314–318

224. Hadziyannis S J, Georgopoulou U, Psalidaki E, Budkowska A. Pre-S1 and Pre-S2 gene-encoded proteins in liver and serum in chronic hepatitis delta infection. J Med Virol 1991; 34: 14–19

225. Krogsgaard K, Kryger P, Aldershvile J et al. δ-Infection and suppression of hepatitis B virus replication in chronic HBsAg carriers. Hepatology 1987; 7: 42–45

226. Krogsgaard K, Aldershvile J, Kryger P et al. Hepatitis B virus DNA, HBeAg and delta infection during the course from acute to chronic hepatitis B virus infection. Hepatology 1985; 5: 778–782

227. Bianchi L, Gudat F. Immunopathology of hepatitis B. In: Popper H, Schaffner F, eds. Progress in liver diseases, vol VI. New York: Grune & Stratton, 1979: pp 371– 392

228. Dienstag J L, Popper H, Purcell R H. The pathology of viral hepatitis types A and B in chimpanzees. A comparison. Am J Pathol 1976; 83: 131–148

229. Edgington T S, Chisari F V. Immunological aspects of hepatitis B virus infection. Am J Med Sci 1975; 270: 213–227

230. Arnold W, Meyer zum Büschenfelde K H, Hess G, Knolle J. The diagnostic significance of intrahepatocellular hepatitis-B surface-antigen (HBsAg), hepatitis-B-core-antigen (HBcAg) and IgG for the classification of inflammatory liver diseases. Klin Wochenschr 1975; 53: 1069–1074

231. Demetris A J, Jaffe R, Sheahan D G et al. Recurrent hepatitis B in liver allograft recipients: Differentiation between viral hepatitis B and rejection. Am J Path 1986; 125: 161–172

232. Lake J R, Wright T L, Liver transplantation for patients with hepatitis B: What have we learned from our results? Hepatology 1991; 13: 796–799

233. Demetris A J, Todo S, Van Thiel D H et al. Evolution of hepatitis B virus liver disease after hepatic replacement. Practical and theoretical considerations. Amer J Path 1990; 137: 667–676

234. Phillips M J, Cameron R, Flowers M A et al. Post-transplant recurrent hepatitis B viral liver disease. Viral-burden, steatoviral, and fibroviral hepatitis B. Am J Pathol 1992; 140: 1295–1308

235. Lau J, Bain V, Davies S et al. High-level expression of hepatitis B viral antigens in fibrosing cholestatic hepatitis. Gastroenterology 1992; 102: 956–962

236. Shafritz D A. Hepatitis B virus DNA molecules in the liver of HBsAg carriers: mechanistic considerations in the pathogenesis of hepatocellular carcinoma. Hepatology 1982; 2: 35S–41S

237. Lau J Y, Bain V G, Davies S E, Alexander G J, Williams R. Export of intracellular HBsAg in chronic hepatitis B virus infection is related to viral replication. Hepatology 1991; 14: 416–421

238. Korenmann J, Baker B, Waggoner J, Everhart J, Di Bisceglie A, Hoofnagle J. Long-term remission of chronic hepatitis B after alpha-interferon therapy. Ann Int Med 1991; 114: 629–634

239. Lok A S F, Lai C L, Wu P C, Leung E K Y, Lam T S. Spontaneous hepatitis B e antigen to antibody seroconversion and reversion in Chinese patients with chronic hepatitis B virus infection. Gastroenterology 1987; 92: 1839–1843

240. Fattovich G, Rugge M, Brollo L et al. Clinical, virologic and histologic outcome following seroconversion from HBeAg to anti-HBe in chronic hepatitis type B. Hepatology 1986; 6: 167–172

241. Anthony P P, Vogel C L, Barker L F. Liver cell dysplasia: a premalignant condition. J Clin Path 1973; 26: 217–223

242. Davies S E, Portmann B C, O'Grady J G, Aldis P M, Chaggar K, Alexander G J M, Williams R. Hepatic histological findings after transplantation for chronic hepatitis B virus infection, including a unique pattern of fibrosing cholestatic hepatitis. Hepatology 1991; 13: 150–157

243. Rizzetto M. The delta agent. Hepatology 1983; 3: 729–737

244. Popper H, Thung S, Gerber M et al. Histologic studies of severe delta agent infection in Venezuelan Indians. Hepatology 1983; 3: 906–912

245. Phillips M J, Blendis L M, Poucell S et al. Syncytial giant-cell hepatitis. Sporadic hepatitis with distinctive pathological features, a severe clinical course, and paramyxoviral features. N Engl J Med 1991; 324: 455–460

246. Thaler H. Post-infantile giant cell hepatitis. Liver 1982; 2: 393–403

247. Spichtin H P, Gudat F, Schmid M, Pirovino M, Altorfer J, Bianchi L. Microtubular aggregates in human chronic non-A, non-B hepatitis with bridging hepatic necrosis and multinucleated hepatocytic giant cells. Liver 1982; 2: 355–360

248. Johnson P J, McFarlane I G, Eddleston A L W F. The natural course and heterogeneity of autoimmune-type chronic active hepatitis. Sem Liver Dis 1991; 11: 187–196

249. Manns M P. Cytoplasmic autoantigens in autoimmune hepatitis: molecular analysis and clinical relevance. Sem Liver Dis 1991; 11: 205–214

250. Mackay I, Taft C, Cowling D. Lupoid hepatitis. Lancet 1956; ii: 1323–1326

251. Homberg J C, Abuaf N, Bernard O et al. Chronic active hepatitis associated with anti-liver/kidney microsome antibody type 1:a second type of "autoimmune hepatitis". Hepatology 1987; 7: 1333–1339

252. Mishiro S. Hoshi Y, Takeda K et al. Non-A, non-B hepatitis specific antibodies directed at host-derived epitope: implication for an autoimmune process. Lancet 1990; 336: 1400–1403

253. Michel G, Ritter A, Gerken G, Meyer zum Büschenfelde K H, Decker R, Manns M P, Anti-GOR and hepatitis C virus in autoimmune liver diseases. Lancet 1992; 339: 267–269

254. Johnson P J, McFarlane I G (Conversion on behalf of the panel). Meeting Report: International Autoimmune Hepatitis Inup. Hepatology 1993; 18: 998–1005

255. Beaune P, Dansette P, Mansuy D et al. Human anti-endoplasmic reticulum autoantibodies appearing in a drug-induced hepatitis are directed against a human liver cytochrome P450 that hydroxylates the drug. Proc Nat Acad Sci USA 1987; 84: 551–555

256. Bourdi M, Larrey D, Nataf J et al. Anti-liver endoplasmic reticulum autoantibodies are directed against human cytochrome P450 IA2. J Clin Invest 1990; 85: 1967–1973

257. Crivelli D, Lavarini C, Chiaberge E et al. Microsomal autoantibodies in chronic infections with HBsAg associated delta agent. Clin Exp Immunol 1983; 54: 232–238

258. Manns M, Gerken G, Kyriatsoulis A, Staritz M, Meyer zum Büschenfelde K H. Characterisation of a new subgroup of autoimmune chronic active hepatitis by autoantibodies against a soluble liver antigen. Lancet 1987; i: 292–294

259. Odièvre A M, Maggiore G, Homberg J C et al. Seroimmunologic classification of chronic hepatitis in 57 children. Hepatology 1983; 3: 407–409

260. Wächter B, Kyriatsoulis A, Lohse A W, Gerken G, Meyer zum Büschenfelde K H, Manns M. Characterization of liver cytokeratin as a major target antigen of anti-SLA antibodies. J Hepatol 1990; 11: 232–239

261. Gerken G, Manns M, Ramadori G et al. Liver membrane autoantibodies in chronic active hepatitis: studies on mechanically and enzymatically isolated rabbit hepatocytes. J Hepatol 1987; 5: 65–74

262. Lefkowitch J, Apfelbaum T, Weinberg L, Forester G. Acute liver biopsy lesions in early autoimmune ("lupoid") chronic active hepatitis. Liver 1984; 4: 379–386

263. Dienes H P, Autschbach F, Gerber M A. Ultrastructural lesion in autoimmune hepatitis and steps of the immune response in liver tissue. Sem Liver Dis 1991; 11: 197–204

264. Treichel U, Poralla T, Hess G, Manns M, Meyer zum Büschenfelde K H. Autoantibodies to human asialoglycoprotein receptor in autoimmune-type chronic hepatitis. Hepatology 1990; 11: 606–612

265. McFarlane I, McFarlane B, Major G, Tolley P, Williams R. Identification of the hepatic asialoglycoprotein receptor (hepatic lectin) as a component of liver specific membrane lipoprotein (LSP). Clin Exp Immunol 1984; 55: 347–354

266. Poralla T, Treichel U, Löhr H, Fleischer B. The asialoglycoprotein receptor as target structure in autoimmune liver diseases. Sem Liver Dis 1991; 11: 215–222

267. Frazer I, Mackay I, Bell J, Becker G. Cellular infiltrate in the liver in autoimmune chronic active hepatitis. Liver 1985; 5: 162–172

268. Autschbach F, Meuer S, Moebius U et al. Hepatocellular expression of lymphocyte function-associated antigen 3 in chronic hepatitis. Hepatology 1991; 14: 223–230

269. Mori T, Mori Y, Yoshida H et al. Cell-mediated cytotoxicity of sensitized spleen cells against target liver cells — in vivo and in vitro study with a mouse model of experimental autoimmune hepatitis. Hepatology 1985; 5: 770–777

270. Mori Y, Mori T, Ueda S et al. Study of cellular immunity in experimental autoimmune hepatitis in mice: transfer of spleen cells sensitized with liver proteins. Clin Exp Immunol 1985; 61: 577–584

271. Ogawa M, Mori Y, Mori T et al. Adoptive transfer of experimental autoimmune hepatitis in mice: cellular interaction between donor and recipient mice. Clin Exp Immunol 1988; 73: 276–282

272. Meuer S C, Moebius U, Manns M et al. Clonal analysis of human T lymphocytes infiltrating the liver in chronic hepatitis B and primary biliary cirrhosis. Europ J Immunol 1988; 18: 1447–1452

273. Autschbach F, Meuer S, Raczek A, Manns M, Meyer zum Büschenfelde K, Dienes H. Components of the effector-target-cell-binding complex in livers from patients with chronic hepatitis. Hepatology 1990; 12: 839 (abstract)

274. Vento S, O'Brien C J, McFarlane B M, McFarlane I G, Eddleston A L W F, Williams R. T-lymphocyte sensitization to hepatocyte antigens in autoimmune chronic active hepatitis and primary biliary cirrhosis. Evidence for different underlying mechanisms and different antigenic determinants as targets. Gastroenterology 1986; 91: 810–817

275. Lobo-Yeo A, Aluiggi L, Mieli-Vergani G, Portmann B, Mowat A P, Vergani D. Preferential activation of helper/inducer T lymphocytes in autoimmune chronic active hepatitis. Clin Exp Immunol 1987; 67: 95–104

276. Paronetto F, Vernace S. Immunological studies in patients with chronic active hepatitis: cytotoxic activity of lymphocytes to autochthonous liver cells grown in tissue culture. Clin Exp Immunol 1975; 19: 99–104

277. Manns M, Meyer zum Büschenfelde K H, Slusarczyk J, Dienes H P. Detection of liver-kidney microsomal autoantibodies by radio immunoassay and their relation to anti-mitochondrial antibodies in inflammatory liver disease. Clin Exp Immunol 1984; 57: 600–608

278. Manns M, Meyer zum Büschenfelde K, Hess G. Autoantibodies against liver-specific membrane lipoprotein in acute and chronic liver diseases: studies on organ-, species- and disease-specificity. Gut 1980; 21: 955–961

279. Hopf U, Meyer zum Büschenfelde K H, Arnold W. Detection of a liver membrane autoantibody in HBsAg-negative chronic active hepatitis. N Engl J Med 1976; 294: 578–582

280. Meyer zum Büschenfelde K H, Hütteroth T H, Manns M, Müller B. The role of liver membrane antigens in autoimmune type liver disease. Springer Sem Immunopathol 1980; 3: 297–316

281. Klingenstein R J, Wands J R. Immunologic effector mechanisms in hepatitis B-negative chronic active hepatitis. Springer Sem Immunopathol 1980; 3: 317–330

282. Mieli-Vergani G, Vergani D, Jenkins P et al. Lymphocyte cytotoxicity to autologous hepatocytes in HBsAg-negative chronic active hepatitis. Clin Exp Immunol 1979; 38: 16–21

283. Eggink H F, Houthoff H J, Huitema S. Wolters G, Poppema S, Gips C H Cellular and humoral immune reactions in chronic active liver disease. II. Lymphocyte subsets and viral antigens in liver biopsies of patients with acute and chronic hepatitis B. Clin Exp Immunol 1984; 56: 121–128

284. Löhr H, Treichel U, Poralla T, Manns M, Meyer zum Büschenfelde K, Fleischer B. The human hepatic asialoglycoprotein receptor is a target antigen for liver-infiltrating T cells in autoimmune chronic active hepatitis and primary biliary cirrhosis. Hepatology 1990; 12: 1314–1320

285. McFarlane B, Sipos J, Gove C, McFarlane I, Williams R. Antibodies against the hepatic asialoglycoprotein receptor perfused in situ preferentially attach to periportal liver cells in the rat. Hepatology 1990; 11: 408–415

286. Löhr H, Manns M, Trautwein C et al. Clonal analysis of liver-infiltrating T cells in patients with autoimmune chronic active hepatitis (AI-CAH). Clin Exp Immunol; 1991; 84: 297–302

287. Robertson D A F, Zhang S L, Guy E C, Wright R. Persistent measles virus genome in autoimmune chronic active hepatitis. Lancet 1987; ii: 9–11

288. Manns M, Griffin K J, Sullivan K F, Meyer zum Büschenfelde K H, Johnson E F. Molecular mimicry between intermediate early protein (IE 175) of herpes simplex virus I and cytochrome P450 db1 (IID6), a major autoantigen in autoimmune hepatitis. Hepatology 1990; 12: 907 (abstract)

289. Brunner G, Klinge O. Ein der chronisch-destruierenden nicht-eitrigen Cholangitis ähnliches Krankheitsbild mit antinukleären Antikörpern (Immuncholangitis). Dtsch Med Wschr 1987; 112: 1454–1458

290. Geubel A P, Baggenstoss S H, Summerskill W H J. Responses to treatment can differentiate chronic active liver disease with cholangitic features from the primary biliary cirrhosis syndrome. Gastroenterology 1976; 71: 444–449

291. Klöppel G, Seifert G, Lindner H, Dammermann R, Sack H J, Berg P A. Histopathological features in mixed types of chronic aggressive hepatitis and primary biliary cirrhosis. Correlations of liver histology with mitochondrial antibodies of different specificity. Virchows Arch (A) 1977; 373: 143–160

292. Carrougher J G, Shaffer R T, Canales L I, Goodman Z D. A 33 year-old woman with an autoimmune syndrome. Sem Liver Dis 1991; 11: 256–262

293. Zimmermann K, Cueni B, Schmid M. Kombinationsform chronisch aggressive Hepatitis/primär biliäre Zirrhose. Schweiz Med Wschr 1977; 107: 1749–1752

294. Okuno T, Seto Y, Okanoue T, Takino T. Chronic active hepatitis with histological features of primary biliary cirrhosis. Dig Dis Sci 1987; 32: 775–779

295. Rubel L R, Seeff L B, Patel V. Primary biliary cirrhosis-primary sclerosing cholangitis overlap syndrome. Arch Path Lab Med 1984; 108: 360–361

296. Sherman S, Nieland N S, Van Thiel D H. Sarcoidosis and primary biliary cirrhosis. Coexistence in a single patient. Dig Dis Sci 1988; 33: 368–374

297. Xerri L, Nosny Y, Minko D et al. Sarcoidosis and primary biliary cirrhosis. Case report with ten years clinical and pathological follow-up (fr.). Gastroent Clin Biol 1989; 13: 513–516

298. Keeffe E B. Sarcoidosis and primary biliary cirrhosis. Literature review and illustrative case. Amer J Med 1987; 83: 977–980

299. Terracciano L, Wurbs D, Klein R, Berg P, Bianchi L. Autoimmune chronic active hepatitis or primary sclerosing cholangitis: the riddle of overlaps. In preparation

300. Doniach D, Walker J D. A unified concept of autoimmune hepatitis. Lancet 1969; i: 813–815

301. Wright R. Drug-induced chronic hepatitis. Springer Sem Immunopathol 1980; 3: 331–338

302. Seeff L. Drug-induced chronic liver disease, with emphasis on chronic active hepatitis. Seminars Liver Dis 1981; 1: 104–115

303. Popper H, Geller S. Pathogenetic considerations in the histologic diagnosis of drug-induced liver injury. In: Fenoglio C, Wolff M, eds. Progress in surgical pathology, vol III. New York: Masson, 1981: pp 233–246

304. Baptista A, Bianchi L, De Groote J et al. Histopathology of the intrahepatic biliary tree. Liver 1988; 3: 161–175

305. Bianchi L. Intrahepatic bile duct damage in various forms of liver disease. In: Brunner H, Thaler H, eds. Hepatology: a Festschrift for Hans Popper. New York: Raven Press, 1985: 295–310

306. Zetterman R K. Autoimmune manifestations of alcoholic liver disease. In: Krawitt E L, Wiesner R H, eds. Autoimmune liver diseases. New York: Raven Press, 1991: pp 247–260

307. Mendenhall C L, Seeff L, Diehl A M et al. Antibodies to hepatitis B virus and hepatitis C virus in alcoholic hepatitis and cirrhosis: Their prevalence and clinical relevance. Hepatology 1991; 14: 581–589

308. Realdi G, Alberti A, Rugge M et al. Seroconversion from hepatitis B e antigen to anti-HBe in chronic hepatitis B virus infection. Gastroenterology 1980; 79: 195–199

309. Hoofnagle J, Dusheiko G, Seeff L, Jones E, Waggoner J, Bales Z. Seroconversion from hepatitis-B-E antigen to antibody in chronic type-B hepatitis. Ann Int Med 1981; 94: 744–748

10

Liver cirrhosis

G. H. Millward-Sadler

Cirrhosis is a stage in the evolution of many chronic liver diseases and a term that implies consequences that are unrelated to the primary aetiology. These consequences are both mechanical, involving intra- and extrahepatic shunting of blood, and functional, leading to failure to perform the physiological roles of the organ. Cirrhosis results from a complex interplay of many factors which include cell death and regeneration, matrix degradation and abnormal matrix formation. These are present in proportions which vary according to the aetiology of the process, its degree of activity and the stage of evolution. The exact point at which a disease process has produced cirrhosis is difficult to define, and the increasing use of needle biopsy for diagnosis and management has magnified this problem. The biopsy is small so that there is considerable potential for sampling error and interpretation may be difficult. Fibrosis can be extensive within the liver without cirrhosis being present, as is seen for example in congenital hepatic fibrosis and schistosomiasis. None the less, many of the complications of cirrhosis may occur when there is only severe fibrosis of the liver.

DEFINITION

There have been many definitions of cirrhosis.[1-4] The most concise and probably the best of these states that cirrhosis is 'a diffuse process characterized by fibrosis and a conversion of normal architecture into structurally abnormal nodules'[3,4] Note that the presence of both fibrosis and nodules are essential to the diagnosis of cirrhosis but regeneration is not, and that the fibrosis and nodules must be present throughout the liver. Needle biopsy diagnosis of cirrhosis must therefore be evaluated with this qualification. Other investigations such as the new imaging techniques will usually be available to indicate the diffuse nature of the process.

Fibrosis is an integral part of cirrhosis and differentiates it from nodular regenerative hyperplasia. Structurally abnormal nodules may be obvious but sometimes can only be inferred from subtle architectural changes such as a disordered or compressed cell plate pattern. Abnormalities in vasculature and blood flow are not included in the definition yet they are very important.[5] These vascular changes, however, are a consequence of the other features present in the definition and not the primary abnormality. Regeneration is also excluded from the definition. True regenerative nodules can be a late occurrence in cirrhosis, and abnormal nodules do not necessarily show features of regeneration. It is important to appreciate that regeneration is a critical factor influencing the evolution of cirrhosis, but it is not essential for its diagnosis.

CLASSIFICATION AND AETIOLOGY

Cirrhosis is most satisfactorily classified by its aetiology (Table 10.1). Some causes can be grouped together under a common pathogenesis, for instance biliary obstruction. The aetiology of the cirrhosis may be unknown, in which case morphological appearances can sometimes indicate the probable aetiology or group of aetiologies. Many morphological classifications have been used but are now superseded by a simple subdivision into micronodular, macronodular and mixed nodularity cirrhosis.[2–4,6] A micronodular cirrhosis has uniform nodules throughout the liver and these are less than 3 mm in diameter. They are separated by definite, but usually indistinct, fine bands of fibrosis. A macronodular cirrhosis has the majority of nodules larger than 3 mm in diameter. The presence of some small nodules is permissible within this category. Mixed nodularity cirrhosis has nodules both smaller and larger than 3 mm in approximately equal proportions. The morphological classification is of greatest value in autopsy studies of the whole liver, less so in wedge or needle biopsies as nodule size is difficult to assess in histological sections.

The aetiological conditions listed in Table 10.1 are separately considered in detail in different chapters throughout this book.

MORPHOLOGY

MACROSCOPIC APPEARANCES

Micronodular cirrhosis

The overall shape and external appearance of the liver in micronodular cirrhosis may not be greatly altered. The nodules on the cut surface are small in size and uniform in appearance but may be difficult to define (Fig. 10.1). The ratio of fibrous matrix to parenchyma is greater than in macronodular cirrhosis and consequently the liver is firm or even hard. Fibrosis is diffusely distributed as fine, indistinct bands between nodules but occasionally these may be broader and define more clearly the nodules on both

Table 10.1 Aetiology of cirrhosis

Drugs and toxins	Alcohol
	Methotrexate
	Isoniazid
	Methyldopa
	Amiodarone
Infections	Hepatitis B
	Hepatitis C
	Schistosomiasis
Autoimmune	Chronic active hepatitis
	Primary biliary cirrhosis
Metabolic	Wilson's disease
	Haemochromatosis
	α_1-antitrypsin deficiency
	Galactosaemia
	Glycogen storage diseases
	Tyrosinaemia
	Urea cycle disorders
	Abetalipoproteinaemia
Biliary obstruction	Atresia
	Cystic fibrosis
	Gallstones
	Strictures
	Sclerosing cholangitis
Vascular	Budd–Chiari syndrome
	Veno-occlusive disease
	Chronic right heart failure
	Hereditary haemorrhagic telangiectasia
Miscellaneous	Neonatal hepatitis syndrome
	Indian childhood cirrhosis
	Intestinal bypass surgery
	Sarcoidosis
Cryptogenic	

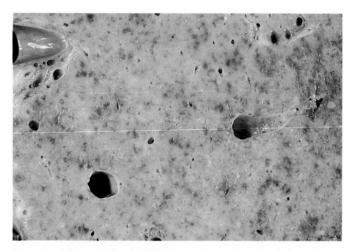

Fig. 10.1 Micronodular cirrhosis in a patient with severe cholestasis due to alcoholic hepatitis. The fibrosis is diffuse with fine fibrous bands and the micronodules are hard to identify.

the cut and the capsular surfaces. In the early stages, the liver may be enlarged, but with advancing disease it shrinks in size. Alcohol is the most frequent association with this micronodular pattern in Europe and North

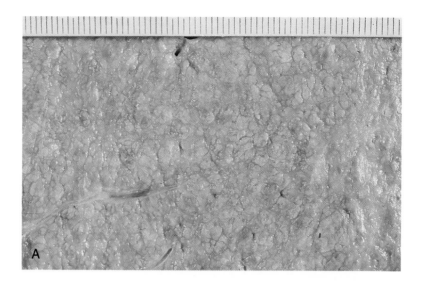

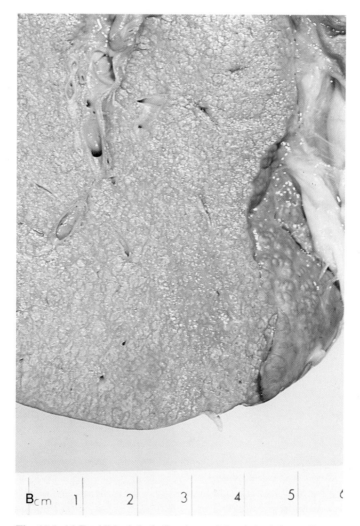

Fig. 10.2 (a) Established alcoholic micronodular cirrhosis has well-defined nodules clearly separated by fibrous bands and a tawny yellow colour due to severe fatty change in hepatocytes. (b) Micronodular cirrhosis in untreated haemochromatosis also has clearly defined nodules but these have a red-brown colour due to excess iron deposition.

America. Other causes include haemochromatosis, biliary obstruction, chronic hepatic venous outflow obstruction, many of the metabolic diseases of infancy and childhood that affect the liver and, rarely, chronic active hepatitis. The macroscopic appearances may help to differentiate these conditions. Alcoholic liver disease shows a diffuse tan or yellow colour due to severe fatty change (Fig. 10.2a) while in haemochromatosis the heavy iron deposition imparts a dark reddish brown colour to the liver (Fig. 10.2b). The cause of the obstruction to the biliary tree (stone, stricture, tumour) (Fig. 10.3) or the hepatic venous outflow (valves, thrombosis, tumour) may be evident on careful dissection of these structures. Obstruction to the venous outflow may also be functional, i.e. secondary to right heart failure, cardiomyopathy or constrictive pericarditis. In such cases the liver, in addition to being hard, is also enlarged and congested. Even then, it may atrophy eventually as it does

in a chronic Budd–Chiari syndrome. There are rarely any distinguishing macroscopic features in cirrhosis due to drugs.

Macronodular cirrhosis

The size of the liver in macronodular cirrhosis is much more variable. It is frequently enlarged but, when associated clinically with liver failure, is usually small and may weigh less than 1000 g. The parenchyma is organized in large bulging nodules which are separated by fibrous bands that vary considerably in width (Fig. 10.4). Early examples may show slender fibrous bands but as the disease progresses these become broader and denser and produce marked grooving and retraction which is visible on the capsular surface (Fig. 10.5). This latter pattern of cirrhosis is the one most frequently found at autopsy as it

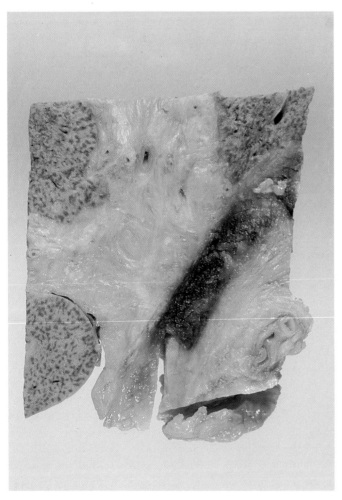

Fig. 10.3 Secondary biliary cirrhosis due to an inoperable cholangiocarcinoma at the confluence of the right and left hepatic bile ducts (Klatskin tumour). Use of expanding metal Wallstents inserted by combined retrograde and percutaneous cholangiography relieved the obstruction and produced considerable symptomatic relief.

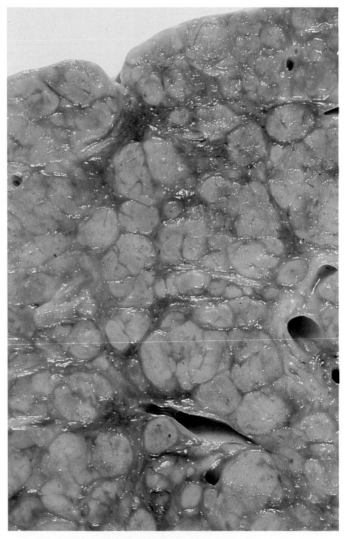

Fig. 10.4 Macronodular cirrhosis due to chronic active hepatitis: note the marked variation in size and shape of the nodules . This is accentuated by the intervening fibrous stroma which varies from broad scars to thin delicate bands of fibrosis tissue.

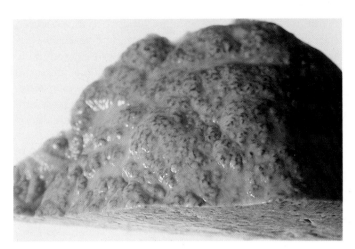

Fig. 10.5 The large nodules in a macronodular cirrhosis are often most easily identified on the capsular surface of the liver.

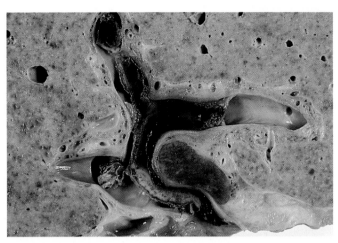

Fig. 10.6 Thrombosis of the main portal vein extending into the major intrahepatic branches. The patient developed a post-transplant cirrhosis from fibrosing cholestatic hepatitis due to recurrence of chronic hepatitis B virus infection.

represents the end stage of almost any form of chronic liver disease and the aetiology can rarely be deduced from the macroscopic appearances. An initially micronodular cirrhosis may progress to a macronodular pattern in patients who survive longer on treatment (e.g. iron depletion therapy in haemochromatosis) or where the aetiological agent is removed (alcohol withdrawal). Diseases which tend to produce a macronodular cirrhosis an initio include chronic viral hepatitis and autoimmune chronic active hepatitis.

Incomplete septal cirrhosis

Macronodular cirrhosis of an incomplete septal pattern is characterized by ill-defined large bulging nodules with only slender fibrous septa, and microscopic examination may be required for its identification. It is most frequently seen in chronic hepatitis B virus (HBV) infection.

Complications

Some of the complications of cirrhosis may be macroscopically visible. Thus, a primary hepatocellular carcinoma may be present. Portal vein thrombosis is a common complication of portal hypertension (Fig. 10.6) and is particularly common when hepatocellular carcinoma invades the vascular tree. Necrosis of nodules can also be identified and is usually present after a vericeal bleed resulting in systemic hypotension (Fig. 10.7). Affected nodules show the classic changes of infarction, becoming bright yellow, and develop a peripheral red zone of new vessel formation. Less significant consequences of cirrhosis that may be macroscopically seen include gallstones in the gallbladder and a patent ductus venosus. Outside the liver, oesophageal and gastric varices are often visible and straw-coloured ascites may be present.

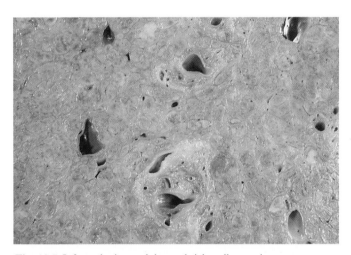

Fig. 10.7 Infarcted micronodules are bright yellow against a background of deeply bile-stained liver. The patient had alcoholic micronodular cirrhosis and died in progressive liver failure with haemorrhage from oesophageal varices.

MICROSCOPIC APPEARANCES

The aetiology of cirrhosis may be apparent on microscopic examination. This is particularly true for hepatitis B virus (HBV) infection, haemochromatosis, Wilson's disease and α_1-antitrypsin deficiency, where specific cytological features can be demonstrated. The aetiology can be reasonably inferred for alcohol and chronic intrahepatic biliary obstruction where combinations of features are suggestive and may even be diagnostic. The detailed microscopic findings are described in the appropriate chapters.

An analysis of the type of architectural distortion can also suggest an aetiology as well as indicate the stage of cirrhosis to which it has progressed. The macro/micronodular classification is not easy to apply in needle biopsy material. It is more helpful to relate the pattern of cirrhosis to the previous normal architecture using trichrome stains for collagen or by staining the elastic tissue of the liver. With these techniques the original portal tracts can, with care, be identified as can some of the larger hepatic veins.

On this basis, cirrhosis nodules may be identified within the acinus and therefore be smaller than the original acinus or may be created by fibrosis that encompasses one or more acini within its boundaries. A more complex histological subdivision of cirrhosis into triadal, paratriadal and atriadal nodules has been proposed.[5] The paratriadal nodules are then further subdivided according to the type of acinus— simple, complex or acinar agglomerate—from which they are derived. This introduces an element of complexity that is difficult to use for standard diagnostic purposes.

Micronodular cirrhosis

Normal acini are approximately 1 mm in diameter and, consequently, 3 mm nodules in a micronodular cirrhotic liver may contain complete acinar units within them. More

commonly, however, the acini are subdivided into nodules, creating a micro-micronodular pattern, and virtually every acinus is affected (Fig. 10.8) This micro-micronodular pattern is most commonly associated with alcohol but drugs and toxins such as methotrexate and carbon tetrachloride, metabolic disturbances such as haemochromatosis, and many of the inherited metabolic childhood causes of cirrhosis can also produce this pattern. In these instances fibrosis connects the smallest portal tracts to their subjacent terminal hepatic venules. Thus, zones 1, 2 and 3 of the acinus have to be transected by fibrovascular septa before abnormal nodules are formed. In typical alcoholic liver disease the fibrosis is focused around the terminal hepatic venules and extends through the sinusoids towards the portal tracts with subacinar areas of parenchyma isolated by these irregular fibrous bridges (Fig. 10.9). All the major hepatic vascular structures (artery, portal vein and hepatic vein) are peripheral to the small nodules so that abnormal patterns of flow are created through the nodule. Gradually these foci link to produce a more diffuse network of fibrosis and eventually a cirrhosis. Fibrosis can also be irregular and focal, as in the early stages of methotrexate-induced injury.[7]

Fibrosis may be dominant in one zone—around the portal tracts (zone 1) in haemochromatosis, or the terminal hepatic venules (zone 3) in alcoholic liver disease—but cirrhosis has not developed if the fibrosis is restricted only to these zones. A pattern of perisinusoidal fibrosis, which can be extensive and diffuse, may be present

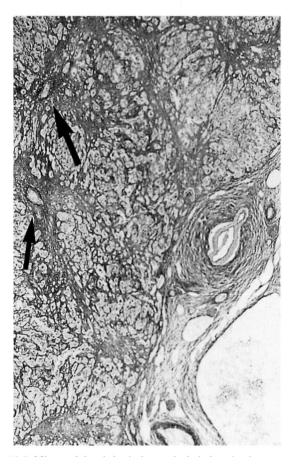

Fig. 10.8 Micronodular cirrhosis due to alcohol: there is a large portal tract lower right. Two terminal hepatic venules are arrowed. The diffuse fibrosis shows irregular bridging of the terminal hepatic venules with each other and with the portal tracts so that a series of small nodules is created. The pericellular fibrosis, so common in alcoholic liver disease, irregularly subdivides these small nodules further. Reticulin.

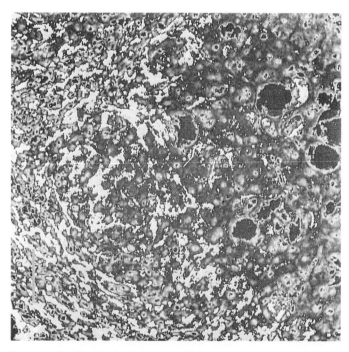

Fig. 10.9 Confocal laser microscopy of the perivenular zone in a 20 μm thick section of liver in alcoholic micronodular cirrhosis. The sinusoidal matrix is blue, hepatocytes light brown and fat purple. The terminal hepatic vein is bottom right. Courtesy Dr W R Roche

and is characteristic of, but not exclusive to, an alcohol aetiology. Hypervitaminosis A, chronic severe passive venous congestion and chronic myelofibrosis are other examples.

In a three-dimensional reconstruction the abnormal fibrous bands are plates of tissue rich in newly formed blood vessels and have been termed 'fibrovascular membranes'.[5] An alternative route for blood flow that does not involve passage through the sinusoids is thus created by these membranes once they bridge portal tracts with hepatic veins. Further circulatory abnormalities arise when blood enters or leaves the parenchyma from these vascularized fibrous septa instead of the normal channels.

This micro-micronodular pattern of cirrhosis seems to be most commonly associated with diseases in which there is a uniform and generalized effect of an hepatotoxic agent or mechanism on the smallest units of the liver. In alcoholic liver disease every acinus has been regularly exposed to high levels of alcohol, and fibrosis can be consistently found in the space of Disse around the terminal hepatic venules. It is interesting in this context that alcohol-induced chronic active hepatitis, which probably proceeds to cirrhosis by a different mechanism, is most commonly associated with a macronodular cirrhosis.[8] In some instances of micronodular cirrhosis, one or two portal tracts may be incorporated into a nodule. This is rare but is occasionally found for instance in early alcoholic liver disease. It can also be associated with a disease more commonly associated with a macronodular cirrhosis, in which the activity is subdividing the nodules more rapidly than usual.

The tiny nodules enlarge as they regenerate, become rounded and develop a pseudocapsule by compression of surrounding connective tissue. Such regenerative nodules can be larger than a simple acinus but less than 3 mm in diameter and lack any acinar substructure. If their expansile growth continues, the nodules become larger than 3 mm in diameter and evolution into a macronodular cirrhosis occurs.

Macronodular cirrhosis

Histologically, three patterns can be identified. These are incomplete septal, multiacinar (multilobular) and regenerative.

Incomplete septal cirrhosis has a pattern characterized by very slender fibrovascular septa that extend from portal tracts into the parenchyma but often do not interconnect with other portal tracts or hepatic veins (Fig. 10.10). Perisinusoidal collagen is not obviously increased. Usually, there is little evidence of cell damage or death, and little or no inflammation is seen in the septa. Abnormal architectural patterns are present and can be identified as a variable mixture of twinned cell plates and dilated sinusoids with compression of the parenchyma between hyperplastic areas. The orientation of the cell plates also changes between and even within areas. These changes probably reflect the

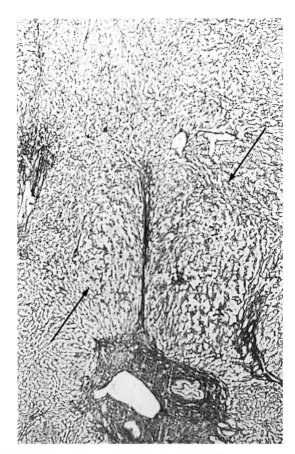

Fig. 10.10 'Incomplete septal' cirrhosis: a slender fibrous spur extending out from the portal tract at the bottom, ends blindly in the parenchyma just to the left of two efferent veins. Abnormal fibrosis is also present left of centre and just to the right of the portal tract. Although it would be difficult to make a diagnosis of cirrhosis on this field alone, note the approximation of large efferent veins to the fibrous bands and also the disorganized cell plate pattern (arrows). With these features present, the diagnosis of cirrhosis should at least be considered and further evidence looked for. Reticulin.

altered blood flows that enter the sinusoids at varying points from the fibrovascular septa.

Distinguishing incomplete septal cirrhosis from non-cirrhotic portal hypertension is a difficult diagnostic problem in liver biopsy interpretation because the morphological criteria that would clearly separate them are not well defined.[9] Morphologically, the emphasis is biased towards fibrosis in incomplete septal cirrhosis, whereas in nodular regenerative hyperplasia it is slight and secondary to the compression of sinusoidal collagens[10] (Figs 10.11 and 10.12)

The major complications of this pattern of cirrhosis derive from portal hypertension, and liver function is usually well preserved. Only rarely are liver function tests abnormal. The prognosis is excellent if portal hypertension can be controlled.

The aetiology of an individual case of incomplete septal cirrhosis is usually not known. Alcohol and 'burnt out' chronic active hepatitis have both been implicated. It is probable that some instances of non-cirrhotic portal hypertension are examples of incomplete septal cirrhosis that

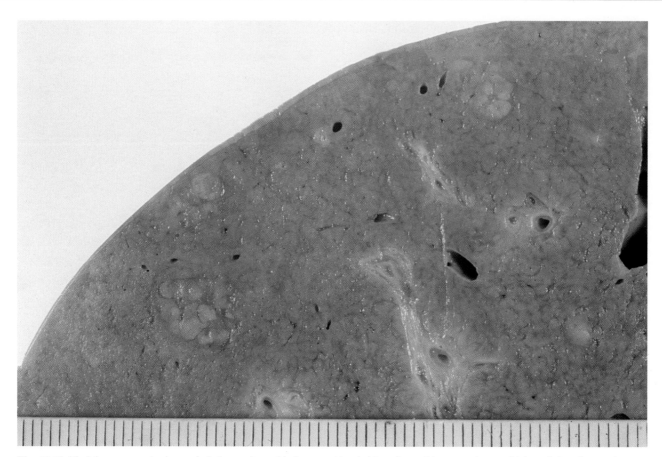

Fig. 10.11 Nodular regenerative hyperplasia in a patient with rheumatoid arthritis and portal hypertension: multiple nodules of parenchyma compress the surrounding liver but it is otherwise normal with no macroscopic evidence of fibrosis.

has not been recognized. It has been suggested that incomplete septal cirrhosis, nodular regenerative hyperplasia, partial nodular transformation and focal nodular hyperplasia are interrelated disorders with a common pathogenesis related to abnormalities in the vascular supply.[10] An

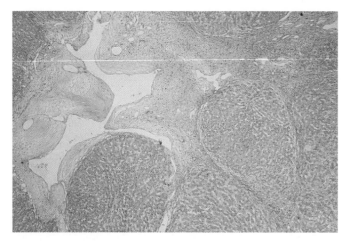

Fig. 10.12 Nodular regenerative hyperplasia may mimic macronodular cirrhosis in a single field. A pseudocapsule has been produced from compression of the surrounding tissues but fibrosis is not otherwise found in the remaining parenchyma. H & E.

'obliterative portal venopathy' is postulated to produce the hyperplastic lesions by inducing non-uniformity of blood supply to the parenchyma.[11–13] The hypothesis is attractive as it unites several entities with similar morphological features but an otherwise poorly understand pathogenesis. It explains the considerable overlap and diagnostic confusion between them and it provides a rational explanation for the lack both of any clinically overt disease and of any inflammatory component. At present it is probably best to retain the concept of incomplete septal cirrhosis but accept it as that end of the spectrum with less emphasis on regeneration and more on fibrosis than is seen in nodular regenerative hyperplasia.

Multiacinar macronodular cirrhosis probably represents an early stage of evolution. The large nodules are defined by abnormal septa but within them some residue of the original architecture can still be identified. This may be represented by one or more minimally distorted portal tracts within the nodule (Fig. 10.13). These can be distinguished from neovascular bundles by the type and pattern of elastic fibres. Original elastic fibres are short, wavy and thick, and have a more random orientation than those in newly formed collagen. These latter fibrils are finer, less intensely stained and tend to be aligned parallel to the septal/parenchymal interface.

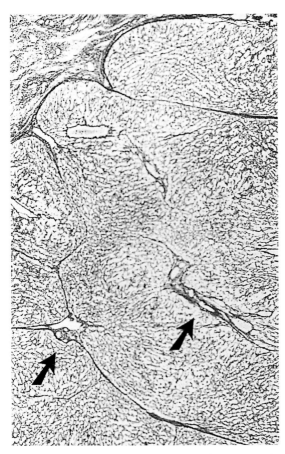

Fig. 10.13 Macronodular cirrhosis: a portal tract is present on the edge of the nodule, top left; slender bands of fibrous tissue are beginning to subdivide a large macronodule but two portal tracts (arrows) are still identifiable and form part of the internal structure of the nodule. Reticulin.

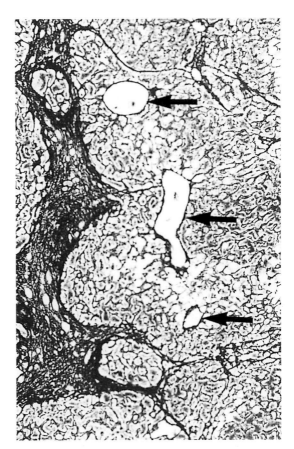

Fig. 10.14 Macronodular cirrhosis: two small nodules of parenchyma have been isolated within the broad scar but a large area of parenchyma is not overtly nodular. There is, however, an excess of efferent veins (arrows) which are also in abnormal proximity to the broad fibrous bands as well as to the multiple other slender fibrous bands. Reticulin.

Cell plates within the nodule are usually single with little evidence of twinning but do not show the regular radial orientation present between portal tracts and hepatic veins of a normal acinus. The abnormal cell plate patterns probably reflect altered blood flow through the nodule that originates from the neovascular septa on the periphery. These septa not only create direct shunts of blood through to the efferent hepatic veins without entering the sinusoids but also permit the blood to enter the sinusoids of the nodule from abnormal directions (Fig. 10.14). This propensity to create an abnormal flow pattern is accentuated by the fact that the new vascular channels are arterially derived and their blood is therefore not only better oxygenated but also at a slightly higher pressure. Although they cannot be regarded as diagnostic on their own, the possibility of a macronodular cirrhosis must be carefully considered when abnormal cell plate patterns and excess efferent veins are present in a needle liver biopsy.

The multiacinar pattern is most easily created when zone 3 of a simple acinus is in close proximity to the large conducting portal tracts. There is only a small sleeve of parenchyma here, the acinulus, which surrounds the tract and is directly supplied by vessels in it (see Ch. 1). According to their calibre, such conducting portal tracts support complex acini (clusters of three or more simple acini with a common vascular stem) and acinar agglomerates (clusters of three or more complex acini). Consequently, fibrosis that bridges zone 3 with the conducting portal tract creates nodules containing the preserved central vascular cores of the simple acini. Depending on the calibre of the bridged portal tract, the macronodule can incorporate elements of complex acini or acinar agglomerates. Such patterns of scarring do not preclude fibrous bridges between the smallest portal tracts and their terminal hepatic venules but, by definition, this is not generalized. None the less, the disease process usually continues to subdivide these macronodules and sometimes can be so active that a micronodular, instead of a macronodular, cirrhosis is produced.

Regenerative activity complicates this pattern even further. Expansion of part of a nodule can occur so that there is compression of cell plates around this focus of regeneration. Such preferential growth probably occurs because of variations in blood supply. The expansile growth leads to nodules within nodules, compression atrophy of cell plates and further distortions of blood flow. Regeneration will gradually expand and enlarge all nodules and parts of nodules so that macronodules are eventually formed.

Regenerative macronodular cirrhosis. In this pattern the nodules are rounded, and may be large and tumour-like. Regenerative activity is usually obvious within the nodule and is identifiable as twinning of cell plates and increased nuclear pleomorphism in hepatocytes. The expansion compresses stroma so that the nodule often has concentric parallel layers of oedematous collagen fibres around it (Fig. 10.15). This regenerative growth rarely, if ever, occurs concentrically around a portal tract or hepatic vein so that these nodules lack these structures and any substructure to the nodule is usually formed by the ingrowth of new fibrovascular septa (Fig. 10.16). Sometimes these septa may contain small bile ductules and mimic portal tracts but they have a different elastic staining pattern, rarely have a true portal vein and are usually extremely small in comparison to most portal tracts. Continuing hepatocellular damage from the original disease process may be evident. In addition, hepatocytes in these nodules may show changes secondary to obstructed bile flow. Feathery degeneration, due to cholate stasis and increased copper and copper-binding protein from impaired copper excretion, are commonly seen, particularly in the periseptal hepatocytes, and Mallory bodies may be present in their cytoplasm. There is no association of these Mallory bodies with excess alcohol consumption and their presence does not indicate that the cirrhosis is of this aetiology.

PATHOGENESIS

There are three major pathological mechanisms that combine to create cirrhosis: cell death, fibrosis and regeneration. The process is usually initiated by cell death but

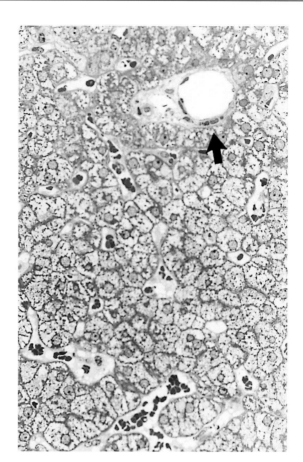

Fig. 10.16 A hypoplastic portal tract (arrow) in a macronodular cirrhosis. A small arteriole and a large venule are present but no biliary radicle. The cell plates show twinning; the sinusoids show increased variation in diameter. Toluidine blue.

only after this has occurred consistently and persistently over a long period of time. Thus, an acute overdose of paracetamol causes severe hepatic necrosis and may kill the patient but it will not produce chronic liver injury in those who survive. In contrast, a small dose of methotrexate which alone is insufficient to cause more than small foci of necrosis, is nevertheless very effective at producing cirrhosis when administered on a daily basis for two or more years. Fibrosis is regarded as a repair mechanism but it is probable that fibrogenesis can also be initiated directly without the intervention of cell death and inflammation. This is probably the mechanism by which prolonged ingestion of vitamin A can induce cirrhosis,[14,15] although it is not certain that proliferation of the perisinusoidal (Ito) cells is a direct consequence of the hypervitaminosis and is not mediated through hepatocellular injury. Fibrosis itself can produce ischaemic and nutrient damage to hepatocytes, by creating a barrier between them and sinusoidal blood.

Regeneration completes the attempted reparative process. Again, this often occurs in response to cell death but other mechanisms can be involved. For example, the dramatic regenerative response that follows surgical resection is out of all proportion to the amount of cell damage caused by

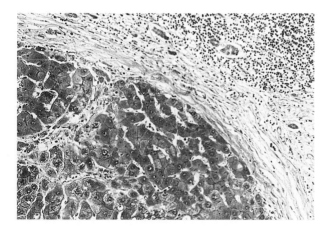

Fig. 10.15 Macronodular cirrhosis at an advanced stage. Part of a broad band of fibrous tissue is present on the right with the edge of a large structureless parenchymal nodule on the left. At the interface, the collagen bundles have become orientated parallel to the edge of the nodule and are compressed together by its expansile growth. H & E

the procedure. The relationships and relative contributions of the factors involved in regeneration are being elucidated but are still poorly understood.[16]

CELL DEATH

Cell damage and death have to occur continuously over a long period of time to induce cirrhosis. In alcoholics, the incidence of cirrhosis increases with duration of excessive drinking but this ranges in individual cases from a few years to several decades.[17] The time required is equally variable in other aetiological categories. For example, in some studies, the administration of methotrexate to patients with psoriasis required an average of 4 years' continuous exposure before cirrhosis supervened,[18,19] but in some cases it took as little as 18 months.[7] There are many forms of injury that can produce cell death. These range from an immunologically-mediated reaction against antigens expressed on the cell membrane, through toxin-induced damage, to an ischaemic necrosis. If any of these insults overwhelms the intracellular homeostatic mechanisms that preserve the redox potential of the cell and/or its intracellular calcium homeostasis, then cell death results.

Immunological mechanisms

This is a large and complicated topic in liver disease, which has been extensively reviewed.[20-23] Humoral immunological mechanisms have little importance, and cellular immune mechanisms are thought to be responsible in most cases. The most important pathway that is morphologically identifiable is the piecemeal necrosis of chronic active hepatitis which produces cirrhosis through lymphocyte toxicity against hepatocytes.[24] Lymphocytes can be identified within the space of Disse in close proximity to hepatocytes (peripolesis) and occasionally entering their cytoplasm (emperipolesis).[25] The mononuclear infiltrate in the biopsy includes an increased number of T-lymphocytes but the proportions and distribution of T-cell subsets varies according to the disease. In chronic HBV infection a preponderance of cytotoxic/suppressor T-cells is found in HBeAg-positive cases[26,27] and of inducer T-cells in those with HBe antibody.[26-28]

Core antigen can be demonstrated on the surface of hepatocytes in chronic HBV infection but only after the elution of IgG from the plasma membrane.[29] Cytotoxic T-lymphocytes recognize the nucleocapsid antigens of the virus (HBcAg and HBeAg) that are expressed on the surface membrane in conjunction with MHC class I glycoprotein. Non-infected hepatocytes express very litttle MHC glycoprotein but this can be induced by viral infections and also by interferon.[30] The close proximity of viral and MHC antigens triggers the sequence that leads to cytotoxic lymphocyte activation. The presence of IgG suggests that the mechanism is antibody dependent. Alternatively, circulating antibody to HBcAg or HBeAg antigens could be protective if it reacted with, and therefore masked, the viral antigens expressed on the surface. There would then be failure of lymphocyte recognition, and viral persistence would be promoted. Similar mechanisms have been postulated for autoimmune chronic active hepatitis though the nature of the surface membrane antigen that acts as a target for cytotoxic lymphocytes is speculative.[24]

Other cellular mechanisms

Macrophages may be the cause of hepatocellular damage in a variety of diseases. Experimentally, hepatocytes are not damaged by endotoxin alone but severe liver-cell damage and necrosis can be induced by endotoxin once macrophages have been recruited into the liver using, for example, dead *Corynebacterium parvum*[31] (Fig. 10.17). These macrophages release a variety of enzymes after exposure to the endotoxin.[32] Damage to hepatocytes can be diminished by treatment with superoxide dismutase[33] which suggests that superoxide formation with lipid peroxidation of membranes is an important route by which cell death is produced.

Toxins

Many chemicals and poisons produce hepatocellular damage but the mechanism varies with each substance (see Ch. 15). For instance, alcohol metabolism involves oxidation to acetate via acetaldehyde with the production of hydrogen ions. These convert NAD to NADH and thus competitively inhibit any other intracellular metabolic function which requires NAD as an hydrogen ion acceptor. This not only inhibits the citric acid cycle but also promotes functions which convert NADH to NAD. Lactate is then preferentially formed instead of pyruvate and hyperlactic acidaemia results.[34]

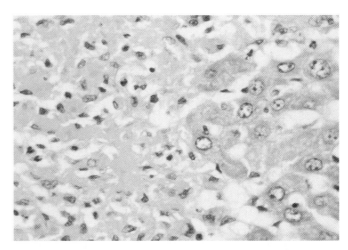

Fig. 10.17 Endotoxin has produced a large confluent zone of coagulative necrosis in liver containing epithelioid granulomas induced by *Corynebacterium parvum*.

Phalloidin interacts with a specific surface membrane receptor which is probably unique to the hepatocyte.[35] Once inside the cell, phalloidin acts to polymerize actin and seems to alter membrane permeability so that large evaginations are seen on electron microscopy.[36]

Carbon tetrachloride, in contrast, produces cell damage after it has been metabolized in the smooth endoplasmic reticulum. Prior enzyme induction by barbiturates increases the severity of the damage,[37] suggesting that it is the metabolites of carbon tetrachloride that are cytotoxic. There is marked loss of ribosomes and considerable membrane damage which could be due to covalent binding of active metabolites to membranes,[38] but is more probably the consequence of lipid peroxidation, secondary to release of halogenated free radicals.[39]

Oxidative stress

Oxidative stress arises from an imbalance between pro-oxidants and antioxidants resulting in a predominance of pro-oxidative processes.[40] Reactive oxygen metabolites are frequently produced as a result of metabolic processes within the cell and their effects are normally counterbalanced by homeostatic reducing mechanisms. A variety of these antioxidants exist in cells, including vitamin E[41] and many protein thiols,[42] but the main one is glutathione (GSH). Glutathione is oxidized to glutathione disulphide (GSSG) and can be regenerated by the enzyme glutathione reductase which interacts with the hydrogen ion donor NADPH. The regeneration of NADPH from NADP can be a rate limiting step[43] which thus compromises the regeneration of GSH from its oxidized disulphide. As glutathione disulphide is rapidly excreted from the hepatocyte, glutathione levels fall and an excess of oxidative metabolites is produced. These can then interact with other critical metabolic pathways that effect membrane lipids,[44] membrane ATPases[45] and DNA.[46] The importance of peroxidation of lipids has been emphasized as lipid peroxides particularly react with membranes, metal ions and metalloproteins. Another major consequence of oxidative stress is the oxidation of other protein thiols that are active in a variety of enzyme systems[47] including those controlling the ATPase-dependent plasma membrane calcium transport[48] and microsomal calcium flux.[49]

Calcium-dependent cytotoxicity

Major disturbance in intracellular calcium homeostasis is so frequent in the process of cell death that it has been proposed as the final common pathway. In an experimental tissue-culture system the degree and severity of cell damage can be regulated by controlling the concentration of calcium in the medium. Cell death is not induced in the absence of calcium ions but occurs rapidly in their presence. Death is associated with a rapid flux of calcium from the supernatant into the cell. This is not a phenomenon that singles out cells that are already dead. The hepatotoxicity of phalloidin can be prevented by pre treatment with cytochalasin B, which binds calcium. When hepatocytes are exposed to phalloidin in a calcium-free medium, death does not occur until calcium ions have been added, and can then be prevented by prior exposure to cytochalasin B.[36] A similar calcium-dependent mechanism has been demonstrated in ischaemic hepatic necrosis. Drugs that modify the transfer of calcium across the cell membrane influence cell death. Chlorpromazine inhibits transfer of calcium across membranes and is protective[50] whereas a calcium ionophore, A23187, which permits rapid transmission of calcium into a cell, is extremely cytotoxic.[51] This evidence suggests that the net influx of calcium into a cell converts severe but reversible damage into an irreversible process resulting in cell death. The mechanism by which this flux finally precipitates cell death is complicated. Calcium crossing the plasma membrane interacts with a calcium receptor protein (calmodulin) and activates various enzymes including phospholipases. Eventually, there is a vast increase in the concentration of calcium in mitochondria, which is thought to disrupt the respiratory cytochromes and thus produce cell death.

Other experimental work has shown that the absence of calcium can potentiate cytotoxicity in some systems. In these situations the loss of protein thiols appears to be more critical than the presence or absence of calcium.[52] The culture of hepatocytes in a calcium-deficient medium can still generate sufficient oxidative stress in cells to produce rapid secondary depletion of GSH and protein thiols.[53] This depletion is prevented by antioxidants such as vitamin E. Protection can also be provided by a metal ion chelator with an affinity for calcium such as EDTA. Even in this system, calcium flux may still be a critical event, related to intracellular changes in the cytosolic and mitochondrial pools that are induced by oxidative stress.[54] Cell damage and death or their products trigger the processes of inflammation, regeneration and repair; the latter involves fibrogenesis and may eventually lead to cirrhosis.

INFLAMMATION

It is not appropriate in this chapter to review inflammation in detail. In cirrhosis, the activity of the disease process is usually judged by the nature, location and extent of the cellular inflammatory infiltrate. Thus, active biliary cirrhosis has many neutrophils clustering around the basement membrane of the peripheral bile ductules, while in alcoholic liver disease neutrophils are present around hepatocytes containing Mallory bodies. This latter process is sometimes referred to as satellitosis.

It is now established that leukotrienes are key mediators in inflammatory liver diseases.[55] Both Kupffer cells and hepatocytes can produce leukotrienes in response to platelet-activating factor and bacterial endotoxin. A compound similar to leukotriene B4 is produced by hepatocytes during alcohol metabolism and this has been postulated as the agent that attracts neutrophils to the liver in alcoholic hepatitis.[56]

REGENERATION

The normal liver consists of a stable population of hepatocytes with a slow turnover rate, but it has a capacity for regeneration that can restore approximately three-quarters of its own mass within six months. Many factors influence this regeneration but the precise triggers which stimulate increased mitotic activity are still uncertain.[16] These hepatic growth regulators can be broadly divided into groups: nutrients and hormones, polypeptide growth factors not necessarily specific to the liver, and serum- or liver-derived growth factors with greater specificity for the liver than other tissues.

Nutrients and hormones

Nutrients

Regeneration depends upon the availability of the basic nutrient building blocks that are usually supplied via portal venous blood from intestinal digestion and absorption. None the less, the effect to specific dietary deficiencies can be difficult to evaluate because of an ability to mobilize these resources from other cells in the body. Fasting has been shown to delay and diminish regeneration in response to partial hepatectomy, but it does not abolish it.[57] It has also been shown that there is an increase in the amino acid pool following partial hepatectomy[58] and enhanced movement of amino acids across the cell membrane.[59] Infusions of a branched-chain-enriched mixture of amino acids have been shown to stimulate regeneration[60] although, generally, infusions of amino acids, lipids or carbohydrate have an inhibitory effect upon the response.[61] However, dietary protein does enhance regeneration as increased mitotic activity can be demonstrated in hepatocytes when the animals are transferred from low-protein to normal or high-protein diets.[62] It has been postulated that this occurs because a population of hepatocytes that require protein to progress to the S phase of the cell cycle builds up during the period of protein deprivation.[63]

Hormones

Virtually all hormones have been shown to influence regeneration in the liver. They include insulin and glucagon, thyroid and adrenal cortical hormones, parathyroid hormone, prolactin, vasopressin, prostaglandins, catecholamines and sex hormones.[16] Of these, the most important seem to

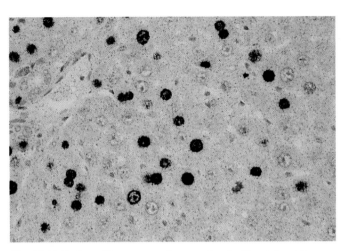

Fig. 10.18 Periportal hepatocytes show uptake of tritiated thymidine, reflecting mitotic activity, 48 hours after partial hepatectomy in a diabetic rat treated with insulin. An identical response is seen in diabetic rats not treated with insulin but is delayed for approximately 12 hours.

be insulin, glucogan and the catecholamines. In the absence of insulin, regeneration is not diminished but it is delayed in onset and takes much longer[64-66] (Fig. 10.18). Conversely, the presence of insulin has the opposite effect.[67] Glucagon acts synergistically with insulin but neither hormone alone or in concert is able to initiate, or by their absence prevent, regeneration.[16]

Various observations suggest that catecholamines are involved in the early stages of liver regeneration and could play a part in the regulation of liver growth. Blood catecholamine levels are known to increase within 2 hours of partial hepatectomy, and DNA synthesis in the regenerating liver is significantly reduced by chemical or surgical sympathetic denervation.[68] The rich sympathetic nerve supply to portal tracts and sinusoids is also greatly increased in liver after regeneration.[69] The response appears to be modulated through tha α-adrenergic receptors as β-blockers do not have any influence. The number of α_1-adrenergic receptors on hepatocytes decreases by 30–40% in the 24 hours after partial hepatectomy while β-receptors increase dramatically.[70,71] Norepinephrine also enhances the effects of epidermal growth factor on DNA synthesis in cultured hepatocytes[72] and counteracts the growth inhibitory effects of transforming growth factor β.[73] Thyroid hormones can also promote regeneration but a combination of tri-iodothyronine, amino acids, glucagon and heparin is even more effective.[74]

Polypeptide growth factors

Several polypeptides have now been identified which are potent but non-tissue-specific mitogens. These include epidermal growth factor, transforming growth factor α, heparin-binding growth factors and insulin-like growth factors.

Epidermal growth factor (EGF) and transforming growth factor α (TGFα)

These two polypeptides are closely related. TGF has approximately 30–40% amino acid sequence homology to EGF and is thought to act through the same receptors as EGF. EGF is synthesized and released by a large number of cells and tissues and is mitogenic in many mesenchymal and epithelial structures including the liver.[75] It is very effective at stimulating liver regeneration and this is considerably enhanced by insulin. Its potency for the liver may be due to the high number of receptors on the hepatocyte plasma membrane and the liver has an extraordinary capacity to clear EGF from the blood.[76] EGF stimulates DNA synthesis in hepatocytes in tissue culture, suggesting that it has a direct effect.[77] This is supported by the preferential accumulation of radioactive label in hepatocyte nuclei of the regenerating liver after giving EGF labelled with radioactive iodine.[78] Although the experimental evidence supports EGE as a major primary hepatic growth regulator, blood levels of EGF do not change much immediately after partial hepatectomy[79] and there is no increase in messenger RNA for EGF receptors for the first 24 hours.[80] The physiological role of EGF in initiating regeneration is therefore uncertain.

TGF α has effects closely related to those of EGF but these may be significantly different. Messenger RNA for TGFα is undetectable in the normal liver but appears within 8 hours of partial hepatectomy and increases rapidly over the next 24 hours in parallel with DNA synthesis.[81] TGFα also directly enhances DNA synthesis in hepatocytes in tissue culture. As these release TGFα into the medium when stimulated by EGE,[82] an early role for EGF in stimulating liver regeneration cannot be excluded. Equally, TGFα could be derived from extrahepatic sources. Either way, TGFα could then act as an autocrine regulator in promoting regeneration.

Other polypeptides

These are mainly the heparin-binding growth factors (HBGF) and the insulin-like growth factors (IGF, somatomedins).

HBGFs have also been termed fibroblast growth factors (FGF) and are mitogens for a wide variety of cell types. There are two main subtypes, HBGF-1 and HBGF-2, and an increase in both is found in hepatocytes at an early, though not the earliest stage in liver regeneration.[83,84] As with TGFα, they may have an autocrine role in helping to amplify the initial regenerative signals.

IGFs are synthesized in the liver in response to growth hormone and represent the probable mechanisms through which growth hormone influences liver regeneration. A time lag of several hours elapses before enhancement of regeneration occurs in response to growth hormone, and

these polypeptides probably have a modulatory rather than an initiating role.[85]

Liver growth factors

Human hepatocyte growth factor (hHGF). This 85 kilodalton (kD) protein is a potent stimulator of DNA synthesis in both rat and human hepatocytes.[86] It has a sequence that is common to part of the hepatopoietin A molecule. It is ten times more effective than other polypeptide growth factors such as EGF,[87] and hHGF levels in the plasma correlate closely with the degree of encephalopathy in patients with fulminant hepatic failure.[88]

Other liver growth factors. A large number of other putatively specific liver growth promoters have been identified, including a hepatocyte growth factor derived from platelets (HGF), two hepatopoietins (HPTA and HPTB), and hepatic stimulating substance (HSS). Their effects have only been identified in tissue culture so that their physiological roles are currently undetermined. Platelet hepatocyte growth factor was identified in rat platelets following the observation that serum from rats was more potent in stimulating regeneration than serum from other species, and that serum was more potent than plasma. It differs in physical characteristics and in biological activity from human hepatocyte growth factor.[89] The hepatopoietins stimulate hepatocytes but not fibroblasts and are found in highest concentration in the serum 24–48 hours after partial hepatectomy. Hepatopoietin A has been identified immunocytochemically in various tissues including pancreatic acinar cells and duodenal Brunner's glands but not in liver and kidney.[90] Hepatopoietin B acts synergistically with HPTA. Hepatocyte stimulating substance is unrelated to other known growth promoters and is heat stable. It is inactive on non-hepatic epithelial tissues but its stimulatory action on adult hepatocytes requires the presence of EGF or serum factors.[91]

Growth inhibitory factors

Even less is known about growth inhibitory factors. It has been suggested that they could represent the normal regulatory mechanism for liver growth. In this model, inhibitory substances would be produced by the normal liver and their relative absence following hepatic resection or significant hepatocellular damage would release hepatocytes from their effects.

Transforming growth factor β (TGFβ) is the most clearly identified candidate. This is a ubiquitous 25 kD polypeptide whose actions in vivo are unknown. In vitro it can either inhibit or stimulate cell proliferation, modulate cell differentiation and regulate numerous cellular functions according to the cell type, culture conditions and presence of other cytokines.[92] However, in an experimental situation,

TGFβ fails to prevent regeneration after hepatectomy[93] so its role would seem to be one of modulation rather than primary control.

Morphology

Regeneration is recognized by the twinning of liver-cell plates, lack of lipofuscin, increased numbers of binucleate or multinucleate hepatocytes, and anisonucleosis. Both multinucleate hepatocytes and enlarged hyperchromatic nuclei increase in number with age. If regeneration is recent, the hepatocytes lack lipofuscin. Twinning of cell plates may be present for some months after regeneration is complete but rarely is as persistent as the cytological changes. As the cell plates double in thickness, a cirrhotic nodule is converted from one merely carved out of the pre-existing parenchyma to a 'regenerative' nodule. The growth of this nodule depends on the rate of regeneration compared with the rate of cell death. A regenerative macronodular cirrhosis eventually results. There are examples of cirrhosis where morphological features of nodular regeneration are not prominent until a late stage. This is particularly true for biliary cirrhosis, both primary and secondary. There are also some circumstances in which regeneration could be directly impaired, as for instance by alcohol and by age. The increased risk of death in acute viral hepatitis when patients are over the age of 30 has been attributed to decreasing regenerative capacity with increasing age.[94] The age-related factors contributing to this phenomenon are unknown and the cause of impaired regeneration is difficult to identify in an individual case.

Cell death may exceed or equal the regenerative activity within a nodule or, alternatively, regeneration may exceed cell death. If cell death is overall in excess of regeneration then rapid clinical deterioration may be expected. This is one of the factors that contributes to the poor survival of alcoholics who continue to drink.[95] Conversely, if regenerative activity exceeds the loss of hepatocytes, then growth of the nodule will occur. This expansile growth compresses the surrounding fibrous stroma and approximates portal tracts. It will also stretch and compress the bile ducts and the vascular channels, including the shunts that have been formed. The compression of vessels by the expanding nodule impedes blood flow, with the most severe effects on the low pressure portal venous system, and thus accentuates portal hypertension. As a result, nodules become increasingly dependent upon hepatic arterial blood flow. Consequently, when hypovolaemic shock occurs from bleeding varices, there is increased risk of cell death due to ischaemia. Obstruction to the biliary tree is associated with proliferation of bile ductules around the nodule and with retention of copper complexed to its binding protein in the hepatocytes.

FIBROSIS

There are many different forms of collagen in the liver and these are all vastly increased in cirrhosis.[96] The types of collagen, the factors controlling the metabolism of each, their relative proportions to each other, the cellular origins and the control mechanisms are currently being intensively studied. It is now clear that the extracellular matrix of the liver includes glycoproteins and proteoglycans as well as the standard collagens. Fibrosis in cirrhosis is not an inert unchanging stromal scaffold but is the product of a dynamic interaction of matrix degradation and matrix formation.

Components of the liver matrix

Collagens

At least 14 different collagens have now been identified. These fall broadly into two categories—fibrillar and basement membrane collagens. Types I, III and V of the fibrillar collagens and types IV and VI of the basement membrane collagens have been identified in the liver. Type I collagen corresponds to the doubly refractile mature collagen in portal tracts and around the walls of hepatic veins, and type III collagen approximates to the reticulin framework of the sinusoids but is also present in portal tracts. Type IV collagen forms the basement membranes around bile ducts, arteries and veins and is distinctive because it forms a two-dimensional lattice.[97] It is also a component of a matrix in the space of Disse which is not normally visualized by routine histological techniques. Type V collagen is closely associated with basement membranes and with the matrix in the space of Disse also. Here it is found along with the collagen-associated protein, fibronectin, around the fibrillar type III collagen.[98,99] Type VI collagen, in contrast, is found in the interstitial matrix of the portal tract. It is absent from basement membranes but is frequently present near blood vessels and it may have a role in anchoring vascular tissue to the perivascular matrix.[100]

Glycoproteins and proteoglycans

The collagens are only one component of the hepatic extracellular matrix; they are intimately complexed and interwoven with glycoproteins and the proteoglycans to form the total supporting structure of the liver.

The glycoproteins include laminin, nidogen, fibronectin, tenascin, undulin and elastin. All types of collagen and glycoproteins are increased in cirrhosis to at least twice the normal amount, but often much more is present. In experimental animal liver injury, the increase in staining for fibronectin and type V collagen suggests that each of these may be important in organizing the bulk of the matrix.[101] A similar role has been proposed for tenascin, based on its discrete localization to connective tissue–parenchymal interfaces.[102]

The proteoglycans have a core protein with a variable number of unbranched carbohydrate side chains composed of repeating sulphated disaccharide units. For heparan sulphate these are iduronic acid-*N*-acetylglucosamine, for dermatan sulphate iduronic acid-*N*-acetylgalactosamine, and for chondroitin sulphate glucuronic acid-*N*-acetylgalactosamine. Hyaluronic acid is different — it lacks a protein core and is formed as a non-sulphated polysaccharide from glucosamine and glucuronic acid. The strong anionic charge on the proteoglycans contributes to their binding to the other constituents of the matrix. Heparan sulphate particularly modulates the proliferative and secretory characteristics of mesenchymal cells[103] and is an essential extracellular component of basement membranes.[104] The proteoglycans also function as adhesion molecules[105] and can act as receptor molecules on cell surfaces.[106] As such they have been identified as an important reservoir for the cytokines, including TGFβ. Heparan sulphate is the predominant proteoglycan in normal liver. In cirrhosis the total proteoglycan content is increased up to five times the normal amount but this is largely due to increases in dermatan and chondroitin sulphates.[107]

The toral matrix in the space of Disse can increase and change its character to the extent that it can be morpho-

NORMAL LIVER

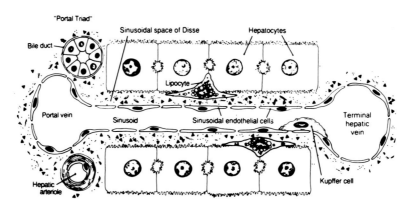

FIBROTIC LIVER

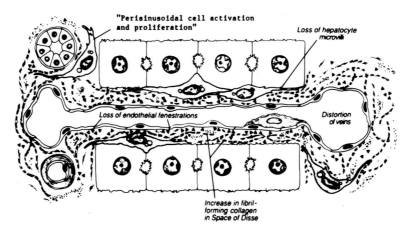

KEY

〰〰〰 Fibril-forming collagens (Types I,III,V)

〰〰〰 Basement membrane collagens (Types IV,VI)

▪▪▴▴ Glycoconjugates (laminin, FN, glycosaminoglycans, tenascin)

Fig. 10.19 Liver fibrosis produces changes in cells and matrix. The process of fibrosis results in the replacement of the normal basement membrane components in the space of Disse (type IV collagen, laminin, heparan sulphate) by fibrillar collagens. This is associated with activation of perisinusoidal cells and loss of both endothelial fenestrations and hepatic microvilli. Reproduced from Freidman et al[96] with permission of the authors and publishers.

logically identified. This is then referred to as 'capillarization of the sinusoids'[108] (Fig. 10.19). Capillarization is a critical and deleterious event and correlates with impaired liver function.[109] In general, abnormal matrix deposition occurs in those parts of the acinus where cell injury and inflammation are greatest. This architectural variation in the distribution of excessive matrix is an early feature and is lost subsequently due to further architectural alterations and increases in matrix deposition.

Function of the extracellular matrix in the liver

As well as providing the structural framework of the liver, there is evidence that the complex matrix in the space of Disse is essential for maintaining the integrity and function of hepatocytes and sinusoidal cells. In most tissue culture environments, hepatocytes rapidly dedifferentiate, but if they are cultured on a gel rich in laminin and containing type IV collagen, heparan sulphate and entactin, they remain polarized and cuboidal and show good preservation of their ultrastructural features.[110] Cell-specific gene expression and protein secretion can also be identified for extended periods.[111–113] Therefore liver injury that disrupts the sinusoidal subendothelial matrix could result in cell dedifferentiation with impairment of liver function. This has been demonstrated in clinical studies — the process of capillarization of sinusoids correlates well with impairment of liver function.[107] The sinusoidal subendothelial matrix also helps to preserve the functions and activities of endothelial cells and perisinusoidal cells. When perisinusoidal cells are maintained on the basement membrane-like gel they remain spherical with extensive filamentous outbranchings and do not proliferate.[114] Similarly, sinusoidal endothelial cells are fenestrated in normal liver but lose their fenestrations in association with sinusoidal capillarization (Fig. 10.19). The size of the fenestrae can be modulated by the nature of the extracellular matrix.[115] This could initiate a vicious cycle of reduced porosity, impaired movement of solutes and macromolecules into the space of Disse, hepatocellular damage and enhanced subendothelial matrix formation.

Cellular origin

In the normal liver, matrix may be produced by hepatocytes, perisinusoidal cells and sinusoidal endothelial cells[116–118] but in cirrhosis the perisinusoidal cell (Ito cell, lipocyte, fat-storing cell) is the primary source for the increased extracellular matrix. There is also evidence that perisinusoidal cells are extensively involved in the degradation of the extracellular matrix.

Perisinusoidal cells

The perisinusoidal cell is present in the subendothelial

space of Disse and sometimes in the perisinusoidal recess between hepatocytes.[119] (see Ch. 1) Characteristically, the cell contains large amounts of vitamin A and can therefore be recognized by its autofluorescence (Fig. 10.20). These cells are present in large numbers in circumstances associated with fibrosis. Transitional forms between them and myofibroblasts have been described.[120–123] Myofibroblasts and transitional forms derived from perisinusoidal cells have been found in the newly formed fibrous tissue in alcoholic liver disease,[124,125] and perisinusoidal cells have been found in the early perivenular fibrosis of alcoholics[120,126] as well as in the fibrosis associated with prolonged severe hypervitaminosis A.[14] These early studies have been supported more recently by others utilizing in-situ hybridization, liver-cell culture techniques and the analysis of gene expression. All these have confirmed hepatic perisinusoidal cells as the major source of extracellular matrix during fibrogenesis.

Immunocytochemical and immunoelectronmicroscopic studies in normal liver have identified types I and IV collagen in perisinusoidal cells, hepatocytes and sinusoidal endothelial cells, and type III collagen and fibronectin in perisinusoidal cells and sinusoidal endothelial cells.[127] These properties are enhanced in the fibrotic liver with hepatocytes additionally displaying positive staining for fibronectin and endothelial cells for laminin.[128] However, in-situ hybridization studies have suggested that in both normal and fibrotic liver the active expression of matrix genes is almost exclusively confined to non-hepatocyte cells. There is marked increase in expression of messenger RNAs for collagens I, III, IV and laminin in these non-parenchymal cells when fibrosis is experimentally induced.[129,130] There is no evidence of collagen formation by hepatocytes, even in fibrotic liver, using these techniques.

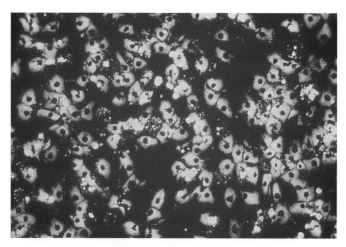

Fig. 10.20 Vitamin A endogenous fluorescence in cultured perisinusoidal cells examined in ultraviolet light. Individual cells appear as bright rings with central non-fluorescent nuclei. Reproduced from Freidman et al[96] with permission of the authors and publishers.

Virtually all cell culture studies agree that the perisinu- soidal cell has the key role in matrix formation. Hepatocytes have been shown to contain small amounts of collagens I and IV with the appropriate messenger RNA[131] and to secrete fibronectin.[123] They also produce the proteo- glycan, heparan sulphate,[133] but do not produce the other proteoglycans which are more commonly found in hepatic fibrosis. Sinusoidal endothelial cells can express type IV collagen immunocytochemically, and their collagen gene expression increases in fibrosis but to a much smaller extent than that in the perisinusoidal cell.[134] In culture, perisinusoidal cells express collagens I, III, IV, laminin and heparin sulphate.[131,135–137]

Cell-matrix interaction

Several receptors for components of the extracellular matrix have now been identified on hepatocyte mem- branes.[138] Amongst these is a family of receptors, the integrins, which possess a recognition site for molecules containing the tripeptide sequence arginine–glycine– aspartic acid (RGD). Laminin, fibronectin, entactin,

tenascin and type I collagen are all known to have RGD sequences. Hepatocytes have integrin receptors for fibronectin and type I collagen[139,140] and non-integrin receptors for laminin and type IV collagen.[141,142] Hepa- tocytes also bind proteoglycans and this binding can be saturated, implying a receptor-mediated interaction.[143] Some of these matrix-associated proteoglycans can bind cytokines — including TGFβ,[104] suggesting that effects on cell function could be mediated by release of cytokines from a reservoir in the matrix. The role of integrins in the interaction of perisinusoidal cells and sinusoidal endothe- lial cells with the matrix is poorly understood. Those receptors that have been characterized on these cells seem to be primarily involved in the clearance of ligands.[144]

Regulation of fibrogenesis

The activation of the perisinusoidal cell is the crucial event in hepatic fibrosis (Fig. 10.21). The requirements of the perisinusoidal cell in tissue culture clearly demonstrate that changes in the extracellular matrix influence the activity of the cell. Perisinusoidal cells grown on uncoated

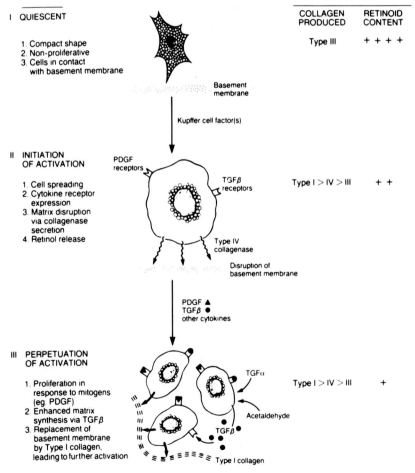

Fig. 10.21 Mechanisms of perisinusoidal cell activation. Reproduced from Freidman et al[96] with permission of the authors and publishers.

plastic show progressive loss of vitamin A and increased collagen, fibronectin and proteoglycan secretion. Conversely, maintenance of perisinusoidal cells on an artificial basement membrane, such as the laminin-rich gel that can be extracted from a murine sarcoma, results in quiescent cells with a well-preserved morphology and low levels of collagen synthesis.[145] Changes in the nature of the extracellular matrix in the space of Disse may therefore be a key factor, if not in initiating, then certainly in amplifying, the enhanced collagen production by the perisinusoidal cell. The changes in the extracellular matrix may be initiated by proteinases that are produced by perisinusoidal cells and Kupffer cells, and a variety of soluble mediators have been identified that are capable of influencing both cell types.

Soluble mediators

These are separated into two broad functional categories of initiation and perpetuation. Thus, it has been suggested that acetaldehyde produced in alcoholic fibrosis is not the crucial factor in activating perisinusoidal cells to produce collagen but it does perpetuate and even enhance that activation.[146] This is supported by tissue culture experiments showing that acetaldehyde is more effective in enhancing type I collagen synthesis if the cells are already activated.[147] Also, perisinusoidal cells in tissue culture do not divide in response to platelet-derived growth factor (PDGF) unless they have been previously exposed to Kupffer cell-conditioned medium, although Kupffer cells do not secrete PDGF and perisinusoidal cells expressing receptors for PDGF do not proliferate in the presence of Kupffer cells. It is postulated that surface receptors for PDGF are induced on perisinusoidal cells by the Kupffer cell-conditioned medium[143] and they can also be shown to increase collagen production.

This activity of Kupffer cell medium has been attributed to the release of cytokines and in particular to TGFβ.[148] The mechanisms controlling the release and activity of cytokines from Kupffer cells are not well elucidated but it is possible that the matrix in the space of Disse may provide an extracellular reservoir for TGFβ which could be released and/or activated by matrix proteinases. Perisinusoidal cells themselves may be capable of producing TGFβ as the messenger RNA for this cytokine has been identified in these cells.[127] TGFβ can also enhance the proliferation of perisinusoidal cells induced by EGF and PDGF.[149] TGFβ would seem to be the most important cytokine so far identified because it can stimulate collagen synthesis, whereas most of the other soluble cytokines simply modulate proliferation of the perisinusoidal cells and have little effect on matrix synthesis. This stimulation of collagen synthesis by TGFβ is influenced by the type of basement membrane. In tissue culture, TGFβ stimulates collagen synthesis when the perisinusoidal cells are maintained on type I collagen but not when they are maintained on type IV collagen.[150] The other cytokines that have been shown to stimulate perisinusoidal cells into mitosis include EGF, TGFα, FGF, insulin-like growth factor, interleukin-1 and tumour necrosis factor α (TNFα). Many of these cytokines are derived from Kupffer cells.

The role of retinoids in activation of perisinusoidal cells seems unclear because of the paradoxical effects of vitamin A. Chronic excess of vitamin A intake is associated with fibrosis and cirrhosis, but cirrhosis from other causes is associated with depletion of hepatic vitamin A.[151] When perisinusoidal cells in tissue culture are activated they show a loss of retinoid, but the addition of exogenous retinoid to the tissue culture medium both inhibits cell proliferation and decreases type I collagen synthesis.[152,153]

Thus, there are a number of interacting soluble factors that enhance or suppress proliferation of perisinusoidal cells and enhance or suppress matrix synthesis, and further modulation results from alterations in the nature of the extracellular matrix.

MATRIX DEGRADATION

Metalloproteinases

The marked excess of matrix in cirrhosis has meant that matrix formation has received most attention and has been considered to be a key event. Matrix degradation by comparison has been ignored but, as has been indicated, could be a key event in activating the perisinusoidal cell into both proliferation and matrix synthesis. In general, matrix may be degraded extracellularly by metalloproteinases and intracellularly by lysosomal cathepsins. The metalloproteinases appear to be important in matrix remodelling in all parts of the body and also play a key role within the liver. These proteinases are subdivided into collagenases which degrade fibrillar collagens, stromelysins which degrade many protein substrates including type IV collagen, gelatin, laminin and fibronectin, and the type IV collagenase/gelatinases which have a specificity indicated by the name. All these enzymes are closely related[154] and their primary structure contains several well-conserved domains.[155] One of these domains is an 80-amino-acid sequence in the propeptide portion of the molecule which is important in enzyme activation; another is a catalytic domain containing the highly conserved zinc-binding site. Additionally, individual metalloproteinases have domains that are specific to them. For instance, the 72 kD type IV collagenase/gelatinase has a fibronectin-like gelatin-binding domain. The current nomenclature and properties of the metalloproteinases are summarized in Table 10.2.

Interstitial collagenase. This proteinase was first identified in 1962 in tadpole tails undergoing morphogenesis[156] but it has since been identified in a wide variety of

Table 10.2 Nomenclature and properties of matrix metalloproteinases. (Reproduced from Friedman et al[96] with permission of the authors and publishers).

Enzyme	Metalloproteinase (MMP) No.	Molecular mass (kD) Pro-enzyme	Active	Substrate specificity
Interstitial collagenase	MMP-1	57, 52	47, 42	Type III>I>II
Neutrophil collagenase	MMP-8	72, 57	70, 50	Type I>II>III
72kD gelatinase/type IV collagenase	MMP-2	72	66	Type IV,?V,VII,X, gelatin
92kD gelatinase/type IV collagenase	MMP-9	92	84	Type IV,V, gelatin
Stromelysin-1	MMP-3	60, 57	45, 28	Type III, IV, V, laminin proteoglycan, casein, fibronectin, gelatins
Stromelysin-2	MMP-10	(53)	47, 28	Type II, IV, V, gelatins, fibronectin
Stromelysin-3	None	—	—	Not known
PUMP-1	MMP-7	28	21, 19	Type IV, laminin, fibronectin, gelatin, casein

cells, including fibroblasts, smooth muscle cells, mononuclear phagocytes and capillary endothelial cells. It is synthesized as a preproenzyme which is then activated by proteinases. The activated enzyme cleaves type I collagen at specific Gly–Ile and Gly–Leu bonds. The collagenase can also degrade type II collagen but has no demonstrable activity against type IV basement membrane collagen.

Interstitial collagenase has been identified in the liver but the cellular origin is uncertain. The earliest studies suggested that Kupffer cells were the source[157] but the techniques used to isolate Kupffer cells resulted in a significant mixture of Kupffer cells with other sinusoidal liver cells. None the less, the identification of this enzyme in peripheral blood monocytes is consistent with Kupffer cells also producing it.[158] The perisinusoidal cell in resting conditions does not produce interstitial collagenase but, in tissue culture, fibroblasts prepared from human liver and exposed to interleukin-1 or tumour necrosis factor α produce messenger RNA for this enzyme.[159]

A neutrophil collagenase which is very similar to interstitial collagenase also exists. This also has a substrate specificity for interstitial collagens but has much greater avidity for degrading type I collagen than type III collagen.[160] The enzyme is released from the cytoplasmic granules of the neutrophil following activation.

Type IV collagenase/gelatinase. Two major proteinases in this category have been described: one is 92 kD and the other 72 kD in size. The larger 92 kD type IV collagenase/gelatinase is synthesized and released predominantly by macrophages and neutrophils.[161,162] As its name implies, it actively degrades gelatin and collagen types IV and V but does not degrade the interstitial fibrillar collagens. The enzyme has been identified in Kupffer cells and is released upon their activation.[163] The 72 kD collagenase/gelatinase is synthesized and released by tumour cells, fibroblasts and osteoblasts, and to a small degree by mononuclear phagocytes. The activated enzyme degrades gelatin, collagen types IV and V and does not cleave the fibrillar collagens. In this respect it is identical to the larger 92 kD proteinase. The cleavage of type IV

collagen is produced by a pepsin-resistant fragment of the molecule which, like interstitial collagenase, cleaves at Gly–Leu and Gly–Ile bonds.[164] The lack of effect of the type IV collagenase on type I and III fibrillar collagens is presumably due to lack of access to these bonds because of the tertiary structure of the fibrillar collagen. In the liver, the perisinusoidal cell produces and releases this enzyme. Perisinusoidal cells in tissue culture have been shown to contain messenger RNA for the enzyme, the enzyme has been immunocytochemically demonstrated in these cells, and extracellular release of the enzyme from the cells into the supernatent has been demonstrated.[165,166]

Stromelysins. Three stromelysins (1, 2 and 3) and a closely related metalloproteinase, PUMP-1, have been identified from a variety of tissues. These enzymes have a broad range of matrix degradation activity but none of them has been clearly identified within liver.

Metalloproteinase inhibitors

Specific tissue inhibitors of metalloproteinases (TIMPs) have been identified and there are other general proteinase inhibitors such as α_2-macroglobulin which can also inhibit their action.

TIMP-1 is a small 28 kD glycoprotein secreted by a wide variety of cell types including fibroblasts. It binds irreversibly to active metalloproteinases of all types. The perisinusoidal cells have been shown to express the gene for TIMP-1, synthesize the immunoreactive protein and release a protein with TIMP-1 activity into the supernatant.[167,168] Regulation of gene expression is influenced by the same growth factors and cytokines that are involved in the regulation of metalloproteinase gene expression.

TIMP-2 is a smaller 21 kD protein with significant homology to TIMP-I and with many similar properties. Its current role in the liver is uncertain, as is the role for the other two TIMP inhibitors which have not yet been well characterized.

α_2-Macroglobulin is a high molecular weight plasma glycoprotein (725 kD) that is able to bind both interstitial collagenase and stromelysin.[169] It is synthesized predominantly by hepatocytes but the perisinusoidal cell also contains messenger RNA for this proteinase scavenger and can synthesize the molecule.[170]

Metalloproteinases, their inhibitors and liver fibrosis

It is apparent that there is a complex interplay of factors involved in the production and maintenance of the liver matrix that is centred around the role of the perisinusoidal cell and is influenced by the metalloproteinases and their inhibitors. Excess matrix may accumulate within the liver following increased formation of interstitial collagens by the perisinusoidal cells, from decreased activity of metalloproteinases in their removal, or by increased inhibition of metalloproteinases. The metalloproteinases, specifically type IV collagenase, could potentially disrupt the normal liver matrix and thus create a micro-environment that would enhance perisinusoidal cell activation and matrix formation.

Interstitial collagenase activity is increased in liver fibrosis. Fibrotic liver from rats treated with carbon tetrachloride degrades type I collagen more readily than does normal liver.[171] This activity seems to be greatest during the development of severe lesions but diminishes with advanced cirrhosis. This increased activity is clearly insufficient to prevent fibrosis, and total interstitial collagenase activity decreases relative to total hepatic collagen content.[172] Interstitial collagenase activity in alcoholic liver disease is increased in fatty liver, shows a further increase in fibrotic liver, but decreases once alcoholic cirrhosis is established.[173] There is little information on the tissue inhibitors of interstitial collagenase in either normal or diseased liver. None the less, a full understanding of the interplay of all these factors could lead to treatments that slow or even halt the progression of chronic liver diseases towards cirrhosis.[94]

COMPLICATIONS AND CLINICAL CONSEQUENCES

With the notable exception of hepatocellular carcinoma, the major clinical consequences of cirrhosis are due to the abnormalities of blood flow and the loss of functional parenchymal mass. The abnormal blood flow creates portal hypertension, contributes to hepatic parenchymal insufficiency and permits infection. The loss of functional parenchymal mass results in impaired protein synthesis, inadequate deactivation of drugs and hormones, jaundice and clotting abnormalities (see Ch. 2). A combination of these disorders can result in hepatic encephalopathy. Hepatocellular carcinoma most commonly arises in patients with a macronodular cirrhosis, especially when

this is associated with the hepatitis B virus, but it may complicate cirrhosis of other aetiologies.

PORTAL HYPERTENSION

Portal hypertension results in splenomegaly, varices and ascites, and it predisposes to portal venous thrombosis. The spleen is usually only moderately enlarged, but features of hypersplenism may occasionally first bring the patient to clinical notice.

Varices

Varices are found at sites of portosystemic venous anastomoses. These include stomach and oesophagus, left kidney and spleen, rectum and anus, and the peri-umbilical soft tissues.[174] The spleen is usually enlarged in the presence of varices but splenomegaly does not necessarily imply that varices are present. Oesophageal varices, though commonly present, are difficult to identify at autopsy except in very gross examples as they are usually collapsed and inconspicuous. Injection techniques are the most reliable way of demonstrating them but transillumination can indicate their presence and is much simpler. Their submucosal location predisposes them to bleeding: prevention or control of this is a major management problem. Injection sclerotherapy is the treatment of choice over drug therapy and oesophageal trans-section but a new interventional radiological technique creating an intrahepatic portosystemic shunt between the portal and hepatic veins is currently being developed (see Ch. 2).

Portal vein thrombosis

This should be suspected when a patient with a known but stable cirrhosis suddenly develops ascites with or without bleeding oesophageal varices. Unless it occurs secondary to portal venous invasion by hepatocellular carcinoma, the macroscopic appearance is no different from venous thrombosis at any other site (Fig. 10.6). Collateral flow is established through a leash of anastomosing small venous channels in the free edge of the lasser omentum. This becomes increasingly prominent with time.

Ascites

Ascitic fluid is a clear, straw-coloured fluid unless infected, when it is turbid or even purulent.[175] In cases of long standing, the serosa of the intestine becomes thickened and pearly-white from deposition of fibrin. Ascites is multifactorial in origin: inadequate albumin synthesis, together with salt and water retention from increased aldosterone levels, make major contributions to its pathogenesis.[176] (see Ch. 2)

Infection

Patients with cirrhosis are at an increased risk of infection and especially those with alcoholic liver disease.[177] One important mechanism in pathogenesis is the large volume of arterial and portal venous blood bypassing Kupffer cells from shunts both around and through the liver. This is estimated at 20% of blood flow to the liver in established cirrhosis but it may be as high as 50% in individual cases.[178,179] Shunting is also a major factor in producing the hypergammaglobulinaemia of patients with cirrhosis. Antibodies develop to intestinal bacteria that are normally removed by the liver but reach the systemic blood circulation in patients with cirrhosis.[180]

Spontaneous bacterial peritonitis. Patients with cirrhosis also have an increased risk of spontaneous bacterial peritonitis.[175,181,182] This only occurs in the presence of ascites but affects about 10–15% of all patients with cirrhosis who develop this complication. Prompt recognition is essential. A high blood neutrophil count is the most important diagnostic pointer, and presence of neutrophils in the ascitic fluid, even in the absence of positive cultures, should be regarded as diagnostic until proved otherwise. The protein content of the infected ascitic fluid is often low at less than 25 g per litre. The prognosis is poor unless the condition is recognized early and treated adequately: a hospital mortality of 40–60% can result.

IMPAIRED PARENCHYMAL FUNCTION

All aspects of normal liver metabolism may be affected, including disturbed glucose hemeostasis, impaired bile salt production, and abnormal amino acid and ammonia metabolism, which in its most severe degree results in hepatic encephalopathy (see Ch. 2). Deficient protein synthesis is one of the most important consequences. Serum albumin concentrations are reduced and this is a major factor in producing oedema and ascites. Albumin is also an important drug-binding protein so that high levels of unbound, and therefore active, drugs and metabolites are found in the circulation. Consequently, patients with cirrhosis are much more sensitive to the action of drugs and this is compounded in many instances by defective clearance. The clotting factors II, IV, VII and X are also made by the liver and their levels are decreased in cirrhosis. This produces a bleeding diathesis manifested by ecchymoses and sometimes by more serious haemorrhage. As the bleeding tendency is secondary to insufficient cell mass, vitamin K is not effective in correcting it.

Impaired inactivation of drugs and hormones results in prolonged actions of these substances. The half-life of pethidine is doubled in patients with cirrhosis while frusemide can precipitate hepatic encephalopathy. Oestrogen metabolism is also impaired, but this is not the full explanation for the gynaecomastia and testicular atrophy that are found in more than 40% of males with cirrhosis, and there is also evidence for decreased testosterone production in these patients.[183] The main oestrogen increases in the serum are in oestrone and oestriol which are metabolically relatively inactive. Deficiencies of bile acid synthesis and excretion lead to gallstone formation and to malabsorption. The metabolism of vitamin D is abnormal and hepatic osteodystrophy may result. Many other phenomena associated with cirrhosis, such as renal dysfunction, parotid enlargement and a variety of skin lesions, are poorly understood and their detailed discussion is available in standard clinical textbooks of hepatology.[184–186]

Infarction of nodules

Infarction of nodules is a common finding at autopsy and almost invariably indicates a period of hypotension, usually from bleeding varices during the terminal illness. The complication reflects the increasing dependence of cirrhotic nodules upon arterial blood flow and consequent susceptibility of these nodules to infarction following a fall in systemic blood pressure. This complication can result in rapid loss of parenchyma and contributes to the clinical downward spiral of patients presenting with bleeding varices and developing hepatic encephalopathy.

HEPATIC ENCEPHALOPATHY

This complex metabolic abnormality has a multifactorial pathogenesis but there are three important prerequisites. These are the shunting of portal venous blood into the systemic circulation, a high protein content in the diet and the presence of bacteria in the gut. Sterilization of the bowel contents with poorly absorbed antibiotics such as neomycin and the reduction of protein intake are two major measures in management that improve this complication. This implies that metabolites and/or toxins, that are produced by bacteria from protein in the intestines, reach the systemic circulation and, directly or indirectly, are involved in the pathogenesis. Inadequate detoxification of such metabolites in the cirrhotic liver may contribute, but even with a normal liver, a surgically created portosystemic anastomosis is sometimes sufficient to produce encephalopathy. The metabolites responsible for hepatic encephalopathy are unknown. Hyperammonaemia is consistently present but it is not universally accepted as a main agent. One possible mechanism involves the production of glutamine from glutamic acid and ammonia which then promotes the formation of the inhibitory neurotransmitter γ-aminobutyric acid (GABA). Other candidates include mercaptans, short chain fatty acids, false neurotransmitters such as octopamine, and lowered levels of branched chain amino acids. There are many methodological problems which seriously impede analysis of the pathogenesis: the topic has recently been reviewed by Fischer[187] and is further considered in chapter 2.

HEPATOCELLULAR CARCINOMA

With increased survival comes an increasing risk of developing hepatocellular carcinoma. Aetiology is one of the major risk-determining factors: hepatocellular carcinoma is rare in patients with primary biliary cirrhosis, medium in alcoholic cirrhosis, and high in cirrhosis due to chronic HBV infection. Nevertheless, the high frequency of alcohol as a cause of cirrhosis in Western Europe and the USA means that it is the most common cause of the cirrhosis underlying hepatocellular carcinoma in these countries. The topic is fully covered in chapter 16.

Once hepatocellular carcinoma develops there is a rapid deterioration in liver function and, because of the tumour's propensity to invade portal and hepatic veins, a rapid increase in portal hypertension. Any patient with a stable compensated cirrhosis who presents with sudden onset of severe ascites and/or severe variceal bleeding that is difficult to control, should be suspected of having developed tumour and the appropriate investigations performed.

EVOLUTION

The natural history of cirrhosis is one of inexorable deterioration with episodes of variceal bleeding secondary to portal hypertension, ascites and increasing hepatocellular dysfunction, as well as an increased risk of sepsis from disordered Kupffer cell function. In addition, there is an increasing risk with time of developing hepatocellular carcinoma. The rate of deterioration is significantly influenced by the activity of the underlying disease process as this determines the extent of cell death: hence the need for abstinence in the alcoholic, effective venesection in haemochromatosis, steroid therapy in autoimmune chronic active hepatitis and interferon therapy in chronic viral hepatitis—even when cirrhosis is present. When the underlying cause has been removed or controlled there is still a slow but inexorable deterioration towards decompensated liver disease that can span 10 or more years. In incomplete septal cirrhosis, where parenchymal damage is minimal and parenchymal function is well preserved, this decompensation is manifest mainly as portal hypertension. For other types of cirrhosis, the outcome for an individual patient is a reflection of the proportional contributions of the volume and distribution of the excess matrix, the regenerative growth of the nodules, the extent of the parenchymal mass lost and the degree of abnormal vascular shunting rendering residual parenchyma and Kupffer cell filtering mechanisms functionally ineffective. With control of the underlying disease process, it is probable that regeneration can paradoxically promote progression towards

decompensated liver disease. Regeneration results in nodule growth, the surrounding stroma is compressed, and the vascular channels and bile ducts are occluded. A cycle of parenchymal cell death is established from impaired nutrient availability, ischaemia, and intracellular cholestasis which initiates more matrix formation and further regenerative activity. Gastrointestinal haemorrhage from bleeding oesophageal varices is particularly potent at accelerating this vicious downward spiral. Hypovolaemic systemic hypotension produces necrosis of nodules which decreases the available cell mass and accelerates the formation of additional matrix. Variceal bleeding and loss of cell mass produce hepatic encephalopathy. Prompt and effective treatment of bleeding varices is therefore essential.

The portosystemic vascular shunts around and within the liver enable both endotoxins and organisms to bypass the filtering mechanism of the liver and then directly enter the systemic circulation. Occult septicaemia has been documented as being commonly present in patients presenting with decompensated chronic liver disease. Rapid identification and successful treatment of infection can be a key factor in determining survival in individual cases. Once cirrhosis is established and is progressing, liver transplantation offers an effective therapy. In appropriately selected patients a 70% 5-year survival can be achieved.[188] The stage of disease at which transplantation becomes a realistic option for consideration will vary with the aetiology and the individual patient. Many of the criteria are still being evaluated. The presence of hepatocellular carcinoma in patients with cirrhosis is now considered to be a contraindication to transplantation because of the high frequency and rapid presentation of the subsequent metastatic disease.

INDIAN CHILDHOOD CIRRHOSIS

First reported by Sen in 1887,[189] this entity was thought to be peculiar to the Indian subcontinent. However, an increasing number of cases have now been reported from elsewhere and in addition some of these have also involved Caucasians.[190–193] In the initial reports it was noted that morbidity and mortality from the disease was high, the age range of affected children was from 6 months to 5 years and there was often a family predilection.[194–197] Clinically the disease was characterized by progressive hepatomegaly and subsequently splenomegaly was a feature and hepatocellular failure was the common cause of death.[194]

The early histological changes comprised steatosis, but subsequently the features comprised ballooning of hepatocytes, focal necrosis, prominent Mallory body formation, marked pericellular fibrosis and an interstitial mixed acute and chronic inflammatory cell infiltrate. There was eventual progression to a micronodular cirrhosis.

While the aetiology of this condition remains uncertain, there is cumulative evidence to suggest that it is due to copper intoxication. Very high liver copper levels have been demonstrated[198–200] and penicillamine therapy seems to be beneficial if started early.[201] Asymptomatic siblings have also tended to have excess liver copper levels.[202] A number of sporadic cases with identical histopathological features have now been reported from outside India and, in some of these, an environmental source of copper has been reported.[190–193] In adults, chronic copper self-intoxication may produce similar clinical and pathological features.[203] It thus seems likely that hepatic copper overload plays a significant part in the aetiology of the condition, but it is not clear whether there is some inherited metabolic defect which increases hepatic susceptibility to injury by this metal.

REFERENCES

1. 5th Pan-American Congress of Gastroenterology. La Habana, Cuba, 1956
2. Leevy C M, Tygstrup N. Standardisation of nomenclature, diagnostic criteria and diagnostic methodology for diseases of the liver and biliary tract. Basel: Karger, 1976
3. Anthony P P, Ishak K G, Nayak N C, et al. The morphology of cirrhosis: definition, nomenclature and classification. Bull W H O 1977; 55: 521–540
4. Anthony P P, Ishak K G, Nayak N C et al. The morphology of cirrhosis. J Clin Pathol 1978; 31: 395–414
5. Rappaport A M, McPhee P J, Fisher M M, Phillips M J. The scarring of the liver acini (cirrhosis). Tridimensional and microcirculatory considerations. Virchows Arch (A) 1983; 402: 107–137
6. Scheuer P J. Liver biopsy in the diagnosis of cirrhosis. Gut 1970; 11: 275–278
7. Ashton R E, Millward-Sadler G H, White J E. Complications in methotrexate treatment of psoriasis with particular reference to liver fibrosis. J Invest Dermatol 1982; 79: 229–232
8. Crapper R M, Bhathal P S, Mackay I R. Chronic active hepatitis in alcoholic patients. Liver 1983; 38: 327–337
9. Levison D A, Kingham J G C, Dawson A M et al. Slow cirrhosis — or no cirrhosis? A lesion causing benign intrahepatic portal hypertension. J Pathol 1982; 137: 253–272
10. Sciot R, Staessen D, van Damme B et al. Incomplete septal cirrhosis: histopathological aspects. Histopathology 1988; 13: 593–603
11. Wanless I R, Godwin T A, Allen F et al. Nodular regenerative hyperplasia of the liver in haematological disorders: a possible response to obliterative portal venopathy. Medicine 1980; 59: 367–379
12. Wanless I R, Lentz J S, Roberts E A. Partial nodular transformation of the liver in an adult with persistent ductus venosus. Review with hypothesis on pathogenesis. Arch Pathol Lab Med 1985; 109: 427–432
13. Wanless I R, Mawdesley C, Adams R. On the pathogenesis of focal nodular hyperplasia of the liver. Hepatology 1985; 5: 1194–1200
14. Jacques E A, Buschman R J, Layden T J. The histopathologic progression of vitamin A-induced hepatic injury. Gastroenterology 1979; 76: 599–602
15. Sarles J, Scheiner C, Sarran M, Giraud F. Hepatic hypervitaminosis A: a familial observation. J Pediatr Gastroenterol Nutr 1990; 10: 71–76
16. Bucher N L R, Strain A J. Regulatory mechanisms in hepatic regeneration. In: Millward-Sadler G H, Wright R, Arthur M J P, eds. Wright's Liver and biliary disease. London: Saunders, 1992: pp 258–274
17. Lelbach W K. Cirrhosis in the alcoholic and its relation to the volume of alcohol abuse. Ann N Y Acad Sci 1975; 252: 85–105
18. Dahl M G C, Gregory M M, Scheuer P J. Methotrexate hepatotoxicity in psoriasis: comparison of different dose regimens. Brit Med J 1972; 1: 654–656
19. Millward-Sadler G H, Ryan T J. Methotrexate-induced liver disease in psoriasis. Br J Dermatol 1974; 90: 661–667
20. Mondelli M, Eddlestone A L W F. Mechanisms of liver cell injury in acute and chronic hepatitis B. Semin Liver Dis 1984; 4: 47–59
21. Thomas H C, Lok A S F. The immunopathology of autoimmune and hepatitis B virus induced chronic hepatitis. Semin Liver Dis 1984; 4: 36–46
22. Paronetto F, Colucci G, Colombo M. Lymphocytes in liver diseases. In: Popper H, Schaffner F, eds. Progress in liver diseases, vol III. New York: Grune & Stratton, 1986: pp 191–208
23. Triger D R, Wright R. Immunological aspects of liver disease. In: Millward-Sadler G H, Wright R, Arthur M J P, eds. Wright's Liver and biliary disease, 3rd edn. London: Saunders, 1992: pp 229–244
24. Jaycna M R, Millward-Sadler G H, Thomas H C. Chronic hepatitis. In: Millward-Sadler G H, Wright R, Arthur M J P, eds. Wright's Liver and biliary disease, 3rd edn., London: Saunders, 1992: pp 787–820
25. Kawanishi H. Morphological association of lymphocytes with hepatocytes in chronic liver disease. Arch Pathol Lab Med 1977; 101: 286–290
26. Pape G R, Rieber E P, Eisenburg J et al. Involvement of the cytotoxic/suppressor T cell subset in liver tissue injury of patients with acute and chronic liver diseases. Gastroenterology 1984; 85: 657–662
27. Mariani E, Facchini A, Miglio F et al. Analysis with OKT monoclonal antibodies of T-lymphocyte subsets present in blood and liver of patients with chronic active hepatitis. Liver 1984; 4: 22–28
28. Montano L, Aranguibel F, Boffill M, Goodall A H, Janossy G, Thomas H C. An analysis of the composition of the inflammatory infiltrate in autoimmune and hepatitis B virus-induced chronic liver disease. Hepatology 1983; 3: 292–296
29. Trevisan A, Realdi G, Alberti A et al. Core antigen-specific immunoglobulin G bound to the liver cell membrane in chronic hepatitis B. Gastroenterology 1982; 82: 218–222
30. Thomas H C, Shipton U, Montano L. The HLA system: its relevance to the pathogenesis of liver disease. Prog Liver Dis 1982; 7: 517–527
31. Ferluga J, Allison A C. Role of mononuclear infiltrating cells in pathogenesis of hepatitis. Lancet 1978; ii: 610–611
32. Tanner A, Keyhani A, Reiner R et al. Proteolytic enzymes released by liver macrophages may promote injury in a rat model of hepatic damage. Gastroenterology 1981; 86: 647–654
33. Arthur M J P, Bentley I S, Tanner A R et al. Oxygen derived free radicals promote hepatic injury in the rat. Gastroenterology 1985; 89: 1114–1122
34. Lieber C S. Pathogenesis and early diagnosis of alcoholic liver injury. N Engl J Med 1978; 288: 888–893
35. Frimmer D. Phalloidin, a membrane specific toxin. In: Keppler D, ed. Pathogenesis and mechanisms of liver cell necrosis. Lancaster: MTP Press, 1973: pp 163–172
36. Kane A B, Young E E, Schanne F A X, Farber J L. Calcium dependence of phalloidin induced liver cell death. Proc Natl Acad Sci USA 1980; 77: 1117–1180
37. Judah J D, McLean A E M, McLean E K. Biochemical mechanisms of liver injury. Am J Med 1970; 49: 609–616
38. Diaz Gomez M I, de Castro C R, d'Acosta N et al. Species difference in carbon tetrachloride-induced hepatotoxicity. The role of carbon tetrachloride activation and lipid peroxidation. Toxicol Appl Pharmacol 1975; 34: 102–114
39. Recknagle R O, Glende E A. Carbon tetrachloride hepato-toxicity: an example of lethal cleavage. Crit Rev Toxicol 1973; 2: 263–297
40. Sies H. Oxidative stress: introductory remarks. In: Sies H, ed. Oxidative stress. London: Academic Press, 1985: pp 1–8
41. Dean R T, Cheeseman K H. Vitamin E protects against free radical damage in lipid environments. Biochem Biophys Res Comm 1987; 148: 1277
42. DiMonte D, Ross D, Bellomo G et al. Alterations in intracellular thiol homeostasis during the metabolism of menadione by isolated hepatocytes. Arch Biochem Biophys 1984; 235: 334–342
43. Reed D J. Regulation of reductive processes by glutathione. Biochem Pharmacol 1986; 35: 7–13

44. Fridovich I. The biology of oxygen radicals. The superoxide radical is an agent of oxygen toxicity: superoxide dismutases provide an important defence. Science 1978; 201: 875–880

45. Jones D P, Thor H, Smith M T et al. Inhibition of ATP-dependent microsomal Ca²⁺ sequestration during oxidative stress and its prevention by glutathione. J Biol Chem 1983; 258: 6390–6393

46. Ueda K, Kobayashi S, Morita J et al. Site specific damage caused by lipid peroxidation products. Biochim Biophys Acta 1985; 824: 341–348

47. Gilbert H F. Biological disulphides: the first messenger? Modulations of phosphofructokinase activity by thiol/disulphide exchange. J Biol Chem 1982; 257: 12086–12091

48. Scherer N M, Deamer D W. Oxidative stress impairs the function of sarcoplasmic reticulum by oxidation of sulfhydryl groups in the Ca²⁺-ATPase. Arch Biochem Biophys 1986; 246: 589–601

49. Thor H, Hartzell P, Svensson S A et al. On the role of thiol groups in the inhibition of liver microsomal Ca²⁺ sequestration by toxic agents. Biochem Pharmacol 1985; 34: 3717–3723

50. Schanne F A X, Pfau R G, Fraber J L. Galactosamine-induced cell death in primary cultures of rat hepatocytes. Am J Pathol 1980; 100: 25–38

51. Schanne F A X, Kane A B, Young E E et al. Calcium dependence of toxic cell death. A final common pathway. Science 1979; 206: 700–702

52. Pascoe G A, Reed D J. Vitamin E protection against chemical-induced cell injury. II. Evidence for a threshold effect of cellular ∞-tocopherol in prevention of adriamycin toxicity. Arch Biochem Biophys 1987; 256: 159–166

53. Thomas C E, Reed D J. Effect of extracellular Ca²⁺ omission on isolated hepatocytes. I. Induction of oxidative stress and cell injury. J Pharmacol Exp Ther 1988; 245: 493–500

54. Thomas C E, Reed D J. Effect of extracellular Ca²⁺ omission on isolated hepatocytes. II. Loss of mitochondrial membrane potential and protection by inhibitors of uniport Ca²⁺ transduction. J Pharmacol Exp Ther 1988; 245: 501–507

55. Keppler D, Hagmann W, Rapp S et al. The relation of leukotrienes to liver injury. Hepatology 1985; 5: 883–891

56. Parez H D, Roll F J, Bissell D M et al. Production of chemotactic activity for polymorphonuclear leukocytes by cultured rat hepatocytes exposed to ethanol. J Clin Invest 1984; 74: 1350–1357

57. Stirling G A, Laughlin J, Washington S L A. Effects of starvation on the proliferative response after partial hepatectomy. Exp Mol Pathol 1973; 19: 44–52

58. Ord M G, Stocken L A. Uptake of amino acid and nucleic acid precursors by regenerating rat liver. Biochem J 1972; 129: 175–181

59. LeCam A, Rey J F, Fehlman M et al. Amino acid transport in isolated hepatocytes after partial hepatectomy in the rat. Am J Physiol 1979; 236: E594–E602

60. Rigotti P, Peters J C, Tranberg K G et al. Effects of amino acid infusions on liver regeneration after hepatectomy in the rat. J Parenter Enteral Nutr 1986; 10: 17–20

61. Talarico K S, Feller D D, Neville E D. Mitotic response to various dietary conditions in the normal and regenerating rat liver. Proc Soc Exp Biol Med 1971; 136: 381–384

62. Schulte-Hermann R. Two-stage control of cell proliferation induced in rat liver by alpha-hexachlorocyclohexane. Cancer Res 1977; 37: 166–171

63. Kallenbach M, Roome N O, Schulte-Hermann R. Kinetics of DNA synthesis in feeding dependent and independent hepatocyte populations of rats after partial hepatectomy. Cell Tiss Kinetics 1983; 16: 321–332

64. Barra R, Hall J C. Liver regeneration in normal and alloxan-induced diabetic rats. J Exp Zool 1977; 201: 93–100

65. Johnston D, Johnson M, Alberti K G M M, Millward-Sadler G H et al. Hepatic regeneration and metabolism after partial hepatectomy in normal rats: effects of insulin therapy. Eur J Clin invest 1986; 16: 376–383

66. Johnston D, Johnson M, Alberti K G M M, Millward-Sadler G H et al. Hepatic regeneration and metabolism after partial hepatectomy in diabetic rats: effects of insulin therapy. Eur J Clin Invest 1986; 16: 384–390

67. Bucher N L R, Patel U, Cohen S. Hormonal factors concerned with liver regeneration. Ciba Foundation Symposium, no. 55 (new series) Hepatotrophic factors. New York: Elsevier, 1978: pp 95–107

68. Cruise J L, Knechtle S J, Bollinger R et al. Alpha-1-adrenergic effects and liver regeneration. Hepatology 1987; 7: 1189–1194

69. Pietralleli R, Chamuleau R A F M, Speranza V et al. Immunocytochemical study of the hepatic innervation in the rat after partial hepatectomy. Histochem J 1987; 19: 327–332

70. Okajima F, Ui M. Conversion of the adrenergic regulation of glycogen phosphorylase and synthase from an alpha to a beta type during primary culture of rat hepatocytes. Arch Biochem Biophys 1982; 213: 658–668

71. Sandnes D, Sand T E, Sager G et al. Elevated level of beta-adrenergic receptors in hepatocytes from regenerating rat liver. Exp Cell Res 1986; 165: 117–126

72. Cruise J L, Cotecchia S, Michalopoulos G K, Norepinephrine decreases EGF binding in primary rat hepatocyte cultures. J Cell Physiol 1986; 127: 39–44

73. Houck K A, Cruise J L, Michalopoulos G K. Norepinephrine modulates the growth-inhibiting effect of transforming growth factor beta in primary rat hepatocyte cultures. J Cell Physiol 1988; 135: 551–555

74. Short J, Brown R F, Husakova A et al. Induction of the DNA synthesis in the liver of the intact animal. J Biol Chem 1972; 247: 1757–1766

75. Marti U, Burwen S J, Jones A L. Biological effects of epidermal growth factor, with emphasis on the gastrointestinal tract and liver: an update. Hepatology 1989; 9: 126–138

76. St Hilaire R J, Hradek G T, Jones A L Hepatic sequestration and biliary secretion of epidermal growth factors: evidence for a high-capacity uptake system. Proc Natl Acad Sci USA 1983; 80: 3797–3801

77. McGowan J A, Strain A J, Bucher N L R. DNA synthesis in primary cultures of adult rat hepatocytes in a defined medium: effects of epidermal growth factor, insulin, glucagon and cyclic AMP. J Cell Physiol 1981; 108: 353–363

78. Raper S E, Burwen S J, Barker M E, Jones A L. Translocation of epidermal growth factor to the hepatocyte nucleus during rat liver regeneration. Gastroenterology 1987; 92: 1243–1250

79. Olsen P S, Boesby S, Kirkegaard P et al. Influence of epidermal growth factor on liver regeneration after partial hepatectomy in rats. Hepatology 1988; 8: 992–996

80. Johnson A C, Garfield S H, Merlino G T, Patsan I. Expression of epidermal growth factor receptor proto-oncogene mRNA in regenerating rat liver. Biochem Biophys Res Commun 1988; 150: 412–418

81. Mead J E, Fausto N. Transforming growth factor alpha may be a physiological regulator of liver regeneration by means of an autocrine mechanism. Proc Natl Acad Sci USA 1989; 86: 1558–1562

82. Fausto N, Mead J E. Regulation of liver growth: Protooncogenes and transforming growth factors. Lab Invest 1989; 60: 4–13

83. Kan M, Huang J, Mansson P E et al. Heparin-binding growth factor type 1 (acidic fibroblast growth factor): A potential biphasic autocrine and paracrine regulator of hepatocyte regeneration. Proc Natl Acad Sci USA 1989; 86: 7432–7436

84. Presta M, Statuto M, Rusnati M et al. Characterization of Mr 25,000 basic fibroblast growth factor form in adult, regenerating and fetal rat liver. Biochem Biophys Res Commun 1989; 164: 1182–1189

85. Caro J F, Poulos J, Ittoop O et al. Insulin-like growth factor 1 binding in hepatocytes from human liver, human hepatoma, and normal regenerating, and fetal rat liver. J Clin Invest 1988; 81: 976–981

86. Strain A J, Ismail T, Tsubouchi H et al. Native and recombinant human hepatocyte growth factors are highly potent promoters of DNA synthesis in both human and rat hepatocytes. J Clin Invest 1991; 87: 1853–1857

87. Gohda E, Tsubouchi H, Nakayama H et al. Purification and partial characterisation of hepatocyte growth factor from plasma of a patient with fulminant hepatic failure. J Clin Invest 1988; 81: 414–419

88. Tsubouchi H, Hirono S, Gouda E et al. Clinical significance of human hepatocyte growth factor in blood from patients with fulminant hepatic failure. Hepatology 1989; 9: 875–881

89. Strain A J, McGowen J A, Bucher N L R. Stimulation of DNA synthesis in primary cultures of adult rat hepatocytes by rat platelet-associated substances. In Vitro 1982; 18: 108–116

90. Zarnegar R, Muga S, Rahija R, Michalopoulos G. Tissue distribution of HPTA: a heparin-binding polypeptide growth factor from hepatocytes. Proc Natl Acad Sci USA 1990; 87: 1252–1256

91. LaBreque D R, Bachur N R. In vitro stimulation of cell growth by hepatic stimulator substances. Am J Physiol 1982; 242: G289–G295

92. Strain A J. Transforming growth factor-beta and inhibition of hepatocellular proliferation. Scand J Gastroenterol 1988; 23(suppl 151): 37–45

93. Russell W E, Coffey J R, Ouellette A J, Moses H L. Type beta transforming growth factor reversibly inhibits the early proliferative response to partial hepatectomy in the rat. Proc Natl Acad Sci USA 1988; 85: 5126–5130

94. Peters R L. Viral hepatitis: a pathologic spectrum. Am J Med Sci 1975; 270: 17–32

95. Powell W J Jr, Klatskin G. Duration of survival in patients with Laennec's cirrhosis: influence of alcohol withdrawal, and possible effects of racent changes in general management of the disease. Am J Med 1968; 44: 406–420

96. Friedman S L, Millward-Sadler G H, Arthur M J P. Liver fibrosis and cirrhosis. In: Millward-Sadler G H, Wright R, Arthur M J, eds. Wright's Liver and biliary disease, 3rd edn. London: Saunders, 1992: pp 821–881

97. Timpl R, Wiedemann H, van Delden V et al. A network model for the organisation of type IV collagen molecules in basement membranes. Eur J Biochem 1981; 120: 203–211

98. Rojkind M, Dunn M A. Hepatic fibrosis. Gastroenterology 1979; 76: 849–863

99. Biempica L, Morecki R, Wu C H et al. Immunocytochemical localisation of type B collagen — a component of basement membrane in human liver. Am J Pathol 1980; 98: 591–692

100. Keene D R, Engvall E, Glanville R W. Ultrastructure of type VI collagen in human skin and cartilage suggests an anchoring function for this filamentous network. J Cell Biol 1988; 107: 1995–2006

101. Schuppan D. Structure of the extracellular matrix in normal and fibrotic liver: collagens and glycoproteins. Semin Liver Dis 1990; 10: 1–10

102. Van Eyken P, Sciot R, Desmet V J. Expression of the novel extracellular matrix component tenascin in normal and diseased human liver: an immunohistochemical study. J Hepatol 1990; 11: 43–52

103. Fritze L M S, Reille C F, Rosenberg R D. An antiproliferative heparan sulfate species produced by postconfluent smooth muscle cells. J Cell Biol 1985; 100: 1041–1049

104. Dziadek M, Fujiwara S, Paulsson M et al. Immunological characterization of basement membrane types of heparan sulfate proteoglycan. EMBO Journal 1985; 4: 1463–1468

105. Elenius K, Salmivirta, Inki P et al. Binding of human syndecan to extracellular matrix proteins. J Biol Chem 1990; 265: 17837–17843

106. Andres J L, Stanley K, Cheifetz S, Massague J. Membrane anchored and soluble forms of betaglucan, a polymorphic proteoglycan that binds transforming growth factor-beta. J Cell Biol 1989; 109: 3137–3145

107. Murata K, Ochiai Y, Akaashio K. Polydispersity of acidic glycosaminoglycan components in human liver and the changes at different stages in liver cirrhosis. Gastroenterology 1985; 89: 1249–1257

108. Schaffner F, Popper H. Capillarization of hepatic sinusoids in man. Gastroenterology 1963; 44: 239–242

109. Orrego H, Medline A, Blendis L M et al. Collagenisation of the Disse space in alcoholic liver disease. Gut 1979; 20: 673–679

110. Friedman S L, Rockey D C, McGuire R F et al. Isolated hepatic lipocytes and Kupffer cells from normal human liver: morphological and functional characteristics in primary culture. Hepatology 1992; 15: 234–243

111. Bissell D M, Arenson D M, Maher J J, Roll F J. Support of cultured hepatocytes by a laminin-rich gel: evidence for a functionally significant subendothelial matrix in normal rat liver. J Clin Invest 1987; 79: 801–812

112. Kleinman H K, McGarvey M L, Hassell J R et al. Basement membrane complexes with biological activity. Biochemistry 1985; 25: 312–318

113. Schuetz E G, Li D, Omiecinski C J et al. Regulation of gene expression in adult rat hepatocytes cultured on a basement membrane matrix. J Hepatol 1988; 134: 309–323

114. Friedman S L, Roll F J, Boyles J et al. Maintenance of differentiated phenotype of cultured rat hepatic lipocytes by basement membrane matrix. J Biol Chem 1989; 264: 10756–10762

115. McGuire R F, Bissell D M, Boyles J et al. Role of extracellular matrix in regulating fenestrations in association with sinusoidal endothelial cells isolated from normal rat liver. Hepatology 1992; 15, 989–997

116. McGee J O'D, Patrick R S. The role of the perisinusoidal cells in hepatic fibrogenesis: an electron microscope study of acute carbon tetrachloride liver injury. Lab Invest 1972; 26: 429–440

117. Langness U, Undenfriend S. Collagen biosynthesis of non-fibroblastic cell lines. Proc Natl Acad Sci USA 1974; 71: 50–51

118. Ross R, Glomsett J. The pathogenesis of atheroscletosis. N Engl J Med 1976; 295: 369–377, 420–425

119. Millward-Sadler G H, Jezequel A M. Normal histology and ultrastructure. In: Millward-Sadler G H, Wright R, Arthur M J P, eds. Wright's Liver and biliary disease, 3rd edn. London: Saunders, 1992: pp 12–42

120. Rudolph R, McClure W J, Woodward M. Contractile fibroblasts in chronic alcoholic cirrhosis. Gastroenterology 1979; 76: 704–709

121. Ballardini G, Esposti S D, Bianchi F B et al. Correlation between Ito cells and fibrogenesis in an experimental model of hepatic fibrosis. A sequential stereological study. Liver 1983; 3: 58–63

122. Minato Y, Hasumura Y, Takeuchi J. The role of fat-storing cells in Disse space fibrogenesis in alcoholic liver disease. Hepatology 1983; 3: 559–566

123. Mak K M, Leo M A, Lieber C S. Alcoholic liver injury in baboons: Transformation of lipocytes to transitional cells. Gastroenterology 1984; 87: 188–200

124. Bhathal P S. Presence of modified fibroblasts in cirrhotic livers in man. Pathology 1972; 4: 139–144

125. Nakano M, Worner T M, Lieber C S. Perivenular fibrosis in alcoholic liver injury: ultrastructure and histologic progression. Gastroenterology 1982; 83: 777–785

126. Okanoue T, Burbige E J, French S W. The role of the Ito cell in perivenular and intralobular fibrosis in alcoholic hepatitis. Arch Path Lab Med 1983; 107: 459–463

127. Geerts A, Geuze J H, Slot J W et al. Immunogold localisation of procollegen III, fibronectin and heparan sulfate proteoglycan on ultrathin frozen sections of the normal rat liver. Histochemistry 1986; 84: 355–362

128. Martinez-Hernandez A. The hepatic extracellular matrix. II. Electron immunohistochemical studies in rats with CCl_4-induced cirrhosis. Lab Invest 1985; 53: 166–186

129. Nakatsukasa H, Nagy P, Evarts R P et al. Cellular distribution of transforming growth factor-beta 1 and procollagen types, I, III, IV transcripts in carbon-tetrachloride-induced rat liver fibrosis. J Clin Invest 1990; 85: 1833–1843

130. Milani S, Herbst H, Schuppan D et al. In situ hybridisation for procollagen types I, III, and IV mRNA in normal fibrotic rat liver: evidence for predominant expression in nonparenchymal liver cells. Hepatology 1989; 10: 84–92

131. Brenner D A, Alcorn J M, Feitelberg S P et al. Expression of collagen genes in the liver. Mol Biol Med 1990; 7: 105–115

132. Ramadori G, Rieder H, Knittel T H et al. Fat storing cells (FSC) of rat liver synthesise and secrete fibronectin. Comparison with hepatocytes. J Hepatol 1987; 4: 190–197

133. Arunsen D M, Friedman S L, Bissell D M. Formation of extracellular matrix in normal rat liver: lipocytes as a major source of proteoglycan. Gastroenterology 1988; 95: 441–447

134. Maher J J, Maguire R F. Extracellular matrix gene expression increases preferentially in rat lipocytes and sinusoidal endothelial cells during hepatic fibrosis in vivo. J Clin Invest 1990; 86: 1641–1648

135. Friedman S L, Roll F J, Boyles J, Bissell D M. Hepatic lipocytes: the principal collagen-producing cells of normal rat liver. Proc Natl Acad Sci USA 1985; 82: 8681–8685

136. Maher J J, Friedman S L, Roll F J, Bissell D M. Immunolocalisation of laminin in normal rat liver and biosynthesis of laminin by hepatic lipocytes in primary culture. Gastroenterology 1988; 94: 1053–1062

137. Senoo H, Hata R-I, Nagai Y, Wake K. Stellate cells (vitamin A storing cells) are the primary site of collagen synthesis in non-parenchymal cells in the liver. Biomed Res 1984; 5: 451–458

138. Maher J J, Bissell D M. Cell matrix interactions in liver. In: Zern M, Reid L, eds. The extracellular matrix and liver disease. New York: Marcel Dekker, 1992: pp

139. Johanssen S, Forsberg E, Lundgren B. Comparison of fibronectin receptors from rat hepatocytes and fibroblasts. J Biol Chem 1987; 262: 7819–7824

140. Gullberg D, Terraccio L, Borg T K, Rubin K. Identification of integrin-like matrix receptors with affinity for interstitial collagens. J Biol Chem 1989; 264: 12686–12694

141. Clement B, Segui-Real B, Savagner P et al. Hepatocyte attachment to laminin is mediated through multiple receptors. J Cell Biol 1990; 110: 185–192

142. Hughes R C, Stamatoglou S C. Adhesive interactions and the metabolic activity of hepatocytes. J Cell Sci 1987; 8: (suppl) 273–291

143. Kirch H C, Lammers M, Gressner A M. Binding of chondroitin sulfate, dermatan sulfate and fat-storing cell-derived proteoglycans to rat hepatocytes. Int J Biochem 1987; 19: 1119–1126

144. Laurent T C, Fraser J R E, Pertoft H, Smedsrod B. Binding of hyaluronate and chondroitin sulphate to liver endothelial cells. Biochem J 1986; 234: 653–658

145. Friedman S L, Arthur M J P. Activation of hepatic lipocytes by Kupffer cell-conditioned medium: direct enhancement of matrix production and stimulation of proliferation via expression of PDGF receptors. J Clin Invest 1989; 84: 1780–1785

146. Friedman S L. Acetaldehyde and alcoholic fibrogenesis: fuel to the fire, but not the spark. Hepatology 1990; 12: 609–612

147. Moshage H, Casini A, Lieber C S. Acetaldehyde selectively stimulates collagen production in cultured rat liver fat-storing cells but not in hepatocytes. Hepatology 1990; 12: 511–518

148. Meyer D H, Bachem M G, Gressner A M. Modulation of hepatic lipocyte proteoglycan synthesis and proliferation by Kupffer cell-derived transforming growth factors type beta 1 and type alpha. Biochem Biophys Res Commun 1990; 171: 1122 –1129

149. Pinzani M, Weber F L, Gesualdo L, Abboud H E, Expression of platelet-derived growth factor (PDGF) in an in vivo model of acute liver inflammation. Hepatology 1990; 12: 920 (abstract)

150. Davis B H. Transforming growth factor beta responsiveness is modulated by the extracellular collagen matrix during hepatic Ito cell culture. J Cell Physiol 1990; 136: 547–553

151. Leo M A, Lieber C S. Hepatic vitamin A depletion in alcoholic liver injury. N Engl J Med 1982; 307: 597–601

152. Davis B H, Pratt B M, Madri J A. Retinol and extracellular collagen matrices modulate hepatic Ito cell collagen phenotype and cellular retinol binding protein levels. J Biol Chem 1987; 262: 10280–10286

153. Davis B H, Vucic A. The effect of retinol on Ito cell proliferation in vitro. Hepatology 1988; 8: 788–793

154. Muller D, Quantin B, Gesnel M C et al. The collagenase gene family in humans consists of at least four members. Biochem J 1988; 253: 187–192

155. Matrisian L M. Metalloproteinases and their inhibitors in matrix remodelling. Trends Genet 1990; 6: 121–125

156. Gross J, Lapiere C M. Collagenolytic activity in amphibian tissues: a tissue culture assay. Proc Natl Acad Sci USA 1962; 48: 1014–1022

157. Bhatnager R, Schade U, Rietschel E T et al. Involvement of prostaglandin E and adenosine 3'5'-monophosphate in lipopolysaccharide-stimulated collagenase release by rat Kupffer cells. Eur J Biochem 1982; 124: 2405–2409

158. Campbell E J, Cury J D, Lazarus C J, Welgus H G. Monocyte procollagenase and tissue inhibitor of metalloproteinases. Identification, characterisation and regulation of secretion. J Biol Chem 1987; 262: 15862–15868

159. Emonard H, Guillouzo A, Lapiere C M, Grimaud J A. Human liver fibroblast capacity for synthesising interstitial collagenase in vitro. Cell Mol Biol 1990; 36: 461–467

160. Hasty K A, Jeffey J J. Hibbs M S, Welgus H G. The collagen substrate specificity of human neutrophil collagenase. J Biol Chem 1987; 262: 10048–10052

161. Hibbs M S, Hasty K A, Seyer J M et al. Biochemical and immunological characterisation of the secreted forms of human neutrophil gelatinase. J Biol Chem 1985; 260: 2493–2500

162. Hibbs M S, Hoidal R, Kang A H. Expression of a metalloproteinase that degrades native type V collagen and denatured collagens by cultured human alveolar macrophages. J Clin Invest 1987; 80: 1644–1650

163. Winwood P J, Kowalski-Saunders P, Arthur M J P. Kupffer cells release a 95kD metalloproteinase with degradative activity against gelatin. Gut 1991; 32: A837–838

164. Selzter J L, Weingarten H, Akers H T et al. Cleavage specificity of type IV collagenase (gelatinase) from human skin. Use of synthetic peptides as model substrates. J Biol Chem 1989; 265: 19583–19586

165. Arthur M J P, Friedman S L, Roll F J, Bissell D M. Lipocytes from normal rat liver release a neutral metalloproteinase that degrades basement membrane (type IV) collagen. J Biol Chem 1989; 84: 1076–1085

166. Arthur M J P, Stanley A, Iredale J P et al. Release of type IV collagenase by cultured human lipocytes: analysis of gene expression, protein synthesis and protease activity. Gastroenterology 1991; 100: A716

167. Arthur M J P. Human hepatic lipocytes synthesise and release TIMP-1: An important inhibitor of matrix metalloproteinase activity. Hapatology 1991; 14: 183A

168. Iredale J P, Murphy G, Hembry R M et al. Human hepatic lipocytes synthesise tissue inhibitor of metalloproteinases-1. Implications for regulation of matrix degradation in liver. J Clin Invest 1992; 90: 282–287

169. Enghild J J, Salvesen G, Brew K, Nagase H. Interaction of human rheumatoid synovial collagenase (matrix metalloproteinase 1) and stromelysin (matrix metalloproteinase 3) with human alpha-2-macroglobulin and chicken ovostatin. J Biol Chem 1989; 264: 8779–8785

170. Andus T, Ramadori G, Heinrich P C. Cultured Ito cells of rat liver express the alpha 2-macroglubulin gene. Eur J Biochem 1987; 168: 641–646

171. Okazaki I, Maruyama K. Collagenase activity in experimental hepatic fibrosis. Nature 1974: 252: 49–50

172. Montfort I, Perez-Tamayo R, Alvizouri A M, Tello E. Collagenase of hepatocytes and sinusoidal liver cells in the reversibility of experimental cirrhosis in the liver. Virchow Arch (B) 1990; 59: 281–289

173. Maruyama K, Feinman L, Okazaki I, Lieber C S. Direct measurement of neutral collagenase activity in hemogenates from baboon and human liver. Biochim Biophys Acta 1981; 658: 121–131

174. MacMathuna P, Westaby D, Williams R. Portal hypertension: pathophysiology, diagnosis and treatment. In: Millward-Sadler G H, Wright R, Arthur M J P, eds. Wright's Liver and biliary disease, 3rd edn. London: Saunders. 1992: pp 1296–1322

175. Crossley I R, Williams R. Spontaneous bacterial peritonitis. Gut 1985; 26: 325–331

176. Moore K, Wilkinson S, Williams R. Ascites and renal dysfunction in liver disease. In: Millward-Sadler G H, Wright R, Arthur M J P, eds. Wright's Liver and biliary disease, 3rd edn. London: W B Saunders, 1992: pp 1346–1371

177. Targan S R, Chow A W, Guze L B. Anaerobic bacteria in spontaneous peritonitis of cirrhosis. Am J Med 1977; 62: 397–403

178. Gross G, Perrier C V. Intrahepatic porta-systemic shunting in cirrhotic patients. N Engl J Med 1975; 293: 1046–1047

179. Groszmann R J, Kravetz D, Parysow O. Intrahepatic arteriovenous shunting in cirrhosis of the liver. Gastroenterology 1977; 73: 201–204

180. Bjorneboe M, Prytz H, Orskov F. Antibodies to intestinal microbes in serum of patients with cirrhosis of the liver. Lancet 1972; i: 58–60

181. Runyon B A. Spontaneous bacterial peritonitis: An explosion of information. Hepatology 1988; 8: 171–175

182. Tito L, Rimola A, Gines P et al. Recurrence and frequency of spontaneous bacterial peritonitis in cirrhosis: Frequency and predictive factors. Hepatology 1988; 8: 27–31

183. Van Thiel D H, Gavaler J S. Hypothalamic–pituitary–gonadal function in liver disease with particular attention to the endocrine effects of chronic alcohol abuse. In: Popper H, Schaffner F, eds. Progress in liver diseases, vol III. New York: Grune & Stratton, 1986: pp 273–282

184. Zakim D, Boyer T D, eds. Hepatology, a textbook of liver disease, 2nd edn. Philadelphia: Saunders, 1990

185. McIntyre N, Benhamou J-P, Bircher J, Rizzetto M, Rodes J, eds. Oxford Textbook of clinical hepatology. Oxford: Oxford University Press, 1991

186. Millward-Sadler G H, Wright R, Arthur M J P, eds. Wright's Liver and biliary disease, 3rd edn. London: Saunders, 1992

187. Fischer J E. Portal-systemic encephalopathy. In: Millward-Sadler G H, Wright R, Arthur M J P, eds. Wright's Liver and biliary disease, 3rd edn. London: Saunders, 1992: pp 1262–1295

188. Wright T L. Medical aspects of liver transplantation. In: Millward-Sadler G H, Wright R, Arthur M J P, eds. Wright's Liver and biliary disease, 3rd edn. London: Saunders, 1992: pp 1417–1438

189. Sen B C. Enlargement of the liver in children. Indian Medical Gazette 1887; 22: 338–343

190. Muller-Hocker J, Meyer U, Wiebecke B et al. Copper storage disease of the liver and chronic dietary copper intoxication in two further German infants mimicking Indian childhood cirrhosis. Path Res Pract 1987; 183: 39–45

191. Lefkowitch J, Honig C, King M, Hagstrom J. Hepatic copper overload and features of Indian childhood cirrhosis in an American sibship. N Engl J Med 1982; 307: 271–277

192. Maggiore G, De Giacomo C, Sessa F, Burgio G. Idiopathic copper toxicosis in a child. J Ped Gastroenterol Nutr 1987; 6: 980–983

193. Adamson M, Reiner B, Olson J, Goodman Z, Plotnick L, Bernardini I, Gahl W. Indian childhood cirrhosis in an American child. Gastroenterology 1992; 102: 1771–1777

194. Nayak N C, Visalakshi S, Singh M, Chawla V, Chandra R K, Ramalingaswami V. Indian childhood cirrhosis – a re-evaluation of its patho-morphologic features and their significance in the light of clinical data and natural history of the disease. Indian J Med Res 1972; 60: 246–259

195. Parekh S R, Patel B D. Epidemiologic survey of Indian childhood cirrhosis. Indian Ped 1972; 9: 431–439

196. Nayak N C, Ramalingaswami V. Indian childhood cirrhosis. In: Popper H, ed. Clinics in Gastroenterology, Vol. 4, No. 2 London: WB Saunders, pp 333–349

197. Nayak N C. Indian childhood cirrhosis – yesterday, today and tomorrow. Indian Ped 1980; 17: 577–580

198. Popper H, Goldfischer S, Sternlieb I, Nayak N C, Madhavan T V. Cytoplasmic copper and its toxic effects – studies in Indian childhood cirrhosis. Lancet 1979; 2: 1205–1208

199. Tanner M S, Portmann B. Indian childhood cirrhosis. Arch Dis Childh 1981; 56: 4–6

200. Tanner M S, Portmann B, Mowat A P, Williams R. Increased hepatic copper concentration in Indian childhood cirrhosis. Lancet 1979; ii: 1203–1205

201. Tanner M S, Bhave S A, Pradhan A M, Pandit A N. Clinical trials of penicillamine in Indian childhood cirrhosis. Arch Dis Childh 1987; 62: 1118–1124

202. Nayak N C, Marwaha N, Kalra V, Roy S, Ghai O P. The liver in siblings of patients with Indian childhood cirrhosis: a light and electron microscopic study. Gut 1981; 22: 295–300

203. O'Donohue J W, Reid M A, Varghese A, Portmann B, Williams R. Micronodular cirrhosis and acute liver failure due to chronic copper self-intoxication. Eur J Gastroenterol Hepatol 1993; 5: 561–562

11

Cholestasis: extrahepatic obstruction and secondary biliary cirrhosis

V. J. Desmet

CHOLESTASIS: GENERAL CONCEPTS

DEFINITIONS OF CHOLESTASIS

The term cholestasis is not strictly defined. Etymologically (χολη bile, and στασις, standstill), it means arrest of bile flow. Cholestasis usually connotes a disturbance in the normal bile secretory mechanisms accompanied by accumulation in the blood of substances normally secreted in the bile.

Bile is a fluid of complex composition, of which water, electrolytes, bile salts, bilirubin, phospholipids, cholesterol and a number of enzymes are the main components. Several exogenous compounds, including many drugs, are eliminated from the body along this pathway, and influence bile composition.[1] Hepatic bile is the secretory product of the liver cells (hepatocellular or canalicular bile flow), to which a bicarbonate-rich solution is added by secretion from the bile-duct cells (duct and ductular bile flow) during its passage through the intrahepatic biliary channels. The latter fraction is modulated by hormones.[2] Hepatocellular or canalicular bile flow appears to be generated by various mechanisms. A fraction of the bile water flow depends on the active secretion of bile acids — the bile-acid-dependent canalicular bile flow; another fraction, of varying importance in different species, represents the so-called bile-acid-independent canalicular bile flow. There is evidence that organic anions, such as bilirubin and bromsulphthalein, share a common transport system separate from that of bile acids.[3]

This multiplicity of hepatocytic excretory mechanisms[4] raises problems in defining cholestasis, since hepatocellular excretory failure may be partial or selective. This is the case in abnormalities such as the Dubin–Johnson syndrome, in which there is marked decrease in the capacity to excrete bromsulphthalein and conjugated bilirubin, with normal or near-normal serum levels of bile acids.[5] Until more is known about the mechanisms of hepatocellular bile formation and the pathogenesis of their defects, the term 'cholestasis' will continue to cover several, not strictly identical, concepts. It is important to be aware of these variants in definition.

The clinical and biochemical definition of cholestasis usually refers to a group of symptoms including jaundice and pruritus, elevated serum levels of conjugated bilirubin, alkaline phosphatase, 5'-nucleotidase, cholesterol, bile acids and IgA,[6] and the appearance in the blood of an abnormal lipoprotein, lipoprotein X. Javitt has stressed the importance of relying on serum bile acid determinations for defining cholestasis, and has called attention to conditions in which there is no associated rise in serum levels of conjugated bilirubin — anicteric cholestasis.[7] Partial obstruction of the bile ducts (for instance, obstruction of one hepatic duct or narrowing of several duct segments) is not associated with hyperbilirubinaemia as long as the liver is otherwise normal. However, pruritus does occur, alkaline phosphatase rises and hypercholesterolaemia may develop.[8]

Aetiological and pathogenetic definitions of cholestasis remain imprecise, because identical or nearly identical syndromes are caused by lesions which may be located at any point along the complex pathway which the excretory products have to take from their site of production inside the liver cell to the duodenal lumen.

Mechanical or obstructive cholestasis usually refers to lesions of the extrahepatic biliary tract (extrahepatic cholestasis), but is occasionally produced by intrahepatic processes which cause jaundice only if the flow is compromised in the majority of the intrahepatic biliary passages. Although mechanical obstructions thus clearly contribute to cholestasis originating within the anatomical confines of the liver, i.e. intrahepatic,[9] the term 'intrahepatic cholestasis' is used by most authors to indicate cholestatic syndromes without demonstrable mechanical obstruction. Such functional intrahepatic cholestasis is ascribed to metabolic alterations provoked by drugs, alcohol, bacterial infections and unknown factors.[10]

From the morphological point of view also, the definition of cholestasis depends on the approach. *Macroscopically*, cholestasis is characterized by a green or greenish-black discoloration or mottling of the liver surface at laparoscopy, laparotomy or autopsy. *Microscopically*, cholestasis was usually defined as microscopically visible accumulation of bile pigment (bilirubinostasis) in the liver tissue in certain preferential locations[11] (Fig. 11.1). However, microscopic bilirubinostasis does not always parallel the usual clinical or functional definition of cholestasis. One problem is technical, since it has been noted that tissue processing and embedding may wash out much of the accumulated bile pigment.[11] Another complication is that microscopic bilirubinostasis does not occur in some animal species, such as the rat, even after ligation of the common bile duct, although functionally this experimental condition qualifies

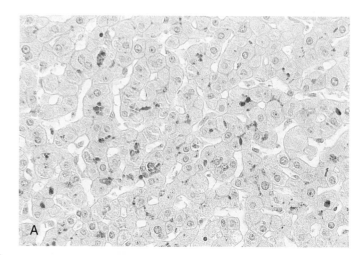

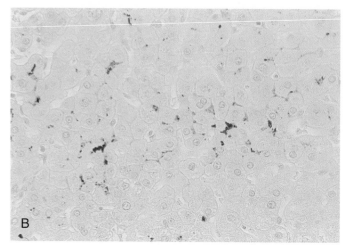

Fig. 11.1 (a,b) Details of perivenular bilirubinostasis. Bilirubin accumulation is visible as hepatocellular granules and mainly intercellular plugs. The latter outline a few canalicular segments. (a) H & E. (b) Hall's bilirubin stain.

fully as an example of cholestasis. Similarly, microscopic bilirubinostasis may be missing in the early stages of incomplete bile duct obstruction (e.g. primary biliary cirrhosis, clinically a cholestatic syndrome).

Changes in staining patterns of *histochemical* preparations incubated for various enzymes (ATPase, alkaline phosphatase, γ-glutamyltransferase) can be recognized as cholestatic patterns that no longer rely on the previous criteria of classic histopathology.[12–14]

Electron microscopically, cholestasis is recognized by a typical pattern of changes in and around the canaliculi, even in the absence of any visible bile pigment accumulation; electron microscopically cholestasis may thus be diagnosed in the absence of light microscopic pigment accumulation or of clinical jaundice.[15] Refinements of ultrastructural investigation, such as the freeze-fracture replica technique,[16] and scanning electron microscopy[17,18] reveal further details of ultrastructural cholestatic changes.

In terms of *molecular biology* and *cell organelle* pathology, various definitions and explanations of non-mechanical cholestasis have been proposed,[10,19-23] among them basolateral membrane changes, cytoskeletal alterations, increased permeability of the paracellular pathway, canalicular membrane changes and disturbed intracellular calcium homeostasis.

For practical clinical and diagnostic purposes, we may summarize as follows:

1. Distinction should be made between:
   a. Conditions with impaired secretion of conjugated bilirubin and exogenous dyes, such as the Dubin–Johnson and Rotor syndromes, which are not really cholestatic although they may cause jaundice with conjugated hyperbilirubinaemia, since bile acid secretory mechanisms are apparently not involved.[3,24]
   b. Conditions with impaired secretion of bile acids, or cholestasis. When this impairment reaches a certain degree of severity, elimination of organic anions (bilirubin, dyes) is impeded and jaundice occurs, since the two excretory pathways, although different, seem to be interrelated.[3,25]

2. Electron microscopy is a more sensitive tool than classic histopathology for revealing cholestatic changes in the liver, since diagnostic alterations can be observed before non-excreted bilirubin becomes visible by light microscopy in tissue sections.[26]

3. Taking into account the possible wash-out of bilirubin by tissue processing, and the absence of bilirubinostasis in the early stages of incomplete bile-duct obstruction, the histopathologist should be aware of the possible presence of a cholestatic condition, even when no bile pigment can be visualized. In this respect, 'cholate stasis' (see below; Figs 11.21, 11.22) is a more reliable diagnostic feature of chronic cholestasis than is bilirubinostasis.[27]

MORPHOLOGICAL SUBSTRATE OF NORMAL BILE SECRETION

Normal bile is a product of both hepatocytes and bile-duct cells. The hepatocyte is a remarkably polarized cell involved in 'internal' secretion of innumerable substances delivered in the blood and in 'external' secretion of bile towards the cholangioles.[28-30] The liver-cell organelles involved in bile secretion have been termed 'the bile secretory apparatus'.[31,32] This was originally conceived as comprising mainly the bile canaliculus, the pericanalicular ectoplasm, lysosomes and the Golgi complex. It appears, however, that the whole liver cell is an impressively integrated complex, with several organelles representing crossroads of internal and external secretory pathways. It may therefore be useful to consider the complete hepatocellular machinery involved in bile production, rather than the more restricted concept of the 'bile secretory apparatus'.[33,34] Furthermore, the volume of the hepatocyte also influences its bile secretory function, in that hypo-osmotic and amino acid-induced cell swelling stimulates taurocholate excretion and bile flow, whereas hyperosmotic cell shrinkage inhibits them.[35,36]

Basolateral membrane; acinar gradient

The sinusoidal domain of the hepatocyte plasma membrane shows irregular microvilli bathed in the fluid of the space of Disse, which has direct communication with the sinusoidal blood through the numerous fenestrations (sieve plates) of the sinusoidal endothelium without interposition of a basement membrane. Such an arrangement favours direct and rapid exchange of metabolites and secretory products between blood and hepatocytes.

Bile acids are considered to represent the prime osmotically active solutes responsible for the generation of bile water flow.[37] The mechanism of transport of bile salts by the hepatocyte includes several successive steps: uptake at the sinusoidal liver-cell membrane, vectorial transcellular transport, and concentrative secretion at the canalicular membrane.

Uptake of bile acids at the sinusoidal pole is predominantly a secondary active, carrier-mediated, sodium-coupled process,[37] energized by the sodium pump or Na^+,K^+-ATPase. This enzyme has been shown to be localized on the sinusoidal and lateral liver-cell membrane.[38] Evidence has been produced for the localization in the plasmalemma of a 48–49 kD sodium-taurocholate cotransporter, which is multisubstrate specific and ontogenetically only reaches full expression approximately one month after birth.[37-40] Bile acid uptake at the sinusoidal domain of the plasmalemma is mainly accomplished by hepatocytes located in zone 1 of the liver acinus.[41] Thus, bile acid transport in the liver follows an intra-acinar gradient, occurring at a decreasing rate away from the portal tract.[42] However, under conditions of increased bile acid load, additional hepatocytes from zones 2 and 3 become recruited to participate in bile acid transport.[43,44]

The basolateral membrane is similarly involved in the uptake of the major fraction of biliary bilirubin, apparently through a carrier-mediated mechanism.[45] Whether uptake, transport, conjugation and secretion of bilirubin are also subject to gradient differences along the acinar axis is not established. However, transport by hepatocytes of organic anions, e.g. bromsulphthalein, depends not only on sinusoidal concentration gradients but is also influenced by albumin, resulting in a more homogeneous distribution within the liver acinus.[42] Plasma-derived proteins and apoproteins are taken up at the sinusoidal membrane either by non-selective fluid pinocytosis or by receptor-mediated endocytosis.[46]

Vesicle-mediated transport

Formation of endocytotic vesicles at the sinusoidal membrane is an obligatory requirement for any transcellular transport by means of 'ferry vesicles'. Hepatocytes have specific membrane receptors for a wide variety of circulating proteins and glycoproteins.[47] Receptor-mediated endocytosis requires specific recognition and binding of the ligand with the receptor in the membrane. The receptors usually concentrate in so-called clathrin-coated pits, which invaginate the cytoplasm.[48]

A vesicle is formed which travels towards the biliary pole of the hepatocyte. Two pathways are recognized:[49] (i) a *direct* pathway, consisting of shuttle vesicles which carry their content directly from the sinusoidal domain towards the canaliculus, emptying themselves in bile through fusion with the canalicular membrane and exocytosis; (ii) an *indirect* pathway consisting of those vesicles which fuse with lysosomes or Golgi components, whereby their content is fully or partially degraded by lysosomal enzymes, with subsequent vesicle-mediated transfer towards the canaliculus.[49]

Vesicle-mediated blood-to-bile transport of dimeric IgA has been shown in rat hepatocytes in vivo[51] and in culture;[52] in man blood-to-bile transport of dimeric IgA occurs primarily in the bile-duct cells and is much smaller overall than in the rat or rabbit.[53] However, recent studies also emphasize a transhepatocytic transfer of IgA from blood to bile in humans.[54] Vesicle-mediated blood-to-bile transfer through rat hepatocytes has been demonstrated also for insulin, epidermal growth factor, asialoglycoproteins, low density lipoproteins[49] and haptoglobin–haemoglobin complexes.[55]

The vesicular transport system can operate even without ligand binding to the receptor. Such a mechanism is of importance for the insertion of glycoproteins and selective membrane constituents in the canalicular domain of the cell membrane,[56,57] thus helping to ensure the integrity of the canalicular domain of the plasmalemma.[58,60]

Mitochondria and peroxisomes

Mitochondria are the power plants of all eukaryotic cells, where energy derived from oxidative metabolism and coupled phosphorylation is captured in the form of ATP, and made available to all energy-requiring functions of the cell, including bile secretory processes (e.g. sodium pump) in the liver cell.

Besides this non-specific role in energy supply, liver-cell mitochondria have a more direct connection with bile secretion in that the side chain oxidation of cholesterol, reducing this molecule to the C_{24} bile acids, occurs in the mitochondrial compartment; in addition peroxisomes are involved in this process, and peroxisomes and mitochondria are functionally integrated.[59,61]

Smooth endoplasmic reticulum

The smooth endoplasmic reticulum (SER) is the site where synthesis of phospholipids takes place, including phospholipids eventually appearing in the bile. It contains 7-α-hydroxylase, which is the rate-limiting enzyme in biotransformation of cholesterol to bile acids, and the enzyme glucuronyltransferase, which conjugates bilirubin to the polar, water-soluble bilirubin diglucuronide.

Studies using the bile acid analogue ^{125}I-cholylglycyltyrosine led to the hypothesis that bile acids coming from the enterohepatic cycle move from the sinusoidal plasma membrane to bile via a pathway that includes the SER and Golgi apparatus.[62–64] Immunoperoxidase studies of taurocholate and ursodeoxycholate have localized these bile acids to vesicles of the SER and Golgi apparatus.[65,66] Furthermore, the SER is the seat of the mixed function oxidase system requiring cytochrome P-450. This is involved in the biotransformation of numerous xenobiotics and carcinogens, forming metabolites which are eliminated with bile. Biotransformation of some xenobiotics that are not cholestatic per se may lead to metabolites with varying degrees of cholestatic potential,[67] depending on individual variations of the enzymatic composition of the SER.[68]

Lysosomes

It has been calculated that acid hydrolases are excreted in bile at a rate corresponding to the daily unloading of 5% of the hepatic lysosomes.[69] Further studies confirmed that several lysosomal enzymes undergo biliary excretion by a specific mechanism apparently independent of bile acid secretion, consistent with the hypothesis of hepatocellular exocytosis of lysosomal contents.[70–72] Lysosomes are involved in the previously described indirect pathway of vesicle-mediated blood-to-bile transfer.

Although the complete physiological significance of lysosomal discharge into bile remains unclear, this mechanism may provide the hepatocyte with a disposal system for indigestible residues accumulating in lysosomes (e.g. copper in Wilson's disease and iron in haemochromatosis).[73,74] Previous experiments using tracer substances led to similar conclusions.[75]

Pericanalicular vesicles

Pericanalicular vesicles with a diameter of more than 100 nm are a normal constituent of the pericanalicular region: they are occasionally found to fuse with the canalicular membrane[76] and are intimately associated with the microfilaments of the pericanalicular web.[77] Studies on isolated rat hepatocyte couplets demonstrated an impressive tubular as well as vesicular configuration of the vesicle system.[78] Their number increases during taurocholate-induced enhancement of bile flow.[51] Some apparently represent ferry vesicles which carry their cargo molecules through the liver cell for excretion into the bile canaliculus.[49,79,80] Studies with fluorescein isothiocyanate-glycocholate suggest that intracellular bile acid transport involves microtubule-dependent vesicular transfer from the Golgi apparatus to the bile canaliculus.[81]

Some of the vesicles seem to derive from the immature face of the Golgi complex, since both structures share the common characteristic of osmication positivity.[82] Possibly, such vesicles take part in biliary bile salt and lipid secretion[83,84] and transport of other cholephilic organic anions.[85] Another part of the vesicles, presumably some of the clathrin-coated ones, may be involved in membrane retrieval and recycling between canaliculus and Golgi complex.[86] Some vesicular structures may be part of a continuous subsurface tubulo-reticular system of the SER, which can be traced to both the sinusoidal and the canalicular membrane and is thought to represent a transcellular transport system.[87]

There is still a need to examine further by appropriate histochemical methods and tracer molecules the contents, origin and destiny of the apparently heterogeneous population of vesicles occurring in the pericanalicular region.[60,88]

Golgi complex

The Golgi apparatus is an extremely complex organelle, composed of a stack of Golgi cisternae, forming an immature(cis-) and mature(trans-) side, Golgi vacuoles and a myriad of vesicles. The liver cell may contain as many as 50 such complexes.[89] The Golgi complex is involved as an obligatory step in secretion in virtually all secretory cells. A role for the hepatocellular Golgi complex in bile secretion was proposed more than half a century ago, but later studies mainly emphasized the involvement of the Golgi system with secretory processes directed towards the sinusoids, such as secretion of albumin, fibrinogen and very low density lipoprotein.

However, in view of the dual ('internal' and 'external') secretory activity of the hepatocyte, one might also expect the liver-cell Golgi complex to exhibit a dual secretory function, with the mature face involved in 'internal' secretion towards the sinusoids and the immature face active in dispatching membrane-enclosed products towards the canaliculus.[90] Evidence has accumulated in recent years in favour of the concept that, in the hepatocyte, the Golgi complex is indeed involved in secretion towards the biliary compartment.[28,51,62,63,91,92] The Golgi complex seems to be involved in intracellular transport of bile acids (at least under high bile acid load) and of lipids.[84] Bile salts have been demonstrated in Golgi vesicles by immunohisto-chemistry using antibodies against natural bile acids.[65]

The Golgi complex further intervenes in post-translational modifications of secretory glycoproteins and in processing of the membranes which envelop secretory products.[93] It plays a role in the flow and reprocessing of membranes during membrane recycling.[94]

Cytoskeleton

The cytoskeleton of the liver cell[95,96] comprises the microfilaments and microtubules. The microfilaments are of different types: thin (actin) and thick (myosin) contractile microfilaments, intermediate microfilaments, and a microtrabecular lattice.[98]

Microfilaments. Contractile microfilaments corresponding to actin are located mainly in the periphery of the liver cell and are concentrated in the pericanalicular zone, forming a pericanalicular web.[77,99–101] They insert into the *zonula adhaerens* portion of the junctional complex, and also extend into the canalicular microvilli where they insert on the inner leaflet of the microvillous membrane, in an alignment adequate for filament sliding.[102]

Thicker filaments were seen between the actin filaments; these appeared to contain Mg^{2+}-ATPase, and seemed to correspond to myosin.[103,104] Later, myosin was demonstrated in the parenchymal cell periphery and around the canaliculus by immunohistochemical techniques.[105] Plasma membrane-associated myosin is drastically reduced after phalloidin treatment, which induces cholestasis.[106] Integrity of the actin–myosin system, as well as the Ca^{2+}–calmodulin system, is essential for normal bile canalicular contraction.[107]

Of the contractile microfilaments, the thin actin microfilaments have mainly been investigated in relation to bile secretion. Four main functions are envisaged: (i) they participate in the translocation of carrier or ferry vesicles and appear to be necessary for adequate secretion of bile acids;[108] (ii) their coordinated contraction around the canaliculus results in a peristalsis-like movement, propelling the secreted bile in the canaliculus;[104–115] (iii) they exert — together with microtubules — a transmembrane control over the topography of intrinsic proteins in the phospholipid bilayer of the cell membranes, thus influencing the protein mosaic and hence the functional differentiation of a particular membrane domain; (iv) they modulate the structure and the tightness of the so-called tight junctions and in this way regulate the permeability of the paracellular pathway.[116]

Intermediate filaments in liver parenchymal cells are of the epithelial keratin type, and comprise the cytokeratins No. 8 and No. 18 of the catalogue of Moll,[117,118] forming an integrated system in the hepatocyte.[119] They form a distinct sheet of matted filaments which envelop the entire hepatocyte and condense around the canaliculus as a 'pericanalicular sheath'.[120] The cortical intermediate filaments are in continuity with the pericanalicular sheath and the filaments located within the cytoplasm. An intact pericanalicular sheath is necessary for an adequate secretory function of hepatocytes;[121] it may serve as an attachment site for contractile microfilaments. It has been speculated that intermediate filaments take part in the bile secretory mechanisms.[122] The intermediate filament part of the cytoskeleton can be studied by the quick-freezing and deep-etching technique.[123]

Microtubules. The microtubules are polymers of a dimer protein tubulin, forming long tubular structures of about 24 nm diameter. Their role in secretory processes has been probed using microtubule inhibitors, e.g. colchicine. Microtubules have been shown to be involved in the blood-bound secretion of several liver-cell products (e.g. albumin, fibrinogen).[97] Further studies have disclosed that they are also required for uptake of bile acids at the sinusoidal pole and the secretion of bile acids and biliary lipids at the canalicular side.[38,84] Microtubules play a role in the intracellular translocation of vesicles containing immunoglobulin A and horseradish peroxidase.[108,124] They are apparently also involved in the canalicular discharge of endogenous and exogenous lysosomal constituents,[125] and in maintaining the structural and functional integrity of the biliary pole of the hepatocyte.[126]

The *microtrabecular lattice*[98] escapes detection by conventional investigative methods, but can be visualized by high voltage electron microscopy. It plays a role in the spatial positioning and movement of intracellular organelles and vesicles; it appears to represent an extremely dynamic system, in connection with the remaining cytoskeletal components, essential for normal intracellular transport functions. Although not yet studied in hepatocytes, it may be assumed to exert a role similar to that in other cells, and thus to be involved in blood-bound and bile-directed secretions.

It has been established that all the components of the cytoskeleton are impressively dynamic structures, subject to rapid modulation and adaptation by means of polymerization and depolymerization of their constituent molecules under the influence of various intracellular factors, of which free Ca^{2+} ions, high-energy compounds and associated proteins should be mentioned.

Hyaloplasm

The hyaloplasm corresponds to the biochemist's 'cytosol' or 'supernatant', and represents an apparently structureless gel, corresponding to the cell's cytoplasm in between the organelles. This cellular compartment was, until recently, less attractive to the morphologist because of its apparent lack of structural organization; however, it is the compartment in which the above-mentioned microtrabecular lattice extends. The hyaloplasm is an important molecular traffic zone; cytosolic binding proteins involved in intracellular transport of bile acids are present in this compartment.[38,127]

Junctional complexes

The junctional complexes are special membrane differentiations which tie the liver cells together on their intercellular domain. Different components have been identified: desmosomes, intermediate junctions, tight junctions and gap junctions.

The *desmosome* (*spot desmosome, macula adhaerens*) is a disc-shaped membrane differentiation where the plasma membranes of two adjacent liver cells lie strictly parallel. On both cytoplasmic sides electron-dense plaques are closely applied to the junctional membrane area. These serve as attachment sites for bundles of intermediate filaments (tonofilaments). The spot desmosome thus serves as a button-like connector between the tonofilament systems of adjacent cells, limits distensibility and prevents excessive deformation and damage from mechanical stress.[128]

The *intermediate junction* (*belt desmosome, zonula adhaerens*) has a comparable structure. It is a continuous belt-like junction immediately below the tight junction. Again, the two plasma membranes show a parallel course, leaving a narrow interspace filled with fine filamentous material. On the cytoplasmic side of the junctional membrane area, a thick mat of intermeshed filaments lies close to the membrane surface. The microfilaments inserting into this mat consist at least in part of fibrous actin.[77,101] The intermediate junction can be viewed as an insertion line for actin microfilaments. Such an arrangement may be functionally important. The regular peristalsis-like contractions of the pericanalicular filamentous web may not only have a propulsive effect on the canalicular content,[111,129] but may also result in a pumping or sucking effect at the level of the intercellular space, so that mechanical forces supplement the osmotic gradient for driving water and solutes through the paracellular pathway of the tight junctions.[28]

The *tight junction* (*zonula occludens*) is the sealing belt which separates the biliary compartment (canaliculus) from the intercellular space. Its structure is more clearly revealed by the freeze-fracture replica technique.[116] This junction is built up by a network of anastomosing junctional lines or fibrils (Fig. 11.2). Each sealing fibril is composed of two firmly attached hemifibrils, located in the plasma membrane of two adjacent hepatocytes. Close analysis reveals that the hemifibrils in each cell membrane are formed by rows of special tight junctional particles inserted in the phospholipid bilayer of the membrane.[130] This sealing element of the canaliculus allows for the formation of steep ionic and osmotic gradients between the lumen and the interspace. The liver cell tight junction is not as 'tight' as the name implies, and is to some extent a 'leaky' tight junction, allowing for a paracellular flux of water and solutes, with selectivity for cations, thus establishing a bio-electrical barrier.[116,131-133]

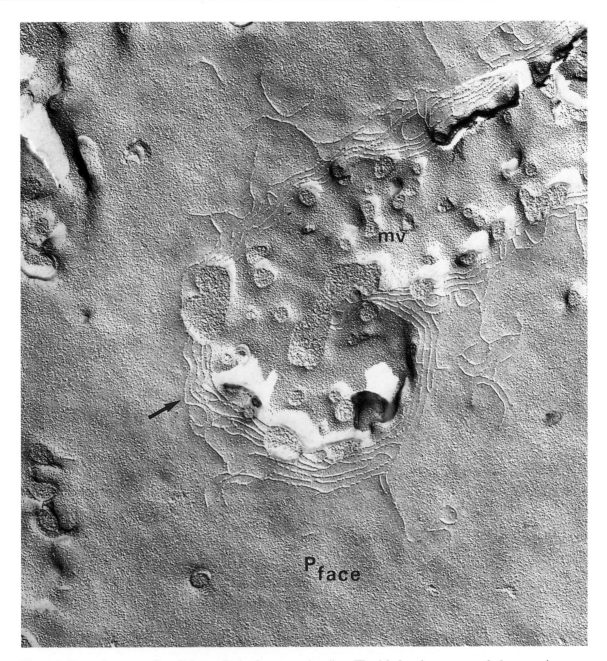

Fig. 11.2 Freeze-fracture replica of bile canaliculus from normal rat liver. The tight junctions appear as 3–6 more-or-less parallel strands or ridges on the so-called P face (protoplasmic leaflet) of the cleaved intercellular membrane (arrow). Bile canalicular microvilli (mv) can be recognized in the canalicular lumen. × 60 000

The liver-cell tight junctions form a varied network, containing points with lower numbers of junctional fibrils, presumably corresponding to spots of higher conductivity.[116,127] Furthermore, this structure is far from static; its architecture may be modulated by various factors resulting in corresponding variations in permeability. Paracellular permeability is subject to a variety of hormonal, metabolic and drug-related influences.[38,135] Components of the cytoskeleton (microfilaments, microtubules) have been shown to influence tight junctional structure and permeability.[136] The tight junctions thus occupy a strategic position: adjacent liver cells exert control not only on the transcellular passage of molecules in transepithelial transport, but also regulate the locks of the paracellular pathway, located at their periphery in the intercellular space. It should be realized, however, that the permeability of the total paracellular pathway depends not only on the tight junctions but also on the configuration of the intercellular space.[137]

The *gap junction* (*nexus*, *macula communicans*) is a different type of membrane differentiation on the intercellular face of the hepatocyte. In the gap junctional area, the two adjacent liver-cell membranes lie strictly parallel, leaving a very narrow interspace or gap of 2 nm. In this area, special proteinaceous particles (connexons) span the entire width of the membrane and fit onto corresponding particles in the adjacent membrane. The centre of the connexon is occupied by a thin hydrophilic channel (1.5 nm), establishing a cell-to-cell communication channel which pierces the phospholipid bilayers of the membranes and at the same time is sealed off from the intercellular space. The gap junction corresponds to the physiologist's low-resistance junction or permeable junction,[138] which is responsible for electrical, ionic and metabolic coupling of neighbouring cells of a tissue. Gap junctional permeability is regulated by local concentrations of free Ca^{2+}.[138]

In the liver cells, gap junctions occur as larger areas on the intercellular domain, but also as small patches between the fibril network of the tight junctions, i.e. very close to the canaliculus. This suggests that part of the intercellular communication is related to the coordination of bile secretory activity between neighbouring liver cells.[75]

Canalicular membrane

The bile canalicular membrane represents a specialized domain on the liver-cell surface.[40,75] The bile canaliculus is formed by a groove (hemicanaliculus) of the lateral plasma membrane (Fig. 11.3). The two hemicanaliculi of adjacent hepatocytes are sealed by tight junctions and express cell adhesion molecule cell-CAM 105.[139] Their location midway in the intercellular plane of a liver-cell muralium creates a chicken-wire-like network, buried in the middle of a one-cell-thick plate.[18,75] Canalicular shape and size may vary to some extent in the normal liver,[140] apparently in relation to secretory activity;[141,142] the normal diameter is about 1 µm.

The canalicular plasma membrane projects into the lumen in the form of numerous finger-like extensions (microvilli) of somewhat variable length and diameter (Fig. 11.3). The spacing of these microvilli is not entirely uniform.[18,143] In the smaller zone 3 canaliculi they appear over the entire canalicular surface; in the broader zone 1 canaliculi there is a preferential location near the margin.[18] Besides finger-like extensions, diverticulum-like evagina-

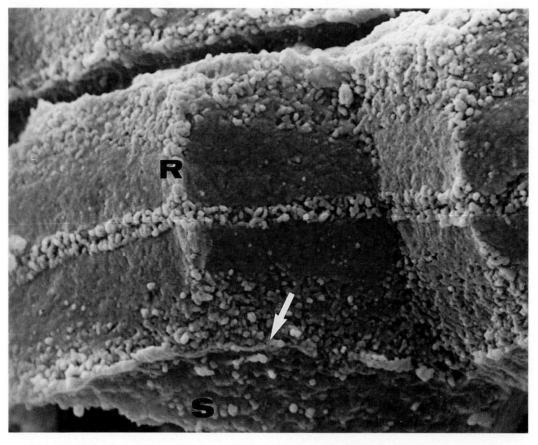

Fig. 11.3 Scanning electron microscopic picture of bile canaliculus in normal rat liver. The picture shows a broken liver-cell plate; the hemicanaliculus lies in the middle of the intercellular domain; it is provided with numerous microvilli, most numerous near the canalicular margin. The intercellular domain is relatively flat, contrasting with the irregular microvilli of the perisinusoidal recess (R). The sinusoidal lumen (S) is separated from the liver cell's sinusoidal domain by a thin veil of endothelial cytoplasm (arrow). × 10 000

tions of the canalicular membrane may be seen, probably representing what have been described as 'intracellular canaliculi'.[18,143]

Techniques for isolation of canalicular subfractions from the liver cell membrane have been progressively refined.[10,144] Biochemically, the canalicular domain is a specially differentiated segment of the liver-cell plasma membrane in terms of phospholipid:cholesterol ratio, content of proteins, presence of specific ectoenzymes and enrichment of glycosphingolipids.[10] At least three different ATP-dependent export carriers exist in the canalicular domain: (i) the canalicular bile salt export carrier; (ii) an export carrier for non-bile-acid organic anions — glutathione conjugates and glucuronides, such as cysteinyl-leukotrienes, bilirubin glucuronide and BSP; and (iii) an export carrier (Gp 170 — gene product of the multidrug resistance gene) for a variety of hydrophobic, mostly basic drugs and organic cations.[38,39,145,146] In addition, bilirubin-diglucuronide transport through the canalicular membrane seems to be carrier-mediated.[147]

The canalicular membrane is covered with a well-developed glycoprotein glycocalyx, demonstrable by ruthenium red staining.[99] It also expresses strong activities of Mg^{2+}-ATPase, 5'-nucleotidase, naphthyl amidase, leucine aminopeptidase, γ-glutamyltranspeptidase and dipeptidyl-peptidase IV.[10] Canalicular specific localization of leucine aminopeptidase was confirmed by immunohistochemistry,[148,149] which also localized the neutral endopeptidase CD10 to liver-cell canaliculi.[150]

Phosphotungstic acid staining on electron microscopy shows that the canalicular domain of the membrane is more akin to membranes of the vacuolar apparatus (Golgi complex and lysosomes) than the rest of the cell membrane.[151] The canalicular membrane contains antigens shared by renal proximal tubules and other epithelia involved in absorption or secretion.[152] Bile salt secretion modulates the phospholipid:cholesterol ratio, and hence the fluidity and permeability of this membrane.[142] By virtue of their detergent activity, bile salts also elute some glycoprotein ectoenzymes from the canalicular membrane, explaining the occurrence in bile of such enzymes as 5'-nucleotidase, phosphodiesterase, γ-glutamyltransferase and alkaline phosphatase.[153-155] Even segments of canalicular membrane may be shed into the canalicular lumen during bile secretion.[51] Loss of membrane components from the canalicular domain may be compensated for by insertion of membrane units derived from Golgi or ferry vesicles.[55,156] Canalicular membrane phospholipids contribute to the phospholipid content of bile.[157,158] The canalicular membrane is thus a crucial structural component involved in bile formation.

From the considerations enumerated above, it is clear that bile secretion is a complex process, implying a highly coordinated activity of numerous liver-cell organelles, if not the liver cell as a whole.

The intra-acinar bile channel or canaliculus (Fig. 11.4)

The bile canalicular network apparently forms a structurally and functionally coherent system; indeed, segments of canaliculi can be isolated as such.[159] Intercellular attachments in the zonulae occludentes, and zonulae and maculae adhaerentes, contribute to the structural cohesion. Its tone is provided by an encircling meshwork of contractile microfilaments inserting on the zonulae adhaerentes; microfilaments running in the axis of microvilli and inserting on the inner leaflet of the microvillous membrane may provide microvillar motility. This arrangement suggests a possible dynamic micro-equivalent at the subcellular level of intestinal villous and peristaltic movements, potentially important in the propagation of fluid flow in the system.[110,111,129,160] Coordination of bile secretory function between the numerous canalicular segments contributed by individual hepatocytes is conceivably important for the canalicular network to function as a whole. Such integration is probably achieved by intercellular communication through maculae communicantes.[161]

The occurrence throughout the liver acinus of a zone 1–zone 3 gradient in the concentration of solutes in the sinusoidal plasma,[162] and the opposite direction of bile flow to that of plasma flow,[163] may further be important in modulating the function of the canalicular network as a whole, since bile secretory activity of individual hepatocytes is partly dependent on solute concentrations in the space of Disse. Further regulating factors are the type and number of carrier molecules,[164] the presence of receptors for hormones and metabolites in the sinusoidal plasma membrane,[47] and innervation of hepatocytes.[165]

Bile ductular (cholangiolar) and bile duct cells

Primary canalicular bile is modified during passage along cholangioles and bile ducts by secretory and absorptive processes.[166,167] Ductular epithelia secrete water, HCO_3^- and IgA. Secretion is under hormonal control. Reabsorption involves water, glucose, glutamate and bile acids. Reabsorpsion of bile acids plays a role in the hypercholeresis induced by ursodeoxycholic acid by the so-called cholehepatic shunt pathway.[38] Recent immunohistochemical studies localizing ursodeoxycholic acid in bile duct cells support this concept.[168] Bile-duct epithelial cells have phenotypic traits which distinguish them from liver parenchymal cells; and display heterogeneity along the different segments of the biliary tree.[169,170]

MORPHOLOGICAL SUBSTRATE OF CHOLESTASIS

Parenchymal changes: acinar gradient

Perivenular bilirubinostasis

Human cholestasis of any aetiology is characterized light

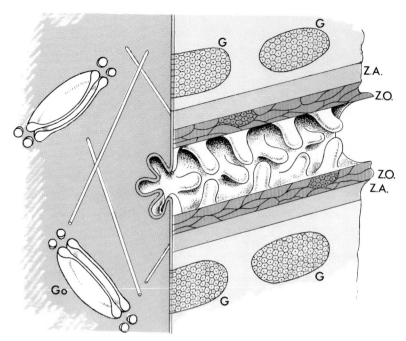

Fig. 11.4 Schematic representation of the biliary pole of the hepatocyte. The picture shows a hemicanaliculus with microvilli, which are more prominent at the margin. The canaliculus is sealed by a tight junction with its characteristic network (zonula occludens) (ZO). In some compartments of the tight junctional network, gap junctions are built in. Next to the tight junction lies the intermediate junction (zonula adhaerens — ZA), which is the attachment site for contractile microfilaments. These form a pericanalicular web and also insert on the inner leaflet of the microvillous membrane. Larger gap junctional areas are represented on the intratrabecular cell surface (G). In the vicinity of the bile canaliculus, the liver-cell cytoplasm contains microtubules, pericanalicular vesicles, lysosomes (the latter two not shown in this drawing) and Golgi complexes (Go).

microscopically by an exclusively or predominantly acinar zone 3 localization of bilirubin deposition in hepatocytes, canaliculi and Kupffer cells. This morphological feature may be more correctly described as 'bilirubinostasis'.[27,171] In severe cholestasis of longer duration, such pigment deposition may extend up to zone 1 around the portal tracts. The predominantly zone 3 localization of 'bilirubinostasis' may be explained by several factors besides the lower O_2 tension in zone 3 of the acinus.[41] Bile acid secretion and corresponding bile water flow is assured by mechanisms different from those responsible for secretion of bilirubin and exogenous dyes.[3,25] Since zone 1 is the main contributor to 'bile-acid-dependent' bile flow, the canaliculi of zones 2 and 3 are perfused with smaller amounts of biliary fluid, which is generated by mechanisms progressively independent of bile acids towards the terminal hepatic venule. Such zonal differences may predispose to a primarily zone 3 distribution of canalicular precipitates during cholestasis.[41] The maximal activity of drug-metabolizing enzymes is located in zone 3, so that some xenobiotics, the toxicity of which is dependent on production of metabolites, may have a major inhibitory effect in this acinar territory.[41] In the case of complete obstruction of distal bile ducts, ductular reabsorption and

hepatocellular re-secretion may assure a higher degree of canalicular flushing in zone 1.[15]

Even in the more cholestatic zone 3, not all canaliculi are equally dilated and filled with bile plugs (Fig. 11.5). This individual behaviour of adjacent canalicular segments may be determined by intermittent variations in blood flow in anastomosing sinusoids[172] and by failure of adequate intercellular coordination through functional closure or even disappearance of the gap junctions as outlined below.[173]

Periportal cholate stasis

Cholestasis of longer duration leads to a peculiar change of hepatocytes in zone 1, termed cholate stasis.[171,174,175] The cells appear swollen and hydropic, while the remaining visible cytoplasm becomes coarsely granular and concentrated in the perinuclear region; gradually more profound cytoskeletal disturbance occurs, with formation of Mallory bodies which are composed of intermediate filaments.[95] Their zone 1 location in cholestatic conditions contrasts with the usual zone 3 location of Mallory bodies in alcoholic liver disease.[176] Progressive accumulation is seen of orcein-positive copper-binding

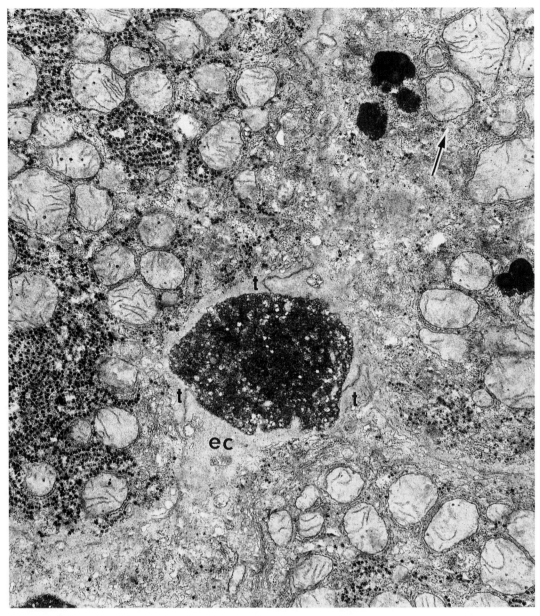

Fig. 11.6 Electron microscopic picture of human cholestatic liver. In the centre of the picture a dilated canaliculus is seen, filled with electron-dense material (bile thrombus). Microvilli have disappeared. The pericanalicular ectoplasm (ec) is thickened. Tight junctions (t) are preserved. Numerous mitochondria show curled or circular cristae (arrow). × 7450

lipoprotein X in cholestasis[208] and in the case of dimeric IgA after intrabiliary injection.[209] However, in a study of bile-duct obstruction in the rat for 2 weeks,[210] it was found that vesicle-mediated transport of horseradish peroxidase proceeded normally in spite of biliary stasis. With presently available morphological techniques, it is still difficult to allocate each individual vesicular structure to its own system: retrograde diacytotic vesicles, coated vesicles, lysosomes, Golgi vesicles or SER profiles.[60]

Lysosomes

Lysosomes, especially secondary lysosomes and auto-

phagic vacuoles, are increased in the hepatocyte in cholestasis. Hepatocytic inclusions interpreted as bile pigment and pseudobile inclusions are more specific for cholestasis than autophagic vacuoles and increased lipofuscin granules (Fig. 11.5), which are encountered in any type of liver injury.

Although definite identification of bilirubin at the ultrastructural level is not yet possible, it is generally assumed that bile pigment inclusions correspond to accumulations of finely granular and fibrillar material, initially devoid of any surrounding membrane. The present interpretation is that intrahepatocytic bile pigment deposition occurs as precipitation of conjugated bilirubin — which has an affinity for non-viable material — in areas of focal cytoplasmic degeneration. These precipitates become sequestered in autophagic vacuoles and are subjected to digestion by lysosomal enzymes, including deconjugation of bilirubin conjugates by β-glucuronidase. This would explain why larger bile-pigment deposits are usually enveloped by a membrane and react histochemically as unconjugated bilirubin. Pseudobile inclusions are membrane-bound vacuoles containing osmiophilic, lamellar and often whorled material (Fig. 11.5). This material resembles phospholipid (and presumably bile salt) liquid crystals. Liver cells containing large numbers of similar inclusions correspond to cells showing feathery degeneration and cholate stasis on light microscopy. Apparently, excessive accumulation of bile constituents, including detergent bile salts, in liver cells exerts a damaging effect on intracellular membranes and finally results in lytic necrosis of affected hepatocytes. In longstanding cholestasis, lysosomes in zone 1 hepatocytes accumulate increasing amounts of copper, complexed with copper-binding protein (metallothionein)[211] (Fig. 11.22).

Golgi complex

As in choleresis, the Golgi complex shows alterations in cholestasis, suggesting its close involvement in bile secretion and its failure.[51] Previous descriptive studies in human cholestasis documented hypertrophy of the Golgi complex, but later morphometric analysis of the Golgi structures in rat liver after bile-duct ligation demonstrated a decreased Golgi complex in periportal hepatocytes and complex changes in the various Golgi components of zone 3 parenchymal cells.[51]

There is an intriguing analogy between the presumably Golgi-derived vacuoles appearing in hypercholeretic states[212] and those observed in some cholestatic conditions.[213,214] These observations remind one of the general problem of distinguishing between physiological adaptation and pathological alteration. A particular type of cholestasis, termed arteriohepatic dysplasia (p. 458), is associated with dilatation of the cis- components of the Golgi complex, suggesting an intracellular secretory block at the level of the Golgi complex.[215] Small granules (very low density lipoprotein), vesicles and stringy material may be found accumulating in Golgi vesicles and cisternae in all forms of cholestasis. Some of the increased vesicular structures in the Golgi area may reflect disturbances in membrane flow and recycling.

Cytoskeleton

The pericanalicular ectoplasm usually appears thickened in cholestasis[15] (Figs 11.5 and 11.6); this is largely the result of cytoskeletal abnormalities. Disturbance of the functional integrity of components of the cytoskeleton may interfere with bile secretion and lead to cholestasis.

Microfilament inhibitors such as cytochalasin B and phalloidin induce cholestasis.[216] The simultaneous development of bile secretory arrest and hypertrophy of the microfilament web suggest that in these conditions the contractile apparatus is the primary target of the cholestatic agent.[28,217,218] In human cholestasis, widening of the pericanalicular ectoplasm has been shown to be due to hypertrophy of the pericanalicular microfilaments.[219–222] The less-evident, thick contractile myosin filaments have not been extensively investigated; evidence was produced for loss of myosin from liver-cell membranes in cholestatic liver.[106] Accumulation of intracytoplasmic vesicles may also be related to disturbance in the arrangement and function of actin microfilaments.[223]

Intermediate filaments and their role in the bile secretory process have been investigated in some recent studies. Taken together, these studies suggest that an intact pericanalicular sheath is important for maintaining canalicular secretion.[121,122,224–226]

Immunohistochemical studies of cytokeratins in human liver specimens from patients with chronic cholestatic liver disease revealed the expression by periportal hepatocytes of 'bile duct cell specific' cytokeratins; this observation supports the concept of 'ductular metaplasia' of hepatocytes in chronic cholestasis.[227] Cytokeratin intermediate filaments have also been studied in relation to Mallory body formation in cholestasis. Griseofulvin administration to mice leads to development of Mallory bodies[228] and also induces cholestasis.[229] Ethinyloestradiol administration to Syrian hamsters produces cholestasis and Mallory bodies, besides a number of additional alterations.[230]

Microtubules are also involved in cholestasis: addition of the antimicrotubular agent colchicine to phalloidin enhances the cholestatic effect of the latter,[231] indicating that disruption of microtubular function is causally involved in bile secretory arrest, presumably by interference with vesicle-mediated transport.

Recent experiments suggest that integrity of contractile microfilaments is required for bile salt uptake and transport, whereas microtubular function seems to be essential for protein uptake.[49,108] The role of the cytoskeleton, especially of the microfilament and intermediate filament components, in choleresis and cholestasis needs to be further defined.[38] In view of the fact that all components of the cytoskeleton seem to form a highly integrated functional system,[98] it should not be too surprising that interference with one of the components of the system may have repercussions on the cytoskeleton as a whole.

Hyaloplasm

The recently discovered microtrabecular lattice of the cell's ground substance[98] seems to be intimately involved in the spatial positioning and movement of intracellular organelles and vesicles; hence, one might expect disturbance of transport functions, such as cholestasis in the liver cell, to be accompanied by dramatic changes in this dynamic system. However, better insight into this new frontier of cell structure and physiology must await broader application of high-voltage electron microscopy.

Junctional complexes

The junctional components that have been most extensively studied in relation to cholestasis are the tight junctions and gap junctions.

Tight junctions. Transmission electron microscopy reveals an increase in tight junctional depth and a more irregular spacing of the close contact points between the membranes of two adjacent hepatocytes, although the tight junctions as such remain preserved even in the case of extreme dilatation of the canaliculus. However, freeze-fracture replicas reveal striking changes in the number and texture of tight junctional fibrils, suggesting an increased permeability of these structures[116,188] (Fig. 11.7). Immunofluorescence studies of ZO-1 (the first- and best-characterized tight junctional protein) indicate that in bile duct-ligated rats the distribution of ZO-1 becomes irregular and discontinuous.[232] Preliminary evidence suggests that ZO-1 mRNA levels increase as a primary hepatic response to bile-duct ligation.[233] Increased permeability was demonstrated by transjunctional passage of tracer molecules which do not cross the tight junctions in normal liver. These tight junctional changes are completely reversible after relief of bile-duct obstruction. Similar changes were observed in liver biopsies from patients with obstructive cholestasis. Morphological evidence of such tight junctional changes and functional evidence of increased permeability have been obtained in several models of experimental intrahepatic cholestasis induced in the rat with ethinyloestradiol, phalloidin, α-naphthyl isothiocyanate and chlorpromazine.[116,234,236] The phalloidin model is of special interest, since it shows that interference with microfilament integrity has repercussions on the arrangement and permeability properties of the tight junctions. The same holds true for the antimicrotubular agents vincristine[237] and vinblastine.[238] It thus appears that the critical canaliculo-sinusoidal barrier, separating the blood from the biliary compartment, undergoes drastic changes in cholestasis, possibly under control of cytoskeletal components. Increased canalicular pressure per se may also influence tight junctions, since these structures are tension sensitive.[239]

Some authors suggest that biliary pressure is a more important determinant than bile acid flux in increasing tight junctional permeability.[240] Increased permeability of tight junctions was proposed as a possible mechanism of cholestasis several years ago.[241] It appears, however, that in some experimental models at least (ethinyloestradiol), tight junctional permeability increase may be the result rather than the cause of cholestasis[242,243] although it may contribute to the cholestatic state in the later phase of the disease process.[244] In other experimental models (α-naphthyl isothiocyanate, carmustine), cholestasis may be primarily caused by an increased tight junctional permeability.[234,235]

A less effective barrier function of the tight junctions under cholestatic conditions may allow for escape of the negatively charged anionic bile salts from the canalicular lumen to the intercellular space, thus blunting the osmotic and electrical gradient necessary for driving water and solutes through the paracellular pathway into the biliary compartment, resulting in arrest of bile flow or cholestasis.[246] In severe and prolonged cholestasis, rupture of tight junctions may occur,[247] this, however, seems to be a late event, not responsible for bile regurgitation in early stages of cholestasis.

Gap junctions. After bile-duct ligation in the rat and obstructive cholestasis in man, disappearance[173,248] or decrease[249] of gap junctions is observed. This may supposedly lead to functional uncoupling of liver parenchymal cells and could explain the heterogeneity of canalicular and cytoplasmic changes observed between individual hepatocytes in cholestasis.[250] Furthermore, uncoupling might serve to protect adjacent liver cells from extension of liver-cell necrosis.[128,251]

Bile canaliculi

Canalicular morphology. The most constant feature described in all forms of cholestasis is dilatation of bile canaliculi with decrease in the number and blunting or distortion of microvilli, occasionally forming microvillous blebs[51] (Fig. 11.8). Similar changes may be induced, however, by choleretic infusions of dehydrocholate.[142]

An increased number of canalicular cross-sections is found, owing to canalicular tortuosity.[17,18,252] Focal dilatations and evaginations of canaliculi lead to varicosity.[18,252] Marginal microvilli seem to be more resistant and remain preserved even in cases of severe canalicular dilatation.[213,253] Occasionally the canalicular membrane appears disrupted with shedding of ectoplasmic material into the lumen.[210,219]

Freeze-fracture replica studies of microvillous membranes reveal lamellar transformation of microvilli and a paucity of intramembrane particles in the transformed region of the canalicular membrane in lithocholic acid-induced cholestasis.[16,254,255] Since the number of intramembranous particles usually parallels the functional activity of a cell membrane,[256] this observation suggests severe damage to the canalicular membrane with corresponding functional impairment.

In rat liver after experimentally induced cholestasis,

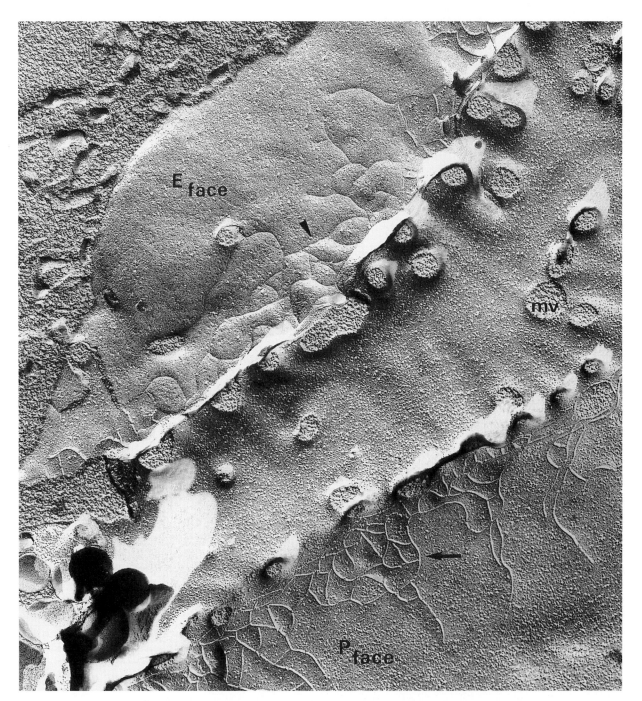

Fig. 11.7 Freeze-fracture replica of bile canaliculus from a rat with ethinyloestradiol-induced cholestasis. The tight junctions (compare with Fig. 11.2 for normal appearance) show a more irregular and loose network of tight junctional fibrils, appearing as ridges on the P face (outer side of protoplasmic leaflet) (arrow) and as grooves on the E face (inner side of extracellular leaflet) (arrowhead) of the intercellular membrane. Some broken-off microvilli (mv) can be recognized in the canalicular lumen. × 72 000 from Desmet V, De Vos R. In: Popper H, Schaffner F, eds. Progress in liver diseases, vol VII. With permission from Grune & Stratton Inc., New York)

enzyme histochemistry reveals increased activity of alkaline phosphatase and 5'-nucleotidase, with a redistribution of the enzymes over all domains of the plasma membrane.[22,257]

Leucine aminopeptidase and γ-glutamyltransferase also show cholestasis-induced changes in activity at the biliary pole of the liver cell; the alterations vary, however,

according to the animal species examined.[14,15,258,259] Similarly, disappearance of the 'ruthenium red-positive glycocalyx has been reported.[260] An unusual change of the canalicular membrane is the appearance of cilia, described in a human case of intrahepatic cholestasis,[219] possibly reflecting a modulation of hepatocytes to bile-duct epithelium,[261] on which surface cilia are regularly observed.[18] A

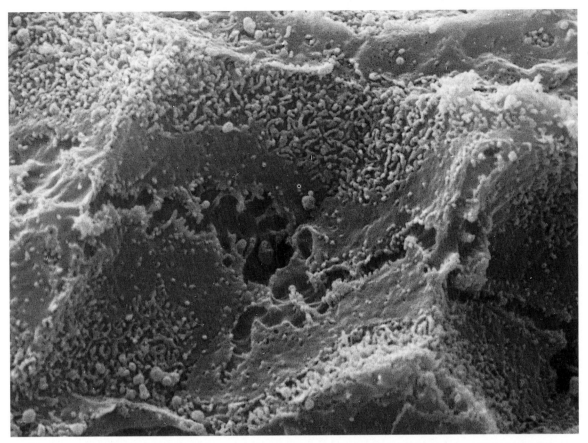

Fig. 11.8 Scanning electron microscopic picture of bile canaliculus in rat liver after 3 days obstruction of the common bile duct. The exposed hemicanaliculus shows a tortuous course, irregular dilatation of the lumen with saccular extensions, and reduced numbers of microvilli. Compare with Fig. 11.3. × 10 000

striking observation is the irregularity and lack of homogeneity in canalicular changes observed in most forms of experimental and human cholestasis[15] (Fig. 11.5). It is not unusual to find normal canaliculi near severely dilated channels.

In longstanding cholestasis, hepatocytes often develop an arrangement that differs from the normal liver-cell plate or muralium. They acquire a tubular arrangement, which on cross-section appears as a dilated canaliculus surrounded by more than two hepatocytes. Such 'cholestatic liver cell rosettes' correspond to so-called 'secondary canaliculi'.[15] Their tubular nature has been demonstrated by computer-assisted three-dimensional reconstruction.[262,263]

Dilated canaliculi in cholestatic liver may appear empty (Fig. 11.5), or be filled with a variety of materials, the most obvious being the typical bile plugs in human liver tissue (Fig. 11.6). Biliary concrements have been noted in all types of cholestasis in many different forms: they may be homogeneous, granular, crystalline, lipid-like, lamellar or whorled. They have been interpreted as representing bilirubin, membrane fragments, extruded pericanalicular ectoplasm or liquid crystals resulting from disturbed

micelle formation. Distinct crystalline precipitates have been observed in lithocholic acid-induced cholestasis in the rat, and interpreted as crystals of lithocholate[16] or free cholesterol.[218,264,265] The composition of bile plugs in human cholestatic liver is complex; they can be shown to contain bilirubin, mainly of the conjugated type. Some, possibly older, deposits show varying degrees of diastase-resistant PAS positivity,[15] suggesting participation of membrane and/or glycocalyx material.

Significance of canalicular changes. The dilatation of the canalicular lumen may be the result of increased intraluminal pressure ('mechanical ileus'), especially in extrahepatic bile duct obstruction, but may also be due to a 'paralytic ileus' of the contractile pericanalicular microfilaments in some types of intrahepatic cholestasis.[15,28,110,160]

The canalicular membrane is the principal target in several models of intrahepatic cholestasis induced by cholestatic bile salts: lithocholate,[266] 3-β-hydroxy-5-cholenoate[213] and allo bile acids.[267] A major change in the lithocholate model is an increase in cholesterol content of the canalicular membrane.[268,269] However, intrahepatic cholestasis can also be associated with a decreased cholesterol content of this membrane, as in cytochalasin B- and norethandrolone-induced cholestasis.[268] It appears that several cholestatic agents, including chlorpromazine,[41] induce changes in the cholesterol:phospholipid ratio of the membrane, decreasing its fluidity and permeability to water, anions and cations.[21] Administration of S-adenosyl-L-methionine can modulate the effect induced by ethinyl-oestradiol.[270] Detergent effects of accumulating bile salts, and possibly abnormal bile salts, may be responsible for elution of ectoenzymes and glycocalyx components.[14,153,154]

Canalicular enlargement correlates with increased serum levels of leucine aminopeptidase, whereas increased serum activity of 5'-nucleotidase correlates with a higher incidence of canaliculi in the sections.[271] Biochemical analysis of liver plasma membrane fractions in various forms of experimental cholestasis shows an increase in alkaline phosphatase and sialic acid, and a decrease in Mg^{2+}-ATPase and 5'-nucleotidase.[272]

The disappearance of microvilli over the roof of the canaliculus with preservation of marginal microvilli has been ascribed to the existence of a 'marginal ridge' or a zone of more resistant cell cortex. However, selective disappearance of microvilli over the roof of the canaliculi could also be due to the insertion of new, non-microvillous membrane segments in this area derived, for example, from movement of Golgi vacuoles into the canaliculus, indicating a disturbance in membrane flow and membrane turnover.[28,212,273]

Diverticula and apparent evaginations of the canalicular lumen are difficult to interpret. It remains unclear whether such profiles represent the stage of fusion of cytoplasmic vacuoles emptying into the canaliculus, or the early formation of retrograde diacytotic vesicles intended to migrate towards the sinusoid and possibly involved in bile regurgitation.[208]

The heterogeneity of canalicular changes in cholestatic liver may be due to several factors. In the rat, it has been shown that lithocholic acid-induced cholestasis produces more focal canalicular changes than extrahepatic bile-duct obstruction.[17,255] Localization of changes along a canalicular segment may result from blockade of intercellular communication through closure or decrease of the gap junctions. Furthermore, it should be realized that cholestasis-induced canalicular changes are far from static. Morphometric analysis of different canalicular types found in rat liver after bile-duct ligation led to the conclusion that new canaliculi are formed,[274] in which the cell adhesion molecule cell-CAM 105 presumably plays a role.[139]

The handicapped liver cell thus appears to adapt by the development of new canaliculi, according to a sequence very similar to the normal differentiation of canaliculi in maturing fetal and neonatal liver.[275] Another factor possibly contributing to the heterogeneity of observed canalicular changes is liver-cell mitosis, known to occur

early after bile-duct obstruction.[276,277] Newly formed hepatocytes presumably establish intercellular junctions and canaliculi at a rapid rate[69] as also occurs in liver-cell cultures.[278,279]

The appearance of 'secondary canaliculi',[15] or 'cholestatic liver-cell rosettes'[262,263] (see Fig. 11.16) can be interpreted as a further sign of adaptation.[280] The ultrastructural and freeze-fracture characteristics of such cholestatic hepatocytes suggest a switch of the parenchymal cell from an isotonic to a hypertonic secretory cell type.[116] From an architectural point of view, this tubular transformation of liver-cell plates represents a regression of the adult mammalian liver architecture to a more primitive type of liver-cell arrangement.[281]

The conjugated nature of the bile pigment in intercellular concretions indicates that this precipitated bilirubin has been conjugated and excreted by the hepatocyte, but that some mechanism is failing to wash it through the channel. This correlates with the existence of different secretory mechanisms for organic anions and bile salts.[38] Bilirubin itself can act as a cholestatic agent when administered to manganese-pretreated rats.[282,283]

The diastase-resistant PAS-positive staining of some bile plugs can be explained by shedding of the glycocalyx,[260] elution of ectoenzymes and other glycoproteins[153] and shedding of ectoplasmic material through ruptured canalicular membranes.[210,219] In lithocholate-induced cholestasis in cultured rat liver cells, shedding of cholesterol-rich membrane fragments from the canalicular domain has been observed.[284] Obstruction of the canalicular lumen by bile plugs and precipitates represents an additional mechanical factor which may aggravate and prolong a cholestatic condition induced by various agents. Canalicular changes thus appear to be caused by interplay of various factors, including increased pressure in the case of extrahepatic obstruction.[285]

Reactive intra-acinar and portal tract changes

Parenchymal inflammation

Human cholestasis of some duration elicits a local mesenchymal cell reaction. Macrophages and mononuclear lymphoid cells accumulate in the sinusoids (Fig. 11.9). The cytoplasm of the macrophages is often abundant and contains inclusions of lipids, bilirubin and lipofuscin, derived from phagocytosis of necrotic liver cells and liberated bile plugs. These cells appear to be in an inactivated state as few express HLA class II antigens.[286] The presence of such pigment-laden macrophages characterizes cholestasis of some duration and intensity, since they are missing in early and mild cholestasis. This local inflammatory reaction is secondary to the liver-cell-damaging effect of retained bile constituents (Fig. 11.10), and must be differentiated from a diffuse hepatitis; the

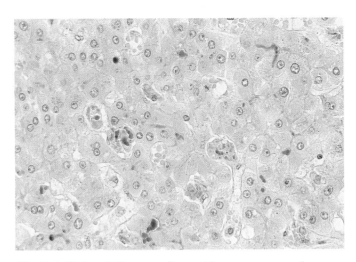

Fig. 11.9 Cholestatic liver parenchyma with numerous macrophages, displaying bulky cytoplasmic masses with bilirubin inclusions. H & E.

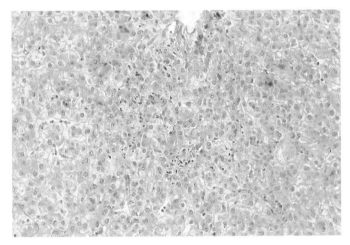

Fig. 11.10 Perivenular area in a liver biopsy from a patient with benign recurrent cholestasis. There is marked cholestasis with bile plugs, and a histiocytic and mononuclear cell infiltration in the cholestatic area. H & E.

main differentiating criterion is its limitation to the cholestatic areas. Inflammation, however, may contribute to cholestasis, since sensitized lymphocytes have been shown to release cholestasis-inducing lymphokines.[287] The latter 'cholestatic factor' was also detected in hepatocytes by immunohistochemistry.[288] Cholestasis further modulates major histocompatibility antigen expression of hepatocytes: in man and in the rat, cholestasis enhances hepatocellular HLA class I antigen expression, thus rendering the liver more vulnerable to immune destruction.[289]

Portal and periportal reactions

The terminal branches of the intrahepatic biliary tree, bile ductules and canals of Hering, have the peculiar property

of increasing in number in many forms of liver disease, especially in cholestasis. These ductules are accompanied by inflammatory infiltrate and fibrosis, the whole being indicated by the term 'ductular reaction'.[2,290] The origin of the increased number of ductules remains subject to debate. Theoretically, three different mechanisms can be envisaged: (i) multiplication of pre-existing ductules by mitotic division of the ductular cells; (ii) generation of ductular structures from proliferation and biliary differentiation of progenitor cells (or stem cells); and (iii) transdifferentiation or metaplasia of periportal hepatocytes into biliary-type cells.

Multiplication of existent biliary epithelium appears to be the main mechanism of the ductular reaction seen in acute cholestasis, for instance that following complete obstruction of the extrahepatic bile duct.[291] The ductular reaction in this case results mainly in elongation, not so much in branching or sprouting of ductules; the factors initiating mitoses of the biliary epithelium are probably multiple, but increased biliary pressure is the one clearly established experimentally.[291]

Derivation of ductules from stimulation of progenitor or stem cells remains highly controversial in the human liver. Although considerable evidence has accumulated in favour of the existence of stem cells in rat liver,[292–298] a less evidence has been produced in man.[2,299] Nevertheless, a recent ultrastructural investigation in human liver showing the ductular reaction has identified a novel small epithelial cell which may play this role since it can differentiate into either liver or bile-duct cells.[300]

Ductular metaplasia of periportal heptocytes[301,302] seems to occur preferentially in chronic cholestatic conditions, for instance primary biliary cirrhosis and primary sclerosing cholangitis.[227] A shift from the hepatocellular to the biliary cell phenotype has been demonstrated for cytokeratins,[227,303] tissue polypeptide antigen,[304] blood group antigens,[305] chromogranin[306] and 'bile duct type' integrins VLA2, 3 and 6.[307] Ductular metaplasia gives rise to so-called atypical ductular proliferation.[2,308] The mechanism inducing ductular metaplasia of periportal hepatocytes appears to be complex, involving pericellular matrix components,[309,310] possibly bile salts[302] and other humoral factors.[311]

The role of the ductular reaction remains incompletely understood. The ductules may provide bypass mechanisms for the drainage of bile in diseases associated with destruction of interlobular bile ducts, like primary biliary cirrhosis.[312] The ductular cells reabsorb bile acids[313] and may thus provide the hepatocytes with a means of avoiding bile acid overload by establishing a chole-hepatic cycling of bile acids.[280]

Ductular reabsorption of biliary constituents in cholestasis is reflected in the occurrence in ductular cells of numerous pinocytotic vesicles, the appearance of vacuoles containing lipid-like material and precipitates interpreted as bile pigment, widening of the intercellular spaces at the basal portion of the ductule, and focal duplication of the basement membrane.[314] Ductular reabsorption of fluid may lead to the formation of inspissated bile concrements obstructing the lumen, thus aggravating the cholestasis.

In cholestasis several changes may occur in these ductules, including focal dilatation of their lumen, decrease in the number and size of microvilli, formation of protruding microvillous blebs, luminal diverticula and curling of mitochondrial cristae.[15] In intra- and extrahepatic cholestasis in the rat, the ductular reaction is the source of the increase in serum γ-glutamyltranspeptidase.[315]

Reabsorption with leakage of bile components into the portal connective tissue leads to a marked inflammatory reaction; polymorphonuclear leucocytes are usually found near the ductules in the oedematous connective tissue at the periphery of the portal tract (Figs 11.11 and 11.12). These morphological features of acute cholangiolitis do not necessarily denote an ascending bacterial cholangitis, but represent a tissue reaction to irritant chemical stimuli.[175,316,317]

Ductular reaction and the accompanying inflammatory reaction play an important role in portal and periportal fibroplasia.[302,318] The neo-ductules are surrounded by a PAS-positive basement membrane which contains collagen type IV and laminin,[319–321] synthesized by the ductular cells themselves.[322] Increased matrix production around proliferating ductules, including collagens and proteoglycans, is also due to stimulation of mesenchymal cells. Close to ductules, myofibroblasts and transitional cell types between perisinusoidal (Ito) cells and myofibroblasts can be observed.[323] These 'activated'

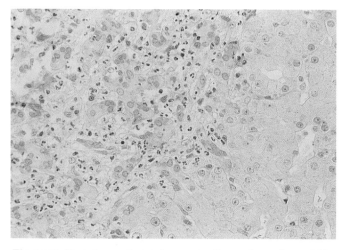

Fig. 11.11 Ductular reaction at the margin of a portal tract (upper left). The portal connective tissue is oedematous and contains many mononuclear and polymorphonuclear leucocytes. Some ductules show continuity with liver-cell plates. The ductules are surrounded by basement membranes. PAS after α-amylase digestion.

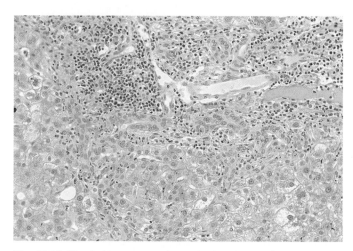

Fig. 11.12 Margin between portal tract (top) and parenchyma (bottom). Note extensive marginal ductular reaction. The inflammatory infiltrate includes many neutrophil leucocytes, especially around the ductules. H & E.

mesenchymal cells have been shown to express α-smooth muscle actin and desmin.[324,325] They are responsible for the production of tenascin in the early stage of ductular reaction,[326,327] followed by deposition of collagens, including type VI collagen,[328] and other matrix components later on.[319] This plays a role in the development of haemodynamic alterations in biliary obstruction.[329]

It is of interest that ductules express transforming growth factor β2, a cytokine known to stimulate perisinusoidal cell and biomatrix production.[330] In this way, ductular reaction is a pacemaker for the development of progressive fibrosis in chronic cholestatic liver disease, eventually resulting in biliary cirrhosis.[302]

Reactive ductular cells express chromogranin and neural cell adhesion molecule, and contain dense-core neuroendocrine-type granules. This finding led to speculation that reactive ductular cells may produce a substance that exerts an autocrine or paracrine regulatory role in the growth of ductules or in the ductular metaplasia of periportal hepatocytes.[306,331] The subsequent demonstration in reactive ductules of parathyroid hormone-like peptide, a factor which modulates cellular growth and differentiation, lends credence to this suggestion.[332]

Ductular reaction and periductular fibrosis is reversible in the early stage. Following removal of the proliferative stimulus (e.g. after relief of bile-duct obstruction) the excess ductular cells are deleted by apoptosis.[318,333] Regression of the ductular reaction is accompanied by regression of the periductular fibrosis,[319] thus facilitating a return of the biliary tree to its original pattern.[280]

Many of the complex series of changes that occur in the liver during prolonged cholestasis are secondary to the cholestatic state. Much of the cellular and tissue damage appears to be due to retention of more hydrophobic, cytotoxic bile acids. Ursodeoxycholic acid appears to protect against such cytotoxic damage of rat hepatocytes in vitro[334] and of rat livers in vivo.[335] It inhibits, at least in part, the biological and toxic effects of the endogenous bile acids by reducing their concentration in and around the liver cells, while ursodeoxycholic acid itself is devoid of toxicity.[336,337] This explains the usefulness of this drug in the treatment of chronic cholestatic disorders.[337–339]

Pathways of bile regurgitation

Since cholestasis represents a bile secretory failure of the liver with concomitant accumulation of bile constituents in the blood, pathways must exist for regurgitation from the biliary compartment into the blood stream. The situation may differ according to whether the cause of cholestasis is a functional disturbance at the level of the hepatocyte, when no hepatocytic bile enters the biliary passages, or whether there is a block along the extrahepatic pathways allowing reabsorption from the duct system. Experimental evidence is mostly derived from studies of extrahepatic bile-duct obstruction.

In the early stages of obstruction, the stagnation of bile in occluded bile ducts is not a static event, but represents a steady state between secretion into and reabsorption from the biliary passages. There is biliary-lymphatic and biliary-venous regurgitation.[313,340] At moderately increased biliary-tract pressure, bile leaks mainly from the small bile ducts into the periportal connective tissue, and water and electrolytes are freely absorbed into the blood stream. This leads to a progressive increase in the concentration of colloid molecules in the interstitial fluid of the portal spaces. As hepatic lymph is formed from this interstitial fluid, the lymph concentration of colloidal or colloid-bound substances (protein-bound bilirubin and bile salts) leaking from the bile ducts will attain high levels. If biliary pressure rises further, bile leakage into the space of Mall becomes limited by the decreased compliance of this part of the liver interstitium. This limits the lymphatic transport of bile constituents.[341,342] At this stage, bile begins to leak from the bile canaliculi into the space of Disse.[340–344] The precise anatomical pathway of bile regurgitation at the canalicular level in intrahepatic as well as extrahepatic cholestasis is still hypothetical.

The extent to which the canalicular tight junctions might be, or might become, permeable to water and small solute molecules, allowing an escape of bile water and solutes from the canaliculi into the blood, remains debatable, although striking changes in the tight junctional network and its permeability suggest the possibility of intercellular escape.[116,188,345] In addition to intercellular escape, transhepatocytic regurgitation offers two further possibilities. A first pathway could be a retrograde diacytotic process with vacuoles pinching off from the bile canaliculus, migrating through the cell and fusing with the sinusoidal cell border.[208,346] This pathway seems to operate for macromolecules, at least for polymeric IgA.[347] A second possible transhepatocytic pathway is a more diffuse and widespread overflow through the cytoplasm towards the liver-cell/blood stream barrier, based on a reversed secretory polarity of the liver cell. Such reversed polarity in cholestasis is supported by the finding of widened intercellular spaces bounded by ATPase- and alkaline phosphatase-positive microvilli, while similar structures disappear from the biliary pole of the hepatocyte and, by the redistribution of the canalicular bile salt, export carrier towards the basolateral membrane.[10,186] Reversed secretory polarity of the hepatocyte may explain regurgitation of bile constituents which never reach the canaliculus and would require active participation of metabolically active liver cells.[9]

Sloughing off of hepatocyte fragments along the length of the cell from the bile canaliculus to the sinusoidal surface may create free communication between the biliary space and the space of Disse.[210] Rupture of dilated canaliculi and liberation of inspissated bile concrements by necrosis of surrounding liver cells is a late event, occurring only after cessation of the cell's secretory activity, and hence cannot play an important role in the pathogenesis of bile regurgitation and jaundice. The released bile concrements, together with cell debris from necrotic liver cells, are engulfed by Kupffer cells.

Increase in the serum level of alkaline phosphatase, originally thought to result from true regurgitation from the biliary compartment, appears to have a different origin. Cholestasis causes an increase in hepatic synthesis of alkaline phosphatase.[189,348,349] Histochemically, the sinusoidal cell membrane becomes strongly positive.[15,257] An important observation in this respect is that the 'high molecular weight isoenzyme' of alkaline phosphatase, which is typically found in the serum of patients with cholestasis, corresponds to alkaline phosphatase of liver-cell origin, either as alkaline phosphatase–lipoprotein complexes,[350] or attached to circulating membrane fragments.[351–353] These vesicular membrane fragments further contain 5'-nucleotidase, L-leucyl-β-naphthylamidase (LAP) and γ-glutamyltransferase, forming a complex 'koinozyme'.[352] It is conceivable that such enzyme-containing membrane fragments are released from the liver cell through the detergent action of locally increased bile-acid concentrations near the liver-cell surface.[354] Shedding of plasma membrane fractions may alter the cell membrane permeability and be responsible for further cell damage and release of intracellular enzymes, thus explaining the striking increase in serum transaminases (aminotransferases) observed in some cases.[355] The reason for the increase in serum levels of phospholipids and free cholesterol is complex and not yet entirely clear.[356]

Lipoprotein X (Lp-X), the circulating transport vehicle

form of the increased phospholipid and free cholesterol seen in cholestatic liver disease, is thought to arise secondarily to regurgitation of a biliary precursor into the plasma. Its final concentration further depends on the activity of lecithin:cholesterol acyltransferase (LCAT).[357] Lp-X is an abnormal serum lipoprotein, originally thought to be specific for cholestasis. It has, however, little diagnostic value.[358]

EXTRAHEPATIC CHOLESTASIS

OVERVIEW OF AETIOLOGICAL FACTORS

The term extrahepatic ('surgical') cholestasis implies mechanical obstruction to large bile ducts outside the liver or within the porta hepatis.[359]

Lithiasis

Gallstones in the common bile duct are the most frequent cause of obstruction. In Western countries most stones in the duct originate from the gallbladder; in certain Oriental countries where recurrent pyogenic cholangitis is prevalent, stones are often found in the duct system even when there are none in the gallbladder.[360]

Tumours

Primary carcinoma of the bile ducts may involve any part of the duct system. Bile-duct carcinoma has a great tendency to infiltrate extensively in the submucosal plane, causing localized sclerosing strictures difficult to differentiate from benign strictures and from sclerosing cholangitis.[360] The tumours are almost invariably adenocarcinomas; squamous cell carcinoma or adenoacanthoma is only occasionally found.

The ampullary area is a common site for carcinomas, which may arise from the mucosa of the lower end of the common duct, the main pancreatic duct, the pancreatic parenchyma, the ampulla itself or, exceptionally, the duodenal mucosa covering the papilla of Vater. Growths arising from any of these sites have the same overall effect, and are often loosely termed cancer of the head of the pancreas or periampullary cancer.[361,362] There is an association between ulcerative colitis and bile-duct carcinoma[360,363] (see Ch. 17).

A bile-duct carcinoma that deserves special mention is the adenocarcinoma of the hepatic duct at its bifurcation within the porta hepatis,[364] since it is easily overlooked and sometimes difficult to diagnose grossly and microscopically; tumours of this type tend to be small and to remain sharply localized, are of the sclerosing type and may be mistaken for a benign stricture.

Rare malignant tumours of the extrahepatic bile ducts include carcinoid, leiomyosarcoma and botryoid sarcoma.[362] Benign tumours of the bile ducts are rare.[365] Cases have been reported of papilloma and papillomatosis (sometimes with subsequent malignant change), adenoma (solid and cystic) and adenomatosis, granular-cell myoblastoma, leiomyoma, apudoma, neurinoma, fibroma, lipoma, adenomyofibroma and hamartoma.

Atresia and choledochal cyst

Atresia of extrahepatic bile ducts and choledochal cyst are discussed in Chapter 3.

Strictures

Benign strictures of the common bile duct almost always follow biliary tract surgery, usually cholecystectomy. Mechanisms include ligation, section or perforation of the duct, prolonged T-tube drainage and rough probing of the duct for calculi. Sclerosing cholangitis is discussed separately in chapter 12.

Rare causes

Enlarged lymph nodes at the porta hepatis only rarely cause extrinsic obstruction. In most cases the nodes are the seat of metastatic tumour, and the ducts are invaded rather than compressed. The same holds true for lymph node enlargement by primary lymphomas. An occasional instance of obstruction by tuberculous lymphadenitis has been reported.

Further rare causes of obstruction reported in the literature include:

1. Inflammatory polyp of the bile duct
2. Intussuscepted cystic duct
3. Choledochal diverticulum
4. Localized, reversible, inflammatory stricture of the common hepatic duct, secondary to cholelithiasis and cholecystitis (Mirizzi syndrome)
5. Parasites in the common bile duct (ascaris, strongyloides, fascioliasis, extrapulmonary paragonimiasis)
6. Congenital diaphragm
7. Blood clot containing liver-cell carcinoma
8. Heterotopic pancreas and heterotopic gastric mucosa in the common bile duct
9. Rupture of hydatid cyst into the bile ducts
10. Aneurysm of the hepatic or gastroduodenal artery
11. Pancreatitis
12. Annular pancreas
13. Pancreatic pseudocyst
14. Metastatic tumour in the pancreas
15. Renal cyst
16. Duodenal ulcer
17. Duodenal diverticulum

18. Foreign bodies (sutures, T-tubes, sponges, bullets, shrapnel).

CHOLANGITIS (CHOLEDOCHITIS)

Cholangitis of the large bile ducts (choledochitis) comprises three forms:[360] simple obstructive cholangitis, recurrent cholangitis (oriental cholangiohepatitis), and sclerosing cholangitis (see Ch. 12).

Simple obstructive cholangitis is by far the most common type in Western countries, and is associated with choledocholithiasis, biliary strictures, stenosis of biliary–enteric anastomoses and biliary fistulas; in short, all forms of intermittent or partial obstruction. It only exceptionally occurs in malignant obstruction of the biliary tree. The chronic form is sometimes referred to as secondary sclerosing cholangitis, to distinguish it from primary sclerosing cholangitis.

The pathogenesis of obstructive cholangitis is still poorly understood; bacteria in portal blood, as found for example in some cases of ulcerative colitis, may be of importance. Ascending bacterial invasion from the intestine is another possible route, which occurs only in the presence of obstruction. Biliary obstruction is therefore an important prerequisite in the pathogenesis of most cases of cholangitis. The rarity of cholangitis in malignant biliary obstruction remains a puzzle; it is speculated that gallstones and inflammatory debris of post-traumatic stricture provide good anchorages for bacterial multiplication.[360,366]

Primary recurrent pyogenic (oriental) cholangitis (oriental cholangiohepatitis) is one of the commonest causes of surgical emergency in South-Eastern and Far-Eastern Asian countries (see Ch. 7). Its aetiology remains unclear. The bile duct is colonized by intestinal bacteria in quantities equalling those in the colon, but the problem of how the enteric bacteria gain such a stronghold in the biliary tract remains unsolved. The ducts are filled with biliary sludge, debris and pus, with stones sometimes lying in the amorphous muddy sludge.[367]

PATHOLOGY OF EXTRAHEPATIC CHOLESTASIS

Macroscopic changes

The liver is enlarged and stained green with bile. It is swollen and its edges are rounded. The intrahepatic bile ducts are dilated (hydrohepatosis). At first they contain dark bile, but later a colourless fluid, the so-called white bile, is found because increased pressure in the ducts finally suppresses secretion of bile by the liver. The already secreted pigment is progressively absorbed or decolorized by leucocytic and bacterial action, and is replaced by a mucous secretion from the glands in the duct wall. In cases of ascending infection proximal to the obstruction, the ducts may contain pus or be surrounded by small abscesses.[359] Careful analysis of the macroscopic aspect of the liver surface, together with the appearance of the gallbladder and other abdominal organs, is useful in the differential diagnosis of cholestasis by laparoscopy.[368]

Microscopic changes

A number of changes are observed in the liver in extrahepatic cholestasis, but it is difficult to elucidate their chronological order in man. Several factors contribute to the problem. It is impossible to carry out serial sampling of the liver in a sufficient number of patients for adequate study. Even if this were done, it would be difficult to assess adequately the nature, degree and variability of the obstructing lesions in humans. In addition, an assessment must be made of the respective parts played by the obstruction and by complicating infection in the production of the histological changes. Although these remarks were made more than a quarter of a century ago,[369] the problem is to a large extent, still with us today. The histological changes will therefore be grouped simply as early and later manifestations.

Early lesions (first weeks)

During the first few days of extrahepatic obstruction there may be little histological change. The earliest changes usually consist of intra-acinar bilirubinostasis, followed by portal oedema and inflammation. The presence of bilirubinostasis alone in some patients with early obstruction causes problems of differentiation from other conditions causing 'simple' or 'pure' cholestasis, such as benign recurrent cholestasis (Summerskill–Tygstrup disease), some forms of drug-induced cholestasis, and postoperative cholestasis.

Microscopic bilirubinostasis usually starts in acinar zone 3.[27,184,370] It is characterized by the appearance of fine bilirubin granules in liver cells and bile plugs or concretions in the intercellular spaces (Fig. 11.1); usually there is some bilirubin impregnation of the liver-cell cytoplasm, only demonstrable in unstained sections or with specific histochemical methods for bilirubin.[11] Intracellular bilirubin granules become coarser with time (Fig. 11.13).

Intercellular bile plugs occur in various forms and distributions; they may appear as thin dots and lines, occasionally delineating a segment of the canalicular network as a dotted or continuous line, or as coarser, inspissated deposits with an irregular surface. Some are located in cholestatic liver-cell rosettes, i.e. they are surrounded by three or more liver cells (see Figs 11.13 and 11.16). Some, probably older, bile concretions are PAS positive. Calcium can be detected cytochemically in bile plugs.[371]

Single liver-cell necroses and acidophil bodies can be found, while mitoses appear in scattered liver cells and

Kupffer cells become more prominent. The perivenular liver cells may exhibit a slightly 'induced' aspect, with peripheral location of organelles and pale pink staining of their cytoplasm, due to hypertrophy of the endoplasmic reticulum.

The portal-tract changes appear with varying speed in different patients, possibly according to the type and location of the obstructing lesion. Rounding and oedema of the portal tracts occurs relatively early in some cases,[372–374] and is more pronounced in the smaller terminal ramifications (Fig. 11.14). In medium-sized portal tracts the oedema may cause a concentric periductal lamellar arrangement of the collagen fibres.[373] Continued increased pressure in the intrahepatic duct system causes dilatation of the bile ducts in the larger portal areas, sometimes with flattening of the lining epithelium.

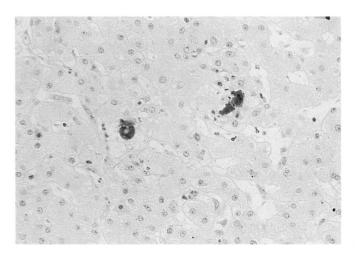

Fig. 11.13 Detail of large intercellular concrements located in hepatocellular tubules. Several adjacent hepatocytes show a rarified and reticular appearance of their cytoplasm, i.e. feathery degeneration. PAS after α-amylase digestion.

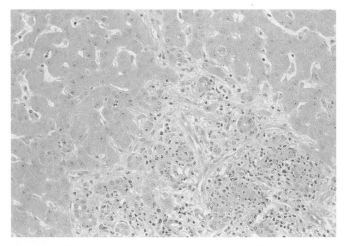

Fig. 11.14 Extrahepatic obstruction with cholangitis. The picture shows a small portal tract with oedematous widening of its connective tissue. Neutrophil leucocytes are present in the connective tissue and between the duct lining cells. H & E.

Bilio-lymphatic reflux[316] is held responsible for the portal oedema, activation of fibroblasts and infiltration of inflammatory cells. Fibroblastic proliferation has been noted early in bile-duct obstruction.[369,373] The portal inflammatory infiltration is composed of mononuclear cells and histiocytes. Neutrophil polymorphonuclear leucocytes are often found close to the ducts in the oedematous terminal portal tracts.

Prominence of ductular structures is followed by real increase in their number, usually at the periphery of the portal area. A slight increase in the number of ductules can be better visualized by immunostaining for cytokeratins.[118,375] Distinction has been made between typical and atypical ductular proliferation,[369] but the distinction is not always easy.[373] In extrahepatic cholestasis, the ductular proliferation is mostly of the 'typical' kind[171,372,376,377] in that the ductules have a recognizable lumen lined by cuboidal cells and surrounded by a basement membrane, best demonstrated in PAS preparations after diastase digestion. The proliferating ductules are almost always accompanied by a neutrophil polymorphonuclear infiltration in close relationship to, and even within, their basement membrane (Fig. 11.10), so-called cholangiolitis.[378,379] Marginal bile-duct proliferation (Fig. 11.11) is one of the most characteristic signs of extrahepatic cholestasis in liver biopsies; in one study it was present in all biopsies examined, and in 82% of all portal areas.[376,380]

Later lesions (several weeks to months)

With continuing obstruction, the acinar and portal changes become more pronounced and show additional components. Intercellular bile plugs increase in number and size and some inspissated concrements may become very large (Fig. 11.13). With time, cholestasis extends towards the acinar zone 1 and may reach the swollen portal tracts (Fig. 11.15).

Rearrangement of hepatocytes is seen, with increasing number of tubular structures surrounded by several liver cells (secondary canaliculi or 'cholestatic liver-cell rosettes')[263,264] (Fig. 11.16); the lumen is of variable width, may appear empty, may contain a precipitate of fluffy bile-stained material, or may be occluded by densely inspissated bile concrements.

Isolated hepatocytes, adjacent to plugs or concrements, or with no topographical relationship to biliary deposits, show an increase in size and rarefaction of their cytoplasm which is reduced to a fine reticular net, sometimes impregnated with bilirubin. This has been termed reticular change or feathery degeneration[378,381] (Fig. 11.13). Feathery degeneration also affects contiguous groups of liver cells, particularly in the lobular periphery. Feathery degeneration results in lytic necrosis of the affected cells or cell groups, leaving empty spaces with some whorled

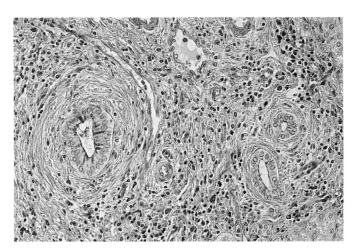

Fig. 11.15 Chronic bile-duct obstruction. The interlobular bile ducts are surrounded by concentric periductal fibrosis. PAS after α-amylase digestion.

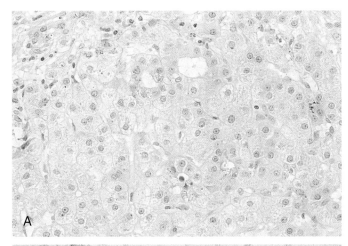

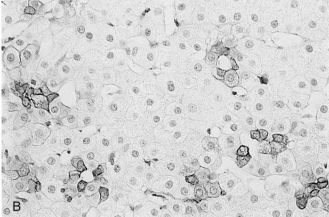

Fig. 11.16 (a,b) Liver parenchyma in chronic bile-duct obstruction, revealing tubular arrangement of hepatocytes (cholestatic liver-cell rosettes). (a) H & E. (b) Cytokeratin immunostain.

membranous material, eventually occupied by invading macrophages and neutrophil leucocytes.

Necrosis of liver cells, lytic or acidophilic, leads to rupture of canaliculi and release of bile plugs and concre-

ments, which become surrounded by a phagocytic, mononuclear cell reaction. In long-standing cholestasis, large bulky macrophages and groups of phagocytic cells may be found, with voluminous cytoplasm, containing recognizable bile plugs and large amounts of PAS-positive ceroid pigment derived from phagocytosed cell debris (Fig. 11.9). In addition to bile- and ceroid-laden macrophages there are, in long-standing cholestasis, single and grouped histiocytes with foamy lipid-laden cytoplasm (Fig. 11.17).

The feathery degeneration of confluent liver-cell groups near portal tracts and their subsequent lytic necrosis is often termed bile infarction or Charcot–Gombault necrosis[382] (Figs. 11.18, 11.19). Larger bile infarcts are diagnostic for extrahepatic cholestasis, although it should be emphasized that smaller areas of such biliary necrosis can occur in intrahepatic forms of cholestasis.[15,175,372] The larger bile infarcts often have a complex appearance; there is lytic necrosis with irregular empty spaces in the centre of

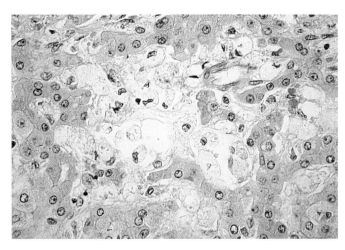

Fig. 11.17 Parenchymal accumulation of foamy histiocytes (xanthomatous cells). H & E.

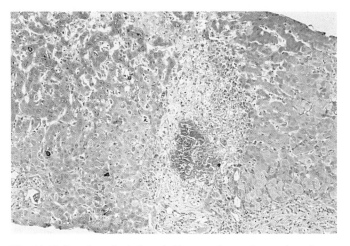

Fig. 11.18 Extrahepatic cholestasis. Paraportal area of parenchymal necrosis with heavy bilirubin impregnation (bile infarct). H & E.

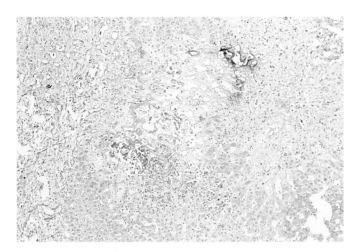

Fig. 11.19 Extrahepatic cholestasis. Bile infarct. Large area of necrosis, occupying the greater part of a liver acinus. The centre of the necrotic zone shows loss of liver cells and bilirubin impregnation of reticulin fibres and cellualr debris. H&E.

an area with heavy bilirubin impregnation of the necrobiotic cells, surrounded by a zone of liver cells with clearer, reticulated cytoplasm representing an earlier stage of feathery degeneration.[302] Bile infarcts appear to be caused by the toxic action of a retained bile constituent, probably bile salts, together with a mechanical cofactor created by the increased biliary pressure.[382] Necrotic areas of bile infarcts are gradually replaced by fibrous scarring (Fig. 11.20).

In cholestasis of long duration, the zone 1 hepatocytes near the swollen portal tracts and septa may show vacuolation and reticular appearance of their cytoplasm, with or without bilirubin impregnation. This apparently corresponds to a less severe variant of feathery degeneration, and has been described as cholate stasis.[383] Long-standing cholestasis is further characterized by the appearance of Mallory bodies in these hepatocytes,[176] together with

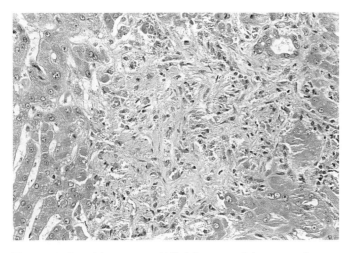

Fig. 11.20 Organizing paraportal bile infarct, containing scattered bilirubin-laden macrophages in the scar tissue. H&E.

deposits of copper and copper-binding protein[175,177] (Figs 11.21 and 11.22). Immunostaining for individual cytokeratins or tissue polypeptide antigen reveals expression

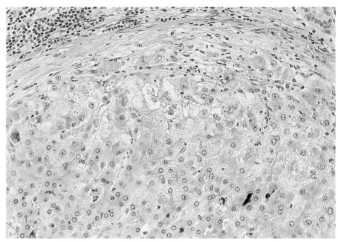

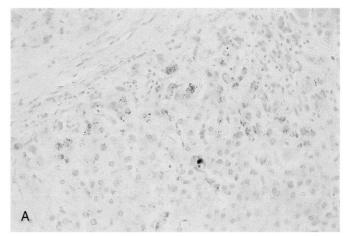

Fig. 11.21 Cholate stasis. Edge of parenchymal nodule in secondary biliary cirrhosis. The paraseptal hepatocytes are swollen, pale and coarsely granular. Some contain Mallory bodies. H&E.

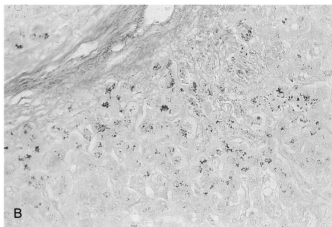

Fig. 11.22 (a,b) Analogous to Fig. 11.21. Paraseptal hepatocytes contain rhodanine-positive (a) and orcein-positive (b) granules, representing copper and copper-binding protein respectively. (a) Rhodanine stain. (b) Orcein stain.

of bile-duct cell 'markers' in periportal hepatocytes, even before the appearance of features of cholate stasis (Fig. 11.23); this observation indicates that such immunocytochemical features are sensitive markers for the existence of chronic cholestasis.[227,304] Siderosis of zone 1 hepatocytes has been reported in extrahepatic cholestasis.[373]

The ductular proliferation extends beyond the limits of the portal tract and invades the parenchyma (Fig. 11.24), most often along the acinar centres towards neighbouring portal tracts (Fig. 11.25). This ductular extension is accompanied by fibroblastic proliferation, creating the accompanying stroma of the outgrowing ductular strands.[320,321,384] The increase in ductular structures is partly brought about by active proliferation of ductular cells, and partly by tubular transformation of liver-cell

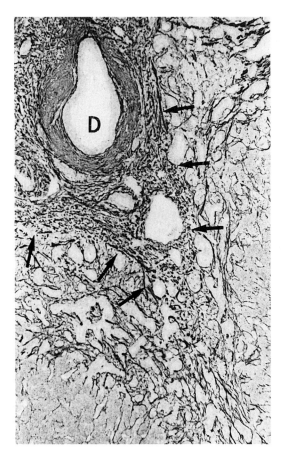

Fig. 11.25 Extrahepatic obstruction and cholangitis. A portal tract is surrounded by extensive ductular reaction. The original portal area can be recognized by the denser appearance of the coarse collagen (arrows). The bile duct (D) is surrounded by dense concentric fibrosis. The neo-ductules invade the parenchymal (especially below right). Reticulin.

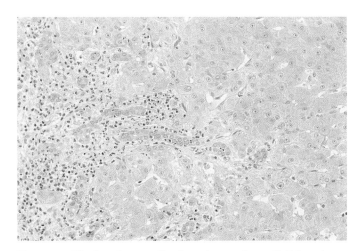

Fig. 11.23 Portal tract in chronic extrahepatic obstruction. Ductules and also periportal hepatocytes express cytokeratin 7 (only found in cells with bile duct cell phenotype in normal liver). Immunostain for cytokeratin 7 on frozen section, counterstained with haematoxylin.

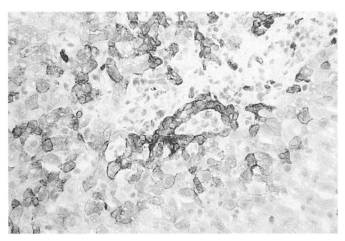

Fig. 11.24 Bile ductules extending from the portal tract (left) into the parenchyma. Note oedema around the ductules, and neutrophils in and around the ductules (cholangiolitis). Patient with extrahepatic obstruction and cholangitis. H & E.

plates in zone 1.[211,301] The ductules may have a narrow lumen and regular cuboidal epithelium; in some cases, usually with more pronounced inflammation, their lumens may be irregularly dilated and their lining cells may show various degenerative changes including anisocytosis, cytoplasmic vacuolation, nuclear pyknosis and epithelial sloughing. In long-standing cholestasis, ductules and transformed hepatocytic tubules show morphological signs of biliary reabsorption in the form of fine vacuolation of their cytoplasm, bilirubin impregnation and lipofuscin accumulation, i.e. a picture of cholate stasis (Fig. 11.26).

The periportal extension of the ductular reaction with its accompanying inflammatory infiltrate, the presence of cholate stasis and the loss of parenchymal cells creates an irregular portal-parenchymal interface, which has been termed 'biliary piecemeal necrosis'.[171,385] The ductular reaction and inflammation may subside in some portal tracts, resulting in periportal fibrosis containing, possibly, sequestrated liver-cell plates at the periphery of the expanded portal tract; this is referred to as 'fibrosing piecemeal necrosis'.[386,387]

Larger interlobular bile ducts may show tortuosity and branching, and occasionally signs of damage to their lining cells or sloughing of the epithelium. The lumen may appear empty, contain a fluffy mucoid or biliary precipitate with or without polymorphonuclear leucocytes, or be occupied by smaller or larger inspissated biliary concrements. In the latter case, the lining epithelium may be flattened.

Biliary concrements can also be observed in the ductular network (Figs 11.26 and 11.27). Their occurrence in septicaemia is discussed later in this chapter. The presence of concrements or microliths in larger ducts is more diagnostic of extrahepatic obstruction than the finding of biliary inspissates in ductules, since the latter

are also found in intrahepatic cholestasis.[175,372] Large concrements in bile ducts may lead to necrosis of the lining epithelium and extravasation of bile. Such portal tract biliary extravasates elicit a phagocytic reaction, often including multinucleated foreign-body giant cells. This is almost pathognomonic for extrahepatic obstructive cholestasis; unfortunately, it is a late phenomenon, usually missing from needle biopsy specimens, and is more often seen in autopsy material.[372,373]

Prolonged increase in biliary pressure may lead to activation of the bile-duct epithelium, especially in larger ducts, resulting in micropapillary projections[374] (Fig. 11.28). The ducts become surrounded by layers of concentric fibrosis, especially if infection is superimposed on the obstruction[373,378,386] (Figs 11.15 and 11.29).

In chronic extrahepatic obstruction, the progressive, concentric, periductal fibrosis may interfere with the ductal blood supply from the periductal capillary plexus,[51] resulting in progressive atrophy and even disappearance of the duct[175] (Fig. 11.30) although usually not to the same extent as in primary intrahepatic bile-duct diseases like primary biliary cirrhosis and primary sclerosing cholangitis. In this way, chronic cholestatic conditions induce a vicious circle, in that the effects of cholestasis result in its aggravation.[280]

The inflammatory infiltrate in the portal tracts is mixed. Mononuclear lymphoid cells predominate in the central part of the portal area, whereas neutrophil leucocytes are usually more prominent among the proliferated ductules at the margins (Figs 11.10 and 11.11). In some cases eosinophils are prominent. Large, pigmented, PAS-positive macrophages accumulate with time in the portal infiltrate, and apparently represent scavenger cells, previously active in the clearing of intra-acinar parenchymal

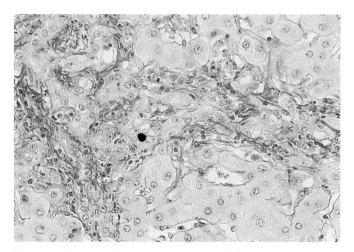

Fig. 11.26 Features of ductular reabsorption of bile constituents in chronic cholestasis. The ductular cells are vacuolated, and contain pigment inclusions (bilirubin and lipofuscin). Note the presence of a small bilirubin concrement in a ductular lumen. Collagen appears in red. Sirius red stain.

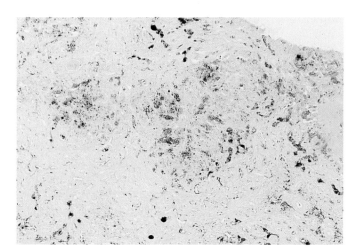

Fig. 11.27 Secondary biliary cirrhosis. View of small parenchymal nodule, surrounded by fibrous septa containing numerous ductular structures. Bile concrements in the ductules, bilirubin in hepatocytes, ductular cells and thrombi, and lipofuscin in ductular cells and hepatocytes show positive reaction (reducing substances), appearing blue in this photomicrograph. Schmorl's stain.

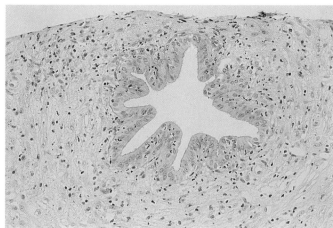

Fig. 11.28 Extrahepatic obstruction and cholangitis. A bile duct in a larger portal tract shows papillary projections of its epithelium and a stellate lumen. Numerous neutrophils permeate between the lining cholangiocytes. The surrounding connective tissue appears oedematous. PAS after α-amylase digestion.

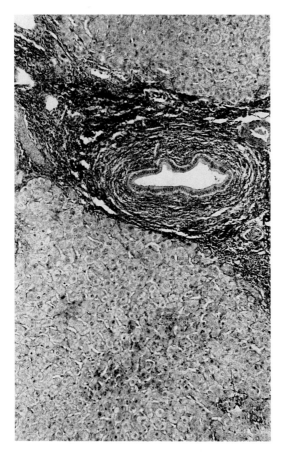

Fig. 11.29 Chronic cholangitis. A large bile duct shows a pale appearance at the base of its lining cells and a thick coat of concentric periductal fibrosis. Cholestasis is seen in the parenchyma (below). Van Gieson.

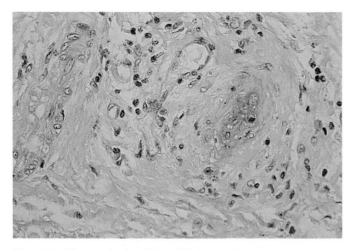

Fig. 11.30 Disappearing interlobular bile duct in chronic extrahepatic bile-duct obstruction. The bile duct lining cells have disappeared, and the bile-duct lumen is collapsed in developing periductal fibrosis. H & E.

debris, migrating to the portal areas. In the later stages of cholestasis, some portal tracts may contain accumulations of lipid-laden histiocytes, with foamy microvacuolated cytoplasm — xanthomatous cells.[27,184,372,378]

Superimposed infection: cholangitis

The presence of neutrophil leucocytes in the portal exudate is not proof of ascending cholangitis, since simple obstruction with biliolymphatic reflux may cause this type of inflammatory reaction. In acute cholangitis, portal oedema and infiltration by neutrophil leucocytes are more pronounced; the infiltration is seen not only around the ductules, but also between the epithelial cells and in the lumens (Fig. 11.24), sometimes with evidence of damage to the lining cells. In severe infection, abscesses form and the ducts are destroyed[389] (Fig. 11.31). In spite of the ascending infection, inflammatory lesions are sometimes confined to the smaller ducts, and the larger ducts in the section are not necessarily inflamed.[175,374] Intra-acinar cholestasis may be disproportionately mild or even absent, but in some cases cholestatic liver-cell rosettes are prominent. In cases of chronic or recurrent cholangitis, there is progressive periportal fibrosis, with concentric periductal lamination of collagen and ductular proliferation (Figs 11.15, 11.25, 11.29).

Unrelated changes

In addition to the histological changes described above there may be unrelated features such as fatty change, hepatocyte swelling due to drug-induced proliferation of endoplasmic reticulum, or ground-glass hepatocytes in patients with hepatitis B surface antigen in the serum. Focal liver-cell necrosis and infiltration by neutrophil polymorphs may result from surgical intervention[390] and must be distinguished from the effects of biliary obstruction.

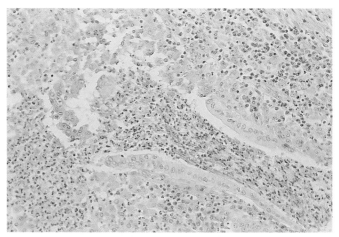

Fig. 11.31 Detail from cholangitic abscess. Note ruptured bile duct filled with pus, and surrounded by inflammatory cells, mainly macrophages and pus cells in the upper and lower part of the figure. H & E.

Reversibility of changes

Relief of bile-duct obstruction leads to regression of the acinar and portal changes with varying speed.[391] Extensive periportal fibrosis and secondary biliary cirrhosis are largely irreversible, although considerable resolution is occasionally seen after relief of obstruction in children.[302,392] Reversibility of the lesions after relief of obstruction has been well established in several experiments in rats, dogs and guinea pigs.[319,393,394] In the later rat studies[319] there was constant recovery from hepatic injury after partial biliary obstruction of up to 8 weeks. As might be expected, the morphological recovery from hepatic damage was faster and more pronounced after shorter periods of biliary obstruction.

Degenerated and necrotic hepatic cells are replaced within a few days by a process of rapid regeneration. Foci of feathery degeneration may persist for long periods. Bile plugs in acinar zone 3 and macrophage pigmentation may persist for several weeks. The proliferation of the ductules subsides.[333] Inflammatory changes in the portal tracts linger for some time, and eventually hyalinized collagen is deposited, resulting in a permanent slight enlargement of the tracts.[381] Full functional recovery of the liver may also take considerable time following relief of bile-duct obstruction.[395–397]

Histological diagnosis of extrahepatic obstruction

Histological differentiation of extrahepatic and intrahepatic cholestasis in needle liver biopsies is sometimes extremely difficult, if not impossible.[15] The major difficulty lies in distinguishing duct obstruction from some types of drug-induced cholestasis and cholestatic viral hepatitis.

The only near-pathognomonic sign is duct rupture and bile extravasation with resulting histiocytic reaction in the portal tracts. As already mentioned, this feature is a late complication of long-standing severe cholestasis, and is seldom seen in biopsy specimens. It is very rarely found also in primary biliary cirrhosis. Features supporting extrahepatic obstruction include oedematous rounding of portal tracts and cholangitis, large periportal bile infarcts, portal accumulations of xanthomatous cells (although these are also seen in primary biliary cirrhosis), bile concrements in ducts (but not ductules), concentric periductal fibrosis and a predominantly neutrophil leucocytic portal infiltrate.[372,373]

It is necessary to evaluate objectively all the histological changes, their mutual intensity and their topography, in order to arrive at a confident diagnosis in as many cases as possible. Unavoidably, in a minority of biopsies, the morphological diagnosis will remain a probability rather than guaranteed certainty. Fortunately, since the 1970s, the differential diagnosis between intra- and extrahepatic cholestasis has come to rely more on modern imaging techniques than on liver biopsy interpretation.

SECONDARY BILIARY CIRRHOSIS

Pathogenesis and morphogenesis

Secondary biliary cirrhosis is a relatively uncommon complication of extrahepatic biliary obstruction, having been reported in 8.6% of a large series by Gibson and Robertson in 1939.[398] The pathogenesis of secondary biliary cirrhosis is controversial with respect to the relative roles of obstruction per se and the common accompanying cholangitis. The latter is particularly seen when the obstruction is incomplete, as is often the case in choledocholithiasis and benign stricture of the common bile duct. That obstruction alone can cause secondary biliary cirrhosis is established in experimental animals subjected to aseptic ligation of the common bile duct,[393,399,400] and in the human by its occurrence in infants with congenital atresia of the extrahepatic bile duct.

The time required for cirrhosis of the liver to develop in unrelieved extrahepatic obstruction is variable. In infants with congenital biliary atresia, irreversible cirrhosis develops after 5–6 months.[304,401] In a series of 60 adults, Scobie & Summerskill[398] found a widely varying mean interval between the onset of biliary obstruction and the confirmation of biliary cirrhosis: 7.1 years in patients with common duct stricture, 4.6 years in those with common duct stones, and 0.8 years in patients with obstruction from malignant lesions. There was no statistical difference between the mean time intervals for patients with stricture and those with stones, but cirrhosis was diagnosed earlier after obstruction in patients with tumour than in those with stricture ($p < 0.05$). Biliary cirrhosis developed less rapidly in patients with symptoms of cholangitis (fever, chills and intermittent jaundice) than in those without (mean durations of 6.7 years and 2.3 years respectively). It was postulated that cholangitis reflected partial or intermittent obstruction, with consequently slower development of cirrhosis, and that the earlier onset of cirrhosis in patients with carcinoma might be due to more complete obstruction as well as to earlier surgical confirmation of cirrhosis because of clinical circumstances.[398] Although secondary biliary cirrhosis thus seems to develop more rapidly in complete (malignant) obstruction, it is most frequently seen as a sequel to benign partial obstruction by gallstones or postoperative strictures of the bile ducts,[359,398] death occurring too early from cachexia and metastases in most cases of malignancy for biliary cirrhosis to develop.

Histologically, cirrhosis is defined as reconstruction of the acinar parenchyma with both extensive fibrosis and regenerative nodules.[402] In this sense, secondary biliary cirrhosis is not a true cirrhosis during much of its evolution,[302] and the term 'biliary fibrosis'[401] is more appropriate until true cirrhosis with nodular regeneration finally develops. The subject is further discussed in Chapter 10.

As mentioned above, the portal tracts in extrahepatic cholestasis show complex changes, presumably related to escape of bile constituents into the portal connective tissue, and the 'ductular reaction' develops.[290] This reaction extends beyond the limits of the portal tracts with concomitant disappearance of zone 1 hepatocytes, creating mesenchymal wedges growing towards neighbouring portal tracts. The original portal connective tissue can still be recognized in preparations stained for collagen as a more densely collagenized area in the middle of an expanding zone rich in loosely woven reticulin fibres, ductules, inflammatory cells and fibroblasts.[379] This cellular fibrosis is potentially reversible.[290,319] Eventually the process develops into perilobular fibrosis, with portal–portal fibrous connections and preserved intrahepatic vascular relationships. This stage corresponds to biliary fibrosis rather than cirrhosis.[302]

Increase in collagen is the result of a disturbance in the balance between the formation of collagen, especially of type I collagen, and its breakdown.[319–321,403] Biochemical studies in rats with bile-duct ligation[404,405] have revealed a progressive increase of type I collagen, and mucopolysaccharides of the connective tissue ground substance are also increased. Lysosomal enzymes involved in collagen breakdown first show an increase after bile-duct obstruction, and then decline.[404]

The combined experimental evidence suggests a close parallel between increase in ductular cells and collagen content, and a sequence whereby, originally, type III collagen is formed in association with enhanced degrading activity (increased collagen turnover and reversible fibrosis), followed by progressive deposition of type I collagen fibres and exhaustion of the breakdown system (irreversible fibrosis).[406] Morphologically, irreversible fibrosis is characterized by dense connective tissue in portal tracts and septa, composed of coarse, hyalinized collagen bundles which are doubly refractile under polarized light, and paucity of mesenchymal and inflammatory cells.[407]

Nodular regeneration remains subdued for a long time in persistent extrahepatic obstruction, although scattered liver-cell regeneration is an early event after experimental bile-duct ligation.[408] Cholestasis may alter programmed liver gene expression, inhibiting normal hepatic regeneration.[409] Weinbren[410] has studied the regenerative capacity of the rat liver in the early as well as the late stage of biliary obstruction. His findings indicated that growth of liver parenchymal cells is not inhibited or diminished by bile-duct obstruction, provided that regeneration is stimulated by partial hepatectomy. If the reactions in man and the rat may be compared, it would seem reasonable to suspect that there is no large-scale destruction of liver cells in bile-duct obstruction and therefore no resultant nodular regeneration of the surviving tissue.[410] However, diffuse regeneration, suggested by thickened liver-cell plates, is common in chronic biliary obstruction and may, together with fibrosis, contribute to portal hypertension even in the absence of cirrhosis.[411]

After prolonged biliary obstruction, there is progressive damage to increasing numbers of liver cells. These already show impairment of maximal biosynthetic activity in the early stages.[412] More extensive loss of parenchymal cells in the peripheral zone of the liver acinus in the later stages leads to the development of periacinar septa, which form intrahepatic vascular shunts and represent a key feature in the derangement of intrahepatic haemodynamics found in cirrhosis.[402,407,413] The establishment of intrahepatic vascular shunting and the ultimate appearance of nodular parenchymal regeneration leads to the final stage of true biliary cirrhosis.[280,302]

Pathology

The liver is at first only slightly increased in size, then becomes considerably enlarged, only to shrink to subnormal proportions in the last stages of the disease.[393] The surface varies in colour from mottled green to green-yellow or dark green. Consistency and granularity vary with the stage of the cirrhosis: the liver feels firm, hard or even wooden, and is smooth, finely granular or nodular. On section, the liver tissue is firm and tough and cirrhosis may be evident. Its colour is yellow, greenish-grey or deep green, stippled with small grey or white areas corresponding to enlarged portal tracts. Small haemorrhages, grey or yellow necrotic patches and even small infarcts may be seen. Bile ducts may sometimes be considerably distended, with light or dark, occasionally inspissated, bile. In some cases the intrahepatic ducts are filled with white, glairy bile under pressure.[393] The large ducts near the hilum are accompanied by an increased amount of connective tissue.

Histologically, the picture also varies with the stage of the disease; it can be summarized as hepatic fibrosis and later cirrhosis, with features of extrahepatic cholestasis. Bile stasis, which is perivenular in the precirrhotic stage of obstruction, may be diffuse or even peripheral once regenerative nodules have developed, and varies widely in degree. Occasionally it is inconspicuous. Microscopic bilirubinostasis may be associated with feathery degeneration of liver cells, bile infarcts and bile lakes. The latter are large masses of pigment in or adjacent to portal tracts. They are surrounded by necrotic liver cells or a mild mesenchymal reaction; such bile lakes are interpreted as extravasates of bile from destroyed bile ducts or as evidence of necrosis of liver cells in zone 1 of the acini.[401] Bile lakes or extravasates are a characteristic sign of an obstructive cause of cirrhosis, but are seldom seen in needle biopsies.[414]

The portal tracts are enlarged and may still appear oedematous. The inflammatory exudate usually continues to include neutrophil leucocytes. Significant from a diagnostic point of view is an increase in the number of ductular structures, especially well-formed ductules with recognizable lumens (Figs 11.10 and 11.11). Biliary microcalculi may be present in these structures and in the ducts (Fig. 11.26). In the late stages of secondary biliary cirrhosis, both ducts and ductules may disappear.[318,414] Remaining ducts are often characterized by concentric periductal fibrosis (Figs 11.15, 11.25, 11.29).

Fibrous connective-tissue septa extend into the parenchyma and ultimately link up with those from adjacent portal tracts (Fig. 11.32). In later stages periacinar (portal–central) septa are found, and even larger scars, resulting from multiacinar collapse, can occasionally be seen.[401] Regenerative nodules are formed from single and multiple acini, often resembling pieces of a jigsaw puzzle[374] or irregular garlands[379] (Fig. 11.33). The nodules are separated by broad serpiginous bands of connective tissue with parallel fibres. There is typically a narrow zone of oedema and ductular proliferation at the junction of parenchyma and septa (Fig. 11.34); the liver

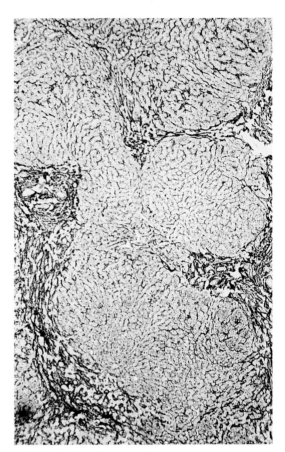

Fig. 11.33 Early secondary biliary cirrhosis. The parenchyma has an irregular configuration, and is surrounded by fibrous septa containing numerous ductular structures. Reticulin.

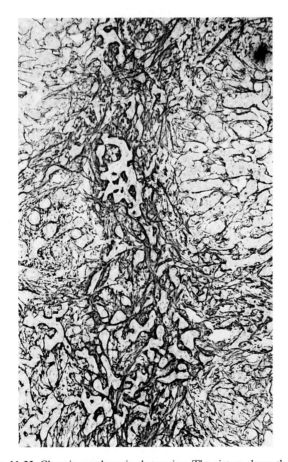

Fig. 11.32 Chronic extrahepatic obstruction. The picture shows the area of fusion of ductular reaction extending from adjacent portal tracts. Reticulin.

cells in this area show cholate stasis. In some cases, zone 1 liver cells contain Mallory bodies, orcein-positive deposits of copper-binding protein and rhodanine-positive granules of copper (Figs 11.21 and 11.22).

Secondary biliary cirrhosis is often complicated by bacterial infection, especially when the obstruction is due to partial or intermittent non-neoplastic obstruction. When the infection is severe, pylephlebitis and cholangitic abscesses may result.[389]

INTRAHEPATIC CHOLESTASIS

Intrahepatic cholestasis is, strictly speaking, a bile secretory failure caused by a mechanism located within the anatomical confines of the liver. The term is also often applied to so-called functional cholestasis. When taken in its strict definition, intrahepatic cholestasis comprises a large group of conditions, which can be separated into diseases in which the apparent cause lies in the hepatocytes or canaliculi (intra-acinar cholestasis), and disorders in which the causative process centres on the intrahepatic biliary passages (extra-acinar cholestasis).

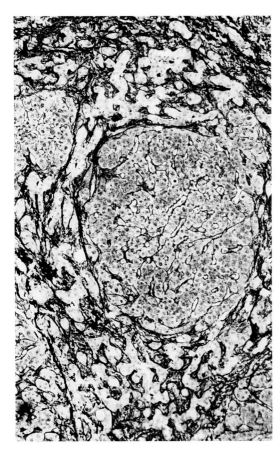

Fig. 11.34 Secondary biliary cirrhosis. A parenchymal nodule is surrounded by fibrosis with numerous plexiform ductular structures. Reticulin.

Table 11.1 Diseases characterized by intrahepatic cholestasis

I. Intra-acinar cholestasis
  A. Congenital disorders
    1. Congenital/familial, cholestatic/hyperbilirubinaemic syndromes
      a. Congenital familial *cholestatic* syndromes
        (i) In infancy and childhood
          — Physiological cholestasis of the newborn
          — Byler syndrome
          — Fatal familial cholestatic syndrome in Greenland Eskimo children
          — Inborn errors, including a defect of bile acid metabolism (for review see[401,402]):
            • cerebrotendinous xanthomatosis
            • Zellweger's syndrome
            • 3β-hydroxy-C_{27}-steroid dehydrogenase/isomerase deficiency
            • Δ^4-3-oxosteroid 5β-reductase deficiency
          — Recurrent cholestasis with lymphoedema
          — Severe familial cholestasis in North American children
          — Cholestasis in α_1-antitrypsin deficiency
        (ii) In adulthood
          — Cholestatic liver disease in PiMZ α_1-antitrypsin deficiency
          — Idiopathic benign recurrent intrahepatic cholestasis
          — Intrahepatic cholestasis of pregnancy
          — Familial benign chronic intrahepatic cholestasis
      b. Congenital/familial *hyperbilirubinaemic* syndromes
        (i) Physiological jaundice of the newborn
        (ii) Unconjugated hyperbilirubinaemic syndromes
          — Crigler–Najjar type I disease
          — Crigler–Najjar type II disease
          — Gilbert's syndrome
        (iii) Conjugated hyperbilirubinaemic syndromes
          — Dubin–Johnson syndrome
          — Rotor's syndrome
    2. Cholestasis in metabolic disorders
      a. Galactosaemia
      b. Fructose intolerance
      c. Tyrosinaemia
      d. Erythropoietic protoporphyria

  B. Acquired disorders
    1. Cholestasis in viral hepatitis
    2. Cholestasis in drug-induced and toxic liver injury
    3. Cholestasis in alcohol-induced liver injury
    4. Postoperative cholestasis
    5. Cholestasis in sepsis, severe haemolysis and shock
    6. Cholestasis in total parenteral nutrition
    7. Inspissated bile syndrome
    8. Cholestasis in passive venous congestion and in sickle cell disease
    9. Cholestasis in amyloidosis
    10. Cholestasis in sarcoidosis
    11. Cholestasis in Hodgkin's disease and lymphoma
    12. Nephrogenic hepatosplenomegaly

II. Extra-acinar cholestasis
  A. 'Vanishing bile duct' disorders
    1 Congenital
      — Extrahepatic bile-duct atresia (Ch. 3)
      — Paucity of interlobular bile ducts (Ch. 3)
        • syndromic form
        • non syndromic form

It must be realized, however, that in several cholestatic disorders a strict distinction between extrahepatic and intrahepatic cholestasis is not possible; examples are atresia of the extrahepatic bile ducts and primary sclerosing cholangitis. In spite of the classic terminology, the disease process leading to bile-duct destruction in so-called 'extrahepatic' biliary atresia also affects the intrahepatic bile ducts. Hence, atresia of the extrahepatic bile ducts is a panbiliary disease, resulting in obstruction of both extra- and intrahepatic bile ducts.[27,304] Primary sclerosing cholangitis (PSC) may affect the extrahepatic ducts (large duct PSC), or only the smaller intrahepatic bile ducts (small duct PSC), or both.[386] Nevertheless, in conventional classification systems, atresia of the extrahepatic bile ducts is usually tabulated under extrahepatic cholestasis, and PSC in the intrahepatic category, thus emphasizing the predominant component in the pathogenesis of cholestasis.

Table 11.1 gives a general overview of diseases belonging to intrahepatic cholestasis.

Table 11.1 (*contd*)

2. Acquired
— Cholestasis in primary biliary cirrhosis (Ch. 12)
— Sarcoidosis with chronic intrahepatic cholestasis (Ch. 17)
— Cholestasis in primary sclerosing cholangitis (Ch. 12)
— Cholestasis in idiopathic adulthood ductopenia (Ch. 12)
— Cholestasis in liver allograft rejection (Ch. 12 and Ch. 18)
— Cholestasis in graft versus host disease (Ch. 12 and Ch. 18)
— Cholestasis in immunodeficiency and opportunistic infections (Ch. 17)
— Cholestasis in drug-induced and toxic cholangitis (Ch. 15)
— Cholestasis in histiocytosis X (Ch. 3)
— Cholestasis in cystic fibrosis (mucoviscidosis) (Ch. 4)

B. Cholestasis in congenital segmental dilatation of intrahepatic bile ducts with lithiasis (Caroli's disease) (Ch. 3)

C. Cholestasis due to space-occupying lesions in the liver (e.g. primary and metastatic malignancies) (Ch. 16)

D. Cholestasis in parasitic infestations of intrahepatic bile ducts (ascariasis, distomiasis) (Ch. 7)

E. Cholestasis in cirrhosis (Ch. 10)

Note: All the conditions under the heading of extra-acinar cholestasis are discussed in other chapters of this book. Clinical features of biliary obstruction may be found in a small proportion of patients with cirrhosis of any cause, and present problems of differentiation from biliary cirrhosis (see Chs 10 and 12). Nodular regenerative hyperplasia and focal nodular hyperplasia (Ch. 16) may also be associated with cholestasis.[417]

INTRA-ACINAR CHOLESTASIS: CONGENITAL/FAMILIAL CHOLESTATIC SYNDROMES

In infancy and childhood

Introductory note

Diseases corresponding to 'intrahepatic cholestasis of childhood' represent an area in which confusion abounds.[418] There is a bewildering variety of patients who demonstrate confusing differences in prognosis and response to therapy.[419] Further confusion may arise by subdivision into disparate syndromes which have been only incompletely characterized. The subdivision is further complicated by the fact that within each syndrome there exists a wide clinical spectrum. Nevertheless, the first step towards understanding is to try to define clearly individual syndromes.[418] The classification that follows is based on recent publications; nevertheless, it must be regarded as an operational classification until elucidation of pathogenetic mechanisms will allow a definite categorization.[420] In the meantime, it suffers from several drawbacks and ambiguities. The problem of differentiating between intrahepatic and extrahepatic cholestasis was already alluded to with regard to extrahepatic bileduct atresia. The same may apply to paucity of the interlobular bile ducts, since at least the non-syndromic variety may also be associated with extrahepatic biliary atresia.[27,304,421,422]

Paucity of interlobular bile ducts of both the syndromic and the non-syndromic varieties poses further problems of classification, which will remain as long as the pathogenesis of these diseases remains unknown. For instance, some neonatal cholestatic disorders, which may be associated with ductopenia[421] (and accordingly could be classified as extra-acinar) have been shown to be due to an inborn error of bile acid metabolism, and hence to be of hepatocellular origin and belonging to the intra-acinar group.[415,416]

Furthermore, some evidence suggested that syndromic paucity of interlobular bile ducts (or Alagille's syndrome) was caused by a primary defect in hepatocellular bile secretory mechanisms, with ductopenia resulting from disuse atrophy.[215] For this reason, Alagille's syndrome was categorized as hepatocellular or 'intra-acinar' cholestasis in the second edition of this book. However, this original suggestion was not supported by subsequent investigations.[423] It may therefore be equally logical to classify cholestatic diseases of unknown aetiology and pathogenesis into either the intra-acinar (parenchymal) or extra-acinar (ductal) variety according to the presence or absence of interlobular bile ducts, as proposed by Alagille et al.[424] In doing so, it is realized that classification according to these histological findings is also inadequate,[418] because variable degrees of paucity of interlobular ducts or ductopenia are observed in a large number of apparently unrelated conditions (for review see[421]). These include the following: infections (cytomegalovirus, rubella, hepatitis B, congenital syphilis); α_1-antitrypsin deficiency; endocrine disorders (hypopituitarism); chromosomal anomalies (trisomy 21, Turner's syndrome); inborn errors of bile acid metabolism; Byler syndrome; Norwegian cholestasis; a miscellaneous group including cystic fibrosis and Ivemark syndrome, and an idiopathic group without associated diseases.

Further problems of classification relate to the fact that several entities (Byler syndrome, benign recurrent or intermittent cholestasis, intrahepatic cholestasis of pregnancy) may occur in either a non-familial or a familial context. The same problem arises when separating adult and childhood diseases. Some forms of 'adult' intrahepatic cholestasis (e.g. benign recurrent or intermittent cholestasis) may occasionally start in early childhood.

With these considerations in mind, it is clear that the classification used in the following discussion should be regarded as an operational one. One merit may be that it allows differentiation of entities with a bad prognosis, namely non-syndromic paucity of interlobular bile ducts, Byler syndrome and Zellweger's syndrome, from the remainder with less sinister outlook. It also represents a first, cataloguing step pending further investigation.

Physiological cholestasis of the newborn

The normal human newborn passes through a period of physiological cholestasis. Serum bile acids are high in normal infants:[425] the subsequent decline to levels of the child and adult demonstrates the progressive maturation of liver function during infancy. Thus, a relative immaturity of hepatic excretory function results in a period of physiological cholestasis during the first 8–10 months of life.[426] In experimental animals also, a cholestatic period can be demonstrated in neonates by histochemical[12] and biochemical[427] investigation. Furthermore, the intrahepatic biliary tree has not yet reached its full development at the time of birth; the intrahepatic bile-duct system requires about 4 additional weeks to reach complete formation.[428] This temporary state of relative immaturity of hepatic excretory function may predispose neonates to overt cholestasis by additional factors, e.g. sepsis or total parenteral nutrition.

Byler syndrome (progressive familial intrahepatic cholestasis; familial intrahepatic cholestasis)

This is an autosomal recessive form of intrahepatic cholestasis progressing to cirrhosis and death in infancy or early childhood.[429] The first reported patients were members of four related Amish sibships bearing the name Byler,[416] but the disease does not appear to be limited to one race or family.[219] About 100 cases have been reported. A series of 33 patients was recently reviewed.[431]

The predominant presenting symptom is pruritus, followed by increasing jaundice with progressive evidence of liver injury and hepatomegaly. Delayed development, rickets, splenomegaly and anaemia are common. Death usually occurs within the first 3 years of life from liver failure or bleeding oesophageal varices. In rare instances patients have survived into the second decade.[431]

The aetiology is unknown. Recent hypotheses included a defect in synthesis or processing of γ-glutamyltranspeptidase, resulting in disordered glutathione homeostasis, or a generalized defect in bile acid transport at the canalicular level. Neither of these pathogenetic hypotheses could be proven.[431] Patients with progressive familial intrahepatic cholestasis have distinctly low values for γ-glutamyltranspeptidase and serum cholesterol compared with most, if not all, other chronic cholestatic conditions.[431,432]

Histopathological changes evolve with the course of the disease. Early stages are characterized by acinar zone 3 bilirubinostasis in hepatocytes and canaliculi, cholestatic liver-cell rosettes and parenchymal giant cell transformation. Features of cholate stasis, with copper overload and development of Mallory bodies, appear in advanced stages. Paucity of interlobular bile ducts is found in the majority of cases,[421,431] whereas remaining ducts may show features of epithelial injury without much inflammation. Ductular reaction occurs at the portal tract periphery in most patients, especially in later stages. Fibrosis is an early finding in acinar zone 3, starting before 2 years of age in most patients; fibrosis extends peripherally, resulting in central–portal bridging fibrosis. In later stages, cirrhosis is found. In some patients hepatocellular carcinoma has developed before 3 years of age.[431]

Electron microscopy reveals classic signs of cholestasis[219,430,433,434] with ruptured segments of the canalicular membrane and shedding of cell organelles into the canalicular lumens. Attention has been drawn to peculiar mitochondrial changes,[435] to pericanalicular microfilamentous hyperplasia and to the development of cilia-like structures on some canalicular membranes.[217,219] Microfilamentous hyperplasia, however, is not unique to this entity (see North American childhood cirrhosis below).

The diagnosis of progressive familial intrahepatic cholestasis should be suspected in a cholestatic infant in whom pruritus is prominent and levels of γ-glutamyltranspeptidase and cholesterol are low. At present, the only known effective treatments for this disease entity are partial cutaneous biliary diversion or orthotopic liver transplantation.[431]

Fatal familial cholestatic syndrome in Greenland Eskimo children

A series of 16 Greenland Eskimo children has been reported with a fatal familial cholestatic syndrome.[436] The patients presented between 1 and 3 months of age with jaundice, pale stools, steatorrhoea and bleeding episodes. They failed to thrive and developed hepatomegaly, pruritus and rickets. Biochemically, they showed conjugated hyperbilirubinaemia, profound hypoprothrombinaemia, thrombocytosis and secondary hyperparathyroidism. The syndrome resulted in death in early childhood. The aetiology is unknown.

A preliminary electron microscopic investigation of liver biopsy specimens revealed only non-specific cholestatic features.[436] A subsequent report detailed the light microscopic features in 28 liver biopsies from 16 of these children.[437] In the early stage, until 5 months of age, changes were restricted to acinar zone 3 bilirubinostasis and cholestatic rosette formation. The intermediate stage, from 5 to 14 months, was characterized by persistent bilirubinostasis which extended towards the portal area; fibrosis developed, first in acinar zone 3, later in zone 1. The late stage, from 17 to 60 months, showed further progression of the lesions: there was an increase in bilirubinostasis, the number of cholestatic liver-cell rosettes, and fibrosis, with development of portal–portal and portal–central fibrous septa, which eventually resulted in cirrhosis in some patients. Of note was the virtual absence of inflammation and the lack of anatomical abnormalities of the intrahepatic bile ducts; no paucity of bile ducts was found.[437]

Although this disease in Greenland Eskimo children has many features in common with Byler disease (progressive familial intrahepatic cholestasis), there are notable differences. The patients were severely ill from early life; jaundice and bleeding episodes were always the first signs; thrombocytosis was an invariable finding; and serum cholesterol and triglyceride levels were normal or low.

Inborn errors, including a defect of bile acid synthesis and metabolism

The classic pathway for bile acid synthesis from cholesterol involves at least nine steps catalysed by 15 different enzymes that are located within various organelles of the hepatocyte. There are now four recognized disorders affecting this biosynthetic pathway.[415,416] Cerebrotendinous xanthomatosis and the peroxisomal disorder termed Zellweger's disease involve defects in the later steps in the pathway, that is side-chain oxidation. Recently two new defects have been characterized involving the enzymes responsible for catalysing the initial reactions in the metabolism of cholesterol: the 3β-hydroxy-C_{27}-steroid dehydrogenase/isomerase deficiency and the Δ^4-3-oxosteroid 5β-reductase deficiency;[416] they are characterized clinically by progressive neonatal cholestasis, although in a number of patients the diagnosis was not made until infancy. One patient was 10 years of age, indicating that late-onset cholestasis may be explained by inborn errors of metabolism.

Liver biopsies revealed marked architectural disarray, hepatocellular and canalicular bilirubinostasis, cholestatic liver-cell rosettes, and extramedullary haematopoiesis. Ultrastructural changes were those of cholestasis in general.[438] The morphological features, thus, were those of non-specific neonatal cholestasis.[27]

Confirmation of the biochemical defect was established from urinary bile acid analysis using the technique of fast atom bombardment ionization mass spectrometry (FAB–MS).[416,439] The cholestasis and liver injury in these patients are considered to occur, either because of the lack of primary choleretic bile acids that are essential to facilitate bile flow and/or the accumulation of atypical primitive bile acids that are potentially hepatotoxic.[439]

The peroxisomal disorders and inborn errors of bile acid synthesis and metabolism are discussed in detail in Chapter 4.

Recurrent cholestasis with lymphoedema (Norwegian cholestasis; Aagenaes syndrome)

Aagenaes et al[440] reported a series of patients with intrahepatic cholestasis from Norway; subsequently, similar cases (in total 21) have been reported from England, France and Sweden.[441] The disease manifests itself in the neonatal period with jaundice, which may clear again in childhood but recur intermittently throughout life. A striking clinical finding in this syndrome is profound lymphoedema of the legs, which begins either in childhood or before puberty; the lymphoedema persists in periods during which jaundice disappears. Hereditary hypoplasia of the lymph vessels has been suggested as a pathogenetic mechanism, because of the frequent occurrence of lymphangiomas and haemangiomas in the same families.[442] Liver biopsy may demonstrate paucity of intrahepatic bile ducts,[421] canalicular bilirubinostasis, some degree of ductular proliferation, and giant cell transformation of hepatocytes. Cirrhosis has been reported in adults with this syndrome, which seems to be of autosomal recessive inheritance.[418]

Severe familial cholestasis in North American Indian children (North American Indian childhood cirrhosis; North American Indian cholestasis)

Weber et al[222] described 14 North American Indian children with a familial type of severe neonatal cholestasis. Jaundice occurred during the neonatal period in 9 children, but disappeared before the end of the first year. Progressive liver damage was documented by the persistence of high levels of alkaline phosphatase, moderate elevation of transaminases, and severe pruritus. Serum bile acids were constantly elevated.

Microscopically, the early stage was characterized by hepatitis with giant cell transformation and bile pigment retention in hepatocytes and canaliculi. Portal fibrosis developed later and was followed by cirrhosis.[418] On electron microscopy the bile canaliculi appeared only slightly dilated, with preservation or only partial loss of microvilli. They were surrounded by a prominent pericanalicular fibrous web of actin-containing microfilaments. This entity was considered to represent a human model of cholestasis induced by microfilament dysfunction.[222]

Neonatal cholestasis in α_1-antitrypsin deficiency (see Ch. 4)

The association of PiZZ phenotype and neonatal cholestasis is well established.[443] Liver biopsy may reveal several morphological patterns besides cholestasis and PAS-positive inclusions in periportal hepatocytes, including hepatocellular damage with giant cell transformation, portal fibrosis with ductular proliferation and ductular hypoplasia.[444] Paucity of interlobular bile ducts has a prevalence of 4–26% in α_1-antitrypsin deficiency.[421]

In adulthood

Cholestatic liver disease in PiMZ α_1-antitrypsin deficiency (see Ch. 4)

In a 5-year prospective study of liver biopsy specimens

from 1055 adults, Hodges et al[445] found a highly significant increase in incidence of PiMZ phenotype in patients with cryptogenic cirrhosis and chronic active hepatitis. The PiMZ patients were mostly elderly and non-alcoholic, without virological or immunological markers. They often had cholestasis and a poor prognosis.

Benign recurrent intrahepatic cholestasis (idiopathic intermittent or recurrent intrahepatic cholestasis; Summerskill-Tygstrup disease)

This rare disorder is usually familial and autosomal recessive in character with poor penetrance.[8] It was first described by Summerskill & Walshe,[446] followed by reports from Tygstrup[447] and De Groote et al.[448] Almost 70 cases have so far been described.[449,450] The syndrome is defined by the following criteria:[449,451]

1. Several episodes of pronounced jaundice with severe pruritus and biochemical signs of cholestasis
2. Bile plugs in the liver biopsy
3. Normal intrahepatic and extrahepatic bile ducts on cholangiography
4. Absence of factors known to produce intrahepatic cholestasis, such as drugs or pregnancy
5. Symptom-free intervals of several months or years.

An attack is usually preceded by a pre-icteric phase of 2–4 weeks, with malaise, anorexia and pruritus, followed by an icteric phase with increasing jaundice without pain or fever. A distinctive pattern of bilirubin and bile acid serum levels may be of diagnostic help.[452]

The aetiology is unknown. Speculation centres on a genetic predisposition, hypersensitivity to an unknown environmental factor or a metabolic disorder of bile-acid metabolism. One study suggests that in these patients a contracted bile acid pool increases the susceptibility of the liver for cholestatic agents.[453] Furthermore, the syndrome may be heterogeneous.[454] A primary disorder of bile ductules has also been suggested, although the ductular alterations are not specific.[455] The syndrome occurs in solitary cases, and occasionally within an isolated community (Cjios island in Greece, Appennines in Italy, Faroe Islands) or within a family. There is a male:female ratio of about 1.7:1. Oral contraceptives or pregnancy may trigger a new cholestatic episode.[449]

De Pagter et al[456] drew attention to the close similarity on clinical, biochemical and histopathological grounds of benign recurrent intrahepatic cholestasis, intrahepatic cholestasis of pregnancy, and cholestasis in patients taking oral contraceptives. Coexistence of these three different forms of recurrent intrahepatic cholestasis was described in the same family, indicating a familial predisposition which, however, seems to be exceptional.[457]

The pathological changes observed in the liver during an attack are the classic ones of cholestasis, at the light and electron microscopical level as well as histochemically.[458,459] These include acinar zone 3 bilirubinostasis (with its ultrastructural and histochemical correlates) and in some cases a mild degree of liver-cell damage and portal mononuclear cell infiltration (Fig. 11.10). There are no morphological features that are pathognomonic. This implies that the disorder remains a diagnostic possibility in any liver biopsy showing signs of zone 3 bilirubinostasis with little or no parenchymal-cell damage or portal infiltration. The disorder cannot be differentiated on morphological grounds alone from other conditions with pure cholestasis, such as drug-induced cholestasis, cholestasis of pregnancy and some instances of early bile-duct obstruction.

The condition is benign in that no long-term sequelae such as fibrosis, cirrhosis or liver failure have been observed, in spite of impressive numbers of repeated attacks; as many as 30 have been recorded. Liver biopsies taken during the silent intervals between the cholestatic episodes appear normal.

(Familial) recurrent intrahepatic cholestasis of pregnancy (see Ch. 17)

This is a disorder characterized by pruritus, with or without moderate cholestatic jaundice, usually occurring in the last trimester of each pregnancy and promptly disappearing post partum.[429] The form without jaundice, pruritus gravidarum, is considered to be a variant of the syndrome. It is believed that recurrent cholestasis of pregnancy is produced in susceptible patients by the known striking increase in endogenous gonadal and placentally derived hormones characteristic of pregnancy. Such patients are also unusually liable to cholestatic jaundice from oral contraceptives.[460] More than 50% of women manifesting the cholestatic syndrome associated with oral contraceptive administration had a previous history of pruritus gravidarum and/or cholestatic jaundice in earlier pregnancies.[461] It is highly probable that oestrogen and progestogen hormones act synergistically in producing this cholestasis, although the exact mechanism remains unclear.[457,460]

Cholestasis of pregnancy, as well as cholestasis due to oral contraceptives, occurs more frequently in certain sibships, and with a strikingly higher incidence in Scandinavia and Chile, suggesting a hereditary predisposition. A hypersensitivity to gonadal steroids has been invoked, possibly due to an inherited defect in the drug-metabolizing enzyme system.[460-463] Reversal of cholestasis may be induced by administration of S-adenosyl-L-methionine.[464] Similar effects were obtained in ethinyl-oestradiol-induced cholestasis in the rat.[270]

Several studies strongly suggest an increased incidence and predisposition to gallstone formation in women who have previously experienced recurrent cholestasis of pregnancy.[461] Although the condition is usually considered benign, further studies have indicated that cholestasis of pregnancy makes fetal prognosis more guarded because of an increased incidence of premature labour, fetal distress and neonatal death.[23,462,463] Cholestasis of pregnancy constitutes the best model of a 'pure' intrahepatic cholestasis, and seems to be restricted to the human species.[457]

The histopathology of the liver in cholestasis of pregnancy is that of a mild perivenular bilirubinostasis.[465] Bile pigment accumulates in some acinar zone 3 areas, with plugs in dilated canaliculi and occasional bilirubin granules in adjacent hepatocytes. The Kupffer cells may be slightly prominent, and contain more PAS-positive granules than normal. The portal tracts are usually normal in size; some show mild infiltration by mononuclear cells, or slight ductular proliferation and an occasional PAS-positive macrophage. The histological differential diagnosis includes all forms of morphologically simple bilirubinostasis: drug-induced cholestasis, benign recurrent intrahepatic cholestasis, intrahepatic cholestasis of Hodgkin's disease, postoperative cholestasis and early extrahepatic bile-duct obstruction.

Familial benign chronic intrahepatic cholestasis

Eriksson & Larsson[466] described 3 adult siblings in a Swedish family that was studied for three generations; they had clinical and laboratory signs of slowly progressive intrahepatic cholestasis, with prolonged increase in serum transaminase, γ-glutamyltransferase and alkaline phosphatase activities. A liver biopsy during jaundice in one of the cases showed changes indistinguishable from extrahepatic obstruction. Asymptomatic intervals were characterized by normal liver histology on light microscopy, but by abnormal bromsulphthalein (BSP) retention, reduced N-demethylation capacity and elevated fasting total serum bile acid levels. The patients were further characterized by a high serum α-lipoprotein level, slight skin hyperpigmentation, facial hypertrichosis, onycholysis, and hypothyroidism. This entity seems to have a relatively benign but progressive course, and appears to be inherited in an autosomal recessive manner. Because of the involvement of skin, hair, nails and cornea, it was speculated that a defect in the metabolism of prekeratin–keratin intermediate filaments of the cytoskeleton might be involved.[466]

INTRA-ACINAR CHOLESTASIS: CONGENITAL/FAMILIAL HYPERBILIRUBINAEMIA SYNDROMES

Physiological jaundice of the newborn

During the first few days of life, the capacity of the liver for bile pigment disposal is not yet completely developed. The reduced hepatic bilirubin clearance, in combination with bilirubin overproduction (accelerated red cell destruction), results in concentrations of plasma unconjugated bilirubin that are higher than those of adults: the so-called physiological hyperbilirubinaemia or jaundice of the newborn. Hepatic uptake, intracellular transport, conjugation and secretion of bilirubin are defective. These functions, including bilirubin UDP-glucuronyltransferase activity, reach adult values during the immediate postnatal period.[467,468]

Unconjugated hyperbilirubinaemia syndromes

Crigler-Najjar syndrome

Congenital deficiency of bilirubin-UDP-glucuronyltransferase leads to a defect in bilirubin conjugation and non-haemolytic unconjugated hyperbilirubinaemia. A complete defect in bilirubin glucuronide formation caused by absence of the conjugating enzyme, *type I*, leads to lifelong severe unconjugated hyperbilirubinaemia. A similar defect exists in a mutant strain of Wistar rats, the Gunn rat. A less severe form, responsive to phenobarbital treatment, is called *type II*.[469,470] Recently, the genetic mutation was identified that is responsible for the absence of the conjugating enzyme bilirubin-UDP-glucuronosyltransferase in a patient with Crigler–Najjar syndrome type I.[471] Immunoblot analysis of microsomes from livers affected by Crigler–Najjar syndrome type I has revealed considerable heterogeneity in the expression of glucuronosyl-transferase isoenzymes among Crigler–Najjar type I patients.[472] Several different genetic mutations are thus likely to be responsible for this clinical syndrome.[473] In both types of Crigler–Najjar disease, light microscopic examination of liver biopsies reveals occasional unexplained bile plugs in an otherwise normal-looking parenchyma.[474]

At the ultrastructural level, several alterations have been reported, including hyperplasia of the smooth endoplasmic reticulum, prominence of the Golgi apparatus, evidence of intracellular and extracellular bile retention, and focal modifications of the sinusoidal domain of the liver-cell plasmalemma. An electron microscopic study of the type II syndrome, using morphometry, failed to confirm a hypertrophy of the smooth endoplasmic reticulum.[475]

Gilbert's syndrome

This syndrome, affecting 3–7% of the adult population, is characterized by only slight or inconstant unconjugated hyperbilirubinaemia and reduced activity of bilirubin-UDP-glucuronyltransferase in the liver.[468,476] Liver biopsy in such patients reveals normal histology. An increased accumulation of lipofuscin-like pigment has been reported,[477] but does not seem to be a constant finding. In some patients, electron microscopy demonstrated hypertrophy of the liver cell's smooth endoplasmic reticulum,[478] but this was not confirmed by morphometry in other patients.[479] A non-human primate model of Gilbert's syndrome has been described.[480]

Conjugated hyperbilirubinaemia syndromes

Dubin-Johnson syndrome

Dubin and Johnson[481] and Sprinz and Nelson[482] described a familial syndrome characterized by chronic or intermittent jaundice and a macroscopically black liver, due to the presence of an unidentified pigment in hepatocytes. The syndrome, inherited in an autosomal recessive pattern, consists of a defect in the hepatocellular secretion of conjugated bilirubin and conjugated bromsulphthalein (BSP), and a diagnostic abnormality of urinary coproporphyrin excretion. The patients have intermittent or chronic fluctuating mild jaundice and bilirubinaemia, with approximately 60% direct-reacting bilirubin, BSP retention, and non-visualization of the gallbladder on oral cholecystography.[468,469]

Macroscopically, the liver surface and biopsy specimens show dark pigmentation, described as green, slate blue, dark grey or black. On light microscopy, liver tissue appears normal except for the presence of coarsely granular, dark, iron-free pigment, observed predominantly in zone 3 hepatocytes with pericanalicular localization. The amounts of pigment are variable; the pigment may disappear following viral hepatitis and reaccumulate over the following months; this suggests that the pigment is the result, rather than the cause, of the hepatic excretory defect.[483]

On electron microscopy, the pigment appears as electron-dense, membrane-bound inclusions, apparently representing pigment-laden lysosomes.[484] The nature and origin of the pigment remain to be determined. Some studies concluded that the pigment is of the melanin type,[485] but later electron spin resonance and spectroscopic studies suggested a different chemical composition.[486,487] Similar abnormalities have been detected in the mutant Corriedale sheep.[488] Recent studies on TR- and EHBR mutant rats, which have a recessively inherited defective bile-canalicular secretion of many non-bile-acid organic anions, suggested that defective canalicular secretion of anionic metabolites of aromatic amino acids may be responsible for the development of the black lysosomal pigment of Dubin–Johnson syndrome.[5]

Rotor's syndrome

This is a benign familial disorder[489] resembling the Dubin–Johnson syndrome. However, the black discoloration of the liver is lacking, plasma BSP kinetics and urinary coproporphyrin excretion are different, and the gallbladder is frequently visualized on oral cholecystography. The inheritance of this rare disorder is autosomal recessive.[468] Macroscopically and microscopically, the liver appears normal.

Cholestasis in metabolic disorders

The metabolic disorders that may be associated with cholestasis (cystic fibrosis, galactosaemia, fructose intolerance, tyrosinaemia and erythropoietic protoporphyria) are discussed in Chapter 4.

Intra-acinar cholestasis: acquired disorders

Several entities listed on page 458 are discussed in other chapters of this book, e.g. viral hepatitis, drug-induced and toxic liver injury and alcohol-induced liver injury. The following discussion is devoted to the remaining conditions.

Postoperative cholestasis

There is a wide spectrum of postoperative hepatic dysfunction, ranging from trivial abnormalities to deep jaundice simulating extrahepatic obstruction or hepatic failure.[490] Many mechanisms may be involved, including bilirubin overload by haemolysis, halothane hepatotoxicity, viral- and drug-induced hepatitis, shock, bacterial infections, bile-duct injury, retained gallstones in the extrahepatic bile ducts, postoperative cholecystitis and pancreatitis.[491]

Benign postoperative intrahepatic cholestasis[492] is a syndrome characterized mainly by a rise in conjugated serum bilirubin, often without other features of cholestasis. It usually occurs within 48 hours after major surgery, sometimes on the first postoperative day. The duration of jaundice is 1–2 weeks. The syndrome is thought to be due to bilirubin overload of the liver. Increased bilirubin production is usually caused by haemolysis of transfused stored blood and resorption of haematomas, and occasionally by the stress or surgery in patients with chronic haemolytic disease (e.g. sickle cell anaemia). In addition to bilirubin overproduction, there must be a reduction in the normal secretory capacity of the liver, since the serum increase in bilirubin is of the conjugated type. In the face of impaired renal function or septicaemia, bilirubin levels may rise much higher.[492–494] Although the pathophysiology is not completely clear, it is thought to be an acquired disorder of hepatic bilirubin transport.[495]

Histologically, the picture is that of simple bilirubinostasis in acinar zone 3, with minimal or absent portal inflammation. In some cases, excess haemolysis is reflected in erythrophagocytosis by Kupffer cells,[493] followed by Kupffer-cell siderosis.

Sepsis, severe haemolysis and shock

Sepsis and severe bacterial infection due to a variety of infecting organisms, either in the postoperative patient or without relation to surgery, may result in a severe degree of jaundice.[496] The conjugated hyperbilirubinaemia in the presence of disproportionately low alkaline phosphatase and cholesterol levels suggests that an isolated defect of excretion of conjugated bilirubin is the cause of the jaundice.[497] However, occasional electron microscopic studies have shown ultrastructural changes of cholestasis.[498]

Histological changes in patients with cholestasis due to sepsis may be non-specific, comprising mild perivenular bilirubinostasis, fatty change in some liver cells and portal inflammatory infiltration.[497] Occasional instances of *E. coli* septicaemia may be characterized by abnormalities in the lining cells of the intrahepatic bile ducts: swelling, pyknosis, and even bile-duct destruction. These lesions are reversible.[499]

In severe septicaemia, increased numbers of ductules and canals of Hering may be observed at the edges of expanded portal tracts; their lumen may be filled with inspissated, PAS-positive, partly bilirubin-stained concrements and polymorphonuclear leucocytes.[175,500,501] Neutrophils in ductules, in the absence of involvement of larger ducts, usually indicate septicaemia rather than bile-duct obstruction with ascending cholangitis.

Bilirubinostasis is often observed in liver biopsies or postmortem specimens from patients with serious illnesses like cardiogenic shock, respiratory failure, postoperative jaundice and sepsis. The pathogenesis of cholestasis in such critically ill patients is complex. Factors that play a role to a variable extent include: (i) inhibition of the hepatocellular $Na^+–K^+$-ATPase at the basolateral membrane due to endotoxin, hypoxic damage and/or drug toxicity; (ii) the febrile state and dehydration; (iii) obstructive effect of proliferated bile ductules; (iv) bile concrement production under the influence of bacterial β-glucuronidase, and (v) effects of leukotrienes and other inflammatory mediators on bile ducts and ductules.[502] Bile ductular bilirubinostasis is a reaction pattern that is highly suggestive of sepsis. However, bile-stained concrements in proliferated ductules are also seen in other conditions like severely necrotizing hepatitis, parenteral nutrition, extrahepatic bile-duct atresia and the terminal stage of cirrhosis.[389,502]

Cholestasis, identified by an increase in serum bile acids, appears to be a universal finding in the *toxic-shock syndrome*, presumably due to hypoperfusion of the liver and a hepatocellular secretory defect due to staphylococcal exotoxin.[503] Histologically, such cases are characterized by suppurative cholangitis.[504] Some forms of septicaemia may be characterized by additional morphological changes. *Leptospirosis* is characterized by focal liver-cell necrosis, bilirubinostasis, which may be severe, and a strikingly high number of liver-cell mitoses.[505]

Total parenteral nutrition (TPN)

Parenteral nutrition is often used in the treatment of critically ill infants and adults. Cholestasis is a frequent but still poorly understood complication.[506] In recent years, the incidence of TPN-associated cholestasis has decreased substantially; at present, hepatobiliary injury in infants appears to occur only with prolonged TPN.[507]

Liver biopsy of infants in this condition reveals hepatocellular and canalicular bilirubinostasis with variable amounts of inflammatory periportal infiltrate, and signs of extramedullary haematopoiesis; steatosis is seen infrequently. Ductular bilirubinostasis may occur after TPN of longer duration.[508] Progressive portal fibrosis has led to cirrhosis and death from liver failure.[506] In adults, similar cholestatic features are observed, as is a higher incidence of steatosis. Parenteral nutrition for more than 1 month has led to the development of chronic inflammation and periportal fibrosis, persisting for months after resumption of a normal diet. Occasionally, the histological picture may mimic that of large bile duct obstruction.[509]

Several mechanisms have been proposed to explain this cholestatic hepatic dysfunction, including toxicity of solutions used for TPN and lack of gastrointestinal stimuli for digestive secretions by interruption of oral intake. Thus, TPN-related cholestasis may be of multifactorial origin: toxicity of TPN itself (fat emulsions, amino acids), gut-derived hepatotoxic substances, and, in young infants, the predisposing condition of physiological cholestasis.[510] The topic was recently reviewed by Balistreri et al.[507]

Inspissated bile syndrome

This is a poorly defined condition, corresponding to a histological picture of perivenular bilirubinostasis with large bile plugs in an otherwise undamaged liver, in the clinical setting of a child with prolonged jaundice in the neonatal period. This is particularly seen in bilirubin overload due to haemolysis caused by ABO or Rhesus incompatibility.[379] In haemolysis, siderosis of Kupffer cells may be seen in addition. It must, however, be emphasized that small bile plugs can be found in the livers of a very high proportion of children dying within a month of birth if the child has been ill for more than a few days with almost any condition.[511] This leads to the conclusion that the inspissated bile syndrome is not an entity, but describes a cholestatic state of undefined complex aetiology and pathogenesis.

Cholestasis in passive venous congestion and sickle cell disease (Ch. 14)

Circulatory failure and shock cause perivenular necrosis in the liver and jaundice in a number of patients.[512] This is due to reduction of the oxygen supply to the liver, especially to acinar zones 3 which represent the peripheral territory of the hepatic acini.[513] Microscopically, there is often cholestasis around the areas of necrosis.[514]

Intrahepatic cholestasis is a rare but lethal complication of sickle cell disease. Sickled red blood cells plug the hepatic sinusoids, causing vascular stasis, Kupffer cell hypertrophy and cholestasis.[515]

Hyperthyroidism; hypothyroidism

Both hyperthyroidism[516] and hypothyroidism[517] may be associated with cholestasis, histologically reflected in simple bilirubinostasis.

Amyloidosis; light-chain deposit disease (Ch. 17)

Cholestatic jaundice may be the presenting symptom of patients with liver amyloidosis.[578] The cholestasis is due to massive amyloid deposition in the space of Disse, atrophy of hepatocytes — mainly in zone 1 — and compression of canaliculi. This clinical variant of amyloidosis is not rare and carries a poor prognosis.[519,520] Intrahepatic cholestasis was also observed in light-chain deposit disease.[521]

Sarcoidosis (Ch. 17)

Chronic intrahepatic cholestasis is one of the expressions of hepatic involvement in sarcoidosis.[522,523] The clinical and biochemical aspects are similar to those of primary biliary cirrhosis and include pruritus, jaundice, hepatomegaly and striking elevations of serum alkaline phosphatase and cholesterol. It is not always easy to differentiate the two conditions and the final diagnosis requires consideration of the complete clinical picture together with the biochemical and serological findings. Mitochondrial antibodies, however, are not found.

Hodgkin's disease and lymphoma (Ch. 17)

Hodgkin's disease may be associated with jaundice, which in the majority of cases is due either to diffuse portal infiltration (45%) or to extrahepatic bile-duct obstruction with (13%) or without (10%) liver involvement; in a minority (2.2%) the cholestasis is apparently of intrahepatic origin and of unknown pathogenesis.[524] A similar intrahepatic cholestasis may be seen with other lymphomas in the absence of bile-duct obstruction or lymphomatous liver involvement.[525] The histological picture is that of simple perivenular bilirubinostasis.

In some cases with hepatic involvement and microscopic portal infiltrates, bile-duct damage and bile-duct loss may be responsible for the development of cholestasis.[526-528]

Nephrogenic hepatosplenomegaly (Stauffer's syndrome)

Nephrogenic hepatosplenomegaly (Stauffer's syndrome) refers to a syndrome of hepatic dysfunction, not due to metastatic tumour, in patients with renal adenocarcinoma.[529] It is characterized by hepatomegaly, retention of bromsulphthalein, and increased serum alkaline phosphatase, the latter possibly secreted by the tumour itself. The hepatic dysfunction disappears after removal of the kidney tumour. The histological picture is that of non-specific reactive hepatitis.[530] Simple zone 3 bilirubinostasis has been observed in other forms as a 'non-metastatic hepatopathy of malignancy',[531] in particular with carcinoma of the kidney[532] and soft tissue sarcoma.[533]

REFERENCES

1. Siegers C P, Watkins III J B. Biliary excretion of drugs and other chemicals. Stuttgart: Gustav Fischer Verlag, 1991: p 563
2. Van Eyken P, Desmet V J. Bile duct cells. In: LeBouton A V, ed. Molecular and cell biology of the liver. Boca Raton: CRC Press, 1993: pp 475–524
3. Sieg A. Bilirubin. In: Siegers C P, Watkins III J B, eds. Progress in pharmacology and clinical pharmacology, vol 8/4. Stuttgart: Gustav Fischer Verlag, 1991: PP 183–199
4. Reichen J, Simon F R. Cholestasis. In: Arias I M, Jakoby W B, Popper H, Schachter D, Shafrits D A, eds. The liver: biology and pathobiology, 2nd edn. New York: Raven Press, 1988: pp 1105–1124
5. Kitamura T, Alroy J, Gatmaitan Z, Inoue M, Mikami T, Jansen P, Arias I M. Defective biliary excretion of epinephrine metabolites in mutant (TR-)rats: relation to the pathogenesis of black liver in Dubin–Johnson syndrome and Corriedale sheep with an analogous excretory defect. Hepatology 1992; 15: 1154–1159
6. Rank J, Wilson I D. Changes in IgA following varying degrees of biliary obstruction in the rat. Hepatology 1983; 3: 241–247
7. Javitt N B. Cholestatic liver disease and its management. Baillière's Clin Gastroenterol 1989; 3: 423–430
8. Schaffner F. Cholestasis. In: Millward-Sadler G H, Wright R, Arthur M J P, eds. Wright's Liver and biliary disease. Pathophysiology, diagnosis and management, vol 1, 3rd edn. London: Saunders, 1992: pp 371–396
9. Desmet V J. Morphologic aspects of intrahepatic cholestasis. In: Gentilini P, Teodori U, Gorini S, Popper H, eds. Intrahepatic cholestasis. New York: Raven Press, 1975: pp 7–23
10. Meier-Abt P J. Cellular mechanisms of intrahepatic cholestasis. Drugs 1990; 40 (suppl 3): 84–97
11. Desmet V, Bullens A, De Groote J. A clinical and histochemical study of cholestasis. Gut 1970; 11: 516–522
12. De Wolf-Peeters C, De Vos R, Desmet V J. Histochemical evidence of a cholestatic period in neonatal rats. Pediatr Res 1971; 5: 704–709
13. Ronchi G, Desmet V. Histochemical study of so-called 'marker enzymes of cholestasis' during extrahepatic bile duct obstruction in the rat. Beitr Pathol 1973; 149: 213–216
14. Busachi C, Mebis J, Broeckaert L, Desmet V. Histochemistry of gamma-glutamyl-transpeptidase in human liver biopsies. Pathol Res Pract 1981; 172: 99
15. Desmet V J. Morphologic and histochemical aspects of cholestasis. In: Popper H, Schaffner F, eds. Progress in liver diseases, vol IV, ch 7. New York: Grune & Stratton, 1972: pp 97–132
16. Miyai K, Mayr W M, Richardson A L. Acute cholestasis induced by lithocholic acid in the rat. A freeze fracture replica and thin section study. Lab Invest 1975; 32: 527–535
17. Layden T J, Schwarz J, Boyer J L. Scanning electron microscopy of the rat liver. Studies on the effect of taurolithocholate and other models of cholestasis. Gastroenterology 1975; 69: 724–738
18. Grisham J W, Nopanitaya W, Compagno J. Scanning electron microscopy of the liver: a review of methods and results. In:

Popper H, Schaffner F, eds. Progress in liver diseases, vol V. New York: Grune & Stratton, 1976: pp 1–23

19. Erlinger S. Pathophysiology of cholestasis. In: Lentze M, Reichen J, eds. Paediatric cholestasis. Novel approaches to treatment. Dordrecht: Kluwer Academic Publishers, 1992: pp 49–54

20. Duffy M C, Boyer J L. Pathophysiology of intrahepatic cholestasis and biliary obstruction. In: Ostrow J D, ed. Bile pigments and jaundice. Molecular, metabolic and medical aspects. New York: Marcel Dekker, 1986: pp 333–372

21. Oelberg D G, Lester R. Cellular mechanisms of cholestasis. Annu Rev Med 1986; 37: 297–317

22. Buscher H P. Cholestase. Berlin: Springer Verlag, 1988: pp 33–71

23. Gleeson D, Boyer J L. Intrahepatic cholestasis. In: McIntyre N, Benhamou J P, Bircher J, Rizzetto M, Rodes J, eds. Oxford Textbook of clinical hepatology, vol 2. Oxford: Oxford University Press, 1991: pp 1087–1107

24. Fevery J, Blanckaert N. Hyperbilirubinemia. In: McIntyre N, Benhamou J P, Bircher J, Rizzetto M, Rodes J, eds. Oxford Textbook of clinical hepatology, vol 2. Oxford: Oxford University Press, 1991: pp 985–991

25. Fevery J, Blanckaert N. Bilirubin metabolism. In: McIntyre N, Benhamou J P, Bircher J, Rizzetto M, Rodes J, eds. Oxford Textbook of clinical hepatology, vol 1. Oxford: Oxford University Press, 1991: pp 107–115

26. Phillips M J, Poucell S, Patterson J, Valencia P. The liver: an atlas and text of ultrastructural pathology. New York: Raven Press, 1987

27. Desmet V J. Pathology of paediatric cholestasis. In: Lentze M, Reichen J, eds. Paediatric cholestasis. Novel approaches to treatment. Dordrecht: Kluwer Academic Publishers, 1992: pp 55–73

28. Desmet V J. Cholestasis: a problem. In: Csomos G, Thaler H, eds. Clinical hepatology. Berlin: Springer Verlag, 1983: pp 299–320

29. Desmet V J. The hepatocyte: structural specialization and functional integration. In: Molino G, Avagnina P, eds. Systematic and quantitative hepatology. Pathophysiological and methodological aspects. Milano: Masson, 1990: pp 43–50

30. McMillan P N, Hixson D C, Hevey K A, Naik S, Jauregui H O. Hepatocyte cell surface polarity as demonstrated by lectin binding. J Histochem Cytochem 1988; 36: 1561–1571

31. Popper H, Schaffner F. Fine structural changes of the liver. Ann Intern Med 1963; 59: 674–691

32. Schaffner F. Morphologic studies on bile secretion. Am J Dig Dis 1965; 10: 99

33. Phillips M J, Poucell S, Oda M. Biology of disease. Mechanisms of cholestasis. Lab Invest 1986; 54: 593–608

34. Desmet V J. Morphology of bile secretion. In: Gentilini P, Arias I M, Arroyo V, Schrier R W, eds. Liver diseases and renal complications. New York: Raven Press, 1990: pp 93–107

35. Häussinger D, Lang F. Cell volume in the regulation of hepatic function: a mechanism for metabolic control. Biochem Biophys Acta 1991; 1071: 331–350

36. Hallbrucker C, Lang F, Gerok W, Häussinger D. Cell swelling increases bile flow and taurocholate excretion into bile in isolated perfused rat liver. Biochem J 1992; 281: 593–595

37. Meier P J. Biliary excretion of bile acids. In: Siegers C P, Watkins III J B, eds. Progress in pharmacology and clinical pharmacology, vol 8/4. Stuttgart: Gustav Fischer Verlag, 1991: pp 159–182

38. Nathanson M H, Boyer J L. Mechanisms and regulation of bile secretion. Hepatology 1991; 14: 551–566

39. Gerok W. Physiology of bile formation. In: Lentze M, Reichen J, eds. Paediatric cholestasis. Novel approaches to treatment. Dordrecht: Kluwer Academic Publishers, 1992: pp 3–19

40. Meier-Abt P J. Molecular mechanisms of bile acid transport in hepatocytes. In: Gentilini P, Arias I M, McIntyre N, Rodes J, eds. Cholestasis. Amsterdam: Excerpta Medica, 1994: pp 61–68

41. Elias E, Boyer J L. Mechanisms of intrahepatic cholestasis. In: Popper H, Schaffner F, eds. Progress in liver diseases, vol VI. New York: Grune & Stratton, 1979: p 457

42. Gumucio J J, Chianale J. Liver cell heterogeneity and liver function. New York: Raven Press, 1988: pp 931–947

43. Dionne S, Russo P, Tuchweber B, Plaa G L, Yousef I M. Cholic acid and chenodeoxycholic acid transport in the hepatic acinus in rats. Effects of necrosis of zone 3 induced by bromobenzene. Liver 1990; 10: 336–342

44. Buscher H P, Schramm V, MacNelly S, Kurz G, Gerok W. The acinar location of the sodium-independent and the sodium-dependent component of taurocholate uptake. A histoautoradiographic study of rat liver. J Hepatol 1991; 13: 169–179

45. Stremmel W, Gerber M A, Glezerow V, Thung S N, Kochwa S, Berk P D. Physicochemical and immunohistological studies of a sulfobromophthalein and bilirubin-binding protein from rat liver plasma membranes. J Clin Invest 1983; 71: 1796–1805

46. Forgac M. Receptor-mediated endocytosis. In: Arias I M, Jakoby W B, Popper H, Schachter D, Shafritz D A, eds. The liver: biology and pathobiology, 2nd edn. New York: Raven Press, 1988: pp 207–225

47. Jones E A, Vierling J M, Steer C J, Reichen J. Cell surface receptors in the liver. In: Popper H, Schaffner F, eds. Progress in liver diseases, vol VI. New York: Grune & Stratton, 1979: p 43

48. Casey C A, Tuma D J. Receptors and endocytosis. In: LeBouton A V, ed. Molecular and cell biology of the liver. Boca Raton: CRC Press, 1993: pp 117–141

49. Jones A L, Renston R H, Burwen S J. Uptake and intracellular disposition of plasma-derived proteins and apoproteins by hepatocytes. In: Popper H, Schaffner F, eds. Progress in liver diseases, vol VII. New York: Grune & Stratton, 1982: p 51

50. Marks D L, LaRusso N F. Vesicle-dependent transport pathways in liver cells. In: Tavoloni N, Berk P D, eds. Hepatic transport and bile secretion. Physiology and pathophysiology. New York: Raven Press, 1993: pp 513–530

51. Jones A L, Schmucker D L, Renston R H, Murakami T. The architecture of bile secretion. A morphological perspective of physiology. Dig Dis Sci 1980; 25: 609–629

52. Gebhardt R. Primary cultures of rat hepatocytes as a model system of canalicular development, biliary secretion, and intrahepatic cholestasis. III. Properties of the biliary transport of immunoglobulin A revealed by immunofluorescence. Gastroenterology 1983; 84: 1462–1470

53. Delacroix D L, Furtado-Barreira G, De Hemptinne B, Goudswaard J, Dive C, Vaerman J P. The liver in the IgA secretory immune system. Dogs, but not rats and rabbits, are suitable models for human studies. Hepatology 1983; 3: 980–988

54. Perez J H, Van Schaik M, Mullock B M, Bailyes E M, Price C P, Luzio J P. The presence and measurement of secretory component in human bile and blood. Clin Chim Acta 1991; 197: 171–188

55. Mullock B M, Hinton R H. Transport of proteins from blood to bile. Trends Biochem Sci 1981; 6: 188–190

56. Mullock B M, Jones R S, Hinton R H. Movement of endocytic shuttle vesicles from the sinusoidal to the bile canicular face of hepatocytes does not depend on occupation of receptor sites. FEBS Lett 1980; 113: 201–205

57. Evans W H. Membrane traffic at the hepatocyte's sinusoidal and canicular surface domains. Hepatology 1981; 1: 452–457

58. Hubbard A L, Stieger B, Bartles J R. Biogenesis of endogenous plasma membrane proteins in epithelial cells. Annu Rev Physiol 1989; 51: 755–770

59. Goldfischer S L. Peroxisomal diseases. In: Arias I M, Jakoby W B, Popper H, Schachter D, Shafritz D A, eds. The liver: biology and pathobiology, 2nd edn. New York: Raven Press, 1988: pp 255–267

60. Boyer J L. The role of vesicle transport and exocytosis in bile formation and cholestasis. in: Gentilini P, Arias I M, McIntyre N, Rodes J, eds. Cholestasis. Amsterdam: Excerpta Medica, 1994: pp 69–78

61. Hofmann A F. Bile acids in liver and biliary disease. In: Millward-Sadler G H, Wright R, Arthur M J P, eds. Wright's Liver and biliary disease, vol 1, 3rd edn. London: Saunders, 1992: pp 288–316

62. Goldsmith M A, Huling S, Jones A L. Hepatic handling of bile salts and protein in the rat during intrahepatic cholestasis. Gastroenterology 1983; 84: 978–986

63. Suchy F J, Balistreri W F, Hung J, Miller P, Garfield S A. Intracellular bile acid transport in rat liver as visualized by electron microscope autoradiography using a bile acid analogue. Am J Physiol 1983; 245: G681–G689

64. Erlinger S. Regulation of bile secretion. In: Gentilini P, Arias I M, McIntyre N, Rodes J, eds. Cholestasis. Amsterdam: Excerpta Medica, 1994: pp 31–42

65. Lamri Y, Roda A, Dumont M, Feldmann G, Erlinger S. Immunoperoxidase localization of bile salts in rat liver cells. Evidence for a role of the Golgi apparatus in bile salt transport. J Clin Invest 1988; 82: 1173–1182

66. Erlinger S. Intracellular events in bile acid transport by the liver. In: Tavoloni N, Berk P D, eds. Hepatic transport and bile secretion. Physiology and pathophysiology. New York: Raven Press, 1993: pp 467–476

67. Tavoloni N, Boyer J L. Relationship between hepatic metabolism of chlorpromazine and cholestatic effects in the isolated perfused rat liver. J Pharmacol Exp Ther 1980; 214: 269–274

68. Caldwell J. Biological implications of xenobiotic metabolism. In: Arias I M, Jakoby W B, Popper H, Schachter D, Shafritz D A, eds. The liver: biology and pathobiology, 2nd edn. New York: Raven Press, 1988: pp 355–362

69. De Duve C, Wattiaux R. Functions of lysosomes. Annu Rev Physiol 1966; 28: 435–492

70. La Russo N F, Fowler S. Coordinate secretion of acid hydrolases in rat bile. Hepatocyte exocytosis of lysosomal protein? J Clin Invest 1979; 64: 948–954

71. La Russo N F, Kost L J, Carter J A, Barham S S. Triton WR-1339, a lysosomotropic compound, is excreted into bile and alters the biliary excretion of lysosomal enzymes and lipids. Hepatology 1982; 2: 209–215

72. Renaud G, Hamilton R L, Havel R J. Hepatic metabolism of colloidal-gold-low-density lipoprotein complexes in the rat: evidence for bulk excretion of lysosomal contents into bile. Hepatology 1989; 9: 380–392

73. Gross J B, Myers B M, Kost L J, Kuntz S M, La Russo N F. Biliary copper excretion by hepatocyte lysosomes in the rat. Major excretory pathway in experimental copper overload. J Clin Invest 1989; 83: 30–39

74. Lévy P, Dumont M, Brissot P, Letreut A, Favier A, Deugnier Y, Erlinger S. Acute infusions of bile salts increase biliary excretion of iron in iron-loaded rats. Gastroenterology 1991; 101: 1673–1679

75. Desmet V J. Anatomy. I. Hepatocyte — canaliculus. In: Bianchi L, Sickinger K, eds. Liver and bile. Lancaster: MTP Press, 1977: pp 3–31

76. Ma M H, Biempica L. The normal human liver cell, cytochemical and structural studies. Am J Pathol 1971; 62: 353–390

77. Phillips M J, Oda M, Mak E, Steiner J W. Fine structure of the biliary tree. In: Taylor W, ed. The hepatobiliary system. Fundamental and pathological mechanisms. New York: Plenum Press, 1976: p 245

78. Sakisaka S, Ng O C, Boyer J L. Tubulovesicular transcytotic pathway in isolated hepatocyte couplets in culture. Effect of colchicine and taurocholate. Gastroenterology 1988; 95: 793–804

79. Ma M H, Laird W A, Scott H. Cytopempsis of horseradish peroxidase in the hepatocyte. J Histochem Cytochem 1974; 22: 160–169

80. Hayakawa T, Cheng O, Ma A, Boyer J L. Taurocholate stimulates transcytotic vesicular pathways labeled by horseradish peroxidase in the isolated perfused rat liver. Gastroenterology 1990; 99: 216–228

81. Kitamura T, Gatmaitan Z, Arias I M. Serial quantitative image analysis and confocal microscopy of hepatic uptake, intracellular distribution and biliary secretion of a fluorescent bile acid analog in rat hepatocyte doublets. Hepatology 1990; 12: 1358–1364

82. Jaeken L, Thines-Sempoux D. A three-dimensional study of organelle interrelationships in regenerating rat liver. 3. Organelles related to bile. Cell Biol Int Rep 1979; 3: 453–462

83. Crawford J M, Berken C A, Gollan J L. Role of the hepatocyte microtubular system in the excretion of bile salt and biliary lipid: implications for intracellular vesicular transport. J Lipid Res 1988; 29: 144–156

84. Coleman R, Rahman K. Review. Lipid flow in bile formation. Biochim Biophys Acta 1992; 1125: 113–133

85. Dumont M, D'hont C, Durand-Schneider A M, Legrand-Defretin V, Feldmann G, Erlinger S. Inhibition by colchicine of biliary secretion of diethylmaleate in the rat: evidence for micro-tubule-dependent vesicular transport. Hepatology 1991; 14: 10–15

86. Alberts B, Bray D, Lewis J, Raff M, Roberts K, Watson J D. Molecular biology of the cell. New York: Garland Publishing, 1983

87. Möller O J, Ostergaard-Thomsen O, Larsen J A. The existence of tubulo-cisternal endoplasmic reticulum in rat hepatocytes. Cell Tissue Res 1983; 228: 13–20

88. Crawford J M, Gollan J L. Transcellular transport of organic anions in hepatocytes: still a long way to go. Hepatology 1991; 14: 192–197

89. Claude A. Growth and differentiation of cytoplasmic membranes in the course of lipoprotein granule synthesis in the hepatic cell. J Cell Biol 1970; 47: 745–766

90. Jaeken L, Thines-Sempoux D. A three-dimensional study of organelle interrelationships in regenerating rat liver. 6. Golgi apparatus. Cell Biol Int Rep 1981; 5: 261–273

91. Jezequel A-M, Bonazzi P, Amabili P, Venturini C, Orlandi F. Changes of the Golgi apparatus induced by diethylmaleate in rat hepatocytes. Hepatology 1982; 2: 856–862

92. Simion F A, Fleischer B, Fleischer S. Two distinct mechanisms for taurocholate uptake in subcellular fractions from rat liver. J Biol Chem 1984; 259: 10874

93. Farquhar M G, Palade G E. The Golgi apparatus (complex) (1954–1981): from artifact to center stage. J Cell Biol 1981; 91: 77s

94. Herzog V. Pathways of endocytosis in secretory cells. Trends Biochem Sci 1981; 6: 319–321

95. French S W, Okanoue T, Swierenga S H H, Marceau N. The cytoskeleton of hepatocytes in health and disease. In: Farber E, Phillips M J, Kaufman N, eds. Pathogenesis of liver diseases. Baltimore: Williams & Wilkins, 1987: pp 95–112

96. French S W, Cadrin M, Kawahara H, Kachi K. Cytoskeleton. In: LeBouton A V, ed. Molecular and cell biology of the liver. Boca Raton: CRC Press, 1993: pp 143–180

97. Feldmann G. The cytoskeleton of the hepatocyte. Structure and functions. J Hepatol 1989; 8: 380–386

98. Porter K R. Cytomatrix. In: Arias I M, Jakoby W B, Popper H, Schachter D, Shafritz D A, eds. The liver: biology and pathobiology, 2nd edn. New York: Raven Press, 1988: pp 29–45

99. Oda M, Price V M, Fisher M M, Phillips M J. Ultrastructure of bile canaliculi, with special reference to the surface coat and the pericanalicular web. Lab Invest 1974; 31: 314–323

100. Phillips M J, Oda M. The bile canalicular web. Fed Proc 1974; 33: 626

101. Phillips M J, Oda M, Mak E, Fisher M M. Bile canalicular structure and function. In: Goresky C A, Fisher M M, eds. Hepatology — research and clinical issues. Vol 2 Jaundice. New York: Plenum Press, 1975: p 367

102. Ishii M, Washioka H, Tonosaki A, Toyota T. Regional orientation of actin filaments in the pericanalicular cytoplasm of rat hepatocytes. Gastroenterology 1991; 101: 1663–1672

103. Oda M, Phillips M J. Electron microscopic cytochemical characterization of bile canaliculi and bile ducts in vitro. Virchows Arch [B] 1975; 18: 109–118

104. Garnett H M, Kemp R B, Gröschel-Stewart U. Inhibitory effects of meralyl and of antibodies directed against smooth-muscle myosin on a calcium adenosine triphosphatase of the plasma membrane from mouse liver cells. Arch Biochem Biophys 1976; 172: 419–424

105. Yasuura S, Ueno T, Watanabe S, Hirose M, Namihisa T. Immunocytochemical localization of myosin in normal and phalloidin-treated hepatocytes. Gastroenterology 1989; 97: 982–989

106. Vonk R J, Yousef I M, Corriveau J P, Tuchweber B. Phalloidin-induced morphological and functional changes of rat liver. Liver 1982; 2: 133–140

107. Watanabe S, Miyazaki A, Hirose M et al. Myosin in hepatocytes is essential for bile canalicular contraction. Liver 1991; 11: 185–189

108. Kacich R L, Renston R H, Jones A L. Effects of cytochalasin D and colchicine on the uptake, translocation, and biliary secretion of horseradish peroxidase and (14C) sodium taurocholate in the rat. Gastroenterology 1983; 85: 385–394

109. Phillips M J, Oshio C, Miyairi M, Smith C R. Intrahepatic cholestasis as a canalicular motility disorder: evidence using cytochalasin. Lab Invest 1983; 48: 203–211

110. Phillips M J, Oshio C, Miyairi M, Watanabe S, Smith C R. What is actin doing in the liver cell? Hepatology 1983; 3: 433–436

111. Phillips M J, Watanabe N. Bile canalicular contractions in vivo. Hepatology 1984; 4: 1050

112. Watanabe S, Miyairi M, Oshio C, Smith C R, Phillips M J. Phalloidin alters bile canalicular contractility in primary monolayer cultures of rat liver. Gastroenterology 1983; 85: 245–253

113. Watanabe N, Tsukada N, Smith C R, Edwards V, Phillips M J. Permeabilized hepatocyte couplets. Adenosine triphosphate-dependent bile canalicular contractions and in circumferential pericanalicular microfilament belt demonstrated. Lab Invest 1991; 65: 203–213

114. French S W. Editorial. Role of canalicular contraction in bile flow. Lab Invest 1985; 53: 245–249

115. Kawahara H, French S W. Role of cytoskeleton in canalicular contraction in cultured differentiated hepatocytes. Am J Pathol 1990; 136: 521–532

116. Desmet V J, De Vos R. Tight junctions in the liver. In: Popper H, Schaffner F, eds. Progress in liver diseases, vol II. New York: Grune & Stratton, 1982: pp 31–50

117. Moll R, Franke W W, Schiller D A, Geiger B, Krepler R. The catalog of human cytokeratins: patterns of expression in normal epithelia, tumors and cultured cells. Cell 1982; 31: 11–24

118. Van Eyken P, Sciot R, Van Damme B, De Wolf-Peeters C, Desmet V J. Keratin-immunohistochemistry in normal human liver. Cytokeratin pattern of hepatocytes, bile ducts and acinar gradient. Virchows Arch [A] 1987; 412: 63–72

119. French S W, Kondo I, Irie T, Ihrig T J, Benson N, Munn R. Morphologic study of intermediate filaments in rat hepatocytes. Hepatology 1982; 2: 29–38

120. Katsuma Y, Marceau N, Ohta M, French S W. Cytokeratin intermediate filaments of rat hepatocytes: different cytoskeletal domains and their three-dimensional structure. Hepatology 1988; 8: 559–568

121. Kawahara H, Marceau N, French S W. Effect of agents which rearrange the cytoskeleton in vitro on the structure and function of hepatocytic canaliculi. Lab Invest 1989; 60: 692–704

122. Kawahara H, Cadrin M, Perry G et al. Role of cytokeratin intermediate filaments in transhepatic transport and secretion. Hepatology 1990; 11: 435–448

123. Furuta K, Ohno S, Gibo Y, Kiyosawa K, Futura S. Three-dimensional ultrastructure of normal rat hepatocytes by quick-freezing and deep-etching method. J Gastroenterol Hepatol 1992; 7: 486–490

124. Goldman I S, Jones A L, Hradek G T, Huling S. Hepatocyte handling of immunoglobulin A in the rat: the role of microtubules. Gastroenterology 1983; 85: 130–140

125. Sewell R B, Barham S S, Zinsmeister A R, LaRusso N F. Microtubule modulation of biliary excretion of endogenous and exogenous hepatic lysosomal constituents. Am J Physiol 1984; 246: G8–G15

126. Durand-Schneider A M, Bouanga J C, Feldmann G, Maurice M. Microtubule disruption interferes with the structural and functional integrity of the apical pole in primary cultures of rat hepatocytes. Eur J Cell Biol 1991; 56: 260–268

127. Sellinger M, Boyer J L. Physiology of bile secretion and cholestasis. In: Popper H, Schaffner F, eds. Progress in liver diseases, vol IX. Philadelphia: Saunders, 1990: pp 237–260

128. Staehelin L A, Hull B E. Junctions between living cells. Sci Am 1978; 238: 140–152

129. Miyairi M, Oshio C, Watanabe S, Smith C R, Yousef I M, Phillips M J. Taurocholate accelerates bile canalicular contractions in isolated rat hepatocytes. Lab Invest 1984; 87: 788–792

130. Montesano R, Friend D S, Perrelet A, Orci L. In vivo assembly of tight junctions in fetal rat liver. J Cell Biol 1975; 67: 310–319

131. Hardison WGM, Lowe P J, Shanahan M. Effect of molecular charge on para- and transcellular access of horseradish peroxidase into rat bile. Hepatology 1989; 9: 866–871

132. Hardison W G M, Dalle-Molle E, Gosink E, Lowe P J, Steinbach J H, Yamaguchi Y. Function of rat hepatocyte tight junctions: studies with bile acid infusions. Am J Physiol 1991; 260: G167–G174

133. Hardison W G M. Hepatocellular tight junctions: role of canalicular permeability in hepatobiliary transport. In: Tavoloni N, Berk P D, eds. Hepatic transport and bile secretion. Physiology and pathophysiology. New York: Raven press, 1993: pp 571–586

134. Lagarde S, Elias E, Wade J B, Boyer J L. Structural heterogeneity of hepatocyte 'tight' junctions: a quantitative analysis. Hepatology 1981; 1: 193–203

135. Yamaguchi Y, Dalle-Molle E, Hardison W G M. Vasopressin and A23187 stimulate phosphorylation of myosin light chain-1 in isolated rat hepatocytes. Am J Physiol 1991; 261: G312–G319

136. Rassat J, Robenek H, Themann H. Alterations of tight and gap junctions in mouse hepatocytes following administration of colchicine. Cell Tissue Res 1982; 223: 187–200

137. Kottra G, Frömter E, Functional properties of the paracellular pathway in some leaky epithelia. J Exp Biol 1983; 106: 217–229

138. Loewenstein W R. Permeable junctions. Cold Spring Harbor Symp Quant Biol 1975; XL: 49–63

139. Mowery J, Hixson D C. Detection of cell-CAM 105 in the pericanalicular domain of the rat hepatocyte plasma membrane. Hepatology 1991; 13: 47–56

140. Cossel L. Die menschliche Leber im Elektronenmikroskop. Jena: Gustav Fischer, 1964: pp 21–31

141. Müller O, Mayer D. Die Circadianperiodik der Gallenkanälchen und der Gallesekretion in der Rattenleber. Acta Histochem Suppl 1975; XIV: 239–246

142. Nemchausky B A, Layden T J, Boyer J L. Effects of chronic choleretic infusions of bile acids on the membrane of the bile canaliculus: a biochemical and morphologic study. Lab Invest 1977; 36: 259–267

143. Motta P, Fumagalli G. Structure of rat bile canaliculi as revealed by scanning electron microscopy. Anat Rec 1975; 182: 499–513

144. Petzinger E. Canalicular transport: experimental models, morphology requirements and transport processes. In: Siegers C P, Watkins III J B, eds. Biliary excretion of drugs and other chemicals. Progress in pharmacology and clinical pharmacology, vol 8/4. Stuttgart: Gustaf Fischer Verlag, 1991: pp 49–87

145. Arias I M. Mechanisms of canalicular secretion. In: Gentilini P, Arias I M, Arroyo V, Schrier R W, eds. Liver diseases and renal complications. New York: Raven Press, 1990: pp 109–117

146. Arias I M. Transhepatic transport, bile secretion and cholestatic mechanisms. In: Gentilini P, Arias I M, McIntyre N, Rodes J, eds. Cholestasis. Amsterdam: Excerpta Medica, 1994: pp 119–128

147. Adachi Y, Kobayashi H, Kurumi Y, Shovji M, Kitano M, Yamamoto T. Bilirubin diglucoronide transport by rat liver canalicular membrane vesicles: stimulation by bicarbonate ion. Hepatology 1991; 14: 1251–1258

148. Roman L M, Hubbard A L. A domain-specific marker for the hepatocyte plasma membrane: localization of leucine amino-peptidase to the bile canalicular domain. J Cell Biol 1983; 96: 1548–1558

149. Roman L M, Hubbard A L. A domain-specific marker for the hepatocyte plasma membrane. II. Ultrastructural localization of leucine aminopeptidase to the bile canalicular domain of isolated rat liver plasma membranes. J Cell Biol 1984; 98: 1488–1496

150. Loke S L, Leung C Y, Chiu K Y, Yau W L, Cheung K N, Ma L. Localization of CD 10 to biliary canaliculi by immunoelectron microscopical examination. J Clin Pathol 1990; 43: 654–656

151. Daems W T, Wisse E, Brederoo P. Electron microscopy of the vacuolar apparatus. In: Dingle J T, Fell H B, eds. Lysosomes in biology and pathology, vol I. Amsterdam: North Holland, 1969: pp 64–112

152. Miettinen A, Linder E. Membrane antigens shared by renal proximal tubules and other epithelia associated with absorption and excretion. Clin Exp Immunol 1976; 23: 568–577

153. Godfrey P P, Warner M J, Coleman R. Enzymes and proteins in bile. Biochem J 1981; 196: 11–16

154. Hatoff D E, Hardison W G M. Bile acid-dependent secretion of alkaline phosphatase in rat bile. Hepatology 1982; 2: 433–439

155. Hirata E, Inoue M, Morino Y. Mechanism of biliary secretion of membranous enzymes: bile acids are important factors for biliary occurrence of gamma-glutamyltransferase and other hydrolases. J Biochem 1984; 96: 289–297

156. Sztul E S, Howell K E, Palade G E. Intracellular and transcellular transport of secretory component and albumin in rat hepatocytes. J Cell Biol 1983; 97: 1582–1591

157. Yousef I M, Bloxam D L, Phillips M J, Fisher M M. Liver cell plasma membrane lipids and the origin of biliary phospholipid. Can J Biochem 1975; 53: 989–997

158. Lowe P J, Barnwell S G, Coleman R. Rapid kinetic analysis of the bile-salt-dependent secretion of phospholipid, cholesterol and a plasma-membrane enzyme into bile. Biochem J 1984; 222: 631–637

159. Phillips M J, Oda M, Mak E, Edwards V, Yousef I, Fisher M M. The bile canalicular network in vitro. J Ultrastruct Res 1976; 57: 163–167

160. Phillips M J, Poucell S. Cholestasis: surgical pathology, mechanisms and new concepts. In: Farber E, Phillips M J, Kaufman N, eds. Pathogenesis of liver diseases. International Academy of Pathology. Monograph 28. Baltimore: Williams & Wilkins, 1987: pp 65–94

161. Watanabe S, Phillips M J. Ca^{2+} causes active contraction of bile canaliculi: direct evidence from microinjection studies. Proc Natl Acad Sci USA 1984; 81: 6164–6168

162. Gumucio J J, Miller D L. Zonal hepatic function: solute–hepatocyte interactions within the liver acinus. In: Popper H, Schaffner F, eds. Progress in liver diseases, vol VII. New York: Grune & Stratton, 1982: pp 17–30

163. Javitt N B. Hepatic bile formation (first of two parts). N Engl J Med 1976; 295: 1464–1468

164. Gumucio D L, Gumucio J J, Wilson J A P, Cutter C, Krauss M, Caldwell R, Chen E. Albumin influences sulfobromophthalein transport by hepatocytes of each acinar zone. Am J Physiol 1984; 246: G86–G95

165. Metz W, Forssmann W G. Comparative morphology of liver innervation. In: Popper H, Bianchi L, Gudat F, Reutter W, eds. Communications of liver cells. Lancaster: MTP Press, 1980: pp 121–127

166. Tavoloni N. The intrahepatic biliary epithelium: an area of growing interest in hepatology. Semin Liver Dis 1987; 7: 280–292

167. Tarsetti F, Lenzen R, Salvi R, Schuler E, Dembitzer R, Tavoloni N. Biology and pathobiology of intrahepatic biliary epithelium. In: Tavoloni N, Berk P D, eds. Hepatic transport and bile secretion. Physiology and pathophysiology. New York: Raven Press, 1993: pp 619–636

168. Lamri Y, Erlinger S, Dumont M, Roda A, Feldmann G. Immunoperoxidase localization of ursodeoxycholic acid in rat biliary epithelial cells. Evidence for a cholehepatic circulation. Liver 1992; 12: 351–354

169. Desmet V J. Morphology and development of the hepatobiliary system. In: Bock K W, Matern S, Gerok W, Schmid R, eds. Hepatic metabolism and disposition of endo- and xenobiotics. Dordrecht: Kluwer Academic Publishers, 1991: pp 3–17

170. Sirica A E. Biology of biliary epithelial cells. In: Boyer J L, Ockner R K, eds. Progress in Liver Diseases, vol X. Philadelphia: Saunders, 1992: pp 63–87

171. Bianchi L. Liver biopsy interpretation in hepatitis. Part I. Presentation of critical morphologic features used in diagnosis (Glossary). Pathol Res Pract 1983; 178: 2

172. McCuskey R S. Hepatic microcirculation. In: Bioulac-Sage P, Balabaud C, eds. Sinusoids in human liver: health and disease. Rijswijk: Kupffer Cell Foundation, 1988: pp 151–164

173. De Vos R, Desmet V J. Morphologic changes of the junctional complex of the hepatocytes in rat liver after bile duct ligation. Br J Exp Pathol 1978; 59: 220–227

174. Popper H. Cholestasis: the future of a past and present riddle. Hepatology 1981; 1: 187–191

175. International Group. Histopathology of the intrahepatic biliary tree. Liver 1983; 3: 161–175

176. Gerber M A, Orr W, Denk H, Schaffner F, Popper H. Hepatocellular hyalin in cholestasis and cirrhosis: its diagnostic significance. Gastroenterology 1973; 64: 89–98

177. Salaspuro M P, Sipponen P, Makkonen H. Occurrence of orcein-positive hepatocellular material in various liver diseases. Scand J Gastroenterol 1976; 11: 677–682

178. Sipponen P. Orcein positive hepatocellular material in long-standing biliary diseases. 1. Histochemical characteristics. Scand J Gastroenterol 1976; 11: 545–552

179. Sipponen P. Orcein positive hepatocellular material in long-standing biliary diseases. 2. Ultrastructural studies. Scand J Gastroenterol 1976; 11: 553–557

180. Irons R D, Schenk E A, Lee J C K. Cytochemical methods for copper. Semiquantitative screening procedure for identification of abnormal copper levels in liver. Arch Pathol Lab Med 1977; 101: 298–301

181. Janssens A R, Bosman F T, Ruiter D J, Van Den Hamer C J. Immunohistochemical demonstration of the cytoplasmic copper-associated protein in the liver in primary biliary cirrhosis: its identification as metallothionein. Liver 1984; 4: 139–147

182. Sokol R J. Lipid peroxidation in cholestasis. In: Lentze M, Reichen J, eds. Paediatric cholestasis. Novel approaches to treatment. Dordrecht: Kluwer Academic Publishers, 1992: pp 75–80

183. Schölmerich J, Straub R. Mechanisms of bile salt toxicity. In: Lentze M, Reichen J, eds. Paediatric cholestasis. Novel approaches to treatment. Dordrecht: Kluwer Academic Publishers, 1992: pp 83–103

184. Desmet V J. Chronic cholestasis. In: Hoofnagle J H, Goodman Z, eds. Liver biopsy interpretation for the 1990's. Thorofare: American Association for the Study of Liver Diseases, 1991: pp 23–38

185. Toda G, Kako M, Oka H, Oda T, Ikeda Y. Uneven distribution of enzymatic alterations on the liver cell surface in experimental extrahepatic cholestasis of rat. Exp Mol Pathol 1978; 28: 10–24

186. Fricker G, Landmann L, Meier P J. Extrahepatic obstructive cholestasis reverses the bile salt secretory polarity of rat hepatocytes. J Clin Invest 1989; 84: 876–885

187. Landmann L, Meier P J, Bianchi L. Bile duct ligation-induced redistribution of canalicular antigen in rat hepatocyte plasma membranes demonstrated by immunogold quantification. Histochemistry 1990; 94: 373–379

188. Landmann L, Rachner C, Stieger B. Morphological aspects of cholestasis. In: Gentilini P, Arias I M, McIntyre N, Rodes J, eds. Cholestasis. Amsterdam: Excerpta Medica, 1994: pp 109–117

189. Kaplan M M, Ohkubo A, Quaroni E G, Sze-Tu D. Increased synthesis of rat liver alkaline phosphatase by bile duct ligation. Hepatology 1983; 3: 368–376

190. Keeffe E B, Scharschmidt B F, Blankenship N M, Ockner R K. Studies of relationship among bile flow, liver plasma membrane Na^+, K^+-ATPase and membrane microviscosity in the rat. J Clin Invest 1979; 64: 1590–1598

191. Jezequel A-M, Librari M-L, Mosca P G, Novelli G. The human liver in extrahepatic cholestasis: ultrastructural morphometric data. Liver 1983; 3: 303–314

192. Witzleben C L. Hepatic ultrastructural effects of cholic acid overload. Exp Mol Pathol 1972; 16: 47–53

193. Van Husen N, Gerlach U, Roessner A, Uchida Y. Mitochondrienmorphologie und Stoffwechsel bei extrahepatischer Obstruktion. Klin Wochenschr 1976; 54: 1107–1108

194. Krähenbühl S, Stucki J, Reichen J. Reduced activity of the electron transport chain in liver mitochondria isolated from rats with secondary biliary cirrhosis. Hepatology 1992; 15: 1160–1166

195. Krähenbühl S, Krähenbühl-Glauser S, Stucki J, Gehr P, Reichen J. Stereological and functional analysis of liver mitochondria from rats with secondary biliary cirrhosis: impaired mitochondrial metabolism and increased mitochondrial content per hepatocyte. Hepatology 1992; 15: 1167–1172

196. Reichen J, Krähenbühl S, Zimmermann H. Impact of cholestasis on hepatic function: retention of cholephiles and their potential targets. In: Gentilini P, Arias I M, McIntyre N, Rodes J, eds. Cholestasis. Amsterdam: Excerpta Medica, 1994: pp 167–175

197. Jezequel A M. Some aspects of ultrastructural pathology. In: Millward-Sadler G H, Wright R, Arthur M J P, eds. Wright's Liver and biliary disease, vol 1, 3rd edn. London: Saunders, 1992: pp 497–518

198. Mathis R K, Watkins I B, Szczepanik-Van Leeuwen P, Lott I T. Liver in the cerebro-hepato-renal syndrome: defective bile acid synthesis and abnormal mitochondria. Gastroenterology 1980; 79: 1311–1317

199. Jezequel A-M, Capurso L, Freddara U, Orlandi F. Cholestasis in man. A re-evaluation of ultrastructural data. II Fegato 1974; 20: 299–314

200. Jones A L, Schmucker D L, Mooney J S, Adler R D, Ockner R K. Morphometric analysis of rat hepatocytes after total biliary obstruction. Gastroenterology 1976; 71: 1050–1060

201. Roels F, Pauwels M, Cornelis A et al. Peroxisomes (microbodies) in human liver. Cytochemical and quantitative studies of 85 biopsies. J Histochem Cytochem 1983; 31 (IA Suppl.): 235–237

202. Schaffner F, Popper H. Causation and consequences of cholestasis: an overview. In: Goresky C A, Fisher M M, eds. Hepatology, research and clinical issues. Vol 2 Jaundice. New York: Plenum Press, 1975: pp 329–349

203. Jones A L, Schmucker D L. Current concepts of liver structure as related to function. Gastroenterology 1977; 73: 833–851

204. Denk H. Hepatic microsomal enzymes and their alterations in pathologic conditions. In: Popper H, Schaffner F, eds. Progress in liver diseases, vol VI. New York: Grune & Stratton, 1979: pp 263–280

205. Nishiura S, Koga A, Yanagisawas J. Effects of bile duct obstruction and decompression on hepatic microsomal mixed function oxidase system in rats. Exp Mol Pathol 1988; 49: 62–74

206. Coquil J F, Berthon B, Chomiki N et al. Effects of taurolithocholate, a Ca^{2+} mobilizing agent, on cell Ca^{2+} in rat hepatocytes, human platelets and neuroblastoma NG 108–15 cell line. Biochem J 1991; 273: 153–160

207. Fevery J, De Groote J, Heirwegh K P M. Quantitation of hepatic bilirubin conjugation. In: Paumgartner G, Preisig R, eds. The liver. Quantitative aspects of structure and function. Basel: Karger, 1973: p 203

208. Felker T E, Hamilton R L, Havel R J. Secretion of lipoprotein-X by perfused livers of rats with cholestasis. Proc Natl Acad Sci USA 1978; 75: 3459–3463

209. Jones A L, Hradek G T, Schmucker D L. Fate of dimeric IgA following retrograde infusion into rat common bile duct. Hepatology 1982; 2: 736

210. Renston R H, Zsigmond G, Bernhoft R A, Burwen S J, Jones A L. Vesicular transport of horseradish peroxidase during chronic bile duct obstruction in the rat. Hepatology 1983; 3: 673–680

211. Desmet V J. Current problems in diagnosis of biliary disease and cholestasis. Semin Liver Dis 1986; 6: 233–245

212. Boyer J L, Itabashi M, Hruban Z. Formation of pericanalicular vacuoles during sodium dehydrocholate choleresis. A mechanism for bile acid transport? In: Preisig R, Bircher J, eds. The liver. Quantitative aspects of structure and function. Aulendorf: Editio Cantor, 1979: p 163

213. Miyai K, Richardson A L, Mayr W, Javitt N B. Subcellular pathology of rat liver in cholestasis and choleresis induced by bile salts. I. Effects of lithocholic, 3 β-hydroxy-5-cholenoic, cholic and dehydrocholic acids. Lab Invest 1977; 36: 249–258

214. Yousef I M, Tuchweber B, Vonk R J, Massé D, Audet M, Roy C C. Lithocholate cholestasis — sulfated glycolithocholate-induced intrahepatic cholestasis in rats. Gastroenterology 1981; 80: 233–241

215. Valencia-Mayoral P, Weber J, Cutz E, Edwards V D, Phillips M J. Possible defect in the bile secretory apparatus in arteriohepatic dysplasia (Alagille's syndrome): a review with observations on the ultrastructure of liver. Hepatology 1984; 4: 691–698

216. Fisher M M, Phillips M J. Cytoskeleton of the hepatocyte. In: Popper H, Schaffner F, eds. Progress in liver diseases, vol VI. New York: Grune & Stratton, 1979: p 105

217. Phillips M J. Recent advances in the electron microscopic evaluation of the liver in cholestasis: In: Javitt N B, ed. Neonatal hepatitis and biliary atresia. Bethesda: Department of Health, Education and Welfare/National Institutes of Health, 1979: p 323

218. Loosli H, Gardiol D, Gautier A. Experimental intrahepatic cholestasis. Virchows Arch [B] 1981; 35: 213–228

219. De Vos R, De Wolf-Peeters C, Desmet V J, Eggermont E, Van Acker K. Progressive intrahepatic cholestasis (Byler's disease): case report. Gut 1975; 16: 943–950

220. Adler M, Chung K W, Schaffner F, Pericanalicular hepatocytic and bile ductular microfilaments in cholestasis in man. Am J Pathol 1980; 98: 603–616

221. Imanari H, Kuroda H, Tamura K. Microfilaments around the bile canaliculi in patients with intrahepatic cholestasis. Gastroenterol Jpn 1981; 16: 168–173

222. Weber A M, Tuchweber B, Yousef I et al. Severe familial cholestasis in North American Indian children: a clinical model of microfilament dysfunction? Gastroenterology 1981; 81: 653–662

223. Watanabe S, Phillips N J. Acute phalloidin toxicity in living hepatocytes: evidence for a possible disturbance in membrane flow and for multiple functions for actin in the liver cell. Am J Pathol 1986; 122: 101–112

224. Ohta M, Marceau N, French S W. Pathologic changes in the cytokeratin pericanalicular sheath in experimental cholestasis and alcoholic fatty liver. Lab Invest 1988; 59: 60–74

225. Kawahara H, Marceau N, French S. Effects of chlorpramazine and low calcium on the cytoskeleton and the secretory function of hepatocytes in vitro. J Hepatol 1990; 10: 8

226. Naramoto A, Ohno S, Furuta K, Itoh N, Nakazawa K, Nakano M, Shigematsu H. Ultrastructural studies of hepatocyte cytoskeletons of phalloidin-treated rats by quick-freezing and deep-etching method. Hepatology 1991; 13: 222–229

227. Van Eyken P, Sciot R, Desmet V J. A cytokeratin immunohistochemical study of cholestatic liver disease: evidence that hepatocytes can express 'bile duct-type' cytokeratins. Histopathology 1989; 15: 125–135

228. Denk H, Franke W W, Eckerstorfer R, Schmid E, Kerjaschki D. Formation and involution of Mallory bodies ('alcoholic hyalin') in murine and human liver revealed by immunofluorescence microscopy with antibodies to prekeratin. Proc Natl Acad Sci USA 1979; 76: 4112–4116

229. Yokoo H, Craig R M, Harwood T R, Cochrane C. Griseofulvin-induced cholestasis in Swiss albino mice. Gastroenterology 1979; 77: 1082–1087

230. Coe I E, Ishak K G, Ross M J. Diethylstilbestrol-induced jaundice in the Chinese and American hamster. Hepatology 1983; 3: 489–496

231. Dubin M, Maurice M, Feldmann G, Erlinger S. Influence of colchicine and phalloidin on bile secretion and hepatic ultrastructure in the rat. Possible interaction between microtubules and microfilaments. Gastroenterology 1980; 79: 646–654

232. Anderson J M, Glade J L, Stevenson B R, Boyer J L, Mooseker M S. Hepatic immunohistochemical localization of the tight junction protein ZO-1 in rat models of cholestasis. Am J Pathol 1989; 134: 1055–1062

233. Fallon M B, Strazzabosco M, Benedetti A, Anderson J M. Common bile duct obstruction in the rat results in elevated hepatic mRNA levels for the tight junction protein ZO-1 (abstract). Hepatology 1990; 12: 401

234. Krell H, Höke H, Pfaff E. Development of intrahepatic cholestasis by alpha-napthyl-isothiocyanate in rats. Gastroenterology 1982; 82: 507–514

235. Elias E, Iqbal S, Knutton S, Hickey A, Coleman R. Increased tight junction permeability: a possible mechanism of oestrogen cholestasis. Eur J Clin Invest 1983; 13: 383–390

236. Adinolfi L E, Utili R, Gaeta G B, Abernathy C O, Zimmerman H J. Cholestasis induced by estradiol-17β-D-glucuronide: mechanisms and prevention by sodium taurocholate. Hepatology 1984; 4: 30–37

237. Rassat J, Robenek H, Themann H. Ultrastructural alterations of the mouse liver following vincristine administration. J Submicrosc Cytol Pathol 1981; 13: 321–335

238. Rassat J, Robenek H, Themann H. Ultrastructural changes in mouse hepatocytes exposed to vinblastine sulfate with special reference to the intercellular junctions. Eur J Cell Biol 1981; 24: 203–210

239. Pitelka D R, Taggart B N. Mechanical tension induces lateral movement of intramembrane components of the tight junction: studies on mouse mammary cells in culture. J Cell Biol 1983; 96: 606–612

240. Toyota N, Miyai K, Hardison W G. Effect of biliary pressure versus high bile acid flux on the permeability of hepatocellular tight junction. Lab Invest 1984; 50: 536–542

241. Forker E L. The effect of estrogen on bile formation in the rat. J Clin Invest 1969; 48: 654–663

242. Robenek H, Rassat J, Grosser V, Themann H. Ultrastructural study of cholestasis induced by longterm treatment with estradiol valerate. I. Tight junctional analysis and tracer experiments. Virchows Arch [B] 1982; 40: 201–215

243. Jaeschke H, Krell H, Pfaff E. No increase of biliary permeability in ethinylestradiol-treated rats. Gastroenterology 1983; 85: 808–814

244. Iqbal S, Mills C O, Elias E. Biliary permeability during ethinyl estradiol-induced cholestasis studied by segmented retrograde intrabiliary injections in rats. J Hepatol 1985; 1: 211–219

245. Krell H, Fromm H, Larson R E. Increased paracellular permeability in intrahepatic cholestasis induced by Carmustine (BCNU) in rats. Gastroenterology 1991; 101: 180–188

246. Boyer J L. New concepts of mechanisms of hepatocyte bile formation. Physiol Rev 1980; 60: 303–326
247. Nishi M. Scanning electron microscope study on the mechanism of obstructive jaundice in rats. Arch Histol Jpn 1978; 41: 411–426
248. Metz J, Aoki A, Merlo M, Forssmann W G. Morphological alterations and functional changes of interhepatocellular junctions induced by bile duct ligation. Cell Tissue Res 1977; 182: 299–310
249. Robenek H, Rassat J, Themann H. A quantitative freeze-fracture analysis of gap and tight junctions in the normal and cholestatic human liver. Virchows Arch [B] 1981; 38: 39–56
250. Desmet V J, De Vos R. Morphology of tight junctions in cholestasis. In: Popper H, Bianchi L, Gudat F, Reutter W, eds. Communications of liver cells. Lancaster: MTP Press, 1980: pp 185–191
251. Desmet V J, De Vos R. Structural analysis of acute liver injury. In: Keppler D, Popper H, Bianchi L, Reutter W, eds. Mechanisms of hepatocyte injury and death. Lancaster: MTP Press, 1984: pp 11–30
252. Compagno J, Grisham J W. Scanning electron microscopy of extrahepatic biliary obstruction. Arch Pathol 1974; 97: 348–351
253. Vial J D, Simon F R, Mackinnon A M. Effect of bile duct ligation on the ultrastructural morphology of hepatocytes. Gastroenterology 1976; 70: 85–92
254. Miyai K, Mayr W, Richardson A. Freeze-fracture study of bile canalicular changes induced by lithocholic acid. Lab Invest 1974; 30: 384
255. Miyai K, Mayr W, Richardson A, Fisher M M. An ultrastructural look at intrahepatic cholestasis. In: Goresky C A, Fisher M M, eds. Hepatology—research and clinical issues. Vol 2 Jaundice. New York: Plenum Press, 1975: p 383
256. Orci L, Perrelet A. Freeze-etch histology. A comparison between thin sections and freeze-etch replicas. Berlin: Springer Verlag, 1975
257. Frederiks W M, Van Noorden C J F, Aronson D C et al. Quantitative changes in acid phosphatase, alkaline phosphatase and 5'-nucleotidase activity in rat liver after experimentally induced cholestasis. Liver 1990; 10: 158–166
258. Hägerstrand I. Enzyme histochemistry of the liver in extrahepatic biliary obstruction. Acta Pathol Microbiol Scand A 1973; 81: 737–750
259. Ronchi G, Desmet V J. Histochemical study of gamma glutamyl transpeptidase (gammaGT) in experimental intrahepatic and extrahepatic cholestasis. Beitr Pathol 1973; 150: 316–321
260. Phillips M J, Oda M, Mak E, Fisher M M, Jeejeebhoy K N. Microfilament dysfunction as a possible cause of intrahepatic cholestasis. Gastroenterology 1975; 69: 48–58
261. Bhathal P S, Christie G S. A fluorescence study of bile duct proliferation induced in guinea pigs by alpha-naphthyl isothiocyanate. Lab Invest 1969; 20: 480–487
262. Nagore N, Howe S, Boxer L, Scheuer P J. Liver cell rosettes: structural differences in cholestasis and hepatitis. Liver 1989; 9: 43–51
263. Nagore N, Howe S, Scheuer P J. The three-dimensional liver. In: Popper H, Schaffner F, eds. Progress in liver diseases, vol IX. Philadelphia: Saunders, 1990: pp 1–10
264. Bonvicini F, Gautier A, Gardiol D. TEM, cytochemistry and SEM of Na-TL-induced acute cholestasis in rats. Experientia 1976; 32: 787
265. Bonvicini F, Gautier A, Gardiol D, Borel G A. Cholesterol in acute cholestasis induced by taurolithocholic acid. A cytochemical study in transmission and scanning electron microscopy. Lab Invest 1978; 38: 487–495
266. Fisher M M. Biochemical basis for toxic liver injury. Lithocholate hepatotoxicity. In: Farber E, Fisher M M, eds. Toxic injury of the liver. Part A. New York: Dekker, 1979: pp 155–192
267. Vonk R J, Tuchweber B, Masse D, Perea A, Audet M, Roy C C, Yousef I M. Intrahepatic cholestasis induced by allo monohydroxy bile acids in rats. Gastroenterology 1981; 80: 242–249
268. Phillips M J, Yousef I M, Kakis G, Oda M, Funatsu K. Biochemical pathology of canalicular membranes in intrahepatic cholestasis. In: Preisig R, Bircher J, eds. The liver. Quantitative aspects of structure and function. Aulendorf: Editio Cantor, 1979: pp 185–191
269. Kakis G, Phillips M J, Yousef I M. The respective roles of membrane cholesterol and of sodium potassium adenosine triphosphatase in the pathogenesis of lithocholate-induced cholestasis. Lab Invest 1980; 43: 73–81
270. Boelsterli U A, Rakhit G, Balazs T. Modulation by S-adenosyl-L-methionine of hepatic Na+, K+-ATPase, membrane fluidity, and bile flow in rats with ethinyl estradiol-induced cholestasis. Hepatology 1983; 3: 12–17
271. Roessner A, Van Husen N, Pauls E, Gerlach U, Themann H. Feinstrukturell-morphometrische Untersuchungen an Leberbiopsien von Patienten mit intrahepatischer Cholestase. I. Korrelation zwischen den morphometrischen Parametern der Gallencapillaren und den serochemischen Cholestasemessgrössen. Virchows Arch [A] 1975; 367: 15–26
272. Simon F R, Arias I M. Alteration of bile canalicular enzymes in cholestasis. J Clin Invest 1973; 52: 765–775
273. Desmet V J. Cholestasis. In: Anthony P P, MacSween R N M, eds. Recent advances in histopathology. No 12. Edinburgh: Churchill Livingstone, 1984: pp 146–158
274. De Vos R, De Wolf-Peeters C, Desmet V J, Bianchi L, Rohr H P. Significance of liver canalicular changes after experimental bile duct ligation. Exp Mol Pathol 1975; 23: 12–34
275. De Wolf-Peeters C, De Vos R, Desmet V J, Bianchi L, Rohr H P. Electron microscopy and morphometry of canalicular differentiation in fetal and neonatal rat liver. Exp Mol Pathol 1974; 21: 339–350
276. MacDonald R, Pechet G. Liver cell regeneration due to biliary obstruction. Arch Pathol 1961; 72: 133–141
277. Stroun J. Précocité de la souffrance hépatocytaire et de l'hyperplasie régénératrice lors d'obstruction biliaire extra-hépatique. Pathol Microbiol 1966; 29: 265–275
278. Gebhardt R, Jung W, Robenek H. Primary cultures of rat hepatocytes as a model system of canalicular development, biliary secretion, and intrahepatic cholestasis. I. Distribution of filipin-cholesterol complexes during de novo formation of bile canaliculi. Eur J Cell Biol 1982; 29: 68–76
279. Feltkamp C A, Van Der Waerden A W H. Junction formation between cultured normal rat hepatocytes. J Cell Sci 1983; 63: 271–286
280. Desmet V J. Modulation of the liver in cholestasis. J Gastroenterol Hepatol 1992; 7: 313–323
281. Elias H, Sherrick J C. Morphology of the liver. New York: Academic Press, 1969
282. Witzleben C, Boyce W H. Bilirubin as a cholestatic agent. IV. Effect of bilirubin and sulfobromophtalein (BSP) on biliary manganese excretion. Arch Pathol 1973; 99: 496–498
283. Veel T, Villanger O, Holthe M R, Skjorten F S, Raeder M G. Intravenous bilirubin infusion causes vacuolization of the cytoplasm of hepatocytes and canalicular cholestasis. Acta Physiol Scand 1991; 143: 421–429
284. Jung W, Gebhardt R, Robenek H. Primary cultures of rat hepatocytes as a model system of canalicular development, biliary secretion and intrahepatic cholestasis. II. Taurolithocholate-induced alterations of canalicular morphology and of the distribution of filipin-cholesterol complexes. Eur J Cell Biol 1982; 29: 77–82
285. Hardison WGM, Weiner R G, Hatoff D E, Miyai K. Similarities and differences between models of extrahepatic biliary obstruction and complete biliary retention without obstruction in the rat. Hepatology 1983; 3: 383–390
286. Collier D S, Pain J A, Wight D G D, Lovat P, Bailey M E. The Kupffer cell in experimental extrahepatic cholestasis in the rat. A light microscopy, immunohistochemical and electron microscopy study. J Pathol 1986; 150: 187–194
287. Mizoguchi Y, Ohnishi F, Monna T, Yamamoto S, Morisawa S. Partial purification of the cholestatic factor derived from the lymphocytes of tuberculin-sensitized guinea pigs. Gastroenterol Jpn 1981; 16: 260–267
288. Yamada S, Takehara K, Takayuki A et al. Immunocytochemical studies on cholestatic factor in human liver with or without cholestasis. Liver 1990; 10: 129–136
289. Calmus Y, Arvieux C, Gane P et al. Cholestasis induces major histocompatibility class I expression in hepatocytes. Gastroenterology 1992; 102: 1371–1377
290. Rubin E, Popper H. The evolution of human cirrhosis deduced from observations in experimental animals. Medicine 1967; 46: 163–183

291. Slott P A, Liu M H, Tavoloni N. Origin, pattern and mechanism of bile duct proliferation following biliary obstruction in the rat. Gastroenterology 1990; 99: 466–477

292. Fausto N, Lemire J M, Shiojiri N. Oval cells in liver carcinogenesis: cell lineages in hepatic development and the identification of facultative stem cells in normal liver. In: Sirica A E, ed. The role of cell types in hepatocarcinogenesis. Boca Raton: CRC Press, 1992: pp 89–108

293. Sell S. Is there a liver stem cell? Cancer Res 1990; 50: 3811–3815

294. Bisgaard H C, Thorgeirsson S S. Evidence for a common cell of origins for primitive epithelial cells isolated from rat liver and pancreas. J Cell Physiol 1991: 147: 333–343

295. Thorgeirsson S S, Evarts R P. Hepatic stem cell compartment in the rat. In: Bock K W, Matern S, Gerok W, Schmid R, eds. Hepatic metabolism and disposition of endo- and xenobiotics. Dordrecht: Kluwer Academic Publishers, 1991: pp 19–26

296. Thorgeirsson S S, Evarts R P. Growth and differentiation of stem cells in adult rat liver. In: Sirica A E, ed. The role of cell types in hepatocarcinogenesis. Boca Raton: CRC Press, 1992: pp 109–120

297. Thorgeirsson S S, Huggett A C, Bisgaard H C. Phenotypic characteristics and neoplastic transformation of primitive epithelial cells derived from rat liver and pancreas. In: Clément B, Guillouzo A, eds. Cellular and molecular aspects of cirrhosis. Colloque INSERM/John Libbey Eurotext, 1992: pp 287–298

298. Sell S. Liver stem cells. Mod Pathol 1994; 7: 105–112

299. Van Eyken P, Desmet V J. Development of intrahepatic bile ducts, ductular metaplasia of hepatocytes, and cytokeratin patterns in various types of human hepatic neoplasms. In: Sirica A E, ed. The role of cell types in hepatocarcinogenesis. Boca Raton: CRC Press, 1992: pp 227–263

300. De Vos R, Desmet V. Ultrastructural characteristics of novel epithelial cell types identified in human pathologic liver specimens with chronic ductular reaction. Am J Pathol 1992; 6: 1441–1450

301. Desmet V J. Modulation of biliary epithelium. In: Bianchi L, Reutter W, eds. Modulation of liver cell expression. Lancaster: MTP Press, 1986: pp 195–214

302. Desmet V J. Cirrhosis : aetiology and pathogenesis:cholestasis. In: Boyer J L, Bianchi L, eds. Liver cirrhosis. Falk Symposium 44. Lancaster: MTP Press, 1987: pp 101–118

303. James J, Lygidakis N J, Van Eyken P et al. Application of keratin immunocytochemistry and Sirius red staining in evaluating intrahepatic changes with acute extrahepatic cholestasis due to hepatic duct carcinoma. Hepatogastroenterology 1989: 36: 151–155

304. Desmet V J, Callea F. Cholestatic syndromes of infancy and childhood. In: Zakim D, Boyer T D, eds. Hepatology. A textbook of liver disease, vol 2, 2nd edn. Philadelphia: Saunders, 1990: pp 1355–1395

305. Nakanuma Y, Sasaki M. Expression of blood group-related antigens in the intrahepatic biliary tree and hepatocytes in normal livers and various hepatobiliary diseases. Hepatology 1989; 10: 174–178

306. Roskams T, Van den Oord J J, De Vos R, Desmet V J. Neuro-endocrine features of reactive bile ductules in cholestatic liver disease. Am J Pathol 1990; 137: 1019–1025

307. Volpes R, Van den Oord J J, Desmet V J. Distribution of the VLA family of integrins in normal and pathological human liver tissue. Gastroenterology 1991; 101: 200–206

308. Nakanuma Y, Ohta G. Immunohistochemical study on bile ductular proliferation in various hepatobiliary diseases. Liver 1986; 6: 205–211

309. Hahn E G, Kirchner J, Schuppan D. Perisinusoidal fibrogenesis and ductular metaplasia of hepatocytes in focal nodular hyperplasia of the liver. J Hepatol 1987; 5: S32

310. Bucher N L R, Robinson G S, Farmer S R. Effects of extracellular matrix on hepatocyte growth and gene expression: implications for hepatic regeneration and the repair of liver injury. Semin Liver Dis 1990; 10: 11–19

311. Hillan K J, Burt A D, George W D, MacSween R N M, Griffiths M R, Bradley J A. Intrasplenic hepatocyte transplantation in rats with experimental liver injury: morphological and morphometric studies. J Pathol 1989; 159: 67–73

312. Yamada S, Howe S, Scheuer P J. Three-dimensional reconstruction of biliary pathways in primary biliary cirrhosis: a computer-assisted study. J Pathol 1987; 152: 317–323

313. Buscher H-P, Miltenberger C, MacNelly G, Gerok W. The histoautoradiographic localization of taurocholate in rat liver after bile duct ligation. J Hepatol 1989; 8: 181–191

314. Sasaki H, Schaffner F, Popper H. Bile ductules in cholestasis. Morphologic evidence for secretion and absorption in man. Lab Invest 1967; 16: 84–95

315. Bulle F, Mavier P, Zafrani E S et al. Mechanism of gamma-glutamyl transpeptidase release in serum during intrahepatic and extrahepatic cholestasis in the rat: a histochemical, biochemical and molecular approach. Hepatology 1990; 11: 545–550

316. Serrao D, Cardoso V. Histodynamic interpretation of biliary epithelio-mesenchymatous reactions in experimental cholestasis. Pathol Eur 1973; 8: 219–234

317. Carlson E, Zukoski C F, Campbell J, Chvapil M. Morphologic, biophysical, and biochemical consequences of ligation of the common biliary duct in the dog. Am J Pathol 1977; 86: 301–320

318. Aronson D C, De Haan J, James J, Bosch K S, Ketel A G, Houtkooper J M, Heijmans H S A. Quantitative aspects of the parenchyma–stroma relationship in experimentally induced cholestasis. Liver 1988; 8: 116–126

319. Abdel-Aziz G, Lebeau G, Rescan P Y et al. Reversibility of hepatic fibrosis in experimentally induced cholestasis in rat. Am J Pathol 1990; 137: 1333–1342

320. Milani S, Herbst H, Schuppan D, Surrenti C, Riecken E O, Stein H. Cellular localization of type I, III and IV procollagen gene transcripts in normal and fibrotic human liver. Am J Pathol 1990; 137: 59–70

321. Milani S, Herbst H, Schuppan D, Kim K Y, Riecken E O, Stein H. Procollagen expression by nonparenchymal rat liver cells in experimental biliary fibrosis. Gastroenterology 1990; 98: 175–184

322. Miyabayashi C, Kojima T, Inoue K, Sasaki H, Muragaki Y, Ooshima A. Ultrastructural localization of type IV collagen, laminin and prolylhydroxylase in biliary epithelial cells of rat liver following ligation of the common bile duct. Gastroenterol Jpn 1987; 22: 354–369

323. Callea F, Mebis J, Desmet V J. Myofibroblasts in focal nodular hyperplasia of the liver. Virchows Arch [A] 1982; 396: 155–166

324. Schmitt-Gräff A, Krüger S, Bochard F, Gabbiani G, Denk H. Modulation of alpha smooth muscle actin and desmin expression in perisinusoidal cells of normal and diseased human livers. Am J Pathol 1991; 138: 1233–1242

325. Pinzani M, Milani S, Grappone C. Cholestasis and fibrogenesis. In: Gentilini P, Arias I M, McIntyre N, Rodes J, eds. Cholestasis. Amsterdam: Excerpta Medica, 1994: pp 129–139

326. Van Eyken P, Sciot R, Desmet V J. Expression of the novel extracellular matrix component tenascin in normal and diseased human liver. An immunohistochemical study. J Hepatol 1990; 11: 43–52

327. Miyazaki H, Van Eyken P, Roskams T, De Vos R, Desmet V J. Transient expression of tenascin in experimentally induced cholestatic fibrosis in rat liver. An immunohistochemical study. J Hepatol 1993; 19: 353–366

328. Griffiths M R, Shepherd M, Ferrier R, Schuppan D, James O F W, Burt A D. Light microscopic and ultrastructural distribution of type VI collagen in human liver: alterations in chronic biliary disease. Histopathology 1992; 21: 335–344

329. Shibayama Y, Nakata K. Haemodynamic alterations and their morphological basis in biliary obstruction. Liver 1992; 12: 175–178

330. Milani S, Herbst H, Schuppan D, Stein H, Surrent C. Transforming growth factors β1 and β2 are differentially expressed in fibrotic liver disease. Am J Pathol 1991; 139: 1221–1229

331. Roskams T, De Vos R, Van den Oord J J, Desmet V. Cells with neuroendocrine features in regenerating human liver. APMIS Suppl 1991; Suppl 23: 32–39

332. Roskams T, Campos R V, Drucker D J, Desmet V J. Reactive human bile ductules express parathyroid hormone-like peptide. Histopathology 1993; 23: 11–20

333. Bhathal P S, Gall J A M. Deletion of hyperplastic biliary epithelial cells by apoptosis following removal of the proliferative stimulus. Liver 1985; 5: 311–325

334. Heuman D M, Pandak W M, Hylemon P B, Vlahcevic Z R. Conjugates of ursodeoxycholate protect against cytotoxicity of

more hydrophobic bile salts: in vitro studies in rat hepatocytes and human erythrocytes. Hepatology 1991; 14: 920–926

335. Poo J L, Feldmann G, Erlinger S et al. Ursodeoxycholic acid limits liver histologic alterations and portal hypertension induced by bile duct ligation in the rat. Gastroenterology 1992; 102: 1752–1759

336. Poupon R, Calmus Y, Poupon R E. Mechanisms of hepatoprotection by ursodeoxycholic acid. In: Lentze M, Reichen J, eds. Paediatric cholestasis. Novel approaches to treatment Dordrecht: Kluwer Academic Publishers, 1992: pp 319–324

337. Poupon R E, Poupon R. Ursodeoxycholic acid for the treatment of cholestatic diseases. In: Boyer J L, Ockner R K, eds. Progress in liver diseases, vol X. Philadelphia: Saunders, 1992: pp 219–238

338. Poupon R E, Balkau B, Eschwège E, Poupon R, UDCA-PBC Study Group. A multicenter, controlled trial of ursodiol for the treatment of primary biliary cirrhosis. N Engl J Med 1991; 324: 1548–1554

339. Lentze M, Reichen J. Paediatric cholestasis. Novel approaches to treatment. In: Lentze M, Reichen J, eds. Dordrecht: Kluwer Academic Publishers, 1992: p 370

340. Bergan A, Taksdal S, Sander J. Transport and conjugation of 14C-Bilirubin during acute and chronic cholestasis in the cholecystectomized dog. Eur J Surg Res 1975; 7: 355–365

341. Szabo G Y, Magyar Z, Jakab F. Bile constituents in blood and lymph during biliary obstruction. I. The dynamics of absorption and transport of ions and colloid molecules. Lymphology 1975; 8: 29–36

342. Szabo G Y, Magyar Z, Szentirmai A, Jakab F, Mihaly K. Bile constituents in blood and lymph during biliary obstruction. II. The absorption and transport of bile acids and bilirubin. Lymphology 1975; 8: 36–42

343. Szabo G, Jakab F, Mihaly K, Szentirmai A. The retention of bile constituents in biliary stasis. Acta Hepatogastroenterol 1976; 23: 415–422

344. Waldeck F. Sekretion und Rückfluss von Galle während und nach chronischer Gallenstauung bei Ratten. Pflugers Arch 1970; 320: 300–317

345. Boyer J L. Tight junctions in normal and cholestatic liver: does the paracellular pathway have functional significance? Hepatology 1983; 3: 614–617

346. Matter A, Orci L, Rouiller C. A study on the permeability barriers between Disse's space and the bile canaliculus. J Ultrastruct Res 1969; 11: 1–71

347. Jones A L, Hradek G T, Schmucker D L, Underdown B J. The fate of polymeric and secretory immunoglobulin A after retrograde infusion into the common bile duct in rats. Hepatology 1984; 4: 1173–1183

348. Kaplan M, Righetti A. Induction of rat liver alkaline phosphatase: the mechanism of the serum elevation in bile duct obstruction. J Clin Invest 1970; 49: 508–516

349. Seetharam S, Sussman N L, Komoda T, Alpers D H. The mechanism of elevated alkaline phosphatase activity after bile duct ligation in the rat. Hepatology 1986; 6: 374–380

350. Brocklehurst D. The alkaline phosphatase–lipoprotein X complex. Clin Chem 1981; 27: 1317–1318

351. De Broe M E, Wieme R G. The cholestatic doublet of alkaline phosphatase; its origin and clinical significance. In: Markert C L, ed. Isozymes III, developmental biology. New York: Academic Press, 1975: pp 799–807

352. De Broe M E, Borgers M, Wieme R J. The separation and characterization of liver plasma membrane fragments circulating in the blood of patients with cholestasis. Clin Chim Acta 1975; 59: 369–372

353. Kihn L, Dinwoodie A, Stinson R A. High-molecular-weight alkaline phosphatase in serum has properties similar to the enzyme in plasma membranes of the liver. Am J Clin Pathol 1991; 96: 470–478

354. Schlaeger R, Haux P, Kattermann R. Studies on the mechanism of the increase in serum alkaline phosphatase activity in cholestasis: significance of the hepatic bile acid concentration for the leakage of alkaline phosphatase from rat liver. Enzyme 1982; 28: 3

355. Gardner B. Marked elevation of serum transaminases in obstructive jaundice. Am J Surg 1966; 111: 575–579

356. Harry D S, McIntyre N. Plasma lipids and lipoproteins. In: McIntyre N, Benhamou J P, Bircher J, Rizzetto M, Rodes J, eds. Oxford Textbook of clinical hepatology, vol 1. Oxford: Oxford University Press, 1991: pp 143–157

357. Sabesin S M. Cholestatic lipoproteins — their pathogenesis and significance. Gastroenterology 1982; 83: 704–709

358. McIntyre N, Rosalki S. Biochemical investigations in the management of liver disease. In: McIntyre N, Benhamou J P, Bircher J, Rizzetto M, Rodes J, eds. Oxford Textbook of clinical hepatology, vol 1. Oxford: Oxford University Press, 1991: pp 293–309

359. Sherlock S. Diseases of the liver and biliary system. 7th edn. Oxford: Blackwell Scientific Publications, 1985

360. Warren K W, Tan E G C. Diseases of the gallbladder and bile ducts. In: Schiff L, ed. Diseases of the liver, 4th edn, ch 38. Philadelphia: Lippincott, 1975: pp 1278–1335

361. Wise L, Pizzimbono C, Dehner L P. Periampullary cancer. A clinico-pathologic study of sixty-two patients. Am J Surg 1976; 131: 141–147

362. Gertsch P, Blumgart L H. Malignant biliary tract obstruction. In: McIntyre N, Benhamou J P, Bircher J, Rizzetto M, Rodes J, eds. Oxford Textbook of clinical hepatology, vol 2. Oxford: Oxford University Press, 1991: pp 1053–1068

363. Miros M, Kerlin P, Walker N, Harper J, Lynch S, Strong R. Predicting cholangiocarcinoma in patients with primary sclerosing cholangitis before transplantation. Gut 1991; 32: 1369–1373

364. Klatskin G. Adenocarcinoma of the hepatic duct at its bifurcation within the porta hepatis. Am J Med 1965; 38: 241–256

365. Burhans R, Myers R T. Benign neoplasms of the extrahepatic biliary ducts. Am Surg 1971; 37: 161–166

366. Dooley J S. Cholangitis and biliary tract infections. In: McIntyre N, Benhamou J P, Bircher J, Rizzetto M, Rodes J, eds. Oxford Textbook of clinical hepatology, vol 2. Oxford: Oxford University Press, 1992: pp 1134–1139

367. Lim J H. Oriental cholangiohepatitis: pathologic, clinical, and radiologic features. Am J Roentgenol 1991; 157: 1–8

368. Beck K. Color atlas of laparoscopy. Philadelphia: Saunders, 1984

369. Shorter R G, Baggenstoss A H. Extrahepatic cholestasis. III. Chronology of histologic changes in the liver. Am J Clin Pathol 1959; 32: 10–17

370. Bianchi L. Liver biopsy interpretation in hepatitis. Part II. Histopathology and classification of acute and chronic viral hepatitis. Differential diagnosis. Pathol Res Pract 1983; 178: 180–213

371. Itoh S, Inomata R, Matsuyama Y, Matsuo S, Gohara S. Calcium staining in diseased liver. J Hepatol 1992; 15: 414–415

372. Bianchi L, Meinecke R. Histologie des Leberpunktates und Ikterus. In: Beck K, ed. Ikterus. Stuttgart: Schattauer Verlag, 1968: pp 351–356

373. Gardiol D, Loup P. Critères histologiques de la cholestase extrahépatique. Acta Hepatosplenol 1971; 18: 253–261

374. Scheuer P J. Liver biopsy interpretation, 4th edn. London: Bailliére Tindall, 1988

375. Treem W R, Krzymowski G A, Cartun R W, Pedersen C A, Hyams J S, Berman M. Cytokeratin immunohistochemical examination of liver biopsies in infants with Alagille syndrome and biliary atresia. J Pediatr Gastroenterol Nutr 1992; 15: 73–80

376. Christoffersen P, Poulsen H. Histological changes in human liver biopsies following extrahepatic biliary obstruction. Acta Pathol Microbiol Scand Suppl 1970; 212: 150–157

377. Poulsen H, Christoffersen P. Histological changes in liver biopsies from patients with surgical bile duct disorders. Acta Pathol Microbiol Scand 1970; 78A: 571–579

378. Gall E A, Dobrogorski O. Hepatic alterations in obstructive jaundice. Am J Clin Pathol 1964; 41: 126–139

379. Thaler H. Leberkrankheiten. Histologie, Pathophysiologie, Klinik, 2nd edn. Berlin: Springer Verlag, 1987

380. Matzen P, Junge J, Christoffersen P, Poulsen H. Reproducibility and accuracy of liver biopsy findings suggestive of an obstructive cause of jaundice. In: Brunner H, Thaler H, eds. Hepatology, a Festschrift for Hans Popper. New York: Raven Press, 1985: pp 285–293

381. Popper H, Schaffner F. Liver, structure and function. New York: McGraw-Hill, 1957

382. Heimann R. Factors producing liver cell necrosis in experimental obstruction of the common bile duct. J Pathol Bacteriol 1965; 90: 479–485

383. Popper H. Morphological and immunological studies on chronic

aggressive hepatitis and primary biliary cirrhosis. In: Smith M, Williams R, eds. Immunology of the liver. London: Heinemann, 1971: pp 17–27

384. Johnstone J M S, Lee E G. A quantitative assessment of the structural changes in the rat's liver following obstruction of the common bile duct. Br J Exp Pathol 1976; 57: 85–94

385. Popper H. General pathology of the liver: light microscopic aspects serving diagnosis and interpretation. Semin Liver Dis 1986; 6: 175–184

386. Ludwig J. New concepts in biliary cirrhosis. Semin Liver Dis 1987; 7: 293–301

387. Desmet V J. General pathology. In: McIntyre N, Benhamou J-P, Bircher J, Rizzetto M, Rodes J, eds. Oxford Textbook of clinical hepatology, vol 1. Oxford: Oxford University Press, 1991: pp 263–269

388. Becker V. Dauerdruckfolge an den Gallengangsepithelien. In: Beck K, ed. Ikterus. Stuttgart: Schattauer Verlag, 1968: pp 362–363

389. Desmet V J. Liver reaction patterns in infections. In: Bianchi L, Maier K-P, Gerok W, Deinhardt F, eds. Infectious diseases of the liver. Dordrecht: Kluwer Academic Publishers, 1990: pp 31–47

390. Christoffersen P, Poulsen H, Skeie E. Focal liver cell necroses accompanied by infiltration of granulocytes arising during operation. Acta Hepato-Splenol 1970; 17: 240–245

391. Yokoi H. Morphologic changes of the liver in obstructive jaundice and its reversibility — with special reference to morphometric analysis of ultrastructure of the liver in dogs. Acta Hepatol Jpn 1983; 24: 1381–1391

392. Bunton G L, Cameron R. Regeneration of liver after biliary cirrhosis. Ann N Y Acad Sci 1963; 111: 412–421

393. Cameron S R, Hou P C. Biliary cirrhosis. Edinburgh: Oliver & Boyd, 1962

394. So S U, Bondar G F. Effect of transient biliary obstruction on liver function and morphology. Can J Surg 1974; 17: 49–58

395. Younes R N, Vydelingum N A, De Rooij P et al. Metabolic alterations in obstructive jaundice: effect of duration of jaundice and bile-duct decompression. HPB Surg 1991; 5: 35–48

396. Melzer E, Krepel Z, Ronen I, Bar-Meir S. Recovery of hepatic clearance and extraction following a release of common bile duct obstruction in the rat. Res Exp Med 1992; 192: 35–40

397. Yaari A, Sikuler E, Keynen A, Ben-Zvi Z. Bromosulfophthalein disposition in chronically bile duct obstructed rats. J Hepatol 1992; 15: 67–72

398. Scobie B A, Summerskill W H J. Hepatic cirrhosis secondary to obstruction of the biliary system. Am J Dig Dis 1965; 10: 135–146

399. Rutherford R B, Biotnott J K, Donohoo J S, Ohlsson E G, Sebor J, Zuidema G D. The production of biliary cirrhosis in Macaca mulatta monkeys. Arch Srug 1970; 100: 55–60

400. Kountouras J, Billing B H, Scheuer P J. Prolonged bile duct obstruction: a new experimental model for cirrhosis in the rat. Br J Exp Pathol 1984; 65: 305–311

401. Foulk W T, Baggenstoss A H. Biliary cirrhosis. In: Schiff L, ed. Diseases of the liver, 4th edn, ch 27. Philadelphia: Lippincott, 1975: pp 940–970

402. Anthony P P, Ishak K G, Nayak N C, Poulsen H, Scheuer P J, Sobin L H. The morphology of cirrhosis: definition, nomenclature and classification. Bull WHO 1977; 55: 521–540

403. Bissell D M. Connective tissue metabolism and hepatic fibrosis: an overview. Semin Liver Dis 1990; 10: iii–iv

404. Koyama K, Muto I, Yamauchi H, Takagi Y, Amezaki T, Sato T. Biochemical study of fibrosis in the rat liver in biliary obstruction. Tohoku J Exp Med 1975; 116: 161–172

405. Gay S, Inouye T, Minick O T, Kent G, Popper H. Basement membrane formation in experimental hepatic injury. Gastroenterology 1976; 71: 907

406. Arthur M J P. Matrix degradation in the liver. Semin Liver Dis 1990; 10: 47–55

407. Popper H. Pathologic aspects of cirrhosis. A review. Am J Pathol 1977; 87: 227–264

408. Kram R. Etude de la régénération du foie et des voies biliaires après ligature du canal cholédoque chez le rat. Rev Belg Pathol Med Exp 1965; 31: 5

409. Tracy T F Jr, Bailey P V, Goerke M E, Sotelo-Avila C, Weber T R.

Cholestasis without cirrhosis alters regulatory liver gene expression and inhibits hepatic regeneration. Surgery 1991; 110: 176–183

410. Weinbren K. The effect of bile duct obstruction on regeneration of the rat's liver. Br J Exp Pathol 1953; 34: 280–289

411. Weinbren K, Hadjis N S, Blumgart L H. Structural aspects of the liver in patients with biliary disease and portal hypertension. J Clin Pathol 1985; 38: 1013–1020

412. Lee E, Ross B D, Haines J R. Effect of experimental bile-duct obstruction on critical biosynthetic functions of the liver. Br J Surg 1972; 59: 564–568

413. Rappaport A M, MacPhee P J, Fisher M M, Phillips M J. The scarring of the liver acini (cirrhosis). Tridimensional and microcirculatory considerations. Virchows Arch [A] 1983; 402: 107–137

414. Baggenstoss A H. Morphological features: their usefulness in the diagnosis, prognosis and management of cirrhosis. Clin Gastroenterol 1975; 4: 227–246

415. Setchell K D R, Street J M. Inborn errors of bile acid metabolism. Semin Liver Dis 1987; 7: 85–99

416. Setchell K D R, Piccoli D, Heubi J, Balistreri W F. Inborn errors of bile acid metabolism. In: Lentze M, Reichen J, eds. Paediatric cholestasis. Novel approaches to treatment. Dordrecht: Kluwer Academic Publishers, 1992: pp 153–158

417. Diaz de Otazu R, Garcia-Campos F, Basterra G, Lopez-Barbarin J M. Nodular regenerative hyperplasia and focal nodular hyperplasia of the liver associated with severe cholestasis. Liver 1986; 6: 30–34

418. Riely C A. Familial intrahepatic cholestatic syndromes. Semin Liver Dis 1987; 7: 119–133

419. Balistreri W F. Neonatal cholestasis. J Pediatr 1985; 106: 171–184

420. Balistreri W F. Interrelationship between the infantile cholangiopathies and paucity of the intrahepatic bile ducts. In: Balistreri W F, Stocker J T, eds. Pediatric hepatology. New York: Hemisphere Publishing Corporation, 1990: pp 1–18

421. Kahn E. Paucity of interlobular bile ducts. Arteriohepatic dysplasia and nonsyndromic duct paucity. In: Abramowsky C R, Bernstein J, Rosenberg H S, eds. Perspectives in pediatric pathology. Transplantation pathology — hepatic morphogenesis. Basel: Karger, 1991: pp 168–215

422. Desmet V J. Vanishing bile duct disorders. In: Boyer J L, Ockner R K, eds. Progress in liver diseases, vol X. Philadelphia: Saunders, 1992: pp 89–121

423. Witzleben C L, Finegold M, Piccoli D A, Treem W R. Bile canalicular morphometry in arteriohepatic dysplasia. Hepatology 1987; 7: 1262–1266

424. Alagille D, Odièvre M, Hadchouel M. Paucity of interlobular bile ducts: recent concepts. In: Kasai M, ed. Biliary atresia and its related disorders. Amsterdam: Excerpta Medica, 1983: pp 59–65

425. Vonk R J, Kuipers F, Smit M J et al. Bile acid metabolism in children. In: Lentze M, Reichen J, eds. Paediatric cholestasis. Novel approaches to treatment. Dordrecht: Kluwer Academic Publishers, 1992: pp 27–37

426. Suchy F J, Bucuvalas J C, Novak D A. Determinants of bile formation during development: ontogeny of hepatic bile acid metabolism and transport. Semin Liver Dis 1987; 7: 77–84

427. Belknap W M, Balistreri W F, Suchy F J, Miller P C. Physiologic cholestasis. II. Serum bile acid levels reflect the development of the enterohepatic circulation in rats. Hepatology 1981; 1: 613–616

428. Van Eyken P, Sciot R, Callea F, Van der Steen K, Moerman P, Desmet V J. The development of the intrahepatic bile ducts in man: a keratin-immunohistochemical study. Hepatology 1988; 8: 1586–1595

429. US Government Printing Office. Diseases of the liver and biliary tract: Standardization of nomenclature, diagnostic criteria, and diagnostic methodology. Fogarty Int Center Proc No. 22, DHEW Publication No. (NIH) 76–725, 1976

430. Clayton R I, Iber F L, Ruebner B H, McKusick V A. Byler disease. Fatal familial intrahepatic cholestasis in an Amish kindred. Am J Dis Child 1969; 117: 112–124

431. Whitington P F, Freese D K, Alonso E M, Fishbein M H, Emond J C. Progressive familial intrahepatic cholestasis (Byler's disease). In: Lentze M, Reichen J, eds. Paediatric cholestasis. Novel approaches to treatment. Dordrecht: Kluwer Academic Publishers, 1992: pp 165–183

432. Chobert M N, Bernard O, Bulle F, Lemonnier A, Guellaen G, Alagille D. High hepatic γ-glutamyltransferase (γGT) activity with normal serum γ-GT in children with progressive idiopathic cholestasis. J Hepatol 1989; 8: 22–25

433. Linarelli L G, Williams C N, Phillips M J. Byler's disease: fatal intrahepatic cholestasis. J Pediatr 1972; 81; 484–492

434. Williams C N, Kaye R, Baker L, Hurwitz R, Senior J R. Progressive familial cholestatic cirrhosis and bile acid metabolism. J Pediatr 1972; 81: 492–500

435. Partin J S, Schubert W K, Partin J C. Unique ultrastructural abnormality of hepatic mitochondria in a patient with Byler-like cholestatic syndrome. Gastroenterology 1975; 69: 852 (Abstract)

436. Nielsen I M, Ornvold K, Jacobsen B B, Ranek L. Fatal familial cholestatic syndrome in Greenland Eskimo children. Acta Paediatr Scand 1986; 75: 1010–1016

437. Ornvold K, Nielsen I M, Poulsen H. Fatal familial cholestatic syndrome in Greenland Eskimo children. A histomorphological analysis of 16 cases. Virchows Arch [A] 1989; 415: 275–281

438. Setchell K D R, Suchy F J, Welsh M B, Zimmer-Nichemias L, Heubi J, Balistreri W F. Δ 4-3-Oxosteroid 5β-reductase deficiency described in identical twins with neonatal hepatitis. A new inborn error in bile acid synthesis. J Clin Invest 1988; 82: 2148–2157

439. Balistreri W F. Fetal and neonatal bile acid synthesis and metabolism — clinical implications. J Inherited Metab Dis 1991; 14: 459–477

440. Aagenaes Ø, Van Der Hagen C B, Refsum S. Hereditary recurrent intrahepatic cholestasis from birth. Arch Dis Child 1968; 43: 646–657

441. Shiraki K, Okaniwa M, Landing B H. Cholestatic syndromes of infancy and childhood. In: Zakim D, Boyer T D, eds. Hepatology. A textbook of liver disease. Philadelphia: Saunders, 1982: pp 1176–1192

442. Sharp H L, Krivit W. Hereditary lymphedema and obstructive jaundice. J Pediatr 1971; 78: 491–496

443. Sveger T. Alpha-1-antitrypsin deficiency in early childhood. Pediatrics 1978; 63: 22–25

444. Hadchouel M, Gautier M. Histopathologic study of the liver in the early cholestatic phase of alpha-1-antitrypsin deficiency. J Pediatr 1976; 89: 211–215

445. Hodges J R, Millward-Sadler G H, Barbatis C, Wright R. Heterozygous MZ alpha-1-antitrypsin deficiency in adults with chronic active hepatitis and cryptogenic cirrhosis. N Engl J Med 1981; 304: 557–560

446. Summerskill W H J, Walshe J M. Benign recurrent intrahepatic 'obstructive' jaundice. Lancet 1959; ii: 686–690

447. Tygstrup N. Intermittent possibly familial intrahepatic cholestatic jaundice. Lancet 1960; i: 1171–1172

448. De Groote J, Goubeau P, Vandenbroucke J. Ictère cholestatique recidivant. Acta Gastroenterol Belg 1960; 23: 747–754

449. Marcellin P, Erlinger S. Benign recurrent cholestasis. Gastroenterol Clin Biol 1985; 9: 679–684

450. Brenard R, Geubel A P, Benhamou J-P. Benign recurrent intrahepatic cholestasis. A report of 26 cases. J Clin Gastroenterol 1989; 11: 546–551

451. Tygstrup N, Jensen B. Intermittent intrahepatic cholestasis of unknown etiology in five young males from the Faroe Islands. Acta Med Scand 1969; 185: 523–530

452. Summerfield J A, Kirk A P, Chitranukroh A, Billing B H. A distinctive pattern of serum bile acid and bilirubin concentration in benign recurrent intrahepatic cholestasis. Hepatogastroenterology 1981; 28: 139–142

453. Bijleveld C M, Vonk R J, Kuipers F et al. Benign recurrent intrahepatic cholestasis: altered bile acid metabolism. Gastroenterology 1989; 97: 427–432

454. Van Berge Henegouwen G P, De Pagter A G F, Brandt K H. Benign recurrent cholestasis. Acta Gastroenterol Belg 1979; 42: 363–368

455. Tygstrup N, Petersen P, Bremmelgaard A. Ultrastructural findings and bile acid patterns in idiopathic intermittent intrahepatic cholestasis. In: Gentilini P, Popper H, Sherlock S, Teodori U, eds. Problems in intrahepatic cholestasis. Basel: Karger, 1979: pp 47–52

456. De Pagter A G F, Van Berghe Henegouwen G P, Ten Bokkel Huininck J A, Brandt K H. Familial benign recurrent intrahepatic cholestasis — interrelation with intrahepatic cholestasis of

pregnancy and from oral contraceptives? Gastroenterology 1976; 71: 202–207

457. Reyes H. The enigma of intrahepatic cholestasis of pregnancy: lessons from Chile. Hepatology 1982; 2: 87–96

458. Biempica L, Gutstein S, Arias I M. Morphological and biochemical studies of benign recurrent cholestasis. Gastroenterology 1967; 52: 521–535

459. Beaudouin M, Feldmann G, Erlinger S, Benhamou J-P. Benign recurrent cholestasis. Digestion 1973; 9: 49–65

460. Adlercreutz H, Tenhunen R. Some aspects of the interaction between natural and synthetic female sex hormones and the liver. Am J Med 1970; 49: 630–648

461. Holzbach R T. Jaundice in pregnancy. Am J Med 1976; 61: 367–376

462. Lunzer M R. Jaundice in pregnancy. Baillière's Clin Gastroenterol 1989; 3: 467–483

463. Burroughs A K. Liver disease and pregnancy. In: McIntyre N, Benhamou J-P, Bircher J, Rizzetto M, Rodes J, eds. Oxford Textbook of clinical hepatology, vol 2. Oxford: Oxford University Press, 1991: pp 1321–1332

464. Frezza M, Pozzato G, Chiesa L, Stramentinoli G, Di Padova C. Reversal of intrahepatic cholestasis of pregnancy in women after high dose S-adenosyl-L-methionine administration. Hepatology 1984; 4: 274–278

465. Haemmerli U P, Wyss H I. Recurrent intrahepatic cholestasis of pregnancy; report of six cases, and review of the literature. Medicine 1967; 46: 299–321

466. Eriksson S, Larsson C. Familial benign chronic intrahepatic cholestasis. Hepatology 1983; 3: 391–398

467. Blanckaert N, Fevery J. Physiology and pathophysiology of bilirubin metabolism. In: Zakim D, Boyer T D, eds. Hepatology. A textbook of liver disease, vol 1, 2nd edn. Philadelphia: Saunders, 1990: pp 254–302

468. Hauser S C, Gollan J. Bilirubin metabolism and hyperbilirubinaemic disorders. In: Millward-Sadler G H, Wright R, Arthur M J P, eds. Wright's Liver and biliary disease. Pathophysiology, diagnosis and management, vol 1, 3rd edn. London: Saunders 1992: pp 317–370

469. Sorrentino D, Jones E A, Berk P D. Familial hyperbilirubinaemia syndromes: kinetic approaches. Baillière's Clin Gastroenterol 1989; 3: 313–336

470. Sinaasappel M, Jansen P L M. The differential diagnosis of Crigler–Najjar disease, types 1 and 2, by bile pigment analysis. Gastroenterology 1991; 100: 783–789

471. Bosma P J, Chowdury N R, Goldhoorn B G et al. Sequence of exons and the flanking regions of human bilirubin-VDP-glucoronosyl-transferase gene complex and identification of a genetic mutation in a patient with Crigler–Najjar syndrome, type I. Hepatology 1992; 15: 941–947

472. Van Es H H G, Goldhoorn B G, Paul-Abrahamse M, Oude Elferink R P J, Jansen P L M. Immunochemical analysis of uridine diphosphate-glucuronosyltransferase in four patients with the Crigler-Najjar syndrome type I. J Clin Invest 1990; 85: 1199–1205

473. Berg C L, Gollan J L. Metabolic liver disease. Curr Opin Gastroenterol 1991; 7: 370–376

474. Crigler J F, Najjar V A. Congenital familial nonhemolytic jaundice with kernicterus. Pediatrics 1952; 10: 169–179

475. Koch M M, Lorenzini I, Freddara U, Jezequel A-M, Orlandi F. Type 2 Crigler–Najjar syndrome. Quantitation of ultrastructural data and evolution under therapy with phenytoin. Gastroenterol Clin Biol 1978; 2: 831–842

476. Watson K J R, Gollan J L. Gilbert's syndrome. Baillière's Clin Gastroenterol 1989; 3: 337–355

477. Barth R F, Grimley P M, Berk P D, Bloomer I R, Howe R B. Excess lipofuscin accumulation in constitutional hepatic dysfunction (Gilbert's syndrome). Arch Pathol 1971; 91: 41–47

478. McGee J O'D, Allan J G, Russell R I, Patrick R S. Liver ultrastructure in Gilbert's syndrome. Gut 1975; 16: 220–224

479. Jezequel A-M, Mosca P G, Koch M M, Orlandi F. The fine morphology of unconjugated hyperbilirubinemia revisited with stereometry. In: Okalicsanyi L, ed. Familial hyperbilirubinemia. Chichester: John Wiley 1981: pp 69–79

480. Portman O W, Chowdhury J R, Chowdhury N R, Alexander M, Cornelius C E, Arias I M. A nonhuman primate model of

Gilbert's syndrome. Hepatology 1984; 4: 175–179

481. Dubin I N, Johnson F B. Chronic idiopathic jaundice with unidentified pigment in liver cells: new clinicopathologic entity with report of 12 cases. Medicine 1954; 33: 155–197

482. Sprinz H, Nelson R S. Persistent nonhemolytic hyperbilirubinemia associated with lipochrome-like pigment in liver cells: report of 4 cases. Ann Intern Med 1954; 41: 952–962

483. Ware A J, Eigenbrodt E H, Shorey J, Combes B. Viral hepatitis complicating the Dubin–Johnson syndrome. Gastroenterology 1972; 63: 331–339

484. Seymour C A, Neale G, Peters T J. Lysosomal changes in liver tissue from patients with the Dubin–Johnson–Sprinz syndrome. Clin Sci Mol Med 1977; 52: 241–248

485. Wegman R, Rangier M, Etévé J, Charbonnier A, Caroli J. Mélanose hépato-splénique avec ictère chronique à bilirubine directe. Sem Hôp Paris 1960; 36: 1761–1781

486. Swartz H M, Sarna T, Varma R R. On the nature and excretion of the hepatic pigment in the Dubin–Johnson syndrome. Gastroenterology 1979; 76: 958–964

487. Swartz H M, Chen K, Roth J A. Further evidence that the pigment in the Dubin–Johnson syndrome is not melanin. Pigment Cell Res 1987; 1: 69–75

488. Arias I, Bernstein L, Toffler R, Cornelius C, Novikoff A B, Essner E. Black liver disease in Corriedale sheep: a new mutation affecting hepatic excretory function. J Clin Invest 1964; 43: 1249–1250

489. Rotor A B, Manahan L, Florentin A. Familial jaundice with direct Van den Bergh reaction. Acta Med Phil 1948; 5: 37–49

490. Hayes P C, Bouchier I A D. Postoperative jaundice. Baillière's Clin Gastroenterol 1989; 3: 485–505

491. Lamont J T, Isselbacher K J. Postoperative jaundice. In: Millward-Sadler G H, Wright R, Arthur M J P, eds. Wright's Liver and biliary disease. Pathophysiology, diagnosis and management, vol 2, 3rd edn. London: Saunders, 1992: pp 1372–1380

492. Schmid M, Hefti M L, Gattiker R, Kistler H J, Senning A. Benign postoperative intrahepatic cholestasis. N Engl J Med 1965; 272: 545–550

493. Kantrowitz P A, Jones W A, Greenberger N J, Isselbacher K. Severe postoperative hyperbilirubinemia simulating obstructive jaundice. N Engl J Med 1967; 276: 591–598

494. Prandi D, Erlinger S, Roche-Sicot J, Husson J, Lortat-Jacob J-L. Benign post-operative intrahepatic cholestasis. Nouv Presse Med 1975; 4: 2165–2168

495. Salmeron J M, Rodes J. Postoperative jaundice. In: McIntyre N, Benhamou J-P, Bircher J, Rizzetto M, Rodes J, eds. Oxford Textbook of clinical hepatology, vol 2. Oxford: Oxford University Press, 1991: pp 1456–1460

496. Zimmerman H J (moderator). Clinical conference: Jaundice due to bacterial infection. Gastroenterology 1979; 77: 362–374

497. Miller D J, Keeton G R, Webber B L, Saunders S J. Jaundice in severe bacterial infection. Gastroenterology 1976; 71: 94–97

498. Theron J J, Pepler W J, Mekel R C P M. Ultrastructure of the liver in Bantu patients with pneumonia and jaundice. J Pathol 1972; 106: 113–117

499. Vyberg M, Poulsen H. Abnormal bile duct epithelium accompanying septicaemia. Virchows Arch [A] 1984; 402: 451–458

500. Banks J G, Foulis A K, Ledingham IMcA, MacSween R N M. Liver function in septic shock. J Clin Pathol 1982; 35: 1249–1252

501. Lefkowitch J H. Bile ductular cholestasis: an ominous histopathologic sign related to sepsis and 'cholangitis lenta'. Hum Pathol 1982: 13: 19–24

502. Lefkowitch J H. Cholestasis in the critically ill. In: Hoofnagle J H, Goodman Z, eds. Liver biopsy interpretation for the 1990's. Clinicopathologic correlations in liver disease. American Association for the Study of Liver Diseases, 1991; pp 65–75

503. Gourley G R, Chesney P J, Davis J P, Odell G B. Acute cholestasis in patients with toxic-shock syndrome. Gastroenterology 1981; 81: 928–931

504. Ishak K G, Rogers W A. Cryptogenic acute cholangitis — association with toxic shock syndrome. Am J Clin Pathol 1981; 76: 619–626

505. MacSween R N M. Liver, biliary tract and exocrine pancreas. In: Anderson J R, ed. Muir's Textbook of pathology. 12th edn. London: Edward Arnold, 1986: pp 20–37

506. Bower R H. Hepatic complications of parenteral nutrition. Semin Liver Dis 1983; 3: 216–224

507. Balistreri W F, Bucuvalas J C, Farrell M K, Bove K E. Total parenteral nutrition-associated cholestasis: factors responsible for the decreasing incidence. In: Lentze M, Reichen J, eds. Paediatric cholestasis. Novel approaches to treatment. Dordrecht: Kluwer Academic Publishers, 1992: pp 191–204

508. Cohen C, Olsen M M. Pediatric total parenteral nutrition: liver histopathology. Arch Pathol Lab Med 1981; 105: 152–156

509. Body I J, Bleiberg H, Bron D, Maurage H, Bigirimana V, Heimann R. Total parenteral nutrition-induced cholestasis mimicking large bile duct obstruction. Histopathology 1982; 6; 787–792

510. Whitington P F. Cholestasis associated with total parenteral nutrition in infants. Hepatology 1985; 5: 693–696

511. Emery I L. Pathology with reference to the bile retention syndrome. Postgrad Med J 1974; 50: 344–347

512. Buhac I, Agrawal A B, Park S K, Lomotan A, Lowen B, Balint J A. Jaundice and bridging centrilobular necrosis of liver in circulatory failure. NY State J Med 1976; 76: 678–683

513. Rappaport A M. The microcirculatory acinar concept of normal and pathological hepatic structure. Beitr Pathol 1976; 157: 215–243

514. Nolte D. Ikterus der Leber bei chronischer Herzinsuffizienz. Virchows Arch Pathol Anat Physiol Klin Med 1966; 341: 37–42

515. Sheehy T W, Law D E, Wade B H. Exchange transfusion for sickle cell intrahepatic cholestasis. Arch Intern Med 1980; 140: 1364–1366

516. Yao J D C, Gross J B, Ludwig J, Purnell D C. Cholestatic jaundice in hyperthyroidism. Am J Med 1989; 86: 619–620

517. Ariza C R, Frati A C, Sierra I. Hypothyroidism-associated cholestasis. JAMA 1984; 252: 2392

518. Rubinow A, Koff R S, Cohen A S. Severe intrahepatic cholestasis in primary amyloidosis — a report of four cases and a review of the literature. Am J Med 1978; 64: 937–946

519. Pirovino M, Altorfer J, Maranta E, Hämmerli U P, Schmid M. Ikterus vom Typ der intrahepatischen Cholestase bei Amyloidose der Leber. Z Gastroenterol 1982; 6: 321–331

520. Calomeni J A, Smith J R. Obstructive jaundice from hepatic amyloidosis in a patient with multiple myeloma. Am J Hematol 1985; 19: 277–279

521. Faa G, Van Eyken P, De Vos R, Fevery J, Van Damme B, De Groote J, Desmet V J. Light chain deposition disease of the liver associated with AL-type amyloidosis and severe cholestasis. J Hepatol 1991; 12: 75–82

522. Rudzki C, Ishak K G, Zimmerman H J. Chronic intrahepatic cholestasis of sarcoidosis. Am J Med 1975; 59: 373–387

523. Bass N M, Burroughs A K, Scheuer P J, James D G, Sherlock S. Chronic intrahepatic cholestasis due to sarcoidosis. Gut 1982; 23: 417–421

524. Bouroncle B A, Old I W Jr, Vazques A G. Pathogenesis of jaundice in Hodgkin's disease. Arch Intern Med 1962; 110: 872–883

525. Groth C G, Hellstrom K, Hofvendahl S, Nordenstam H, Wengle B. Diagnosis of malignant lymphoma at laparotomy disclosing intrahepatic cholestasis. Acta Chir Scand 1972; 138: 186–189

526. Cavalli G, Casali A M, Lambertini F, Busachi C. Changes in the small biliary passages in the hepatic localization of Hodgkin's disease. Virchows Arch [A] 1979; 384: 295–306

527. Lefkowitch J H, Falkow S, Whitlock R T. Hepatic Hodgkin's disease simulating cholestatic hepatitis with liver failure. Arch Pathol Lab Med 1985; 109: 424–426

528. Hubscher S G, Lumley M A, Elias E. Vanishing bile duct syndrome: a possible mechanism for intrahepatic cholestasis in Hodgkin's lymphoma. Hepatology 1993; 17: 70–77

529. Stauffer M H. Nephrogenic hepatosplenomegaly. Gastroenterology 1961; 40: 694

530. Strickland R C, Schenker S. The nephrogenic hepatic dysfunction syndrome: a review. Am J Dig Dis 1977; 22: 49–55

531. Reddy A N, Grosberg S J, Wapnick S. Intermittent cholestatic jaundice and nonmetastatic prostatic carcinoma. Arch Intern Med 1977; 137: 1616–1618

532. Jakobovits A W, Crimmins F B, Sherlock S, Erlinger S, Rambaud J. Cholestasis as a paraneoplastic manifestation of carcinoma of the kidney. Aust NZ J Med 1981; 11: 64–67

533. Shahara A I, Panella T J, Fitz J G. Paraneoplastic hepatopathy associated with soft tissue sarcoma. Gastroenterology 1992; 103: 330–332

12

Diseases of the intrahepatic bile ducts

B. C. Portmann   R. N. M. MacSween

This chapter deals with the different diseases in which there is injury to the intrahepatic bile ducts. These are summarized in Table 12.1; a number are discussed elsewhere in this volume and appropriate cross-references are given. We shall emphasize those histological features which characterize the early stages of the diseases in which there are distinctive bile-duct lesions that may be identified in liver biopsies. In some of these conditions, especially primary biliary cirrhosis, liver allograft rejection and graft-versus-host disease, the interlobular bile ducts, up to a diameter of 100 µm, are damaged and progressively disappear from the liver — the so-called vanishing or disappearing bile-duct disorders. In others, these structures may be affected together with larger intrahepatic and extrahepatic bile ducts; this is particularly true of primary sclerosing cholangitis which is discussed here as it shares many clinico-pathological features with primary biliary cirrhosis. In children and in adults, progressive destruction and loss of bile ducts lead to portal–portal bridging fibrosis and eventual development of a biliary cirrhosis. Thus, in their later stages, these various diseases have many pathological features in common. These closely resemble the changes seen with secondary biliary cirrhosis and which have been fully reviewed in the preceding chapter. In contrast to extrahepatic biliary obstruction, chronic intrahepatic bile-duct lesions may evolve over many years without obvious morphological cholestasis or *bilirubinostasis*. This period of evolution is characterized by profound changes at the interface between portal tracts and parenchyma — *cholate stasis* and *biliary piecemeal necrosis* — which are attributable to the effects of the prolonged impairment of bile excretion. Although some of these features have been described in Chapter 11, it seems pertinent to review them briefly as, in the absence of characteristic bile-duct lesions, their recognition is essential to distinguish biliary from other forms of chronic liver disease.

Table 12.1 Diseases of the intrahepatic bile ducts

Neonates and children
   Ductal plate malformation (infantile polycystic disease, congenital hepatic fibrosis, Caroli's disease — Ch. 3)
   Extrahepatic biliary atresia (Ch. 3)*
   Paucity of the interlobular bile ducts
      Syndromic (Alagille's syndrome) and non-syndromic (Ch. 3)
      α_1-Antitrypsin deficiency (Ch. 4)
   Cystic fibrosis (Chs. 4 and 17)
   Sclerosing cholangitis*
      Primary, with or without ulcerative colitis
      Acquired (immunodeficiency, Langerhans cell histiocytosis)

Adults
1. Destruction and progressive loss of bile ducts
   Primary biliary cirrhosis
   Sclerosing cholangitis*
      Primary or idiopathic: with or without ulcerative colitis
      Acquired:
         Opportunistic (primary or secondary immunodeficiency — AIDS)*
         Ischaemic (arterial cytotoxic infusion)*
         Toxic (treated hydatid cyst)
   Idiopathic adulthood ductopenia
   Hepatic allograft rejection (Ch. 18)
   Graft-versus-host disease (Ch. 18)
   Suppurative cholangitis usually with biliary obstruction (Chs. 7 and 11)*
   Sarcoidosis (Ch. 17)
   Hodgkin's disease (Ch. 17)

2. Usually reversible injury'to bile ducts
   Extrahepatic obstruction (Ch. 11)*
   Viral hepatitis, especially HCV, cytomegalovirus (Chs. 6 and 7)
   Drug reactions (Ch. 15)
   Septicaemia, endotoxic shock and toxic shock syndrome
   Parasitic infestation (Ch. 7)*
   Oriental recurrent pyogenic cholangitis (Chs. 7 and 10)*

*Extrahepatic bile ducts additionally and/or preferentially affected

PATHOLOGICAL FEATURES SECONDARY TO IMPAIRED BILE FLOW

The mechanisms of bile secretion and cholestasis have been described in detail in Chapter 11. As already stressed, there may be a striking discrepancy between morphological (microscopic) and clinical cholestasis. Morphological cholestasis or bilirubinostasis[1] is not only a result of mechanical biliary obstruction but a common feature of parenchymal damage of various aetiologies in which complex metabolic alterations at the level of the hepatocyte produce an abnormally thick bile which becomes inspissated in the canaliculi of acinar zone 3.[2] Conversely, conditions which are clinically cholestatic and considered as primarily biliary diseases may progress without evident bilirubinostasis on biopsy. This is mainly the case in incomplete obstruction of the biliary passages as occurs in primary biliary cirrhosis and primary sclerosing cholangitis. In these disorders, the patient experiences pruritus and there are biochemical signs of cholestasis such as raised serum alkaline phosphatase, 5'-nucleotidase, γ-glutamyltransferase and cholesterol, whereas conjugated bilirubin remains often normal or only marginally raised until the disease is very advanced. Morphologically, this pre-icteric phase is charac-terized by cholate stasis and biliary piecemeal necrosis which affects the periportal areas and, later, the periseptal areas or periphery of cirrhotic nodules.

CHOLATE STASIS

The term cholate stasis acknowledges the fact that the cytological alterations are thought to be caused by the intracellular detergent action of retained bile acids.[3] Cells in acinar zone 1 are preferentially affected as it is here that there is most bile acid transport in normal liver.[4] The hepatocytes are swollen and rounded with a distinct border and a clear cytoplasm which may contain web-like membranous and perinuclear granular remnants (Fig. 12.1a). They often contain copper and its binding protein, a polymerized form of metallothionein which accumulates in lysosomes where it is readily demonstrated by Shikata's orcein stain as black/brown granules.[5] This indirect method, unlike the rhodanine stain for copper, is not influenced by fixation;[6] it is therefore a useful diagnostic tool since, at an early stage, the demonstration of orcein-positive granules in the periportal regions is the best indicator of cholestasis (Fig. 12.1b).[7] As the lesion progresses, the thread-like reticular cytoplasm — *feathery degeneration* — acquires a greenish-brown tinge from impregnation with bilirubin, and bile pigment may later accumulate (Fig. 12.1c). During the process, there is cytoskeletal injury and this may culminate in the formation of Mallory bodies (Fig. 12.1d).[8] This is thought to reflect a toxic effect of bile acids, and possibly copper, on the microtubules with consequent aggregation of intermediate microfilament proteins. Mallory bodies in chronic cholestasis are identical morphologically and chemically to the ones observed in alcoholic liver disease,[9,10] but differ in their intra-acinar location.

BILIARY PIECEMEAL NECROSIS[11,12]

This implies a disruption of the parenchymal limiting plates by a complex process which, in addition to cholate stasis, comprises liver-cell necrosis, inflammation, fibroplasia and ductular proliferation in variable combinations (Figs 12.2a and b). The limiting plates become irregular with separation of hepatocytes, sprouting and proliferation of bile ductules and deposition of loose fibrous tissue which contrasts sharply with the compact collagen of the original portal tract or, later, of the central core of the fibrous septa. In contrast to the changes of cholate stasis, some liver-cell plates become thinner with a darker staining cytoplasm. These cells acquire phenotypic characteristics of duct cells, in particular the expression of cytokeratin 7 and 19,[13] and merge imperceptibly with the so-called proliferating ductules which develop at the periphery of the portal areas. These neo-ductules, lined by cuboidal or flattened cells, seem to arise from 'ductular metaplasia' of periportal hepatocytes,[14] and to a lesser extent from a proliferation of pre-existing

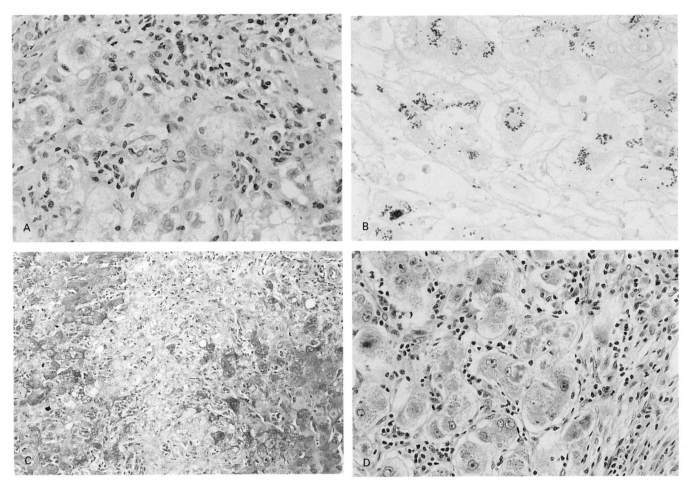

Fig. 12.1 Cholate stasis in primary biliary cirrhosis. (a) Distended and rounded hepatocytes with a clear cytoplasm containing web-like eosinophilic remnants are intermingled with ductular epithelium. H & E. (b) The hepatocytes contain orcein-positive copper-associated protein. Shikata's orcein. (c) Later stage with an extensive accumulation of feathery cells, some of which are hepatocytes and others macrophages. PAS. (d) Cholestatic phase with accumulation of bilirubin pigment and formation of Mallory bodies. H & E.

cholangioles, although the relative role of these two mechanisms may vary with the degree of biliary obstruction[15] or the duration of cholestasis.[16] The possibility of proliferation from cholangiolar stem cells has recently been suggested (see Ch. 1 and review by Burt & MacSween[17]). There is an associated inflammatory infiltrate which is usually less dense and of different cellular composition from that observed in the lymphocytic piecemeal necrosis of chronic active hepatitis (see Ch. 9).[18] In the biliary type, neutrophil polymorphs are conspicuous and may predominate. They can be numerous and are closely associated with the proliferated ductules (Fig. 12.2c); this cholangiolitis represents a tissue reaction to retention or leakage of bile rather than a true bacterial infection.[19] There is a variable accumulation of cholesterol/lipid-laden macrophages with a foamy or microvesicular appearance — xanthomatous cells.

The neo-ductules and their associated inflammation, the so-called *ductular reaction*, play an important role in portal and periportal fibroplasia, as discussed in the preceding chapter (p. 443). Surrounded by PAS-positive basement membrane, the reactive ductules are invariably set in a loose connective tissue matrix which contains type IV collagen and laminin in addition to interstitial collagens (types I, III and V). In cholestatic liver disease in man it is still uncertain whether ductular, mesenchymal cells or both are committed to matrix protein synthesis.[20] It is of interest that in the two chronic cholestatic disorders — namely paucity of the intrahepatic bile ducts (Alagille's syndrome) and chronic liver allograft rejection — in which ductular proliferation is inconspicuous, periportal fibrosis is also not a feature.

In common with chronic extrahepatic biliary obstruction, progressive fibrosis at the limiting plate produces gradual enlargement of the portal areas followed by portal–portal bridging with fibrous septa and eventually the development of a micronodular cirrhosis with parenchymal regeneration and distortion. Until very advanced, the process spares the basic acinar architecture with terminal hepatic venules and portal tracts maintaining an almost normal

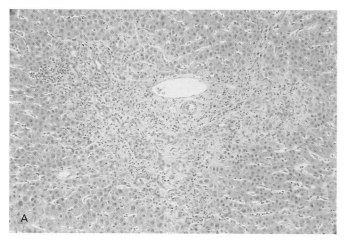

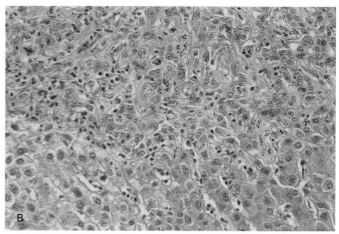

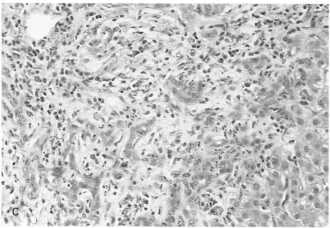

Fig. 12.2 Primary biliary cirrhosis: biliary piecemeal necrosis. (a) There is no bile duct in the portal tract; the periportal parenchyma is disturbed due to loose connective tissue containing a mixed inflammatory cell infiltrate which separates the liver-cell plates (b) some of which show tubular transformation. (a) H & E; (b) Masson's trichrome. (c) Ductular proliferation is more marked in this case and closely associated with a predominantly neutrophil infiltrate. H & E.

anatomical relationship, hence the term *monolobular cirrhosis*. This provides a hint as to the biliary aetiology of the lesion but may lead to difficulty in deciding morphologically when a true cirrhosis has been estabilshed (Fig. 12.3a). The features of cholate stasis and the deposition of oedematous collagen matrix produce a striking peripheral 'halo' which further points to the biliary nature of the lesion (Figs 12.3b–d).

Finally, it must be stressed that biliary features, including copper-associated protein deposition and Mallory bodies, may occur focally in advanced cirrhosis of any aetiology, at times involving entire nodules. These changes, which probably reflect the profound architectural distortion and subsequent interference with bile flow, may be misleading in biopsy specimens if a correct aetiological diagnosis has not previously been made.

PRIMARY BILIARY CIRRHOSIS

Primary biliary cirrhosis (PBC) is a disease which mostly affects middle-aged women. Although the first description by Addison & Gull was in 1851,[21] and its recognition as a distinct entity by Hanot was in 1876,[22] the term PBC was first introduced by Dauphinee & Sinclair in 1949.[23] Ahrens and his colleagues (1950)[24] clearly separated biliary cirrhosis

into primary and secondary types on the basis of the destruction of smaller intrahepatic bile radicles in the former and large duct obstruction in the latter. The term PBC is inaccurate, for only in the later stages is a true cirrhosis established, and a presymptomatic, or symptomatic but precirrhotic stage may last for many years. The term chronic non-suppurative destructive cholangitis[25] more accurately describes the initial lesions. Nevertheless, the term PBC is almost invariably used to describe the entire spectrum of the disease.

CLINICAL FEATURES

Diagnostic histopathological lesions may be found only in the early stages; consequently familiarity with the clinical aspects of the disease is essential in establishing the diagnosis in subsequent stages. For more detailed accounts the reader is referred to recent surveys.[26–28]

The peak incidence is in the 40–60 age group, reported ages at diagnosis having ranged from 23 to 78 years. There is an overall female to male preponderance of 9–10 to 1, but this may be less in older age groups. The disease is generally similar in both sexes,[29] except that males were found to have less pruritus and pigmentation, and a higher incidence of hepatocellular carcinoma.[30] Although PBC occurs worldwide and has been found in all races, there is some geographical variation in incidence with few cases reported from the Indian and African continents. In the United Kingdom the annual incidence is 5.8–10.6 patients per million per year with a prevalence rate of 40–52 patients per million.[31,32] In a combined European study[33] the overall prevalence was 23 per million, but with regional variations ranging from <10 to >60 per million. In a study

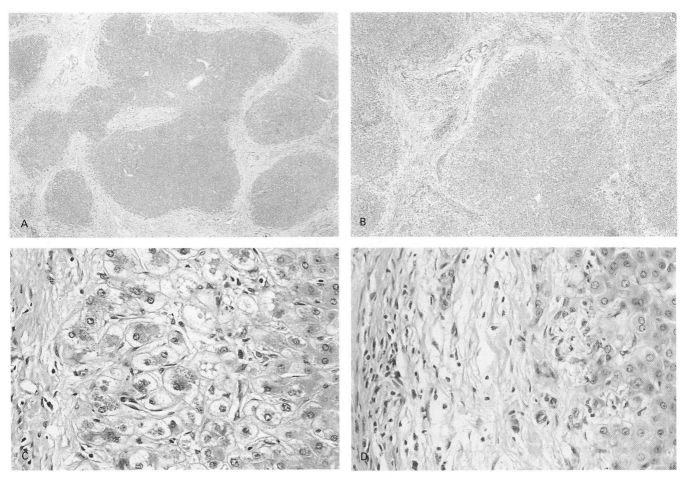

Fig. 12.3 Biliary cirrhosis. (a) Irregularly shaped parenchymal areas, some having a normally positioned hepatic venule, are delineated by serpiginous bands of oedematous connective tissue. H & E. (b) Note the peripheral 'halo' which surrounds the nodules in this case. H & E. The peripheral 'halo' may be predominantly cellular as in (c) or fibrous as in (d). H & E.

from Sweden in 1990, a point prevalence of 151 per million was reported.[34] An increased awareness of the condition and the diagnosis of asymptomatic patients seem to account for the apparent rise in incidence and prevalence of PBC in recent years.[35]

Insidious in onset, the presenting features are usually intense pruritus and lethargy with increasing skin pigmentation and eventually cholestatic jaundice, although icterus may not develop for months or sometimes years after the initial symptoms. Some patients first present with jaundice, and in a very few instances hepatic decompensation may bring the patient to clinical notice. Portal hypertension may become manifest before a true cirrhosis is established.[36,37] Xanthomas/xanthelasma occur in 30% of patients. The incidental finding of hepatomegaly (sometimes massive), a raised serum alkaline phosphatase or of circulating antimitochondrial antibodies may result in the recognition of patients who are asymptomatic.[38,39] They may remain asymptomatic for some years and experience a normal life expectancy,[40,41] although an increased mortality is shown for those in whom symptoms subsequently develop.[42,43] Symptomatic patients may survive for

10–15 years but the onset of jaundice heralds clinical deterioration with a worsening prognosis. Death is usually due to hepatocelluar failure, with bleeding from oesophageal varices in approximately 30% of cases; non-hepatic causes of death are found in less than 20% of the patients.[44] Predicting the prognosis has became a major issue, with the use of liver transplantation as the only treatment option in patients with advanced disease. Several models based on multiple regression analysis of clinical, biochemical[45] and histopathological[46,47] variables have been proposed, and in these the serum bilirubin levels and the presence of fibrosis/cirrhosis are the most significant risk factors. These statistical models have proved useful in determining the optimal timing and in assessing the efficacy of liver transplantation in PBC.[48,49]

Associated conditions

The co-existence of PBC with other diseases which are themselves associated with immunological abnormalities is not uncommon.[50] Features of Sjögren's syndrome or the 'sicca complex' of dry eyes and dry mouth may be found in more than half the patients;[50-53] this led to the postulate that a common mechanism may be responsible for damaging epithelial-lined ducts in lacrimal and salivary glands and in the liver.[54] PBC may be associated with all or some of the features of the CREST syndrome: Calcinosis, Raynaud's phenomenon, oEsophageal dysfunction, Sclerodactyly and Telangiectasis,[50,55] to which anticentromere antibodies and keratoconjunctivitis sicca were later added.[56] Other reported associations include seropositive and seronegative arthritis,[57,58] autoimmune thyroiditis,[59] renal tubular acidosis,[60,61] coeliac disease,[62,63] and vasculitis.[64] Rare, possibly coincidental, associations include interstitial pulmonary fibrosis,[65] pulmonary haemorrhage and glomerulonephritis,[66] multiple sclerosis,[67,68] ulcerative colitis,[69] and systemic lupus erythematosus,[70] the latter being difficult to interpret, since as many as 26% of patients with PBC may have anti-double stranded DNA antibodies.[71] Patients with PBC (in common with other chronic cholestatic syndromes) also develop osteoporosis[26] and there is progressive bone loss in the course of the disease leading to severe osteoporosis.[72]

Laboratory tests

Liver function tests show a mild elevation of bilirubin (34–68 μmol/l; 2–4 mg/dl), accompanied by a striking and disproportionate elevation of the alkaline phosphatase to levels three to five times normal, although a normal value does not preclude the diagnosis.[73] There is a moderate elevation of serum transaminase levels (100–150 iu/l). Serum immunoglobulins of all three major classes are elevated, but elevation of IgM is most consistent with mean increases in excess of 150% of normal.[74]

The most helpful diagnostic test is the demonstration of serum antimitochondrial antibodies (AMA).[75] AMA are found in more than 95% of patients' sera[76,77] by immunofluorescence using various mammalian tissues as substrates. The majority of the cases who are negative at presentation will become positive later or will be found positive by other methods such as complement fixation, immunodiffusion, or enzyme linked immunosorbent assay (ELISA[78]). Antimitochondrial antibodies are heterogeneous, and sophisticated immunological methods using purified antigens derived from subcellular fractions have allowed the characterization of nine AMA types which have different disease associations: of these, anti-M2, anti-M4, anti-M8 and anti-M9 are found in PBC patients. Anti-M2, directed against components of dehydrogenase multienzyme complexes on inner mitochondrial membranes, is found in all patients and is thus a specific marker for PBC.[78-80] AMA profiles determined at early stages may have a prognostic significance,[79] anti-M2/anti-M9 having identified patients with a more benign course, whereas the presence of anti-M4 and/or anti-M8 may herald a more rapidly progressive disease course.[81] However, other workers have not been able to confirm the prognostic value of the AMA profile.[82]

AETIOLOGY AND PATHOGENESIS

The aetiology and pathogenesis of PBC remain obscure.[26] In contrast with many autoimmune disorders, a clear association with class I HLA antigens has not been demonstrated but, recently, an increased frequency of certain class II HLA haplotypes has been shown in PBC patients.[83-85] Reports of a familial predisposition to PBC and of an increased prevalence of autoantibodies in relatives of PBC patients further suggest that genetic factors play a role.[86,87] The finding of AMA in relatives of PBC patients suggests the presence of active PBC.[86] Many features indicate that there may be an autoimmune component, notably the association with other autoimmune diseases, the presence of AMA and various other autoantibodies,[50,88] circulating immune complexes with activation of complement,[89-91] impairment of cell-mediated immunity,[92] alteration of T-cell subsets[93-95] and disturbance of serum immunoregulatory factors.[96,97] However, many of these features reflect a failure, in PBC patients, to adequately suppress immune responses, and their pathogenetic implications have not been shown.

In PBC there is enhanced expression on bile-duct epithelium of MHC class I antigens[98] and aberrant expression of MHC class II antigens.[99,100] The latter is also found in primary sclerosing cholangitis, in extrahepatic obstruction and other forms of chronic liver disease[101,102] and may be an epiphenomenon. However, aberrant expression of MHC class II antigens is important in the induction of immune responses and might enable these cells to present 'self-antigens' to sensitized T-lymphocytes and thus provoke autosensitization in response to some extraneous factor. Immunohistochemical studies of liver biopsies suggest a role for cytotoxic T-cells in the pathogenesis of the bile-duct destruction,[103-105] although natural killer cell and antibody dependent cytotoxicity may contribute.[20] In PBC, increased expression of intercellular adhesion molecule 1(ICAM-1) has been demonstrated in bile duct cells,[106] which also show an induced expression of heat–shock proteins.[107] The similarity of the bile-duct damage in PBC with that observed in graft-versus-host disease[108] and allograft rejection[109] adds circumstantial support to the bile-duct destruction being immunologically mediated.

The nature of the initiating factor and of the antigen(s) to which the patients become sensitized remains unknown. Sensitization to various bile antigens occurs in other liver diseases[110,111] and these antigens await further characterization.[112] There is little evidence that AMAs play a major role in the pathogenesis of bile-duct destruction,[80,113] although component E2 of the mitochondrial pyruvate dehydrogenase complex has recently been demonstrated on the membrane of cultured biliary epithelial cells from

PBC patients.[114,115] One hypothesis still in favour is that AMAs are induced by initial exposure to a precipitating infectious agent(s) which expresses mitochondrial cross-reacting epitopes. Recently, atypical mycobacterial infection has been added as a possible candidate following the demonstration of a high prevalence of anti-M2 antibodies in the serum of patients with tuberculosis.[116] A histological lesion resembling that of PBC has been induced in mice inoculated with human mycoplasma-like organisms.[117] The possibility of overlap of sarcoidosis and PBC has been raised by virtue of a small number of patients in whom features of both diseases have co-existed (see Ch. 17).[118–120]

PATHOLOGICAL FEATURES

The histopathology of PBC has been extensively reviewed.[121–123] The initial injury affects interlobular bile ducts 40–80 μm in diameter,[124] the smaller ones disappearing first.[125] The actual size of the affected ducts may be difficult to estimate as they tend to enlarge following rupture of their basement membranes. The early lesions are focal within the liver and segmental within the duct system. They might therefore not be sampled by liver biopsy needles, and pathologists should be aware that non-specific portal inflammation can be found in early liver biopsies from patients with a clinical diagnosis of PBC. There is a chronic inflammatory cell infiltrate within the portal tracts and this is intimately related to the bile ducts (Fig. 12.4a). The infiltrate is usually confined to the portal tract, and in the early stages, even if there is spillover to involve the periportal parenchyma, there is very little liver-cell necrosis.

The involved bile ducts show distinctive abnormalities (Fig. 12.4b). The epithelium becomes swollen with an irregular luminal border, and may become stratified with some poorly developed papillary ingrowths. In this hyper-

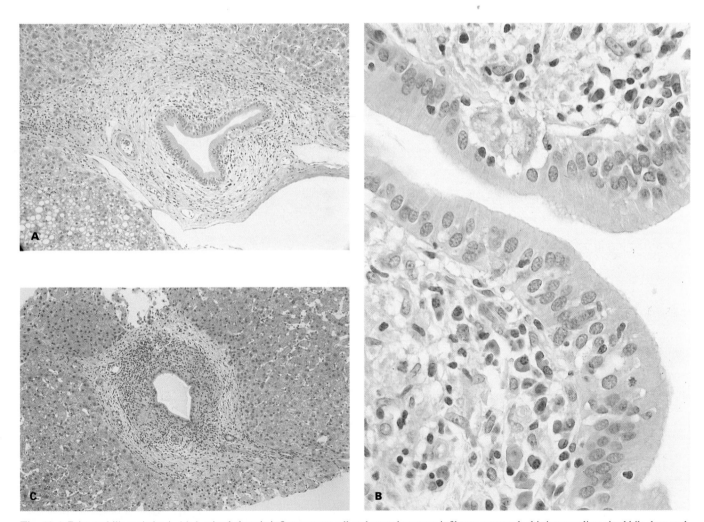

Fig. 12.4 Primary biliary cirrhosis (a) A mixed chronic inflammatory cell and granulomatous infiltrate surrounds this intermediate sized bile duct and there is focal disruption of the basement membrane H & E. (b) At a higher magnification note that the inflammatory cell infiltrate extends into hyperplastic biliary epithelium and there is focal dissolution of the epithelium. H & E. (c) In this case note the bile duct is completely surrounded by an epithelioid cell granulomatous reaction and there is focal disruption of the epithelium H & E.

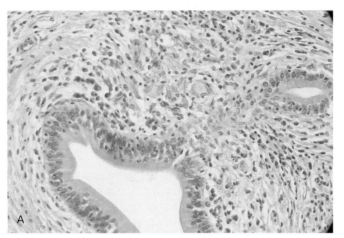

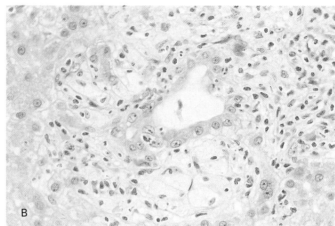

Fig. 12.5 Primary biliary cirrhosis. (a) Site of rupture of a bile duct showing a granulomatous reaction in which multinucleate cells are present (same case as shown in Figs 12.4a & b). H & E. (b) Foamy macrophages have accumulated near this damaged and ectatic bile duct. H & E.

plastic epithelium, individual cells appear more eosinophilic than normal and there is a reduction or loss of their PAS-positive supranuclear granules. The basement membrane is focally disrupted and lymphocytes and plasma cells infiltrate the epithelium and appear within cytoplasmic vacuoles. The lesions could be described as an erosion of the ductal basement membrane with 'piecemeal necrosis' of the bile-duct epithelium. In serial sections, rupture of the bile ducts can be demonstrated, and at these sites a macrophage reaction characterized by aggregates of ceroid-laden phagocytes and some foamy, multinucleate giant cells is found, probably a reaction to escaped bile (Figs 12.5a and b).

In the smaller portal tracts there is usually a chronic inflammatory cell infiltrate but this may show varying patterns in the same biopsy. In some, the inflammatory cells are predominantly lymphocytic and well-formed germinal centres may be present (Fig. 12.6a); in some, focal lymphocytic aggregates are found and the involved bile duct is surrounded by a mixed mononuclear cell infiltrate in which

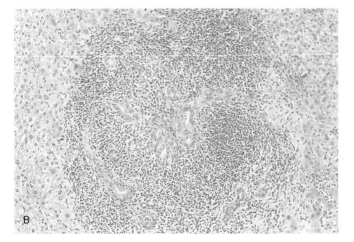

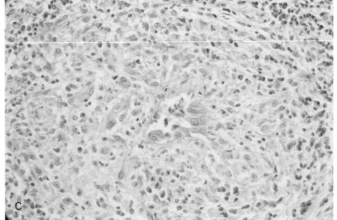

Fig. 12.6 Primary biliary cirrhosis. Variations which may characterize the bile-duct lesions. (a) A lymphocytic aggregate with a germinal centre is present beside a damaged duct surrounded by an epithelioid granulomatous reaction. H & E. (b) Focally dense, chronic inflammatory cell infiltrates are closely associated with hyperplastic bile ducts, the number of which appears to be excessive. H & E. (c) Degenerate bile-duct epithelium surrounded by an epithelioid granulomatous reaction with some plasma cells. H & E.

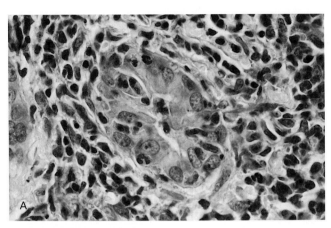 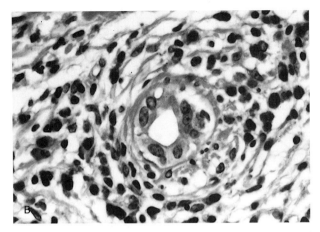

Fig. 12.7 Primary biliary cirrhosis. Involvement of small bile ducts (a) Note the swollen bile-duct epithelium and the presence of neutrophil polymorphs around and within the duct. H & E. (b) Note the surrounding loose connective tissue in which there is a mixed infiltrate of plasma cells and lymphocytes. H & E.

plasma cells are conspicuous and macrophages and eosinophils are also found (Fig. 12.6b); in others, a focal aggregate of epithelioid cells is present and sometimes an epithelioid granulomatous reaction surrounds the duct (Figs 12.6a and c). The bile-duct epithelium shows degenerative changes similar to those already described; some-

times neutrophil polymprohs may be seen intra-epithelially or within the duct lumen and, less commonly, they may be the predominant cell type (Fig. 12.7a). In the smallest portal tracts, there is also a chronic inflammatory cell infiltrate and bile ducts of 20–30 μm in diameter are affected from an early stage of the disease. There is periductal oedema with separation of the investing connective tissue bands; lymphocytes and plasma cells surround the ducts and may extend into the epithelium which shows degenerative changes (Fig. 12.7b).

Serial sections may demonstrate the complete destruction of bile-duct radicles, the only remnant of which is a small amorphous deposit of PAS-positive material within a lymphocytic aggregate; such vestigial remnants are often

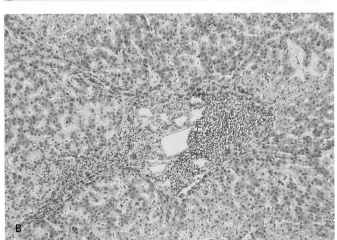

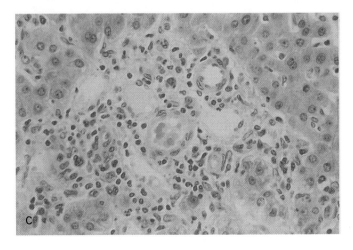

Fig. 12.8 Evidence of ductopenia in primary biliary cirrhosis. (a) High power view of same portal tract as shown in Fig. 12.2a; some focal condensation of fibrous tissue is present to the left of the hepatic artery at the site of which a bile duct was probably present. H & E. (b) In this portal tract a lymphocytic aggregate is present at the presumed site of the bile duct. Masson's trichrome. (c) Small chronically inflamed portal tract in which a number of hepatic arteries are present, but no bile duct. H & E.

absent and only a focal lymphocytic aggregate remains to identify the site from which a bile duct has disappeared (Figs 12.8a and b). In the small portal tracts, the distinctive feature is that bile ducts are often conspicuously absent; only very rarely may fibrous whorls be seen replacing them. In an elegant histometric study Nakanuma & Ohta highlighted this early disappearance of small bile ducts.[125] They drew attention to the fact that bile ducts are normally accompanied by a hepatic artery branch and that the expected ratio of the diameter of the duct to that of the corresponding artery is approximately 0.75. In any portal tract, hepatic artery branches unaccompanied by a bile duct are a useful marker of ductopenia (Figs 12.8a and c). It has to be borne in mind, however, that similar findings occur in a number of other ductopenic syndromes, e.g. primary sclerosing cholangitis (see Fig. 12.19).

Parenchymal changes are mild initially; focal epithelioid granulomas may be found in approximately 25% of biopsies. Focal Kupffer cell hyperplasia and intrasinusoidal infiltration by lymphocytes and macrophages (Fig. 12.9) may be a conspicuous feature of diagnostic help in small biopsies. Hepatocyte hyperplasia, with twin-cell liver plates and

focal compression of adjacent parenchyma, is best appreciated in a reticulin preparation (Fig. 12.10).[126] This regenerative response is more marked in the perivenular zone. Early parenchymal hyperplasia has been substantiated by increased uptake of bromodeoxyuridine,[127] and when prominent the lesion has been reported as nodular regenerative hyperplasia.[128–130] It is probably an important factor both in the hepatomegaly of PBC and in producing portal hypertension which may sometimes be clinically significant before cirrhosis is established.[35–37]

Progression of the liver injury

The lesions which have been described in the preceding paragraphs are those which are characteristic of PBC and on which a definitive histological diagnosis can be made. The subsequent progression of the disease is the result of:

1. The 'toxic' effect of bile retention which occurs proximal to damaged and lost bile ducts and leads to cholate stasis and biliary piecemeal necrosis. The features are common to biliary cirrhosis of whatever aetiology, but, in

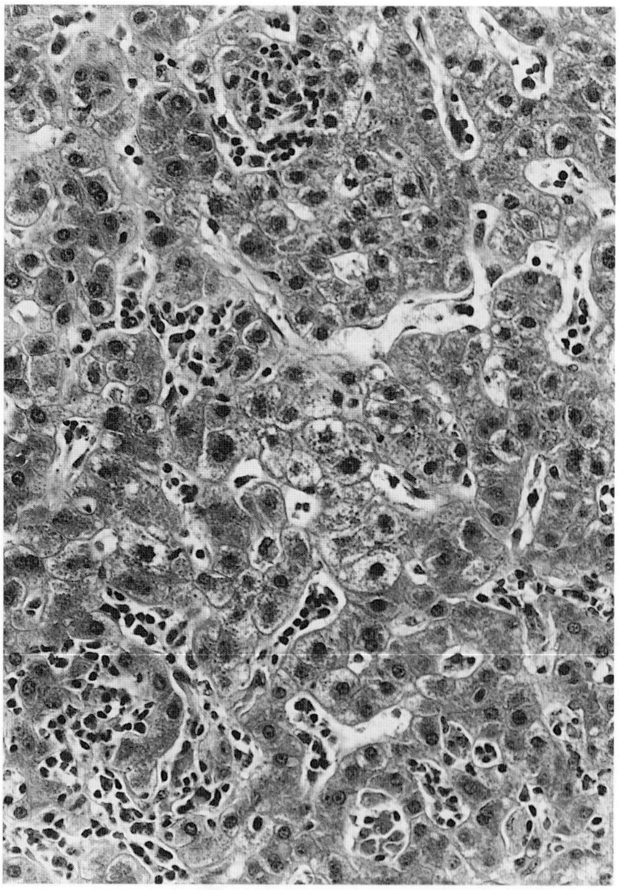

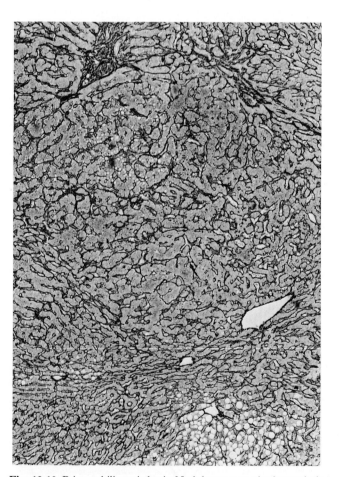

Fig. 12.9 Primary biliary cirrhosis. Parenchymal changes in the early stages; note the presence of some small, poorly-defined macrophage granulomas, some focal liver-cell necrosis and prominent intrasinusoidal aggregates of mononuclear cells. H&E.

Fig. 12.10 Primary biliary cirrhosis. Nodular regenerative hyperplasia with twin-cell plates producing some compression of the surrounding parenchyma. Gordon & Sweets' reticulin.

contrast to the secondary biliary cirrhosis (see Ch. 11) resulting from extrahepatic obstruction, the picture in PBC is not complicated by changes of acute cholangitis, bile lakes or bile infarcts.

2. The extension of the necro-inflammatory process to involve the hepatocytes, possibly as part of the same immunological process as that involving the duct system.[12,122,131]

3. The microcirculatory and architectural disturbances produced by progressive fibrosis and which, as in cirrhosis of whatever aetiology, contribute to the final end-stage liver.

There is marked individual variation in the rate of progression of the disease, but sooner or later liver injury occurs with increased chronic inflammation in portal tracts, extension of the process to involve periportal parenchyma, fibro-inflammatory septum formation, disturbance of architecture, cholestasis, regenerative activity and eventual development of an established cirrhosis.

Extension of the lesion to the periportal parenchyma takes the form of biliary piecemeal necrosis but, in a substantial number of cases, lymphocytic piecemeal necrosis resembling that seen in autoimmune chronic active hepatitis (CAH) is also present or may even dominate the picture.[12,132] In this situation the differential diagnosis may be difficult, especially when characteristic bile-duct lesions are no longer present and overlapping features also occur clinically. At this stage, copper-associated protein deposition[7] and conspicuous ductular proliferation favour a diagnosis of PBC, whereas swollen hepatocytes occurring singly or in rosettes and surrounded by lymphocytes are more often seen in CAH. Lymphocytic piecemeal necrosis seen in early biopsies has a tendency to subside in the later stages of the disease.[12] In most instances, the dense mononuclear cell infiltrates are then centrally situated in the portal tracts and fibrous septa, but at the periportal and periseptal margins a paler staining zone shows sparse, mixed inflammatory cells and proliferated ductules set in a loose fibrous matrix (Figs 12.11a and b). In some patients, usually those with hypercholesterolaemia, lipid-laden macrophages (xanthoma cells) or lipid-laden hepatocytes (pseudoxanthoma cells) may be present singly or as discrete aggregates (Fig. 12.12), usually in the periportal areas.

In time the periportal inflammation extends along the terminal distribution of the portal tracts; portal–portal linkages are formed and polyhedral 'classic lobules' may be defined — a monolobular pattern of fibrosis. At the interface between septa and parenchyma there is continuing biliary piecemeal necrosis with copper-associated protein deposition (Figs 12.11a and b) and later bilirubinostasis. The accumulation of copper, which increases with the duration of cholestasis, is probably due to a combination of impaired biliary secretion and some increased uptake by the liver.[133,134] It does not appear to contribute significantly to the liver injury in PBC.[132,133] The degree

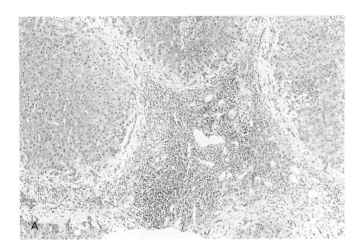

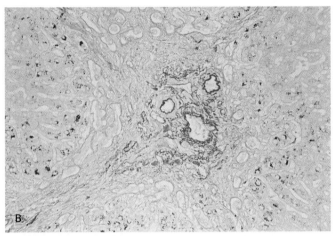

Fig. 12.11 Primary biliary cirrhosis, stage 3. (a) Characteristic portal–septal fibrous expansion in which, centrally, there is chronic inflammation and fibrosis while there are clear margins ('halo, effect) indicating continuing biliary piecemeal necrosis. H & E. (b) Orcein staining highlights the original boundaries of the portal tract with its abundant elastic content and copper-associated granules within what is now the parenchymal limiting plate. Shikata's orcein

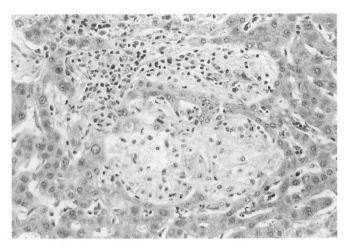

Fig. 12.12 Periportal aggregates of xanthoma cells in primary biliary cirrhosis. Masson's trichrome.

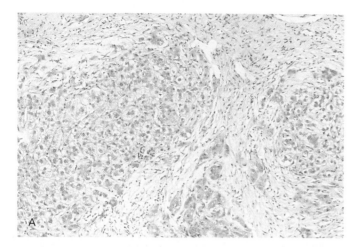

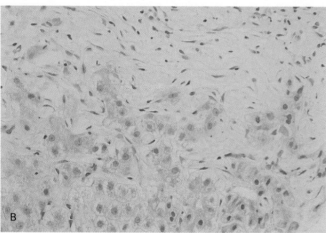

Fig. 12.13 Fibrous piecemeal necrosis in primary biliary cirrhosis stage 4. (a) Inflammation is now minimal and the margins of the septa mostly comprise loose fibrous tissue which extends between the disrupted liver-cell plates. H & E. (b) The peripheral liver-cell plates seem to end blindly in the fibrous matrix of the septum. H & E.

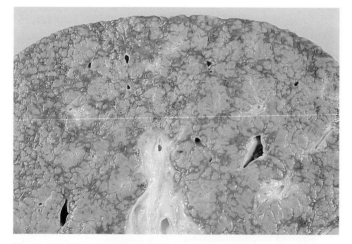

Fig. 12.14 Primary biliary cirrhosis. Coronal section through the hilar region of a liver with primary biliary cirrhosis. The cirrhosis is of a regular micronodular pattern with marked bile staining affecting the periphery of the nodules.

of ductular proliferation tends to become less marked with time, and a layer of loose oedematous fibrous tissue produces the 'halo effect' characteristic of advanced biliary disorders (Fig. 12.3b, 12.11a). When ductular proliferation remains the predominant feature, the term *ductular piecemeal necrosis* has been applied,[12] a pattern which might reflect a more rapidly progressive and fibrogenic lesion.[12,137,138] Canalicular bilirubinostasis with concretions eventually appears, but may occasionally be an early feature.[139] Mallory bodies are present in about 25% of cases.[8,140]

Progressive disturbance of the liver architecture and nodular regenerative activity heralds an established cirrhosis. However, because of the focal nature of the disease from its earliest onset, the liver removed at transplantation or at autopsy may show areas in which nodularity is inconspicuous and architectural disturbance is slight. In some instances, stages 2, 3 or 4 may be observed in different areas of the same liver. At times the inflammatory process subsides and the parenchymal limiting plate appears either remodelled or still indented with irregular hepatocytic plates which seem to end blindly in the oedematous margins of the fibrous septum (Figs 12.13a and b). This so-called *fibrous piecemeal necrosis* probably represents the scarring stage of biliary piecemeal necrosis.[12] Macroscopically, the cirrhosis is predominantly micronodular and of a relatively regular appearance (Fig. 12.14); the liver size is usually greater than that seen in posthepatitic type cirrhosis following viral or autoimmune chronic active hepatitis, but a shrunken macronodular cirrhosis may also be observed. Microscopically, the cirrhosis may be difficult to distinguish from cirrhosis of other aetiology. Primary biliary cirrhosis should be suspected, however, on the following features: (i) virtual absence of medium and small sized bile ducts; (ii) focal lymphocytic aggregates in portal areas; (iii) peripheral cholestasis and, in particular, cholate stasis with Mallory bodies and copper accumulation; (iv) a biliary or monolobular pattern of fibrosis; (v) partial or focal preservation of an acinar architecture. In a few instances the diagnostic bile-duct lesions may persist at the cirrhotic stage and granulomas may also be seen. The histological distinction between PBC and primary sclerosing cholangitis is discussed later. The main clinicopathological features of the two conditions are compared in Table 12.2.

Hepatocellular carcinoma has been reported as a terminal complication in a very small number of patients with PBC,[141–144] exceptionally at a precirrhotic stage;[145] the small number possibly reflects the female preponderance of PBC and the relatively short duration of the truly cirrhotic stage. There are reports also of an increased incidence of extrahepatic malignancies, notably breast cancer,[146–148] the incidence of which was found to be 4.4 times that predicted for the general population.[149]

Table 12.2 Comparison of clinicopathological features in primary biliary cirrhosis and primary sclerosing cholangitis. Compiled from references 12,28,187

Feature	Primary biliary cirrhosis	Primary sclerosing cholangitis
Clinical		
Sex, M/F	1/9	2/1
Age	Middle-age	Children–Adult
Symptomatic	> 65%	> 80%
Pruritus	> 70%	> 70%
Cholangitis	Absent	< 15%
Hyperpigmentation	> 50%	< 25%
Xanthelasma	< 20%	< 5%
Laboratory tests		
Alkaline phosphatase	+ + + +	+ + + +
Bilirubin	+ to + + +	+/+ +
Raised immunoglobulin M	+ + + +	+ +
AMA	> 95%	Absent or low-titre
Other autoantibodies	< 30%	Children > adults
HLA association	Not certain	B8, DR3, DR2, DRw52a
Associated diseases		
Inflammatory bowel disease	< 4%	> 65%
Sicca syndrome	> 65%	< 2%
Arthritis	> 15%	< 10%
Thyroid disease	> 15%	< 2%
Cholangiography	Often normal	Diagnostic
Histological features (needle biopsy)		
Granulomatous cholangitis	30–50%	Very rarely
Fibro-obliterative cholangitis	Absent	> 10%
Cholestasis	Late	Variable
Copper-associated granules	> 80%	> 70%

Histological staging of PBC

In the foregoing account no attempt has been made to divide the evolution of PBC into successive stages.[25,150–152] The stages proposed in various studies are summarized in Table 12.3. Because the evolution of PBC is variable within the liver there is considerable overlap between the stages described. Furthermore, there is individual variation in the progression of the disease; some patients progress for some time but, in our experience, may then remain at the same stage for years. In addition, there is frequently a poor correlation between the clinical state of the patient and the apparent histological staging, such that some asymptomatic patients may already have extensive hepatic fibrosis. Clinically, the development of jaundice is

a bad prognostic sign. Histologically, the presence of portal–portal bridging fibrosis has been shown to correlate conversely with survival,[46] and in a large series of sequential biopsies, the presence of cirrhosis, extensive cholestasis, prominent Mallory bodies and halo formation were more frequent in specimens taken within two years of death.[12] These studies were unable to confirm an earlier report that the presence of granulomas, irrespective of the stage, indicated a more favourable outlook.[153]

Except for the demonstration of an established cirrhosis, the histological staging has been of little assistance in assessing the likely prognosis in PBC. The numerous controlled trials of treatments have been mainly evaluated according to patients' survival. At the present time there is no widely accepted treatment regime, although prednisolone,[154] cyclosporin,[155,156] colchicine[157] and ursodeoxycholic acid[158] may have beneficial effects, at least in relieving symptoms if not in delaying disease progression.

CHRONIC ACTIVE HEPATITIS/PBC — MIXED TYPE

The histological features which differentiate between PBC and autoimmune chronic active hepatitis are summarized on page 387 and in the above account. They have also been previously reviewed.[123] In our own experience, comprising large series of PBC and chronic active hepatitis, histopathological differentiation of the two conditions presents a problem in about 15% of cases. The overlap may be confined to histological appearances, i.e. misleading bile-duct damage or predominantly lymphocytic piecemeal necrosis in cases which have all the clinical features of chronic active hepatitis or PBC respectively. In a few instances, the overlap extends to the clinical and serological data.[159] In this situation, a treatment trial has been advocated, a response to corticosteroids being expected in autoimmune CAH but not in PBC.

Berg and his colleagues have proposed a classification of PBC into subgroups according to the AMA pattern.[77,159] In an experience of over 500 patients they found anti-M2 activity in all patients, together with anti-M8 in 40%, and together with both anti-M8 and anti-M4 in 20%. Klöppel et al[137] noted that, in these mixed types, there was more severe liver injury with distinctive features of both PBC and autoimmune chronic active hepatitis. In contrast to

Table 12.3 Histological staging of PBC

Author	Stage 1	Stage 2	Stage 3	Stage 4
Rubin et al[25]	Damage to intrahepatic bile ducts	Ductular proliferation	Ductular proliferation	Cirrhosis
Scheuer[150]	Florid duct lesion	Ductular proliferation	Scarring	Cirrhosis
Popper & Schaffner[151]	Cholangitis	Ductular proliferation and destruction	Precirrhotic stage	Cirrhosis
Ludwig et al[152]	Portal hepatitis	Periportal hepatitis	Bridging necrosis or fibrosis or both	Cirrhosis

'pure' PBC cases, moreover, there was a more intense periportal parenchymal involvement with bridging necrosis and an earlier progression to cirrhosis; ductular proliferation was intense and more prominent than usually found in autoimmune chronic active hepatitis. The possibility that the presence of anti-M8 or anti-M4 may indicate a more rapidly progressive course of the disease,[81,82,159] has already been discussed but this interesting finding may be of limited value in evaluating individual cases.[160]

IMMUNE CHOLANGITIS (AUTOIMMUNE CHOLANGIOPATHY)

This term was first applied to 3 patients, 2 being mother and daughter, who presented with clinico-pathological features of PBC, but were AMA-negative and had high titres of serum antinuclear antibodies (ANA).[161] A further series of 15 patients was reported with a similar presentation and antibody profile and with histological features of PBC[162] and, in a single case report, Carrougher et al[163] detailed the clinical and histological features of this autoimmune syndrome. Ben-Ari et al[164] have recently described 4 patients (3 female) with overlapping features of PBC and autoimmune chronic active hepatitis, referring to this entity as autoimmune cholangiopathy. The 4 patients were AMA-negative but had high titre ANA and the liver biopsy showed bile-duct lesions resembling PBC. In 3 of the 4 patients there was a rapid clinical and biochemical remission in response to prednisolone.

Antinuclear antibodies with different antigenic specificities are frequently found in PBC[88,159,165] but none are specific and, in one large series, although ANA-positive patients (29%) had significantly lower titres of AMA,[166] they did not differ in any other respect from those without ANA. We have seen similar patients in whom the liver biopsy showed bile-duct lesions resembling PBC and with a marked periportal lymphocytic piecemeal necrosis and intra-acinar inflammation (Fig. 12.15). Whether AMA-negative/ANA-positive autoimmune cholangiopathy represents a distinct subgroup of patients who will respond to immunosuppressive treatment,[164] awaits further confirmation.

PRIMARY SCLEROSING CHOLANGITIS

Primary sclerosing cholangitis (PSC), first reported by Delbet (1924),[167] is a disorder characterized by non-specific inflammatory fibrosis in the wall of the biliary tree leading to irregular stenosis and ectasia, usually of both the intra- and extrahepatic bile ducts.[168–170] However, intrahepatic disease can occur in the absence of extrahepatic involvement — *small duct primary sclerosing cholangitis*.[171] Furthermore, within the liver, small duct and large duct involvement may occur independently but, with

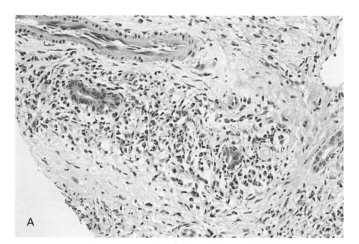

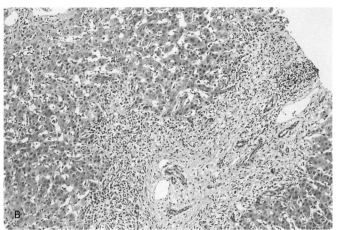

Fig. 12.15 Immune cholangitis. Liver biopsy from a male aged 19 with high titre ANA and a negative AMA test. (a) Bile-duct lesion: there is periductal oedema and inflammation, predominantly plasma cells with some eosinophils; the bile-duct epithelium is damaged and some intra-epithelial lymphocytes are present. H & E. (b) There is portal tract inflammation with bile-duct injury; note, in addition, the marked periportal inflammation with piecemeal necrosis and an intra-acinar (lobular) hepatitis. H & E.

progression of the disease, all segments of the biliary tree may be affected.[172] The disease has to be distinguished from the secondary sclerosing cholangitis which may follow biliary surgery, cholelithiasis or congenital biliary abnormalities, as well as from sclerosing bile-duct carcinoma which may produce similar clinico-pathological features. As a consequence, the classic diagnostic criteria included: (i) absence of previous biliary tract surgery; (ii) absence of choledocholithiasis; (iii) diffuse involvement of the extrahepatic biliary tract; and (iv) exclusion of cholangiocarcinoma. However, with the recognition of small duct disease, diffuse involvement of the extrahepatic biliary tract is no longer a prerequisite, and there is mounting evidence that a strict adherence to the first two criteria would underestimate the frequency and clinico-pathological spectrum of the disease.[173] In reality, a proportion of patients who underwent recurrent biliary surgery had

PSC, and choledocholithiasis develops in a third of otherwise classic PSC cases.[174] Exclusion of a cholangiocarcinoma is not simple; cholangiographic appearances may be difficult to interpret against the background of a markedly distorted biliary tree.[175] Furthermore, a reasonably long follow-up does not exclude malignancy as cholangiocarcinoma may develop *de novo* after years in up to 10% of patients with PSC.[176,177]

There is a tendency to separate sclerosing cholangitis into a *primary* or *idiopathic* form, of which 70–80% of cases are associated with ulcerative colitis, and an *acquired* form (p. 496) in which infectious, toxic or ischaemic causes are recognized. Although this distinction might prove useful for further studies on pathogenesis and for the development of specific treatments, it must be stressed that the two subgroups are often indistinguishable clinically and radiologically as well as morphologically.[178]

CLINICAL FEATURES

Seventy five per cent of patients are less than 50 years old at the time of diagnosis, but the disease can affect any age group[179,180] and is now well recognized in infancy[181] and in childhood.[182] There is a male preponderance of 2–3 to 1. Patients asymptomatic with respect to their hepatobiliary disease, 5–25% in some series,[183] are discovered because of an isolated rise in alkaline phosphatase found as part of regular screening of patients with chronic inflammatory bowel disease.[184] The classic presentation is with fatigue, vague upper abdominal pain, intermittent or progressive jaundice and, less commonly, with recurrent attacks of cholangitis.[185,186] In the majority of patients, including those who are asymptomatic at the time of diagnosis,[187] the disease will progress and biliary cirrhosis develops with progressive liver failure, deepening jaundice and death within 5–17 years of diagnosis. However, follow-up studies show a considerable variation in clinical course[177,188–191] with survival in one patient of up to 30 years.[192] As with PBC, a number of studies using multivariate analysis have been carried out to identify prognostic factors which might indicate the need to proceed to liver transplantation. Chapman[193] reviewed these and noted that age and raised serum bilirubin levels usually indicated a poor prognosis. There are no means of identifying the 10% or more of patients who are at risk of developing a cholangiocarcinoma.

Liver function tests show cholestasis with a pattern similar to that seen in PBC except that the alkaline phosphatase levels are usually higher and there is no marked increase in serum IgM levels in PSC.[186] As in PBC, a normal alkaline phosphatase does not preclude the diagnosis.[194] AMA is not present in PSC, but circulating antibodies against neutrophil nuclei are frequently present and low titre antinuclear and anti-smooth muscle antibodies are found in one-third of the patients;[180] these were mainly of IgM class in one series.[195] The prevalence of antibodies is higher in children, in whom serum IgG is also often elevated.[182]

Associated disorders

Primary sclerosing cholangitis may occur alone, but in 54–75% of patients[177,178] or more,[179] it is associated with chronic inflammatory bowel disease, mainly ulcerative colitis. Conversely, PSC may occur in approximately 3–7.5% of patients with ulcerative colitis.[196,197] These figures vary considerably in different series, probably reflecting patient selection and differences in the diagnostic methods applied.[198] Primary sclerosing cholangitis may also be associated with Crohn's disease.[177] The prevalence may be similar to that in ulcerative colitis, and colonic involvement is usually present in affected patients.[199] The term pericholangitis was previously synonymous both clinically and histologically with the liver involvement in chronic inflammatory bowel disease (see Ch. 17). The term covered a range of portal and biliary tract changes but, with the advent of cholangiography, it was applied to other patients with abnormal liver function tests and a normal ERCP. The term small duct primary sclerosing cholangitis is now used for this subgroup.[171]

The pancreatic duct may be involved causing chronic pancreatitis[179,200–202] which may dominate the clinical picture.[203] Pancreatic involvement may be associated with the sicca complex[204] or Sjögren's syndrome.[205,206] Less commonly reported clinical associations include retroperitoneal and mediastinal fibrosis, Riedel's thyroiditis, orbital pseudotumour,[207–210] coeliac disease,[211–212] and hypereosinophilic syndrome.[213,214] There are single reports of associated Peyronie's disease,[215] angioimmunoblastic lymphadenopathy,[216] massive intra-abdominal lymphadenopathy,[217] systemic lupus erythematosus,[218] systemic sclerosis,[219] lupus anticoagulant,[220] Budd–Chiari syndrome,[221] autoimmune haemolytic anaemia with hyperthyroidism,[222] and sarcoidosis;[223] the majority of these reported associations appear to be coincidental. There is a predisposition to osteoporosis, and severe bone rarefaction is common in advanced PSC.[224] The high incidence of a complicating cholangiocarcinoma has already been mentioned. There are also reports of hepatocellular carcinoma in PSC, in one case the fibrolamellar variant.[225,226]

RADIOLOGICAL FEATURES

Primary sclerosing cholangitis has been diagnosed with increasing frequency since the mid 1970s owing to a greater clinical awareness and a wider use of either endoscopic retrograde cholangiopancreatography (ERCP)[227] or Chiba skinny-needle percutaneous transhepatic cholangiography (PTC). Cholangiography, the most important radiological diagnostic test, demonstrates irregular areas

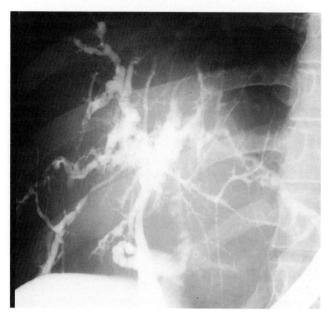

Fig. 12.16 ERCP film in primary sclerosing cholangitis. Note the markedly distorted extra- and intrahepatic biliary tree with variable beading, stenosis, and thinning of the ducts.

of stricture and beading of the bile ducts which, in 80% of patients, involve both intra- and extrahepatic ducts (Fig. 12.16).[179,228] Diverticular outpouchings may be seen[170] and, in a few cases, cholangiectases may mimic the changes seen in Caroli's disease.[229] Later, decreased intrahepatic branching produces a 'pruned tree' appearance which may resemble the attenuated pattern seen in primary biliary cirrhosis and other forms of cirrhosis.[230] Localized stricture with marked progression in sequential cholangiograms, and excessive duct dilatation suggest the development of cholangiocarcinoma, but the diagnosis of tumour is difficult and is often only made at autopsy or when the liver is removed at transplantation.[231]

AETIOLOGY AND PATHOGENESIS

The various factors responsible for the acquired forms of sclerosing cholangitis (p. 496) have all been considered as potential causes of PSC, but none has yet been convincingly implicated. In view of the frequent association with ulcerative colitis, chronic portal toxaemia and bacteraemia from the diseased colon have been proposed, but not supported by appropriate data.[173,321] Furthermore, chronic inflammatory bowel disease does not cause PSC; the two diseases occur independently. No differences have been demonstrated between PSC occurring in association with chronic inflammatory bowel disease and that occurring in its absence.[184] The interval between the onset of the bowel disease and the onset of biliary tract disease varies widely; the chronic inflammatory bowel disease may become symptomatic some years after PSC has been diagnosed and, conversely, PSC may become symptomatic years after

colectomy. However, their frequent association suggests that chronic inflammatory bowel disease and PSC have some aetiopathogenetic factor in common.

Evidence of a genetic predisposition is provided by reports of familial cases,[204,233,234] and of a close association of PSC with HLA-B8 and DR3 phenotypes,[235-238] and with DR2 in those who are HLA-DR3 negative.[239] The HLA-B8 DR3 phenotype is not increased in patients with ulcerative colitis per se, but its presence in a patient with ulcerative colitis confers a tenfold increase in the relative risk of developing sclerosing cholangitis. More recently a close association between HLA-DRW52 and primary sclerosing cholangitis has been demonstrated.[240] Both DRW-52 and DR2 encode a leucine residue at position 38 of the DRβ chain and it has been postulated that it is this feature of the DR molecule which confers susceptibility to PSC.[241]

Humoral immune abnormalities recorded in PSC include: hypergammaglobulinaemia,[177] non-organ specific[195,242] and anti-neutrophil antibodies[243,244] (which are more prevalent in children[182,245,246]), increased levels of circulating immune complexes[247] (of which clearance by fixed macrophages could be impaired) and activation of the complement system.[248] Cellular abnormalities include lymphocyte sensitization to biliary antigens,[110] an increased CD4 : CD8 ratio of circulating T-cells,[249,250] (perhaps not in children[245]), and a predominance of T-lymphocytes in the portal tract infiltrate.[250,251] Although some of these abnormalities may be secondary, they suggest that immune mechanisms may play a role in perpetuation of the bile-duct lesion. Increased expression of intercellular adhesion molecule 1 (ICAM-1)[106] and of heat-shock protein[107] by biliary epithelial cells has been documented in PSC. As mentioned for PBC, aberrant expression of HLA-DR antigens on the surface membrane of bile-duct epithelium is not specific for PSC[101,102] but may enable the biliary epithelial cells to present antigens to sensitized T-lymphocytes. In PSC, genetically predisposed individuals appear to become sensitized to triggering antigens, the nature of which remains unknown. There has been speculation on the role of viruses,[252] in that PSC exhibits many morphological resemblances to biliary atresia which may be induced in weanling mice, and possibly also in humans, by infection with reovirus type 3.[253,254] However, only a minority of patients with PSC had significantly elevated titres of serum antibody to reovirus type 3 and the virus could not be detected in liver tissue.[255] An association with cytomegalovirus, frequent in AIDS-related sclerosing cholangitis (p. 301), has not been found in PSC.[256]

PATHOLOGICAL FEATURES

The distinctive bile-duct lesion in PSC is a fibro-obliterative one characterized by an 'onion-skin' type of periductal fibrosis around medium-sized or larger bile ducts, with degeneration and atrophy of the epithelial lining and

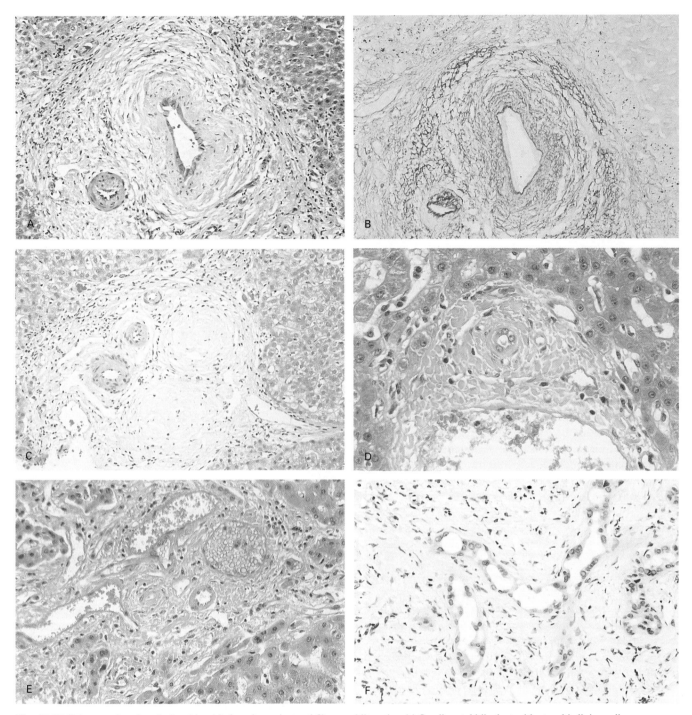

Fig. 12.17 Primary sclerosing cholangitis with ductal scarring and fibrous obliteration (a) Small septal bile duct with atrophic lining cells surrounded by dense hyaline collagen. H & E. (b) Same field as (a) to show the elastic content of the periductal collagen; note granular copper-associated protein deposits within periportal hepatocytes. Orcein. (c) Complete obliteration of bile ducts which are replaced by dense fibrous whorls; note the prominence of adjacent arterial branches. H & E. (d) and (e) In this case with ulcerative colitis who had a negative ERCP, the liver biopsy shows fibro-obliterative lesions of the small bile ducts with virtually no lumen discernible in (e). H & E. (f) In this case there is periductal fibrosis; the luminal margin is irregular and lined by epithelial cells with an atrophic degenerative appearance. H & E.

eventual replacement of the bile duct by fibrous cords (Figs 12.17a–c). These lesions, accompanied by reduced numbers of interlobular bile ducts, are virtually diagnostic of PSC. However, due to the large size of the ducts involved the lesions may be present in less than 40% of biopsy specimens. The small interlobular bile ducts may also be af-fected and replaced by fibrous scars (Figs 12.17d–f), either in addition to the involvement of larger ducts or alone in the rare variant confined to the intrahepatic biliary tree.[257] Thus, examination of the peripheral parenchyma obtained in needle biopsies may reveal portal tract changes which are either non-specific, but suggestive of a pathological

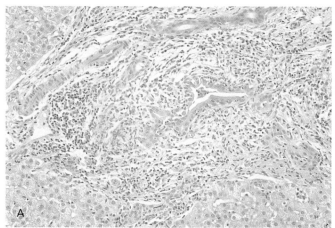

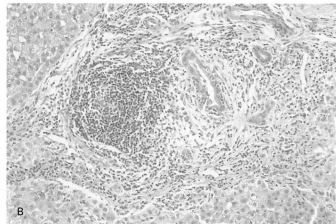

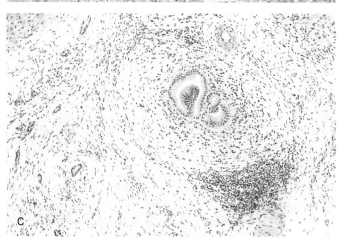

Fig. 12.18 Primary sclerosing cholangitis. Ductal lesion and portal inflammation. (a and b) Two portal areas from the same biopsy specimen. A dense chronic inflammatory cell infiltrate surrounds the bile duct and inflammatory cells extend into the bile-duct epithelium raising the differential diagnosis of primary biliary cirrhosis; note a lymphoid follicle in (b). H & E. (c) Hyperplastic, tortuous bile duct with surrounding concentric fibrosis and a chronic inflammatory cell infiltrate with lymphocytic aggregates; there is also oedema of the remainder of the portal area and a sparse inflammatory cell infiltrate. H & E.

process involving the major bile ducts, or which are characteristic of small duct PSC[258] which may not invariably be associated with involvement of the extrahepatic bile ducts.

By analogy with PBC, the histological changes may be divided into four stages. In stage 1 the changes are confined within the boundaries of portal tracts. These contain a diffuse mixed inflammatory cell infiltrate of lymphocytes, plasma cells and neutrophils, and this tends to be more intense around the bile ducts (Fig. 12.18a). Lymphoid follicles or aggregates may be present (Fig. 12.18b), but granulomas are only very occasionally found.[180] Small bile ducts may show degenerative epithelial changes (Figs 12.17d and e) and may be surrounded by a ring of oedematous or hyaline fibrosis (Fig. 12.18c).

In stage 2, portal tracts are swollen with disruption of the parenchymal limiting plates. The histological picture varies, presumably depending on the severity of biliary obstruction,[259] the degree of superimposed cholangitis, and the activity of the immune-mediated processes. Biliary piecemeal necrosis with focal ductular proliferation may predominate. Sometimes, dense portal tract inflammation is associated with lymphocytic piecemeal necrosis and the appearance mimics autoimmune chronic active hepatitis. This may cause diagnostic problems when hyperglobulinaemia and autoantibodies are present. In many instances, the inflammation seems to have subsided, the mildly fibrotic portal tracts have a stellate shape due to short and thin radiating septa and there is a slight excess of ductules and a few granules of copper-associated protein. Unless periductal fibrosis, cholangitis and focal ductopenia are present, the changes are not diagnostic, but are suggestive enough to indicate ERCP examination.

Further progression of the disease is characterized by increasing portal fibrosis with the formation of portal–portal linking septa (stage 3) and eventual development of cirrhosis (stage 4). As the disease advances, the inflammation has a tendency to subside leaving a combination of portal–septal fibrosis and oedema, focal ductular proliferation, periseptal biliary piecemeal necrosis with copper accumulation, Mallory bodies, 'halo' formation and progressive reduction in the number of bile ducts as described for PBC. Bile ducts disappear, their former site being indicated by either small aggregates of lymphocytes or macrophages as in PBC or rounded scars which are much more common in PSC (Fig. 12.17c). As in PBC, the presence of an unaccompanied hepatic artery branch is an indication of bile-duct loss (Fig 12.19a & b). Occasionally the portal tract contain unusually prominent hepatic artery branches (Fig. 12.17c), which may reflect either an increased number of vessels or increased tortuosity of the peribiliary plexus as a result of the disappearance of the bile ducts.

The distinction between PSC and PBC on histological appearances alone may be difficult;[123] it was reliable in only 28% of a series of 318 patients who had one of these two syndromes.[186] The distinction is even more difficult on the basis of a single biopsy and where the size of the

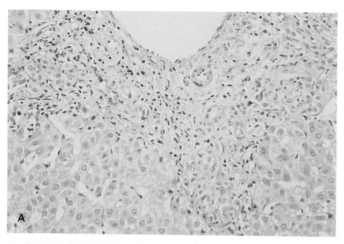

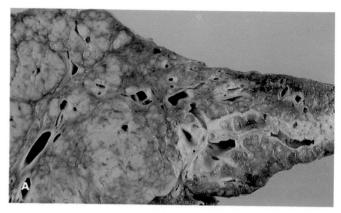

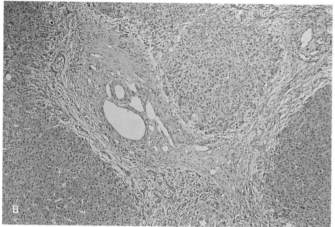

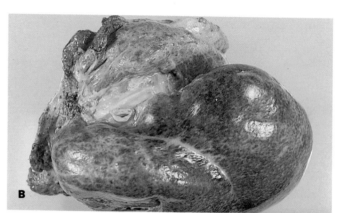

Fig. 12.19 Primary sclerosing cholangitis with disappearance of bile ducts. (a) There is a moderately intense chronic inflammatory cell infiltrate of the portal tract and two unaccompanied hepatic artery branches are seen; compare with Figs 12.2a and 12.8a. H & E. (b) Cirrhotic stage. A portal–portal fibrous septum is devoid of a bile duct and there is an unaccompanied hepatic artery branch; note the hyaline scars and the periseptal biliary piecemeal necrosis with a 'halo' effect. H & E.

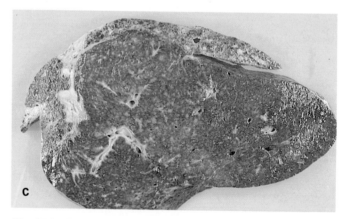

Fig. 12.20 Primary sclerosing cholangitis with cirrhosis. (a) This liver shows a markedly and irregularly dilated duct almost reaching the capsular surface of an atrophic left lobe. (b) Inferior aspect of a grossly deformed liver showing massive expansion of left and caudate lobes contrasting with the markedly atrophic, cirrhotic right lobe. (c) Coronal section of the liver shown in (b); the cirrhotic right lobe is stretched at the periphery of the massively expanded caudate and left lobes which histologically showed stage 2 disease with marked features of regeneration and cholestasis.

portal tracts contained in the biopsy specimen may determine the pattern of the histological lesions seen. Cholestasis is an early and more frequent finding in PSC than in PBC.[187] Periductal fibrosis or duct replacement by fibrous cords with or without superimposed acute cholangitis favour PSC, whereas granulomas are mostly found in PBC (Table 12.2).

Livers obtained at transplantation have allowed more detailed examination of the large intrahepatic ducts and of the extrahepatic biliary tree, whose pathology more closely reflects the changes seen radiologically.[170,260] Macroscopically, there are annular scars or fibrous cords which alternate with tubular or saccular cholangiectases, including luminal fibrous webs (Fig. 12.20a), ulceration of large ducts with or without cholangitic abscesses, and intrahepatic stones. Large perihilar scars may show yellow discolouration due to the presence of xanthomatous aggregates, at times simulating a desmoplastic tumour. In

general the pattern of cirrhosis is more irregular than that of PBC, reflecting the larger calibre of the ducts involved (Fig. 12.20b). Obliteration of segmental or main left or right hepatic ducts may occasionally lead to a segmental or

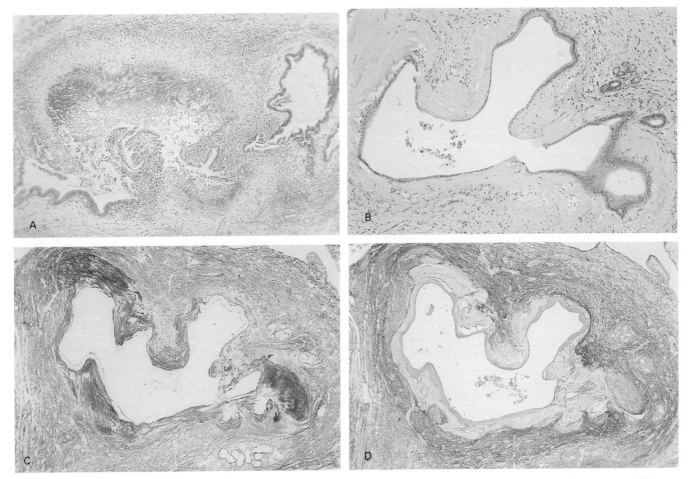

Fig. 12.21 Primary sclerosing cholangitis. (a) Ulceration with bilirubin impregnation and inflammatory reaction in the wall of a large septal bile duct. H&E. (b–d) A distorted septal duct with variably atrophic epithelial lining is stained with H&E in (b), Gordon & Sweets' reticulin (c), and Shikata's orcein (d) to illustrate the uneven distribution and composition of the periductal scarring.

'hemi-cirrhosis' respectively (Figs 12.20b and c). Histological examination of these livers may confirm ulceration of large bile ducts with bile impregnation and a xanthogranulomatous reaction in the surrounding tissue (Fig. 12.21).

In a few patients with undisputed PSC on cholangiography the changes are unexpectedly mild on liver biopsy. Conversely, there is a subgroup of patients with ulcerative colitis in whom histological features of PSC may be present or even advanced, but in whom ERCP examination is normal.[172,252] The apparent discrepancy between radiological and histological appearances at either end of the lesion spectrum emphasizes the heterogeneity of PSC, and the necessity for performing both cholangiography and liver biopsy to reach a reliable diagnosis; indeed, each of the techniques provides information on essentially different segments of the biliary system.[170,261]

ACQUIRED SCLEROSING CHOLANGITIS

Acquired forms of sclerosing cholangitis in which the radiological findings are similar to those of PSC are increasingly identified. The condition may occur in patients with primary or acquired immunodeficiency syndromes and in whom biliary infection is probably involved in the pathogenesis. In AIDS patients, acalculous cholecystitis, sclerosing cholangitis and/or papillary stenosis (AIDS cholangiopathy)[262] is now well recognized[263–265] and cryptosporidiosis and/or cytomegalovirus infection co-exist in up to 80% of patients (see Ch. 7). A few cases have been reported in children with congenital immunodeficiency syndromes,[266–268] occasionally in siblings.[269–271] Sclerosing cholangitis has occurred following rupture of hydatid cysts into the biliary tree,[272] more often as a complication of surgical treatment in which the cysts had been injected with scolicidal solutions such as 2% formaldehyde or 20% sodium chloride.[273,274] In these patients, leakage through a cystic-biliary connection is supposed to produce a caustic sclerosing cholangitis[275] similar to that induced experimentally.[276] Sclerosing cholangitis has also been observed in up to 56% of patients receiving intra-arterial infusion of fluorodeoxyuridine (FUDR) for palliative treatment of liver metastases from colorectal adenocarcinoma[277–280] (see also Ch. 15). The cholangitis was assumed to be caused by the toxic effect of FUDR;[279,280] an ischaemic aetiology was later considered,[281] and was supported by the demonstration of obliterative changes in the periductal arteries in these livers;[282] bile-duct scarring has also been produced experimentally by ethanol embolization of the hepatic artery in monkeys.[283] Langerhans cell histiocytosis (histiocytosis X) may produce a picture of sclerosing cholangitis, both in children[284,285] and adults.[286] This seems to follow infiltration of the bile ducts by Langerhans cell granulomatous tissue.

Finally, mention should be made of a radiological and clinical syndrome identical to PSC which may develop secondary to extrahepatic portal vein obstruction. The change is thought to be the result of choledochal varices, part of the collateral system bypassing the portal venous block, but these have yet to be demonstrated morphologically.[287]

IDIOPATHIC ADULTHOOD DUCTOPENIA

Several authors[288-291] have identified patients who present in adult life with a chornic cholestatic and disappearing bile duct syndrome leading to biliary cirrhosis but in whom the clinical, radiological and immunological features do not satisfy the criteria for either PSC or PBC. The patients are AMA-negative, have an essentially normal cholangiogram and lack the known disease associations such as ulcerative colitis. The group, described as having idiopathic adulthood ductopenia,[291] might be heterogeneous. Most of the patients were younger than the lower age limit encountered in PBC, making a diagnosis of AMA-negative PBC unlikely; some may represent small duct PSC without associated ulcerative colitis while others may be virus-induced, in particular by hepatitis C virus. A few patients were related,[290,292] and one patient presented with chronic recurrent cholestasis.[293]

BILE-DUCT INJURY IN THE LIVER ALLOGRAFT

Although the first successful liver transplant in man was carried out in 1963,[294] it was not until the late 1970s that the interlobular bile ducts were recognized as one of the main targets of the immune attack in allograft rejection.[295-297] A detailed account of liver allograft pathology is presented in Chapter 18. This section emphasizes the injury to the interlobular bile ducts.

In acute or cellular rejection, there is an accumulation of large lymphocytes, immunoblasts, neutrophils, eosinophils and a few plasma cells in portal tracts, and to a much lesser extent in the perivenular regions; there is a frequent endotheliitis or venulitis of portal and less often hepatic venules.[298-300] The small interlobular bile ducts may be obscured by the cell infiltrate or exhibit variable nuclear crowding, cytoplasmic vacuolation, pleomorphism and eosinophilic transformation of their epithelial lining cells; there is nuclear irregularity and hyperchromatism[301] (Fig. 12.22a). At times, neutrophils are numerous within the wall and lumen of ducts. The lesion then resembles a suppurative cholangitis, but in this morphological context it seems to be part of, and reflects a more severe form of, the rejection process (Fig. 12.22b). In most instances, cellular rejection is successfully treated with steroids and the duct lesion is reversible. Occasional cases run an acute or subacute course to complete duct loss — *acute vanishing bile duct syndrome*.[302] This may be associated with the features of severe cellular rejection, advanced ductopenia and foam cell arteritis or arteriopathy, the latter changes classically considered to be the hallmarks of 'chronic' rejection.

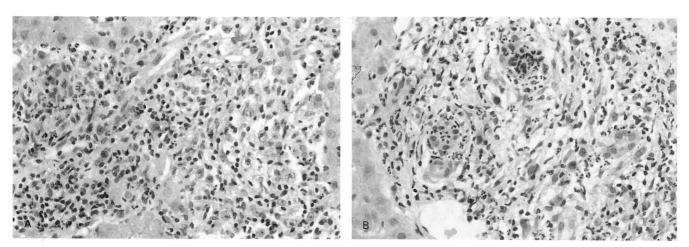

Fig. 12.22 Acute rejection of liver allograft. Two portal tracts from the same biopsy specimen. (a) A severe, predominantly mononuclear cell infiltrate is present and obscures the portal tract structures, in particular the bile duct which is difficult to identify. H & E. (b) Marked cholangitic component with clusters of neutrophils overlying small bile ducts. H & E.

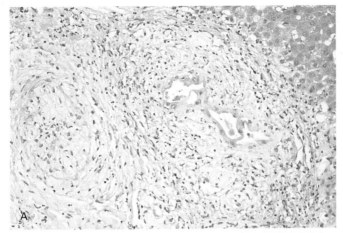

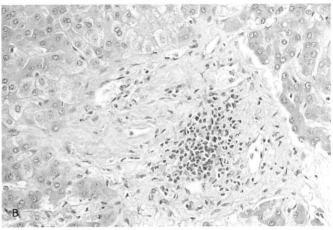

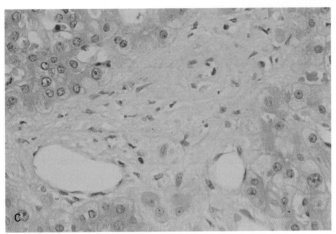

Fig. 12.23 Chronic (ductopenic) allograft rejection. (a) The lumen of the hepatic artery branch is virtually occluded by subintimal accumulation of foamy macrophages; the bile duct on the right shows degenerative changes with epithelial atrophy and is surrounded by a light mixed inflammatory cell infiltrate. H&E. (b) This portal tract is devoid of a bile duct and there is a small residual collection of lymphocytes. H&E. (c) Advanced stage: the portal tract is difficult to identify as such, due to the disappearance of its bile duct and an attenuation of the arterial branches; inflammation is now inconspicuous. H&E.

Chronic rejection is usually preceded by cellular rejection, but this need not necessarily be severe. Clinically, it takes the form of persistent graft dysfunction, in particular progressive cholestasis, which is unresponsive to additional immunosuppression and develops in the absence of demonstrable biliary tract obstruction. Histologically, the interlobular bile ducts show variable degrees of epithelial degeneration (Fig. 12.23a); they become distorted, apparently being compressed by small amounts of surrounding collagen and eventually disappear completely from the graft (Fig. 12.23b,c) — *vanishing bile duct syndrome* or *ductopenic rejection*.[302–304] Cellular infiltration is usually scanty and becomes inconspicuous with time. There is usually intense cholestasis in acinar zone 3. Focal ductular proliferation may be seen early on, but it is characteristically absent later, in contradistinction to the changes associated with large duct obstruction or other ductopenic syndromes. Foam cell arteritis or arteriopathy (Ch. 18; Fig 12.23a), which most often accompanies ductopenic rejection, is rarley observed in needle biopsy specimens due to the large calibre of the arteries involved. Its presence is suspected when the biopsy specimen reveals a persistent, probably ischaemic perivenular cell dropout.[305] Perhaps as a corollary to the lack of ductular prolif-

eration, periportal fibrosis is minimal in chronic rejection. However, conspicuous perivenular fibrosis may occur with central–central, and later central–portal bridging septa. In rare cases periportal ductular proliferation and fibrosis are prominent, usually as a result of a superimposed stricture or of cholangiodestruction and/or cholangitis of the major bile ducts. The pathogenesis of ductopenic rejection is discussed in chapter 18.

In addition to immune rejection, injury to the interlobular bile ducts may result from viral infection, in particular *de novo* or reactivation of hepatitis C and cytomegalovirus infection, and from disease recurrence in patients with liver transplants for end-stage PBC.[306] Persistence of AMA in the serum is common after transplantation, irrespective of any allograft lesion.[307] Furthermore, PBC and rejection share many histological features, and a diagnosis of recurrent PBC rests on the demonstration of classic granulomatous destructive cholangitis (see Fig. 18.16). Until now, this has been observed in a few patients only[306,308,309,310] and the immunosuppressive regime, in particular cyclosporin A, appears to prevent such an event.[308,312] This is consistent with two multicentre trials which have shown a beneficial effect of this drug in naturally occurring PBC.[155,156] There is also some evidence that steroids may be protective.[311]

BILE-DUCT INJURY IN GRAFT-VERSUS-HOST DISEASE

In graft-versus-host disease (GVHD) transferred donor lymphocytes act as immunocompetent cells and aggressively attack the tissues of the host, principally the skin, the gastrointestinal tract and the liver.[313,314] In acute GVHD, jaundice develops in approximately 50% of patients.[315] A chronic form of GVHD, reminiscent of an autoimmune disorder, is characterized by general wasting with skin involvement, lachrimal and salivary gland injury and liver dysfunction with persistent elevation of serum alkaline phosphatase.[316] Chronic GVHD may follow the acute form with or without a clinically quiescent phase or may present *de novo* more than 100 days after grafting, indicating that acute and chronic GVHD may have a different pathogenesis.[317,318]

In acute GVHD, liver biopsy initially shows mild lymphocyte infiltration in both portal tracts and acinar parenchyma with acidophilic necrosis of single hepatocytes which may be difficult to distinguish from hepatitis due to other causes.[319-321] As the disease progresses bile ducts of 25–40 μm in diameter show degenerative atrophic changes with loss of their normal regular appearance. There is cytoplasmic vacuolation of epithelial cells and occasional single cell eosinophilic necrosis; some nuclei become hyperchromatic and there is considerable variation in their shape and size (Fig. 12.24a). The bile-duct damage is similar to allograft rejection but the portal tracts have a less intense chronic inflammatory cell infiltrate. Endotheliitis is present in approximately 10% of cases,[320] and lymphocytes in close contact with bile-duct cells have been demonstrated ultrastructurally.[322] In chronic GVHD, although the liver changes are basically the same, bile-duct damage and distortion are more severe and progressive ductopenia may be observed,[316] similar to that of chronic allograft rejection. However, obliterative endarteritis has not been reported in GVHD (Fig. 12.24b). In a few instances the lesion seems to have progressed to cirrhosis.[323-325] Finally, it is of interest to mention that GVHD has been occasionally recorded after liver transplantation,[326] probably as a result of a clonal expansion of lymphocytes transplanted with the donor organ. In theory the bile ducts should not be attacked in such a setting as they are bound to share the phenotype of the transplanted lymphocytes.[327]

OTHER DISORDERS ASSOCIATED WITH INTRAHEPATIC BILE-DUCT LESIONS

ACUTE AND CHRONIC VIRAL HEPATITIS

A hepatitis-associated bile-duct lesion was first reported by Poulsen & Christoffersen[328] and subsequent studies by these workers and by others have shown that this lesion is most commonly found in chronic hepatitis C and also in autoimmune chronic active hepatitis.[329-333] The distinctive lesions (Fig. 12.25a,b) affect bile ducts of less than 50 μm in diameter and are characterized by prominent swelling and vacuolation of the bile-duct epithelium with piling up of irregularly spaced and hyperchromatic nuclei.

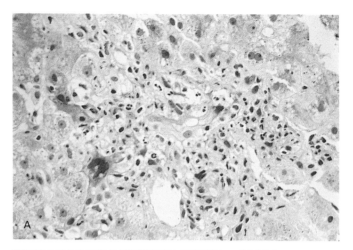

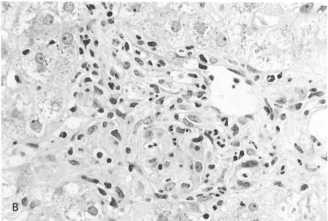

Fig. 12.24 Graft-versus-host disease. (a) Distorted bile duct showing epithelial atrophy with both surrounding and infiltrating mononuclear cells. Marginal bile ducts also show degenerative changes. H & E. (b) Duct epithelium is swollen and the lumen is virtually obliterated; intra-epithelial lymphocytes are surrounded by a vacuole; there are also intraluminal inflammatory cells. H & E.

The lumen may be considerably narrowed and there may be reduplication of the epithelial basement membrane (Fig. 12.25b). The surrounding inflammatory cell infiltrate often includes lymphocytic aggregates with or without a follicular arrangement. The lesion may involve only a segment of the duct circumference; duct destruction may occur but rupture is unusual, granulomas are not found and there is no evidence of progressive bile-duct loss. Vyberg,[334] using serial three-dimensional studies, described a diverticular variant of the hepatitis-associated bile-duct lesions. The aetiopathogenesis of the lesions is not known, and viral injury or immunological mechanisms have been postulated. Using in situ hybridization, Nouri Aria et al[335] have detected HCV genome in bile-duct epithelium as well as in hepatocytes. However, in contrast to what is found in PBC and PSC, aberrant expression of HLA-DR antigens cannot be demonstrated in damaged bile ducts in HCV infection, suggesting that different mechanisms are responsible for the bile-duct injury.[336] Vyberg[334] commented on their similarity to the benign lympho-epithelial lesion

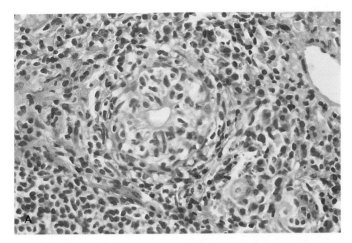

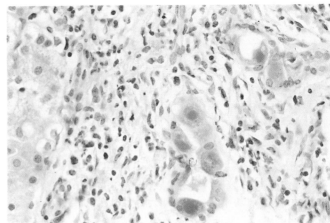

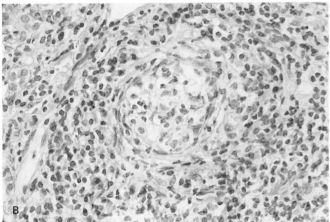

Fig. 12.26 Neonatal hepatitis. Cytomegalovirus inclusions in the epithelial lining of a small bile duct. H&E.

Fig. 12.25 Hepatitis-associated bile-duct lesion. (a) There is an intense chronic inflammatory cell infiltrate in the portal tract; the bile-duct epithelium is swollen and stratified producing reduction of the luminal diameter; the epithelial cell cytoplasm is vacuolated and intra-epithelial inflammatory mononuclear cells are present. H&E. (b) Serial section from the same case showing virtual obliteration of the lumen; there appears to be some reduplication of the basement membrane. PAS. By courtesy of Prof. H. Poulsen.

which is seen in autoimmune lymphocytic sialadenitis (Sjögren's syndrome), and in which an association with chronic hepatitis C has recently been reported.[337]

The prevalence of bile-duct lesions varies from 0–90% in various series;[338–341] this probably reflects differences in timing of the biopsy in relation to the clinical disease, the number of post-transfusion as compared with sporadic cases of hepatitis C infection, and variations in the criteria used to diagnose bile-duct injury. The approximate frequency is 10–15% in acute viral hepatitis, 20–25% in chronic viral hepatitis and 25–30% in chronic autoimmune hepatitis. The presence of these bile duct lesions has been associated with a chronic course in acute non-A/non-B hepatitis[342,343] but it is not an independent prognostic variable. Conflicting reports have been published on the significance of bile-duct lesions as predictors of progression to cirrhosis in chronic active hepatitis.[344,345]

Reversible injury to bile-duct epithelium in cytomegalovirus (CMV) hepatitis is not unusual, particularly in the neonatal period (Fig. 12.26). That obliterative cholangitis due to CMV might be a precursor of paucity of intrahepatic bile ducts in infants (Ch. 3) has been claimed in a single case report,[346] but not supported by further evidence. A close association exists between CMV infection and both GVHD[347] and liver allograft rejection.[348] Although CMV infection has been shown to increase the risk of ductopenic rejection[347] there is still doubt as to whether the virus, which has been shown to persist in the chronically rejected liver graft,[349] is there as an innocent bystander or as a trigger of cholangiodestruction.[350]

DRUG AND TOXIN-INDUCED INJURY

Various drugs may produce a cholestatic type of reaction which, when prolonged, closely resembles the clinical syndrome and serum biochemical abnormalities of PBC. These are reviewed in chapter 15; see also Tables 15.11 and 15.12. The portal tract changes, however, are usually much less prominent than in PBC, with a mild to moderate inflammatory infiltrate which is often rich in eosinophils and neutrophils. The small bile ducts may show variable vacuolation or eosinophilic degeneration with nuclear pyknosis, and signs of regeneration with mitotic activity (Fig. 12.27a). The number of ducts may be markedly reduced,[351] and although the lesions are generally reversible, progressive duct loss is increasingly recognized in this situation.[352–354] Granulomatous destructive cholangitis indistinguishable from the lesion of PBC is exceptionally recorded,[355] but small collections of foamy macrophages may occur at the site of apparent bile-duct rupture. A granulomatous reaction with eosinophils may be seen, particularly in patients presenting signs of hypersensitivity (Fig. 12.27b). Bilirubinostasis is a constant finding. In some cases there may also be considerable portal tract oedema, with biliary piecemeal necrosis, ductular proliferation and periductular inflam-

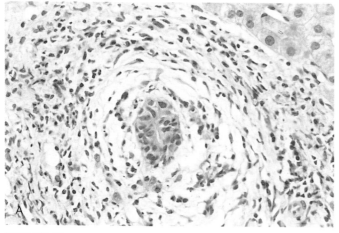
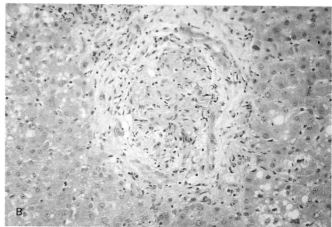
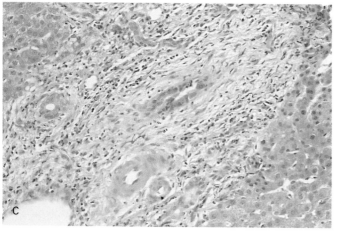
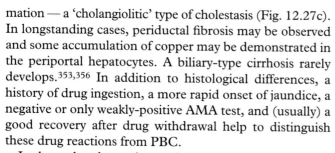

Fig. 12.27 Drug-induced bile-duct injury. (a) Imipiramine-induced jaundice: the small bile duct shows epithelial atypia with nuclear pleomorphism and crowding; there is marked periductal oedema with a light mixed inflammatory cell infiltrate. H & E. (b) Carbamazepine (Tegretol): there is a granulomatous reaction in the portal tract with marked oedema of the portal tract fibrous tissue and a neutrophil polymorph reaction; the damaged bile duct shows epithelial degeneration and a surrounding and infiltrative neutrophil polymorph reaction. H & E. (c) Chronic jaundice due to chlorpromazine: there is a continuing inflammatory reaction of the portal tract with a periportal ductular reaction; there is some periductal fibrosis, the epithelium shows degenerative change and there is a related neutrophil polymorph reaction. H & E.

mation — a 'cholangiolitic' type of cholestasis (Fig. 12.27c). In longstanding cases, periductal fibrosis may be observed and some accumulation of copper may be demonstrated in the periportal hepatocytes. A biliary-type cirrhosis rarely develops.[353,356] In addition to histological differences, a history of drug ingestion, a more rapid onset of jaundice, a negative or only weakly-positive AMA test, and (usually) a good recovery after drug withdrawal help to distinguish these drug reactions from PBC.

In the authors' experience, duct damage may be readily overlooked in drug-induced cholestatic injury and histopathologists should be aware of this type of injury. Similar lesions have been produced experimentally or accidentally by toxic substances such as α-naphthylisothiocyanate, dibutylin-dichloride and 4,4'-diaminodiphenylmethane (Epping jaundice). In paraquat poisoning, eosinophilic shrinkage of duct epithelium, nuclear pyknosis and epithelial detachment from the basement membrane have been noted (see Fig. 15.18) with a very scanty inflammatory reaction.[357,358]

SUPPURATIVE CHOLANGITIS

Bacterial cholangitis complicating extrahepatic obstruction is discussed in Chapter 11.

Primary recurrent pyogenic (Oriental) cholangitis

This is a common condition in the Far East but cases also occur in Oriental immigrants to Western countries[359,360] The essential lesion is dilatation and inflammation of the extra- and intrahepatic bile ducts unassociated with cholecystitis and gallstones. The disease may affect only one lobe and there may be segmental atrophy.[361] Intrahepatic stones may form but these are of a different composition to classic gallstones.[362] The symptoms vary from vague right-sided epigastric pain and fever to severe pain radiating to the back and right scapula, vomiting, jaundice and rigors. Patients may present as an acute abdominal emergency. In some patients the acute attacks are due to secondary infection and respond to antibiotic treatment; in others biliary tract decompression has to be performed; in a few cases endotoxic shock may develop. The liver is enlarged and tender and the gallbladder may be distended and palpable.[360] The patients are usually underweight and come from the lower socio-economic groups. They are in the 20–50 year-old age group and males are affected as frequently as females. The diagnosis can be established radiologically and by CT scan, and interventional treatment can be instituted.[361,363] The aetiology is obscure but it has been reported in some patients in association with opisthorchiasis and ascariasis. In many patients no aetiological agent may be discovered.

It is difficult to explain why this condition is uncommon in tropical Africa in spite of the fact that infestation with parasites is rife. Liver flukes are common in the Far East and certainly account for some cases, but it is unclear why ascariasis so rarely causes liver lesions in Africa. There is a reported association between the cholangitis and morphine addiction; morphia causes spasm of the sphincter of Oddi and this might result in obstruction and dilatation of the proximal bile duct with secondary infection.[364] In a recent study disturbance of common bile-duct motor activity was demonstrated in some patients with recurrent pyogenic cholangitis; this was thought to be secondary to inflammation of the ampulla of Vater but could be a factor in precipitating the recurrent attack of cholangitis.[365]

A review of 141 patients from Korea[366] suggested that the acute cholangitis was caused by parasitic infestation of the biliary tract, from below in most cases; the authors suggested the name 'oriental infestational cholangitis' as an alternative. They proposed a sequence of changes which starts with infestation and leads to sclerosing cholangitis with segmental narrowing and ectasia of the common bile duct. The formation of stasis calculi leads to obstruction and dilatation involving first one hepatic duct and later, the other. Eventually, bilateral hepatic duct ectasia, with or without calculi, results. Secondary infection may lead to multiple pericholangiolar abscesses, culminating in the clinical picture of acute septic shock.

Secondary infection in this condition is common. The organism most frequently involved is *E. coli* but other organisms including *S. typhi* have been described. The source of secondary infection is considered to be the colon and the route of infection is via the portal vein. The wall of the gallbladder is oedematous but signs of inflammation are not usually present. Occasionally the gallbladder may contain white bile. Secondary biliary cirrhosis may occur. Other complications include perforation of the gallbladder with biliary peritonitis, or extension of infection to the pleura and base of the right lung. Biliary–enteric fistula and thrombophlebitis of the hepatic or portal veins have also been reported. Pulmonary hypertension due to repeated microemboli from the liver has been described.[367]

SEPTICAEMIA: SEPTIC/ENDOTOXIC SHOCK

Septicaemia from any cause may produce a suppurative cholangitis. In one female patient with *E. coli* septicaemia and severe cholestasis, liver histology showed reversible bile-duct damage characterized by epithelial swelling with nuclear pleomorphism, hyperchromasia or pyknosis. Duct cells protruded into the lumen which was variably narrowed or dilated.[368]

In septic/endotoxic shock, jaundice is frequently present; possible mechanisms are discussed in Chapter 11. The biopsy shows a striking and characteristic cholangiolitis (Fig. 12.28a–c), the portal tracts being surrounded by dilated cholangioles which extend into the periportal zone and contain PAS-positive concretions; neutrophil polymorphs are present within and surrounding the ductules.[369,370] This is an important lesion to recognize, in that the picture of an acute cholangiolitis without a suppurative cholangitis suggests septicaemia rather than duct obstruction.[369] In longstanding cases or at autopsy, the portal tracts are ringed by the bile-containing dilated cholangioles (Fig. 12.28d), a pattern often encountered in biopsy specimens from liver allografts. Similar striking cholangiolar bile retention may sometimes be seen at autopsy after submassive liver-cell necrosis of viral or drug aetiology, and in decompensated cirrhosis, when it could reflect a superadded sepsis.

'TOXIC SHOCK' SYNDROME

The toxic shock syndrome is thought to be due to an exotoxin produced by *Staphylococcus aureus* and in some cases was associated with the use of vaginal tampons; in other cases skin infection was present but in many no source of infection could be defined. There is a high mortality rate. The patients present with multi-system involvement — vomiting and diarrhoea, myalgia, impaired renal function, thrombocytopenia, mental deterioration and jaundice with elevated aminotransferases.[371,372] Jaundice was a feature in 50% of patients; histologically there was a severe cholangitis and cholangiolitis with an intense mural, luminal and periductal infiltrate of neutrophil polymorphs (Fig. 12.29). The lesion was attributed to chemical irritation, probably resulting from exotoxin excretion in the bile, combined with liver hypoperfusion.

PARASITIC INFESTATION (see Ch. 7)

At the stage of bile-duct invasion by the adult worms *Fasciola hepatica* and *Ascaris lumbricoides*, a cholangitis develops which is characterized by a heavy periductal inflammatory cell infiltrate particularly rich in eosinophils. Epithelial hyperplasia with adenomatous proliferation and mucous gland metaplasia affecting larger intrahepatic ducts is more common and more prominent in clonorchiasis and opisthorchiasis. Their association with intrahepatic bile-duct carcinoma is addressed in Chapter 16. The development of a sclerosing cholangitis after rupture or scolicidal fluid injection of hydatid cyst is discussed on page 496.

HODGKIN'S DISEASE

Liver involvement in Hodgkin's disease is discussed in Chapter 17. A syndrome of idiopathic intrahepatic cholestasis has been recognized in patients with Hodgkin's disease and non-Hodgkin's lymphoma.[373,374] Hubscher and his colleagues[375] have recently reported 3 patients with Hodgkin's disease who had severe progressive cholestasis and in

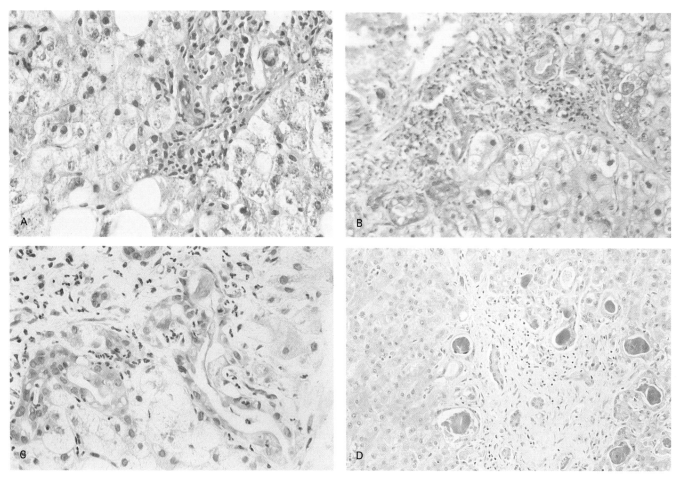

Fig. 12.28 Cholangiolar cholestasis associated with septicaemia. (a) Biopsy 6 days post-operative showing some mild increased prominence of cholangioles (canals of Hering). Masson's trichrome. (b) Biopsy 7 days later showing marked prominence of the cholangioles with a related cholangiolitis. Masson's trichrome. (c) Same biopsy as (b) showing the cholangiolar swelling, the presence of a bile concretion and an intense acute cholangiolitis. H & E. (d) Autopsy case showing dilated periportal cholangioles with numerous bile concretions. H & E.

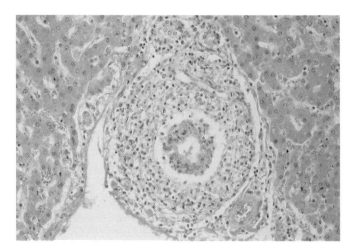

Fig. 12.29 Toxic shock syndrome. Autopsy liver showing intense acute inflammatory cell infiltrate of the portal tract with a cholangitis. H & E.

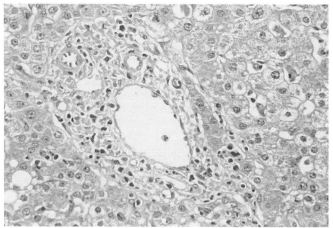

Fig. 12.30 Hodgkin's disease with cholestatic syndrome. There is a mild chronic inflammatory cell infiltrate of the portal tract in which, however, no bile duct is present. H & E.

whom liver biopsy showed progressive ductopenia. We have seen occasional similar cases (Fig. 12.30). The mechanisms of the injury are not known but such a disappearing bile duct syndrome may be one explanation for intrahepatic cholestasis in patients with Hodgkin's disease.

NEONATAL AND CHILDHOOD DISORDERS
(see Ch. 3)

In extrahepatic biliary atresia the small intrahepatic bile ducts may show evidence of damage with progressive reduction in number and eventual complete disappearance in advanced cases. The liver lesions associated with α_1-antitrypsin deficiency may include progressive ductopenia (Ch. 4). In juveniles and young adults with a ZZ phenotype, the cirrhosis may be biliary in type and, on occasion, features of cholate stasis with hydropic swelling of hepatocytes, copper accumulation and Mallory bodies may occur.

REFERENCES

1. Bianchi L. Liver biopsy interpretation in hepatitis. Part I. Presentation of critical morphologic features used in diagnosis (Glossary). Pathol Res Pract 1983; 178: 2–19
2. Gleeson D, Boyer J L. Intrahepatic cholestasis. In: McIntyre N, Benhamou J P, Bircher J, Rizzetto M, Rodes J, eds. Oxford Textbook of clinical hepatology, vol 2. Oxford: Oxford University Press, 1991: pp 1087–1107
3. Popper H, Schaffner F. The pathophysiology of cholestasis. Hum Pathol 1970; 1: 1–24
4. Gumucio J J, Miller D L. Zonal hepatic function: solute-hepatocyte interactions within the liver acinus. In: Popper H, Schaffner F, eds. Progress in liver diseases, vol VII. New York: Grune & Stratton, 1982: pp 17–30
5. Salaspuro M, Sipponen P. Demonstration of an intracellular copper-binding protein by orcein staining in long-standing cholestatic liver diseases. Gut 17: 787–790
6. Portmann B C. Histochemistry in diagnostic assessment of liver biopsy. In: Filipe M I, Lake B D, eds. Histochemistry in pathology, 2nd edn. Edinburgh: Churchill Livingstone 1990: pp 221–234
7. Guarascio P, Yentis F, Cevikbas U, Portmann B, Williams R. Value of copper-associated protein in diagnostic assessment of liver biopsy. J Clin Pathol 1983; 36: 18–23
8. Gerber M A, Orr W, Denk H, Schaffner F, Popper H. Hepatocellular hyalin in cholestasis and cirrhosis: its diagnostic significance. Gastroenterology 1973; 64: 89–98
9. Denk M, Lackinger E. Cytoskeleton in liver diseases. Semin Liver Dis 1986; 6: 199–211
10. Burt A D, Stewart J A, Aitchison M, MacSween R N M. Expression of tissue polypeptide antigen (TPA) in fetal and adult liver: changes in liver disease. J Clin Pathol 1987; 40: 719–724
11. Popper H. Morphological and immunological studies on chronic aggressive hepatitis and primary biliary cirrhosis. In: Smith M, Williams R, eds. Immunology of the liver. London: Heinemann, 1971: 17–27
12. Portmann B, Popper H, Neuberger J, Williams R. Sequential and diagnostic features in primary biliary cirrhosis, based on serial histologic study in 209 patients. Gastroenterology 1985; 88: 1777–1790
13. Van Eyken P, Sciot R, Desmet V J. A cytokeratin immunohistochemical study of cholestatic liver disease: evidence that hepatocytes can express "bile duct-type" cytokeratin. Histopathology 1989; 15: 125–136
14. Nakanuma Y, Ohta G. Immunohistochemical study on bile ductular proliferation in various hepatobiliary diseases. Liver 1989; 6: 205–211
15. Slott P A, Liu M H, Tavoloni N. Origin, pattern and mechanism of bile duct proliferation following biliary obstruction in the rat. Gastroenterology 1990; 99: 466–477
16. Desmet V J. Current problems in diagnosis of biliary disease and cholestasis. Semin Liver Dis 1986; 6: 133–245
17. Burt A D, MacSween R N M. Bile duct proliferation — its true significance. Histopathology 1993; 23: 590–596
18. Baptista A, Bianchi L, De Groote J et al. The diagnostic significance of periportal hepatic necrosis and inflammation. Histopathology 1988; 12: 569–579
19. International Group. Histopathology of the intrahepatic bile ducts. Liver 1983; 3: 161–175
20. MacSween R N M, Burt A D. Pathology of the intrahepatic bile ducts. In: Anthony P P, MacSween R N M, eds. Recent advances in histopathology, no 14. Edinburgh: Churchill Livingstone, 1989: pp 161–183
21. Addison T, Gull W. On a certain affection of the skin — vitiligoidea α-plana, β-tubersoa. Guy's Hospital Reports, 2nd series 1851; 7: 265–277
22. Hanot V (ed). Étude sur une forme de cirrhose hypertrophique du foie (Cirrhose hypertrophique avec icterè chronique). Paris: J B Ballière, 1876
23. Dauphinee J A, Sinclair J C. Primary biliary cirrhosis. Can Med Ass J 1949; 61: 1–6
24. Ahrens E H Jr, Payne M A, Kunkel H G, Eisenmenger W J, Blondheim S H. Primary biliary cirrhosis. Medicine 1950; 29: 299–364
25. Rubin E, Schaffner F, Popper H. Primary biliary cirrhosis. Chronic non-suppurative destructive cholangitis. Am J Pathol 1965; 46: 387–407
26. Kaplan M M. Primary biliary cirrhosis. N Engl J Med 1987; 316: 521–528
27. Mackay I R, Gershwin M E. Primary biliary cirrhosis: Current knowledge, perspectives, and future directions. Semin Liver Dis 1989; 9: 149–157
28. Vierling J M. Primary biliary cirrhosis. In Zakim D, Boyer T D, eds. Hepatology: a textbook of liver disease, vol 2. Philadelphia: W B Saunders, 1990: pp 1158–1205
29. Rubel L R, Rabin L, Seeff L B, Licht H, Cuccherini B A. Does primary biliary cirrhosis in men differ from primary biliary cirrhosis in women? Hepatology 1984; 4: 671–677
30. Lucey M R, Neuberger J M, Williams R. Primary biliary cirrhosis in men. Gut 1986; 27: 1373–1376
31. Hislop W S. Primary biliary cirrhosis: an epidemiological study. Brit Med J 1980; ii: 1069–1070
32. Triger D R. Primary biliary cirrhosis: an epidemiological study. Brit Med J 1980; ii: 772–775
33. Triger D R, Berg P A, Rodes J. Epidemiology of primary biliary cirrhosis. Liver 1984; 4: 195–200
34. Danielsson A, Boqvist L, Uddenfeldt P. Epidemiology of primary biliary cirrhosis in a defined rural population in the Northern part of Sweden. Hepatology 1990; 11: 458–464
35. Myszor M, James O F W. The epidemiology of primary biliary cirrhosis in North-east England: an increasingly common disease? Quart J Med 1990; 75: 377–385
36. Kew M C, Varma R R, Dos Santos H A, Scheuer P J, Sherlock S. Portal hypertension in primary biliary cirrhosis. Gut 1971; 12: 830–834
37. Navasa M, Parés A, Bruguera M, Caballería J, Bosch J. Rodés J. Portal hypertension in primary biliary cirrhosis. Relationship with histological features. J Hepatol 1987; 5: 292–298
38. Long R G, Scheuer P J, Sherlock S. Presentation and course of asymptomatic primary biliary cirrhosis. Gastroenterology 1977; 72: 1204–1207
39. Fleming R C, Ludwig J, Dickson E R. Asymptomatic primary biliary cirrhosis. Mayo Clin Proc 1978; 53: 587–593
40. James O, Macklon A F, Watson A J. Primary biliary cirrhosis — a revised clinical spectrum. Lancet 1981; i: 1278–1281
41. Beswick D R, Klatskin G, Boyer J L. Asymptomatic primary biliary cirrhosis. A progress report on long-term follow-up and natural history. Gastroenterology 1985; 89: 267–271

42. Balasubramaniam K, Grambsch P M, Wiesner R H, Lindor K D, Dickson E R. Diminished survival in asymptomatic primary biliary cirrhosis. A prospective study. Gastroenterology 1990; 98: 1567–1571

43. Mitchison H C, Lucey M R, Kelly P J, Neuberger J M, Williams R, James O F W. Symptom development and prognosis in primary biliary cirrhosis: a study in two centers. Gastroenterology 1990; 99: 778–784

44. Goudie B M, Burt A D, Macfarlane G J et al. Risk factors and prognosis in primary biliary cirrhosis. Am J Gastroenterol 1989; 84: 713–716

45. Dickson E R, Grambsch P M, Fleming T R, Fisher L D, Longworthy N. Prognosis in primary biliary cirrhosis: model for decision making. Hepatology 1989; 10: 1–10

46. Roll J, Boyer J L, Barry D, Klatskin G. The prognostic importance of the clinical and histologic features in asymptomatic primary biliary cirrhosis. N Engl J Med 1983; 308: 1–7

47. Christensen E, Neuberger J, Crowe J et al. Beneficial effect of azathioprine and prediction of prognosis in primary biliary cirrhosis. Gastroenterology 1985; 5: 1084–1091

48. Neuberger J, Altman D, Christensen E, Tygstrup N, Williams R. Use of a prognostic index in evaluation of liver transplantation for primary biliary cirrhosis. Transplantation 1986; 41: 713–716

49. Markus B, Dickson E R, Grambsch P et al. Efficacy of liver transplantation in patients with primary biliary cirrhosis. N Engl J Med 1989; 320: 1709–1713

50. Culp K S, Fleming C R, Duffy J, Baldus W P, Dickson E R. Autoimmune associations in primary biliary cirrhosis. Mayo Clin Proc 1982; 57: 365–370

51. Tsianos E V, Hoofnagle J H, Fox P C et al. Sjögren's syndrome in patients with primary biliary cirrhosis. Hepatology 1990; 11: 730–734

52. Uddenfeldt A, Danielsson A, Forssell A, Holm M, Östberg Y. Features of Sjögren's syndrome in patients with primary biliary cirrhosis. J Int Med 1991; 230: 443–448

53. Golding P L, Brown R, Mason A M S, Taylor E. "Sicca complex" in liver disease. Br Med J 1970; iv: 340–342

54. Epstein O, Thomas H C, Sherlock S. Primary biliary cirrhosis is a dry gland syndrome with features of chronic graft-versus-host (GVH) disease. Lancet 1980; i: 1166–1168

55. Reynolds T B, Dension E K, Frankl H D, Lieberman F L, Peters R L. Primary biliary cirrhosis with scleroderma, Raynaud's phenomenon and telangiectasia. Am J Med 1971; 50: 302–312

56. Powell F C, Schroeter A L, Dickson E R. Primary biliary cirrhosis and the CREST syndrome: a report of 22 cases. Quart J Med 1987; 62: 75–82

57. Marx W J, O'Connell D J. Arthritis of primary biliary cirrhosis. Arch Int Med 1979; 139: 213–216

58. Modena V, Marengo C, Amoroso A et al. Primary biliary cirrhosis and rheumatic diseases. A clinical, immunological and immunogenetical study. Clin Exp Rheum 1986; 4: 129–134

59. Crowe J P, Christensen E, Butler J et al. Primary biliary cirrhosis: The prevalence of hypothyroidism and its relationship to thyroid auto-antibodies and sicca syndrome. Gastroenterology 1980; 78: 1437–1441

60. Golding P L, Smith M, Williams R. Multi-system involvement in chronic liver disease. Am J Med 1973; 55: 772–782

61. Pares A, Rimola A, Bruguera M, Mas E, Rodes J. Renal tubular acidosis in primary biliary cirrhosis. Gastroenterology 1981; 80: 681–686

62. Logan R F A, Ferguson A, Finlayson N D C, Weir D G. Primary biliary cirrhosis and coeliac disease: an association? Lancet 1978; i: 230–233

63. Gabrielsen T O, Hoel P S. Primary biliary cirrhosis associated with coeliac disease and dermatitis herpetiformis. Dermatologica 1985; 170: 31–34

64. Mutimer D J, Bassendine M F, Crook P, James O F W. Vasculitis in primary biliary cirrhosis — response to prednisolone. Q J Med 1990; 75: 509–514

65. Weissman E, Becker N H. Interstitial lung disease in primary biliary cirrhosis. Am J Med Sci 1983; 285: 21–27

66. Bissuel F, Bizollon T, Dijoud F et al. Pulmonary hemorrhage and glomerulonephritis in primary biliary cirrhosis. Hepatology 1992; 16: 1357–1361

67. Taub W H, Lederman R J, Tuthill R J, Falk G W. Primary biliary cirrhosis in a patient with multiple sclerosis. Am J Gastroenterol 1989; 84: 415–417

68. Pontecorvo M J, Levinson J D, Roth J A. A patient with primary biliary cirrhosis and multiple sclerosis. Am J Med 1992; 92: 433–436

69. Bush A, Mitchison H, Walt R et al. Primary biliary cirrhosis and ulcerative colitis. Gastroenterology 1987; 92: 2009–2013

70. Hall S, Axelsen P H, Larson D E, Bunch T W. Systemic lupus erythematosus developing in patients with primary biliary cirrhosis. Ann Int Med 1984; 100: 388–389

71. Jain S, Markham R, Thomas H C et al. Double stranded DNA binding capacity of serum in acute and chronic liver diseases. Clin Exp Immunol 1976; 26: 35–41

72. Eastell R, Dickson E R, Hodgson S F, Wiesner R H et al. Rates of vertebral bone loss before and after liver transplantation in women with primary biliary cirrhosis. Hepatology 1991; 14: 296–300

73. Mitchison H C, Bassendine M F, Hendrick A. Positive antimitochondrial antibody but normal alkaline phosphatase: Is this primary biliary cirrhosis? Hepatology 1986; 6: 1279–1284

74. MacSween R N M, Horne C H W, Moffat A J, Hughes H M. Serum protein levels in primary biliary cirrhosis. J Clin Pathol 1972; 25: 789–792

75. Walker J G, Doniach D, Roitt I M, Sherlock S. Serological tests in diagnosis of primary biliary cirrhosis. Lancet 1965; i: 827–831

76. Goudie R B, MacSween R N M, Goldberg D M. Serological and histological diagnosis of primary biliary cirrhosis. J Clin Pathol 1966; 19: 527–538

77. Berg P A, Klein R. Clinical and prognostic relevance of different mitrochondrial antibody profiles in primary biliary cirrhosis (PBC). Mol Aspects Med 1985; 8: 235–248

78. Berg P A, Klein R. Heterogeneity of antimitochondrial antibodies. Semin Liver Dis 1989; 9: 103–116

79. Gershwin M E, Coppel R L, Mackay I R. Primary biliary cirrhosis and mitochondrial autoantigens — insights from molecular biology. Hepatology 1988; 8: 147–151

80. Bassendine M F, Fussey S P M, Mutimer D J, James O F W, Yeaman S J. Identification and characterization of four M2 mitochondrial auto-antigens in primary biliary cirrhosis. Semin Liver Dis 1989; 9: 124–131

81. Berg P A, Klein R. Antimitochondrial antibodies in primary biliary cirrhosis and other disorders: definition and clinical relevance. Dig Dis Sci 1992; 10: 85–101

82. Palmer J M, Yeaman S J, Bassendine M F, James O F W. M4 and M9 autoantigens in primary biliary cirrhosis — a negative study. J Hepatol 1993; 18: 251–254

83. Gores G J, Moore S B, Fisher L D, Powell F C, Dickson E R. Primary biliary cirrhosis: association with class II major histocompatibility complex antigens. Hepatology 1987; 7: 889–892

84. Manns M P, Bremm A, Schneider P M et al. HLA DRw8 and complement C4 deficiency as risk factors in primary biliary cirrhosis. Gastroenterology 1991; 101: 1367–1373

85. Underhill J, Donaldson P, Bray G, Doherty D, Portmann B, Williams R. Susceptibility to primary biliary cirrhosis is associated with the HLA-DR8-DQB1 *0402 haplotype. Hepatology 1992; 16: 1404–1408

86. Caldwell S H, Leung P S C, Spivey J R et al. Antimitochondrial antibodies in kindreds of patients with primary biliary cirrhosis: anti-mitochondrial antibodies are unique to clinical disease and are absent in asymptomatic family members. Hepatology 1992; 16: 889–905

87. Tsuji H, Murai K, Agagi K, Fujishima M. Familial primary biliary cirrhosis associated with impaired concanavalin A-induced lymphocyte transformation in relatives. Dig Dis Sci 1992; 37: 353–360

88. Berg P A, Klein R. Autoantibodies in primary biliary cirrhosis. Semin Immunopathol 1990; 12: 85–99

89. Wands J R, Dienstag J L, Bhan A L, Feller E R, Isselbacher K J. Circulating immune complexes and complement activation in primary biliary cirrhosis. N Engl J Med 1978; 298: 233–237

90. Lindgren S, Laurell A-B, Ericsson S. Complement components and activation in primary biliary cirrhosis. Hepatology 1984; 4: 9–14

91. Bodenheimer H C, Charland C, Thayer W R, Schaffner F, Staples P J. Effects of penicillamine on serum immunoglobulins and immune complex-reactive material in primary biliary cirrhosis. Gastroenterology 1985; 88: 412–417

92. James S P, Vierling J M, Strober W. The role of the immune response in the pathogenesis of primary biliary cirrhosis. Semin Liver Dis 1981; 1: 322–337

93. Routhier G, Epstein O, Janossy G et al. Effects of cyclosporin A on suppressor and inducer T lymphocytes in primary biliary cirrhosis. Lancet 1980; ii: 1223–1226

94. Bhan A K, Dienstag J L, Wands J R, Schlossman S F, Reinherz E L. Alterations of T-cell subsets in primary biliary cirrhosis. Clin Exp Immunol 1982; 47: 351–358

95. MacSween R N M, Burt A D. The cellular pathology of primary biliary cirrhosis. Mol Aspects Med 1985; 8: 269–292

96. MacLean C A, Goudie B M, MacSween R N M, Sandilands G P. Serum Fcδ receptor-like molecules in primary biliary cirrhosis: a possible immunoregulatory mechanism. Immunology 1984; 53: 315–324

97. Ekdahl K N, Lööf L, Nyberg A, Nilsson U R, Nilsson B. Defective Fcδ receptor-mediated clearance in patients with primary biliary cirrhosis. Gastroenterology 1991; 101: 1076–1082

98. Nagafuchi Y, Scheuer P J. Hepatic β_2-microglobulin distribution in primary biliary cirrhosis. J Hepatol 1986; 2: 73–80

99. Ballardini G, Mirakian R, Bianchi F B, Pisi E, Doniach D, Botazzo G F. Aberrant expression of HLA-DR antigens on bile duct epithelium in primary biliary cirrhosis: relevance to pathogenesis. Lancet 1984; ii: 1009–1013

100. Spengler U, Pape G R, Hoffman R M et al. Differential expression of MHC class II subregion products on bile duct epithelial cells and hepatocytes in patients with primary biliary cirrhosis. Hepatology 1988; 8: 459–462

101. van den Oord J J, Sciot P, Desmet V J. Expression of MHC products by normal and abnormal bile duct epithelium. J Hepatol 1986; 3: 310–317

102. Chapman R W, Kelly P M A, Heryet A, Jewell D P, Fleming K A. Expression of HLA-DR antigens on bile duct epithelium in primary sclerosing cholangitis. Gut 1988; 29: 870–877

103. Yamada G, Hyodo I, Tobe K et al. Ultrastructure and immunocytochemical analysis of lymphocytes infiltrating bile duct epithelia in primary biliary cirrhosis. Hepatology 1986; 6: 385–391

104. Colucci G, Schaffner F, Paronetto F. In situ characterization of the cell surface antigens of the mononuclear cell infiltrate and bile duct epithelium in primary biliary cirrhosis. Clin Immunol Immunopathol 1986; 41: 35–42

105. Krams S M, Van de Water J, Coppel R L et al. Analysis of hepatic T lymphocyte and immunoglobulin deposits in patients with primary biliary cirrhosis. Hepatology 1990; 12: 306–313

106. Adams D H, Hubscher S G, Shaw J et al. Increased expression of intercellular adhesion molecule 1 on bile ducts in primary biliary cirrhosis and primary sclerosing cholangitis. Hepatology 1991; 14: 426–431

107. Broome U, Scheynius A, Hultcrantz R. Induced expression of heat-shock protein on biliary epithelium in patients with primary sclerosing cholangitis and primary biliary cirrhosis. Hepatology 1993; 18: 298–303

108. Bernuau D, Feldmann G, Degott C, Gisselbrecht C. Ultrastructural lesions of bile ducts in primary biliary cirrhosis. A comparison with the lesions observed in graft versus host disease. Hum Pathol 1981; 12: 782–793

109. Fennell R H. Ductular damage in liver transplant rejection. Its similarity to that of primary biliary cirrhosis and graft-versus-host disease. In: Sommers S C, Rosen P P, eds. Pathol Ann 16 (Part 2). New York: Appleton-Century-Crofts, 1981: pp 289–294

110. McFarlane I G, Wojcicka B M, Tsantoulas D C, Portmann B, Eddleston A L W F, Williams R. Leucocyte migration inhibition in response to biliary antigens in primary biliary cirrhosis, sclerosing cholangitis, and other chronic liver disease. Gastroenterology 1979; 76: 1333–1340

111. Vento S, O'Brien C J, McFarlane B M, McFarlane I G, Eddleston A L W F, Williams R. T-lymphocytes' sensitization to hepatocyte antigens in autoimmune chronic active hepatitis and primary biliary cirrhosis. Gastroenterology 1986; 91: 810–817

112. Onishi S, Maeda T, Iwasaki S et al. A biliary protein identified by immunoblotting stimulates proliferation of peripheral blood T lymphocytes in primary biliary cirrhosis. Liver 1991; 11: 32–328

113. Berg P A, Klein R. Leader: Antimitochondrial antibodies in primary biliary cirrhosis. A clue to its etiopathogenesis? J Hepatol 1992; 15: 6–9

114. Joplin R, Lindsay J G, Johnson G D, Stain A, Neuberger J. Membrane dihydrolipoamide acetyltransferase (E2) on human biliary epithelial cells in primary biliary cirrhosis. Lancet 1992; 339: 93–94

115. Van de Water J, Turchany J J, Leung P S C et al. Molecular mimicry in primary biliary cirrhosis. Evidence for epithelial expression of a molecule cross-reactive with pyruvate dehydrogenase complex-E2. J Clin Invest, 1993; 91: 2653–64

116. Klein R, Berg P A. Demonstration of antibodies against the pyruvate dehydrogenase complex (M2) in sera from patients with tuberculosis. Hepatology 1992; 16: 556 (abstract)

117. Johnson L, Wirostko E, Wirostko W. Primary biliary cirrhosis in the mouse: induction by human mycoplasma-like organism. Int J Exp Pathol 1990; 71: 701–712

118. Stanley N N, Fox R A, Whimster W F, Sherlock S, Jones D G. Primary biliary cirrhosis or sarcoidosis or both. N Engl J Med 1972; 287: 1282–1284

119. Fagan E A, Moore-Gillon J C, Turner-Warwick M. Multi-organ granulomas and mitochondrial antibodies. N Engl J Med 1983; 308: 572–575

120. Maddrey W C. Sarcoidosis and primary biliary cirrhosis: Associated disorders? N Engl J Med 1983; 308: 588–590

121. MacSween R N M, Sumithran E. Histopathology of primary biliary cirrhosis. Semin Liver Dis 1981; 1: 282–292

122. Schaffner F, Popper H. Clinical-pathologic relations in primary biliary cirrhosis. In: Popper H, Schaffner F, eds. Progress in liver diseases, vol VII. New York: Grune & Stratton, 1982: pp 529–554

123. Scheuer P J. Liver biopsy interpretation, 4th edn. London: Bailliere Tindall, 1987

124. Yamada S, Howe S, Scheuer P J. Three-dimensional reconstruction of biliary pathways in primary biliary cirrhosis: a computer-assisted study. J Pathol 1987; 152: 317–323

125. Nakanuma Y, Ohta G. Histometric and serial section observation of the intrahepatic bile ducts in primary biliary cirrhosis. Gastroenterology 1979; 76; 1326–1332

126. Portmann B, MacSween R N M. Diseases of the intrahepatic bile ducts. In: MacSween R N M, Anthony P P, Scheuer P J, eds. Pathology of the liver, 2nd edn. Edinburgh: Churchill Livingstone, 1987: pp 424–453

127. Tarao K, Shimizu A, Ohkawa S et al. Increased uptake of bromodeoxyuridine by hepatocytes from early stages of primary biliary cirrhosis. Gastroenterology 1991; 100: 725–730

128. Chazouilleres O, Andreani T, Legendre C, Poupon R, Darnis F. Hyperplasie nodulaire régénérative du foie et cirrhose biliaire primitive. Une association fortuite? Gastroenterol Clin Biol 1986; 10: 764–766

129. Nakanuma Y, Ohta G. Nodular regenerative hyperplasia of the liver in primary biliary cirrhosis of early histological stages. Am J Gastroenterol 1987; 82: 8–10

130. Colina F, Pinedo F, Solis J A, Moreno D, Nevado M. Nodular regenerative hyperplasia of the liver in early histological stages of primary biliary cirrhosis. Gastroenterology 1992; 102: 1319–1324

131. Popper H. The problem of histologic evaluation of primary biliary cirrhosis. Virchows Arch (A) 1978; 379: 99–102

132. Popper H, Paronetto F. Clinical, histologic, and immunologic features in primary biliary cirrhosis. Springer Sem Immunopathol 1980; 3: 339–354

133. Janssens A R, van den Hamer C J A. Kinetics of ^{64}copper in primary biliary cirrhosis. Hepatology 1982; 2: 822–827

134. Winge D R. Normal physiology of copper metabolism. Semin Liver Dis 1984; 4: 239–251

135. Epstein O, Arborgh B M A, Sagiv M, Wroblewski R, Scheuer P J. Is copper hepatotoxic in primary biliary cirrhosis? J Clin Pathol 1981; 34: 1071–1075

136. Walshe J M. Copper: its role in the pathogenesis of liver disease. Semin Liver Dis 1984; 4: 252–263

137. Klöppel G, Seifert G, Lindner R, Dammermann R, Sack H J, Berg P A. Histopathological features in mixed types of chronic aggressive hepatitis and primary biliary cirrhosis. Virchows Arch (A) 1977; 373: 143–160

138. Nakanuma Y, Hoso M, Mizuno Y, Unoura M. Pathologic study of primary biliary cirrhosis of early histologic stages presenting with cholestatic jaundice. Liver 1988; 8: 319–324

139. Nakanuma Y, Saito K, Unoura M. Semiquantitative assessment of cholestasis and lymphocytic piecemeal necrosis in primary biliary cirrhosis: a histologic and immunohistochemical study. J Clin Gastroenterol 1990; 12: 357–362

140. MacSween R N M. Mallory's (alcoholic) hyaline in primary biliary cirrhosis. J Clin Pathol 1973; 26: 340–342

141. Krasner N, Johnson P J, Portmann B, Watkinson G, MacSween R N M, Williams R. Hepatocellular carcinoma in primary biliary cirrhosis: report of four cases. Gut 1979; 20: 255–258

142. Kapelman B, Schaffner F. The natural history of primary biliary cirrhosis. Semin Liver Dis 1981; 1: 273–281

143. Melia W N, Johnson P J, Neuberger J, Zaman S, Portmann B, Williams R. Hepatocellular carcinoma in primary biliary cirrhosis. Detection by α-fetoprotein estimation. Gastroenterology 1984; 87: 660–663

144. Nakanuma Y, Terada T, Doishita K, Miwa A. Hepatocellular carcinoma in primary biliary cirrhosis: an autopsy study. Hepatology 1990; 11: 1010–1016

145. Gluskin L E, Guariglia P, Payne J A, Banner B F, Economou P. Hepatocellular carcinoma in a patient with precirrhotic primary biliary cirrhosis. J Clin Gastroenterol 1985; 7: 441–444

146. Viteri A, Vernace S J, Schaffner F. Extrahepatic malignancy in chronic liver disease: report of six cases. Gastroenterology 1976; 71: 1075–1078

147. Mills P R, Boyle P, Quigley E M M et al. Primary biliary cirrhosis: an increased incidence of extrahepatic malignancy? J Clin Pathol 1982; 35: 541–543

148. Goudie B M, Burt A D, Macfarlane G J et al. Breast cancer in primary biliary cirrhosis. Br Med J 1985; ii: 1597–1598

149. Wolke A M, Schaffner F, Kapelman B, Sacks H S. Malignancy in primary biliary cirrhosis. High incidence of breast cancer in affected women. Am J Med 1984; 76: 1075–1078

150. Scheuer P J. Primary biliary cirrhosis. Proc Roy Soc Med 1967; 60: 1257–1260

151. Popper H, Schaffner F. Non-suppurative destructive chronic cholangitis and chronic hepatitis. In: Popper H, Schaffner F, eds. Progress in liver diseases, vol III. New York: Grune & Stratton, 1970: pp 336–354

152. Ludwig J, Dickson E R, McDonald G S. Staging of chronic non-suppurative cholangitis (syndrome of primary biliary cirrhosis). Virchows Arch (A) 1978; 379: 103–112

153. Lee R G, Epstein O, Jauregui H, Sherlock S, Scheuer P J. Granulomas in primary biliary cirrhosis: a prognostic feature. Gastroenterology 1981; 81: 983–986

154. Mitchison H C, Palmer J M, Bassendine M F, Watson A J, Record C O, James O F W. A controlled trial of prednisolone treatment in primary biliary cirrhosis. Three-year results. J Hepatol 1992; 15: 336–344

155. Wiesner R H, Ludwig J, Lindor K D et al. A controlled trial of cyclosporin in the treatment of primary biliary cirrhosis. N Engl J Med 1990; 322: 1419–1424

156. Lombard M, Portmann B, Neuberger J et al. Cyclosporin A treatment in primary biliary cirrhosis. Result of a long-term placebo controlled trial. Gastroenterology 1993; 104: 519–526

157. Kaplan M M, Alling D W, Zimmerman H J et al. A prospective trial of colchicine for primary biliary cirrhosis. N Engl J Med 1986; 315: 1448–1454

158. Poupon R E, Balkau B, Eschwege E and the UDCA-PBC Study Group. A multicenter, controlled trial of ursodiol for the treatment of primary biliary cirrhosis. N Engl J Med 1991; 324: 1548–1554

159. Berg P A, Klein R. Autoantibody patterns in primary biliary cirrhosis. In: Krawitt E L, Wiesner R H, eds. Autoimmune liver diseases. New York: Raven Press, 1991: pp 123–142

160. Okuno T, Seto Y, Okanoue T, Takino T. Chronic active hepatitis with features of primary biliary cirrhosis. Dig Dis Sci 1987; 32: 775–779

161. Brunner G, Klinge O. Ein der chronisch-destruierenden nicht-eitrigen Cholangitis ähnliches Krankheitsbild mit antinukleären Antikörpern (Immuncholangitis). Dtsch Med Wochschr 1987; 112: 1454–1458

162. Michieletti P, Wanless I R, Katz A, et al Antimitochondrial antibody negative primary biliary cirrhosis: a distinctive syndrome of autoimmune cholangitis. Gut 1994; 35: 260–265

163. Carrougher J G, Schaffer R T, Canales L I, Goodman Z A. A 33 year old woman with an autoimmune syndrome. Semin Liver Dis 1991; 11: 252–262

164. Ben-Ari Z, Dhillon A P, Sherlock S. Autoimmune cholangiopathy: part of the spectrum of autoimmune chronic active hepatitis? Hepatology 1993; 18: 10–15

165. Pawlotsky J-M, Andre C, Metreau J-M, Beaugrand M, Zafrani E-S, Dhumeaux D. Multiple nuclear dot antinuclear antibodies are not specific for primary biliary cirrhosis. Hepatology 1992; 16: 127–131

166. Lassoued K, Brenard R, Degos F et al. Antinuclear antibodies directed to a 200-kilodalton polypeptide of the nuclear envelope in primary biliary cirrhosis. A clinical and immunological study of a series of 150 patients with primary biliary cirrhosis. Gastroenterology 1990; 99: 181–186

167. Delbet P. Rétrécissement du cholédoque cholecystoduodénostomie. Bull Soc Nat Chir 1924; 50: 1144–1146

168. Thorpe M E, Scheuer P J, Sherlock S. Primary sclerosing cholangitis, the biliary tree, and ulcerative colitis. Gut 1967; 8: 435–448

169. MacSween R N M. Primary sclerosing cholangitis. In: Anthony P P, MacSween R N M, eds. Recent advances in histopathology. Edinburgh: Churchill Livingstone, 1984: pp 158–167

170. Ludwig J, MacCarty R L, LaRusso N F, Krom R A F, Wiesner R H. Intrahepatic cholangiectases and large-duct obliteration in primary sclerosing cholangitis. Hepatology 1986; 6: 560–568

171. Ludwig J. New concepts in biliary cirrhosis. Semin Liver Dis 1987; 7: 293–301

172. Wee A, Ludwig J. Pericholangitis in chronic ulcerative colitis: primary sclerosing cholangitis of the small bile ducts? Ann Intern Med 1985; 102: 581–587

173. Warren K W, Anthanassiades S, Monge J I. Primary sclerosing cholangitis. A study of forty-two cases. Am J Surg 1966; 111: 23–38

174. Pokorny C S, McCaughan G W, Gallager N D, Selby W S. Sclerosing cholangitis and biliary tract calculi — primary or secondary? Gut 1992; 33: 1376–1380

175. Miros M, Kerlin P, Walker N, Harper J, Lynch S, Strong R. Predicting cholangiocarcinoma in patients with primary sclerosing cholangitis before transplantation. Gut 1991; 32: 1369–1373

176. Rosen C B, Nagorney D M, Wiesner R H et al. Cholangiocarcinoma complicating primary sclerosing cholangitis. Ann Surg 1991; 213: 21–25

177. Aadland E, Schrumpf E, Fausa O et al. Primary sclerosing cholangitis: A long-term follow-up study. Scand J Gastroenterol 1987; 22: 655–664

178. Sherlock S. Pathogenesis of sclerosing cholangitis: the role of immune factors. Semin Liver Dis 1991; 11: 5–10

179. Wiesner R H, LaRusso N F. Clinicopathological features of the syndrome of primary sclerosing cholangitis. Gastroenterology 1980; 79: 200–206

180. Chapman R W G, Arborgh B M A, Rhodes J M, Summerfield J A, Dick R, Scheuer P J. Primary sclerosing cholangitis: a review of its clinical features, cholangiography and hepatic histology. Gut 1980; 21: 870–877

181. Amedee-Manesme O, Bernard O, Brunelle F et al. Sclerosing cholangitis with neonatal onset. J Paediatr 1987; 111: 225–229

182. El-Shabrawi M, Wilkinson M L, Portmann B et al. Primary sclerosing cholangitis in childhood. Gastroenterology 1987; 92: 1226–1235

183. Helzberg J H, Petersen J M, Boyer J L. Improved survival with primary sclerosing cholangitis. A review of clinicopathologic features and comparison of symptomatic and asymptomatic patients. Gastroenterology 1987; 92: 1869–1875

184. Rabinovitz M, Gavaler J S, Schade R R, Dindzans V J, Chien M-C, van Thiel D H. Does primary sclerosing cholangitis occurring in association with inflammatory bowel disease differ from that occurring in the absence of inflammatory bowel disease? a study of sixty-six subjects. Hepatology 1990; 11: 7–11

185. Schrumpf E, Fausa O, Kolmannskog F, Eglio K, Ritland S, Gjone E. Sclerosing cholangitis in ulcerative colitis. a follow-up study. Scand J Gastroenterol 1982; 17: 33–39

186. Wiesner R H, LaRusso N F, Ludwig J, Dickson E R. Comparison of the clinicopathologic features of primary sclerosing cholangitis and primary biliary cirrhosis. Gastroenterology 1985; 88: 108–114

187. Porayko M K, Wiesner R H, LaRusso N F et al. Patients with asymptomatic primary sclerosing cholangitis frequently have progressive disease. Gastroenterology 1990; 98: 1595–1602

188. Lebovics E, Palmer M, Woo J, Schaffner F. Outcome of primary sclerosing cholangitis. Analysis of long-term observation in 38 patients. Arch Intern Med 1987; 147: 729–731

189. Wiesner R H, Grambsch P M, Dickson E R et al. Primary sclerosing cholangitis: Natural history, prognostic factors and survival analysis. Hepatology 1989; 10: 430–436

190. Farrant J M, Hayllar K M, Wilkinson M L, Karani J, Portmann B C, Westaby D, Williams R. Natural history and prognostic variables in primary sclerosing cholangitis. Gastroenterology 1991; 100: 1710–1717

191. Porayko M K, LaRusso N F, Wiesner R H. Primary sclerosing cholangitis: A progressive disease? Semin Liver Dis 1991; 11: 18–25

192. Goudie B M, Birnie G G, Watkinson G, MacSween R N M. A case of long-standing primary sclerosing cholangitis. J Clin Pathol 1983; 36: 1298–1301

193. Chapman R W. Aetiology and natural history of primary sclerosing cholangitis — a decade of progress? Gut 1991; 32: 1433–1435

194. Balasubramaniam K, Wiesner R H, LaRusso N R. Primary sclerosing cholangitis with normal serum alkaline phosphatase activity. Gastroenterology 1988; 95: 1395–1398

195. Zauli D, Schrumpf E, Crespi C, Cassani F, Fausa O, Aadland E. An autoantibody profile in primary sclerosing cholangitis. J Hepatol 1987; 5: 14–18

196. Olsson R, Danielsson A, Jarnerot G et al. Prevalence of primary sclerosing cholangitis in patients with ulcerative colitis. Gastroenterology 1991; 100: 1319–1323

197. Rasmussen H H, Fallingborg J, Mortensen P B et al. Primary sclerosing cholangitis in patients with ulcerative colitis. Scand J Gastroenterol 1992; 27: 732–736

198. Fausa O, Schrumpf E, Elgjo K. Relationship of inflammatory bowel disease and primary sclerosing cholangitis. Semin Liver Dis 1991; 11: 31–39

199. McGarity B, Bansi D S, Robertson D A F, Millward-Sadler G H, Shepherd H A. Primary sclerosing cholangitis: an important and prevalent complication of Crohn's disease. Eur J Gastroenterol Hepatol 1991; 3: 361–364

200. Epstein O, Chapman R W G, Lake-Bakaar G, Foo A Y, Rosalki S B, Sherlock S. The pancreas in primary biliary cirrhosis and primary sclerosing cholangitis. Gastroenterology 1982; 83: 1177–1182

201. Gurian L E, Keeffe E B. Pancreatic insufficiency associated with ulcerative colitis and pericholangitis. Gastroenterology 1982; 82: 581–585

202. Børkje B, Vetvik K, Odegaard S, Schrumpf E, Larssen T B, Kolmannskog F. Chronic pancreatitis in patients with sclerosing cholangitis and ulcerative colitis. Scand J Gastroenterol 1985; 20: 539–542

203. Kawaguchi K, Koike M, Tsuruta K, Tabata I, Fujita N. Lymphoplasmacytic sclerosing pancreatitis with cholangitis: A variant of primary sclerosing cholangitis extensively involving the pancreas. Hum Pathol 1991; 22: 387–395

204. Waldram R, Kopelman H, Tsantoulas D, Williams R. Chronic pancreatitis, sclerosing cholangitis and sicca complex in two siblings. Lancet 1975; i: 550–552

205. Sjögren I, Wengle B, Korsgren M. Primary sclerosing cholangitis associated with fibrosis of the submandibular glands and the pancreas. Acta Medica Scand 1979; 205: 139–141

206. Montefulso P P, Geiss A C, Bronzo R L et al. Sclerosing cholangitis, chronic pancreatitis, and Sjögren's syndrome: A syndrome complex. Am J Surg 1984; 147: 822–826

207. Bartholomew L G, Cain J C, Woolner L B, Utz D C. Sclerosing cholangitis. Its possible association with Riedel's thyroiditis and fibrous retroperitonitis. N Engl J Med 1963; 267: 8–12

208. Comings D E, Skubi K B, van Eyes J, Motulsky A G. Familial multifocal fibrosclerosis. Findings suggesting that retroperitoneal fibrosis, mediastinal fibrosis, sclerosing cholangitis, Riedel's thyroiditis, and pseudotumor of the orbit may be different manifestations of a single disease. Ann Intern Med 1967; 66: 884–892

209. Thompson B W, Read R C. Sclerosing cholangitis and other intra-abdominal fibrosis. Am J Surg 1974; 128: 777–781

210. Laitt R D, Hubscher S G, Buckels J A, Darby S, Elias E. Sclerosing cholangitis associated with multifocal fibrosis: a case report. Gut 1992; 33: 1430–1432

211. Hay J E, Wiesner R H, Shorter R G, LaRusso N F, Baldus W P. Primary sclerosing cholangitis and celiac disease. A novel association. Ann Intern Med 1988; 109: 713–717

212. Schrumpf E. Association of primary sclerosing cholangitis and celiac disease: fact or fancy? Hepatology 1989; 10: 1020–1021

213. Mir-Madjlessi S H, Sivak M V, Farmer R G. Hypereosinophilia, ulcerative colitis, sclerosing cholangitis, and bile duct carcinoma. Am J Gastroenterol 1986; 81: 483–485

214. Scheurlen M, Mork H, Weber P. Hypereosinophilic syndrome resembling inflammatory bowel disease with primary sclerosing cholangitis. J Clin Gastroenterol 1992; 14: 59–63

215. Viteri A L, Hardin W J, Dyck W P. Peyronies' disease and sclerosing cholangitis in a patient with ulcerative colitis. Dig Dis Sci 1979; 24: 490–491

216. Bass N M, Chapman R W, O'Reilly A, Sherlock S. Primary sclerosing cholangitis associated with angioimmunoblastic lymphadenopathy. Gastroenterology 1983; 85: 420–424

217. Alberti-Flor J J, Kalemeris G, Dunn G D, Avant G R. Primary sclerosing cholangitis associated with massive intra-abdominal lymphadenopathy. Am J Gastroenterol 1986; 81: 55–60

218. Alberti-Flor J J, Jeffers L, Schiff E R. Primary sclerosing cholangitis occurring in a patient with systemic lupus erythematosus and diabetes mellitus. Am J Gastroenterol 1984; 70: 889–891

219. Fraile G, Rodriguez-Garcia J L, Moreno A. Primary sclerosing cholangitis associated with systemic sclerosis. Postgrad Med J 1991; 67: 189–192

220. Kirby D F, Blei A T, Rosen S T et al. Primary sclerosing cholangitis in the presence of lupus anticoagulant. Am J Med 1986; 83: 1077–1080

221. Karatapanis T, McCormich P A, Burroughs A K. Ulcerative colitis complicated by Budd–Chiari syndrome and primary sclerosing cholangitis. Eur J Gastroenterol Hepatol 1992; 4: 683–686

222. Moeller D D. Sclerosing cholangitis associated with autoimmune hemolytic anaemia and hyperthyroidism. Am J Gastroenterol 1985; 80: 122–125

223. Schep G N, Scully L J. Primary sclerosing cholangitis and sarcoidosis: An unusual combination. Case report and review of the literature. Can J Gastroenterol 1990; 4: 489–494

224. Hay J E, Lindor K D, Wiesner R H et al. The metabolic bone disease of primary sclerosing cholangitis. Hepatology 1991; 14: 257–261

225. Snook J A, Kelly P, Chapman R W, Jewell D P. Fibrolamellar hepatocellular carcinoma complicating ulcerative colitis with primary sclerosing cholangitis. Gut 1989; 30: 243–245

226. Ismail T, Angrisani L, Hubscher S, McMaster P. Hepatocellular carcinoma complicating primary sclerosing cholangitis. Br J Surg 1991; 78: 360–361

227. Elias E, Summerfield J D, Dick R, Sherlock S. Endoscopic retrograde cholangiopancreatography in the diagnosis of jaundice associated with ulcerative colitis. Gastroenterology 1974; 67: 907–911

228. MacCarty R L, LaRusso N F, Wiesner R H, Ludwig J. Primary sclerosing cholangitis: Findings on cholangiography and pancreatography. Radiology 1983; 149: 39–44

229. Geneve J, Dubuc N, Mathieu D, Zafrani E S, Dhumeaux D, Métreau J M. Cystic dilatation of intrahepatic bile ducts in primary sclerosing cholangitis. J Hepatol 1990; 11: 196–199

230. Chen L V, Goldberg H I. Sclerosing cholangitis: Broad spectrum of radiographic features. Gastrointest Radiol 1984; 9: 39–47

231. Rosen C B, Nagorney D M. Cholangiocarcinoma complicating primary sclerosing cholangitis. Semin Liver Dis 1991; 11: 26–30

232. Eade M N, Brooke B N. Portal bacteraemia in cases of ulcerative colitis submitted to colectomy. Lancet 1969; i: 1008–1009

233. Quigley E M M, LaRusso N F, Ludwig J, MacSween R N M, Birnie G G, Watkinson G. Familial occurrence of primary sclerosing cholangitis and ulcerative colitis. Gastroenterology 1983; 85: 1160–1165

234. Silber G H, Finegold M J, Wagner M L, Klish W J. Sclerosing cholangitis and ulcerative colitis in a mother and her son. J Pediatr Gastroenterol Nutr 1987; 6: 147–152

235. Chapman R W G, Varghese Z, Graul R, Patel G, Kokinon N, Sherlock S. Association of primary sclerosing cholangitis with HLA-B8. Gut 1983; 24: 38–41

236. Schrumpf E, Fausa O, Forre O, Dobloug J H, Ritland S, Thorsby E. HLA antigens and immunoregulatory T cells in ulcerative colitis associated with hepatobiliary disease. Scand J Gastroenterol 1982; 17: 187–191

237. Asquith P, Mackintosh P, Stokes P L et al. Histocompatibility antigens in patients with inflammatory bowel disease. Lancet 1974; i: 113–115

238. Donaldson P T, Farrant J M, Wilkinson M L, Hayllar K, Portmann B, Williams R. Dual association of HLA DR2 and DR3 with primary sclerosing cholangitis. Hepatology 1991; 13: 129–133

239. Prochazka E J, Terasaki P I, Park M S, Goldstein L I, Busuttil R W. Association of primary sclerosing cholangitis with HLA-DRW52a. N Engl J Med 1990; 322: 1842–1844

240. Farrant J M, Doherty D G, Donaldson P T et al. Amino acid substitutions at position 38 of the DR polypeptide confer susceptibility to and protection from primary sclerosing cholangitis. Hepatology 1992; 16: 390–395

241. Chapman R W, Cottone M, Selby W S, Shepherd H A, Sherlock S, Jewell D P. Serum autoantibodies, ulcerative colitis and primary sclerosing cholangitis. Gut 1986; 27: 86–91

242. Lo S K, Fleming K A, Chapman R W. Prevalence of anti-neutrophil antibody in primary sclerosing cholangitis and ulcerative colitis using an alkaline phosphatase technique. Gut 1992; 33: 1370–1375

243. Seibold F, Weber P, Klein R, Berg P A, Wiedmann K H. Clinical significance of antibodies against neutrophils in patients with inflammatory bowel disease and primary sclerosing cholangitis. Gut 1992; 33: 657–662

244. Mieli-Vergani G, Lobo-Yeo, McFarlane B M, McFarlane I G, Mowat A P, Vergani D. Different immune mechanism leading to autoimmunity in primary sclerosing cholangitis and autoimmune chronic active hepatitis of childhood. Hepatology 1989; 9: 198–203

245. Lo S K, Chapman R W G, Cheeseman P et al. Antineutrophil antibody: a test for autoimmune primary sclerosing cholangitis in childhood? Gut 1993; 34: 199–202

246. Bodenheimer H C, LaRusso N F, Thayer W P Jr et al. Elevated circulating immune complexes in primary sclerosing cholangitis. Hepatology 1983; 3: 150–154

247. Minuk G Y, Angus M, Brickman C M et al. Abnormal clearance of immune complexes from the circulation of patients with primary sclerosing cholangitis and ulcerative colitis. Gastroenterology 1985; 88: 166–170

248. Senaldi G, Donaldson P, Magrin S et al. Activation of the complement system in primary sclerosing cholangitis. Gastroenterology 1989; 97: 1430–1434

249. Lindsor K D, Wiesner R H, Katzmann J A et al. Lymphocyte subsets in primary sclerosing cholangitis. Dig Dis Sci 1987; 32: 720–725

250. Snook J A, Chapman R W, Sachdev G K et al. Peripheral blood and portal tract lymphocyte populations in primary sclerosing cholangitis. J Hepatol 1989; 9: 36–40

251. Whitside T L, Lasky S, Si L, van Thiel D H. Immunologic analysis of mononuclear cells in liver tissue and blood of patients with primary sclerosing cholangitis. Hepatology 1985; 5: 468–474

252. Ludwig J, Barham S S, LaRusso N F, Elveback L R, Wiesner R H, McCall J T. Morphologic features of chronic hepatitis associated with primary sclerosing cholangitis and ulcerative colitis. Hepatology 1981; 1: 632–640

253. Bangaru B, Morecki R, Glaser J H, Gartner L M, Horwitz M S. Comparative studies of biliary atresia in the human newborn and reovirus-induced cholangitis in weanling mice. Lab Invest 1980; 43: 456–462

254. Glaser J H, Morecki R. Reovirus type 3 and neonatal cholestasis. Semin Liver Dis 1987; 7: 100–107

255. Minuk G Y, Rascanin N, Paul R W, Lee P W K, Buchan K, Kelly J K. Reovirus type 3 infection in patients with primary sclerosing cholangitis. J Hepatol 1987; 5: 8–13

256. Mehal W Z, Hattersley A T, Chapman R W, Fleming K A. A survey of cytomegalovirus (CMV) DNA in primary sclerosing cholangitis (PSC) liver tissue using a sensitive polymerase chain reaction (PCR) based assay. J Hepatol 1992; 15: 396–399

257. Bhathal P S, Powell L W. Primary intrahepatic obliterating cholangitis: a possible variant of "sclerosing cholangitis". Gut 1969; 10: 886–893

258. Ludwig J. Small-duct primary sclerosing cholangitis. Semin Liver Dis 1991; 11: 11–17

259. Lefkowitch J H. Primary sclerosing cholangitis. Arch Intern Med 1982; 142: 1157–1160

260. Harrison R F, Hubscher S G. The spectrum of bile duct lesions in end-stage primary sclerosing cholangitis. Histopathology 1991; 19: 321–327

261. Shepherd H A, Selby W S, Chapman R W G et al. Ulcerative colitis and persistent liver dysfunction. Q J Med 1983; 208: 503–513

262. Cello J P. Acquired immunodeficiency syndrome cholangiopathy: spectrum of disease. Am J Med 1989; 86: 539–546

263. Bonacini M. Hepatobiliary complication in patients with human immunodeficiency virus infection. Am J Med 1992; 92: 404–411

264. Bouche H, Housset C, Dumont J L et al. AIDS-related cholangitis; diagnostic features and course in 15 patients. J Hepatol 1993; 17: 34–39

265. Forbes A, Blanshard C, Gazzard B. Natural history of AIDS related sclerosing cholangitis: A study of 20 cases. Gut 1993; 34: 116–121

266. Naveh Y, Mendelsohn H, Spira G, Auslaender L, Mandel H, Berant M. Primary sclerosing cholangitis associated with immunodeficiency. Am J Dis Child 1983; 137: 114–117

267. DiPalma J A, Strobel C T, Farrow J G. Primary sclerosing cholangitis associated with hyperimmunoglobulin M immunodeficiency (dysgammaglobulinemia). Gastroenterology 1986; 91: 464–468

268. Davis J J, Heyman M B, Ferrel L, Kerner J, Kerlan R, Thaler M M. Sclerosing cholangitis associated with cryptosporidiosis in a child with a congenital immunodeficiency disorder. Am J Gastroenterol 1987; 82: 1196–1202

269. Record C O, Eddleston A L W F, Shilkin K B, Williams R. Intrahepatic sclerosing cholangitis associated with a familial immunodeficiency. Lancet 1973; ii: 18–20

270. Dayer E, Roux-Lombard P, Huber O, Dayer J-M. Chronic sclerosing cholangitis and recurrent pulmonary infections in two brothers associated with cellular immunodeficiency and increased cytokine production. Ped Allergy Immunol 1991; 2: 87–92

271. Matamoros N, Ciria L, Julia M R, Infante D, Martinez Ibanez V, Portmann B, Webster A D B. Familial sclerosing cholangitis and

immunodeficiency — recurrence after liver transplantation. Gut 1994; (in press)

272. Van Steenbergen W, Fevery J, Broeckaert L et al. Hepatic echinococcosis ruptured into the biliary tract. J Hepatol 1987; 4: 133–139

273. Cohen-Solal J L, Eroukmhanoff P, Desoutter P, Loisel J C, Kohlmann G, Flabeau F. Cholangite sclérosante survenue apres traitement chirurgical d'un kyste hydatique du foie. Sem Hop 1983; 59: 1623–1624

274. Terés J Gomez-Moll J, Bruguera M, Visa J, Bordas J M, Pera C. Sclerosing cholangitis after surgical treatment of hepatic echinococcal cyst. Report of three cases. Am J Surg 1984; 148: 694–697

275. Belghiti J, Benhamou J-P, Houry S, Grenier P, Huguier M, Fékété F. Caustic sclerosing cholangitis. Arch Surg 1966; 121: 1162–1165

276. Houry S, Languille O, Hugier M, Benhamou J-P, Belghiti J, Msika S. Sclerosing cholangitis induced by formaldehyde solution injected into the biliary tree of rats. Arch Surg 1990; 125: 1059–1061

277. Hohn D, Rayner A A, Exonomou J S, Ignoffo R J, Lewis B J, Stag R J. Toxicities and complications of implanted pump hepatic arterial and intravenous Floxuridine infusion. Cancer 1986; 57: 465–470

278. Herrmann G, Lorenz M, Kirkowa-Reiman M et al. Morphological changes after intra-arterial chemotherapy of the liver. Hepato-Gastroenterology 1987; 34: 5–9

279. Shea W J, Demas B E, Goldberg H I et al. Sclerosing cholangitis associated with hepatic arterial FUDR chemotherapy: radiographic-histologic correlation. Am J Roentgenol 1986; 146: 717–721

280. Doria M I, Shepard K V, Levin B, Riddell R H. Liver pathology following hepatic arterial infusion chemotherapy. Hepatic toxicity with FUDR. Cancer 1986; 58: 855–861

281. Dikengil A, Siskind B N, Morse S S, Swedlund A, Bober-Sorcinelli K E, Burrell M I. Sclerosing cholangitis from intra-arterial floxuridine. J Clin Gastroenterol 1986; 8: 690–693

282. Ludwig J, Kim C H, Wiesner R H, Krom R A F. Floxuridine-induced sclerosing cholangitis: An ischemic cholangiopathy? Hepatology 1989; 9: 215–218

283. Doppman J L, Girton M E. Bile duct scarring following ethanol embolization in the hepatic artery: An experimental study in monkeys. Radiology 1984; 152: 621–626

284. Leblanc A, Hadchouel M, Jehan P, Odièvre M, Alagille D. Obstructive jaundice in children with histiocytosis X. Gastroenterology 1961; 80: 134–139

285. Rand E B, Whitington P F. Successful orthotopic liver transplantation in two patients with liver failure due to sclerosing cholangitis with Langerhans cell histiocytosis. J Pediatr Gastroenterol Nutr 1992; 15: 202–207

286. Thompson H H, Pitt H A, Lewin K J, Longmire W P Jr. Sclerosing cholangitis and histiocytosis X. Gut 1984; 25: 526–530

287. Dilawari J B, Chawla Y K. Pseudosclerosing cholangitis in extrahepatic portal vein obstruction. Gut 1992; 33: 272–276

288. Galambos J T, Brooks W S Jr. Atypical biliary cirrhosis — or sclerosing cholangitis. J Clin Gastroenterol 1980; 2: 43–52

289. Nakanuma Y, Ohta G, Takeshita H et al. Florid duct lesions and extensive bile duct loss of the intrahepatic biliary tree in chronic liver disease other than primary biliary cirrhosis. Acta Pathol Jpn 1983; 33: 1095–1104

290. Haratake J, Horie A, Ishii N, Okuno F. Familial intrahepatic cholestatic cirrhosis in young adults. Gastroenterology 1985; 89: 202–209

291. Ludwig J, Wiesner R H, LaRusso N F. Idiopathic adulthood ductopenia. A cause of chronic cholestatic liver disease and biliary cirrhosis. J Hepatol 1988; 7: 193–199

292. Zafrani E S, Metreau J-M, Douvin C et al. Idiopathic biliary ductopenia in adults: a report of five cases. Gastroenterology 1990; 99: 1823–1828

293. Faa G, van Eyken P, Demelia L, Vallebona E, Costa V, Desmet V J. Idiopathic adulthood ductopenia presenting with chronic recurrent cholestasis. A case report. J Hepatol 1991; 12: 14–20

294. Starzl T E, Marchioro T L, von Kaula K N, Hermann G, Brittain R S, Waddell W R. Homotransplantation of the liver in humans. Surg Gynecol Obstet 1963; 117: 659–676

295. Calne R Y, McMaster P, Portmann B, Wall W J, Williams R. Observations on preservation, bile drainage and rejection in 64 human orthotopic liver allografts. Ann Surg 1977; 186: 282–290

296. Portmann B, Williams R. Histopathology of the transplanted liver. In: Williams R, Cantoni L, eds. Recenti progressi in epatologia. Milan: Casa Editrice Ambrosiana, 1979: pp 369–381

297. Fennell R H, Roddy H J. Liver transplantation: the pathologist's perspective. In: Sommers S C, Rosen P P, eds. Pathol Ann. NY: Appleton-Century-Crofts, 1972: 14 (part 2), pp 155–182

298. Snover D C, Sibley R K, Freese D K et al. Orthotopic liver transplantation: A pathological study of 63 serial liver biopsies from 17 patients with special reference to the diagnostic features and natural history of rejection. Hepatology 1984; 4: 1212–1222

299. Demetris A J, Lasky S, Van Thiel D H, Starzl T E, Dekker A. Pathology of hepatic transplantation. A review of 62 adult allograft recipients immunosuppressed with a cyclosporin/steroid regimen. Am J Pathol 1985; 118: 151–161

300. Wight D G D, Portmann B. Pathology of liver transplantation. In: Sir Roy Calne, ed. Liver transplantation, 2nd edn. London: Grune & Stratton, 1987: pp. 385–435

301. Vierling J M, Fennell R H. Histopathology of early and late human hepatic allograft rejection: evidence of progressive destruction of interlobular bile ducts. Hepatology 1985; 5: 1076–1085

302. Ludwig J, Wiesner R H, Batts K P, Perkins J D, Krom R A F. The acute vanishing bile duct syndrome (acute irreversible rejection) after orthotopic liver transplantation. Hepatology 1987; 7: 476–483

303. Portmann B, Neuberger J, Williams R. Intrahepatic bile duct lesions. In: Calne R Y, ed. Liver transplantation. London: Grune & Stratton, 1983: pp 279–287

304. Wiesner R H, Ludwig J, van Hoek B, Krom R A F. Current concepts in cell-mediated hepatic allograft rejection leading to ductopenia and liver failure. Hepatology 1991; 14: 721–729

305. Ludwig J, Gross J B, Perkins J D, Moore S B. Persistent centrilobular necroses in hepatic allografts. Hum Pathol 1990; 21: 656–661

306. Neuberger J, Portmann B, MacDougall B R D, Calne R Y, Williams R. Recurrence of primary biliary cirrhosis after liver transplantation. N Engl J Med 1982; 306: 1–4

307. Haagsma E B, Manns M, Klein R et al. Subtypes of antimitochondrial antibodies in primary biliary cirrhosis before and after orthotopic liver transplantation. Hepatology 1987; 7: 129–133

308. Polson R J, Portmann B, Neuberger J, Calne R Y, Williams R. Evidence for disease recurrence after transplantation for primary biliary cirrhosis. clinical and histologic follow-up studies. Gastroenterology 1989; 97: 715–725

309. Hubscher S G, Elias E, Buckels A C, Mayer A D, McMaster P, Neuberger J M. Primary biliary cirrhosis. Histological evidence of disease recurrence after liver transplantation. J Hepatol 1993; 18: 173–184

310. Balan V, Batts K P, Porayo M K, Krom R A F, Ludwig J, Wiesner R H. Histologic evidence for recurrence of primary biliary cirrhosis after liver transplantation. Hepatology 1992; 18: 1392–1398

311. Portmann B, Neuberger J M. Recurrence of primary disease following liver transplantation. In: Williams R, Portmann B, Tan K-C, eds, The practice of liver transplantation. London: Churchill Livingstone 1994; in press.

312. Wong P Y N, Portmann B, O'Grady J G et al. Recurrence of primary biliary cirrhosis after liver transplantation following FK506-based immunosuppression. J Hepatol 1993; 17: 284–287

313. Woodruff J M, Hansen J A, Good R A, Santos G W, Slavin R E. The pathology of the graft-versus-host reaction (GVHR) in adults receiving bone marrow transplants. Transpl Proc 1976; 8: 675–684

314. McDonald G B, Shulman H M, Wolford J L, Spencer G D. Liver disease after human bone marrow transplantation. Semin Liver Dis 1987; 7: 210–229

315. Thomas E D, Storb R, Clift R A et al. Bone-marrow transplantation (second of two parts). N Engl J Med 1975; 292: 895–902

316. Graze P R, Gale R P. Chronic graft-versus-host disease: a syndrome of disordered immunity. Am J Med 1979; 66: 611–620

317. Shulman H M, Sullivan K M, Weiden P L et al. Chronic graft-versus-host syndrome in man. A long-term clinicopathologic study of 20 Seattle patients. Am J Med 1980; 69: 204–217

318. Snover D C. Acute and chronic graft-versus-host disease: histopathological evidence for two pathogenic mechanisms. Hum Pathol 1984; 15: 202–205

319. Sloane J P, Farthing M J G, Powles R L. Histopathological changes in the liver after allogeneic bone marrow transplantation. J Clin Pathol 1980; 33: 334–350

320. Snover D C, Weisdorf S A, Ramsay N K, McGlave P, Kersey J H. Hepatic graft-versus-host disease: a study of the predictive value of liver biopsy in diagnosis. Hepatology 1984; 4: 123–130

321. Shulman H M, Sharma P, Amos D, Fenster L F, McDonald G B. A coded histologic study of hepatic graft-versus-host disease after human bone marrow transplantation. Hepatology 1988; 8: 463–470

322. Bernuau D, Gisselbrecht C, Devergie A et al. Histological and ultrastructural appearance of the liver during graft-versus-host disease complicating bone marrow transplantation. Transplantation 1980; 29: 236–244

323. Knapp A B, Crawford J M, Rappeport J M, Gollan J L. Cirrhosis as a consequence of graft-versus-host disease. Gastroenterology 1987; 92: 513–519

324. Stechschulte D J Jr, Fishback J L, Emami A, Bhatia P. Secondary biliary cirrhosis as a consequence of graft-versus-host disease. Gastroenterology 1990; 98: 223–225

325. Rhodes D F, Lee W M, Wingard J R et al. Orthotopic liver transplantation for graft-versus-host disease following bone marrow transplantation. Gastroenterology 1990; 99: 536–538

326. Burdick J F, Vogelsang G B, Smith W J et al. Graft-vs.-host disease after liver transplantation. N Engl J Med 1988; 318: 689–691

327. Alexander G, Portmann B. Graft-vs.-host disease after liver transplantation. Hepatology 1990; 11: 144–145

328. Poulsen H, Christoffersen P. Abnormal bile duct epithelium in liver biopsies with histological signs of viral hepatitis. Acta Path Microbiol Scand 1969; 76: 383–390

329. Christoffersen P, Dietrichson O, Faber V, Poulsen H. The occurrence and significance of abnormal bile duct epithelium in chronic aggressive hepatitis. Acta Path Microbiol Scand Sect A 1972; 80: 294–302

330. Poulsen H, Christoffersen P. Abnormal bile duct epithelium in chronic aggressive hepatitis and cirrhosis. A review of morphology and clinical, biochemical, and immunologic features. Hum Pathol 1972; 3: 217–225

331. Schmid M, Pirovino M, Altorfer J, Gudat F, Bianchi L. Acute hepatitis non-A, non-B: are there any specific light microscopic features? Liver 1982; 2: 61–67

332. Bianchi L. Intrahepatic bile duct damage in various forms of liver diseases. In: Brunner H, Thaler H, eds. Hepatology: A Festschrift for Hans Popper. New York: Raven Press, 1985: pp 295–310

333. Ludwig J, Czaja A J, Dickson E R, LaRusso N F, Wiesner R H. Manifestations of nonsuppurative cholangitis in chronic hepatobiliary diseases: morphologic spectrum, clinical correlations and terminology. Liver 1984; 4: 105–116

334. Vyberg M. Diverticular bile duct lesion in chronic active hepatitis. Hepatology 1989; 10: 774–780

335. Nouri Aria K T, Sallie R, Sangar F, et al. Detection of hepatitis C virus genoma in liver tissue by in situ hybridisation. J Clin Invest 1993; 91: 2226–2234

336. Danque P O V, Bach N, Schaffner F, Gerber M A, Thung S N. HLA-DR expression in bile duct damage in hepatitis C. Modern Pathol 1993; 6: 327–332

337. Haddad J, Deny P, Munz-Gotheil C et al. Lymphocytic sialadenitis of Sjögren's syndrome associated with chronic hepatitis C virus liver disease. Lancet 1992; 339: 321–323

338. Scheuer P J, Ashrafzadeh P, Sherlock S, Brown D, Dusheiko G M. The pathology of hepatitis C. Hepatology 1992; 15: 567–571

339. Bach N, Thung S N, Schaffner F. The histological features of chronic hepatitis C and autoimmune chronic hepatitis: a comparative analysis. Hepatology 1992; 15: 572–577

340. Gerber M A, Krawczynski K, Alter M J et al. Histopathology of community acquired chronic hepatitis C. Modern Pathol 1992; 5: 438–486

341. Lefkowitch J H, Schiff E R, Davis G L et al. Pathological diagnosis of chronic hepatitis C: a multicenter comparative study with chronic hepatitis B. Gastroenterology 1993; 104: 595–603

342. Kryger P, Christoffersen P. The Copenhagen Hepatitis Acuta Programme. Light microscopic morphology of acute hepatitis non-A, non-B. A comparison with hepatitis type A and B. Liver 1982; 2: 200–206

343. Schmid M, Pirovino M, Altorfer J, Gudat F, Bianchi L. Acute heapitis non-A, non-B: are there any specific light microscopic features? Liver 1982; 2: 61–67

344. Dietrichson O, Christoffersen P. The prognosis of chronic aggressive hepatitis. A clinical and morphological follow-up study. Scand J Gastroenterol 1977; 12: 289–295

345. Di Bisceglie A M, Goodman Z D, Ishak K G, Hoofnagle J H, Melpolder J J, Alter H J. Long-term clinical and histopathological follow-up of chronic post-transfusion hepatitis. Hepatology 1991; 14: 969–974

346. Finegold M J, Carpenter R J. Obliterative cholangitis due to cytomegalovirus: a possible precursor of paucity of intrahepatic bile ducts. Hum Pathol 1982; 13: 662–665

347. Beschorner W E, Pino J, Boitnott J K, Tutschka P J, Santos G W. Pathology of the liver with bone marrow transplantation. Effects of busulfan, carmustine, acute graft-versus-host disease and cytomegalovirus infection. Am J Pathol 1980; 99: 369–385

348. O'Grady J G, Alexander G J M, Sutherland S et al. Cytomegalovirus infection and donor/recipient HLA antigens: interdependent cofactors in the pathogenesis of vanishing bile duct syndrome after liver transplantation. Lancet 1988; ii: 301–305

349. Arnold J C, Portmann B C, O'Grady J G, Naoumov N V, Alexander G J M, Williams R. Cytomegalovirus infection persists in the liver graft in the vanishing bile duct syndrome. Hepatology 1992; 16: 285–292

350. Wright T L. Cytomegalovirus infection and the vanishing bile duct syndrome. Culprit or innocent bystander? Hepatology 1992; 16: 494–496

351. Gregory D H, Zaki G F, Sarosi G A, Carey J B. Chronic cholestasis following prolonged tolbutamide administration. Arch Pathol 1967; 84: 194–201

352. Manivel J C, Bloomer J R, Snover D C. Progressive bile duct injury after thiabendazole administration. Gastroenterology 1987; 93: 245–249

253. Degott C, Feldmann G, Larrey D. Drug-induced prolonged cholestasis in adults: a histological semiquantitative study demonstrating progressive ductopenia. Hepatology 1992; 15: 244–251

354. Forbes G N, Jeffrey G P, Shilkin K B, Reed W D. Carbamazepine hepatotoxicity: another cause of the vanishing bile duct syndrome. Gastroenterology 1992; 102: 1385–1388

355. McMaster K R, Henniger G R. Drug induced granulomatous hepatitis. Lab Investigation 1981; 44: 61–73

356. Walker C O, Combes B. Biliary cirrhosis induced by chlorpromazine. Gastroenterology 1985; 511: 631–640

357. Matsumoto T, Matumori H, Kuwabara N, Fukuda Y, Ariwa R. A histopathological study of the liver in paraquat poisoning. An analysis of fourteen autopsy cases with emphasis on bile duct injury. Acta Pathol Japn 1980; 30: 859–870

358. Mullick F G, Ishak K G, Mahabir R, Stromeyer F W. Hepatic injury associated with paraquat toxicity in humans. Liver 1981; 1: 209–211

359. Cook J, Hou P C, Ho H C, McFadzean A J S. Recurrent pyogenic cholangitis. Br J Surg 1954; 42: 188–203

360. Kashi H, Lam F, Giles G R. Recurrent pyogenic

cholangiohepatitis. Ann Roy Coll Surg Eng 1989; 71: 387–389

361. Chan F L, Man S W, Leong L L, Fan S T. Evaluation of recurrent pyogenic cholangitis with CT: analysis of 50 patients. Radiology 1989; 170: 165–169

362. Ti T K, Yuen R. Chemical composition of biliary calculi in relation to pattern of biliary disease in Singapore. Br J Surg 1985; 72: 556–558

363. Fan S T, Choi T K, Wong J. Recurrent pyogenic cholangitis: current management. World J Surg 1991; 15: 248–253

364. Hwang S. Cholelithiasis in Singapore. Part I. A necropsy study. Gut 1970; 11: 141–148

365. Khuroo M S, Zargar S A, Yattoo G N et al. Oddi's sphincter motor activity in patients with recurrent pyogenic cholangitis. Hepatology 1993; 17: 13–58

366. Seel D J, Park Y K. Oriental infestational cholangitis. Am J Surg 1983; 146: 366–370

367. Lai K S, McFadzean A J S, Yeung R. Microembolic pulmonary hypertension in pyogenic cholangitis. Brit Med J 1968; 1: 22–24

368. Vyberg M, Poulsen H. Abnormal bile duct epithelium

accompanying septicaemia. Virchows Arch (A) 1984; 71: 1075–1078

369. Banks J G, Foulis A K, Ledingham I McA, MacSween R N M. Liver function in septic shock. J Clin Pathol 1982; 35: 1249–1252

370. Lefkowitch J H. Bile ductular cholestasis: an ominous histopathologic sign related to sepsis and "cholangitis lenta". Hum Pathol 1982; 13: 19–24

371. Gourley G R, Chesney P J, Davis J P, Odell G B. Acute cholestasis in patients with toxic-shock syndrome. Gastroenterology 1981; 81: 928–931

372. Ishak K G, Rogers W A. Cryptogenic acute cholangitis — association with toxic shock syndrome. Am J Clin Pathol 1981; 76: 619–626

373. Lieberman D A. Intrahepatic cholestasis due to Hodgkin's disease: an elusive diagnosis. J Clin Gastroenterol 1986; 8: 304–307

374. Birrer M J, Young R C. Differential diagnosis of jaundice in lymphoma patients. Semin Liver Dis 1987; 3: 269–277

375. Hubscher S G, Lumley M A, Elias E. Vanishing bile duct syndrome: a possible mechanism for intrahepatic cholestasis in Hodgkin's lymphoma. Hepatology 1993; 17: 70–77

13

Diseases of the gallbladder

D. Weedon

The gallbladder is a pear-shaped hollow viscus, closely attached to the liver and covered to a variable extent by peritoneum reflected off the liver. It measures approximately 10 cm in length and 3–4 cm in width, with a capacity of 50 ml or more. The gallbladder is divided into a fundus, body and a neck, the latter leading into the cystic duct. Hartmann's pouch, a dilatation in the region of the neck, is considered to be a pathological variation.

The mucosa is lined by tall columnar cells which, on electron microscopy, have a microvillous border.[1] The columnar cells are strongly immunoreactive for epithelial membrane antigen and for low molecular weight keratin using the CAM 5.2 antibody.[2] Small tubulo-alveolar glands may be found in different parts of the wall in the region of the neck. The lamina propria (submucosa) abuts directly on to the muscular layer. The adventitia or subserosa is composed of loosely arranged collagen and elastic tissue with variable amounts of adipose tissue. Small ducts resembling bile ducts are sometimes found in the adventitia adjacent to the liver. The function of these, Luschka's ducts, is uncertain, but for the most part they do not seem to communicate with the lumen of the gallbladder.[3]

The arterial supply is by the cystic artery, a branch of the right hepatic artery. The cystic artery usually bifurcates near the neck into a superficial and a deep branch, although these may arise separately from the right hepatic artery. Aberrant vascular patterns are not unusual. Many of the veins pass directly into the liver, although sometimes there is a well-formed cystic vein which empties into the portal vein. Lymph drainage is into the cystic or the superior pancreatico-duodenal glands. Sympathetic nerves arise mainly from the coeliac ganglia, while parasympathetic nerves are branches of the vagus nerve. Paraganglia have been reported in the adventitia.[4]

CONGENITAL ABNORMALITIES

Embryologically, the gallbladder and cystic duct arise from the caudal part of the hepatic diverticulum, an outpouching of gut endoderm. Congenital anomalies of the gallbladder can be considered under seven separate headings:

(i) anomalies in shape and form;
(ii) agenesis and hypoplasia;
(iii) duplication;
(iv) triplication;
(v) anomalies of position;
(vi) anomalies of the cystic duct;
(vii) miscellaneous anomalies.

Anomalies in shape and form

Some of the variations in shape and size of the gallbladder are best regarded as variations in the normal anatomy, rather than true congenital anomalies. The *Phrygian cap deformity*, which is found in 4% of routine cholecystograms, has been regarded as congenital by some, while others believe it is an acquired characteristic.[5] It consists of an angulation of the distal portion of the fundus of the gallbladder.

Diverticula are usually solitary outpouchings of the wall.[6] They may become separated from the rest of the gallbladder to form fundal cysts, having no communication with the lumen of the gallbladder.[7] *Cysts* may also be found in the body of the gallbladder; most are acquired and develop from Rokitansky–Aschoff sinuses. Congenital cysts are a rare occurrence.[8]

Multiseptate gallbladders are divided into a variable number of communicating chambers by multiple thin septa.[9] This deformity may result from incomplete cavitation of the developing gallbladder bud. *Hour-glass deformities* are usually acquired, while the congenital form is closely related to the septate gallbladder of transverse type.[10]

Agenesis and hypoplasia

Agenesis is thought to result from a failure of development of the ventrocaudal sacculation of the hepatic diverticulum. A vestigial or hypoplastic structure may result if the gallbladder anlage fails to recanalize after the solid phase. Over 200 cases of gallbladder agenesis have been reported.[11,12] The cystic duct is usually absent as well and there is poor development of the gallbladder fossa on the undersurface of the liver. The incidence of choledocholithiasis is increased in these patients. Other congenital anomalies may also be present.[13] Agenesis of the gallbladder may be diagnosed without resort to surgery, using imaging techniques.[14]

Duplication

Congenital duplication of the gallbladder has been described in animals since ancient times. Over 200 cases have been reported in humans.[15,16] The most common type of duplicated gallbladder is where the cystic duct and the accessory cystic duct enter the common bile duct separately (H-type). The individual cystic ducts may also unite to form a common cystic duct which then drains into the common bile duct (Y-type). Duplicated gallbladders may share a common peritoneal investment. The duplicated gallbladder is only marginally predisposed to disease when compared with the single organ. Also included under the duplications are bi-lobed and septate gallbladders.[17] A septate gallbladder has a longitudinal or transverse septum dividing it into two chambers.[10]

Triplication

This is a very rare anomaly which may be further subdivided on the basis of the arrangement of the cystic ducts.[11]

Anomalies of position

Malposition of the gallbladder is a rare anomaly. The positions reported include the left upper quadrant of the abdomen, either with or without situs inversus, in an intrahepatic position, retroplacement including retroperitoneal,[18] suprahepatic including above the diaphragm, in a transverse position within the falciform ligament, lesser sac or abdominal wall.[11] Usually included in this group are so-called wandering (floating) gallbladders where the gallbladder has a long mesentery or has no firm attachment to the liver.[19] Minor malposition of the gallbladder is often found as an acquired phenomenon in patients with cirrhosis of the liver.[20]

Anomalies of the cystic duct

The cystic duct is absent in most cases of agenesis of the gallbladder. Rarely, the duct may be absent in the presence of a gallbladder. Other anomalies include duplication of the duct and variations in the drainage of the cystic duct.

Miscellaneous

Included in this group are anomalies of the hepatic ducts and accessory bile ducts.[21] The accessory bile ducts are aberrant ducts draining individual segments of the liver.[22] They may drain into the right hepatic, common hepatic, cystic or common bile duct. Ducts have also been described connecting the liver and gallbladder, usually in the region of its neck.[23]

ECTOPIC AND METAPLASTIC TISSUES

Ectopic tissues are only rarely found within the gallbladder wall. The most common of these is *liver tissue*.[24] Ectopic liver may be attached by a broad mesenteric stalk to the serosa of the posterior wall of the gallbladder, or be found as an intramural or mucosal nodule.[25] The nodules are round to oval in shape and from 0.5 to 1.5 cm in diameter.

Ectopic *pancreatic tissue* may include islets of Langerhans in addition to exocrine pancreas.[26] The nodules of heterotopic pancreatic tissue are usually less than 1 cm in diameter. Acute pancreatitis may involve the ectopic tissue while the pancreas itself is uninvolved.[27] *Adrenal and thyroid tissue* have also been reported in the wall of the gallbladder.[11]

Heterotopic islands of *gastric mucosa* complete with chief and parietal cells may be found anywhere in the gallbladder (Fig. 13.1), although the region of the neck and the fundus are the most common sites.[28,29] The cystic and common bile ducts have also been involved.[30] Lesions may be polypoid, plaque-like or macroscopically indiscernible. The gastric mucosa may replace the normal mucosa, or be situated deep into it as an intramural nodule. Adjacent peptic ulceration is surprisingly uncommon.[31] These rare cases with well-developed foci of gastric body mucosa should be distinguished from the not uncommon finding of *antral or gastric surface epithelium*. The latter changes are presumed to have developed as a metaplastic process (Fig. 13.2). They may be an incidental finding in up to two-thirds of gallbladders removed for cholecystitis. Metaplastic gastric mucosa is found in a much older group of patients than those with heterotopic gastric mucosa.[32] Enterochromaffin cells, goblet cells and, less commonly, Paneth cells may be found in association with metaplastic antral or superficial gastric mucosa.[33] In metaplasia of the superficial gastric type, the epithelium is taller than the normal columnar epithelium of the gallbladder. Sometimes islands of this epithelium are confined to the apical areas of the mucosal folds while the basal regions contain antral or normal mucosa. Immunofluorescence studies have detected a small-intestinal-mucin antigen in areas of antral metaplasia, suggesting, perhaps, that all forms of glandular metaplasia in the gallbladder are intestinal in type.[34]

Although goblet cells are not uncommon in gallbladder epithelium, either randomly distributed or in association with metaplastic gastric epithelium, the presence of true *intestinal metaplasia* with secretory or non-secretory columnar cells with a high brush border combined with goblet, enterochromaffin and Paneth cells is very rare.[35] Intestinal epithelium may also be found in papillomas of the gallbladder. Goblet cell metaplasia and marked hyperplasia of mucous glands are often seen in the vicinity of carcinomas of the gallbladder.[36]

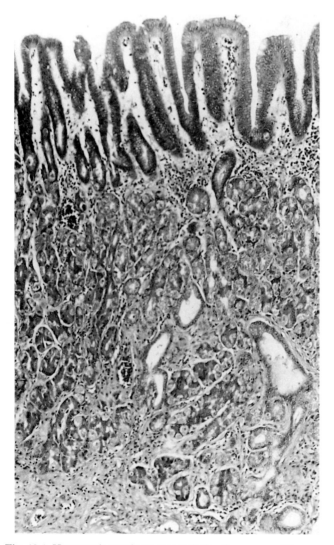

Fig. 13.1 Heterotopic gastric mucosa replacing the mucosa of the gallbladder. H & E.

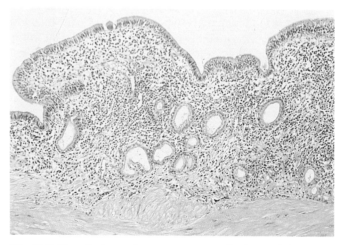

Fig. 13.2 Metaplastic antral-type mucosa occurring in association with severe chronic cholecystitis. H & E.

Squamous metaplasia is occasionally seen adjacent to squamous cell carcinomas, particularly in 'porcelain' gallbladder.

NON-INFLAMMATORY DISEASES

VASCULAR DISEASES

Primary vascular disease involving the cystic artery or its branches is quite rare. There are reports of their involvement by polyarteritis nodosa, allergic granulomatosis, rheumatoid vasculitis and 'focal arteritis' of unspecified type.[11] Polyarteritis nodosa may involve the vessels of the gallbladder as a localized phenomenon or as part of disseminated disease.[37]

Other abnormalities of the gallbladder vasculature include the rare cystic artery aneurysm, and rupture of the cystic artery as a complication of a penetrating duodenal ulcer, trauma or erosion of an impacted calculus in the gallbladder neck. Thrombosis of the cystic artery and vein is rare in the absence of other pathology in the area, although it may be seen in a small number of patients with acalculous cholecystitis following trauma or other surgical procedures. Embolization of the cystic artery has been documented only rarely.[38] Varices of the cystic vein may develop in the presence of portal hypertension.[39] They are usually asymptomatic and clinically insignificant.[40]

TORSION (VOLVULUS)

Approximately 300 cases of torsion of the gallbladder have been reported;[41] it is more common in the elderly.[42] Torsion may occur as an acute event or be recurrent (chronic torsion). Pre-operative diagnosis from cholecystitis is usually difficult.[43] Torsion results from abnormal mobility associated with one or two different anatomical abnormalities: either the gallbladder possesses a mesentery or, less commonly, it may lie free in the peritoneal cavity connected to the biliary system only by the cystic duct and vessels. Increased mobility may follow atrophy of fat in the elderly with downward displacement of abdominal viscera. Torsion may exceed 180° (complete), thereby compromising the blood supply.[44] Microscopic examination in complete torsion shows pronounced haemorrhage; if sufficient time has elapsed, signs of infarction will be present.

TRAUMA

Because of its protected site, the gallbladder is uncommonly injured following abdominal trauma. Two major types of trauma may occur: penetrating injuries resulting from stabbing, gun shots or technical procedures on the liver or biliary tract; and blunt abdominal trauma, associated with kicks, crushing or motor vehicle accidents.[45] Penetrating injuries are more common.[46]

Trauma may result in contusions, avulsion, lacerations, rupture, perforation with fistula formation, bile peritonitis, displacement, bile duct injury or haemobilia. Acute cholecystitis, often acalculous, may develop two or three weeks after major injury in up to 0.5% of cases.[47] Gangrene leading to perforation is sometimes present. The aetiology of the post-traumatic cholecystitis is probably multifactorial. Suggested causes include shock, sepsis, dehydration, transfusions and local vascular factors.

HAEMOBILIA

The terms 'haemocholecyst' and 'haematocele' of the gallbladder have been used for the finding of blood and clots of non-traumatic origin within the gallbladder. Haemobilia refers to bleeding into the biliary tract from any cause. It is being seen increasingly as a complication of diagnostic procedures involving the liver and the bile ducts — iatrogenic haemobilia.[48] The liver is the most frequent source of the bleeding in haemobilia, although gallbladder causes are responsible in about 20% of cases.[49] In these latter cases, the bleeding mostly results from the erosion of stones into the vasculature of the gallbladder, usually the cystic artery itself. Minor haemobilia is more frequent, but is usually ignored.[50]

HYDROPS AND MUCOCELE

Hydrops is characterized by a large distended gallbladder, the lumen of which is filled with clear material. If the contents are mucoid, the term mucocele is used. In children, hydrops is usually associated with a wide range of infectious diseases, particularly Kawasaki syndrome, and is reversible.[51] In adults, however, hydrops and mucoceles are usually secondary to obstruction of the ampulla or cystic duct by an impacted calculus and occur without any inflammation. Ultrasonography is useful in making the diagnosis.[52] A mucocele may also develop in the allograft cystic duct remnant in the recipient of a liver transplant.[53]

The organ is distended and sometimes elongated. It may contain up to 1500 ml of fluid. The wall is pale and usually thickened in adults, but thin in many of the acute cases (Fig. 13.3). On microscopic examination the mucosa is usually flattened. There is often partial fibrous replacement of the muscularis in the longstanding cases in adults. There is usually only a sparse chronic inflammatory cell infiltrate in the wall.

FOREIGN BODIES

Three categories of foreign bodies are recognized in the biliary tract: operative residuals, penetrating objects and

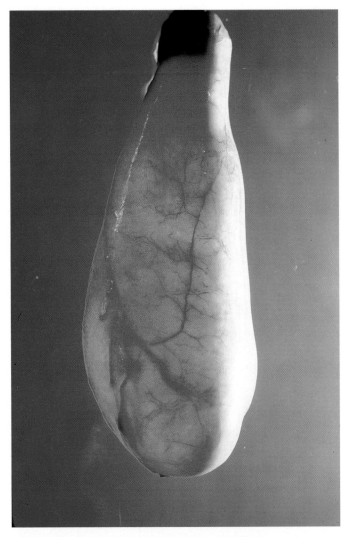

Fig. 13.3 Hydrops of the gallbladder. The wall is thin; a stone is impacted in the neck. Transillumination has been used.

ingested material.[54] Operative residuals, mostly non-absorbable suture material used on the cystic duct stump or cystic artery or for closing cholecystostomy incisions, account for nearly half of the foreign bodies reported. The ligatures may also act as a nidus for stone formation. Penetrating objects include missile and bullet fragments. Many types of ingested food matter and foreign bodies have been reported in the biliary tract. Patients with enteric–biliary anastomoses are particularly susceptible to the reflux of food into the biliary tract.[55] Foreign bodies may be present for a long time before they produce biliary tract symptoms.

CHOLESTEROLOSIS

Cholesterolosis is found in about 10% of patients coming to autopsy and in nearly 20% of surgically removed gallbladders. In about half of these cases the deposits are diffuse while in the remainder they are localized and often recognized only on careful inspection, or on histological examination. The peak incidence is in the fifth and sixth decades of life.[56] There is a female preponderance. Improvement in symptoms following cholecystectomy suggests that cholesterolosis may produce clinical manifestations, even in the absence of concomitant cholelithiasis.

The aetiology of cholesterolosis is unknown but most theories suggest that the accumulation of cholesterol esters results from altered uptake of cholesterol from the bile. Elfving and colleagues believe that mucosal hyperplasia is the primary event, resulting in an increased mucosal surface area leading to increased cholesterol absorption.[57]

On gross examination, the mucosa shows yellow, granular or punctate deposits studded over the mucosa (Fig. 13.4). In severe cases the summits of the mucosal ridges are extensively involved, imparting the appearance of yellow linear streaks. The term 'strawberry gallbladder' has led many students to believe mistakenly that the intervening mucosa is hyperaemic. The mucosa may be quite bile-stained, reflecting the dark and viscous bile that is sometimes present in these patients. Stones, usually of cholesterol type, are present in more than one-half of the surgical cases.

Microscopy shows that the mucosa is almost invariably hyperplastic. Foamy, lipid-laden macrophages with small dark nuclei are found in the elongated villous processes of the mucosa. Initially they involve the tips, but later they fill the entire villous process, even spilling over into the submucosa. Fat globules may also be seen in the base of the overlying epithelial cells while the luminal aspect of these cells may contain PAS-positive mucosubstances and, less commonly, lipochrome pigments. Although mild inflammation is sometimes present, it is interesting to note that cholesterolosis is not usually seen in the very inflamed

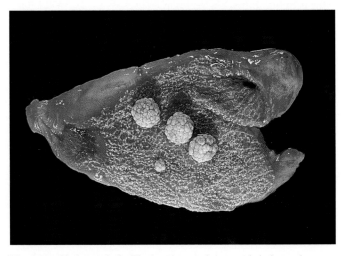

Fig. 13.4 Cholesterolosis. The lumen contains several cholesterol stones.

gallbladder, possibly because of extrusion of the foamy macrophages through the ulcerated tips of the inflamed mucosal villi. Electron microscopy has shown that the cholesterol vacuoles within the macrophages show great variation in size.[58]

Cholesterol polyps, although not true neoplasms, account for between 60 and 90% of gallbladder polyps. They are found in approximately 10% of all cases with diffuse cholesterolosis, but they are also found, not infrequently, in its absence. They are small, pedunculated lesions from 0.4 to 1.0 cm in diameter and are connected to the mucosa by a fine filamentous stalk.[59] They are usually multiple, with 3–10 or more being present. The polyps have a vascular connective tissue stalk. The stroma is usually packed with numerous foamy macrophages. Cholesterol polyps have been implicated in the aetiology of acute pancreatitis.[60] It has been postulated that detached cholesterol polyps impact in the sphincter of Oddi, leading to obstruction of pancreatic secretions.

INFLAMMATORY DISEASES — CHOLECYSTITIS

Cholecystitis is an important cause of morbidity, particularly in industrialized countries. The annual incidence of acute cholecystitis has been put at 60 cases per 100 000 population.[61] Chronic cholecystitis is much more common, although this term is sometimes applied indiscriminately to any cholecystectomy specimen containing a few chronic inflammatory cells. Cholelithiasis is present in at least 90% of cases of acute cholecystitis, and in 95% of chronic cases. Those without stones (acute acalculous cholecystitis) form an important group which will be considered separately.

ACUTE CHOLECYSTITIS

Acute cholecystitis is found in from 5 to 10% of cholecystectomy specimens, although this figure will be higher in those institutions in which early surgery is used in the treatment of acute cholecystitis. There is a female preponderance, with a mean age close to 60 years. Clinical symptoms include abdominal pain, particularly in the right upper quadrant, nausea, vomiting, flatulence and fever. The routine use of ultrasonography has enhanced the clinical diagnosis of acute cholecystitis.[62]

Obstruction of the cystic duct, most often resulting from a stone, appears to be the most important factor in the aetiology and pathogenesis of acute cholecystitis.[63] The presence of lithogenic bile has also been important in the prairie dog model.[64] The role of bacteria in the aetiology of acute calculous cholecystitis has been controversial, with conflicting reports. Although some have suggested that bacterial growth is probably secondary to what is initially aseptic inflammation, recent studies have cultured organisms from 80% of gallbladders removed within two days from the onset of symptoms.[65]

The formalin-fixed, partly shrunken specimen usually examined by the pathologist does not reflect the congested, oedematous and distended organ seen by the surgeon (Fig. 13.5). Complications such as focal gangrene or perforation may be superimposed. If the acute episode has developed in a gallbladder which was already the seat of longstanding chronic cholecystitis with much fibrosis, it may be of normal or even smaller size. The lumen will contain a variable mixture of bile, pus and sometimes haemorrhagic fluid. A solitary stone is more common in acute cholecystitis than in the chronic form, and this may be impacted in Hartmann's pouch.[66] In severe cases necrotic slough may be adherent to the mucosa.

On microscopic examination, changes will depend on the duration and severity of the inflammatory process. There is usually marked oedema of the wall in the early

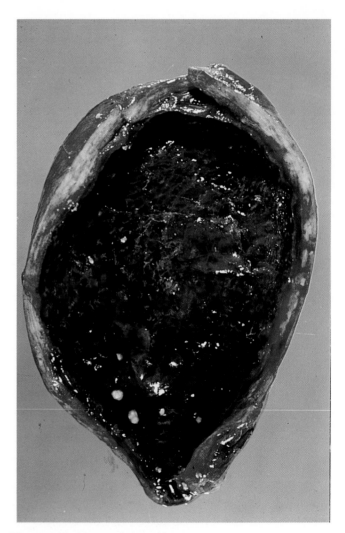

Fig. 13.5 Florid acute cholecystitis.

stages, involving particularly the adventitia. This is accompanied by an outpouring of fibrin and sometimes haemorrhage. There may be mucosal ulceration and even necrosis. The neutrophil response is variable and is usually most marked between the third and fifth days. Fibroblasts appear early and their activity is quite pronounced by the 10th day. There may be changes of pre-existing chronic cholecystitis. There is a tendency for pathologists to 'downgrade' the inflammatory process compared with the operative assessment of the surgeon.[67] This comes about because the neutrophil response is often scanty and transient, and the fibroblastic response is well developed in the adventitia at an early stage. The term 'organizing acute cholecystitis' is preferable to chronic cholecystitis for these cases.

The overall mortality for acute cholecystitis is approximately 4%,[62] although higher rates are sometimes reported in patients over 70 years of age.[68] Early operation within the first 48–72 hours has reduced mortality and morbidity by avoiding serious complications such as perforation.

Empyema

Empyema refers to the presence of macroscopically identifiable pus in the lumen of the gallbladder. It results from infection of the gallbladder with superimposed obstruction of the cystic duct, usually by a stone.[69] It is found in 5–10% of cases of acute cholecystitis. Organisms, particularly *E. coli* and *Klebsiella* sp., can be cultured from the contents in about 70% of cases.[70] Perforation of the gallbladder is a common complication of empyema.

Gangrenous cholecystitis

Traditionally, gangrenous cholecystitis has been regarded as a complication of severe acute cholecystitis or as a consequence of torsion of the gallbladder. The infarction which is associated with severe inflammation is thought to be secondary to obstruction and distension of the gallbladder and the consequent thrombosis of vessels.[71] The incidence of gangrenous cholecystitis varies widely in different series. It probably complicates about 15–20% of cases of acute cholecystitis; perforation supervenes in about 25%.[72] The mortality approaches 10% overall, and is highest in those with perforation.

The gallbladder is usually enlarged and the wall thickened and dark (Fig. 13.6). The mucosa is often friable and discoloured. The infarction may be limited to the mucosa and superficial muscularis or involve the full thickness of the wall. Sometimes there is only minimal inflammation present, confined to the adventitia. Cases such as this add support to the concept of an ischaemic aetiology in some instances.[73]

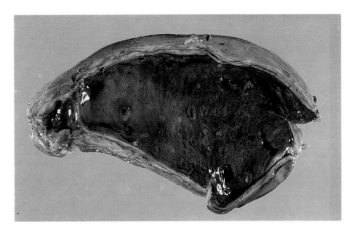

Fig. 13.6 Acute gangrenous cholecystitis.

Perforation

Perforation occurs in approximately 5–10% of cases of acute cholecystitis (both calculous and acalculous forms), particularly in those with gangrenous change.[74] Traditionally, perforations have been classified into free perforation, perforation with localized pericholecystic abscess formation and perforation into the intestine with fistula formation.[75] Perforation into the liver is a fourth category.[76] Positive cultures are found in 80% or more of cases, with *E. coli* the most common organism isolated. The perforation is most usually at the fundus of the gallbladder. Perforation may be accompanied by haemorrhage and even haemoperitoneum.[77] Bile peritonitis is an important complication of free perforation of the gallbladder. The mortality with perforation of the gallbladder is approximately 20% and is highest for free perforations.[78]

CHRONIC CHOLECYSTITIS

The incidence of chronic cholecystitis depends very much on the criteria used in making the diagnosis. There is a female preponderance of approximately 3:1 or more, with a peak incidence in the fifth and sixth decades. The usual symptoms are of intermittent biliary colic, nausea, flatulence, or ill-defined 'dyspeptic' symptoms.

The macroscopic appearances of the gallbladder will depend on the variable factors of obstruction, inflammation and fibrosis. The gallbladder may be shrunken and fibrotic, or distended. Gallstones are present in about 95% of cases. They are usually multiple and faceted, although sometimes only a solitary stone is present. The microscopic appearances are variable. Rokitansky–Aschoff sinuses are usually present and sometimes these contain inspissated bile. Bile granulomas are occasionally related to these sinuses (Fig. 13.7). There is variable fibrosis of the wall, although this is not always

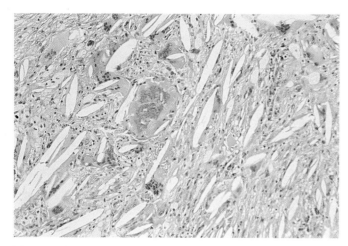

Fig. 13.7 Cholegranuloma with macrophages, giant cells and cholesterol clefts. H & E.

prominent. There may be severe endarteritis obliterans of vessels, and a variable chronic inflammatory cell infiltrate.

An attempt has been made to classify chronic cholecystitis into two types: a primary form in which there is no history or evidence of previous cholecystitis and a secondary type in which there are changes of previous acute cholecystitis.[79] In the secondary form the wall is usually thicker, the inflammatory infiltrate more marked, and changes of endarteritis obliterans sometimes quite prominent. Antral metaplasia of the mucosa is a common finding in chronic cholecystitis. Goblet cells and argentaffin cells may also be present.

The term *chronic follicular cholecystitis* should be used for those rare variants of chronic cholecystitis in which there are lymphoid follicles in the mucosa, often with hyperplastic germinal centres.[80] There may be a few follicles also in the adventitia. There is a greater incidence of this form in patients with typhoid fever, although Salmonella infections account for only a small number of the cases now seen.[81]

The pathogenesis of chronic cholecystitis is related to the associated cholelithiasis, which results in a low grade chronic inflammatory reaction with eventual fibrosis, contraction and loss of function. At times, cystic duct obstruction producing acute cholecystitis is a precursor. Positive bile cultures have been found in 20–30% of patients with chronic cholecystitis and cholelithiasis.[82]

MISCELLANEOUS TYPES OF CHOLECYSTITIS

Acalculous cholecystitis

Acalculous cholecystitis, which accounts for 10% of cases of acute cholecystitis, may be found in a wide variety of clinical settings.[83,84] It may complicate severe trauma, surgery, childbirth, burns, bacterial sepsis, hyperalimentation, the acquired immunodeficiency syndrome,[85] bone marrow transplantation[86] and systemic disease, particularly diabetes mellitus.[87,88] When trauma, burns or surgery are involved, they precede the onset of the cholecystitis by a mean period of 14 days. Although acalculous cholecystitis is found at all ages, including childhood, it is particularly common in debilitated patients over the age of 65 years. It is more common in males.

The gross and microscopic features are indistinguishable from those seen in acute cholecystitis of calculous type, except for the higher incidence of gangrene, empyema and perforation.[88,89] The morbidity and mortality are also higher in the acalculous variant.

Platelet-activating factor and prostaglandins have been implicated in the pathogenesis of some cases.[90] This might explain the higher incidence of gangrene seen in acalculous cholecystitis. Other factors which may have aetiological significance include stasis and increased viscosity and lithogenicity of bile.[91] Bacteria can be cultured in about 70% of cases.[89]

Emphysematous cholecystitis

Acute emphysematous cholecystitis (Fig. 13.8) is a rare form of cholecystitis characterized by the presence of gas in the wall and lumen of the gallbladder.[92] The clinical diagnosis can be made by plain radiography or computed tomography of the abdomen rather than by ultrasonography.[93,94] *Clostridium perfringens* has been isolated in nearly half of the cases, with *E. coli*, *Klebsiella*, or a mixed growth sometimes cultured. Clinically, it is correlated with diabetes mellitus, male sex, and age over 50 years. Gangrene of the wall is present in most cases and the contents are usually frankly purulent. The mucosa may separate completely, forming a cast. Colonies of microorganisms are often seen within the necrotic mucosa or in mural abscesses. It is now considered that gangrene of the wall is a facilitating factor for the proliferation of the gas-forming organisms.

Eosinophilic cholecystitis

The term eosinophilic cholecystitis should be restricted to those cases in which the mural infiltrate is virtually a pure infiltrate of eosinophils. The term should not be used for those gallbladders in which eosinophils are merely a prominent component of an otherwise polymorphic infiltrate. These latter cases represent a stage in the evolution of an episode of cholecystitis. Eosinophils may be prominent in the inflammatory infiltrate in acalculous cholecystitis.[95] Eosinophilic cholecystitis is usually a localized phenomenon without any clinical history of systemic allergy or peripheral eosinophilia. Rare cases have been associated with eosinophilic enteritis, parasitic infestation, antibiotic therapy[96] or a history of atopy.[97,98] The infiltrate may extend through the wall, but is usually prominent in the muscularis, associated with separation of the muscle

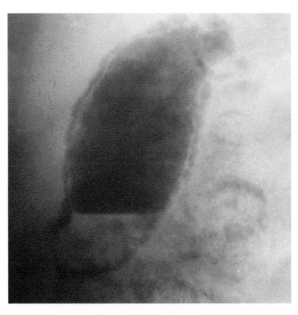

Fig. 13.8 Emphysematous cholecystitis. Plain X-ray to show gas in the wall and a fluid level in the lumen.

bundles. Eosinophils may also be found in the cystic duct lymph node.

Xanthogranulomatous cholecystitis

Xanthogranulomatous cholecystitis is a form of chronic cholecystitis that results from extravasation of bile into the wall of the gallbladder with a subsequent inflammatory response.[99,100] Lipid from the bile is ingested by macrophages which assume the appearance of xanthoma cells. Giant cells of foreign body or Touton type and fibroblasts are also present. Progressive organization occurs, leading to the formation of dense fibrous tissue. Dystrophic calcification is a late complication in some cases. Adenocarcinoma of the gallbladder may also develop in gallbladders with xanthogranulomatous cholecystitis.[101] Ceroid granuloma is a related entity.[102] It results from the oxidation of lipid in the bile to a yellow-brown pigment which is engulfed by macrophages. A localized inflammatory lesion is present.

The term *melanosis of the gallbladder* refers to the presence of a lipofuscin-like pigment in mucosal epithelial cells and less commonly in the underlying submucosa (Fig. 13.9). The pigment stains positively with the Masson–Fontana method.[103] Unlike ceroid granulomas and xanthogranulomatous cholecystitis there is no significant inflammatory reaction in melanosis of the gallbladder.

'Porcelain' gallbladder

Dystrophic calcification, 'porcelain' gallbladder, is found in approximately 0.5% of cholecystectomy specimens.[104]

The aetiology of the disease is uncertain, but is most likely a consequence of chronic inflammation and fibrosis of the wall. It may follow xanthogranulomatous cholecystitis (unpublished observation). Carcinomas have been reported in about 20% of 'porcelain' gallbladders.[105]

The gallbladder is usually contracted with a somewhat thickened wall (Fig. 13.10). There may be a bluish discoloration of the mucosa, associated with some brittleness of the wall. On microscopy, the wall is extensively fibrosed with hyalinization of the collagen. The calcification is usually in broad bands, although a rare form with small mucosal concretions has been described (Fig. 13.11). The mucosal epithelium is often absent in severe cases of 'porcelain' gallbladder. There is now some evidence to suggest that carcinoma is less likely in these

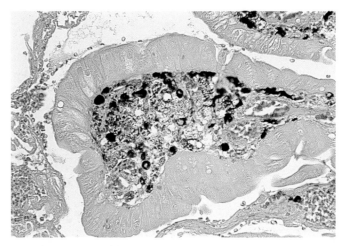

Fig. 13.9 A mucosal villous projection containing pigment-laden macrophages. Masson–Fontana stain.

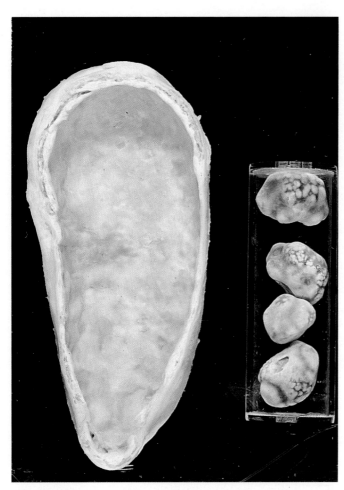

Fig. 13.10 'Porcelain' gallbladder. The four stones from the lumen are mounted separately.

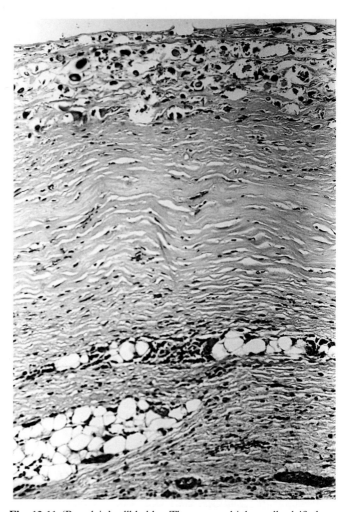

Fig. 13.11 'Porcelain' gallbladder. There are multiple small calcified concretions in the mucosa. H & E.

cases where the mucosa has been replaced by fibrous tissue.[106]

SPECIFIC INFECTIONS OF THE GALLBLADDER

Bacterial. Localization of *Salmonella typhi* in the gallbladder is a common event in typhoid fever, although acute cholecystitis is an uncommon complication of this colonization. When cholecystitis occurs, perforation may supervene. The gallbladder may harbour *Salmonella* in chronic carrier states, although one-third of these patients have no past history of typhoid fever. Chronic cholecystitis is frequently present in these carriers, and occasionally this takes the form of chronic follicular cholecystitis.[107] *Salmonella* may also be isolated from gallstones in carriers.

Asymptomatic carriers of *Vibrio cholerae* may also occur. There are no specific features in the cholecystitis which may develop in up to 1% of convalescent cholera patients. Several species of *Campylobacter* have been implicated in the aetiology of cholecystitis.[108] Sporadic cases of *tuberculosis* of the gallbladder have been reported from India and

Europe. There may be miliary lesions, confluent caseating granulomas or spread from tuberculous foci of other organs. Acute acalculous cholecystitis is a rare complication of systemic *brucellosis*.[109]

Fungal. Although Hermanek has reported fungi on histological examination in approximately 10% of cholecystectomy specimens,[110] this could not be confirmed in a personal study by the author. Fungal infections of the gallbladder are very rare, except in debilitated patients.[111] Infections with *Candida albicans*, *Torulopsis glabrata*, *Aspergillus* and actinomyces have been reported. There has been one case of granulomatous cholecystitis from *Torulopsis*.[112]

Viral. Obstruction of the cystic duct by enlarged cells infected with cytomegalovirus has been reported in nearly 10% of patients, following orthotopic liver transplantation.[113] This virus may also be found in epithelial, endothelial and connective tissue cells of the gallbladder in patients with the acquired immunodeficiency syndrome. Such patients may present with the clinical features of an ascending cholangitis.[114–116]

Protozoal. There are many reports in the European literature of biliary tract dysfunction associated with infestation of the gallbladder and common bile duct with *Giardia lamblia*.[11] Infestation is more frequent in patients with achlorhydria, malabsorption or IgA deficiency. Giardiasis has been incriminated in the aetiology of several cases of cholecystitis with mucosal ulceration. The gallbladder may be involved by rupture or direct extension of an amoebic abscess of the liver. *Cryptosporidium* has been found in the gallbladder and biliary tract of several patients with the acquired immunodeficiency syndrome.[117] Cholecystitis may accompany this infestation.[118]

Helminth infestations. Infestation of the gallbladder with parasites of the phylum *Platyhelminthes* is uncommon, although the common bile duct is involved much more often. Granulomas have been reported in association with the ova of *Schistosoma mansoni* and *haematobium*, *Fasciola hepatica*, *Paragonimus westermani* and *Ascaris lumbricoides*.[11] Eosinophils and fibrosis are usually present. Calcification of the granulomas in schistosomiasis may produce a characteristic appearance on abdominal radiographs.[119] Cholelithiasis, with pigment stones and even cholecystitis, may result from infestation of the common duct by the trematodes *Fasciola hepatica* and *Clonorchis sinensis*. Adenocarcinoma of the cystic duct has been associated with opisthorchis infestation.[120] Hydatid disease usually involves the common duct as a complication of the rupture of hydatid cyst of the liver. The gallbladder is only rarely involved. The biliary tract is the most frequent ectopic location of *Ascaris lumbricoides*, although only rarely do they reach the gallbladder itself. Remnants of ascaris, its larvae or ova are often found in the centre of stones in some parts of the world.[121]

CHOLELITHIASIS

Although the majority of gallstones are clinically silent, they are nevertheless an important cause of morbidity. Approximately 20% of adults in Western countries will have formed gallstones by the time they die.

CLINICAL FEATURES

There is an increasing incidence of gallstones with age, although they have also been reported in infants and children.[122] There is an overall female preponderance of approximately 2 : 1, although there is a more equal sex incidence for pigment stones. There is sometimes a family history of gallstones. Cholesterol gallstones are found in association with obesity, diabetes mellitus, Crohn's disease of the terminal ileum, and following terminal ileal resection, jejuno-ileal bypass surgery, truncal vagotomy and pregnancy.[123] Black pigment stones are associated with chronic haemolysis, including heart valve replacement, cirrhosis, chronic alcoholism, total parenteral nutrition and advanced age.[124-126] Brown pigment stones, which are common in Oriental persons, usually occur as a result of infection of bile with enteric bacteria. They may also occur in primary sclerosing cholangitis and in association with a juxtapapillary duodenal diverticulum.[124]

Flatulence, epigastric or right upper quadrant pain, intolerance of fatty foods and biliary colic may all be found in symptomatic patients, although they are not diagnostic of cholelithiasis. Only a minority of gallstones give rise to symptoms. In one study, the 15-year cumulative probability of developing biliary pain or complications with cholelithiasis was only 18%.[127] Once biliary pain occurs, the chances of further trouble are much higher.

Over 70% of gallstones are radiolucent; and of radioopaque ones, about two-thirds are of black pigment type. Ultrasound, which will detect stones larger than 3 mm in diameter, is being used with increasing frequency to diagnose cholelithiasis. Computed tomography can be used to predict the composition of gallstones.[128]

MORPHOLOGICAL TYPES OF GALLSTONES

There are two major types of gallstones: cholesterol and pigment stones.

Cholesterol stones. These account for nearly 80% of all gallstones in the Western world. Cholesterol stones are composed of at least 50% by weight of crystalline cholesterol monohydrate. Because most cholesterol stones also contain bile pigments, calcium salts and a mucoprotein or pigment matrix, they have been known in the past as *mixed cholesterol stones*. Mixed stones are usually multiple, round or faceted, and less than 2 cm in diameter. Sometimes a gallbladder will contain stones of greatly different sizes, suggesting the presence of two or more generations of stones (Fig. 13.12). In one report, there were said to have been 36 329 stones in the gallbladder.[129] Approximately 10% of cholesterol stones are essentially

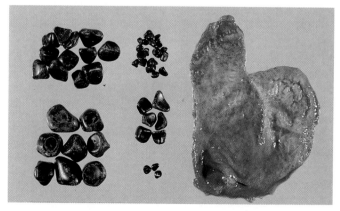

Fig. 13.12 Cholelithiasis. There are probably several different generations of stones present.

pure cholesterol. Such stones are cream to yellow radiolucent stones. They are usually larger than the mixed cholesterol stones, measuring up to 4 cm in diameter. There is a radial arrangement of the crystals on the cut surface.

Pigment stones. These account for nearly 20% of all stones, although they are much more common in some Asian countries.[130] Two types of pigment stone are recognized: black stones and brown stones.[124] Both contain, primarily, calcium bilirubinate, either polymerized (black stones) or as the precipitated salt (brown stones).[131] Brown stones also contain calcium palmitate and some cholesterol, while black stones also contain calcium carbonate or calcium phosphate, or both. *Black stones* form mainly in the gallbladder. They are amorphous with a powdery consistency and an irregular outline. *Brown stones* are orange-brown in colour, often laminated and soft in consistency. They are usually formed in the bile ducts in association with infection.[132]

PATHOGENESIS OF GALLSTONES

A detailed account of the pathogenesis of gallstones is beyond the scope of this chapter. The subject will be considered only in broad outline.

There are three distinct, but interdependent stages in the formation of cholesterol stones. (i) the formation of bile saturated with cholesterol (lithogenic bile); (ii) nucleation; (iii) crystal retention and cohesion (growth of the stone).[131,133,134] The lithogenicity of bile depends not only on the absolute concentration of cholesterol, but also on the amount of bile salts and lecithin, which have limited capacity to solubilize cholesterol. Bile saturation with cholesterol originates in the liver, not from bile undergoing changes in the gallbladder. The fact that persons without cholelithiasis often secrete lithogenic bile indicates that factors other than cholesterol saturation of bile are important in the pathogenesis of cholesterol stones.[135] Nucleation is one such process. It involves the aggregation of cholesterol crystals from carrier vesicles in the bile, usually around particles such as mucus, calcium salts, bacteria, parasitic ova or detached cells from the mucosa of the gallbladder. The bile contains both inhibitors and accelerators of nucleation.[136] Mucous glycoproteins are powerful nucleating agents. The growth of gallstones is poorly understood but it is likely that factors such as gallbladder motility and inflammation influence the growth of cholesterol stones.[137] The healthy gallbladder absorbs cholesterol and desaturates bile, protective factors that may be lost with chronic cholecystitis.[133]

The earliest phase in the development of both cholesterol and pigment stones is the formation of biliary sludge composed of mucus and cholesterol vesicles or calcium bilirubinate.[131] Sludge may disappear or proceed to gallstone formation. The recognition of biliary sludge as a precursor of stone formation is relatively recent. It appears to represent a stage between nucleation and growth of the stone, although further studies are needed to ascertain its significance.

Pigment stones result from the precipitation of calcium salts of bilirubin and other anions.[138] Brown stones are associated with infections of the biliary tract by bacteria with high levels of β-glucuronidase and phospholipase activity that result in the precipitation of calcium bilirubinate and calcium palmitate.[132] Black stones may be associated with the increased secretion of conjugated bilirubin, as in haemolytic states. Their pathogenesis in other circumstances is not well understood. They are not usually related to infection. The calcium bilirubinate that precipitates is polymerized to a greater extent in black than brown stones. The precipitation of the other calcium salts that constitute black stones may be influenced by local gallbladder factors.[124] The nucleation of pigment stones probably involves mucus as well as bacteria and bacterial glycocalyx.[139] Parasite ova are sometimes found in the centre of pigmented stones in the Orient.

PATHOLOGY

In cholelithiasis, the gallbladder may show any one of a number of changes. It may be normal, particularly in children. It often shows mild hypertrophy of the muscularis with some loss of the mucosal papillary folds, this latter change becoming marked in obstructive cases leading to mucocele formation or acute cholecystitis. The incidence of chronic cholecystitis depends on the criteria used for the diagnosis. A few chronic inflammatory cells are almost invariable in adults with cholelithiasis. Cholelithiasis can be found in association with a wide range of disease processes in the gallbladder including acute cholecystitis, empyema, cholesterolosis, adenomyomatosis, 'porcelain' gallbladder, and even malignancy.

An ultrastructural study of the mucosal epithelium in cholelithiasis has found a markedly reduced volume density of lysosomes compared with gallstone-free subjects.[140] However, the volume of mucin secretory granules was similar in both groups.

Special variants of gallstones include 'floating' stones, which have a lower specific gravity than bile-containing contrast medium. They can be detected in about 1% of cholecystograms. They have no special significance. Gas-containing stones can be detected as stellate radiolucencies within the gallbladder. The gas may be the result of anaerobic bacterial action. The efficacy of lithotripsy increases with increasing content of gas in the stones.[141]

BILIARY FISTULAS AND GALLSTONE ILEUS

Fistulas between the biliary and gastrointestinal tracts are usually secondary to longstanding calcareous biliary tract disease. They result from the formation of adhesions between the gallbladder or common duct and the intestine with subsequent necrosis of the walls of the adherent organs, as a result of further inflammation or pressure from a gallstone. In about 5% of cases penetrating peptic ulcer is responsible for the fistula,[142] while in a similar number of cases a wide range of disease processes may be involved.[143] These include trauma, Crohn's disease of the gut, and carcinoma of either the biliary tract or intestines.

More than half the fistulas are cholecystoduodenal in type, followed by cholecystocolic and choledochoduodenal fistulas. Multiple structures may be involved, the commonest being the cholecysto-duodeno-colic fistula.[144] Fistulas between the gallbladder and common bile duct (cholecystobiliary) account for about 1% of internal biliary fistulas.[145] External biliary fistulas, opening spontaneously on to the cutaneous surface, are now quite uncommon.[146]

Fistulas are more common in females than males. The diagnosis is usually made by finding air in the biliary tract on radiological examination, or by barium studies. Gallstone ileus may complicate a biliary fistula in about 20% of cases.[147] The mortality of internal biliary fistulas may be as high as 15%.[148]

As a general rule, the gallbladder is thickened and chronically inflamed. Dense adhesions are often present. Stones are present in up to 90% of cases, usually in the gallbladder, but sometimes in the common bile duct or even the duodenum, jejunum or ileum. In one composite review,[149] the gallbladder was involved in 88% of cases and the common bile duct in 11%, while the enteric component was the duodenum in 69%, colon in 26% and the stomach in 4.4% of cases.

Gallstone ileus complicates about 20% of cases of biliary–enteric fistula and about 0.3% of cases of cholelithiasis.[147] It has been estimated that only 10% of gallstones entering the intestines cause obstruction, as those less than 2.5 cm in diameter usually pass naturally.[150] The average diameter of impacted stones varies from 3 to 4.5 cm, and the average weight is just over 20 g. More than one stone is sometimes present.[151] The ileum is the site of impaction in 65–80% of cases.[151] This is usually within 30 cm of the ileo-caecal valve. The jejunum is involved in approximately 20% of cases and the large bowel, usually the sigmoid colon, in up to 5%. The duodenum may also be involved, particularly the duodenal bulb (Bouveret's syndrome).[152] The stomach and appendix are rare sites of impaction. Gallstones need to be distinguished from enteroliths, particularly in the appendix.

Cholecystenteric fistulas, usually of cholecystoduodenal type, are assumed to have been present in most cases. Spontaneous closure of fistulas is well documented, and this may explain the absence of fistulas in some patients with gallstone ileus. Recurrent gallstone ileus may occur in about 5% of cases.[153]

LIMY BILE

Limy (milk of calcium) bile is characterized by the presence in the gallbladder or common bile duct of excessive amounts of calcium carbonate, often mixed with other calcium salts.[154,155] This has the appearance of inspissated cream-grey to yellow-green material. Limy bile may cast a shadow on a plain abdominal X-ray, almost indistinguishable from a normal cholecystogram. Its pathogenesis is still controversial, although stasis gallbladder appears to precede its formation in the gallbladder.[156]

HYPERPLASTIC DISEASES OF THE GALLBLADDER

ADENOMYOMATOSIS

No other entity in the gallbladder is subject to as much confusion as adenomyomatosis. It may be defined as a hyperplastic lesion of the gallbladder characterized by excessive proliferation of surface epithelium with invaginations into the thickened muscularis or beyond.[157] The term adenomyomatosis should not be used synonymously with the microscopic presence of a few Rokitansky–Aschoff sinuses, although sometimes the distinction can be quite subjective, particularly if only one section is available for study. Adenomyomatosis may be generalized (diffuse), segmental or localized (adenomyoma) in type.[158,159] When it is localized, the fundus is usually involved (Fig. 13.13). The term *cholecystitis glandularis proliferans* has been used in the past for what is now called adenomyomatosis of generalized type.[160] The incidence of this condition has varied from 1 to 33%, depending on the source of material and the criteria used for diagnosis.[157,161]

Adenomyomatosis is more common in females and there is an increased incidence with age.[162] It may be asymptomatic, although there is evidence that it can produce symptoms even in the absence of cholelithiasis.[163,164] This applies particularly to fundal adenomyomas. Cholelithiasis is also present in about half the cases. The diagnosis may be made by cholecystography or ultrasonography.

Generalized adenomyomatosis is characterized by outpocketings of the mucosa into the muscularis, which is three to five times the normal thickness (Fig. 13.14). They may extend into the adventitia. Some of these sinuses are

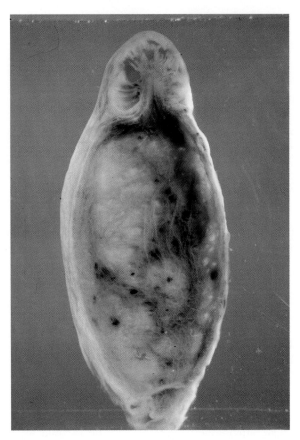

Fig. 13.13 Adenomyoma of the fundus. A number of bile-filled Rokitansky–Aschoff sinuses are visible in the body of the gallbladder.

dilated and contain pigment debris. There may also be an increase in the height of the mucosal folds. Mild chronic inflammation or focal bile granulomas may also involve the wall. In the segmental type, a thickened circumferential band or segment of the gallbladder wall with the morphological features of adenomyomatosis is found.[165] Subtypes have been identified on the basis of the site of this involvement.[166] The localized adenomyoma is a small nodule, devoid of a capsule, usually situated in the muscularis at the fundus. Sometimes they are entirely subserosal in position. Adenomyomas average 1.5 cm in diameter.[167] They are composed of glands admixed with interlacing bundles of smooth muscle. The overlying mucosa may show papillary folds and invaginations. Rarely, atypical epithelial hyperplasia may extend into the invaginated glands of adenomyomatosis. In these circumstances it may be difficult to distinguish the changes from adenocarcinoma. There are only a few reports of gallbladder carcinoma actually arising in adenomyomatosis.[168]

The aetiology of adenomyomatosis is controversial. It is generally regarded as an acquired phenomenon akin to diverticular disease of the colon and resulting from increased luminal pressure, perhaps secondary to neuromuscular incoordination or to partial obstruction of the cystic duct by stones, folds or abnormal smooth muscle bands. Smooth muscle hypertrophy has been found in the neck of the gallbladder in patients with fundal adenomyomas.[169]

MUCOSAL HYPERPLASIA

Mucosal hyperplasia has been neglected by most authors.[170] It may be a primary process, or occur in association with other diseases such as cholesterolosis, adenomyomatosis and metachromatic leucodystrophy. Primary

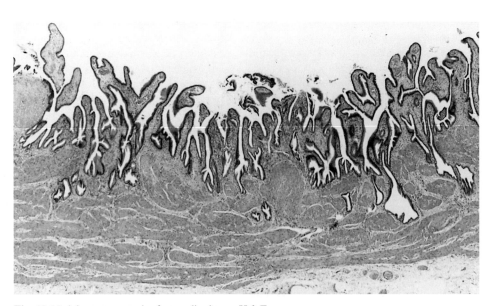

Fig. 13.14 Adenomyomatosis of generalized type. H & E.

hyperplasia which appears capable of producing symptoms is an uncommon process.[171,172] The two most important forms are villous hyperplasia and adenomatous hyperplasia (Fig. 13.15). In both types the mucosa may appear thickened or velvety, sometimes with an uneven surface. This change is often unrecognized on macroscopic examination. Villous hyperplasia has thin, tall, papillary folds covered by tall, regular columnar cells. These projections sometimes ramify. This type of mucosal hyperplasia is often a precursor to the development of cholesterolosis.[57] Adenomatous hyperplasia is associated with marked antral metaplasia of the mucosa. Sometimes micropolyps are formed.

ATYPICAL HYPERPLASIA

In atypical hyperplasia (dysplasia) the mucosa is flat or has small papillary projections (Fig. 13.16). There is some pseudostratification of the epithelium with disorganization

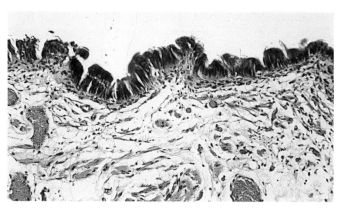

Fig. 13.16 Atypical hyperplasia of the mucosa. H & E.

of the epithelial architecture.[173] Loss of cell polarity, nuclear corwding, hyperchromatism and mitoses are also present. Metaplastic changes frequently accompany the dysplasia.[174] If atypical hyperplasia is found, the pathologist should carefully examine the gallbladder to ensure that no foci of invasive carcinoma have been missed. Foci of atypical hyperplasia or the more severe changes of carcinoma-in-situ are found quite frequently adjacent to invasive carcinoma of the gallbladder.[173] The term carcinoma-in-situ has usually been applied to atypical changes occurring in adenomatous polyps, in the absence of stalk invasion. It has also been applied to severe atypia of the mucosa, although it is often a matter of opinion whether the changes should be interpreted as atypical hyperplasia or carcinoma-in-situ.[175,176] Morphometry has been used to assist in this distinction.[177] There have been reports of patients with carcinoma-in-situ, in whom generalized metastases have subsequently developed. This illustrates the need for caution in making the diagnosis and the necessity to examine the gallbladder carefully in such cases.

TUMOURS OF THE GALLBLADDER

BENIGN TUMOURS

Mucosal polyps

Cholesterol polyps account for more than 80% of mucosal polyps found in the gallbladder. They have already been considered in the section on cholesterolosis. *Inflammatory polyps* are rare, firm, sessile polyps 0.5–1.0 cm in diameter.[178] They may be solitary or multiple, with up to five or more polyps present. They are composed of heavily inflamed granulation and fibrous tissue with surface ulceration. The predominant inflammatory cell is the lymphocyte. They are thought to represent a residual localized inflammatory process following an episode of cholecystitis.

Adenomatous polyps (adenomas) are uncommon lesions, occurring anywhere in the gallbladder. They are usually

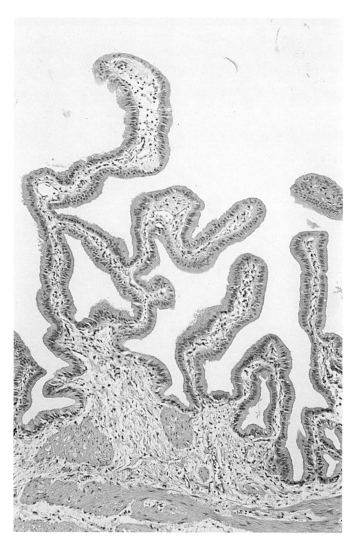

Fig. 13.15 Villous hyperplasia of the mucosa. H & E.

pedunculated but may be sessile. They measure from 0.5 to 2 cm in diameter, or more. Several lesions are found in one-third of cases. Three histological types of adenoma are recognized: papillary, tubular and tubulopapillary.[179] The papillary adenomas (also called papillomas) have a branching structure with a fibrous stroma and covering of tall columnar cells. The tubular variant has a proliferation of glands within the substance of the polyp. The risk of malignant transformation of these polyps is very small although foci of cytological atypia are sometimes seen in the sessile polyps that occur in a gallbladder which is the seat of extensive metaplasia.[180,181] One study reported 'adenomatous residues' in 19% of invasive carcinomas, suggesting a transition of benign adenomas into carcinoma.[182]

Multicentric papillomatosis is a rare entity characterized by numerous papillary tumours involving the mucosa of the gallbladder and usually other parts of the biliary tract.[183] The polyps vary in size and configuration. Adenocarcinomatous transformation has been reported.[183]

Benign mesenchymal tumours

Benign mesenchymal tumours of the gallbladder are rare, and usually resemble their counterparts in other sites. Those reported include fibroma, fibroadenoma, leiomyoma, neurofibroma,[184] haemangioma,[185] lipoma, amputation neuroma,[186] paraganglioma,[187] granular cell myoblastoma[188] and lymphangioma.[11] Amputation neuromas are not uncommon after cholecystectomy. Their role in producing symptoms is controversial. They are firm, grey nodules 1–3 cm in diameter. There are prominent nerve bundles, arranged in different directions, with a background of collagenous stroma.

MALIGNANT TUMOURS

Carcinoma of the gallbladder

Carcinoma of the gallbladder ranks fifth in order of frequency of tumours of the gastrointestinal tract. The annual incidence per 100 000 of the population is approximately 2.5 cases. The average age of patients is about 65 years, while up to 75% are females. Presenting symptoms include abdominal pain, nausea, vomiting, jaundice and weight loss.[189] A correct pre-operative diagnosis is made in less than 10% of patients, and in up to 20% the diagnosis is made subsequently by the pathologist.[190] Ultrasound has not led to a marked improvement in the pre-operative diagnosis.[191,192] The serum carbohydrate antigen 19.9 (CA 19.9) is a useful tumour marker, although further experience with it is needed.[193] Gallstones are present in about 70%. Occasionally there is an underlying 'porcelain' gallbladder, or an anomalous

connection between the common duct and the pancreatic duct.[194]

Adenocarcinoma. Approximately 80% of carcinomas of the gallbladder are adenocarcinomas, although this figure is higher if some poorly differentiated carcinomas are included in this group. The tumours may be bulky, localized nodular growths, thickened plaques, or macroscopically indiscernible. The entire organ is involved in nearly 80% of cases, while the tumour is limited to the gallbladder in less than 20% of all patients.[195] The histological appearances are variable from tumour to tumour and sometimes within the same lesion. This applies to the differentiation, spacing of the glands and degree of stromal desmoplasia.

Several variants of adenocarcinoma are recognized.[179] The papillary variant usually grows as a bulky intraluminal mass (Fig. 13.17). It has a better prognosis than other types.[196] The mucinous (colloid) variant tends to occur in older patients and produces diffuse thickening of the wall;[197] perforation is more common than with other types and signet-ring

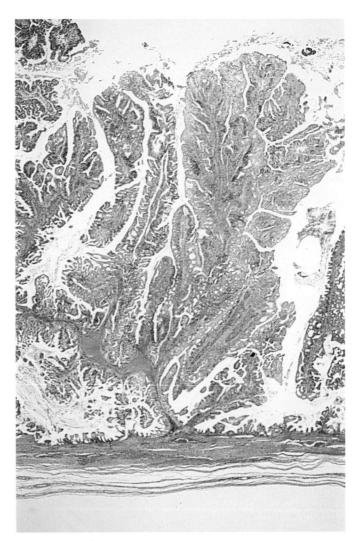

Fig. 13.17 Papillary adenocarcinoma of the gallbladder. There is no obvious invasion of the wall in this area. H & E.

cells are sometimes present. Other rare variants include a giant cell adenocarcinoma, an intestinal type adenocarcinoma[198] and one with choriocarcinoma-like areas.[199,200]

Squamous cell carcinoma. These comprise about 4% of all carcinomas of the gallbladder.[201] They are usually widely infiltrating tumours, although distant metastases are often delayed. In about 2% of carcinomas of the gallbladder, there are mixtures of adenocarcinoma and squamous cell carcinoma (adenosquamous carcinoma).

Undifferentiated carcinoma. About 5% of gallbladder carcinomas are regarded as undifferentiated or anaplastic tumours.[202] They are usually bulky tumours replacing the gallbladder and infiltrating widely into adjacent structures. An anaplastic, small cell carcinoma with oat-cell morphology has been described.[199,203]

Complications and spread of carcinoma of gallbladder

Complications include fistula formation, perforation, superimposed cholecystitis and empyema. The tumour may spread by lymphatics, vascular channels, intraperitoneal seeding, perineural spaces, intraductal growth and direct extension.[204] Lymph nodes may be involved in from 35 to 80% of patients at the time of surgery. Massive direct extension to the liver and adjacent viscera occurs early, but disseminated systemic metastases occur later. Sometimes the rapidity of a patient's death fails to correspond to the extent of the disease found at autopsy. In these cases, death is often due to bronchopneumonia. Five-year survival rates continue to be about 5%, although radical surgery has marginally improved these figures.[191] Survival is usually limited to those with papillary tumours, or those with localized disease in whom the tumour was an incidental finding by the pathologist on subsequent examination of a cholecystectomy specimen (Fig. 13.18). DNA ploidy of the tumour cells does not appear to be a prognostic indicator.[191]

Sarcoma and carcinosarcoma

Sarcomas constitute approximately 1.5% of malignant tumours of the gallbladder.[205,206] There is a marked female preponderance and a high incidence of gallstones. They are aggressive tumours with a poor prognosis, survival usually being measured in months. The tumours are sometimes quite bulky. They spread in the first instance to the liver, omentum and regional lymph nodes, but distant metastases may also occur. Before a diagnosis of sarcoma or carcinosarcoma is made, a pleomorphic spindle cell carcinoma or poorly differentiated adenocarcinoma must be excluded. At least 20 cases of carcinosarcoma and 5 of malignant mixed tumour have been reported.[11,207,208] In carcinosarcomas, the carcinomatous

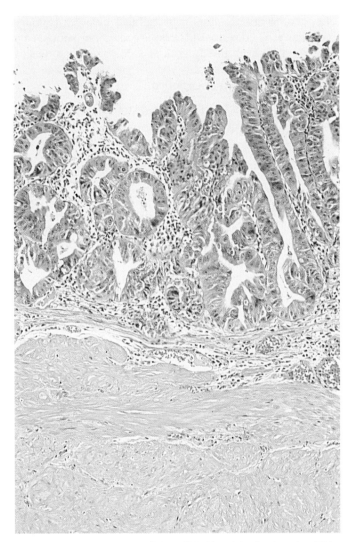

Fig. 13.18 Adenocarcinoma of the gallbladder with microinvasion. This lesion was an incidental finding by the pathologist and was not detected clinically. H & E.

component is usually adenocarcinoma with variable amounts of squamous cell carcinoma. The sarcomatous part is usually of spindle cell or chondrosarcomatous type.

The older literature contains many cases reported simply as 'polymorphous', 'round cell', 'spindle cell' or 'fusocellular' sarcoma. About 20 cases of leiomyosarcoma have been reported.[11,209] Other rare sarcomas reported include angiosarcoma,[210,211] osteogenic sarcoma, neurofibrosarcoma and fibrosarcoma. Rhabdomyosarcoma of the gallbladder is very rare, although the botryoid type is the most common neoplasm of the extrahepatic biliary ducts in childhood.[212]

Malignant melanoma

Approximately 20 cases of primary melanoma of the gallbladder have been documented.[213] Because a primary lesion may be difficult to distinguish from a secondary one, certain criteria should be fulfilled before a primary melanoma is diagnosed. Primary lesions should be solitary, arise from the mucosa as a polypoid tumour and display 'junctional' melanocytic activity at the edge and have other primary sites excluded.

Carcinoid tumour

Carcinoid tumours are rare, usually small, white to yellowish nodules. They are usually solitary, although multiple tumours have been recorded. Histologically, they resemble the carcinoid tumour found in other sites. In a small number of cases the cells show cytological atypia with frequent mitoses. Metastatic spread to lymph nodes occurs in these cases. The term 'endocrine cell carcinoma' has been suggested for such cases.[214,215] A composite tumour showing both adenocarcinoma and endocrine cell carcinoma has been reported.[214,216]

Lymphoma

Although involvement of the gallbladder in patients with known malignant lymphoma is well established, primary lymphoma of the gallbladder is very rare. One case of pseudolymphoma and two of myeloma involving the gallbladder have been reported.[11] A case of angiotropic lymphoma has recently been reported.[217]

Secondary tumours

Involvement of the gallbladder by metastatic tumour has been recorded in 0.025% of all autopsies, and in 5.8% of patients dying with carcinoma.[11] The primary tumours have most often been in the stomach, pancreas, breast, colon, kidney[218] or lung. Metastatic melanoma also occurs in the gallbladder.[219]

INVOLVEMENT OF THE GALLBLADDER IN OTHER DISEASES

Cystic fibrosis

The gallbladder is abnormally small in about one-third of patients coming to autopsy.[220] The lumen contains thick, pale mucus, or viscid green bile. There is an increased incidence of cholelithiasis.[221] The mucosa has numerous epithelial-lined cysts that often project into the lumen. They contain residual mucoid material that contains a sulphomucin.

Crohn's disease and ulcerative colitis

There is an increased incidence of cholelithiasis in patients with Crohn's disease involving the terminal ileum, and in those who have had ileal resections. This is related to a reduction in the circulating bile salt pool. Crohn's disease of the gallbladder has also been reported.[222] Patients with chronic ulcerative colitis have an increased risk of developing carcinoma of the bile ducts, but carcinoma of the gallbladder has also been reported.[223]

Metachromatic leucodystrophy

Hyperplasia of the mucosa and polypoid masses containing macrophages filled with metachromatic sulphatides may be found in this condition.[224] (see also Ch. 4).

Diabetes mellitus

There is a twofold to threefold increase in the incidence of cholesterol gallstones in patients with diabetes mellitus. Impaired gallbladder emptying and the secretion of a more lithogenic bile may both contribute to this increased incidence.[225]

Acute hepatitis

The wall of the gallbladder is temporarily thickened in patients with acute hepatitis of both viral and alcoholic aetiology.[226] This thickening can be detected by ultrasound. It probably results from submucosal oedema.

REFERENCES

1. Evett R D, Higgins J A, Brown A L. The fine structure of normal mucosa in human gallbladder. Gastroenterology 1964; 47: 49–60
2. Frierson H F. The gross anatomy and histology of the gallbladder, extrahepatic bile ducts, Vaterian system, and minor papilla. Am J Surg Pathol 1989; 13: 146–162
3. Elfving G. Crypts and ducts in the gallbladder wall. Acta Pathol Microbiol Scand [A] 1960; 49 (suppl 135): 1–45
4. Fine G, Raju U B. Paraganglia in the human gallbladder. Arch Pathol Lab Med 1980; 104: 265–268
5. Meyer W H, Carter R F, Meeker L H. The 'Phrygian Cap' deformity of gallbladder. Am J Roentgenol 1937; 37: 786–789
6. Breslaw L. Gallbladder diverticula: an interesting congenital anomaly. Am J Gastroenterol 1960; 34: 260–265
7. Sworn M J, Gay P. A fundal cyst of the gallbladder. Med J Aust 1975; 2; 307–308
8. Jacobs E, Ardichvili D, D'Avanzo E, Penneman R, Van Gansbeke D. Cyst of the gallbladder. Dig Dis Sci 1991; 36: 1769–1802
9. Oliva I O, Moran M R, Sanchez F L, Alonso A G. Multiseptate gallbladder. Int Surg 1985; 70: 83–84
10. Deutsch A A, Engelstein D, Cohen M, Kunichevsky M, Reiss R. Septum of the gallbladder. Postgrad Med J 1986; 62: 453–456
11. Weedon D. Pathology of the gallbladder. New York: Masson, 1984
12. Jackson R J, McClellan D. Agenesis of the gallbladder. A cause of false-positive ultrasonography. Am Surg 1989; 55: 36–40
13. Wilson J E, Deitrick J E. Agenesis of the gallbladder: case report and familial investigation. Surgery 1986; 99: 106–109
14. Sugrue M, Gani J, Sarre R, Watts J. Ectopia and agenesis of the gall-bladder: a report of two sets of twins and review of the literature. Aust N Z J Surg 1991; 61: 816–818

15. Udelsman R, Sugarbaker P H. Congenital duplication of the gallbladder associated with an anomalous right hepatic artery. Am J Surg 1985; 149: 812–815

16. Diaz M J, Fowler W, Hnatow B J. Congenital gallbladder duplication: preoperative diagnosis by ultrasonography. Gastrointest Radiol 1991; 16: 198–200

17. Harlaftis N, Gray S W, Skandalakis J E. Multiple gallbladders. Surg Gynecol Obstet 1977; 145: 928–934

18. Feldman L, Venta L. Percutaneous cholecystostomy of an ectopic gallbladder. Gastrointest Radiol 1988; 13: 256–258

19. Morse J M D, Lakshman S, Thomas E. Gallbladder ectopia simulating pancreatic mass on CT. Gastrointest Radiol 1985; 10: 111–113

20. Gore R M, Ghahremani G G, Joseph A E, Nemcek A A, Marn C S, Vogelzang R L. Acquired malposition of the colon and gallbladder in patients with cirrhosis: CT findings and clinical implications. Radiology 1989; 171: 739–742

21. Walia H S, Abraham T K, Bareka A. Gall-bladder interposition: a rare anomaly of the extrahepatic ducts. Int Surg 1986; 71: 117–121

22. Goor D A, Ebert P A. Anomalies of the biliary tree. Report of a repair of an accessory bile duct and review of the literature. Arch Surg 1972; 104: 302–309

23. Kihne M J, Schenken J R, Moor B J, Karrer F W. Persistent cholecystohepatic ducts. Arch Surg 1980; 115: 972–974

24. Tejada E, Danielson C. Ectopic or heterotopic liver (choristoma) associated with the gallbladder. Arch Pathol Lab Med 1989; 113: 950–952

25. Natori T, Hawkin S, Aizawa M, Asai T, Kameda Y, Ikuyohashi K. Intra-cholecystic ectopic liver. Acta Pathol Jpn 1986; 36: 1213–1216

26. Ben-Baruch D, Sandbank Y, Wolloch Y. Heterotopic pancreatic tissue in the gallbladder. Acta Chir Scand 1986; 152: 557–558

27. Qizilbash A H. Acute pancreatitis occurring in heterotopic pancreatic tissue in the gallbladder. Can J Surg 1976; 19: 413–414

28. Runge P M, Schwartz J N, Seigler H F, Woodard B H, Shelburne J D. Gallbladder with ectopic gastric mucosa. Ultrastructural analysis. Arch Pathol Lab Med 1978; 102: 209–211

29. Adam R, Fabiani B, Bismuth H. Hematobilia resulting from heterotopic stomach in the gallbladder neck. Surgery 1989; 105: 564–569

30. Evans M M, Nagorney D M, Pernicone P J, Perrault J. Heterotopic gastric mucosa in the common bile duct. Surgery 1990; 108: 96–100

31. Lamont N, Winthrop A L, Cole F M, Langer J C, Issenman R M, Finkel K C. Heterotopic gastric mucosa in the gallbladder: a cause of chronic abdominal pain in a child. J Pediatr Surg 1991; 26: 1293–1295

32. Kozuka S, Hachisuka K. Incidence by age and sex of intestinal metaplasia in the gallbladder. Hum Pathol 1984; 15: 779–784

33. Albores-Saavedra J, Nadji M, Henson D E, Ziegels-Weissman J, Mones J M. Intestinal metaplasia of the gallbladder: a morphologic and immunocytochemical study. Hum Pathol 1986; 17: 614–620

34. De Boer W G R M, Ma J, Rees J W, Nayman J. Inappropriate mucin production in gall bladder metaplasia and neoplasia — an immunohistological study. Histopathology 1981; 5: 295–303

35. Laitio M. Intestinal, gastric body- and antral-type mucosal metaplasia in the gallbladder. Beitr Pathol 1976; 159: 271–279

36. Kozuka S, Kurashina M, Tsubone M, Hachisuka K, Yasui A. Significance of intestinal metaplasia for the evolution of cancer in the biliary tract. Cancer 1984; 54: 2277–2285

37. Ito M, Sano K, Inaba H, Hotchi M. Localized necrotizing arteritis. A report of two cases involving the gallbladder and pancreas. Arch Pathol Lab Med 1991; 115: 780–783

38. Moolenaar W, Kreuning J, Eulderink F, Lamers C B H W. Ischaemic colitis and acalculous necrotizing cholecystitis as rare manifestations of cholesterol emboli in the same patient. Am J Gastroenterol 1989; 84: 1421–1422

39. West M S, Garra B S, Horii S C et al. Gallbladder varices: imaging findings in patients with portal hypertension. Radiology 1991; 179: 179–182

40. Rosen I E, Wilson S R. Varices of the gallbladder. J Can Assoc Radiol 1980; 31: 73–74

41. Stieber A C, Bauer J J. Volvulus of the gallbladder. Am J Gastroenterol 1983; 78: 96–98

42. McHenry C R, Byrne M P. Gallbladder volvulus in the elderly: an emergent surgical disease. J Am Geriatr Soc 1986; 34: 137–139

43. Ingwang R, Belsham P, Scott H, Barker S, Bearn P. Torsion of the gall-bladder: rare, unrecognized or under-reported? Aust NZ J Surg 1991; 61: 717–719

44. Whipple R D, Sabo R R. Acute torsion of the gallbladder. Am J Surg 1979; 137: 798–799

45. Wiener I, Watson L C, Wolma F J. Perforation of the gallbladder due to blunt abdominal trauma. Arch Surg 1982; 117: 805–807

46. McNabney W K, Rudek R, Pemberton L B. The significance of gallbladder trauma. J Emerg Med 1990; 8: 277–280

47. Herlin P, Ericsson M, Holmin T, Jonsson P-E. Acute acalculous cholecystitis following trauma. Br J Surg 1982; 69: 475–476

48. Sandblom P. Iatrogenic hemobilia. Am J Surg 1986; 151: 754–758

49. Sandblom P. Hemobilia. In: Schiff L, Schiff E R, eds. Diseases of the liver, 5th edn. Philadelphia: Lippincott, 1982: 1595–1602

50. Sandblom P, Mirkovitch V. Minor hemobilia. Clinical significance and pathophysiological background. Ann Surg 1979; 190: 254–264

51. Wheeler R A, Najmaldin A S, Soubra M, Griffiths D M, Burge D M, Atwell J D. Surgical presentation of Kawasaki disease (mucocutaneous lymph node syndrome). Br J Surg 1990; 77: 1273–1274

52. Neu J, Arvin A, Ariagno R L. Hydrops of the gallbladder. Am J Dis Child 1980; 134: 891–893

53. Zajko A B, Bennett M J, Campbell W L, Koneru B. Mucocele of the cystic duct remnant in eight liver transplant recipients: findings at cholangiography, CT, and US. Radiology 1990; 177: 691–693

54. Ban J G, Hirose F M, Benfield J R. Foreign bodies of the biliary tract: report of two patients and a review of the literature. Ann Surg 1972; 176: 102–107

55. Gooding G A. Food particles in the gallbladder mimic cholelithiasis in a patient with a cholecystojejunostomy. J Clin Ultrasound 1981; 9: 346–347

56. Salmenkivi K. Cholesterosis of the gall-bladder. A clinical study based on 269 cholecystectomies. Acta Chir Scand 1964; 128 (suppl 324): 1–93

57. Elfving G, Palmu A, Teir H. Cholesterolosis and mucosal hyperplasia of gallbladder. Ann Chir Gynaecol Fenn 1968; 57: 28–30

58. Nevalainen T, Laitio M. Ultrastructure of gallbladder with cholesterolosis. Virchows Arch [B] 1972; 10: 237–242

59. Christensen A H, Ishak K G. Benign tumors and pseudotumors of the gallbladder. Report of 180 cases. Arch Pathol 1970; 90: 423–432

60. Parrilla Paricio P, Garcia Olmo D, Pellicer Franco E, Prieto Gonzalez A, Carrasco Gonzalez L, Bermejo Lopez J. Gallbladder cholesterolosis: an aetiological factor in acute pancreatitis of uncertain origin. Br J Surg 1990; 77: 735–736

61. Gunn A A. Acute cholecystitis. Practitioner 1981; 225: 491–497

62. Hidalgo L A, Capella G, Pi-Figueras J et al. The influence of age on early surgical treatment of acute cholecystitis. Surg Gynecol Obstet 1989; 169: 393–396

63. Schein C J. Acute cholecystitis. New York: Harper & Row, 1972

64. Roslyn J J, DenBesten L, Thompson J E Jr, Silverman B F. Role of lithogenic bile and cystic duct occlusion in the pathogenesis of acute cholecystitis. Am J Surg 1980; 140: 126–130

65. Claesson B E B, Holmlund D E W, Matzsch T W. Microflora of the gallbladder related to duration of acute cholecystitis. Surg Gynecol Obstet 1986; 162: 531–535

66. Carveth S W, Priestley J T, Gage R P. Size and number of gallstones in acute and chronic cholecystitis. Mayo Clin Proc 1959; 34: 371–374

67. Gagic N, Frey C F, Gaines R. Acute cholecystitis. Surg Gynecol Obstet 1975; 140: 868–874

68. Edlund G, Ljungdahl M. Acute cholecystitis in the elderly. Am J Surg 1990; 159: 414–416

69. Thornton J R, Heaton K W, Espiner H J, Eltringham W K. Empyema of the gallbladder — reappraisal of a neglected disease. Gut 1983; 24: 1183–1185

70. Fry D E, Cox R A, Harbrecht P J. Empyema of the gallbladder: a complication in the natural history of acute cholecystitis. Am J Surg 1981; 141: 366–369

71. Fry D E, Cox R A, Harbrecht P J. Gangrene of the gallbladder: a complication of acute cholecystitis. South Med J 1981; 74: 666–668

72. Hallendorf L C, Dockerty M B, Waugh J M. Gangrenous cholecystitis: a clinical and pathologic study of 100 cases. Surg Clin North Am 1948; 28: 978–998

73. Matz L R, Lawrence-Brown M M D. Ischaemic cholecystitis and infarction of the gallbladder. Aust NZJ Surg 1982; 52: 466–471

74. Essenhigh D M. Perforation of the gallbladder. Br J Surg 1968; 55: 175–178

75. Niemeier O W. Acute free perforation of the gallbladder. Ann Surg 1934; 99: 922–924

76. Syme R G. Management of gallstone ileus. Can J Surg 1989; 32: 61–64

77. Atkins P. Haemoperitoneum associated with a ruptured gallbladder. Br Med J 1967; 4: 602

78. Tsai C-J, Wu C-S. Risk factors for perforation of gallbladder. A combined hospital study in a Chinese population. Scand J Gastroenterol 1991; 26: 1027–1034

79. Edlund Y, Zettergren L. Histopathology of the gallbladder in gallstone disease related to clinical data. Acta Chir Scand 1959; 116: 450–460

80. Estrada R L, Brown N M, James C E. Chronic follicular cholecystitis. Radiological, pathological and surgical aspects. Br J Surg 1960; 48: 205–209

81. Hatae Y, Kikuchi M. Lymph follicular cholecystitis. Acta Pathol Jpn 1979; 29: 67–72

82. Bergan T, Dobloug I, Liavag I. Bacterial isolates in cholecystitis and cholelithiasis. Scand Gastroenter 1979; 14: 625–631

83. Frazee R C, Nagorney D M, Mucha P Jr. Acute acalculous cholecystitis. Mayo Clin Proc 1989; 64: 163–167

84. Savoca P E, Longo W E, Zucker K A, McMillen M M, Modlin I M. The increasing prevalence of acalculous cholecystitis in outpatients. Results of a 7-year study. Ann Surg 1990; 211: 433–437

85. Aaron J S, Wynter C D, Kirton O C, Simko V. Cytomegalovirus associated with acalculous cholecystitis in a patient with acquired immune deficiency syndrome. Am J Gastroenterol 1988; 83: 879–881

86. Pitkaranta P, Haapiainen R, Taavitsainen M, Elonen E. Acalculous cholecystitis after bone marrow transplantation in adults with acute leukaemia. Case report. Eur J Surg 1991; 157: 361–364

87. Glenn F. Acute acalculous cholecystitis. Ann Surg 1979; 189: 458–465

88. Johnson L B. The importance of early diagnosis of acute acalculous cholecystitis. Surg Gynecol Obstet 1987; 164: 197–203

89. Coelho J C U, Campos A C L, Moreira M, Moss A A Jr, Villanova Artigas G. Acute acalculous cholecystitis. Int Surg 1991; 76: 146–148

90. Kaminski D L, Andrus C H, German D, Deshpande Y G. The role of prostanoids in the production of acute acalculous cholecystitis by platelet activating factor. Ann Surg 1990; 212: 455–461

91. Flancbaum L, Majerus T C, Cox E R. Acute posttraumatic acalculous cholecystitis. Am J Surg 1985; 150: 252–256

92. Mentzer R M, Golden G T, Chandler J G, Horsley J S. Emphysematous cholecystitis — an important clinical variant of acute cholecystitis. Rev Surg 1974; 31: 454–456

93. Andreu J, Perez C, Caceres J, Llauger J, Palmer J. Computed tomography as the method of choice in the diagnosis of emphysematous cholecystitis. Gastrointest Radiol 1987; 12: 315–318

94. Topp S W, Edlund G. Ultrasonic nonvisualization of the gallbladder in emphysematous cholecystitis. Acta Chir Scand 1988; 154: 153–155

95. Dabbs D J. Eosinophilic and lymphoeosinophilic cholecystitis. Am J Surg Pathol 1993; 17: 497–501

96. Parry S W, Pelias M E, Browder W. Acalculous hypersensitivity cholecystitis: hypothesis of a new clinicopathologic entity. Surgery 1988; 104: 911–916

97. Kerstein M D, Sheahan D G, Gudjonsson B, Lewis J. Eosinophilic cholecystitis. Am J Gastroenterol 1976; 66: 349–352

98. Russell C O H, Dowling J P, Marshall R D. Acute eosinophilic cholecystitis in association with hepatic echinococcosis. Gastroenterology 1979; 77: 758–760

99. Dao A H, Wong S W, Adkins R B Jr. Xanthogranulomatous cholecystitis. A clinical and pathologic study of twelve cases. Am Surg 1989; 55: 32–35

100. Franco V, Aragona F, Genova G, Florena A M, Stella M, Campesi G. Xanthogranulomatous cholecystitis. Histopathological study and classification. Pathol Res Pract 1990; 186: 383–390

101. Benbow E W. Xanthogranulomatous cholecystitis. Br J Surg 1990; 77: 255–256

102. Amazon K, Rywlin A M. Ceroid granulomas of the gallbladder. Am J Clin Pathol 1980; 73: 123–127

103. Weedon D, Moore A W E, Graff J. Melanosis of the gall bladder. Pathology 1980; 12: 265–267

104. Cornell C M, Clarke R. Vicarious calcification involving the gallbladder. Ann Surg 1959; 149: 267–272

105. Berk R N, Armbuster T G, Saltzstein S L. Carcinoma in the porcelain gallbladder. Radiology 1973; 106: 29–31

106. Shimizu M, Miura J, Tanaka T, Itoh H, Saitoh Y. Porcelain gallbladder: relation between its type by ultrasound and incidence of cancer. J Clin Gastroenterol 1989; 11: 471–476

107. Mallory T B, Lawson G M. Chronic typhoid cholecystitis. Am J Pathol 1931; 7: 71–75

108. Verbruggen P, Creve U, Hubens A, Verhaegen J. *Campylobacter fetus* as a cause of acute cholecystitis. Br J Surg 1986; 73: 46

109. Morris S J, Greenwald R A, Turner R L, Tedesco F J. Brucella-induced cholecystitis. Am J Gastroenterol 1979; 71: 481–484

110. Hermanek P. Zur Mykologie der Galle bzw. Gallenblase II. Mitteilung. Histologische Untersuchungen. Arch Klin Chir 1965; 310: 137–159

111. Morris A B, Sands M L, Shiraki M, Brown R B, Ryczak M. Gallbladder and biliary tract candidiasis: nine new cases and review. Rev Infect Dis 1990; 12: 483–489

112. Warren G H, Marsh S. Granulomatous torulopsis glabrata cholecystitis in a diabetic. Am J Clin Pathol 1982; 78: 406–410

113. Coleman D V, Field A M, Gardner S D, Porter K A, Starzl T E. Virus-induced obstruction of the ureteric and cystic duct in allograft recipients. Transplant Proc 1973; 5: 95–98

114. Agha F P, Nostrant T T, Abrams G D, Mazanec M, Van Moll L, Gumucio J J. Cytomegalovirus cholangitis in a homosexual man with acquired immune deficiency syndrome. Am J Gastroenterol 1986; 81: 1068–1072

115. Iannuzzi C, Belghiti J, Erlinger S, Menu Y, Fekete F. Cholangitis associated with cholecystitis in patients with acquired immunodeficiency syndrome. Arch Surg 1990; 125: 1211–1213

116. Cappell M S. Hepatobiliary manifestations of the acquired immune deficiency syndrome. Am J Gastroenterol 1991; 86: 1–15

117. Guarda L A, Stein S A, Cleary K A, Ordonez N G. Human cryptosporidiosis in the acquired immune deficiency syndrome. Arch Pathol Lab Med 1983; 107: 562–566

118. Kahn D G, Garfinkle J M, Klonoff D C, Pembrook L J, Morrow D J. Cryptosporidial and cytomegaloviral hepatitis and cholecystitis. Arch Pathol Lab Med 1987; 111: 879–881

119. Fataar S, Bassiony H, Satyanath S, Rudwan A, Al Ansari A G. Radiologically visible gallbladder calcification due to schistoomiasis. Brs J Radiol 1990; 63: 706–709

120. Chainuvati T, Paosawadhi A, Sripranoth M, Manasatith S, Viranuvatti V. Carcinoma of the cystic duct associated with opisthorchiasis. Southeast Asian J Trop Med Public Health 1976; 7: 482–486

121. Yellin A E, Donovan A J. Biliary lithiasis and helminthiasis. Am J Surg 1981; 142: 128–134
122. Bailey P V, Connors R H, Tracy T F Jr, Sotelo-Avila C, Lewis J E, Weber T R. Changing spectrum of cholelithiasis and cholecystitis in infants and children. Am J Surg 1989; 158: 585–588
123. Diehl A K. Epidemiology and natural history of gallstone disease. Gastroenterol Clin North Am 1991; 20: 1–19
124. Trotman B W. Pigment gallstone disease. Gastroenterol Clin North Am 1991; 20: 111–126
125. Conte D, Barisani D, Mandelli C et al. Cholelithiasis in cirrhosis: analysis of 500 cases. Am J Gastroenterol 1991; 86: 1629–1632
126. King D R, Ginn-Pease M E, Lloyd T V, Hoffman J, Hohenbrink K. Parenteral nutrition with associated cholelithiasis: another iatrogenic disease of infants and children. J Pediatr Surg 1987; 22: 593–596
127. Gracie W A, Ransohoff D F. The innocent gallstone is not a myth. N Engl J Med 1982; 307: 798–800
128. Brakel K, Lameris J S, Nijs H G T, Terpstra O T, Steen G, Blijenberg B C. Predicting gallstone composition with CT: in vivo and in vitro analysis. Radiology 1990; 174: 337–341
129. Schenken J R, Coleman F C. Cholelithiasis. Report of a case with 36,329 stones in the gallbladder. Gastroenterology 1945; 4: 344–346
130. Soloway R D, Trotman B W, Ostrow J D. Pigment gallstones. Gastroenterology 1977; 72: 167–182
131. Donovan J M, Carey M C. Physical-chemical basis of gallstone formation. Gastroenterol Clin North Am 1991; 20: 47–66
132. Akiyoshi T, Nakayama F. Bile acid composition in brown pigment stones. Dig Dis Sci 1990; 35: 27–32
133. Hofmann A F. Pathogenesis of cholesterol gallstones. J Clin Gastroenterol 1988; 10 (suppl 2): S1–S11
134. Cooper A D. Metabolic basis of cholesterol gallstone disease. Gastroenterol Clin North Am 1991; 20: 21–47
135. Strichartz S D, Abedin M Z, Abdou S, Roslyn J J. Increased biliary calcium in cholesterol gallstone formation. Am J Surg 1988; 155: 131–136
136. Swobodnik W, Wenk H, Janowitz P et al. Total biliary protein, mucus glycoproteins, cyclic-AMP, and apolipoproteins in the gallbladder bile of patients with cholesterol stones and stone-free controls. Scand J Gastroenterol 1991; 26: 771–778
137. Everson G T. Gallbladder function in gallstone disease. Gastroenterol Clin North Am 1991; 20: 85–110
138. Ostrow J D. The etiology of pigment gallstones. Hepatology 1984; 4: 215s–222s
139. Stewart L, Smith A L, Pellegrini C A, Motson R W, Way L W. Pigment gallstones form as a composite of bacterial microcolonies and pigment solids. Ann Surg 1987; 206: 242–250
140. Sahlin S, Ahlberg J, Einarsson K, Henriksson R, Danielsson A. Quantitative ultrastructural studies of gallbladder epithelium in gallstone free subjects and patients with gallstones. Gut 1990; 31: 100–105
141. Vakil N, Everbach E C. Gas in gallstones: quantitative determinations and possible effects on fragmentation by shock waves. Gastroenterology 1991; 101: 1628–1634
142. Ayyash K, Jadallah F. Choledochoduodenal fistula: a rare complication of duodenal ulcer. Acta Chir Scand 1989; 155: 423–425
143. ReMine W H. Biliary-enteric fistulas: natural history and management. Adv Surg 1973; 7: 69–94
144. Pangan J C, Estrada R, Rosales R, Cholecystoduodenocolic fistula with recurrent gallstone ileus. Arch Surg 1984; 119: 1201–1203
145. Csendes A, Carlos Diaz J, Burdiles P, Maluenda F, Nava O. Mirizzi syndrome and cholecystobiliary fistula: a unifying classification. Br J Surg 1989; 76: 1139–1143
146. Birch B R P, Cox S J. Spontaneous external biliary fistula uncomplicated by gallstones. Postgrad Med J 1991; 67: 391–392
147. Glenn F, Reed C, Grafe W R. Biliary enteric fistula. Surg Gynecol Obstet 1981; 153: 527–531
148. Safaie-Shirazi S, Zike W L, Printen K J. Spontaneous enterobiliary fistulas. Surg Gynecol Obstet 1973; 137: 769–772
149. Hicken N F, Coray Q B. Spontaneous gastrointestinal biliary fistulas. Surg Gynecol Obstet 1946; 82: 723–730
150. Raiford T S. Intestinal obstruction due to gallstones (gallstone ileus). Ann Surg 1961; 153: 830–838
151. Clavien P-A, Richon J, Burgan S, Rohner A. Gallstone ileus. Br J Surg 1990; 77: 737–742
152. Ah-Chong K, Leong Y P. Gastric outlet obstruction due to gall stones (Bouveret syndrome). Postgrad Med J 1987; 63: 909–910
153. Buetow G W, Glaubitz J P, Crampton R S. Recurrent gallstone ileus. Surgery 1963; 54: 716–724
154. Meyerowitz B R. Lime water bile. J R Coll Surg Edin 1960; 5: 308–312
155. Gya D, Sali A, Vitetta L, Eu P, Arkles B. Limy bile cholecystitis: an in vitro study and a case report. Aust N Z J Surg 1990; 60: 998–1000
156. Naryshkin S, Trotman B W, Raffensperger E C. Milk of calcium bile. Evidence that gallbladder stasis is a key factor. Dig Dis Sci 1987; 32: 1051–1055
157. Ram M D, Midha D. Adenomyomatosis of the gallbladder. Surgery 1975; 78: 224–229
158. Jutras J A, Longtin J M, Levesque H P. Hyperplastic cholecystoses. Am J Roentgenol 1960; 83: 795–827
159. Berk R N, van der Vegt J H, Lichtenstein J E. The hyperplastic cholecystoses: cholesterolosis and adenomyomatosis. Radiology 1983; 146: 593–601
160. Le Quesne L R, Ranger I. Cholecystitis glandularis proliferans. Br J Surg 1957; 44: 447–458
161. Williams I, Slavin G, Cox A, Simpson P, de Lacey G. Diverticular disease (adenomyomatosis) of the gallbladder: a radiological-pathological survey. Br J Radiol 1986; 59: 29–34
162. Jutras J A, Levesque H P. Adenomyoma and adenomyomatosis of the gallbladder. Radiologic and pathologic correlations. Radiol Clin North Am 1966; 4: 483–500
163. Meguid M M, Aun F, Bradford M L. Adenomyomatosis of the gallbladder. Am J Surg 1984; 147: 260–262
164. Kang J Y, Williamson R C N. Does adenomyosis of the gall-bladder cause symptoms? J Gastroenterol Hepatol 1990; 5: 204–205
165. Halpert R D, Bedi D G, Tirman P J, Gore D C. Segmental adenomyomatosis of the gallbladder. A radiologic, sonograhic, and pathologic correlation. Am J Surg 1989; 56: 570–572
166. Aguirre J R, Bohier R O, Guraieb S. Hyperplastic cholecystoses; a new contribution to the unitarian theory. Am J Roentgenol 1969; 107: 1–13
167. Young T E. So-called adenomyoma of the gallbladder. Am J Clin Pathol 1959; 31: 423–427
168. Paraf F, Potet F. Gallbladder carcinoma arising in adenomyomatosis. Am J Gastroenterol 1988; 83: 1439
169. Beilby J O W. Diverticulosis of the gallbladder. The fundal adenoma. Br J Exp Pathol 1967; 48: 455–461
170. Elfving G, Lehtonen T, Teir H. Clinical significance of primary hyperplasia of gallbladder mucosa. Ann Surg 1967; 165: 61–69
171. Yamamoto M, Nakajo S, Ito M, Tahara E. Primary mucosal hyperplasia of the gallbladder. Acta Pathol Jpn 1988; 38: 393–398
172. Albores-Saavedra J, Defortuna S M, Smothermon W E. Primary papillary hyperplasia of the gallbladder and cystic and common bile ducts. Hum Pathol 1990; 21: 228–231
173. Albores-Saavedra J, Alcantara-Vasquez A, Cruz-Ortiz H, Herrera-Goepfert R. The precursor lesions of invasive gallbladder carcinoma. Hyperplasia, atypical hyperplasia and carcinoma-in-situ. Cancer 1980; 45: 919–927
174. Yamamoto M, Nakajo S, Tahara E. Dysplasia of the gallbladder. Its histogenesis and correlation to gallbladder adenocarcinoma. Pathol Res Pract 1989; 185: 454–460
175. Bivins B A, Meeker W R, Weiss D L, Griffen W O. Carcinoma-in-situ of the gallbladder. A dilemma. South Med J 1975; 68: 297–300
176. Albores-Saavedra J, Angeles-Angeles A, de Jesus Manrique J, Henson D E. Carcinoma in situ of the gallbladder. A clinicopathologic study of 18 cases. Am J Surg Pathol 1984; 8: 323–333
177. Nakajo S, Yamamoto M, Tahara E. Morphometric analysis of

gallbladder adenocarcinoma: discrimination between carcinoma and dysplasia. Virchows Arch [A] 1989; 416: 133–140

178. Christensen A H, Ishak K G. Benign tumours and pseudotumours of the gallbladder. Report of 180 cases. Arch Pathol 1970; 90: 423–432

179. Albores-Saavedra J, Henson D E, Sobin L H. Histological typing of tumours of the gallbladder and extrahepatic bile ducts. WHO international histological classification of tumours, 2nd edn. Berlin: Springer-Verlag, 1991

180. Yamamoto M, Nakajo S, Tahara E. Histological classification of epithelial polypoid lesions of the gallbladder. Acta Pathol Jpn 1988; 38: 181–192

181. Aldridge M C, Bismuth H. Gallbladder cancer: the polyp-cancer sequence. Br J Surg 1990; 77: 363–364

182. Kozuka S, Tsubone M, Yasui A, Hachisuka K. Relation of adenoma to carcinoma in the gallbladder. Cancer 1982; 50: 2226–2234

183. Neumann R A, Li Volsi V A, Rosenthal N S, Burrell M, Ball T J. Adenocarcinoma in biliary papillomatosis. Gastroenterology 1976; 70: 779–782

184. Morizumi H, Sano T, Hirose T, Hizawa K. Neurofibroma of the gallbladder seen as a papillary polyp. Acta Pathol Jpn 1988; 38: 259–268

185. Jones W P, Keller F S, Odrezin G T, Kelly D R. Venous hemangioma of the gallbladder. Gastrointest Radiol 1987; 12: 319–321

186. Sano T, Hirose T, Kagawa N, Hizawa K, Saito K. Polypoid traumatic neuroma of the gallbladder. Arch Pathol Lab Med 1985; 109: 574–576

187. Wolff M. Paraganglioma of the gallbladder. Arch Surg 1973; 107: 493

188. Yamaguchi K, Kuroki S, Daimaru Y, Hashimoto H, Enjoji M. Granular cell tumor of the gallbladder. Report of a case. Acta Pathol Jpn 1985; 35: 687–691

189. Jones R S. Carcinoma of the gallbladder. Surg Clin North Am 1990; 70: 1419–1428

190. Ohlsson E G, Aronsen K F. Carcinoma of the gallbladder. A study of 181 cases. Acta Chir Scand 1974; 140: 475–480

191. Donohue J H, Nagorney D M, Grant C S, Tsushima K, Ilstrup D M, Adson M A. Carcinoma of the gallbladder. Does radical resection improve outcome? Arch Surg 1990; 125: 237–241

192. Silk Y N, Douglass H O Jr, Nava H R, Driscoll D L, Trartarian G. Carcinoma of the gallbladder. The Roswell Park experience. Ann Surg 1989; 210: 751–757

193. Nishino H, Satake K, Kim E-C et al. Primary carcinoma of the gallbladder. Am Surg 1988; 54: 487–491

194. Kinoshita H, Nagata E, Hirohashi K, Satai K, Kobayashi Y. Carcinoma of the gallbladder with an anomalous connection between the choledochus and the pancreatic duct. Report of 10 cases and review of the literature in Japan. Cancer 1984; 54: 762–769

195. Arnaud J-P, Graf P, Gramfort J-L, Adloff M. Primary carcinoma of the gallbladder. Review of 25 cases. Am J Surg 1979; 138: 403–406

196. Hisatomi K, Haratake J, Horie A, Ohsato K. Relation of histopathological features to prognosis of gallbladder cancer. Am J Gastroenterol 1990; 85: 567–572

197. Brandt-Rauf P W, Branwood A W. An unusual case of gallbladder cancer in an automotive worker. Cancer J for Clinicians 1980; 30: 333–336

198. Albores-Saavedra J, Nadji M, Henson D E. Intestinal-type adenocarcinoma of the gallbladder. A clinicopathologic and immunocytochemical study of seven cases. Am J Surg Pathol 1986; 10: 19–25

199. Albores-Saavedra J, Cruz-Ortiz H, Alcantara-Vazques A, Henson D E. Unusual types of gallbladder carcinoma. A report of 16 cases. Arch Pathol Lab Med 1981; 105: 287–293

200. Abu-Farsakh H, Fraire A E. Adenocarcinoma and (extragonadal) choriocarcinoma of the gallbladder in a young woman. Hum Pathol 1991; 22: 614–615

201. Karasawa T, Itoh K, Komukai M, Ozawa U, Sakurai I, Shikata T. Squamous cell carcinoma of gallbladder. Report

of two cases and review of literature. Acta Pathol Jpn 1981; 31: 299–308

202. Guo K-J, Yamaguchi K, Enjoji M. Undifferentiated carcinoma of the gallbladder. A clinicopathologic, histochemical, and immunohistochemical study of 21 patients with a poor prognosis. Cancer 1988; 61: 1872–1879

203. Cavazzana A O, Fassina A S, Tollot M, Ninfo V. Small cell carcinoma of gallbladder. An immunocytochemical and ultrastructural study. Pathol Res Pract 1991; 187: 472–476

204. Fahim R B, McDonald J R, Richards J C, Ferris D O. Carcinoma of the gallbladder. A study of its modes of spread. Ann Surg 1962; 156: 114–124

205. Yasuma T, Yanaka M. Primary sarcoma of the gallbladder — report of three cases. Acta Pathol Jpn 1971; 21: 285–304

206. Vaittinen E. Sarcoma of the gall-bladder. Ann Chir Gynaecol Fenn 1972; 61: 185–189

207. Born M W, Ramey W G, Ryan S F, Gordon P E. Carcinosarcoma and carcinoma of the gallbladder. Cancer 1984; 53: 2171–2177

208. Ishihara T, Kawano H, Takahashi M et al. Carcinosarcoma of the gallbladder. A case report with immunohistochemical and ultrastructural studies. Cancer 1990; 66: 992–997

209. Newmark H III, Kliewer K, Curtis A, DenBesten L, Enenstein W. Primary leiomyosarcoma of gallbladder seen on computed tomography and ultrasound. Am J Gastroenterol 1986; 81: 202–204

210. Kumar A, Lal B K, Singh M K, Kapur B M L. Angiosarcoma of the gallbladder. Am J Gastroenterol 1989; 84: 1431–1433

211. White J, Chan Y-F. Epithelioid angiosarcoma of the gallbladder. Histopathology 1994; 24: 269–271

212. Mihara S, Matsumoto H, Tokunaga F, Yano H, Ota M, Yamashita S. Botryoid rhabdomyosarcoma of the gallbladder in a child. Cancer 1982; 49: 812–818

213. Zhang Z, Myles J, Pai R P, Howard J M. Malignant melanoma of the biliary tract: a case report. Surgery 1991; 109: 323–328

214. Yamamoto M, Nakajo S, Miyoshi N, Nakai S, Tahara E. Endocrine cell carcinoma (carcinoid) of the gallbladder. Am J Surg Pathol 1989; 13: 292–302

215. McLean C A, Pedersen J S. Endocrine cell carcinoma of the gallbladder. Histopathology 1991; 19: 173–176

216. Wada A, Ishiguro S, Tateishi R, Ishikawa O, Matsui Y. Carcinoid tumor of the gallbladder associated with adenocarcinoma. Cancer 1983; 51: 1911–1917

217. Laurino L, Melato M. Malignant angioendotheliomatosis (angiotropic lymphoma) of the gallbladder. Virchows Arch (A) 1990; 417: 243–246

218. Satoh H, Iyama A, Hidaka K, Nakashiro H, Harada S, Hisatsugu T. Metastatic carcinoma of the gallbladder from renal carcinoma presenting as intraluminal polypoid mass. Dig Dis Sci 1991; 36: 520–523

219. Goldin E G. Malignant melanoma metastatic to the gallbladder. Case report and review of the literature. Am Surg 1990; 56: 369–373

220. Esterly J R, Oppenheimer E H. Observations in cystic fibrosis of the pancreas. I. The gallbladder. Bull Johns Hopkins Hosp 1962; 110: 247–254

221. Angelico M, Gandin C, Canuzzi P et al. Gallstones in cystic fibrosis: a critical reappraisal. Hepatology 1991; 14: 768–775

222. McClure J, Banerjee S S, Schofield P S. Crohn's disease of the gallbladder. J Clin Pathol 1984; 37: 516–518

223. Joffe N, Antonioli D A. Primary carcinoma of the gallbladder associated with chronic inflammatory bowel disease. Clin Radiol 1981; 32: 319–324

224. Burgess J H, Kalfayan B, Slungaard R K, Gilbert E. Papillomatosis of the gallbladder associated with metachromatic leukodystrophy. Arch Pathol Lab Med 1985; 109: 79–81

225. Stone B G, Gavaler J S, Belle S H et al. Impairment of gallbladder emptying in diabetes mellitus. Gastroenterology 1988; 95: 170–176

226. Sharma M P, Dasarathy S. Gallbladder abnormalities in acute viral hepatitis: a prospective ultrasound evaluation. J Clin Gastroenterol 1991; 13: 697–700

14

Vascular disorders

I. R. Wanless

Non-cirrhotic portal hypertension: nomenclature and pathophysiology

Portal veins
  Normal variations and congenital anomalies
  Acquired disease of large portal veins (portal vein thrombosis)
  Acquired disease of small portal veins
  Pathology of portal vein disease

Hepatic veins
  Normal variations and congenital anomalies
  Hepatic vein thrombosis
  Veno-occlusive disease
  Other venous lesions

Sinusoids
  Normal sinusoidal structure
  Sinusoidal capillarization and pericellular fibrosis
  Sinusoidal dilatation
  Peliosis hepatis
  Toxic microvascular injury
  Other sinusoidal lesions

Arteries
  Normal variations and congenital anomalies
  Diseases of the hepatic arteries
  Hepatic ischaemia

Nodular hyperplasia
  Diffuse nodular hyperplasia (nodular regenerative hyperplasia)
  Diffuse nodular hyperplasia in cirrhosis
  Lobar or segmental atrophy and hyperplasia
  Focal nodular hyperplasia

Vascular disease in cirrhosis

Vascular lesions in the liver are most commonly encountered as an integral component of cirrhosis. This chapter deals mainly with hepatic vascular disease in the absence of cirrhosis. Although lesions of portal veins, hepatic veins, sinusoids, and arteries are described separately, they often occur together. Obstruction to the flow of blood at one level often leads to secondary lesions up- and downstream from the initial lesion. Toxins affecting the endothelium of hepatic venules may also involve portal venules and sinusoids.

This chapter reviews anatomical lesions and pathophysiology; the normal physiology and pharmacology of the hepatic circulation have been reviewed elsewhere.[1–4] Historical and embryological aspects can be found in several sources.[2,5–7]

NON-CIRRHOTIC PORTAL HYPERTENSION: NOMENCLATURE AND PATHOPHYSIOLOGY

Portal hypertension arises because of obstruction to hepatic blood flow. The lesion most commonly associated with vascular obstruction is cirrhosis, a lesion that arises when parenchymal fibrosis follows hepatocellular necrosis. Primary injury to hepatic veins may lead to portal hypertension, but the accompanying parenchymal congestion causes hepatocellular necrosis so that cirrhosis develops. Primary injury to portal veins also causes portal hypertension, but portal vein obstruction causes only mild parenchymal atrophy without necrosis, so that cirrhosis does not occur.

Patients with portal hypertension are broadly divided into those with either pre-sinusoidal or post-sinusoidal obstruction on the basis of pressure measurements or clinical findings. The validity of the assumptions underlying this nomenclature has been questioned.[8] However, it is usually true that, in the absence of cirrhosis, varices and splenomegaly are features of portal vein disease while ascites and hepatomegaly are features of hepatic vein disease.

Patients with *pre-sinusoidal non-cirrhotic portal hypertension*

535

have usually been classified according to clinical or radiological features rather than by anatomical lesions or pathogenetic mechanisms. The classification used is largely dependent on the method of investigation. Splanchnic arteriograms viewed in the venous phase allow rather crude identification of the portal vein up to the second- or third-order branches. This technique allows division of cases into extrahepatic block and intrahepatic block. The term *cavernous transformation*, often considered as synonymous with extrahepatic block, refers to the presence of abundant collateral veins in the region of the original portal vein or to multiple tortuous channels within that vein.[9]

Idiopathic portal hypertension is defined as non-cirrhotic portal hypertension in the absence of known cause of liver disease and with a patent extrahepatic portal vein.[10,11] This may be synonymous with intrahepatic portal vein block, although the lesions have not always been well documented. 'Hepatoportal sclerosis' is a term suggested by Mikkelsen et al[12] to describe fibrous intimal thickening of the portal vein or its branches in patients with non-cirrhotic portal hypertension. 'Non-cirrhotic portal fibrosis' is the term chosen by a panel of Indian experts for the lesions in such patients.[13] Although these three terms are nearly synonymous, there have been differences in their application. Some cases with non-cirrhotic portal hypertension have been defined by the presence of hepatocellular nodules and called 'nodular regenerative hyperplasia' or 'partial nodular transformation'.

The hepatic pathology in patients with non-cirrhotic portal hypertension has not been fully documented. This is because clinical manifestations occur long after vascular lesions have lost their specific histological features, and liver biopsies are often inadequate to establish with confidence the presence of vascular lesions. Lesions in large vessels can be documented adequately only at autopsy.

The difficulty in appreciating portal vein lesions has caused some to wonder if sinusoidal lesions may be sufficient to cause portal hypertension.[14,15] This idea is supported by the occasional finding of portal hypertension in patients with sinusoidal compression or cellular infiltration as in steatosis,[16] acute hepatitis,[17] leukaemia,[18] mastocytosis,[19] Gaucher's disease,[18] and agnogenic myeloid metaplasia.[20] However, portal hypertension in agnogenic myeloid metaplasia and in polycythaemia rubra vera correlates with portal vein lesions and not with sinusoidal infiltration.[21] Furthermore, the rarity of clinical portal hypertension in amyloidosis despite massive sinusoidal deposition[22] makes it unlikely that mild or moderate disease confined to the sinusoids produces clinical portal hypertension. It is possible that undocumented portal venous lesions are responsible for the portal hypertension occasionally found in these various conditions.

It has also been suggested that splenomegaly[23] and vascular malformations[24] may produce sufficiently high portal flow for clinically significant portal hypertension to develop in the absence of hepatic vascular obstruction. The poor correlation of spleen size and portal flow with portal pressure and the variable response to splenectomy are against splenomegaly as a sufficient causative factor.[21,25] This subject has been reviewed in detail.[26]

PORTAL VEINS

Portal vein disease is conveniently divided into hypoplasia, thrombosis, and local portal tract disease. A pathogenetic classification of portal vein disease is presented in Table 14.1. Large vessel disease is most commonly a result of thrombosis while small vessel disease may be caused either by propagation of thrombus or local portal tract inflammation. In idiopathic portal hypertension small vessel lesions are dominant but large vein lesions are usually found when sought.[12,13,27] In my opinion, most cases of idiopathic portal hypertension have been a result of primary large portal vein thrombosis. This possibility has often been discounted because of the failure to recognize that large thrombi usually recanalize (see below), leaving a patent portal vein trunk and permanent obliteration of the distal small branches.

Table 14.1 Pathogenetic classification of portal vein disease

Pathogenesis	Comments and examples
1. *Primary agenesis or hypoplasia*	This is seen in childhood 'cavernous transformation' and in patent ductus venosus. Hypoplasia of small portal veins is present in congenital hepatic fibrosis.
2. *Thrombosis* a. thrombosis of large portal veins	This includes some cases of 'cavernous transformation' and extrahepatic portal vein block. It may be secondary to inflammation, hypercoagulable states, or stasis.
b. thrombosis of small portal veins (i) propagation from large portal vein thrombosis	This explains residual small portal vein obliteration after large portal vein thrombosis. The large portal veins are often recanalized. This includes many cases of idiopathic portal hypertension.
(ii) primary emboli or thrombi	This is theoretically possible but hard to differentiate from 2b(i).
3. *Local portal tract disease*	This includes some cases of idiopathic portal hypertension.
a. primary portal phlebitis	Granulomatous vasculitis, schistosomiasis, vinyl chloride, and other toxins
b. primary arteritis	Polyarteritis nodosa, rheumatoid arteritis, systemic lupus erythematosus
c. primary duct disease	Primary biliary cirrhosis, primary sclerosing cholangitis, bacterial cholangitis
d. primary portal tract disease, site uncertain or variable	Sarcoidosis, lymphoma

NORMAL VARIATIONS AND CONGENITAL ANOMALIES

The portal vein diameter is 0.6–1.2 cm in normal adults[28] and up to 1.9 cm in patients with portal hypertension.[29]

Hypoplasia or atresia of the portal vein may be developmental or secondary to neonatal disease.[30] Portal vein atresia has been found in two cases with the multiple focal nodular hyperplasia syndrome.[31,32] Congenital absence of the portal vein has been reported in patients with oculoauriculo-vertebral dysplasia (Goldenhar syndrome)[33] and with biliary atresia.[34] Odièvre et al[35] found that non-hepatic malformations, often of a vascular nature, occurred in many children with non-cirrhotic portal hypertension. A mass of *ectopic liver* tissue may obstruct the portal vein.[36] Portal vein *aneurysm* is a rare congenital anomaly or response to portal hypertension, usually occurring in the extrahepatic vein.[37] Many rare anomalies of the portal vein can be explained by abnormal persistence of portions of the vitelline veins.[38] The most common of these anomalies, *preduodenal portal vein*, often with anomalous origin of the hepatic artery, has been associated with biliary atresia.[39,40] *Anomalous pulmonary venous drainage* into a portal or hepatic vein has been reported,[41,42] usually in association with cardiac and other anomalies.

Intrahepatic shunts connecting large portal veins to hepatic veins or vena cava may occur as congenital anomalies[43] or secondary to portal hypertension, post-traumatic fistula, or rupture of a portal vein aneurysm.[44–46] Many reported cases had a single large channel between the right portal vein and vena cava.[47] Others had multiple peripheral intrahepatic shunts.[48] The largest intrahepatic shunt, the *ductus venosus*, almost always closes within days of birth. When the ductus remains patent there may be hypoplasia of the portal venous tree, nodular hyperplasia of the parenchyma, and portosystemic encephalopathy[49,50] (Fig. 14.1).

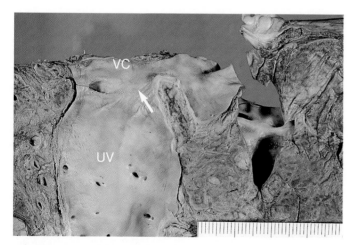

Fig. 14.1 Patent ductus venosus (arrow) connecting the umbilical portion of the left portal vein (UV) with the inferior vena cava (VC). From Wanless et al.[50]

The two adult patients I have seen with patent ductus venosus also had atrial septal defect.

Patent umbilical vein, associated with dilated peri-umbilical veins, abdominal bruit, hypoplasia of intrahepatic portal veins, and atrophy of the liver with little or no hepatic fibrosis, has been called Cruveilhier–Baumgarten disease.[51] When the dilated veins are secondary to portal hypertension, the condition has been defined as Cruveilhier–Baumgarten syndrome.[51] In retrospect, it is likely that the reported patients with Cruveilhier–Baumgarten disease also had portal hypertension, either from portal vein thrombosis or congenital hypoplasia of the intrahepatic portal veins,[52] so that the distinction between the disease and the syndrome is of little value. Recent evidence indicates that the prominent peri-umbilical circulation in Cruveilhier–Baumgarten syndrome is usually fed by dilated para-umbilical veins rather than a patent umbilical vein.[51,53]

ACQUIRED DISEASE OF LARGE PORTAL VEINS (PORTAL VEIN THROMBOSIS)

Thrombosis of the portal vein is usually associated with the presence of a hypercoagulable state, vascular injury, or stasis (Table 14.2). Associated hypercoagulable states have included pregnancy, use of oral contraceptives, protein C deficiency, and myeloproliferative disorders. Some putative 'myeloproliferative disorders' could only be diagnosed with special techniques such as measurement of red cell mass or detection of spontaneous erythroid colony formation or other abnormalities on bone marrow culture.[54,55]

Table 14.2 Causes of portal vein thrombosis

	References
Hypercoagulable states	
Polycythaemia rubra vera	21, 54, 304
Agnogneic myeloid metaplasia	21, 54
Idiopathic thrombocytosis	10, 20, 54
Paroxysmal nocturnal haemoglobinuria	54, 305
Chronic myeloid leukaemia	306
Subclinical myeloproliferative disease	54
Undefined (e.g. history of thrombotic disease)	305
Oral contraceptive therapy	307
Pregnancy	30
Protein C deficiency	308
Antithrombin III deficiency	309
Stasis or mass lesion	
Cirrhosis	56, 58, 63, 310
Hepatocellular carcinoma	56, 305
Carcinoma of pancreas	311, 312
Splenectomy	313
Vascular injury	
Umbilical sepsis	306
Pylephlebitis	8, 304, 314, 315
Trauma	316, 317
Catheterization	318
Oesophageal sclerotherapy	319, 320
Schistosomiasis	85
Inflammatory bowel disease	321–323

Inflammation of the portal vein (pylephlebitis) can be induced by:

1. infection, especially appendicitis, diverticulitis, or omphalitis;
2. chemical injury initiated by pancreatitis, bile leak from transcutaneous biliary drainage, oesophageal sclerotherapy, or infusion of hyperosmolar glucose into the umbilical vein; and
3. surgical or accidental trauma.

Stasis is a cause of portal vein thrombosis in cirrhosis, primary or secondary neoplasms, and retroperitoneal fibrosis. There is evidence of portal vein thrombosis in 0.6–40% of patients with cirrhosis.[27,56–58] Portal vein obstruction with tumour and/or thrombus occurs in 23–70% of patients with hepatocellular carcinoma[27,56,59–61] and in 5–8% of patients with metastatic tumour in the liver.[56,62] Thrombosis in the presence of cirrhosis or hepatic neoplasm may precipitate hepatic decompensation, variceal bleeding, or ascites.[63]

The relative importance of these causal factors varies geographically. In Western countries and Japan, cirrhosis is the cause of portal vein thrombosis in 20–60% of cases[57,58] and myeloproliferative disorders account for up to half of cases.[54] The high prevalence of non-cirrhotic portal hypertension and extrahepatic portal vein block in India may be related to the high incidence of omphalitis and of dehydration in some regions of that country.[64]

Recanalization after thrombosis of large portal veins has been documented by ultrasound and by histological examination.[57,65,66] Thrombosis in large portal veins usually propagates to small veins which are less likely to recanalize. The transient nature of thrombotic occlusion in large vessels may explain why it has been so difficult to establish the importance of portal vein thrombosis in the genesis of non-cirrhotic portal hypertension when block is confined to the small intrahepatic branches, as seen in idiopathic portal hypertension. In the neonate, umbilical vein infection may induce fibrosis so that the portal vein fails to enlarge as the body grows. This may explain why extrahepatic portal vein block is more common in children than in adults.

ACQUIRED DISEASE OF SMALL PORTAL VEINS

Patients with portal hypertension because of obliteration of small portal veins may also have evidence of systemic microvascular disease as seen in rheumatoid arteritis,[67,68] myeloproliferative diseases,[21] systemic lupus erythematosus,[69] polyarteritis nodosa,[70] systemic sclerosis,[71] and monoclonal gammopathies,[72] or exposure to vasculo-toxic chemicals, such as azathioprine, vinyl chloride, 'toxic oil', or arsenic[73] (Table 14.4).* Obliteration of small portal veins may also occur early in the course of primary biliary cirrhosis,[74]

---

* It is curious that Banti believed that arsenic was the only effective treatment for patients affected by his disease.

primary sclerosing cholangitis, and sarcoidosis,[75,76] causing portal hypertension before the development of cirrhosis.

The genesis of portal hypertension in these various conditions can be explained by the concept of *menage à foie*.[77] This is the development of injury to one portal structure because of inflammation primarily directed at a neighbouring portal tract structure. Thus, local portal venous obliteration may be secondary to arteritis (Fig. 14.2) or to ductal inflammation, as in primary sclerosing cholangitis and primary biliary cirrhosis. The obliteration is usually confined to small portal veins because they are closely approximated to the inflamed small arteries or ducts (Fig. 14.3). However, even first- and second-order portal vein branches may be obliterated by portal inflammation.[78]

Portal vein obliteration may be caused by interstitial disease in sarcoidosis (Fig. 14.4), mineral oil granulomas,[79] and following exposure to Thorotrast. Emboli or local

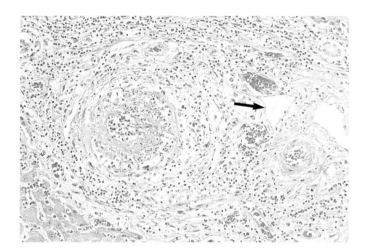

Fig. 14.2 Acute polyarteritis nodosa (left) with marked inflammation of the adjacent portal vein wall (arrow). H & E.

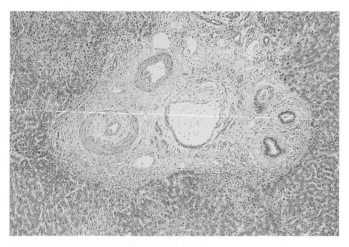

Fig. 14.3 Healed arteritis and adjacent organized portal vein thrombosis. Haematoxylin–phloxine–saffron.

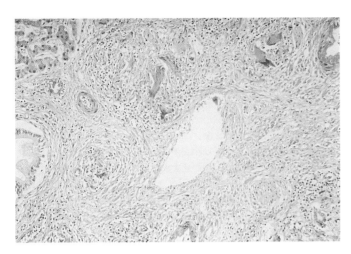

Fig. 14.4 Sarcoidosis with involvement of the portal vein. Haematoxylin–phloxine–saffron.

thromboses are important in schistosomiasis and possibly in normal ageing and in congestive heart failure.[80] Idiopathic granulomatous vasculitis involving portal or hepatic venules is rare.[74]

Ducts may also be injured by inflammation primarily involving the arteries and other portal tract structures. This could explain the elevated alkaline phosphatase commonly present in patients with temporal or rheumatoid arteritis,[67,81] nodular regenerative hyperplasia,[80] idiopathic portal hypertension,[82] and sarcoidosis.[83]

Schistosomiasis

Schistosomiasis deserves special mention as the most common cause of portal hypertension in the world (see Ch. 7). In some endemic regions there is evidence of hepatic schistosomiasis in up to 18% of the population.[84] Eggs deposited in rectal veins float into the small portal veins where a transient eosinophilic infiltrate is followed by a granulomatous reaction. The veins are obliterated with fibrous tissue and a PAS-positive egg cuticle is seen in one third of surgical wedge biopsies.[85] Clusters of small eggs are seen with *S. japonicum*, and larger single eggs with a lateral spine are seen with *S. mansoni* (Fig. 14.5). Although the primary lesion is in small portal veins, secondary proximal thrombosis causes dense fibrosis of the main perihilar portal tracts, so-called Symmers' pipe-stem fibrosis.[85-87] This lesion is easily seen by ultrasonography, allowing detailed demographic studies.[88,89] After treatment, ultrasound evidence of portal vein disease abates in the majority of cases.

PATHOLOGY OF PORTAL VEIN DISEASE

After thrombosis followed by organization, large veins may have subtle white intimal plaques or mural calcification. When recanalization is less complete the lumen may be obliterated or contain complex webs (Fig. 14.6). Portal

veins larger than 200 μm in diameter have eccentric intimal fibrous thickening which may be layered, suggesting recurrent thrombosis. Small veins are commonly involved by extension of thrombus from larger vessels. After organiza-

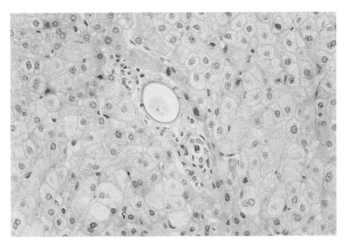

Fig. 14.5 *Schistosoma japonicum* egg in portal vein. H & E.

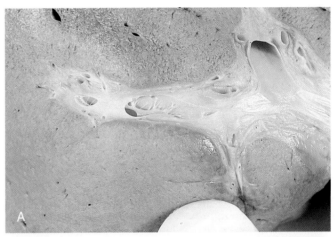

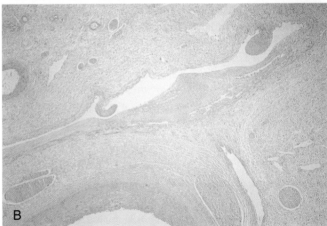

Fig. 14.6 Portal vein thrombosis after splenectomy. (a) Portal vein web from organized portal vein thrombosis illustrating near-total recanalization. Many peripheral portal veins were obliterated. (b) The webs are intimal fibrous tags. Haematoxylin–phloxine–saffron.

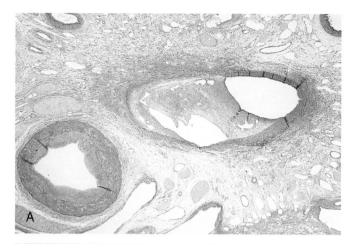

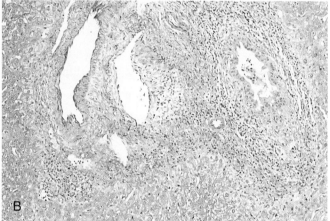

Fig. 14.7 Organized portal vein thrombosis showing partial fibrous occlusion in (a) large and (b) medium-sized portal veins after thrombosis. The original wall is often not recognizable in small veins after thrombosis. Elastic–trichrome.

tion, veins less than 200 μm in diameter disappear as the wall becomes incorporated into fibrous scar, while larger veins may have residual wall, best seen with the elastic–trichrome or Movat stains (Fig. 14.7).

Some small portal veins remain patent and become dilated if the supplying portal veins are patent, because the elevated portal pressure is transmitted to the small veins.[90,91] These dilated veins often expand outside the portal tract stroma into the adjacent parenchyma giving an 'ectopic' appearance (Fig. 14.8). It is a common error for the eye to recognize these 'supernormal' veins and to ignore the more subtle absence of veins. When evaluating the extent of obliteration of small portal veins, a quantitative approach is necessary because histologically identical lesions, but fewer in number, occur in elderly subjects without clinical portal hypertension.[92]

Multiple dilated collateral veins appear within the large and medium-sized portal tracts. These dilated vessels, grossly recognized as cavernous transformation,[93] arise in part by enlargement of normal collateral portal venous channels and in part by dilatation of the artery-fed peribiliary plexus[94] (see Ch.1). The number of small portal tract vessels is increased in extrahepatic portal vein obstruction and in cirrhosis but is decreased in idiopathic portal hypertension,[95] suggesting that more severe injury to the small portal veins has occurred in the latter disease.

Specific causes of portal vein obstruction are suggested by finding chronic cholangitis, paucity of bile ducts, mineral oil or Thorotrast deposits, sarcoid granulomas, schistosome eggs, or healed arteritis.

Vascular occlusion causes remodelling of the parenchyma. Acute thrombosis of a small portal vein results in a pseudo-infarct (of Zahn—Fig. 14.9);[96] obstruction of the portal vein trunk leads to diffuse atrophy of the liver.[97] Partial recanalization or compensatory arterial dilatation allows regeneration of parts of the liver, especially near the hilum. The result may be a localized depression on the capsular surface, atrophy of a lobe,[98] partial nodular transformation, or nodular regenerative hyperplasia (see below). The Zahn infarct is a region of hepatocellular atrophy which has a congested appearance because of the enlarged sinusoidal

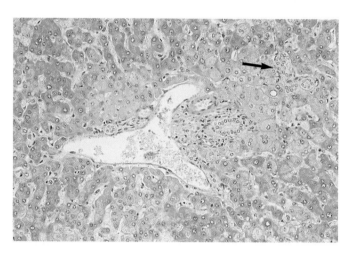

Fig. 14.8 Ectopic portal vein in a patient with non-cirrhotic portal hypertension. The portal vein is dilated and spills out into the adjacent parenchyma. An adjacent small portal tract has no vein (arrow). Haemotoxylin-phloxine-saffron.

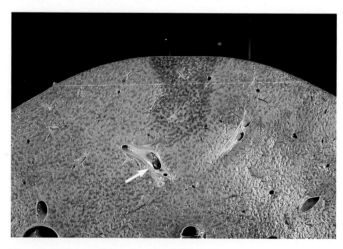

Fig. 14.9 Infarct of Zahn with acute portal vein thrombus (arrow).

volume. Many agents causing lesions in small portal veins, such as arsenic, vinyl chloride and Thorotrast, also cause mild hepatocellular necrosis leading to incomplete septal cirrhosis,[99] possibly because they are capable of causing veno-occlusive disease[100] with secondary congestive parenchymal damage.

HEPATIC VEINS

Hepatic vein lesions should be classified according to the anatomical distribution of the lesion and the apparent pathogenesis whenever possible.[101] Classification of individual cases may be inexact for many reasons. Although thrombosis is important in the pathogenesis of most venous lesions, the thrombotic component in small veins may be organized so quickly that it is seldom apparent histologically. The site of origin may be in doubt since thrombosis often begins in vessels of one size, propagates to larger or smaller vessels[102] and may recanalize almost completely.

The term *Budd–Chiari syndrome* is usually applied to the clinical manifestations of hepatic venous outflow obstruction secondary to hepatic vein thrombosis but sometimes to suprahepatic obstruction of the inferior vena cava and to disease affecting small hepatic vein branches. The term should be used with circumspection because of its variable definition.

NORMAL VARIATIONS AND CONGENITAL ANOMALIES

There is considerable variation in the large hepatic veins, with accessory or absent veins seen in 10–14% of individuals.[39,103–105] Collateral drainage between anatomical segments is often sufficient to ameliorate hepatic necrosis after hepatic vein obstruction and to lessen peripheral oedema after thrombosis of the inferior vena cava.[106,107] The inferior right hepatic vein often forms collaterals because it enters the vena cava caudal to the main hepatic veins.

HEPATIC VEIN THROMBOSIS

Clinical findings

There is a broad clinical spectrum associated with hepatic vein thrombosis. The classic findings are hepatomegaly, ascites, abdominal pain, and varying degrees of hepatic dysfunction.[108] Splenomegaly and ascites are each found at presentation in approximately two-thirds of patients.[109] The majority of patients present with subacute findings which lead to hepatic failure with median survival less than 2 years in the absence of surgical therapy.[108,110–112] Fulminant hepatic failure may be the initial presentation when there is obstruction of all major hepatic veins.[113] Patients with sparing of one large vein may have only hepatomegaly and mild or transient liver test abnormalities; such patients are not easily diagnosed in life and the

venous lesions may be discovered as an incidental finding at autopsy. Oesophageal varices are found in half of patients and bleed in approximately 20%.[114] Bleeding varices are usually accompanied by cirrhosis or portal vein thrombosis.[115] The latter occurs secondarily in 20%. Extension of thrombus to small mesenteric veins may cause bowel infarction.

The differential diagnosis includes constrictive pericarditis, which should be distinguished on clinical grounds as biopsy findings may be similar to those of hepatic vein obstruction.[116] Aggressive attempts to establish the diagnosis should be made, as some of the underlying diseases require therapy, and surgical intervention often leads to prolonged survival.[109,117,118]

Aetiology and pathogenesis

Three-quarters of patients in American, British, and French series with Budd–Chiari syndrome have a recognized predisposing factor belonging to Virchow's triad[119,120] (Table 14.3). Such factors are less common in children and in Japanese adults.[109,121] The most common factor is a hypercoagulable state, especially polycythaemia rubra vera, paroxysmal nocturnal haemoglobinuria, oral contraceptive use, pregnancy, and the presence of anticardiolipin antibodies.[112,122] Recently, other abnormalities of the coagulation system have been associated, such as antithrombin III deficiency and protein C deficiency. A large proportion of those with no obvious risk factor appear to have a subclinical blood dyscrasia characterized by spontaneous erythroid colony formation in vitro.[55,123] Pregnancy and oral contraceptive therapy may unmask latent hypercoagulable states.[123] Hypercoagulable states are often associated with thrombosis in arteries and veins of other organs, or in the allograft after liver transplantation.[124]

Vascular injury and stasis are other causes. The high prevalence in some developing countries suggests that infection, toxins,[109] or dehydration may have a role, especially in children[125] and postpartum women. In North America the common causes are polycythaemia (10%), paroxysmal nocturnal haemoglobinuria (7%), oral contraceptives (9%), pregnancy (10%), tumours (9%), and infections (9%).[112] In India, the most commonly associated conditions are amoebic abscess (18%), pregnancy (15%), and hepatic neoplasm (13%).[126,127]

Tumours involving the vena cava or hepatic veins may present with hepatic outflow obstruction (Table 14.3). Hepatocellular carcinoma involves the major hepatic veins in 6–23% of cases.[59,61] Most patients with hepatic vein involvement by this tumour also have portal vein involvement.[61]

Budd–Chiari syndrome may be associated with a radiological appearance suggesting membranous obstruction or stricture of the inferior vena cava.[128–130] While some early investigators believed these lesions to be developmental

Table 14.3 Causes of hepatic vein thrombosis

	References
Hypercoagulable states	
Polycythaemia vera	119
Agnogenic myeloid metaplasia	21
Paroxysmal nocturnal haemoglobinuria	101, 102, 324
Promyelocytic leukaemia	325, 326
Chronic myeloid leukaemia	114
Subclinical myeloproliferative disease	123
Undefined (e.g. history of thrombotic disease)	111
Oral contraceptive therapy	119, 327–329
Pregnancy	126
Lupus anticoagulant or anticardiolipin antibodies	132, 330–333
Idiopathic thrombocytopenic purpura	119
Protein C deficiency	101, 334
Antithrombin III deficiency	335, 336
Stasis or mass lesion	
Membranous obstruction of inferior vena cava	
(see text)	125, 131
Congenital anomalies	109, 337
Cirrhosis	111
Congestive heart failure	111
Constrictive pericarditis	338, 339
Superior vena cava obstruction	340
Atrial myxoma	341
Sickle-cell disease	342
Hepatocellular carcinoma	343, 344
Renal cell carcinoma	345
Adrenal carcinoma	346
Hodgkin's disease	232
Wilms' tumour	347, 348
Leiomyosarcoma or leiomyoma	344, 349–351
Metastatic neoplasm	344
Hydatid cyst	352
Hepatic abscess, pyogenic or amoebic	108, 353
Haematoma	354
Vascular injury	
Trauma	115, 124, 355–357
Ventriculo-atrial shunt	358
Catheterization	359
Sclerotherapy	319
Amyloidosis	360
Vasculitis or tissue inflammation	109
Tuberculosis	361
Fungal vasculitis	362, 363
Behçet's disease	364
Sarcoidosis	185, 365
Idiopathic granulomatous venulitis	186
Filariasis	366
Associations with uncertain mechanism	
Inflammatory bowel disease	111, 367, 368
Mixed connective tissue disease	369
Protein-losing enteropathy	370, 371
Multiple myeloma	372

anomalies causing hepatic vein thrombosis,[125,131] recent histological[121,127] and sequential radiological studies[132] suggest that these caval lesions are secondary to extension of hepatic vein thrombosis. Compression of the vena cava by an enlarged caudate lobe may precipitate this extension.[125,133] Hepatocellular carcinoma occurs in 36–46% of patients with membranous obstruction of the vena cava and less often in hepatic vein obstruction with patent vena cava.[128,134,135]

The initial site of thrombosis cannot be determined from examination of established Budd–Chiari syndrome. However, my experience with subclinical hepatic vein thrombosis found incidentally at autopsy suggests that thrombi begin in sinusoids or terminal hepatic venules and propagate towards the large hepatic veins. The frequency of primary thrombosis in small hepatic vein branches is probably underestimated because this lesion is clinically silent until propagation to several large hepatic veins has occurred.[136]

Pathology

The acute lesions after hepatic vein thrombosis are dilatation of veins and sinusoids, and variable degrees of necrosis (Fig. 14.10). The sinusoids are congested and red blood cells infiltrate the space of Disse.[137] Acute or organizing thrombus is occasionally seen within small hepatic[112] or portal veins.[121] As disease advances, the sinusoids become collagenized and dilated and hepatocytes become atrophic and are lost. The small hepatic veins disappear as they are incorporated into septa which eventually link hepatic veins to form cirrhosis with relative sparing of the portal triads, so-called 'reversed lobulation' (Fig. 14.11).

The liver remodels in a fashion dependent on the pattern of venous involvement. The left lobe is hypertrophied when the left vein is relatively spared. The caudate lobe becomes hypertrophied when the caudate lobe veins, which enter the vena cava directly, remain patent. Small regions of regeneration and hypertrophy commonly occur to form nodules or a ribbon of healthy hepatocytes surrounding the larger portal systems.[138,139] Lesions grossly similar to Zahn infarcts may be seen with localized hepatic vein thrombosis.[140]

Fibrous thickening and stenosis of the hepatic portion of the inferior vena cava is found in approximately 50% of cases of Budd–Chiari syndrome. The thickened region may form a thin valve-like membrane or may be several centimetres in length. Histologically, these lesions show thrombus in various stages of organization, often with calcification, and with no evidence of a pre-existing congenital membrane.[121]

Clinico-pathological correlation

A normal biopsy, especially early in the course, does not exclude the diagnosis. However, most patients have evidence of histological chronicity soon after the onset of clinical symptoms, suggesting that recurrence and extension of thrombosis is the rule. Hepatic vein thrombosis presenting in the postpartum period does not usually have histological evidence of chronicity.[127]

Histological diagnosis can be difficult in chronic disease because congestion and reversed lobulation are focal and may not be seen in a small biopsy. Hepatic vein thrombosis should be considered in any cirrhotic liver with si-

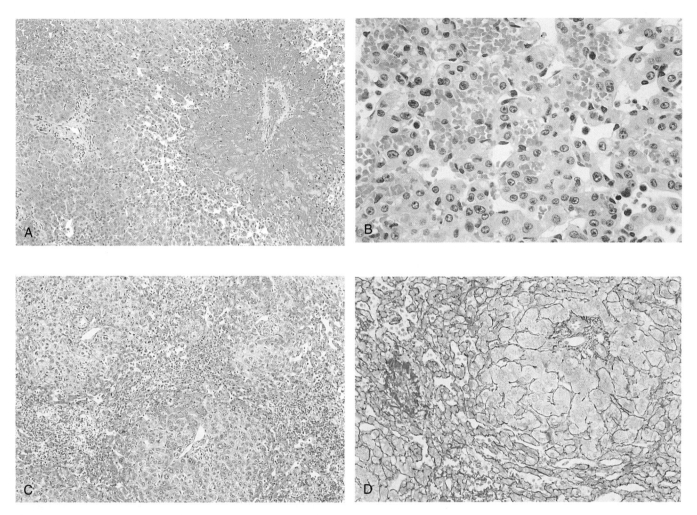

Fig. 14.10 Hepatic vein thrombosis (acute Budd–Chiari syndrome). (a) Marked zone 3 sinusoidal congestion and hepatocellular necrosis. H & E. (b) Insudation of red cells into the hepatocyte plates. H & E. (c) Atrophy and necrosis with evacuation of hepatocellular plates and nodular transformation. Note that the portal veins are patent in the nodules and obliterated in the atrophic region. Masson's trichrome. (d) Nodular transformation with occluded hepatic venule (left). Reticulin stain.

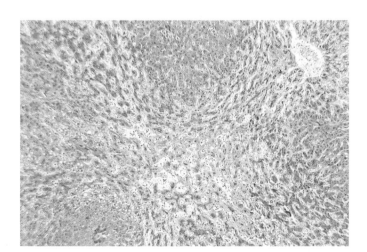

Fig. 14.11 Chronic hepatic vein thrombosis with zone 3 sinusoidal fibrosis, early septum formation, and 'reversed lobulation'. Masson's trichrome.

nusoidal dilatation or prominent dilated vascular channels. Organized thrombi or fibrous obliteration of small hepatic veins may be histologically identical to the lesions of chronic veno-occlusive disease.[136,141] Haemosiderosis may occur, especially when there is co-existent paroxysmal nocturnal haemoglobinuria.[107]

Many surgeons use the liver biopsy to guide therapy, with necrosis suggesting the need for a shunt procedure and extensive fibrosis favouring the need for transplantation.[115,120] Although the risk of bleeding from the biopsy site is significant, the benefit in therapeutic guidance may justify the procedure even in the presence of coagulopathy and ascites. Accurate assessment requires at least two biopsies from different lobes because of the marked regional variation in severity found in this condition.[113] Histological and clinical improvement is often seen after a decompression procedure such as meso-caval shunt.[142] Repeat biopsies after therapy are recommended; CT guidance is useful to ensure that the specimens are obtained from the same sites on the repeat occasion. The appearance of regenerative nodules on imaging studies may be misinterpreted as malignancy.[143]

VENO-OCCLUSIVE DISEASE

Veno-occlusive disease (VOD) is characterized by fibrous occlusion of small hepatic veins less than 1 mm in diameter with secondary hepatic congestion.[140,144]

Aetiology and clinical findings

Hepatic injury presenting as abdominal pain and ascites after ingestion of plants or extracts of *Senecio* species was described in humans long before the actual vascular lesions were recognized.[145–147] This disease, known variously as Senecio disease, serous hepatosis, heliotrope toxicosis, and Pictou cattle disease,[148,149] has been reported in humans and livestock from many parts of the world. The apparent cause of the condition is ingestion of pyrrolizidine alkaloids derived mostly from *Senecio* species, *Crotalaria* species, *Heliotropium lasiocarpum*,[150] or *Symphytum* species (comfrey).[151] Hepatotoxic pyrrolizidine alkaloids have been found in more than 150 species of plants and there are several thousand potentially toxic species.[152] Alkaloid preparations of this type have been shown to produce marked hepatic congestion and venular endothelial necrosis in many rodents and ruminants. The pattern of toxicity in rats depends on the dose, with diffuse hepatocellular necrosis and pulmonary vascular injury occurring at doses higher than those producing VOD.[153] Hepatic tumours have been produced in rats.[154]

Reports of human toxicity have followed ingestion of the alkaloids in herbal teas or in epidemics caused by contaminated grain. The disease usually affects young children but adults are also susceptible. The onset may be acute or insidious. Acute disease is characterized by rapid onset of abdominal pain, hepatomegaly and ascites, usually without jaundice, splenomegaly, or fever. Chronic disease may be indistinguishable from cirrhosis of other causes, with features of portal hypertension or hepatic failure.

An epidemic of VOD occurred in India after consumption of cereal contaminated with a *Crotalaria* species.[155] Of 188 cases found among 486 villagers, 49% died within 5 years, mostly in the first 6 months.[156] A similar outbreak occurred in Afghanistan, affecting 23% of the local population after consumption of bread contaminated with *Heliotropium* plants.[157] Herbal tea made from *Heliotropium* is used in India for the treatment of psoriasis and other skin conditions.[127,150]

After bone marrow transplantation, symptomatic VOD occurs in up to 54% of patients.[158,159] The lesions are thought to be caused by the hepatic radiation and intense chemotherapy preceding the transplantation. Patients usually present in the three weeks after therapy with weight gain, thrombocytopenia, jaundice, hepatic failure, and increased aminotransferases and alkaline phosphatase. Ascites is present in 23% and peripheral oedema in 63% of patients.[159] Liver disease contributed to death in 25% of patients with symptomatic VOD.[159]

Hepatic radiation[160,161] and chemotherapeutic drugs given without bone marrow transplantation have been implicated (Table 14.3 and Fig. 14.12).[161–170] Azathioprine therapy has been associated with VOD, presenting insidiously with cholestasis or ascites after renal transplantation and, rarely, after azathioprine treatment of other conditions.[169] There is a striking male predominance among patients with VOD after azathioprine therapy.[171] Other associations include immunodeficiency states,[172] tyrosinaemia,[173] and cystinosis with cysteamine therapy.[165]

The pathogenesis of the lesions is believed to be a primary injury to the endothelial cells of sinusoids and small venules.[159,171,174] The mechanism of endothelial injury after cytotoxic drugs may involve depletion of cellular

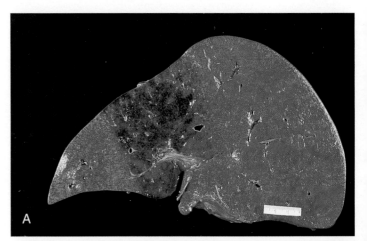

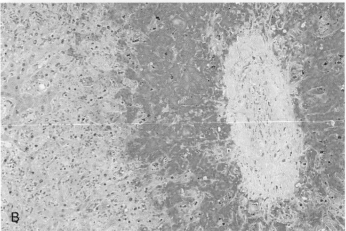

Fig. 14.12 Veno-occlusive disease with peripheral oedema and ascites 3 weeks after bone marrow transplantion. (a) Congestion involves the midportion of the liver. Microscopic lesions were confined to veins less than 0.5 mm in diameter. (b) A small hepatic vein contains macrophages and fibrous tissue. Masson's trichrome.

glutathione.[174,175] Patients with VOD related to a variety of insults may improve after cessation of the offending agent[166,168,171,176] or after portacaval shunt.[177,178]

Pathology

The early lesion is subintimal oedema and haemorrhage involving the small hepatic veins. Most affected veins are less than 300 μm in diameter. Thrombosis is usually not recognized, but fibrin deposits are often present on ultrastructural and immunochemical examination of acute lesions.[161,179] Sinusoidal congestion and hepatocellular necrosis may be severe with sparing of only a few periportal hepatocytes. In mild cases there may be patchy congestion in zone 3. Cholestasis is often prominent in chemotherapy-induced lesions.[169] The venous lesion heals with concentric or eccentric intimal fibrosis, fibrous obliteration, and occasionally multiple lumens. Angiomatoid endothelial proliferation has been described.[180] Zone 3 hepatocytes atrophy and sinusoidal fibrosis develops. Patients surviving for years may develop 'congestive cirrhosis' with relative sparing of the portal tracts.[140,144] Regenerative nodules similar to those of nodular regenerative hyperplasia may be seen.[162,168,169,172,181] Obliteration of small portal veins has been seen in some patients with VOD after irradiation,[161] and peliosis hepatis has been reported in renal transplant recipients with VOD.[162]

After high-dose drug therapy, the lesions may develop within days of intensive therapy so that the veins are not fibrotic and the importance of the venous injury may not be recognized amid the intense haemorrhage.[163] Dacarbazine has been associated with acute thrombosis of small and medium-sized hepatic veins. Reaction to this drug may have an allergic component, as it typically occurs shortly after beginning the second course of therapy and is associated with eosinophils in portal tracts and hepatic vein walls and peripheral blood eosinophilia.[163]

Differential diagnosis

If the vascular lesions are missed on needle biopsy, marked congestion of sinusoids suggests VOD if the history is appropriate, with a differential diagnosis of constrictive pericarditis[116] congestive heart failure, and hepatic vein thrombosis. In VOD, secondary thrombosis may propagate to involve the large hepatic veins.[146] Conversely, thrombosis of large hepatic veins is often accompanied by fibrous obliteration of small hepatic veins with an appearance identical to VOD.[136,141] Thus, occasional patients are difficult to classify histologically.

Fibrous obliteration of small hepatic veins is frequently found in alcoholic and non-alcoholic cirrhosis.[182–184] In cirrhosis, the obliterated veins are usually incorporated into fibrous septa so that VOD-like lesions are only occasionally recognized. The occluded veins are present in small

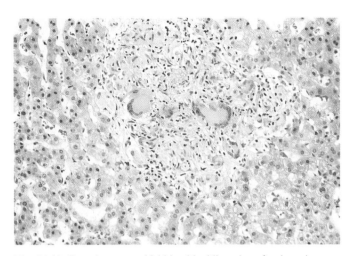

Fig. 14.13 Granulomatous phlebitis with obliteration of an hepatic venule. Portal veins were also involved. The patient was a young man with vasculitic rash and hepatomegaly. H & E. Courtesy of Dr E Keystone.

numbers in cirrhosis (< 2/cm²) compared with veno-occlusive disease (23/cm²).[184]

OTHER VENOUS LESIONS

Small hepatic veins have been involved in inflammatory lesions in a variety of conditions including sarcoidosis,[185] idiopathic granulomatous vasculitis (Fig. 14.13),[186] and virus-associated haemophagocytic syndrome.[187]

SINUSOIDS

NORMAL SINUSOIDAL STRUCTURE (see Ch. 1)

Sinusoids are lined by modified endothelial cells containing fenestrations 50–300 nm in diameter which allow passage of lipoproteins and other large molecules but provide a barrier to blood cells. The fenestrations are dynamic, responding to pharmacological agents and the quality of matrix in the space of Disse.[188] Normally there is almost no basement membrane under the endothelium, and the space of Disse contains scanty collagen.[189,190] The endothelial cells participate in the metabolism of macromolecules such as glycosaminoglycans and lipoproteins.[189,191] Kupffer cells reside in the lumen and are anchored to the underlying sinusoidal wall. Perisinusoidal (Ito) cells are stellate cells found in the space of Disse with processes that embrace the sinusoids. At rest, these cells contain 95% of the hepatic vitamin A;[192] they are specialized fibroblasts which produce collagen in response to liver injury (see Ch. 10). When activated, they have contractile properties that may control sinusoidal blood flow. Natural killer cells (pit cells) and mast cells may also be found in small numbers within the space of Disse.

SINUSOIDAL CAPILLARIZATION AND PERICELLULAR FIBROSIS

In alcoholic cirrhosis and in alcoholic liver disease with mild pericellular fibrosis there is a decrease in sinusoidal fenestrations, deposition of subendothelial basement membrane and collagen, loss of hepatocellular microvilli, increased expression of endothelial factor VIII, and binding of *Ulex europaeus* I (UEA I) lectin to endothelial cells.[193,194] These findings are typical of non-hepatic capillaries and are known as capillarization.[191,195] Permeability of the sinusoidal wall may be significantly impaired by these changes, although the clinical significance is uncertain. Linear sinusoidal deposition of IgA is found in most biopsies from alcoholics and diabetics, and to a lesser degree in other diseases and in normal controls.[196] Sinusoidal binding of UEA I lectin or increased expression of factor VIII may be useful findings when small biopsies are otherwise not diagnostic of cirrhosis.[191,194]

Pericellular fibrosis is commonly seen in alcoholic liver disease, chronic passive congestion, Budd–Chiari syndrome, diabetes type I,[190] steatohepatitis of obesity and diabetes type II,[197–199] Gaucher's disease, congenital syphilis, and vitamin A toxicity. Vitamin A toxicity is characterized by marked enlargement of perisinusoidal cells, progressive collagenization of the space of Disse and, eventually, fibrous septum formation and micronodular cirrhosis.[200,201] Vitamin A toxicity is silent unless complications of portal hypertension supervene.[202]

SINUSOIDAL DILATATION

Sinusoidal dilatation occurs when there is increased pressure in the hepatic veins, atrophy of hepatocytes, or disruption of the sinusoidal reticulin fibres. Increased pressure in cardiac failure, constrictive pericarditis, and hepatic vein thrombosis cause sinusoidal dilatation which is accentuated by secondary atrophy in zone 3 (Fig. 14.14). Erythrocytes may extravasate into the space of Disse and between hepatocytes.[137,203] Hyaline globules may be seen in zone 3 hepatocytes in the presence of ischaemia and cardiac failure.[204,205] Sinusoidal dilatation with atrophy also occurs after portal vein obstruction, as seen in Zahn infarcts, nodular hyperplasia, and adjacent to neoplasms. Nodular regenerative hyperplasia occasionally occurs in chronic passive congestion,[206] probably because of co-existent portal or hepatic vein obstruction.

Sinusoidal dilatation may be seen as a result of non-specific malnutrition in wasting illnesses such as malignancy, tuberculosis, and AIDS[207,208] and as a paraneoplastic lesion associated with renal cell carcinoma[209,210] and Hodgkin's disease.[211]

Sinusoidal dilatation after oral contraceptive therapy or in pregnancy usually occurs in zones 1 and 2.[212,213] It is accompanied by mild sinusoidal fibrosis best seen by electron

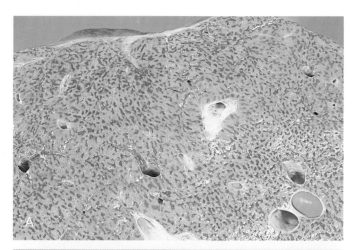

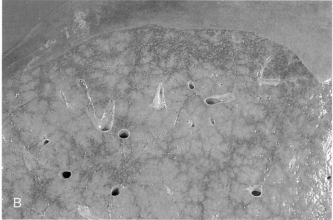

Fig. 14.14 Chronic passive congestion with (a) diffuse 'nutmeg' pattern, and (b) diffuse nodular hyperplasia pattern.

microscopy.[213,214] Sinusoidal dilatation induced by steroids and wasting illnesses may be a precursor to peliosis hepatis.

In sickle-cell disease there is often a mild elevation of aminotransferases, chronic cholestasis or, rarely, progressive hepatic failure.[215] Hepatic dysfunction does not appear to correlate temporally with crisis involving other organs.[216,217] Biopsies usually show sinusoids packed with sickled red cells and erythrophagocytosis (Fig. 14.15). Pericellular fibrosis is occasionally prominent.

PELIOSIS HEPATIS

Peliosis hepatis is defined by the presence of cystic blood-filled spaces in liver, spleen, lymph nodes, and other organs (Fig. 14.16).[218] Although the term was originally applied to macroscopic lesions (peliosis=dusky or purple), microscopic lesions are now often called peliosis. Microscopic peliosis hepatis is often confused with extreme sinusoidal dilatation or with 'evacuation of the liver-cell plates', a lesion seen after zonal hepatocellular dropout but without loss of the normal reticulin fibres that support the plates. To be called peliosis hepatis, lesions should have

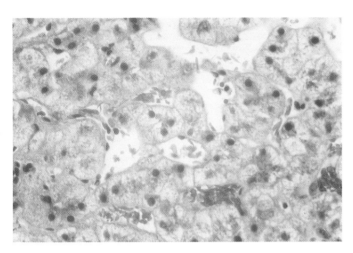

Fig. 14.15 Sickle-cell disease. Sinusoids are dilated and contain sickled red cells. There is slight sinusoidal fibrosis. Masson's trichrome.

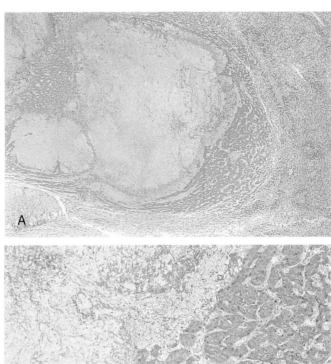

Fig. 14.17 Peliosis hepatis which produced fatal bleeding in a male of 18 who had had prolonged treatment with androgenic steroids for Fanconi's syndrome: the peliotic cavities are sharply defined (a), and at the interface with the liver parenchyma there is an acellular coagulum and some fibrin (b). Masson's trichrome. Courtesy of Dr H Cameron.

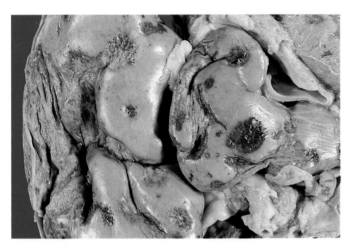

Fig. 14.16 Peliosis hepatis in a patient who received testosterone replacement therapy for 8 years after hypophysectomy. The capsular surface shows cavities up to many centimetres in diameter. Courtesy of Dr D V Brunsden.

evidence of lysis of these fibres (Fig. 14.17). This lysis may follow intrinsic weakness of the fibres of the wall (*phlebectatic type*) or may accompany focal hepatocyte necrosis (*parenchymal type*).[219,220] Initially the spaces may have no endothelial lining but re-endothelialization probably occurs rapidly. Thus, classification of lesions on the basis of the presence or absence of endothelium is not warranted.[221] Lesions are randomly distributed without zonal preference.

It is appropriate to classify peliosis hepatis according to the apparent aetiology as this correlates with distinctive histological and clinical features. Macroscopic lesions are usually induced by anabolic, oestrogenic, or adrenocortical steroids and are often associated with splenic peliosis. Macroscopic peliosis hepatis has also been reported with a variety of chronic diseases such as malnutrition,[222] leukaemia,[223] tuberculosis,[218] leprosy,[224] vasculitis,[225] and AIDS.[226] Microscopic lesions occur in patients receiving

thiopurines for renal transplantation, liver transplantation, or various malignancies.[227–229] Other associated drugs are listed in Table 14.4.

The peliotic lesions found in AIDS[230] are often caused by the rickettsial organism *Rochalimaea henselae* which causes cutaneous bacillary angiomatosis.[231] These lesions have a myxoid stroma which has a bluish haze on H&E and contains clumps of organisms which stain with the Warthin–Starry technique. Patients often have peliosis of the spleen and lymph nodes and cutaneous angiomatous lesions. Hepatosplenomegaly and increased alkaline phosphatase are usually present and respond to antibiotics. This lesion should be distinguished from sinusoidal dilatation and Kaposi's sarcoma, which also occur in AIDS.[208]

In 'hairy cell' leukaemia, peliosis of liver and spleen may be the result of sinusoidal wall injury induced by tumour cells.[223] Peliosis hepatis also occurs within neoplasms such as adenoma and hepatocellular carcinoma (Fig. 14.18). Peliosis hepatis of minor degree has rarely been associated with Hodgkin's disease,[232] angioimmunoblastic lymphaden-

Table 14.4 Microvascular disease related to drugs and toxins

	Obliterative portal venopathy	Sinusoidal fibrosis	Veno-occlusive disease*	Peliosis hepatis	Angiosarcoma	References
6-Thioguanine			++	+		227
Azathioprine	+	+	+	+		14, 162, 167, 171, 228
6-Mercaptopurine	+	+	+	+		14
BCNU			+			373
Hepatic radiation	+		++			161
Dacarbazine			++			163
Flurodeoxyuridine (intra-arterial)	+		+			170
Methotrexate		+		+		374
Senecio alkaloids		+	++			150
Cysteamine			+			165
Thorotrast	++	++	++	++	+	375, 376
Arsenic	++	+	+	+	+	99, 100, 375
Copper	+	+				377
Vinyl chloride monomer	++	++			+	375
Vitamin A	+	++		+		200
'Toxic oil'	+	+				378
Anabolic and oestrogenic steroids; medroxyprogesterone				++	+	379
Corticosteroids				+		380
Tamoxifen				+		381

*Other drugs associated with VOD include busulfan, dimethylbusulfan, cytosine arabinoside, cyclophosphamide, indicine-*N*-oxide, mustine-HCl, adriamycin, urethane, vincristine, mitomycin-C, and etoposide.[159,382]

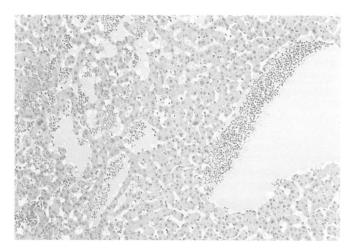

Fig. 14.18 Peliosis hepatis within a hepatic adenoma associated with oral contraceptive use; an endothelial lining is present. H & E.

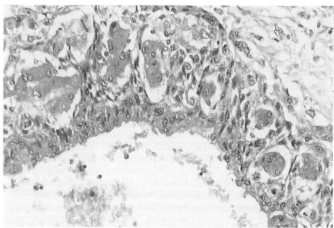

Fig. 14.19 Angiosarcoma with peliotic cavity lined by neoplastic cells. H & E.

opathy,[233] myeloproliferative disorders[234] and Waldenstrom's macroglobulinaemia with light chain deposition.[235]

Peliotic cysts lined by dysplastic or frankly malignant endothelial cells are seen in association with angiosarcoma (Fig. 14.19). Livers with angiosarcoma also may have portal fibrosis and poorly formed nodules of hepatocytes.[236] These nodules have been considered to be the result of hepatocellular dysplasia but may be nodular hyperplasia secondary to portal vascular obliteration.

Although peliosis hepatis is usually of no clinical signifi-cance, macroscopic peliosis of liver or spleen may rupture spontaneously or after trauma.[237,238] The lesions may also be associated with cholestasis,[222,227] hepatic failure,[222,230] and, rarely, portal hypertension.[239]

TOXIC MICROVASCULAR INJURY

Drugs and other toxins, especially alkylating agents, may cause a variety of histological lesions involving the microvasculature (Table 14.4 and Ch. 15). These lesions include veno-occlusive disease, sinusoidal fibrosis, peliosis hepatis, obliterative portal venopathy, and nodular regenerative hyperplasia. Some patients have presented with portal hypertension.[240,241] Although patients are categorized according to the dominant clinical or histological finding, several lesions often occur together.[227,242] The dominant lesion appears to depend on host factors and drug dosage as well as the particular agent. The lesions are more common when the drugs are used in antineoplastic regimens than with lower immunosuppressive doses. High-dose therapy tends to give acute or subacute VOD while low-dose therapy gives chronic lesions of VOD, non-cirrhotic portal hypertension, nodular regenerative hyperplasia, or sinusoidal fibrosis. As previously mentioned, males appear to be more susceptible than females to azathioprine-induced lesions.[171]

OTHER SINUSOIDAL LESIONS

Hepatic amyloidosis (see Ch. 17) is characterized by deposits within vessel walls, portal stroma, and in the space of Disse.[243] Diffuse sinusoidal wall thickening may be so marked as to cause atrophy and disappearance of hepatocytes. Rarely, one may see only small sinusoidal nodules of amyloid.[244] In AA disease, amyloid is found in portal vessels in 90% and in sinusoids in 37% of cases. In AL disease, deposits are found in portal vessels in 87% and in sinusoids in 75%.[243,245] Diffuse deposition causes hepatomegaly, cholestasis,[246] and, rarely, portal hypertension.[22]

Light chain disease may be associated with cholestasis and deposition of light chains in sinusoids and portal tracts. The deposits are PAS positive and may also be congophilic.[247]

Infiltration of sinusoids by cells may be of diagnostic value but rarely causes clinical effects unless it is massive. *Lymphoid infiltration* is seen in viral and autoimmune hepatitis, phenytoin (and other) hepatotoxicity (see Ch. 15), allograft rejection, leukaemia, and lymphoma. Extramedullary haematopoiesis is seen in myeloproliferative disorders;[248] characteristic cells are seen in *mastocytosis*, *Gaucher's disease*, and metastatic infiltration by carcinomas and other tumours. *Primary angioformative tumours* (haemangiosarcoma and epithelioid haemangioendothelioma) characteristically grow along the sinusoidal wall replacing the original endothelium and causing hepatocellular atrophy and peliosis hepatis.

In disseminated intravascular coagulation and eclampsia, fibrin deposits may be seen in small portal veins, the media or lumen of arterioles, and sinusoids. Sinusoidal fibrin and secondary necrosis are most prominent in zone 1. When this lesion is severe, widespread infarction and rupture of the liver may occur. Sinusoidal microthrombi have been noted in the antiphospholipid syndrome.[249]

Ischaemic injury of the sinusoidal endothelial cells of the allograft is commonly seen immediately after liver transplantation and may be important in some cases of early graft dysfunction.[250,251] The endothelial cells are rounded up and may either recover or detach.

ARTERIES

NORMAL VARIATIONS AND CONGENITAL ANOMALIES (see Ch. 3)

Unlike the portal and hepatic veins, the hepatic artery exhibits considerable variation (Fig. 14.20), which may lead to inadvertent ligation with secondary duct strictures or allograft failure.[252,253] A variety of vascular anomalies may be found in the liver with diverse clinical presentations. Abnormal origin of the hepatic artery is frequent with biliary atresia.[39] Haemangiomas and focal nodular hyperplasia may present as a mass lesion. Arteriovenous malformations of the spleen or liver may cause high portal blood flow and portal hypertension.[24,254] Intrahepatic arteriovenous fistulae in Osler–Weber–Rendu disease may be associated with high output cardiac failure, portal or pulmonary hypertension, and ascites.[255,256]

DISEASES OF THE HEPATIC ARTERIES

The hepatic artery is susceptible to diseases found in other arteries. Atherosclerosis, hyaline arteriosclerosis, thrombotic and atheromatous embolism, transplant arteriopathy, cryoglobulinaemia, monoclonal gammopathies, and amyloidosis may involve hepatic arteries but are rarely of clinical significance.[257] Arterial injury may occur with polyarteritis nodosa, Takayasu's arteritis, rheumatoid arteritis,[258] septic embolus, tuberculosis, syphilis, local infection, pancreatitis, or trauma. The histological appearance of these lesions is the same as in other organs. For example, temporal arteritis may be associated with giant cell arteritis in the liver.[81] Complications of inflammatory arterial lesions include aneurysmal dilatation, arterial rupture, arteriovenous fistula,[259] infarction, ischaemic biliary stricture, biliary cysts, rupture of the bile duct or gallbladder, hydrops of the gallbladder, and haemobilia.[67,70,260–262] Aneurysms most commonly involve the extrahepatic arteries.[263] Arteritis involving small arteries and arterioles is easily missed and may heal without a trace of the original vessel. Such lesions cause portal fibrosis and obliteration of portal veins and ducts.

Since the advent of percutaneous biliary drainage procedures several complications have become frequent clinical events. These include arteriovenous fistula, pseudoaneurysm, and portobiliary fistula with secondary peritoneal haemorrhage or haemobilia.[264,265] Percutaneous drainage tracts are lined by granulation tissue, usually with cytolysis secondary to direct bile exposure and organized thrombi in adjacent portal veins. Veins draining arteriovenous fistulae may resemble arteries because of marked medial hyperplasia.[259]

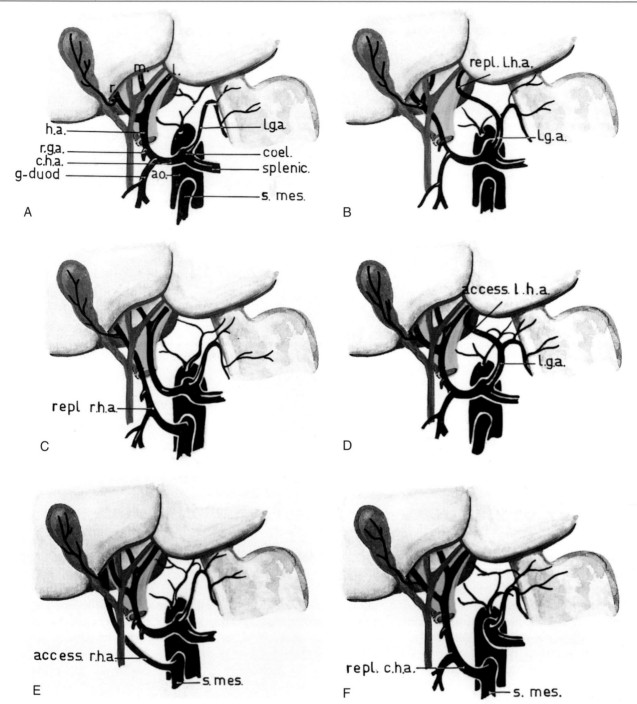

Fig. 14.20 Variations in hepatic arterial blood supply and collaterals after Michels[252] and Netter[252a] Abbreviations as follows: h.a. = hepatic artery; c.h.a., r.h.a., m.h.a. and l.h.a. = common, right, middle and left hepatic artery; r.g.a. and l.g.a. = right and left gastric artery; g.duod. = gastroduodenal artery; ao. = aorta; s.mes. = superior mesenteric artery; coel. = coeliac axis. (a) Commonest patterns of arterial supply—55% of dissections. (b) Replaced (repl.) left hepatic artery—10%. (c) Replaced (repl.) right hepatic artery—11%. (d) Accessory (access.) left hepatic artery originating from left gastric artery—8%. (e) Accessory (access.) right hepatic artery originating from superior mesenteric artery—7% (f) Replaced (repl.) common hepatic artery—2.5%.

HEPATIC ISCHAEMIA

Ischaemic necrosis may have a generalized zone 3 distribution or the circumscribed geographic pattern of an infarct, in which there is involvement of at least two contiguous acini.[266] The parenchyma is protected against ischaemia by its double blood supply. Most individuals can tolerate hepatic artery ligation without infarction.[267] Large infarcts are usually accompanied by obstruction of both artery and portal vein but in 20% of cases there is portal vein thrombosis alone and in 40% there is no identifiable vascular lesion[261,266,268,268a] (Fig. 14.21).

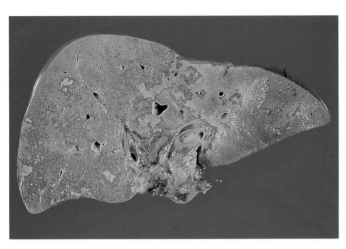

Fig. 14.21 Multiple infarcts after shock.

Zone 3 necrosis is much more common than infarction. The former occurs after shock[269] when arterial flow and portal vein oxygen saturation are decreased simultaneously. Although hepatic necrosis in shock is usually a zone 3 lesion, zone 2 may rarely be the site of maximum necrosis.[270] A polymorphonuclear infiltrate may be prominent in the healing phase, followed by perivenular fibrosis and rarely calcification.[271] Co-existent atrophy of zone 3 hepatocytes suggests chronic right heart failure.[269] Zone 3 ischaemic necrosis may be very difficult to distinguish from toxic injury caused by acetaminophen or cocaine.[272]

The cirrhotic liver is susceptible to ischaemia because portal flow is impeded and the parenchyma is largely dependent on arterial flow. Infarction of individual nodules in the cirrhotic liver commonly occurs after variceal haemorrhage.

Infarction in pregnancy may arise because of one or more events related to eclampsia, disseminated intravascular coagulation, hypovolaemic shock, or thrombosis of the hepatic artery, portal vein, or hepatic veins.[273] In pre-eclampsia and eclampsia there may be fibrinoid necrosis of arteries in many organs (see Ch. 17).

Ischaemia occurring in the hepatic allograft is discussed in Chapter 18.

NODULAR HYPERPLASIA

Nodular hyperplasia is defined by the presence of non-neoplastic nodules that are not delimited by fibrous septa (Fig. 14.22)[80]. The cells of the nodules are often arranged in double-cell plates. The cells of the surrounding parenchyma are atrophic. The nodules usually measure 1 mm in diameter and have a central portal tract.

The term nodular hyperplasia has many synonyms, especially 'nodular transformation'[80,274]. Several anatomic patterns are recognized, as described below.

Nodular hyperplasia may be difficult to distinguish histologically from low-grade dysplastic lesions[274, 275].

Nodular hyperplasia is usually a regenerative response occurring after circulatory stress. Portal vein obstruction causes widespread hepatocellular atrophy and secondary hepatic artery dilatation[275a]. Increased arterial flow and possibly hepatotropic factors, cause hepatocellular hyperplasia with the formation of nodules. Other stimuli, such as hepatic vein thrombosis, lead to increased arterial flow and nodular hyperplasia, although the histological appearance is less uniform because of the variable degree of congestion, necrosis, and fibrosis. Nodular hyperplasia is the hepatic analogue of the irregular parenchyma seen in kidneys with senile nephrosclerosis or specific glomerular diseases.

DIFFUSE NODULAR HYPERPLASIA (NODULAR REGENERATIVE HYPERPLASIA)

The term 'nodular regenerative hyperplasia' was originally applied to livers which had diffuse nodular hyperplasia but with minimal or no parenchymal fibrosis (Fig. 14.22). The term 'diffuse nodular hyperplasia' is less specific and may be applied to livers with fibrous septa or cirrhosis (see below).

Nodular regenerative hyperplasia occurs in up to 5% of the elderly population, but with higher prevalence in patients with certain systemic diseases that are associated with vascular disease, such as polycythemia, rheumatoid arthritis, and polyarteritis nodosa[80, 276]. Symptomatic patients are usually discovered because of œsophageal varices, splenomegaly, or moderate elevation of alkaline phosphatase; ascites is not uncommon.

The term 'partial nodular transformation' has been used for non-cirrhotic livers with large nodules situated in the perihilar region (Figs 14.23 and 14.24)[80, 277]. The main portal vein usually has evidence of healed thrombosis. Diffuse nodular hyperplasia is present in both the hilar and peripheral tissue, with more severe atrophy in the latter. This pattern was explained by coexistent obstruction of portal veins and small hepatic veins in several examples seen by the author. When viewed microscopically, partial nodular transformation may be indistinguishable from nodular regenerative hyperplasia.

DIFFUSE NODULAR HYPERPLASIA IN CIRRHOSIS

In cirrhotic livers, nodules bounded by fibrous septa often contain smaller nodules not surrounded by septa, a pattern called 'nodules within nodules' by Rubin et al.[278,279]. This represents co-existent nodular hyperplasia and cirrhosis and is usually associated with superimposed portal vein thrombosis. Most livers with incomplete septal cirrhosis have this combination of lesions; such livers can be classified according to the extent of fibrous septum formation, eg. fibrous 'septation' (grade 1,2, or 3) with nodular hyperplasia (grade 1,2,

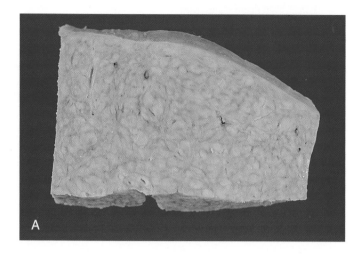

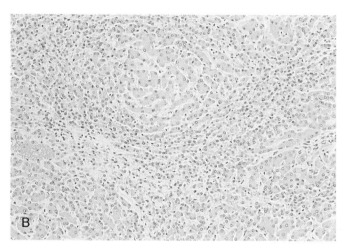

Fig. 14.22 Nodular regenerative hyperplasia. The patient had acute polyarteritis nodosa in many organs (same patient as Fig. 14.2.) (a) Most nodules are 1 mm in diameter, the size of a normal acinus. (b) Microscopic appearance with normal or atrophic cells in adjacent acini. H&E.

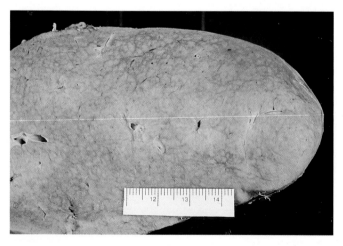

Fig. 14.23 Nodular hyperplasia with a diffuse micronodular pattern (nodular regenerative hyperplasia) as well as deep masses of larger confluent nodules in a pattern of partial nodular transformation. The patient had long-standing 'idiopathic portal hypertension'.

or 3). Only if septa are absent should a diagnosis of nodular regenerative hyperplasia be made; large samples of liver may be necessary for an accurate diagnosis to be established.

LOBAR OR SEGMENTAL ATROPHY AND HYPERPLASIA

Atrophy involving one or more lobes, usually the left, occurs in about 13% of cirrhotic livers, in 50% of livers with non-cirrhotic portal hypertension, and rarely in other livers[98, 280, 281]. This atrophy usually occurs following portal vein thrombosis but also after hepatic vein thrombosis, unilateral duct obstruction, or as a congenital anomaly[282]. Deep segmentation (hepar lobatum) occurs after vascular lesions, especially in syphilis and metastatic carcinoma[283]. Loss of tissue in one lobe is accompanied by compensatory hyperplasia of the other lobes, a pattern called 'the atrophy-hypertrophy complex'[283a].

Insufficient attention has been paid to the terminology of lobar atrophy. The term is usually applied to the gross appearance of shrinkage of a lobe irrespective of the histology. The histological appearance may be that of a decrease in size of hepatocytes, as seen after portal vein obstruction and manifested by infarcts of Zahn or nodular transformation; this is true atrophy. Alternatively, there may be fibrous obliteration of the hepatocellular parenchyma, as seen after chronic hepatic vein obstruction; this is not atrophy and requires another term, such as focal parenchymal extinction (see below)[279].

FOCAL NODULAR HYPERPLASIA

Focal nodular hyperplasia is a localized region of hyperplasia within otherwise normal liver (Fig. 14.25)[284]. The lesions have a central stellate fibrous region containing a large arterial malformation. The spider-like branches of the artery supply the component nodules. The arterial lesions may be a developmental anomaly that provides focal hyperaemia; the nodular hyperplasia may be a secondary response analogous to hypertrophy of the arms or legs occurring secondary to vascular malformations in those limbs[284]. Nodules similar to focal nodular hyperplasia occur in Osler-Weber-Rendu disease[285] and rarely in tissue adjacent to haemangiomas[286].

Most focal nodular hyperplasia lesions are discovered incidentally during investigation of other problems. When the lesions are multiple, there is a high probability of associated lesions, most commonly hepatic haemangiomas, meningioma, astrocytoma, and arterial dysplasia in various organs[32].

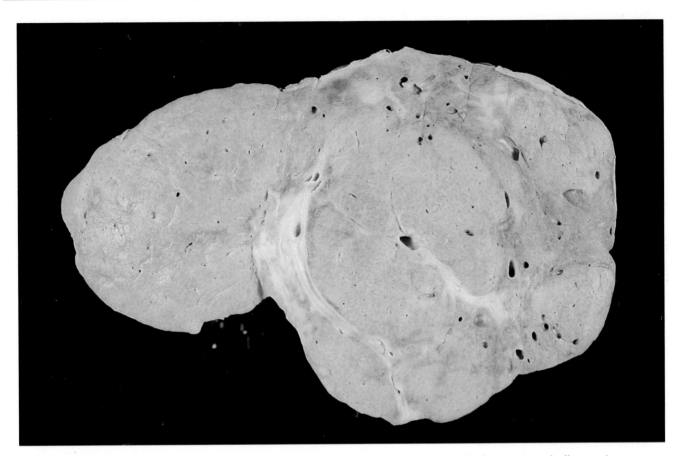

Fig. 14.24 Partial nodular transformation in a patient with sarcoidosis. The largest obliterated portal veins were 1 mm in diameter (same case as in Fig. 14.4). There was also granulomatous involvement and obliteration of some small hepatic vein branches.

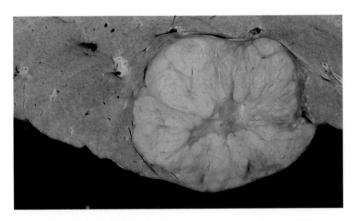

Fig. 14.25 Focal nodular hyperplasia with characteristic central fibrous region and radiating fibrous cords.

VASCULAR DISEASE IN CIRRHOSIS

Hepatocellular necrosis precedes the development of cirrhosis. However, necrosis per se is not sufficient, as rapid regeneration may allow restitution of normal liver architecture.[287] Cirrhosis only develops if there is concomitant fibrous obliteration of the microvasculature. Mechanisms

of obliteration include thrombosis[288] and inflammatory activation of perisinusoidal cells.[289]

Post-thrombotic obliteration of small hepatic veins can be found in most cirrhotic livers, and lesions are especially frequent in alcoholic liver disease.[182,183] Hepatic vein thrombosis occurring in the cirrhotic liver causes a regional increase in fibrosis with decrease in nodule size and widening of fibrous septa (Fig. 14.26). When the thrombus is poorly recanalized, there is total loss of the affected parenchyma, a lesion called focal parenchymal extinction[285] or confluent hepatic fibrosis.[290] Portal vein thrombosis also occurs in established cirrhosis (see above) and may be an important complication leading to progression of portal hypertension or hepatic failure.

As cirrhosis develops, necrotic acinar parenchyma is replaced with scar tissue which includes vascular channels that effectively shunt blood from the portal venous circulation to the systemic venous circulation.[291] Other shunts of lesser importance develop between hepatic arteries and hepatic veins.[292] Although most intrahepatic porto-systemic shunts are microscopic, approximately 25% of cirrhotic patients have 1–2 mm diameter shunts visible on transhepatic portography.[293] Large portal vein to hepatic vein (or to inferior vena cava) shunts occasionally develop

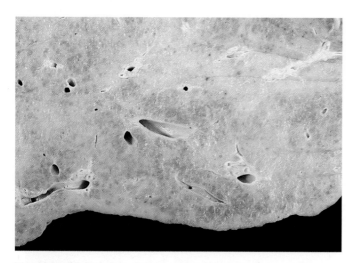

Fig. 14.26 Cirrhotic liver showing regional heterogeneity caused by hepatic vein thrombosis. Regions containing small cirrhotic nodules and accentuation of fibrosis alternate with 'veno-centric' clusters of larger cirrhotic nodules.

spontaneously; they are associated with severe encephalopathy which may respond to embolization therapy.[47,294] Spontaneous splenorenal shunts also occur in patients with cirrhosis or portal vein block.[295,296] Dilated paraumbilical veins form significant collaterals in 11–25% of patients with portal hypertension,[297–299] explaining periumbilical bruits and the rare caput medusa.

Intrapulmonary shunts occur in approximately 20% of patients with cirrhosis or non-cirrhotic portal hypertension,[300] often in association with clubbing and hypoxia. Severe hypoxia is becoming a frequent indication for liver transplantation.[301] The mechanism of the shunts is not certain but they are probably a pulmonary manifestation of the generalized vasodilation found in patients with portal hypertension (see Ch. 2). Pulmonary hypertension occurs in 2% of patients with portal hypertension, with or without cirrhosis.[302] The pulmonary lesion is plexogenic arteriopathy, the result of spasm-induced arterial necrosis that occurs in certain individuals in response to increased pulmonary blood flow (and pressure).[303]

REFERENCES

1. Ballet F. Hepatic circulation: potential for therapeutic intervention. Pharmacol Ther 1990; 47: 281–328
2. Rappaport A M, Wanless I R. Physioanatomic considerations. In: Schiff L, Schiff E R, eds. Diseases of the liver, 7th edn. Philadelphia: J B Lippincott, 1993: pp 1–41
3. Bomzon A, Blendis L M, eds. Cardiovascular complications of liver disease. Boca Raton: CRC Press, 1990
4. Okuda K, Benhamou J P, eds. Portal hypertension. Clinical and physiological aspects. Tokyo: Springer-Verlag, 1991
5. Child C G III. The hepatic circulation and portal hypertension. Philadelphia: W B Saunders, 1954
6. Hunt A H. A contribution to the study of portal hypertension. Edinburgh: Livingstone, 1958
7. Marks C. The portal venous system. Springfield: CC Thomas, 1973
8. Wanless I R. The pathophysiology of non-cirrhotic portal hypertension: a pathologist's perspective. In: Boyer J L, Bianchi L, eds. Falk Symposium 44: Liver cirrhosis. Proceedings of the VIIth International Congress of Liver Diseases. Lancaster: MTP Press, 1987: pp 293–311
9. Williams A O, Johnston G W. Cavernous transformation of the portal vein in rhesus monkeys. J Pathol Bacteriol 1965; 90: 613–618
10. Klemperer P. Cavernous transformation of the portal vein. Its relation to Banti's disease. Arch Pathol Lab Med 1928; 6: 353–377
11. Okuda K, Kono K, Ohnishi K et al. Clinical study of eighty-six cases of idiopathic portal hypertension and comparison with cirrhosis with splenomegaly. Gastroenterology 1984; 86: 600–610
12. Mikkelsen W P, Edmondson H A, Peters R L, Redeker A G, Reynolds T B. Extra- and intrahepatic portal hypertension without cirrhosis (hepatoportal sclerosis). Ann Surg 1965; 162: 602–618
13. Nayak N C. Pathology of noncirrhotic portal fibrosis of India. In: Okuda K, Omata M, eds. Idiopathic portal hypertension. Tokyo: University of Tokyo Press, 1983: pp 37–47
14. Nataf C, Feldmann G, Lebrec D et al. Idiopathic portal hypertension (perisinusoidal fibrosis) after renal transplantation. Gut 1979; 20: 531–537
15. Tandon B N, Lakshminarayanan R, Bhargava S, Nayak N C, Sama S K. Ultrastructure of the liver in non-cirrhotic portal fibrosis with portal hypertension. Gut 1970; 11: 905–910
16. Vidins E I, Britton R S, Medline A, Blendis L M, Israel Y, Orrego H. Sinusoidal calibre in alcoholic and nonalcoholic liver disease: diagnostic and pathogenic implications. Hepatology 1985; 5: 408–414
17. Valla D, Flejou J F, Lebrec D et al. Portal hypertension and ascites in acute hepatitis: clinical, hemodynamic and histological correlations. Hepatology 1989; 10: 482–487
18. Blendis L M, Banks D C, Ramboer C, Williams R. Spleen blood flow and splanchnic haemodynamics in blood dyscrasia and other splenomegalies. Clin Sci 1970; 38: 73–84
19. Grundfest S, Cooperman A M, Ferguson R, Benjamin S. Portal hypertension associated with systemic mastocytosis and splenomegaly. Gastroenterology 1980; 78: 370–373
20. Shaldon S, Sherlock S. Portal hypertension in the myeloproliferative syndrome and the reticuloses. Am J Med 1962; 32: 758–764
21. Wanless I R, Peterson P, Das A, Boitnott J K, Moore G W, Bernier V. Hepatic vascular disease and portal hypertension in polycythemia vera and agnogenic myeloid metaplasia: a clinicopathological study of 145 patients examined at autopsy. Hepatology 1990; 12: 1166–1174
22. Melkebeke P, Vandepitte J, Hannon R, Fevery J. Huge hepatomegaly, jaundice, and portal hypertension due to amyloidosis of the liver. Digestion 1980; 20: 351–357
23. Williams R, Parsonson A, Somers K, Hamilton P J S. Portal hypertension in idiopathic tropical splenomegaly. Lancet 1966; i: 329–333
24. Donovan A J, Reynolds T B, Mikkelsen W P, Peters R L.

Systemic–portal arteriovenous fistulas: pathologic and hemodynamic observations in two patients. Surgery 1969; 66: 474–482

25. Ohnishi K, Saito M, Sato S et al. Portal hemodynamics in idiopathic portal hypertension (Banti's syndrome). Gastroenterology 1987; 92: 751–758

26. Morali G A, Blendis L M. Splenomegaly in portal hypertension: causes and effects. In: Okuda K, Benhamou J P, eds. Portal hypertension. Clinical and physiological aspects. Tokyo: Springer-Verlag, 1991: pp 85–99

27. Douglass B E, Baggenstoss A A, Hollinshead W H. The anatomy of the portal vein and its tributaries. Surg Gynecol Obstet 1950; 91: 562–576

28. Kage M, Arakawa M, Fukuda K, Kojiro M. Pathomorphologic study on the extrahepatic portal vein in idiopathic portal hypertension. Liver 1990; 10: 209–216

29. Doust B, Pearce J. Gray-scale ultrasonic properties of the normal and inflamed pancreas. Radiology 1976; 120: 653–657

30. Webb L J, Sherlock S. The aetiology, presentation and natural history of extrahepatic portal venous obstruction. Q J Med 1979; 48: 627–639

31. Everson R B, Museles M, Henson D E, Grundy G W. Focal nodular hyperplasia of the liver in a child with hemihypertrophy. J Pediat 1976; 88: 985–987

32. Wanless I R, Albrecht S, Bilbao J et al. Multiple focal nodular hyperplasia of the liver associated with vascular malformations of various organs and neoplasia of the brain: a new syndrome. Mod Pathol 1989; 2: 456–462

33. Barton J W III, Keller M S. Liver transplantation for hepatoblastoma in a child with congenital absence of the portal vein. Pediatr Radiol 1989; 20: 113–114

34. Woodle E S, Thistlethwaite J R, Emond J C, Whitington P F, Vogelbach P, Yousefzadeh D K, Broelsch C E. Successful hepatic transplantation in congenital absence of recipient portal vein. Surgery 1990; 107: 475–479

35. Odièvre M, Pige G, Alagille D. Congenital abnormalities associated with extrahepatic portal hypertension. Arch Dis Childh 1977; 52: 383–385

36. Matley P J, Rode H, Cywes S. Portal vein obstruction by ectopic liver tissue. J Pediatr Surg 1989; 24: 1163–1164

37. Ohnishi K, Nakayama T, Saito M et al. Aneurysm of the intrahepatic branch of the portal vein. Report of two cases. Gastroenterology 1984; 86: 169–173

38. Shawker T H, Miller D. The persistent vitelline vein segment. Embryologic and ultrasound features. J Ultrasound Med 1988; 7: 681–685

39. Yamagiwa I, Ohta M, Obata K, Washio M. Case report of biliary atresia associated with preduodenal portal vein, ventricular septal defect and bilobed spleen. Z Kinderchir 1988; 43: 108–109

40. Carmi R, Magee C A, Neill C A, Karrer F M. Extrahepatic biliary atresia and associated anomalies — etiologic heterogeneity suggested by distinctive patterns of associations. Am J Med Genet 1993; 45: 683–693

41. Bullaboy C A, Johnson D H, Azar H, Jennings R B Jr. Total anomalous pulmonary venous connection to portal system: a new therapeutic role for prostaglandin E1? Pediatr Cardiol 1984; 5: 115–116

42. Duff D F, Nihill M R, McNamara D G. Infradiaphragmatic total anomalous pulmonary venous return. Review of clinical and pathological findings and results of operation in 28 cases. Br Heart J 1977; 39: 619–626

43. Chagnon S F, Vallee C A, Barge J, Chevalier L J, Le Gal J, Blery M V. Aneurysmal portahepatic venous fistula: report of two cases. Radiology 1986; 159: 693–695

44. Takayasu K, Moriyama N, Shima Y. Spontaneous portal-hepatic venous shunt via an intrahepatic portal vein aneurysm. Gastroenterology 1984; 86: 945–948

45. Tsukuda M, Yokomizo Y, Shima Y. Intrahepatic portal vein aneurysm with portal-hepatic venous shunt: case report. Acta Radiol Jpn 1988; 48: 304–307

46. Araki T, Ohtomo K, Kachi K et al. Magnetic resonance imaging of macroscopic intrahepatic portal-hepatic venous shunts. Gastrointest Radiol 1991; 16: 221–224

47. Park J H, Cha S H, Han J K, Han M C. Intrahepatic portosystemic venous shunt. Am J Roentgenol 1990; 155: 527–528

48. Mori H, Hayashi K, Fukuda T et al. Intrahepatic portosystemic venous shunt: occurrence in patients with and without liver cirrhosis. Am J Roentgenol 1987; 149: 711–714

49. Ohnishi K, Hatano H, Nakayama T, Kohno K, Okuda K. An unusual portal–systemic shunt, most likely through a patent ductus venosus. A case report. Gastroenterology 1983; 85: 962–965

50. Wanless I R, Lentz J S, Roberts E A. Partial nodular transformation of liver in an adult with persistent ductus venosus. Arch Pathol Lab Med 1985; 109: 427–432

51. Armstrong E L, Adams W L, Tragerman L J, Townsend E W. The Cruveilhier–Baumgarten syndrome: review of the literature and report of two additional cases. Ann Intern Med 1942; 16: 113–149

52. Leger L, Lemaigre G, Richarme J, Chapuis Y. La maladie de Cruveilhier–Baumgarten: cas particulier d'hypertension portale essentielle. Presse Med 1966; 74: 1031–1036

53. Lafortune M, Constantin A, Breton G, Legare A G, Lavoie P. The recanalized umbilical vein in portal hypertension. A myth. Am J Roentgenol 1985; 144: 549–553

54. Valla D, Casadevall N, Huisse M G et al. Etiology of portal vein thrombosis in adults: a prospective evaluation of primary myeloproliferative disorders. Gastroenterology 1988; 94: 1063–1069

55. Pagliuca A, Mufti G J, Janossa-Tahernia M et al. In vitro colony culture and chromosomal studies in hepatic and portal vein thrombosis — possible evidence of an occult myeloproliferative state. Q J Med 1990; 76: 981–989

56. Albacete R A, Matthews M J, Saini N. Portal vein thromboses in malignant hepatoma. Ann Intern Med 1967; 67: 337–348

57. Belli L, Sansalone C V, Aseni P, Romani F, Rondinara G. Portal thrombosis in cirrhosis. A retrospective analysis. Ann Surg 1986; 302: 286–291

58. Okuda K, Ohnishi K, Kimura K et al. Incidence of portal vein thrombosis in liver cirrhosis. An angiographic study of 708 patients. Gastroenterology 1985; 89: 279–286

59. Shimokawa Y et al. C P characteristics of gross anatomy of HCC according to the Nokashima–Okuda classification. Acta Hepatol Jpn 1975; 16: 752

60. Okuda K, Musha H, Yoshida T et al. Demonstration of growing casts of hepatocellular carcinoma in the portal vein by celiac angiography: the thread and streaks sign. Radiology 1975; 117: 303–309

61. Nakashima T, Okuda K, Kojiro M et al. Pathology of hepatocellular carcinoma in Japan. 232 consecutive cases autopsied in ten years. Cancer 1983; 51: 863–877

62. Atri M, de Stempel J, Bret P M, Illescas F F. Incidence of portal vein thrombosis complicating liver metastasis as detected by duplex ultrasound, J Ultrasound Med 1990; 9: 285–289

63. Hunt A H, Whittard B R. Thrombosis of the portal vein in cirrhosis hepatis. Lancet 1954; i: 281–284

64. Sarin S K. Non-cirrhotic portal fibrosis. Gut 1989; 30: 406–415

65. Benhamou J P. Transient portal hypertension. In: Okuda K, Benhamou J P, eds. Portal hypertension. Clinical and physiological aspects. Tokyo: Springer-Verlag, 1991: pp 363–364

66. Knockaert D C, Robaeys G K, Cox E J, Marchal G J. Suppurative pylethrombosis: a changing clinical picture. Gastroenterology 1989; 97: 1028–1030

67. Reynolds W J, Wanless I R. Nodular regenerative hyperplasia of the liver in a patient with rheumatoid vasculitis: a morphometric study suggesting a role for hepatic arteritis in the pathogenesis. J Rheumatol 1984; 11: 838–842

68. Thorne C, Urowitz M, Wanless I R, Roberts E, Blendis L M. Liver disease in Felty's syndrome. Am J Med 1982; 73: 35–40

69. Kuramochi S, Tashiro Y, Torikata C, Watanabe Y. Systemic lupus erythematosus associated with multiple nodular hyperplasia of the liver. Acta Pathol Jpn 1982; 32: 547–560

70. Nakanuma Y, Ohta G, Sasaki K. Nodular regenerative hyperplasia of the liver associated with polyarteritis nodosa. Arch Pathol Lab Med 1984; 108: 133–135

71. Russell M L, Kahn H J. Nodular regenerative hyperplasia of

the liver associated with progressive systemic sclerosis: a case report with ultrastructural observation. J Rheumatol 1983; 10: 748–752

72. Wanless I R, Solt L, Kortan P, Deck J H N, Gardiner G W, Prokipchuk E J. Nodular regenerative hyperplasia of the liver associated with macroglobulinemia: A clue to the pathogenesis. Am J Med 1981; 70: 1203–1209

73. Banti G. Splenomegalie mit Lebercirrhose. Beitr Path Anat 1898; 24: 21–33

74. Nakanuma Y, Ohta G, Doishita K, Maki H. Granulomatous liver disease in the small hepatic and portal veins. Arch Pathol Lab Med 1980; 104: 456–458

75. Berger I, Katz M. Portal hypertension due to hepatic sarcoidosis. Am J Gastroenterol 1973; 59: 147–151

76. Devaney K, Goodman Z D, Epstein M S, Zimmerman H J, Ishak K G. Hepatic sarcoidosis-clinicopathologic features in 100 patients. Am J Surg Pathol 1993; 17: 1272–1280

77. Wanless I R. Understanding non-cirrhotic portal hypertension: menage à foie (editorial). Hepatology 1988; 8: 192–193

78. Shimada H, Nihmoto S, Matsuba A, Nakagawara G. Acute cholangitis: a histopathologic study. J Clin Gastroenterol 1988; 10: 197–200

79. Wanless I R, Geddie W R. Lipogranulomata in liver and spleen: An autopsy series. Arch Pathol Lab Med 1985; 109: 283–286

80. Wanless I R. Micronodular transformation (nodular regenerative hyperplasia) of the liver: a report of 64 cases among 2500 autopsies and a new classification of benign hepatocellular nodules. Hepatology 1990; 11: 787–797

81. Rousselet M C, Kettani S, Rohmer V, Saint-André J P. A case of temporal arteritis with intrahepatic arterial involvement. Pathol Res Pract 1989; 185: 329–331

82. Nakanuma Y, Nonomura A, Hayashi M et al. Pathology of the liver in 'idiopathic portal hypertension' associated with autoimmune disease. The Ministry of Health and Welfare Disorders of Portal Circulation Research Committee. Acta Pathol Jpn 1989; 39: 586–592

83. Murphy J R, Sjogren M H, Kikendall J W, Peura D A, Goodman Z. Small bile duct abnormalities in sarcoidosis. J Clin Gastroenterol 1990; 12: 555–561

84. Homeida M, Ahmed S, Dafalla A, Suliman S, Eltom I, Nash T, Bennett J L. Morbidity associated with Schistosoma mansoni infection as determined by ultrasound: a study in Gezira, Sudan. Am J Trop Med Hyg 1988; 39: 196–201

85. Andrade Z A, Peixoto E, Guerret S, Grimaud J A. Hepatic connective tissue changes in hepatosplenic schistosomiasis. Hum Pathol 1992; 23: 566–573

86. Cheever A W, Andrade Z A. Pathological lesions associated with Schistosoma mansoni infection in man. Trans R Soc Trop Med Hyg 1967; 61: 626–639

87. Nash T E, Cheever A W, Ottesen E A, Cook J A. Schistosome infections in humans: perspectives and recent findings. Ann Intern Med 1982; 97: 740–754

88. Homeida M A, El Tom I, Nash T, Bennett J L. Association of the therapeutic activity of praziquantel with the reversal of Symmers' fibrosis induced by Schistosoma mansoni. Am J Trop Med Hyg 1991; 45: 360–365

89. Doehring-Schwerdtfeger E, Mohamed-Ali G, Abdel-Rahim I M, et al. Sonomorphological abnormalities in Sudanese children with Schistosoma mansoni infection: a proposed staging-system for field diagnosis of periportal fibrosis. Am J Trop Med Hyg 1989; 41: 63–69

90. Fukuda K, Kage M, Arakawa M, Nakashima T. Portal vein or hepatic vein? A curious aberrant vasculature in the liver with idiopathic portal hypertension. Acta Pathol Jpn 1985; 35: 885–897

91. Eckhauser F E, Appelman H D, Knol J A, Strodel W E, Coran AG, Turcotte J G. Noncirrhotic portal hypertension: differing patterns of disease in children and adults. Surgery 1983; 94: 721–728

92. Wanless I R, Bernier V, Seger M. Intrahepatic portal sclerosis in patients without history of liver disease: an autopsy study. Am J Pathol 1982; 106: 63–70

93. Terada T, Hoso M, Nakanuma Y. Development of cavernous

94. vasculatures in livers with hepatocellular carcinoma. An autopsy study. Liver 1989; 9: 172–178

94. Terada T, Ishida F, Nakanuma Y. Vascular plexus around intrahepatic bile ducts in normal livers and portal hypertension. J Hepatol 1989; 8: 139–149

95. Terada T, Hoso M, Nakanuma Y. Microvasculature in the small portal tracts in idiopathic portal hypertension. A morphological comparison with other hepatic diseases. Virchows Archiv (A) 1989; 415: 61–67

96. Horrocks P, Tapp E. Zahn's 'infarcts' of the liver. J Clin Pathol 1966; 19: 475–478

97. Putnam C W, Porter K A, Starzl T E. Hepatic encephalopathy and light and electron micrographic changes of the baboon liver after portal diversion. Ann Surg 1976; 184: 155–161

98. Watanabe M, Umekawa Y, Ueki K, Hirakawa H, Fukumoto S, Shimada Y. Laparoscopic observation of hepatic lobe atrophy. Endoscopy 1989; 21: 234–236

99. Nevens F, Fevery J, Van Steenbergen W, Sciot R, Desmet V, De Groote J. Arsenic and non-cirrhotic portal hypertension. A report of eight cases. J Hepatol 1990; 11: 80–85

100. Labadie H, Stoessel P, Callard P, Beaugrand M. Hepatic venoocclusive disease and perisinusoidal fibrosis secondary to arsenic poisoning. Gastroenterology 1990; 99: 1140–1143

101. Ludwig J, Hashimoto E, McGill D B, van Heerden J A. Classification of hepatic venous outflow obstruction: ambiguous terminology of the Budd–Chiari syndrome. Mayo Clinic Proc 1990; 65: 51–55

102. Valla D, Dhumeaux D, Babany G et al. Hepatic vein thrombosis in paroxysmal nocturnal hemoglobinuria: a spectrum from asymptomatic occlusion of hepatic venules to fatal Budd–Chiari syndrome. Gastroenterology 1987; 93: 569–575

103. Makuuchi M, Hasegawa H, Yamazaki S, Bandai Y, Watanabe G, Ito T. The inferior right hepatic vein: ultrasonic demonstration. Radiology 1983; 148: 213–217

104. Cosgrove D O, Arger P H, Coleman B G. Ultrasonic anatomy of hepatic veins. J Clin Ultrasound 1987; 15: 231–235

105. Mukai J K, Stack C M, Turner D A et al. Imaging of surgically relevant hepatic vascular and segmental anatomy. Part 1. Normal anatomy. Am J Roentgenol 1987; 149: 287–292

106. Takayasu K, Moriyama N, Muramatsu Y et al. Intrahepatic venous collaterals forming via the inferior right hepatic vein in 3 patients with obstruction of the inferior vena cava. Radiology 1985; 154: 323–328

107. Ou Q J, Hermann R E. Hepatic vein ligation and preservation of liver segments in major resections. Arch Surg 1987; 122: 1198–1200

108. Parker R G F. Occlusion of the hepatic veins in man. Medicine 1959; 38: 369–402

109. Gentil-Kocher S, Bernard O, Brunelle et al. Budd–Chiari syndrome in children: report of 22 cases. J Pediatr 1988; 113: 30–38

110. Tavill A S, Wood E J, Creel L, Jones E A, Gregory M, Sherlock S. The Budd–Chiari syndrome. Correlation between hepatic scintigraphy and the clinical, radiological and pathological findings in 19 cases of hepatic venous outflow obstruction. Gastroenterology 1975; 68: 509–518

111. Averbuch M, Aderka D, Winer Z, Levo Y. Budd–Chiari syndrome in Israel: predisposing factors, prognosis, and early identification of high-risk patients. J Clin Gastroenterol 1991; 13: 321–324

112. Mitchell M C, Boitnott J K, Kaufman S, Cameron J L, Maddrey W C. Budd–Chiari syndrome: etiology, diagnosis and management. Medicine 1982; 61: 199–218

113. Bismuth H, Sherlock D J. Portasystemic shunting versus liver transplantation for the Budd–Chiari syndrome. Ann Surg 1991; 214: 581–589

114. Wang Z, Zhu Y, Wang S et al. Recognition and management of Budd–Chiari syndrome. A report of 100 cases. J Vasc Surg 1989; 10: 149–156

115. Millikan W J Jr, Henderson J M, Sewell C W et al. Approach to the spectrum of Budd–Chiari syndrome: which patients require portal decompression? Am J Surg 1985; 149: 167–176

116. Arora A, Tandon N, Sharma M P, Acharya S K. Constrictive

pericarditis masquerading as Budd–Chiari syndrome. J Clin Gastroenterol 1991; 13: 178–181

117. Martin L G, Henderson J M, Millikan W J Jr, Casarella W J, Kaufman S L. Angioplasty for long-term treatment of patients with Budd–Chiari syndrome. Am J Roentgenol 1990; 154: 1007–1010

118. Orloff M J, Girard B. Long term results of treatment of Budd–Chiari syndrome by side to side portacaval shunt. Surg Gynecol Obstet 1989; 168: 33–41

119. Klein A S, Sitzmann J V, Coleman J, Herlong F H, Cameron J L. Current management of the Budd–Chiari syndrome. Ann Surg 1990; 212: 144–149

120. Henderson J M, Warren W D, Millikan W J Jr, Galloway J R, Kawasaki S, Stahl R L, Hertzler G. Surgical options, hematologic evaluation, and pathologic changes in Budd–Chiari syndrome. Am J Surg 1990; 159: 41–50

121. Kage M, Arakawa M, Kojiro M, Okuda K. Histopathology of membranous obstruction of the inferior vena cava in the Budd–Chiari syndrome. Gastroenterology 1992; 102: 2081–2090

122. Asherson R A, Khamashta M A, Hughes G R. The hepatic complications of the antiphospholipid antibodies (editorial). Clin Exp Rheumatol 1991; 9: 341–344

123. Valla D, Casadevall N, Lacombe N et al. Primary myeloproliferative disorders and hepatic vein thrombosis: a prospective study of erythroid colony formation in vitro in 20 patients with Budd–Chiari syndrome. Ann Intern Med 1985; 103: 329–334

124. Campbell D A, Rolles K, Jameson N et al. Hepatic transplantation with perioperative and long term anticoagulation as treatment for Budd–Chiari syndrome. Surg Gynecol Obstet 1988; 166: 511–518

125. Okuda K, Ostrow J D. Clinical conference: Membranous type of Budd–Chiari syndrome. J Clin Gastroenterol 1984; 6: 81–88

126. Khuroo M, Datta D V. Budd–Chiari syndrome following pregnancy. Report of 16 cases, with roentgenologic, hemodynamic and histologic studies of the hepatic outflow tract. Am J Med 1980; 68: 113–121

127. Bhusnurmath S R. Budd–Chiari syndrome. In: Okuda K, ed. 2nd International Conference on Budd–Chiari Syndrome. Kyoto: Annual Report of the Ministry of Health of Japan, 1991: pp 280–293

128. Simson I. Membranous obstruction of the inferior vena cava and hepatocellular carcinoma in South Africa. Gastroenterology 1982; 82: 171–178

129. Wang Z G. Recognition and management of Budd–Chiari syndrome. Experience with 143 patients. Chin Med J 1989; 102: 338–346

130. Chang C H, Lee M C, Shieh M J, Chang J P, Lin P J. Transatrial membranotomy for Budd–Chiari syndrome. Ann Thorac Surg 1989; 48: 409–412

131. Hirooka M, Kimura C. Membranous obstruction of the hepatic portion of the inferior vena cava: surgical correction and etiological study. Arch Surg 1970; 100: 656–663

132. Terabayashi H, Okuda K, Nomura F, Ohnishi K, Wong P. Transformation of inferior vena caval thrombosis to membranous obstruction in a patient with the lupus anticoagulant. Gastroenterology 1986; 91: 219–224

133. Mori H, Hayashi K, Amamoto Y. Membranous obstruction of the inferior vena cava associated with intrahepatic portosystemic shunt. Cardiovasc Intervent Radiol 1986; 9: 209–213

134. Okuda K. Membranous obstruction of the inferior vena cava: etiology and relation to hepatocellular carcinoma. Gastroenterology 1982; 82: 376–379

135. Kew M C, McKnight A, Hodkinson J, Bukofzer S, Esser J D. The role of membranous obstruction of the inferior vena cava in the etiology of hepatocellular carcinoma in Southern African blacks. Hepatology 1989; 9: 121–125

136. Girardin M S, Zafrani E S, Prigent A, Larde D, Chauffour J, Dhumeaux D. Unilobar small hepatic vein obstruction: possible role of progestogen given as oral contraceptive. Gastroenterology 1983; 84: 630–635

137. Leopold J G, Parry T E, Storring F K. A change in the sinusoid-trabecular structure of the liver with hepatic venous outflow block. J Pathol 1970; 100: 87–98

138. de Sousa J M, Portmann B, Williams R. Nodular regenerative hyperplasia of the liver and the Budd–Chiari syndrome. Case report, review of the literature and reappraisal of pathogenesis. J Hepatol 1991; 12: 28–35

139. Castellano G, Canga F, Solis-Herruzo J A, Colina F, Martinez-Montiel M P, Morillas J D. Budd–Chiari syndrome associated with nodular regenerative hyperplasia of the liver. J Clin Gastroenterol 1989; 11: 698–702

139a. Wanless I R. Regenerative nodules in Budd–Chiari syndrome. Hepatology 1994; 19: 1391

140. Bras G, Brandt K H. Vascular disorders. In: MacSween R N M, Anthony P P, Scheuer P J, eds. Pathology of the liver, 2nd edn. Edinburgh: Churchill Livingstone, 1987; pp 478–502

141. Alpert L I. Veno-occlusive disease of the liver associated with oral contraceptives: case report and review of literature. Hum Pathol 1976; 7: 709–718

142. Cameron J L, Herlong H F, Sanfey H et al. The Budd–Chiari syndrome. Treatment by mesenteric-systemic venous shunts. Ann Surg 1983; 198: 335–346

143. Simon D C, Olsen J O. The development of regenerative nodules in Budd–Chiari syndrome demonstrated by liver scan. Clin Nucl Med 1985; 10: 374–375

144. Bras G, Hill K R. Veno-occlusive disease of the liver. Essential pathology. Lancet 1956; ii: 161–163

145. Willmot F C, Robertson G W. Senecio disease, or cirrhosis of the liver due to senecio poisoning. Lancet 1920; ii: 848–849

146. Selzer G, Parker R G F. Senecio poisoning exhibiting as Chiari's syndrome. A report of 12 cases. Am J Pathol 1951; 27: 885–907

147. Bras G, Jelliffe D B, Stuart K L. Veno-occlusive disease of the liver with non-portal type of cirrhosis, occurring in Jamaica. Arch Pathol 1954; 57: 285–300

148. Adami J G. Pictou cattle disease. Montreal Med J 1902; 31: 105–117

149. Cushny A R. On the action of senecio alkaloids and the causation of the hepatic cirrhosis of cattle (Pictou, Molteno, or Winton disease). J Pharmacol Exp Ther 1910–11; 2: 531–548

150. Culvenor C C, Edgar J A, Smith L W, Kumana C R, Lin H J. Heliotropium lasiocarpum Fisch and Mey identified as cause of veno-occlusive disease due to a herbal tea (letter). Lancet 1986; i: 978

151. Bach N, Thung S N, Schaffner F. Comfrey herb tea-induced hepatic veno-occlusive disease. Am J Med 1989; 87: 97–99

152. Smith L W, Culvenor C C J. Plant sources of hepatotoxic pyrrolizidine alkaloids. J Nat Prod 1981; 44: 129–144

153. Shubat P J, Banner W, Huxtable R J. Pulmonary vascular responses induced by the pyrrolizidine alkaloid monocrotaline in rats. Toxicon 1987; 25: 995–1002

154. Hirono I, Mori H, Haga M. Carcinogenic activity of Symphytum officinale. J Nat Cancer Inst 1978; 61: 865–869

155. Tandon B N, Tandon H D, Tandon R K, Narndranathan M, Joshi Y K. An epidemic of veno-occlusive disease of liver in central India. Lancet 1976; ii: 271–272

156. Tandon B N, Joshi Y K, Sud R, Koshy A, Jain S K, Tandon H D. Follow-up of survivors of epidemic veno-occlusive disease in India (letter). Lancet 1984; i: 730

157. Mohabbat O, Younos M S, Merzad A A, Srivastava R N, Sediq G G, Aram G N. An outbreak of hepatic veno-occlusive disease in north-western Afghanistan. Lancet 1976; ii: 269–271

158. McDonald G B, Sharma P, Matthews D E, Shulman H M, Thomas E D. The clinical course of 53 patients with venocclusive disease of the liver after marrow transplantation. Transplantation 1985; 39: 603–608

159. McDonald G, Hinds M S, Fisher L D et al. Veno-occlusive disease of the liver and multiorgan failure after bone marrow transplantation: a cohort study of 355 patients. Ann Intern Med 1993; 118: 255–267

160. Reed G B, Cox A J Jr. The human liver after radiation injury. A form of veno-occlusive disease. Am J Pathol 1966; 48: 597–611

161. Fajardo L F, Colby T V. Pathogenesis of veno-occlusive liver disease after radiation. Arch Pathol Lab Med 1980; 104: 584–588

162. Liano F, Moreno A, Matesanz R et al. Veno-occlusive hepatic

disease of the liver in renal transplantation: is azathioprine the cause? Nephron 1989; 51: 509–516

163. Ceci G, Bella M, Melissari M, Gabrielli M, Bocchi P, Cocconi G. Fatal hepatic vascular toxicity of DTIC. Is it really a rare event? Cancer 1988; 61: 1988–1991

164. Shulman H M, McDonald G B, Matthews D et al. An analysis of hepatic venocclusive disease and centrilobular hepatic degeneration following bone marrow transplantation. Gastroenterology 1980; 79: 1178–1191

165. Avner E D, Ellis D, Jaffe R. Veno-occlusive disease of the liver associated with cysteamine treatment of nephropathic cystinosis. J Pediatr 1983; 102: 793–796

166. D'Cruz C A, Wimmer R S, Harcke H T, Huff D S, Naiman J L. Veno-occlusive disease of the liver in children following chemotherapy for acute myelocytic leukemia. Cancer 1983; 52: 1803–1807

167. Katzka D A, Saul S H, Jorkasky D, Sigal H, Reynolds J C, Soloway R D. Azathioprine and hepatic venocclusive disease in renal transplant patients. Gastroenterology 1986; 90: 446–454

168. Read A E, Wiesner R H, LaBrecque D R et al. Hepatic veno-occlusive disease associated with renal transplantation and azathioprine therapy. Ann Intern Med 1986; 104: 651–655

169. Weitz H, Gokel J M, Loeschke K, Possinger K, Eder M. Veno-occlusive disease of the liver in patients receiving immunosuppressive therapy. Virchows Arch (A) 1982; 395: 245–256

170. Nakhleh R E, Wesen C, Snover D C, Grage T. Venoocclusive lesions of the central veins and portal vein radicles secondary to intraarterial 5-fluoro-2'-deoxyuridine infusion. Hum Pathol 1989; 20: 1218–1220

171. Haboubi N Y, Ali H H, Whitwell H L, Ackrill P. Role of endothelial cell injury in the spectrum of azathioprine-induced liver disease after renal transplant: light microscopy and ultrastructural observations. Am J Gastroenterol 1988; 83: 256–261

172. Mellis C, Bale P M. Familial hepatic veno-occlusive disease with probable immune deficiency. J Pediatr 1976; 88: 236–242

173. Jevtic M M, Thorp F K, Hruban Z. Hereditary tyrosinemia with hyperplasia and hypertrophy of juxtaglomerular apparatus. Am J Clin Pathol 1974; 61: 423–437

174. DeLeve L D, Kaplowitz N. Selective susceptibility of hepatic endothelial cells to dacarbazine toxicity, a model for hepatic veno-occlusive disease. Hepatology 1991; 14: 161A

175. Shulman H M, Luk K, Deeg H J, Shuman W B, Storb R. Induction of hepatic veno-occlusive disease in dogs. Am J Pathol 1987; 126: 114–125

176. Kumana C R, Ng M, Lin H J, Ko W, Wu P C, Todd D. Hepatic veno-occlusive disease due to toxic alkaloid herbal tea (letter). Lancet 1983; ii: 1360–1361

177. Eisenhauer T, Hartmann H, Rumpf K W, Helmchen U, Scheler F, Creutzfeldt W. Favourable outcome of hepatic veno-occlusive disease in a renal transplant patient receiving azathioprine, treated by portacaval shunt. Report of a case and review of the literature. Digestion 1984; 30: 185–190

178. Murray J A, LaBrecque D R, Gingrich R D, Pringle K C, Mitros F A. Successful treatment of hepatic venocclusive disease in a bone marrow transplant patient with side-to-side portacaval shunt. Gastroenterology 1987; 92: 1073–1077

179. Shulman H M, Gown A M, Nugent D J. Hepatic veno-occlusive disease after bone marrow transplantation: immunohistochemical identification of the material within occluded central venules. Am J Pathol 1987; 127: 549–558

180. Burkhardt A, Klöppel G. Unusual obliterative disease of the hepatic veins in an infant. Virchows Arch (A) 1977; 375: 225–232

181. Snover D C, Weisdorf S, Bloomer J, McGlave P, Weisdorf D. Nodular regenerative hyperplasia of the liver following bone marrow transplantation. Hepatology 1989; 9: 443–448

182. Goodman Z D, Ishak K G. Occlusive venous lesions in alcoholic liver disease: a study of 200 cases. Gastroenterology 1982; 83: 786–796

183. Burt A D, MacSween R N M. Hepatic vein lesions in alcoholic liver disease: retrospective biopsy and necropsy study. J Clin Pathol 1986; 39: 63–67

184. Nakanuma Y, Ohta G, Doishita K. Quantitation and serial section observations of focal veno-occlusive lesions of hepatic veins in liver cirrhosis. Virchows Arch (A) 1985; 405: 429–38

185. Russi E W, Bansky G, Pfaltz M, Spinas G, Hammer B, Senning A. Budd–Chiari syndrome in sarcoidosis. Am J Gastroenterol 1986; 81: 71–75

186. Young I D, Clark R N, Manley P N, Groll A, Simon J B. Response to steroids in Budd–Chiari syndrome caused by idiopathic granulomatous venulitis. Gastroenterology 1988; 94: 503–507

187. Hoagland M H, Zinkham W H, Hutchins G M. Generalized venocentric lesions in the virus-associated hemophagocytic syndrome. Hum Pathol 1986; 17: 195–198

188. McGuire R F, Bissell D M, Boyles J, Roll F J. Role of extracellular matrix in regulating fenestrations of sinusoidal endothelial cells isolated from normal rat liver. Hepatology 1992; 15: 989–997

189. De Leeuw A M, Brouwer A, Knook D L. Sinusoidal endothelial cells of the liver: fine structure and function in relation to age. J Electron Microsc Tech 1990; 14: 218–236

190. Bernuau D, Guillot R et al. Ultrastructural aspects of the liver perisinusoidal space in diabetic patients with and without microangiopathy. Diabetes 1982; 31: 1061–1067

191. Babbs C, Haboubi N Y, Mellor J M, Smith A, Rowan B P, Warnes T W. Endothelial cell transformation in primary biliary cirrhosis: a morphological and biochemical study. Hepatology 1990; 11: 723–729

192. Wanless I R. The cellular distribution of vitamin A in the liver. Liver 1983; 3: 403–409

193. Taguchi K, Asano G. Neovascularization of pericellular fibrosis in alcoholic liver disease. Acta Pathol Jpn 1988; 38: 615–626

194. Tsui M S, Burroughs A, McCormick P A, Scheuer P J. Portal hypertension and hepatic sinusoidal Ulex lectin binding. J Hepatol 1990; 10: 244–250

195. Schaffner F, Popper H. Capillarization of hepatic sinusoids in man. Gastroenterology 1963; 44: 239–242

196. Nagore N, Scheuer P J. Does a linear pattern of sinusoidal IgA deposition distinguish between alcoholic and diabetic liver disease? Liver 1988; 8: 281–286

197. Falchuk K R, Fiske S C, Haggitt R C, Federman M, Trey C. Pericentral hepatic fibrosis and intracellular hyalin in diabetes mellitus. Gastroenterology 1980; 78: 535–541

198. Le Bail B, Bioulac-Sage P, Senuita R, Quinton A, Saric J, Balabaud C. Fine structure of hepatic sinusoids and sinusoidal cells in disease. J Electron Microsc Tech 1990; 14: 257–282

199. Latry P, Bioulac-Sage P, Echinard E et al. Perisinusoidal fibrosis and basement membrane-like material in the livers of diabetic patients. Hum Pathol 1987; 18: 775–780

200. Zafrani E S, Bernuau D, Feldmann G. Peliosis-like ultrastructural changes of the hepatic sinusoids in human chronic hypervitaminosis A: report of 3 cases. Hum Pathol 1984; 15: 1166–1170

201. Russell R M, Boyer J L, Bagheri S A, Hruban Z. Hepatic injury from chronic hypervitaminosis A resulting in portal hypertension and ascites. N Engl J Med 1974; 291: 435–440

202. Bioulac-Sage P, Quinton A, Saric J, Grimaud J A, Mourey M S, Balabaud C. Chance discovery of hepatic fibrosis in patient with asymptomatic hypervitaminosis A. Arch Pathol Lab Med 1988; 112: 505–509

203. Kanel G C, Ucci A A, Kaplan M M, Wolfe H J. A distinctive perivenular hepatic lesion associated with heart failure. Am J Clin Pathol 1980; 73: 235–239

204. Klatt E C, Koss M N, Young T S, Macauley L, Martin S E. Hepatic hyaline globules associated with passive congestion. Arch Pathol Lab Med 1988; 112: 510–513

205. Holdstock G, Millward-Sadler G H. Hepatic changes in systemic disease. In: Wright R, Alberti K G M M, Karran S, Millward-Sadler G H, eds. Liver and biliary disease. London: W B Saunders, 1979: p 862

206. Steiner P E. Nodular regenerative hyperplasia of the liver. Am J Pathol 1959; 35: 943–953

207. Bruguera M, Aranguibel F, Ros E, Rodés J. Incidence and clinical significance of sinusoidal dilatation in liver biopsies. Gastroenterology 1978; 75: 474–478

208. Welch K, Finkbeiner W, Alpers C E et al. Autopsy findings in the acquired immune deficiency syndrome. JAMA 1984; 252: 1152–1159

209. Delpre G, Ilic B, Papo J, Streifler C, Gefel A. Hypernephroma with nonmetastatic liver dysfunction (Stauffer syndrome) and hypercalcemia. Am J Gastroenterol 1979; 72: 239–247

210. Aoyagi T, Mori I, Ueyama Y, Tamaoki N. Sinusoidal dilatation of the liver as a paraneoplastic manifestation of renal cell carcinoma. Hum Pathol 1989; 20: 1193–1197

211. Bain B J, Coghlan S J, Chong K C, Roberts S J. Hepatic sinusoidal ectasia in association with Hodgkin's disease. Postgrad Med J 1982; 58: 182–184

212. Winckler K, Poulsen H. Liver disease with periportal sinusoidal dilatation. A possible complication to contraceptive steroids. Scand J Gastroenterol 1975; 10; 699–704

213. Spellberg M A, Mirro J, Chowdhury L. Hepatic sinusoidal dilatation related to oral contraceptives. Am J Gastroenterol 1979; 72: 248–252

214. Balazs M. Sinusoidal dilatation of the liver in patients on oral contraceptives. Electron microscopical study of 14 cases. Exp Pathol 1988; 35: 231–237

215. Bauer T W, Moore G W, Hutchins G M. The liver in sickle cell disease: a clinicopathologic study of 70 patients. Am J Med 1980; 69: 833–837

216. Omata M, Johnson C S, Tong M, Tatter D. Pathological spectrum of liver diseases in sickle cell diseases. Dig Dis Sci 1986; 31: 247–256

217. Mills L R, Mwakyusa D, Milner P F. Histopathologic features of liver biopsy specimens in sickle cell disease. Arch Pathol Lab Med 1988; 112: 290–294

218. Zak F G. Peliosis hepatis. Am J Pathol 1950; 26: 1–15

219. Zafrani E S. An additional argument for a toxic mechanism of peliosis hepatis in man. Hepatology 1990; 11; 322–323

220. Yanoff M, Rawson A J. Peliosis hepatis. An anatomic study with demonstration of two varieties. Arch Pathol 1964; 77: 159–165

221. Wold L E, Ludwig J. Peliosis hepatis: two morphologic variants? Hum Pathol 1981; 12; 388–389

222. Simon D M, Krause R, Galambos J T. Peliosis hepatis in a patient with marasmus. Gastroenterology 1988; 95: 805–809

223. Zafrani E S, Degos F, Guigui B et al. The hepatic sinusoid in hairy cell leukemia. An ultrastructural study of 12 cases. Hum Pathol 1987; 18: 801–807

224. Furata M, Asmaoto H, Kitachi M. A case of peliosis hepatis appearing in a patient with lepromatous leprosy. Nippon Rai Gakkai Zasshi 1982; 51: 22–27

225. Delas N, Faurel J P, Wechsler B, Adotti F, Leroy D, Lemerez M. Association of peliosis and necrotizing vasculitis (letter). Nouv Presse Med 1982; 11; 2787

226. Scoazec J Y, Marche C, Girard P M et al. Peliosis hepatis and sinusoidal dilation during infection by the human immunodeficiency virus (HIV). An ultrastructural study. Am J Pathol 1988; 131: 38–47

227. Larrey D, Freneaux E, Berson A et al. Peliosis hepatis induced by 6-thioguanine administration. Gut 1988; 29: 1265–1269

228. Degott C, Rueff B, Kreis H, DuBoust A, Potet F, Benhamou J P. Peliosis hepatis in recipients of renal transplants. Gut 1978; 19: 748–753

229. Scheuer P J, Schachter L A, Mathur S, Burroughs A K, Rolles K. Peliosis hepatitis after liver transplantation. J Clin Pathol 1990; 43: 1036–1037

230. Czapar C A, Weldon-Linne C M, Moore D M, Rhone D P. Peliosis hepatis in the acquired immunodeficiency syndrome. Arch Pathol Lab Med 1986; 110: 611–613

231. Perkocha L A, Geaghan S M, Yen T S B et al. Clinical and pathological features of bacillary peliosis hepatis in association with human immunodeficiency virus infection. N Engl J Med 1990; 323: 1581–1586

232. Bhaskar K V S, Joshi K, Banerjee C K, Rao R K S, Verma S C. Peliosis hepatis in Hodgkin's disease: an infrequent association (letter). Am J Gastroenterol 1990; 85: 628–629

233. Cadranel J F, Cadranel J, Buffet C et al. Nodular regenerative hyperplasia of the liver, peliosis hepatis, and perisinusoidal fibrosis. Association with angioimmunoblastic lymphadenopathy and severe hypoxemia. Gastroenterology 1990; 99; 268–273

234. Lioté F, Yeni P, Teillet-Thiebaud F et al. Ascites revealing peritoneal and hepatic extramedullary hematopoiesis with peliosis in agnogenic myeloid metaplasia: case report and review of the literature. Am J Med 1991; 90: 111–117

235. Voinchet O, Degott C, Scoazec J Y, Feldmann G, Benhamou J P. Peliosis hepatis, nodular regenerative hyperplasia of the liver, and light-chain deposition in a patient with Waldenstrom's macroglobulinemia. Gastroenterology 1988; 95: 482–486

236. Thomas L B, Popper H, Berk P D, Selikoff I, Falk H. Vinyl-chloride-induced liver disease. From idiopathic portal hypertension (Banti's syndrome) to angiosarcoma. N Engl J Med 1975; 292: 17–22

237. Hayward S R, Lucas C E, Ledgerwood A M. Recurrent spontaneous intrahepatic hemorrhage from peliosis hepatis. Arch Surg 1991; 126: 782–783

238. Kubosawa H, Konno A, Komatsu T, Ishige H, Kondo Y. Peliosis hepatis. An unusual case involving the spleen and lymph nodes. Acta Pathol Jpn 1989; 39: 212–215

239. Chawla S K, Patel H D, Mahadevia S D, LoPresti P A. Portal hypertension in peliosis hepatis: report of the first case. Am J Proctol Gastroenterol Colon Rect Surg 1980; 31: 11–17

240. Yanagisawa N, Sugaya H, Yunomura K, Harada T, Hisauchi T. A case of idiopathic portal hypertension after renal transplantation. Gastroenterol Jpn 1990; 25: 643–648

241. Fonseca V, Havard C W. Portal hypertension secondary to azathioprine in myasthenia gravis. Postgrad Med J 1988; 64: 950–952

242. Olsen T S, Fjeldborg O, Hansen H E. Portal hypertension without liver cirrhosis in renal transplant recipients. APMIS Suppl 1991; 23: 13–20

243. Buck F S, Koss M N. Hepatic amyloidosis: morphologic differences between systemic AL and AA types. Hum Pathol 1991; 22: 904–907

244. French S W, Schloss G T, Stillwan A E. Unusual amyloid bodies in human liver. Am J Clin Pathol 1981; 75: 400–402

245. Looi L M, Sumithran E. Morphologic differences in the pattern of liver infiltration between systemic AL and AA amyloidosis. Hum Pathol 1988; 19: 732–735

246. Rubinow A, Koff R S, Cohen A S. Severe intrahepatic cholestasis in primary amyloidosis: a report of four cases and a review of the literature. Am J Med 1978; 64: 937–946

247. Faa G, Van Eyken P, De Vos R et al. Groote J, Desmet V J. Light chain deposition disease of the liver associated with AL-type amyloidosis and severe cholestasis. J Hepatol 1991; 12: 75–82

248. Pereira A, Bruguera M, Cervantes F, Rozman C. Liver involvement at diagnosis of primary myelofibrosis: a clinicopathological study of twenty-two cases. Eur J Haematol 1988; 40: 355–361

249. Inam S, Sidki K, al-Marshedy A R, Judzewitsch R. Addison's disease, hypertension, renal and hepatic microthrombosis in 'primary' antiphospholipid syndrome. Postgrad Med J 1991; 67: 385–388

250. Kakizoe S, Yanaga K, Starzl T E, Demetris A J. Evaluation of protocol before transplantation and after reperfusion biopsies from human orthotopic liver allografts: considerations of preservation and early immunological injury. Hepatology 1990; 11: 932–941

251. McKeown C M, Edwards V, Phillips M J, Harvey P R, Petrunka C N, Strasberg S M. Sinusoidal lining cell damage: the critical injury in cold preservation of liver allografts in the rat. Transplanatation 1988; 46: 178–191

252. Michels N A. Newer anatomy of liver—variant blood supply and collateral circulation. JAMA 1960; 172: 125–132

252a Netter F H. Ciba collections of medical illustrations, vol 3. Digestive system, part III: Liver, biliary tract and pancreas. New York: Colorpress, 1964

253. Halasz N A. Cholecystectomy and hepatic artery injuries. Arch Surg 1991; 126: 137–138

254. Van Way C W, Crane J M, Riddell D H, Foster J H. Arteriovenous fistula in the portal circulation. Surgery 1971; 70: 876–890

255. Brohée D, Franken P, Fievez M, Baudoux M et al. High-output right ventricular failure secondary to hepatic arteriovenous microfistulae. Selective arterial embolization treatment. Arch Intern Med 1984; 144: 1282–1284

256. Danchin N, Thisse J Y, Neimann J L, Faivre G. Osler–Weber–Rendu disease with multiple intraheptic arteriovenous fistulas. Am Heart J 1983; 105: 856–859

257. Liu G, Butany J, Wanless I R, Cameron R, Greig P, Levy G. The vascular pathology of human hepatic allografts. Hum Pathol 1993; 24: 182–188

258. Hocking W G, Lasser K, Ungerer R, Bersohn M, Palos M, Spiegel T. Spontaneous hepatic rupture in rheumatoid arthritis. Arch Intern Med 1981; 141: 792–794

259. Hashimoto E, Ludwig J, MacCarty R L, Dickson E R, Krom R A. Hepatoportal arteriovenous fistula: morphologic features studied after orthotopic liver transplantation. Hum Pathol 1989; 20: 707–709

260. Parangi S, Oz M C, Blume R S et al. Hepatobiliary complications of polyarteritis nodosa. Arch Surg 1991; 126: 909–912

261. Haratake J, Horie A, Furuta A, Yamato H. Massive hepatic infarction associated with polyarteritis nodosa. Acta Pathol Jpn 1988; 38: 89–93

262. Doppman J L, Dunnick N R, Girton M, Fauci A S, Popovsky M A. Bile duct cysts secondary to liver infarcts: report of a case and experimental production by small vessel hepatic artery occlusion. Radiology 1979; 130: 1–5

263. Song H Y, Choi K C, Park J H, Choi B I, Chung Y S. Radiological evaluation of hepatic artery aneurysms. Gastrointest Radiol 1989; 14: 329–333

264. Rankin R N, Vellet D A. Portobiliary fistula: occurrence and treatment. Can Assoc Radiol J 1991; 42: 55–59

265. Okuda K, Musha H, Nakajima Y et al. Frequency of intrahepatic arteriovenous fistula as a sequela to percutaneous needle puncture of the liver. Gastroenterology 1978; 74: 1204–1207

266. Wooling K R, Baggenstoss A H, Weir J F. Infarction of the liver. Gastroenterology 1951; 17: 479–493

267. Brittain R S, Marchioro T L, Hermann G, Waddell W, Starzl T E. Accidental hepatic artery ligation in humans. Am J Surg 1964; 107: 822–832

268. Chen V, Hamilton J, Qizilbash A. Hepatic infarction. Arch Pathol Lab Med 1976; 100: 32–36

268a. Saegusa M, Takano Y, Okudaira M. Human hepatic infarction: histopathological and postmortem angiological studies. Liver 1993; 13: 239

269. Arcidi J M Jr, Moore G W, Hutchins G M. Hepatic morphology in cardiac dysfunction. A clinicopathologic study of 1000 subjects at autopsy. Am J Pathol 1981; 104: 159–166

270. Bynum T E, Boitnott J K, Maddrey W C. Ischemic hepatitis. Dig Dis Sci 1979; 24: 129–135

271. Shibuya A, Unuma T, Sugimoto T et al. Diffuse hepatic calcification as a sequela to shock liver. Gastroenterology 1985; 89: 196–201

272. Wanless I R, Dore S, Gopinath N et al. Histopathology of cocaine hepatotoxicity: report of four patients. Gastroenterology 1990; 98: 497–501

273. Dammann H G, Hagemann J, Runge M, Kloppel G. In vivo diagnosis of massive hepatic infarction by computed tomography. Dig Dis Sci 1982; 27: 73–79

274. Stromeyer F W, Ishak K G. Nodular transformation (nodular 'regenerative' hyperplasia) of the liver. Hum Pathol 1981; 12: 60–71

275. Lui A F K, Hiratzka L F, Hirose F M. Multiple adenomas of the liver. Cancer 1980; 45: 1001–1004

275a. Lautt W W, Legare D J, Daniels T R. The comparative effect of administration of substances via the hepatic artery or portal vein on hepatic arterial resistance, liver blood volume and hepatic extraction in cats. Hepatology 1984; 4: 927–932

276. Nakanuma Y. Nodular regenerative hyperplasia of the liver: retrospective survey in autopsy series. J Clin Gastroenterol 1990; 12: 460–465

277. Sherlock S, Feldman C A, Moran B, Scheuer P J. Partial nodular transformation of the liver with portal hypertension. Am J Med 1966; 40: 195–203

278. Wanless I R, Wong F, Greig P, Blendis L M, Levy G, Heathcote E J. Hepatic vein thrombosis occurring in the cirrhotic liver: prevalence and significance for the pathogenesis of cirrhosis. Hepatology 1993; 18: 112A

279. Rubin E, Krus S, Popper H. Pathogenesis of postnecrotic cirrhosis in alcoholics. Arch Pathol 1962; 73: 288–299

280. Benz E J, Baggenstoss A H, Wollaeger E E. Atrophy of the left lobe of the liver. Arch Pathol 1950; 42; 315–330

281. Lehmann H, Kaiserling E, Schlaak M. Left hepatic lobe atrophy and partial Budd–Chiari syndrome in a patient with alcoholic liver cirrhosis. Hepatogastroenterology 1982; 29: 3–5

282. Janev S. Abnormalities of the site of the stomach in agenesis or hypoplasia of the left lobe of the liver. Radiol Diagn 1977; 18: 487–492

283. Qizilbash A, Kontozoglou T, Sianos J, Scully K. Hepar lobatum associated with chemotherapy and metastatic breast cancer. Arch Pathol Lab Med 1987; 111: 58–61

283a. Hadjis N S, Blumgart L H. Clinical aspects of liver atrophy. J Clin Gastroenterol 1989; 11: 3–7

284. Wanless I R, Mawdsley C, Adams R. On the pathogenesis of focal nodular hyperplasia of the liver. Hepatology 1985; 5: 1194–1200

285. Wanless I R, Gryfe A. Nodular transformation of the liver in hereditary hemorrhagic telangiectasia. Arch Pathol Lab Med 1986; 110: 331–335

286. Ndimbie O K, Goodman Z D, Chase R L, Ma C K, Lee M W. Hemangiomas with localized nodular proliferation of the liver. A suggestion on the pathogenesis of focal nodular hyperplasia. Am J Surg Pathol 1990; 14: 142–150

287. Karvountzis G G, Redeker A G, Peters R L. Long term follow-up studies of patients surviving fulminant viral hepatitis. Gastroenterology 1974; 67: 870–877

288. Wanless I R. An hypothesis for the pathogenesis of cirrhosis based on vascular pathology of liver in pre-cirrhotic states. Mod Pathol 1994; 7: 136A

289. McClain C, Hill D, Schmidt J, Diehl A M. Cytokines and alcoholic liver disease. Semin Liver Dis 1993; 13: 170–182

290. Ohtomo K, Baron R L, Dodd G D et al. Confluent hepatic fibrosis in advanced cirrhosis—appearance at CT. Radiology 1993; 188: 31–35

291. Popper H. Pathologic aspects of cirrhosis. Am J Pathol 1977; 87: 228–264

292. Ohnishi K, Chin N, Sugita S et al. Quantitative aspects of portal–systemic and arteriovenous shunts within the liver in cirrhosis. Gastroenterology 1987; 93: 129–134

293. Ohnishi K, Chin N, Saito M et al. Portographic opacification of hepatic veins and (anomalous) anastomoses between the portal and hepatic veins in cirrhosis—indication of extensive intrahepatic shunts. Am J Gastroenterol 1986; 81: 975–978

294. Horiguchi Y, Kitano T, Imai H et al. Intrahepatic portal-systemic shunt: its etiology and diagnosis. Gastroenterol Jpn 1987; 22: 496–502

295. Dilawari J B, Raju G S, Chawla Y K. Development of large splenoadrenorenal shunt after endoscopic sclerotherapy. Gastroenterology 1989; 97: 421–426

296. Dilawari J B, Chawla Y K. Spontaneous (natural) splenoadrenorenal shunts in extrahepatic portal venous obstruction: a series of 20 cases. Gut 1987; 28: 1198–1200

297. Burcharth F. Percutaneous transhepatic portography. I. Technique and application. Am J Roentgenol 1979; 132: 177–182

298. Schabel S I, Rittenberg G M, Javid L H, Cunningham J, Ross P. The 'bull's-eye' falciform ligament: a sonographic finding of portal hypertension. Radiology 1980; 136: 157–159

299. Okuda K, Matsutani S. Portal–systemic collaterals: anatomy and clinical implications. In: Okuda K, Benhamou J P, eds. Portal hypertension. Clinical and physiological aspects. Tokyo: Springer-Verlag, 1991: pp 51–62

300. Krowka J K. Hepatopulmonary syndrome: an evolving perspective in the era of liver transplantation. Hepatology 1990; 11: 138–142

301. Krowka M J. Hepatopulmonary syndrome. Transplant Proc 1993; 25: 1746–1747

302. Hadengue A, Lebrec D, Benhamou J-P. Pulmonary arterial hypertension in patients with portal hypertension. In: Okuda K, Benhamou J-P, eds. Portal hypertension. Clinical and physiological aspects. Tokyo: Springer-Verlag, 1991: pp 401–411

303. Wanless I R. Coexistent pulmonary and portal hypertension: Yin and Yang. Hepatology 1989; 10: 255–257

304. Simonds J P. Chronic occlusion of the portal vein. Arch Surg 1936; 33: 397–424

305. McDermott W V, Bothe A, Clouse M E, Bern M M. Noncirrhotic portal hypertension in adults. Am J Surg 1981; 141: 514–518

306. Thompson E N, Sherlock S. The aetiology of portal vein thrombosis with particular reference to the role of infection and exchange transfusion. Q J Med 1964; 33: 465–480

307. Capron J P, Lemay J L, Muir J F, Dupas J L, Lebrec D, Gineston J L. Portal vein thrombosis and fatal pulmonary thromboembolism associated with oral contraceptive treatment. J Clin Gastroenterol 1981; 3: 295–298

308. Orozco H, Guraieb E, Takahashi T et al. Deficiency of protein C in patients with portal vein thrombosis. Hepatology 1988; 8: 1110–1111

309. Odegard Q R, Abildgaard U. Antifactor Xa activity in thrombophilia. Studies in a family with AT-III deficiency. Scand J Haematol 1977; 18: 86–90

310. Chang H P, McFadzean A J S. Thrombosis and intimal thickening in the portal system in cirrhosis of the liver. J Pathol Bacteriol 1965; 89: 473–480

311. Die Goyanes A, Pack G T, Bowden L. Cancer of the body and tail of the pancreas. Rev Surg 1971; 28: 153–175

312. McDermott W V Jr. Portal hypertension secondary to pancreatic disease. Ann Surg 1960; 152: 147–150

313. Bilbao J I, Rodriguez-Cabello J, Longo J, Zornoza G, Paramo J, Lecumberri F J. Portal thrombosis: percutaneous transhepatic treatment with urokinase—a case report. Gastrointest Radiol 1989; 14: 326–328

314. Lin C S. Suppurative pylephlebitis and liver abscess complicating colonic diverticulitis: report of two cases and review of literature. Mt Sinai J Med 1973; 40: 48–55

315. Slovis T L, Haller J O, Cohen H L, Berdon W E, Watts F B Jr. Complicated appendiceal inflammatory disease in children: pylephlebitis and liver abscess. Radiology 1989; 171: 823–825

316. Whipple A O. The problem of portal hypertension in relation to the hepatosplenopathies. Ann Surg 1945; 122: 449–475

317. Maddrey W C, Sen Gupta K P, Basu Mallik K C, Iber F L, Basu A K. Extrahepatic obstruction of the portal venous system. Surg Gynecol Obstet 1968; 127: 989–998

318. Lauridsen U B, Enk B, Gammeltoft A. Oesophageal varices as a late complication to neonatal umbilical vein catheterization. Acta Paediatr Scand 1978; 67: 633–636

319. Hunter G C, Steinkirchner T, Burbige E J, Guernsey J M, Putnam C W. Venous complications of sclerotherapy for esophageal varices. Am J Surg 1988; 156: 497–501

320. Thatcher B S, Sivak M V, Ferguson D R, Petras R E. Mesenteric venous thrombosis as a possible complication of endoscopic sclerotherapy. Am J Gastroenterol 1986; 81: 126–129

321. Talbot R W, Heppell J, Dozois R R, Baert R W Jr. Vascular complications of inflammatory bowel disease. Mayo Clin Proc 1986; 61: 140–145

322. Capron J P, Remond A, Lebrec D, Delamarre J, Dupas J L, Lorriaux A. Gastrointestinal bleeding due to chronic portal vein thrombosis in ulcerative colitis. Dig Dis Sci 1979; 24: 232–235

323. Aronson A R, Steinheber F U. Portal vein thrombosis in ulcerative colitis. N Y State J Med 1971; 71: 2310–2311

324. Leibowitz A I, Hartmann R C. The Budd-Chiari syndrome and paroxysmal nocturnal haemoglobinuria. Br J Haematol 1981; 48: 1–6

325. Riccio J A, Colley A T, Cera P J. Hepatic vein thrombosis (Budd-Chiari syndrome) in the microgranular variant of acute promyelocytic leukemia. Am J Clin Pathol 1989; 92: 366–371

326. Chillar R K, Paladugu R R. Hepatic vein thrombosis (acute Budd-Chiari syndrome) in acute leukemia. Am J Med Sci 1981; 282: 153–156

327. Lewis J H, Tice H L, Zimmerman H J. Budd-Chiari syndrome associated with oral contraceptive steroids. Review of treatment of 47 cases. Dig Dis Sci 1983; 28: 673–683

328. Maddrey W C. Hepatic vein thrombosis (Budd–Chiari syndrome): possible association with the use of oral contraceptives. Semin Liver Dis 1987; 7: 32–39

329. Valla D, Le G M, Poynard T, Zucman N, Rueff B, Benhamou J P. Risk of hepatic vein thrombosis in relation to recent use of oral contraceptive: a case–control study. Gastroenterology 1986; 90: 807–811

330. Pomeroy C, Knodell R G, Swaim W R, Arneson P, Mahowald M L. Budd-Chiari syndrome in a patient with the lupus anticoagulant. Gastroenterology 1984; 86: 158–161

331. Asherson R A, Thompson R P, MacLachlan N, Baguley E, Hicks P, Hughes G R. Budd–Chiari syndrome, visceral arterial occlusions, recurrent fetal loss and the 'lupus anticoagulant' in systemic lupus erythematosus. J Rheumatol 1989; 16: 219–224

332. Farrant J M, Judge M, Thompson R P. Thrombotic cutaneous nodules and hepatic vein thrombosis in the anticardiolipin syndrome. Clin Exp Dermatol 1989; 14: 306–308

333. Nakamura H, Uehara H, Okada T et al. Occlusion of small hepatic veins associated with systemic lupus erythematosus with the lupus anticoagulant and anti-cardiolipin antibody. Hepato-gastroenterology 1989; 36: 393–397

334. Couffinhal T, Bonnet J, Benchimol D, Dos Santos P, Besse P, Bricaud H. A case of the Budd–Chiari syndrome attributed to a deficit in protein C. Eur Heart J 1991; 12: 266–269

335. Das M, Carroll S. Antithrombin III deficiency: an etiology of Budd–Chiari syndrome. Surgery 1985; 97: 242–245

336. McClure S, Dincsoy H P, Glueck H. Budd–Chiari syndrome and antithrombin III deficiency. Am J Clin Pathol 1982; 78: 236–241

337. Correa de Araujo R, Bestetti R B, Oliveira J S M. An unusual case of Budd–Chiari syndrome—a case report. Angiology 1988; 39: 193–198

338. Lorenzo M J, Gual Corts M, Morato Griera J. The syndrome of Budd–Chiari associated with constrictive pericarditis and complete thrombosis of the inferior vena cava. Rev Clin Esp 1979; 152: 407–410

339. Paul O, Castleman B, White P D. Chronic constrictive pericarditis: a study of 53 cases. Am J Med Sci 1948; 216: 361–377

340. Fonkalsrud E W, Linde L M, Longmire W P J. Portal hypertension from idiopathic superior vena caval obstruction. JAMA 1966; 196: 115–118

341. Feingold M L, Litwak R L, Geller S S, Baron M M. Budd–Chiari syndrome caused by a right atrial tumor. Arch Intern Med 1971; 127: 292–295

342. Sty J R. Ultrasonography: hepatic vein thrombosis in sickle cell anemia. Am J Pediatr Hematol–Oncol 1982; 4: 213–215

343. Reynolds T B. Budd–Chiari syndrome. In: Schiff L, Schiff E R, eds. Diseases of the Liver, 7th edn. Philadelphia: JB Lippincott, 1993; pp 1091–1098

344. Fortner J G, Kallum B O, Kim D K. Surgical management of hepatic vein occlusion by tumor. Arch Surg 1977; 112: 727–728

345. Spapen H D, Volckaert A, Bourgain C, Braeckman J, Van Belle S J. Acute Budd–Chiari syndrome with portosystemic encephalopathy as first sign of renal carcinoma. Br J Urol 1988; 62: 274–275

346. Carbonnel F, Valla D, Menu Y et al. Acute Budd–Chiari syndrome as first manifestation of adrenocortical carcinoma. J Clin Gastroenterol 1988; 10: 441–444

347. Jose B, Narayan P I, Pietsch J B et al. Budd–Chiari syndrome secondary to hepatic vein thrombus from Wilm's tumor. Case report and literature review. J Ky Med Assoc 1989; 87: 174–176

348. Kinmond S, Carter R, Skeoch C H, Morton N S. Nephroblastoma presenting with acute hepatic encephalopathy. Arch Dis Child 1990; 65: 542–543

349. Imakita M, Yutani C, Ishibashi-Ueda H, Hiraoka H, Naito H. Primary leiomyosarcoma of the inferior vena cava with Budd–Chiari syndrome. Acta Pathol Jpn 1989; 39: 73–77

350. Lee P K, Teixeira O H, Simons J A et al. Atypical hepatic vein leiomyoma extending into the right atrium: an unusual cause of the Budd–Chiari syndrome. Can J Cardiol 1990; 6: 107–110

351. Pollanen M, Butany J, Chiasson D. Leiomyosarcoma of the inferior vena cava. Arch Pathol Lab Med 1987; 111: 1085–1087

352. Koshy A, Bhusnurmath S R, Mitra S K, Mahajan K K, Datta D V, Aikat B K, Bhagwat A G. Hydatid disease associated with hepatic outflow tract obstruction. Am J Gastroenterol 1980; 74: 274–278

353. Aikat B K, Bhusnurmath S R, Chhuttani P N, Datta D V. Hepatic vein obstruction—a retrospective analysis of 72 autopsies and biopsies. Ind J Med Res 1978; 67: 128–144

354. Nicoloff D M, Fortuny I E, Pewall R A. Acute Budd–Chiari syndrome secondary to intrahepatic hematoma following blunt abdominal trauma: treatment by open intracardiac surgery. J Thorac Cardiovasc Surg 1964; 47: 225–229

355. Klein M D, Philippart A I. Posttraumatic Budd–Chiari syndrome with late reversibility of hepatic venous obstruction. J Pediatr Surg 1979; 14: 661–663

356. Hales M R, Scatliff J H. Thrombosis of the inferior vena cava and hepatic veins (Budd-Chiari syndrome). Ann Intern Med 1966; 65: 768–781

357. Chamberlain D W, Walter J B. The relationship of Budd–Chiari syndrome to oral contraceptives and trauma. Can Med Assoc J 1969; 101: 618

358. O'Shea P A. Inferior vena cava and hepatic vein thrombosis as a rare complication of ventriculoatrial shunt. J Neurosurg 1978; 48: 143–145

359. Estrada V, Gutierrez F M, Cortes M, Garcia-Gonzalez C, Estrada R V. Budd–Chiari syndrome as a complication of the catheterization of the subclavian vein (letter). Am J Gastroenterol 1991; 86: 250–251

360. Paliard P, Bretagnolle M, Collet P, Vannieuwenhyse A, Berger F. Inferior vena cava thrombosis with Budd–Chiari syndrome during the course of hepatic and digestive amyloidosis. Gastroenterol Clin Biol 1983; 7: 919–922

361. Victor S, Jayanthi V, Madanagopalan N. Budd–Chiari syndrome in a child with hepatic tuberculosis. Ind Heart J 1989; 41: 279

362. Vallaeys J H, Praet M M, Roels H J, Van Marck E, Kaufman L. The Budd–Chiari syndrome caused by a zygomycete. A new pathogenesis of hepatic vein thrombosis. Arch Pathol Lab Med 1989; 113: 1171–1174

363. Young R C. The Budd–Chiari syndrome caused by Aspergillus. Two patients with vascular invasion of the hepatic veins. Arch Intern Med 1969; 124: 754–757

364. al-Dalaan A, al-Balaa S, Ali M A et al. al-Fadda M. Budd–Chiari syndrome in association with Behçet's disease. J Rheumatol 1991; 18: 622–626

365. Natalino M R, Goyette R E, Owensby L C, Rubin R N. The Budd–Chiari syndrome in sarcoidosis. JAMA 1978; 239: 2657–2658

366. Victor S. In: Okuda K, ed. 2nd International Conference on Budd–Chiari Syndrome. Kyoto: Annual Report of the Ministry of Health of Japan, 1991

367. Maccini D M, Berg J C, Bell G A. Budd–Chiari syndrome and Crohn's disease. An unreported association. Dig Dis Sci 1989; 34: 1933–1936

368. Brinson R R, Curtis W D, Schuman B M, Mills L R. Recovery from hepatic vein thrombosis (Budd–Chiari syndrome) complicating ulcerative colitis. Dig Dis Sci 1988; 33: 1615–1620

369. Cosnes J, Robert A, Levy V G, Darnis F. Budd–Chiari syndrome in a patient with mixed connective-tissue disease. Dig Dis Sci 1980; 25: 467–469

370. Shani M, Theodor E, Frand M, Goldman B. A family with protein-losing enteropathy. Gastroenterology 1974; 66: 433–445

371. Tsuchiya M, Oshio C, Asakura H, Ishii H, Aoki I, Miyairi M. Budd–Chiari syndrome associated with protein-losing enteropathy. Gastroenterology 1978; 75: 114–117

372. Tsuji H, Murai K, Kobayashi K et al. Multiple myeloma associated with Budd–Chiari syndrome. Hepato gastroenterology 1990; 37 (supplement 2): 97–99

373. McIntyre R E, Magidson J G, Austin G E, Gale R P. Fatal veno-occlusive disease of the liver following high-dose 1, 3-bis(2-chloroethyl)-1-nitrosourea (BCNU) and autologous bone marrow transplantation. Am J Clin Pathol 1981; 75: 614–617

374. Brick J E, Moreland L W, Al-Kawas F, Chang W W L, Layne R D, DiBartolomeo A G. Prospective analysis of liver biopsies before and after methotrexate therapy in rheumatoid patients. Semin Arthritis Rheum 1989; 19: 31–44

375. Popper H, Thomas L B, Telles N C, Faek H, Selikoff I J. Angiosarcoma in man induced by vinyl chloride, thorotrast, and arsenic: comparison of cases with unknown etiology. Am J Pathol 1978; 92: 349–376

376. Okuda K, Omata M, Itoh Y, Ikezaki H, Nakashima T. Peliosis hepatis as a late and final complication of thorotrast liver disease. Report of five cases. Liver 1981; 1: 110–122

377. Pimental J C, Menezes A P. Liver disease in vineyard sprayers. Gastroenterology 1977; 72: 275–283

378. Solis-Herruzo J A, Vidal J V, Colina F, Santalla F, Castellano G. Nodular regenerative hyperplasia of the liver associated with the toxic oil syndrome: report of five cases. Hepatology 1986; 6: 687–693

379. Nadell J, Kosek J. Peliosis hepatis. Twelve cases associated with oral androgen therapy. Arch Pathol Lab Med 1977; 101: 405–410

380. Taxy J B. Peliosis: a morphological curiosity becomes an iatrogenic problem. Hum Pathol 1978; 9: 331–340

381. Loomus G N, Aneja P, Bota R A. A case of peliosis hepatis in association with tamoxifen therapy. Am J Clin Pathol 1983; 80: 881–883

382. McDonald G B, Sharma P, Matthews D E, Shulman H M, Thomas E D. Venocclusive disease of the liver after bone marrow transplantation: diagnosis, incidence and predisposing factors. Hepatology 1984; 4: 116–122

15

Hepatic injury due to drugs and toxins

H. J. Zimmerman   K. G. Ishak

Many chemical agents can produce hepatic injury. Some are intrinsic toxins; others are drugs which produce liver damage as an idiosyncratic reaction. Acute injury may consist mainly of parenchymal damage (cytotoxic or cytolytic injury), arrested bile flow and jaundice (cholestatic injury), or be a mixture of the two. The damage may be acquired as a toxicological phenomenon, therapeutic misadventure, or be induced experimentally. This chapter deals with the forms of injury produced by various chemical agents in man as seen by light microscopy. Electron microscopy is useful in experimental hepatotoxicology, and sheds light on mechanisms of injury[1] but has limited direct relevance to clinical hepatology.

IMPORTANCE OF CHEMICAL HEPATIC INJURY

The relative importance of hepatic injury due to various types of exposure to toxins has changed considerably over the years. Acute toxic injury, formerly an occupational and domestic hazard, is now mainly a domestic one. Chlorinated hydrocarbons are an uncommon, but still encountered, cause of injury in the home.[2] Poisoning by phosphorus has almost disappeared from the USA but remains a problem in parts of the world where suicidal or accidental ingestion of rodenticides or fire crackers containing it still occur.[3–5] Mushroom poisoning accounts for several hundred cases of hepatic injury per year, most of them in Europe.[6–8] A recently emerged cause of hepatotoxicity, outstripping all others in England and of growing importance in the USA, is the suicidal ingestion of paracetamol.[9–11]

To most clinicians and pathologists, hepatic injury caused by adverse reactions to medicinal agents is more important than that caused by other substances. Nevertheless, adverse reactions to drugs have ranked numerically as a relatively minor cause of acute hepatic disease. Less than 5% of instances of jaundice in several series,[12,13] have been attributed to drug reactions. More recent analysis suggests that 10% of cases of apparent 'hepatitis' are due to drug-induced injury, the figure rising to over 40% in patients above the age of 50.[6] As a cause of severe hepatic necrosis, drug-induced injury also assumes an important role. Up to 25% of cases of fulminant hepatic failure may be the result of adverse reactions to medicinal agents.[14]

Drugs also are an important cause of chronic hepatic disease. They have been held responsible for instances of chronic active hepatitis, fatty liver, cirrhosis and several vascular and neoplastic lesions of the liver.[15-19] Of increasing concern is the risk of acquiring chronic hepatic disease, particularly hepatic neoplasms, as a result of prolonged occupational exposure to toxic chemicals[20,21] and of the ingestion of mycotoxins and other natural hepatotoxins.[22-25] Some drugs, e.g. anabolic and contraceptive steroids, have been incriminated in the causation of hepatic tumours.[26-30]

CLASSIFICATION OF HEPATOTOXIC AGENTS

There are two main categories of agents that can produce hepatic injury (Table 15.1). One consists of intrinsic hepatotoxins, i.e. they are predictable or true hepatotoxins; the others are idiosyncratic hepatotoxins, i.e. their toxicity is non-predictable, and they produce hepatic injury in the small proportion of exposed individuals who are unusually susceptible.[15,18,19,31-33]

INTRINSIC HEPATOTOXINS

Intrinsic hepatotoxins are recognized by the high incidence of hepatic injury in individuals exposed to them, the production of a similar lesion in experimental animals, and the dose-dependence of the phenomena. There appear to be two types of intrinsic hepatotoxins, which we have categorized as direct and indirect (Fig. 15.1). These categories are approximately equivalent to the toxipathic and trophopathic forms of hepatic injury, respectively, of Himsworth.[34]

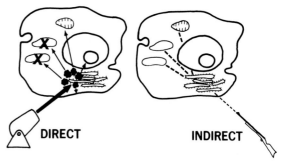

Fig. 15.1 Sketch depicting difference between direct and indirect hepatotoxins: direct destroy structural basis of metabolism, indirect produce selective biochemical lesion which results in structural injury. From Zimmerman.[18]

Table 15.1 Classification of hepatotoxic agents and major characteristics of each group

Category of Agent	Incidence	Experimental reproducibility	Dose-dependent	Mechanism	Histological lesion	Examples[*]
Intrinsic toxicity						
Direct	High	Yes	Yes	Direct physicochemical destruction by peroxidation of:		
Cytotoxic	High	Yes	Yes	hepatocytes	Necrosis and/or steatosis	Carbon tetrachloride phosphorus
Cholestatic	High	Yes	Yes	ductal cells	Cholestasis Duct destruction	Paraquat
Indirect						
Cytotoxic	High	Yes	Yes	Interference with specific pathways or producing selective lesions in: hepatocytes	Necrosis and/or steatosis	See Table 15.2
Cholestatic	High	Yes	Yes	ductal cells	Cholestasis Duct destruction	Methylene dianiline
Host idiosyncrasy						
Immunological (Hypersensitivity)	Low	No	No	Drug allergy	Necrosis or cholestasis	
Metabolic	Low	No	No	Production of hepatotoxic metabolites?	Necrosis or cholestasis	Phenytoin, PAS, sulphonamides, HALO[+], CPZ, PBZ INH, VPA, HALO[+]

[*] PAS = Para-aminosalicylic acid; HALO = halothane; CPZ = chlorpromazine; PBZ = phenylbutazone; INH = isoniazid; VPA = valproic acid
[+] Features suggestive of both hypersensitivity and metabolic idiosyncrasy

Direct hepatotoxins

These agents, or their metabolic products, injure the hepatocyte and its organelles by a direct physicochemical affect, i.e. peroxidation of the membrane lipids or other chemical changes that lead to distortion or destruction of the membranes. We would epitomize direct hepatotoxicity as destruction of the structural basis of hepatocyte metabolism, whereas indirect hepatotoxicity is the secondary effect of changes in key metabolites or in the structure, metabolism or function of hepatocytes.[18]

Direct hepatotoxins include carbon tetrachloride (CCl_4), some other chlorinated aliphatic hydrocarbons and the white allomorph of phosphorus. The category does not include modern medicinal agents, although at one time CCl_4 and chloroform ($CHCl_3$) were employed in clinical medicine. Direct hepatotoxins characteristically produce cytotoxic injury by damaging or destroying hepatocytes, although they may also injure Kupffer and perisinusoidal cells. At least one direct toxin, paraquat, produces cholestasis;[35] it causes bile-duct destruction, probably by peroxidative injury.

Indirect hepatotoxins

Agents in this category produce hepatic injury by interference with a specific metabolic pathway or process or by selective damage to cell components. The hepatic damage produced by indirect hepatotoxins may be mainly cytotoxic and expressed as steatosis or necrosis, or mainly cholestatic and expressed as arrested bile flow.

Cytotoxic indirect hepatotoxins

Cytotoxic indirect hepatotoxins cause injury by interfering with metabolic pathways or molecules essential for parenchymal cell integrity (Table 15.2). In this group are drugs, botanical hepatotoxins and compounds that are mainly of experimental interest. The lesions induced by these agents lead to steatosis, necrosis or both.[18]

Hepatic steatosis is usually the result of defective egress of lipid from the liver. The physiological lesion is deficient or defective synthesis of the apoprotein moiety of the very low density lipoprotein (VLDL) or defective assembly of triglyceride with apoprotein to form the VLDL needed to transport the lipid from the liver to the depots (Fig. 15.2). Increased mobilization of lipids from the depots and increased synthesis and decreased oxidation of fatty acids by the hepatocyte may contribute to the pathogenesis of steatosis. Some of the mechanisms for the steatogenic effects of several indirect hepatotoxins are depicted in Figure 15.2, and some of the physiological lesions are listed in Table 15.2. Ethionine competes with methionine for available adenosine triphosphate (ATP), interferes with the utilization of methionine, and ethylates compounds that should be methylated.[36, 37] The resultant

Table 15.2 Putative biochemical lesions produced by indirect hepatotoxins

Biochemical lesion	Histological lesion	Agent†
A. Attachment to membrane receptors	Necrosis Peliosis	Phalloidin
B. Covalent binding of active metabolite to:		
1. Cytosol molecules		
a. Alkylation	Necrosis +/- steatosis	DMN* and other nitrosamines Thioacetamide
b. Arylation	Necrosis +/- steatosis	Acetaminophen Bromobenzene AFB* Amanitine PAs*
2. Nuclear molecules (**DNA**)		
a. Alkylation	Carcinoma	Ethionine DMN* and other nitrosamines Thioacetamide Vinyl chloride
b. Arylation	Carcinoma, sarcoma	AFB*, PAs*
C. Binding or blockade of **tRNA**	Steatosis	Tetracycline, Puromycin
D. Cofactor depletion		
1. ATP	Steatosis, cirrhosis, carcinoma	Ethionine
2. UTP	Necrosis, steatosis	Galactosamine
E. Thiol group binding	Necrosis, steatosis, carcinoma	Arsenicals inorganic

* AFB = Aflatoxin B; DMN = dimethylnitrosamine; PAs = pyrrolizidine alkaloids
+ Individual agents may lead to other biochemical lesions as well

deficient synthesis of the apoprotein moiety and defective assembly of the VLDL needed to remove lipid from the liver leads to steatosis.[36] Puromycin also causes steatosis by interfering with protein synthesis. It blocks synthesis by attachment to the ribosomes in place of the normally attached activated tRNA. This leads to the formation of incomplete proteins truncated by a terminal puromycin molecule.[37] Tetracycline in high doses also leads to rapid inhibition of movement of lipid from the liver and to steatosis. It may be speculated that this is related to the known ability of tetracycline to interfere with protein synthesis, through binding of tRNA or interference with some other element of the complex system of synthesis of the VLDL. Other effects that may contribute to steatogenesis include impaired mitochondrial oxidation of fatty acids.[38]

Alcohol also warrants classification as an indirect hepatotoxin.[18] It leads to fatty change (see Ch 8) by a number of adverse effects on hepatocyte metabolism.[39] It also can lead

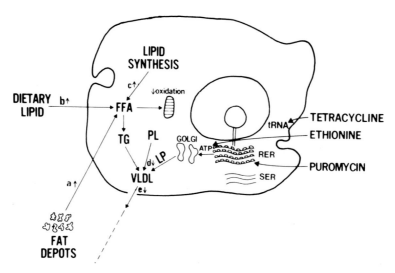

Fig. 15.2 Diagrammatic representation of lesions in lipid metabolism that can lead to hepatic steatosis. Fat in liver comes from peripheral depots (a), diet (b) and hepatic synthesis (c). Steatosis can result from increased mobilization of fatty acids from depots (a), decreased egress from liver (e) as a consequence of deficient or defective formation of apoprotein of very low density lipoprotein (VLDL), or impaired union (d) of apoprotein with phospholipid and triglyceride. Inhibition of synthesis of apoprotein results from selective lesions, e.g. ethionine leading to ATP depletion, tetracycline binding to transfer RNA, puromycin blocking access of activated amino acids to RER. From Zimmerman.[18]

to necrosis, perhaps by the necrogenic effect of acetaldehyde[39] and by increasing the oxygen requirements of hepatocytes.[40]

A number of compounds produce necrosis by selective biochemical lesions (Table 15.2). Depletion of uridine triphosphate (UTP), alkylation and arylation of macromolecules, or selective attachment (of the toxins or their metabolites) to membranes are among the reactions that may be responsible.[18,41–43]

Cholestatic indirect hepatotoxins

Cholestatic indirect hepatotoxins produce jaundice or impaired liver function by selective interference with hepatic mechanisms for excretion of substances into the canaliculus or uptake from the blood. In this category are icterogenin (an alkaloid of the plant *Lippia rhemani*), the

C-17 alkylated anabolic and contraceptive steroids, and lithocholic acid.[18,44,45] We also include in this category agents that can produce hyperbilirubinaemia by selective interference with the sinusoid/hepatocyte uptake or with the conjugation of bilirubin. Examples of such agents are flavaspidic acid, cholecystographic dyes, rifampicin and novobiocin. The cholestatic effects of ethinyloestradiol apparently include inhibition of uptake of bile acids at the sinusoidal membrane.[45,46]

IDIOSYNCRATIC HEPATIC INJURY

Agents that injure the liver of only specially susceptible individuals also appear to fall into two categories. The mechanism for the injurious action of one group appears to be hypersensitivity; the mechanism for the other

Table 15.3 Features that distinguish intrinsic hepatotoxins from those that produce hepatic injury as idiosyncratic reactions

Basis for hepatic injury	Characteristics			
	Experimental reproducibility	Dose dependence	Incidence in humans	Latent period
Intrinsic hepatotoxicity (true, predictable hepatotoxic agents)	Yes*	Yes	High**	Often short and relatively consistent
Idiosyncratic reaction* (non-predictable hepatotoxic agents)	No***	No	Low	Often long and variable

* May apply only to some species
**Depends on dose
***When due to metabolic idiosyncrasy, may be reproducible experimentally in specially manipulated models

appears to be a metabolic aberration of the host that permits production or accumulation of damaging amounts of hepatotoxic metabolites (Table 15.3). Some drugs seem able to produce hepatic injury by either mechanism. Thus, the majority of cases of liver damage induced by isoniazid appear to result from toxic metabolites,[47] but in a minority of cases the liver damage is accompanied by fever and eosinophilia and may be presumed to result from hypersensitivity.[18]

Hypersensitivity-related

Immunological idiosyncrasy ('allergy') is the presumptive mechanism for the hepatic injury which develops after a relatively fixed sensitization period of 1–5 weeks, recurs promptly on re-administration of the agent, and tends to be accompanied by fever, rash and eosinophilia, and by an eosinophil-rich or granulomatous inflammatory infiltrate in the liver. These features, however, provide only circum-

Table 15.4 Morphological types of toxic hepatic injury

Type of injury	Agent or comment [d]
Acute	
Cytotoxic	
Necrosis[a]	
Zonal	
Zone 3	CCl_4, acetaminophen, halothane
Zone 2	Ngaione, frusemide
Zone 1	Allylformate, albitocin
Massive	TNT, some drugs
Diffuse (panacinar)	Some drugs [b]
Focal	Some drugs [b]
Degeneration (ballooning, acidophilic)	
Acidophilic bodies (apoptosis)	Large number of agents
Steatosis	
Microvesicular	Ethionine, tetracycline, phosphorus, ethanol
Macrovesicular	Ethanol, MTX
Cholestatic	
Hepatocanalicular ('pericholangitic')	CPZ, erythromycin estolate, organic arsenicals
Canalicular ('bland')	C-17 alkylated anabolic and contraceptive steroids
Vascular	
Hepatic vein injury (VOD)	PAs, antineoplastic agents
Peliosis hepatis [c]	See Chronic lesions
Hepatic vein thrombosis	Contraceptive steroids
Chronic	
Parenchymal lesions	
Chronic necro-inflammatory disease (chronic hepatitis)	Oxyphenisatin, methyldopa, nitrofurantoin, dantrolene, clometacine, papaverine, sulphonamides, PTU
Subacute necrosis	Drugs listed under chronic necro-inflammatory disease
Steatosis	Ethanol, MTX, glucocorticoids, antineoplastic agents
Phospholipidosis	Amphophilic compounds
Cirrhosis	CCl_4, AF, PAs
Cholestatic lesions	
Chronic intrahepatic cholestasis (resembles primary biliary cirrhosis)	CPZ, haloperidol, imipramine, organic arsenicals, thiobendazole, tolbutamide
Biliary sclerosis	Floxuridine by hepatic artery perfusion
Vascular lesions	
Hepatic vein thrombosis	OCs, antineoplastic agents
Veno-occlusive disease	PAs, antineoplastic agents, X-ray, OCs, anabolic steroids
Peliosis hepatis	Medroxyprogesterone, vinyl chloride, As, Th-O, AZA-T
Other sinusoidal lesions	
Sinusoidal dilatation	OCs
Perisinusoidal fibrosis	As, vitamin A, $CuSO_4$, Th-O, antineoplastic agents, AZA-T
Hepatoportal sclerosis (portal vein and perisinusoidal)	As, $CuSO_4$, Th-O, antineoplastic agents
Granulomas	Many drugs (see Table 15.8)
Neoplasms	
Adenoma	OCs, anabolic steroids
Carcinoma	Anabolic steroids, OCs, Th-O, vinyl chloride
Angiosarcoma	Th-O, vinyl chloride, As, $CuSO_4$, anabolic steroids, oestrogen (?), OCs

[a] Degenerative changes including acidophilic bodies, hyalinization, and ballooning precede necrosis
[b] Small doses of toxic agents and drugs can lead to focal necrosis
[c] Pelisis hepatis may be produced in experimental animals as an acute lesion by phalloidin, or occurs in humans as chronic lesions induced by anabolic and contraceptive steroids
[d] TNT = trinitrotoluene; CPZ = chlorpromazine; DMN = dimethylnitrosamine; PAs = pyrrolizidine alkaloids; MTX = methotrexate; AF = aflatoxin; INH = isoniazid; As = arsenic; PTU = propylthiouracil; Th-O = Thorotrast; AZA-T = azathioprine; OCs = oral contraceptives; DES = diethylstilboestrol

stantial evidence for hypersensitivity as the cause of hepatic disease. Efforts to demonstrate a role for humoral or cell-mediated immunity in clinical cases have yielded variable results. Furthermore, efforts to establish an immunological basis for drug-induced hepatic disease are hampered by the probability that the putative antigen may be an unknown metabolite of the suspected drug. Nevertheless, the cirumstantial evidence seems sufficiently compelling to support the view that hypersensitivity plays an important role in the hepatic injury provoked by some drugs.[15]

Metabolic aberration: toxic metabolite dependent

Some drugs produce hepatic injury in low incidence, which is not accompanied by features that point to hypersensitivity as the mechanism. These are characterized by a variable duration of exposure prior to onset of injury, and delay of recurrence on challenge. Evidence to support early views that hepatotoxic metabolites might be responsible for this type of injury, however, had been scanty until the convincing demonstration for such a role by the metabolites of isoniazid and iproniazid.[43] There is also reason to believe that valproic acid, an anticonvulsant, produces its hepatic injury by a hepatotoxic metabolite.[48,49]

MORPHOLOGICAL FORMS OF TOXIC HEPATIC INJURY

The main types of morphological change in the liver produced by chemicals, drugs and other agents are listed in Table 15.4. Definition of the forms of injury produced by the intrinsic hepatotoxins has been relatively simple, since the hepatic damage can be reproduced in experimental animals.[18,50] Characterization of the forms of idiosyncratic injury, however, has been more difficult, and has depended on collation of material from reports of individual and groups of cases.

ACUTE HEPATIC INJURY

Toxic agents may lead to cytotoxic injury or to cholestatic injury. There is some relationship between the type of hepatotoxin and the form of injury. Most intrinsic toxins produce mainly cytotoxic injury, and in only a few is the injury mainly cholestatic.[18] Idiosyncratic injury caused by some drugs is cholestatic and by others is cytotoxic.[51] Some drugs characteristically produce a mixed type of injury in which both cytotoxic and cholestatic injury are prominent.[18]

Cytotoxic injury

Degeneration, necrosis and steatosis of hepatocytes can occur in various combinations.[19,51] Indeed, toxic hepatic damage can cause virtually all of the morphological lesions known in hepatology.

Necrosis (Table 15.5)

This may be zonal, diffuse or massive. In general, but with some notable exceptions to which reference is made, the necrosis produced by intrinsic hepatotoxins is zonal, while that produced by idiosyncratic injury is usually diffuse and, when extreme, massive.

Zonal necrosis may be in zone 3 (perivenular), zone 1 (periportal) or zone 2 (midzonal) of the hepatic acinus. These correspond roughly to the central, peripheral, and mid-zone of the classic (anatomical) lobule (see Ch. 1). Perivenular necrosis is the characteristic lesion produced by a number of intrinsic toxins (Figs 15.3–15.5). Some are mainly of experimental interest.[18,50] Relevant to human disease are CCl_4 (Fig. 15.3), $CHCl_3$, copper salts, pyrrolizidine alkaloids, tannic acid, the toxins of *Amanita phalloides* (Fig. 15.5) and others.[18] In overdose, paracetamol becomes an intrinsic hepatotoxin that can cause

Table 15.5 Toxins[a] that produce hepatic necrosis[b] with or without steatosis[c]

Necrosis	Necrosis and steatosis
Albitocin (PP)	Aflatoxins (PV, PP)
Alloxan (PP)	L-Amanitin (PV)
Allyl compounds (PP)	Arsenic compounds (inorganic) (PV, M)
Aniline (M)	Bromobenzene (PV)
Beryllium (MZ)	Carbon tetrachloride (PV)
Chlorinated benzenes (M or PV)	Chlorinated diphenyls (M)
Dioxane (M)	Chlorinated naphthalene (M)
Diphtheria toxin (PV)	Chloroform (PV)
Ferrous sulphate (PP)	Chloroprene (PV)
Manganese compounds (PP)	2-Chloropropane (PV)
Ngaione (MZ)	DDT (PV)
Paracetamol (PV)	Dichloropropane (PV)
Paraquat (PV)[d]	Dimethylnitrosamine (PV)
Phalloidin (PV)	Dinitrobenzone (PV, M)
P. vulgaris endotoxin (PP)	Dinitrotoluene (PV, M)
Rubratoxin (PV)	Ethylene dibromide (PV)
Selenium (M)	Ethylene dichloride (PV)
Sporidesmin (PP)	Galactosamine (D)
Thioacetamide (PV)	Iodoform (PV)
Urethane (PV)	Islandicum (PV)
	Luteoskyrin (PV)
	Methylchloroform (PV)
	Naphthalene (PV)
	Pyrrolizidine alkaloids (PV)
	Synthaline (PP)
	Tannic acid (PV)
	Tetrachloroethane (PV, M)
	TNT (PV, M)

(a) Partial list. See Rouiller[50] for other agents
(b) PV = perivenular, acinar zone 3; PP = periportal, acinar zone 1; MZ = midzonal, acinar zone 2; M = massive/panacinar necrosis; D = diffuse necrosis
(c) From Zimmerman[18] (modified)
(d) Acute injury is necrosis; later lesion is destruction of interlobular bile ducts and cholestasis

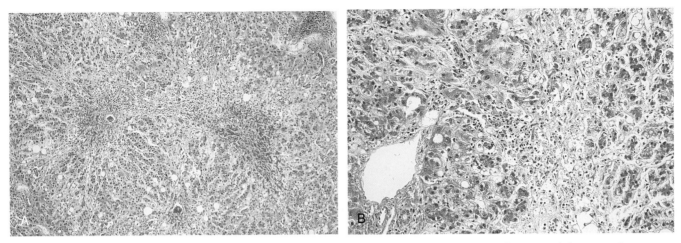

Fig. 15.3 Carbon tetrachloride toxicity. Both figures **A, B** from same case. (**A**) Bridging zone 3 necrosis. Note focal steatosis in preserved parenchyma. H & E. (**B**) There is drop out of liver cells in zone 3 and neutrophilic infiltration of the residual stroma. H & E.

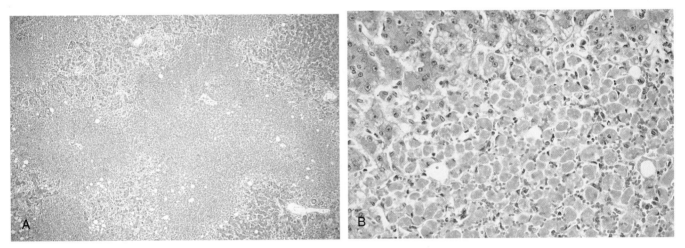

Fig. 15.4 Paracetamol (acetaminophen) toxicity. (**A**) Confluent coagulative necrosis involving zones 3 and 2. H & E. (**B**) Coagulated hepatocytes are shrunken, eosinophilic, more or less rounded and have lost their nuclei. H & E.

perivenular necrosis (Fig. 15.4). The central necrosis induced by some agents (pyrrolizidine alkaloids, aflatoxin B in some species) is accompanied by injury to the hepatic veins or venules, adding a haemorrhagic component to the necrosis.[18,50,52] In the idiosyncratic injury caused by halothane and other halogenated anaesthetics (Fig. 15.6), the necrosis is often perivenular and strikingly similar to that of CCl$_4$ or CHCl$_3$.[18,53–55] Some instances of halothane injury, however, are in the peripheral periportal zone and some are non-zonal.

A few agents characteristically produce periportal necrosis (Fig. 15.7); in this category are known toxins such as phosphorus,[3] poisonous doses of ferrous sulphate,[15] allyl alcohol and its esters,[56] the endotoxin of *Proteus vulgaris*,[34] as well as adverse reactions to some drugs. A few agents produce midzonal necrosis in experimental animals. These include ngaione, beryllium, frusemide, and, in

hyperthyroid animals, CCl$_4$ and CHCl$_3$.[18,49,57] Midzonal necrosis, however, is a rare lesion in humans.

The zonality of necrosis appears to be related to the mechanism of injury. The zone 3 location of the lesion induced by CCl$_4$,[58] by bromobenzene,[59] and by paracetamol[60] appears to reflect the concentration in that zone of the enzyme system responsible for the conversion of these agents to hepatotoxic metabolites.[60] The periportal necrosis produced by allyl formate has been attributed to the location in that zone of the enzyme (alcohol dehydrogenase) which converts the compound to its toxic metabolite, acrolein.[56] The recent demonstration that allyl alcohol is metabolized in the perivenular zone at least as well as in the peripheral zone, however, casts some doubt on the hypothesis.[61]

Diffuse necrosis, which is the usual form caused by idiosyncratic injury, resembles that produced by viral

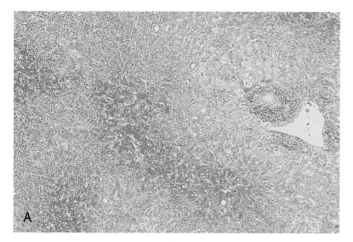

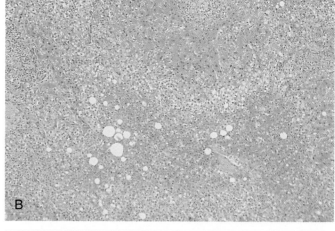

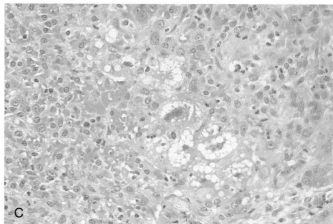

Fig. 15.5 Mushroom toxicity. All figures from same case. (**A**) Bridging zone 3 necrosis with marked sinusoidal congestion. Masson' trichrome. (**B**) Haematoxylin and eosin-stained section. (**C**) Higher magnification showing drop-out of liver cells and stromal inflammation. Note mocrovesicular steatosis of residual hepatocytes. H & E.

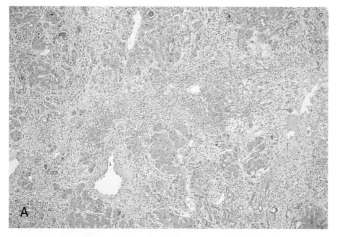

Fig. 15.6 Halothane injury. All figures from same case. (**A**) Bridging zone 3 necrosis. H & E (**B**) A bridge of necrosis ('central to portal'). Note periportal cholangiolar proliferation and the moderate inflammatory response. H & E (**C**) There is drop-out of liver cells in zone 3, ceroid pigment accumulation in hypertrophied Kupffer cells, and mononuclear cell infiltration. H & E.

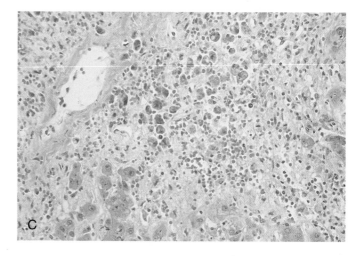

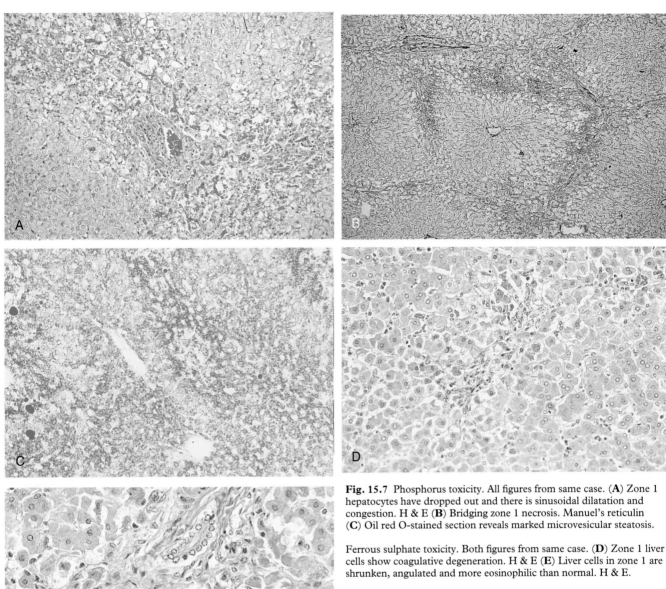

Fig. 15.7 Phosphorus toxicity. All figures from same case. (**A**) Zone 1 hepatocytes have dropped out and there is sinusoidal dilatation and congestion. H & E (**B**) Bridging zone 1 necrosis. Manuel's reticulin (**C**) Oil red O-stained section reveals marked microvesicular steatosis.

Ferrous sulphate toxicity. Both figures from same case. (**D**) Zone 1 liver cells show coagulative degeneration. H & E (**E**) Liver cells in zone 1 are shrunken, angulated and more eosinophilic than normal. H & E.

hepatitis (Figs 15.8 and 15.9); although the injury may be more intense in zone 3.[19] The experimental necrosis produced by the intrinsic toxin galactosamine is diffuse rather than zonal.[62] The extreme form of diffuse injury is massive necrosis (Fig. 15.8). The idiosyncratic injury caused by halothane and other haloalkane anaesthetics differs from that caused by other drugs in that the necrosis is often in zone 3 and strikingly similar to that of CCl_4 or $CHCl_3$.[53–55]

Massive necrosis, in which many entire acini are destroyed, seems to be an extreme form of diffuse necrosis and should be distinguished from the zonal type. Indeed, zonal necrosis, even when severe, usually leaves a surviving rim of hepatocytes; even when the entire acinus is wiped out, the architectural arrangement remains. In true massive necrosis, however, there is parenchymal collapse with loss of the normal architecture.

Degeneration

Degeneration of hepatocytes precedes necrosis; in the zone destined to undergo necrosis, or at its periphery, hepatocytes show hydropic degeneration of 'ballooning', eosinophilic degeneration and 'free' sinusoidal, acidophilic bodies. The free acidophilic body, a characteristic lesion of

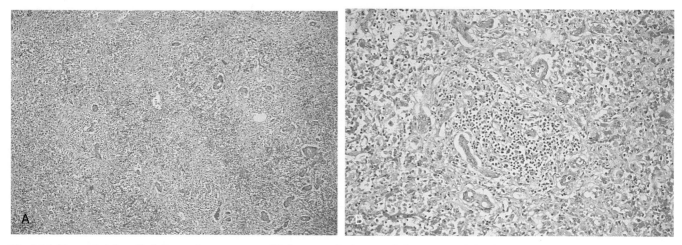

Fig. 15.8 Phenytoin injury. Both figures from same case. (**A**) Acute massive hepatocellular necrosis. H & E. (**B**) Portal area is moderately inflamed. Note periportal ductular proliferation with neutrophil infiltration. All liver cells (zone 1) have dropped out. H & E.

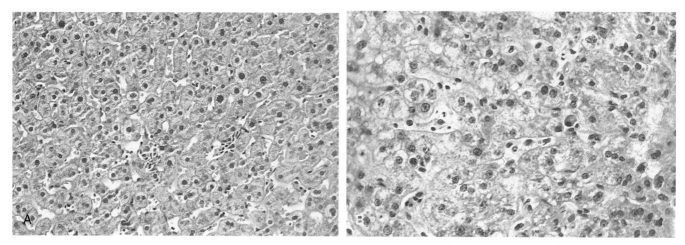

Fig. 15.9 Phenytoin injury. Both figures from same case. (**A**) Two small foci of necrosis. H & E. (**B**) Sinusoidal acidophilic body and mild ballooning of hepatocytes. H & E.

viral hepatitis, may also result from parenchymal injury induced by a number of drugs and other chemicals. The acidophilic body of drug-induced injury (Figs 15.9 and 15.10) may differ from that of viral hepatitis by being irregular in shape and containing a nuclear remnant. Formation of the acidophilic body has been called *apoptosis* and the body an *apoptotic body*.[63]

The Mallory body ('alcoholic hyalin') is a dramatic form of hyaline degeneration of hepatocytes (Fig. 15.11) seen in alcoholic liver disease and a number of other diseases.[64] These include Indian childhood cirrhosis, Wilson's disease, chronic cholestatic diseases such as primary biliary cirrhosis, liver damage after intestinal bypass for obesity and hepatocellular carcinoma[64] (see Ch. 9). In Western societies alcoholic hepatitis remains the clinical setting in which the Mallory body is most regularly found.

The relative importance of malnutrition and of the toxicity of ethanol in producing the hepatic disease of alcoholics remains uncertain. There is little doubt, however, that ethanol is an intrinsic hepatotoxin; the liver disease is, at least in part, a form of hepatotoxicity, and the Mallory body is its characteristic, histological marker. Furthermore, the recent reports of Mallory bodies in patients with liver damage produced by perhexilene maleate,[65-67] amiodarone,[68-70] and nifedipine,[71] and in mice given toxic doses of griseofulvin[72] and in hamsters given stilboestrol[73] confirm it as a histological marker of toxicity (Table 15.6). Indeed, the injury produced by perhexilene maleate and amiodarone resembles that of alcoholic hepatitis; the term non-alcoholic steatohepatitis (NASH) has been introduced for this pattern of injury and the topic is discussed on p. 582.

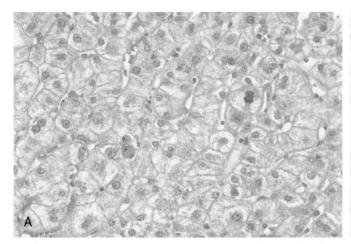

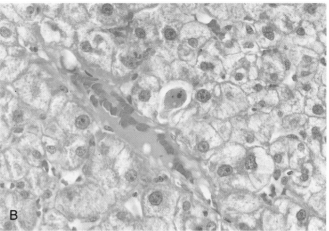

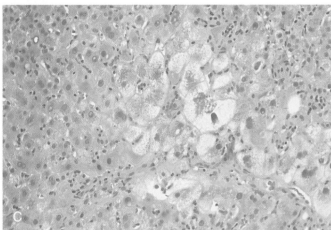

Fig. 15.10 Injury following treatment with sulphamethoxazole–trimethoprim (Septra). Both from same case. (**A**) Two apoptotic bodies (left) and mitotic figure (right). H & E. (**B**) Apoptotic (acidophilic) body (center) contains nuclear fragments. H & E. (**C**) Sulphasalazine injury. Ballooning degeneration. H & E.

Table 15.6 Drugs that produce Mallory bodies, phospholipidosis or both

	Mallory bodies	Phospholipidosis
Amiodarone	+	+
Coralgil[a]	+	+
Perhexiline maleate	+	+
Chlorphentramine[b]	−	+
Thioradazine[b]	−	+
Nifedipine[c]	+	−
Stilboestrol[c]	+	−
Glucocorticoids[c]	+	−
Ethanol[d] (alcoholic liver disease)	+	−

[a] Trade name for 4,4'diethylaminoethoxydexoestrol
[b] Amphophilic drugs, many of which can lead to phospholipidosis
[c] Very few instances
[d] Alcoholism leads to Mallory bodies in humans. Alcohol per se does not do so in experimental animals

Steatosis

Steatosis can be produced by a large number of agents (Table 15.7). Although the zonality of steatosis has not commanded the attention of zonal necrosis, there are differences in the zonal distribution of fat of different toxic aetiologies. Phosphorus leads mainly or initially to accumulation of fat in the periportal zone, while tetracycline and alcohol lead predominantly or initially to perivenular steatosis.[18]

Two main types of fatty change occur — *microvesicular* and *macrovesicular*.[19,74] In the microvesicular form the hepatocytes are filled with many tiny fat droplets that do not displace the nucleus. Tetracycline (Fig. 15.12b) produces this lesion,[75] and a similar hepatic lesion occurs in Reye's syndrome and in fatty liver of pregnancy.[74] Hepatic injury caused by alcohol in some instances,[76] valproic acid[48] and salicylates[77] also leads to the accumulation of fine lipid droplets in liver cells. Microvesicular steatosis in Thai children has been ascribed to aflatoxins and has been produced in monkeys by aflatoxin B_1.[78] Dimethylformamide has also been reported to lead to

Table 15.7 Agents that produce steatosis[a]

Alcohol	Dicholoroethylene	Methyl
Antimony	Dimethylhydrazine	chlorobromide
L-Asparaginase (Colaspase)	Ethionine	Methyl dichloride
Azacytidine	Ethyl bromide	Orotic acid
Azaserine	Ethyl chloride	Phosphorus[b]
Azauridine	Flectol H	Puromycin
BAL	Hydrazine	Rare earths[c]
Barium salts	Hypoglycin	Safrole
Bleomycin	Methotrexate	Tetracycline
Borates	Methyl bromide	Thallium compounds
Carbon disulphide	Methyl chloride	Uranium compounds
Chromates		Warfarin

[a] Partial list of agents that produce fatty liver in animals or humans
[b] Phosphorus causes mainly fatty liver; may be some periportal necrosis as well
[c] Only rare earths of low atomic number produce fatty liver

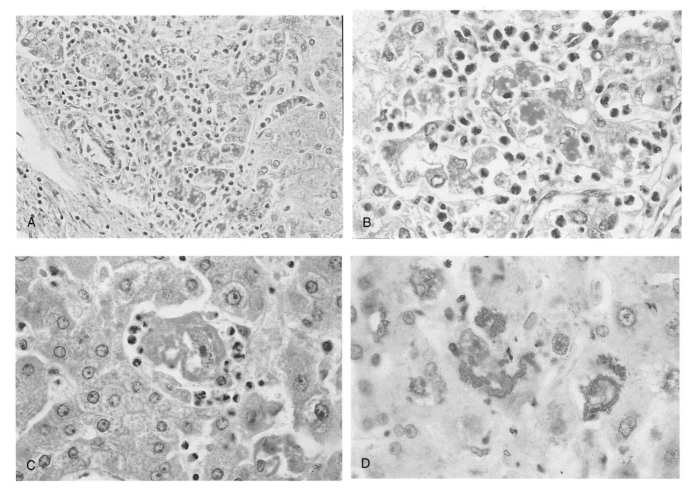

Fig. 15.11 Amiodarone injury. All figures from same case. (**A**) Zone 1 liver cells contain Mallory bodies and are surrounded by neutrophils. H & E. (**B**) High power view of Mallory bodies. (**C**) Neutrophil 'satellitosis', the Mallory body is rope-like and includes the nucleus of a lysed liver cell. H & E. (**D**) Mallory bodies (light brown) are demonstrated by immunostaining for ubiquitin.

microvesicular steatosis as an occupational toxicity,[79] and cocaine abuse has also been reported to lead to the lesion.[80] Macrovesicular steatosis, in which the hepatocyte contains a large fat droplet that displaces the nucleus to the periphery, is characteristic of alcohol abuse, methotrexate injury and a number of other agents (Fig. 15.12). Necrosis and steatosis may occur together. For some toxins (CCl_4, $CHCl_3$, tannic acid) the necrosis is dominant, while for others (amanitin, phosphorus) the steatosis is more prominent.

Phospholipidosis is an additional form of lipid accumulation that may be drug-induced.[81,82] It differs strikingly in pathogenesis and characteristics from the two classic forms of steatosis. A lesion first recognized in Japan in 1969[81] to be the result of administration of the 'coronary vasodilator' 4,4'-diethylaminoethoxyhexoestrol (Coralgil®), it has been recorded by Japanese authors in over 100 patients.[81,82] It is characterized by enlarged, foamy hepatocytes as seen by light microscopy

(Fig. 15.13A,B) and by lamellated or crystalloid inclusions, seen by electron microscopy[1,81,82] (Fig. 15.13C). There are similar changes in Kupffer cells and in cells at extrahepatic sites.[82] The lesion, which resembles that of several inborn disorders of phospholipid metabolism,[81] is accompanied by a characteristic clinical syndrome and can lead to cirrhosis.[82] Recently, amiodarone has been reported[68] to produce phospholipidosis (Fig. 15.13) and a number of amphophilic compounds produce similar ultrastructural changes in experimental animals.[82] The full-blown lesion is a chronic change which requires several months to develop, but early changes occur after only several doses.

Patterns of inflammatory response in cytotoxic injury

Necrosis induced by most drugs is accompanied by relatively slight inflammatory infiltration. In general, it appears to be less prominent than the inflammatory response

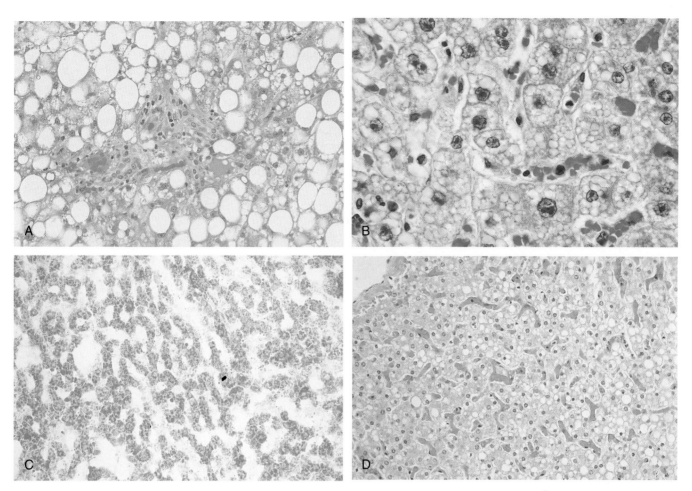

Fig. 15.12 (**A**) Methotrexate injury. Macrovesicular steatosis. H & E. (**B**) Tetracycline injury. Microvesicular steatosis. H & E. (**C**) Same case illustrated in Fig. 15.13**B**. Liver cells show marked small droplet steatosis. Oil red O stain. (**D**) Asparaginase injury. Lipid vacuoles in liver cells are of medium size. H & E.

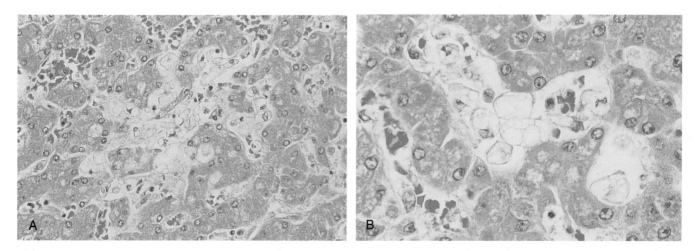

Fig. 15.13 Amiodarone-induced phospholipidosis. (**A**) Cluster of foam cells. H & E. (**B**) Same case illustrated in Fig. 15.11**A**. Foam cells in hepatic sinusoid. H & E. (**C**) Electron micrograph of hepatocytes in aminodarone-associated phospholipidosis showing two membrane-bound lysosomal structures (asterisks) in a hepatocyte. These structures are composed of densely-packed concentric membranous arrays with a fingerprint pattern and are identical to those described in phospholipidosis (Lullman et al).[82] Note also altered mitchondria (m) with reduced cristae and increased matrix density and vesiculated smooth ER (arrowheads). Lead citrate, × 36 900. Courtesy of Dr M J Philips.

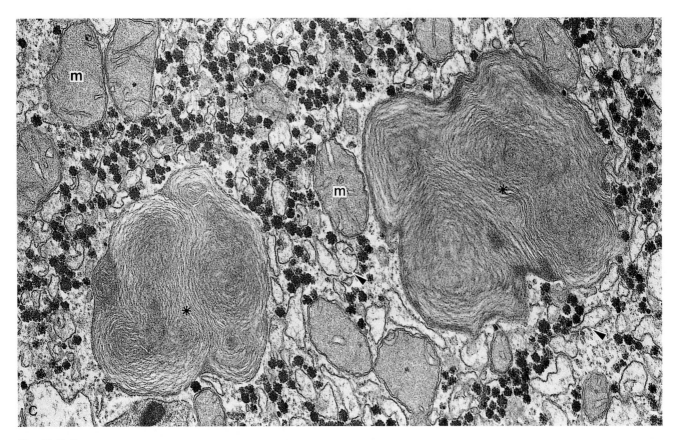

Fig. 15.13 C

to necrosis of equal severity caused by viral hepatitis.[19,83] However, the cytotoxic injury induced by some drugs, e.g. phenytoin and paraminosalicylic acid, usually leads to a striking infiltration of mononuclear cells with or without eosinophils. The mononuclear infiltrate may be diffusely distributed throughout the parenchyma or aggregated around areas of necrosis, and there are usually prominent aggregates in the portal areas.[19] The inflammation accompanying phenytoin-induced injury may resemble infectious mononucleosis (Fig. 15.14). It may include granulomas or granulomatoid lesions. Some drugs may cause granulomas (Fig. 15.15) with or without other manifestations of hepatic injury (Table 15.8). Indeed, approximately 30% of instances of hepatic granulomas were attributed to medicinal agents.[84] More than 60 drugs have been incriminated in the production of hepatic granulomas.[85] Note should also be made of the occurrence of sarcoid-like granulomas in the liver, lungs and other organs as a result of chronic occupational exposure to heavy metals such as beryllium[86] and copper.[87]

The character of the inflammatory response bears some relation to the apparent pathogenesis of the injury. Eosinophilic or granulomatous inflammation in a patient with drug-induced hepatic injury is generally taken as evidence

Table 15.8 Drugs that can lead to hepatic granulomas[*]

Allopurinol	Papaverine
Aspirin	Penicillin
Bacille Calmette–Guerin (BCG)	Phenazone
Carbamazepine	Phenprocoumon
Carbutamide	Phenylbutazone
Cephalexin	Phenytoin
Chlorpromazine	Prajmalium
Chlorpropamide	Procainamide
Contraceptive steroids	Procarbazine
Dapsone	Quinidine
Diazepam	Quinine
Diltiazem	Ranitidine
Disopyramide	Succinylsulphathiazole
Dimethicone	Sulphadiazine
Feprazone	Sulphadimethoxine
Glibenclamide	Sulphadoxine–pyrimethamine
Gold	Sulphamethoxazole–trimethoprim
Green-lipped mussel (Seatone)[†]	Sulphanilamide
Halothane	Sulphasalazine
Isoniazid	Sulphathiazole
Metolazone	Sulphonamide, unspecified
Mineral oil	Tocainide
Nitrofurantoin	Tolbutamide
Oxacillin	Trichlormethiazide
Oxyphenbutazone	

[*] Ishak & Zimmerman[85]; [†] Ahern et al[433]

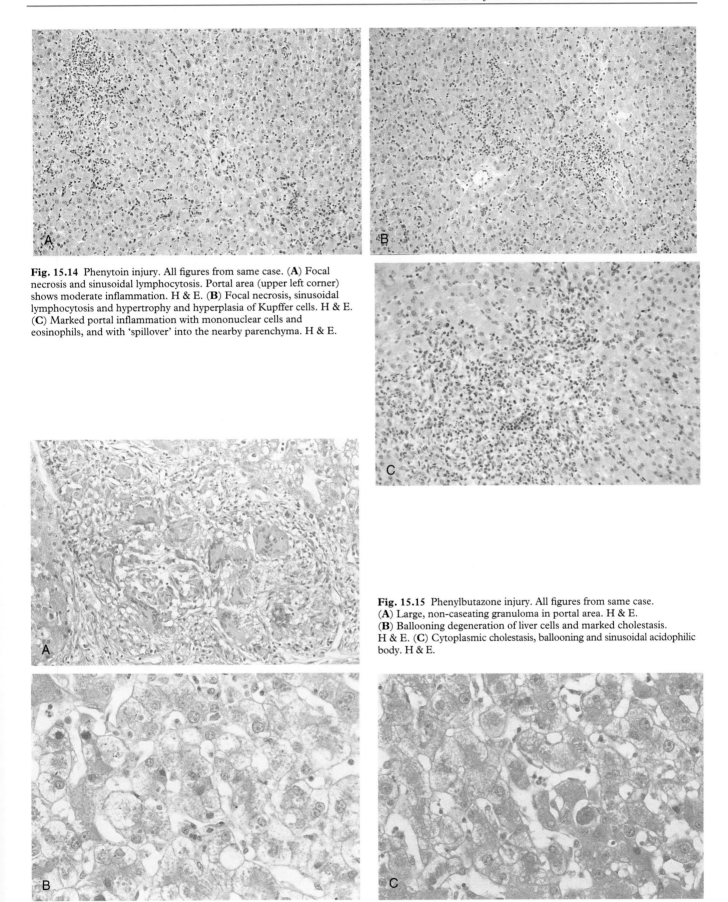

Fig. 15.14 Phenytoin injury. All figures from same case. (**A**) Focal necrosis and sinusoidal lymphocytosis. Portal area (upper left corner) shows moderate inflammation. H & E. (**B**) Focal necrosis, sinusoidal lymphocytosis and hypertrophy and hyperplasia of Kupffer cells. H & E. (**C**) Marked portal inflammation with mononuclear cells and eosinophils, and with 'spillover' into the nearby parenchyma. H & E.

Fig. 15.15 Phenylbutazone injury. All figures from same case. (**A**) Large, non-caseating granuloma in portal area. H & E. (**B**) Ballooning degeneration of liver cells and marked cholestasis. H & E. (**C**) Cytoplasmic cholestasis, ballooning and sinusoidal acidophilic body. H & E.

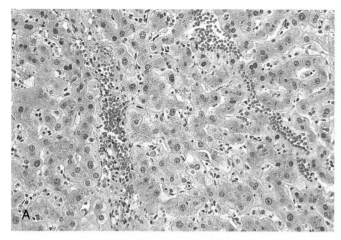

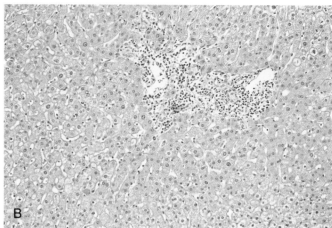

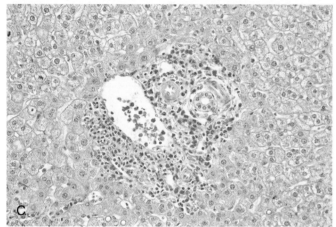

Fig. 15.16 Erythromycin estolate injury. All figures from same case. (**A**) Marked cholestasis in zone 3. Note acidophilic body, mild to moderate balloning and anisonucleosis. H & E. (**B**) Portal area is infiltrated with a moderate number of inflammatory cells. There is one acidophilic body (lower left). H & E. (**C**) Moderate portal inflammation with many eosinophils. Note mitoses to left. H & E.

disease and cirrhosis, so acute cholestatic disease can, at times, produce a chronic cholestatic lesion which mimics primary biliary cirrhosis.[15,19,32,88,90] Another form of ductal injury, drug-induced sclerosing cholangitis, is discussed with chronic lesions.

Patterns of inflammatory response in cholestatic injury

Inflammation mainly localized to the portal areas has a special relevance to cholestatic injury. In some forms of drug-induced intrahepatic cholestasis (chlorpromazine or

that the mechanism for injury is hypersensitivity.[19] Prominence of eosinophils in the sinusoids is usually a reflection of peripheral eosinophilia.[88]

Cholestatic injury

Some agents lead to injury that appears to spare the parenchyma and to cause only, or mainly, arrested bile flow.[15,18,19,32] The histological manifestation of cholestatic injury consists mainly of bilirubin casts in the canaliculi and, at times, in cholangioles. Cholestatic injury induced by some agents (e.g. chlorpromazine, erythromycin estolate) is more likely to be accompanied by a minor degree of parenchymal injury and by more portal inflammation (Fig. 15.16) than that induced by others (e.g. anabolic and contraceptive steroids)[15,18,19] (Fig. 15.17). The type of injury caused by chlorpromazine, we have called *hepato-canalicular* cholestasis; that caused by steroids, we have called *canalicular*. A third form of intrahepatic cholestasis (Table 15.9) which we have called *ductal* or *cholangio-destructive* is exemplified by the ductal injury (Fig. 15.18) of paraquat poisoning.[35,89] Sequelae of cholestatic injury can occur. Just as acute cytotoxic injury can lead to chronic

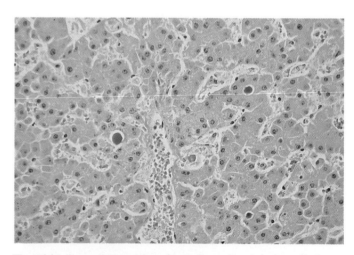

Fig. 15.17 Oxymetholone injury. Marked cytoplasmic and canalicular cholestasis in zone 3.

Table 15.9 Types of cholestatic jaundice caused by drugs (examples)

Features	Canalicular jaundice	Hepatocanalicular jaundice	Ductal	Cholangiodestructive
	(C-17 alkylated steroids — anabolic, contraceptives)	(Chloropromazine)	(Benoxaprofen)	(Paraquat, floxuridine)
Clinical evidence of hypersensitivity	0	Frequent	0	0
Biochemical features				
AST-ALT	(1–8×)	(2–10×)	2–10×	2–10×
Alkaline phosphatase	(1–3×)	(3–10×)		
Histological features				
Bile casts	+	+	+[b]	+
Portal inflammation	0	++(especially early)	+	+
Duct destruction	0	+	0	+
Association[a]				
Adenoma	+	0	0	0
Carcinoma	+	0	0	0
Chronic cholestasis	±	+	±	0 or +[c]
Peliosis hepatis	+	+	0	±
Other terms	Bland cholestasis Steroid jaundice	Cholangiolitic Sensivity cholestasis		Biliary sclerosis[d]

[a] As a possible consequence
[b] In canaliculi, ductules and interlobular ducts
[c] No chronic cholestasis in paraquat poisoning, because death is usually due to pulmonary fibrosis but chronic cholestasis is typical of FUDR injury
[d] A lesion caused by floxuridine resembles sclerosing cholangitis; referred to as biliary sclerosis
+ = occurs; 0 = does not occur; ± = uncertain

erythromycin estolate) there is a prominent portal tract infiltrate often rich in eosinophils. According to Scheuer,[19] the portal inflammatory lesion is prominent only early in the illness. Intrahepatic cholestasis accompanied by portal inflammation has been called the 'cholangiolitic' or 'hypersensitivity' type of cholestasis. In the intrahepatic cholestasis induced by anabolic or contraceptive steroids, there is little or no portal tract inflammation. This has been called the 'bland' or 'steroid' type (Fig. 15.17). Some degree of overt hepatocyte injury is more characteristic of the hypersensitivity than of the 'bland' type of injury. As cited in the preceding paragraph, we have termed the hypersensitivity type 'hepatocanalicular' and the bland type 'canalicular' injury.[18]

Mixed injury

Some drugs produce a mixed form of hepatic injury with features of both hepatocellular and cholestatic jaundice (Fig. 15.19). Injury which is predominantly hepatocellular but with a cholestatic component may be called *mixed-hepatocellular*, and that which is predominantly cholestatic but with a significant hepatocellular component may be called *mixed cholestatic* or *mixed hepatocanalicular*.[18]

SUBACUTE HEPATIC INJURY

There are two main forms of subacute toxic liver injury. One, subacute hepatic necrosis, lies midway between acute hepatic necrosis and cirrhosis in clinical and histological features. This term has been applied to a form of viral hepatitis characterized by bridging necrosis,[91] conveying the concept of severity rather than duration. The other, the subacute form of veno-occlusive disease (VOD), is described in a later section.

Subacute hepatic necrosis was a dread occupational disease of the defence industries during both world wars, a consequence of prolonged exposure to tetrachlorethane, trinitrotoluene, chlorinated biphenyl-chloronaphthalene mixtures or dinitrobenzene.[15,34,92,93] This occupationally acquired disease is now virtually obsolete. Subacute

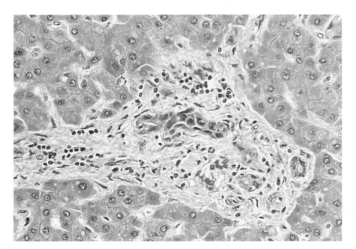

Fig. 15.18 Paraquat toxicity. Bile-duct degeneration. H & E.

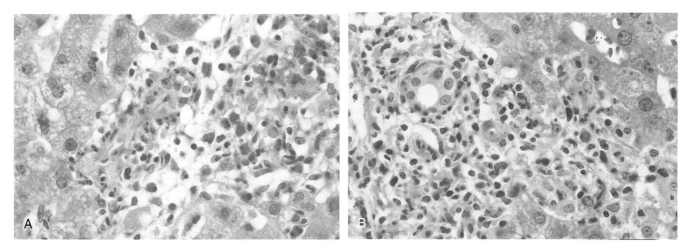

Fig. 15.19 Phenytoin injury. Both figures from same case. (**A**) Acute cholangiolitis and portal inflammation with many neutrophils. H & E, × 450 (**B**) Acute cholangitis (left upper corner). H & E, × 450.

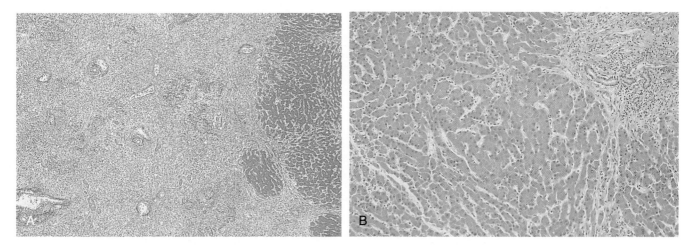

Fig. 15.20 Isoniazid injury. Both figures from same case. (**A**) Subacute hepatic necrosis. Area of multiacinar necrosis and residual parenchyma (right). Masson trichrome. (**B**) Residual parenchyma shows thick liver plates indicative of regeneration. H & E.

hepatic necrosis can, however, also result from long-term administration of isoniazid[94,95] or methyldopa[96,97] and was seen in recipients of cinchophen.[98,99] The histological features include varying degrees of necrosis, fibrosis and regeneration (Fig. 15.20).

In patients with a brief (2–3 weeks) clinical course of industrial, subacute hepatic necrosis the changes largely comprised extensive necrosis and collapse with relatively little cirrhosis.[92,93] The liver in these circumstances was remarkably shrunken, weighing as little as 500 g. Patients with a prolonged course of several months or more, usually had macronodular cirrhosis, with areas of extensive necrosis, with or without fibrosis, and areas of surviving or regenerated parenchyma. Architectural distortion leading to a macronodular cirrhosis had resulted from collapse of parenchyma in some areas and fibrous distortion of acinar morphology in others. Similar features can be seen in drug-induced subacute hepatic necrosis.

Fat was prominent in surviving cells in those exposed to occupational toxins, and its prominence seemed inversely proportional to the rate of necrosis. Fatty change has not been a prominent feature of drug-induced necrosis.

CHRONIC HEPATIC INJURY

A number of chronic lesions can result from the subtle, continued or repeated injury of prolonged exposure to hepatotoxic agents or drugs, or can be a sequel to acute injury. These lesions may be parenchymal, cholestatic, vascular, neoplastic, or granulomatous (Table 15.4). The parenchymal lesions include chronic active hepatitis, steatosis, phospholipidosis, non-alcoholic steatohepatitis and cirrhosis. The cholestatic lesions include prolonged intrahepatic cholestasis with a syndrome resembling primary biliary cirrhosis and one resembling sclerosing cholangitis.[45]

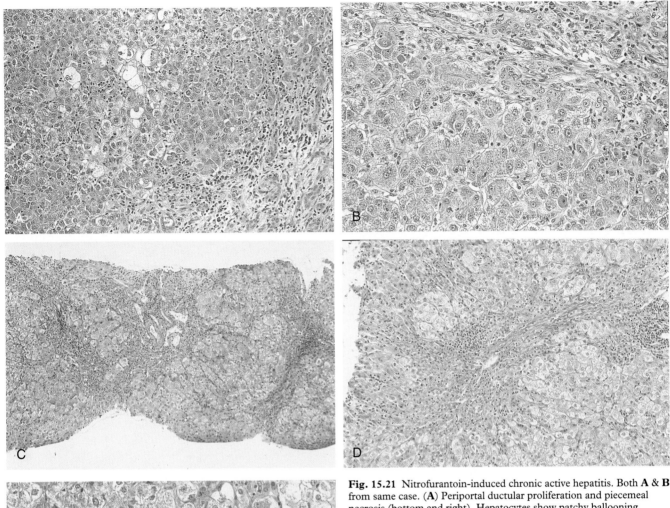

Fig. 15.21 Nitrofurantoin-induced chronic active hepatitis. Both **A** & **B** from same case. (**A**) Periportal ductular proliferation and piecemeal necrosis (bottom and right). Hepatocytes show patchy ballooning degeneration. H & E. (**B**) Scattered acidophilic bodies and mild to moderate ballooning in periportal area. H & E. Pemoline-induced chronic active hepatitis. Figures **C-E** from same case.
(**C**) Architectural distortion caused by bridging fibrosis. Masson
(**D**) Portal–portal bridging fibrosis, marked portal inflammation and piecemeal necrosis. H & E. (**E**) Higher magnification of periportal piecemeal necrosis. H & E.

Parenchymal lesions

Chronic active hepatitis

A number of drugs have been incriminated in the production of chronic necro-inflammatory disease that resembles chronic active hepatitis.[19,100–107] The lesion is characterized by dramatic portal and periportal inflammation composed of lymphocytes, plasma cells and, often, eosinophils (Fig. 15.21). A cardinal histological characteristic is the extension of the inflammation, often accompanied by fibrous strands, into the periportal area, surrounding individual degenerating cells and groups of cells — piecemeal necrosis.

The entity resembles autoimmune chronic active hepatitis ('lupoid hepatitis') in its histological and clinical features. There is a striking female preponderance among patients. A majority of patients have serological features considered to be autoimmune markers. These include antinuclear antibodies, smooth muscle antibodies, and anti-single-strand DNA antibodies; several other antibodies against

Table 15.10 Drugs that appear to lead to chronic active hepatitis

Amineptine	Fenofibrate	Nitrofurantoin	Pemoline
Clometacine	Isoniazid[2]	Oxyphenisatin	Propylthiouracil[1]
Dantrolene	Isoxonine	Papaverine	Sulfonamide[1]
Diclofenac	Methyldopa	Paracetamol[2]	Ticrynafen

[1] Only one or two instances of chronic hepatitis attributed to sulfonamide or propylthiouracil have been reported
[2] Chronic disease attributed to these drugs probably reflects continued toxic injury rather than the immune type of CAH

cell organelles have been noted.[107,108] Frequently, there is also marked hyperglobulinaemia. Drugs that have been incriminated in this lesion are listed in Table 15.10.

Several drugs (propylthiouracil, sulphonamides) have been implicated less convincingly in the production of this entity, and several others can lead to a smouldering, subtle necrosis accompanied by little inflammation and no autoimmune serological markers (isoniazid, paracetamol). There is no evidence that any of these lesions have persisted after the drug has been withdrawn.

Steatosis

Chronic steatosis is mostly macrovesicular. The steatosis of chronic valproate injury, however, is usually microvesicular.[48,109,110] Macrovesicular steatosis can be produced by several drugs including ethanol, glucocorticoids, and a number of antineoplastic agents, most notably methotrexate and asparaginase.[18,111] (Fig. 15.12) Glucocorticoid-induced steatosis appears to have no sequelae; methotrexate steatosis can proceed to cirrhosis; and asparaginase fatty liver may be accompanied by necrosis.

Phospholipidosis (Fig. 15.13)

This form of lipid accumulation differs strikingly in pathogenesis and appearance from the two classic forms of steatosis. First recognized in Japan[81,82] in patients taking a drug used to treat coronary disease (4,4'-diethyldiaminoethoxyhexoestrol — Coralgil), it has been seen in patients taking perhexiline maleate[82,112] or amiodarone.[68,70] It has been reproduced in experimental animals taking amphophilic compounds.[82] Indeed, the amphophilic character of the drugs appears to account for the accumulation of phospholipids in lysosomes of hepatocytes and other cells. The drug traps by binding to phospholipids as well as by inhibiting hydrolysis of the phospholipids by the phospholipase A of the lysosomes.[82,113,114]

The lesions are characterized by enlarged, foamy or granular hepatocytes.[68,115] Electron microscopy shows the cells to be filled with dramatically abnormal, lamellated lysosomes (Fig. 15.13C) that permit ready identification of the lesions.[68,81,82] There are similar changes in Kupffer cells and in cells at extrahepatic sites.[81,82,116–118]

The phospholipidosis reported from Japan[81,82] and that seen in recipients of amiodarone[68–70,117,118] and perhexiline maleate[65–67,119] is accompanied by a high incidence of cirrhosis. Whether the cirrhosis is a consequence of the accumulation of phospholipids or the result of other cytological injury is not clear. That other cytological injury can occur is shown by the non-alcoholic steatohepatitis ('pseudo-alcoholic' liver disease) with Mallory bodies and associated changes that occurs in some recipients of Coralgil, perhexiline maleate or amiodarone.[65–71,80,119–122] The pathogenesis of the phospholipidosis and Mallory body change by the same drug, however, appears to be distinct. Mallory bodies may be seen without the phospholipidosis, and vice versa, in recipients of these three drugs.[70,122] Furthermore, there are drugs that can produce either lesion or both (Table 15.6).

The lesions may be relatively acutely produced, but the syndrome is a chronic one. Often accompanied by Mallory bodies, it may merge with and present with the syndrome of non-alcoholic steatohepatitis.[68,70,122] Clinical manifestations of phospholipidosis per se consist of hepatomegaly alone or with other manifestations of hepatic disease that overlap with those of non-alcoholic steatohepatitis. The neuropathy, pulmonary manifestations, thyroid dysfunction, skin changes and wasting due to systemic phospholipidosis are usually more prominent than the hepatic manifestations.[123]

Non-alcoholic steatohepatitis (pseudo-alcoholic liver disease)

The clinical features that accompany these lesions, when due to drugs, usually reflect both the pseudo-alcoholic liver disease and the usually associated phospholipidosis. They may include wasting, lassitude, hepatomegaly, ascites, and peripheral neuropathy. Biochemical changes consist of mildly elevated (twofold to fourfold) transaminase levels.[122] Liver biopsy shows Mallory bodies, relatively slight steatosis, and a portal mononuclear cell inflammation.[68,70,116] The phospholipid-laden cells may be recognized on light microscopy or may require electron microscopy (Fig. 15.13) to identify the morphological marker, the abnormal lysosomes.[1,68,70,122,123] The drugs chiefly responsible for the entity have been perhexiline maleate[112,119,124] and amiodarone.[68–70,116,122,123] The Mallory body lesions have been produced without phospholipidoses by diethylstillboestrol in hamsters[73] and in a patient being treated for prostatic carcinoma,[125] and by nifedipine.[71]

Fibrosis

Changes ranging from portal and periportal fibrosis to frank cirrhosis occur in patients with chronic active hepatitis,[102–107] with methotrexate injury[126,127] and with

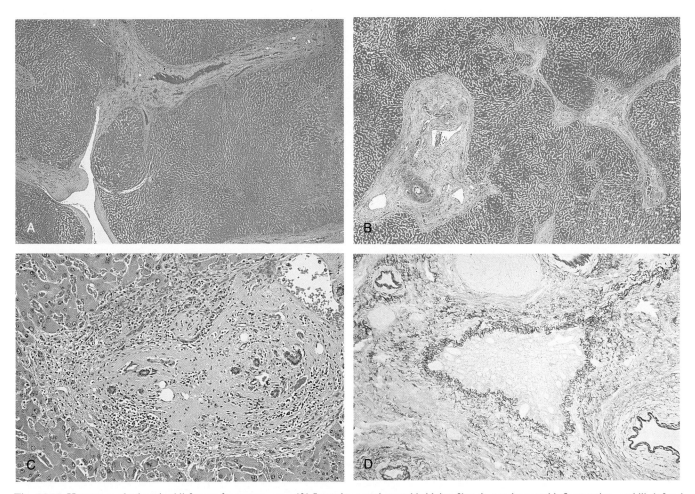

Fig. 15.22 Hepatoportal sclerosis. All figures from same case. (**A**) Irregular portal–portal bridging fibrosis, patchy portal inflammation, and ill-defined nodularity of the parenchyma. H & E. There was no known cause for this lesion, as is often true of hepatoportal sclerosis. The lesion is typical of that seen after long-term exposure to inorganic trivalent arsenic. (**B**) Markedly expanded acellular portal area (left) and portal–portal fibrous bridge (right). Masson trichrome. (**C**) Expanded portal area lacks portal vein branches with a diameter corresponding to its size. There is patchy infiltration with lymphocytes and plasma cells. H & E. (**D**) Occluded portal vein branch is readily identified by an elastic stain. Orcein.

phospholipidosis/non-alcoholic steatohepatitis.[69] Strategic deposition of collagen in the periportal area and space of Disse, accompanied by reduction of portal vein calibre even without cirrhosis, can also lead to portal hypertension (Fig. 15.22). This non-cirrhotic portal hypertension has been termed 'hepatoportal sclerosis'.[128-130]

Instances of non-cirrhotic portal hypertension have been attributed to chronic exposure to inorganic arsenicals,[130] to vinyl chloride[20] and to copper sulphate[131] as well as to alcoholic liver disease.[132] A form of non-cirrhotic portal hypertension can result from vitamin A intoxication[133] (Fig. 15.23). Several protocols employed to treat neoplastic disease have led to non-cirrhotic portal hypertension by producing hepatoportal sclerosis[134] or nodular regenerative hyperplasia of the liver.[135]

Periportal fibrosis occurs in drug-induced chronic active hepatitis[102-107] and in the chronic cholestasis that may follow acute cholestasis induced by chlorpromazine[88] and a number of other drugs (Table 15.11).

Table 15.11 Drugs incriminated in chronic cholestasis*

Aceprometazine (with meprobamate)
Ajmaline and related drugs
Amitryptyline
Ampicillin†
Barbiturate
Carbamazepine
Carbutamide
Chlorpromazine
Cimetidine
Cyproheptadine
Haloperidol
Imipramine
Methyltestosterone
Norandrostenolone
Phenytoin
Prochlorperazine
Thiabendazole
Tiopronin
Tolbutamide
Troleandomycin
Xenelamine

* De Gott et al[90]; †Cavanzo et al[552]

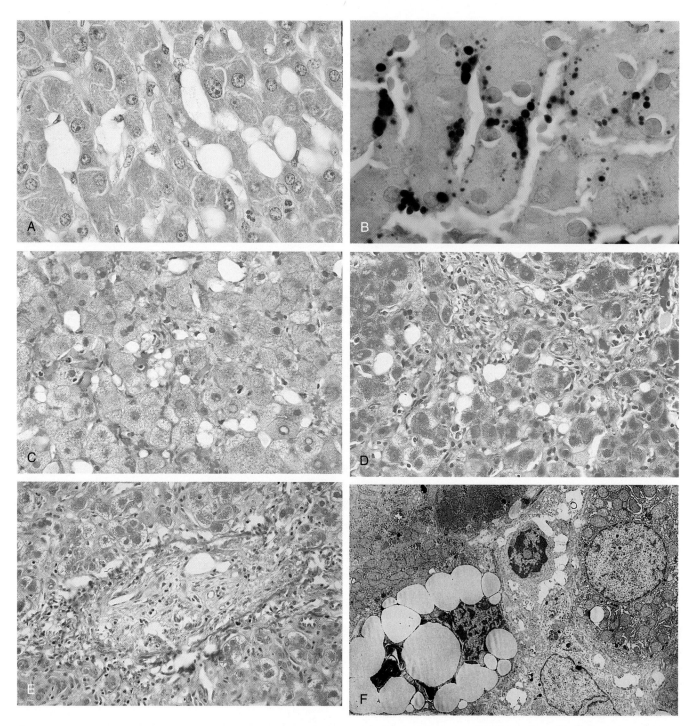

Fig. 15.23 Hypervitaminosis A. All figures from same case. (**A**) Markedly hypertrophied perisinusoidal cells (Ito cells) consist of clusters of faintly outlined fat vacuoles and distorted eccentrically-located nuclei. H & E. (**B**) Perisinusoidal location of Ito cells is demonstrated by use of lipid stain. Osmium tetroxide post-fixation. (**C**) Perisinusoidal fibrosis. Vacuoles represent perisinusoidal cells jammed in spaces of Disse. Masson trichrome. (**D**) More extensive fibrosis in zone 3. Masson. (**E**) Occluded terminal hepatic venule. Masson' trichrome. (**F**) Markedly hypertrophied perisinoidal cell (lower left) contains numerous lipid vacuoles and an eccentrically-located nucleas with scalloped margins. Electron micrograph, ×14 000.

Methotrexate has led to periportal fibrosis when used in the treatment of leukaemia,[136,137] and to both periportal and intra-acinar fibrosis and possibly to cirrhosis when used in the long-term therapy of psoriasis and, rarely, of rheumatoid arthritis[126,127] (Fig. 15.24). Alcoholic liver disease[132] and hypervitaminosis A[133] can lead to zone 3 fibrosis; in the latter condition there is also marked hypertrophy of the perisinusoidal cells (Ito cells) that store the vitamin A, atrophy of liver cells and dilatation of sinusoids (Fig. 15.23).

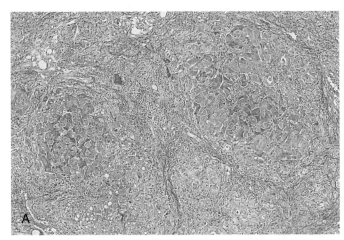

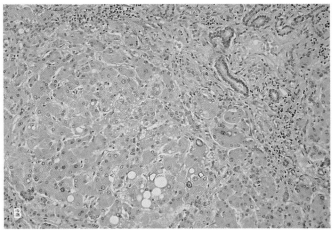

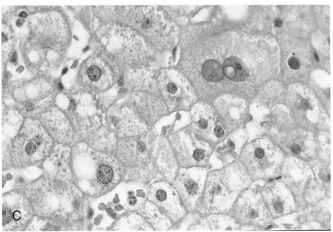

Fig. 15.24 Methotrexate-induced micronodular cirrhosis. (**A**) Masson' trichrome. (**B**) Same case illustrated in (**A**) Segment of micronodule reveals mild portal inflammation, patchy steatosis, glycogenated nuclei and moderate anisonucleosis. H & E. (**C**) Methotrexate-induced anisonucleosis. H & E.

Cirrhosis

Chemical hepatic injury can lead to all of the known morphological types of cirrhosis. Macronodular and micronodular cirrhosis,[34,138] congestive 'hepatopathy' resembling cardiac cirrhosis,[52,139–141] and a biliary cirrhosis-like lesion[88,142–147] can all result from toxin- or drug-induced liver damage.

Macronodular or micronodular cirrhosis may be a sequel to continued or often-repeated subtle injury, the result of subacute necrosis, or of chronic necro-inflammatory disease.[17] Cirrhosis of the macronodular type following a single episode of necrosis has been cited[15] but is rare, if it occurs at all. Massive, but non-lethal, necrosis may leave architectural distortion but rarely leads to cirrhosis.[34,138] In general, a single episode of zonal necrosis in experimental animals (e.g. CCl_4 poisoning), even when extensive, is followed by complete histological restitution in surviving animals.[34,138] Given at intervals too short to permit recovery from each dose, CCl_4 can lead to cirrhosis.[138]

Many of the known hepatotoxins can lead to cirrhosis in experimental animals.[50] Presumably, they could also do so in humans, although epidemiological evidence to support this possibility is limited. Occupational exposure to CCl_4,

tetrachlorethane, dimethylnitrosamine, and trinitrotoluene has been incriminated in instances of cirrhosis.[15,18,50] Inorganic arsenical compounds employed in the past for the treatment of leukaemia and psoriasis have also been incriminated.[148,149] In a sense, history has repeated itself in the modern era as instances of cirrhosis have resulted from the use of methotrexate to treat these diseases (Fig. 15.24).[127] The most important paths to cirrhosis as the result of drug-induced injury are the lesions of chronic active hepatitis[102–107] (Fig. 15.21), subacute necrosis (Fig. 15.20)[98] and phospholipidosis/non-alcoholic steatohepatitis[68,70,112,119] (Figs 15.11 and 15.13). The role of fungal and plant toxins in the production of cirrhosis in humans remains inconculsive, although probable in some settings.[18]

'*Congestive cirrhosis*' may be a sequel to veno-occlusive disease, hepatic vein thrombosis or congestive cardiac failure.[52,139–141] Primary biliary cirrhosis may be mimicked by chronic intrahepatic cholestasis (Fig. 15.25) occurring as a sequel to acute intrahepatic cholestasis.[142–147] An obstructive biliary cirrhosis type of injury might be a consequence of the biliary sclerosis produced by hepatic artery infusion of floxuridine for treatment of metastatic carcinoma of the liver[150,151] (Fig. 15.26).

Cholestatic lesions

Chronic intrahepatic cholestasis

A syndrome that resembles primary biliary cirrhosis has followed acute cholestasis due to chlorpromazine, prochlorperazine, amitryptyline, imipramine, organic arsenicals,

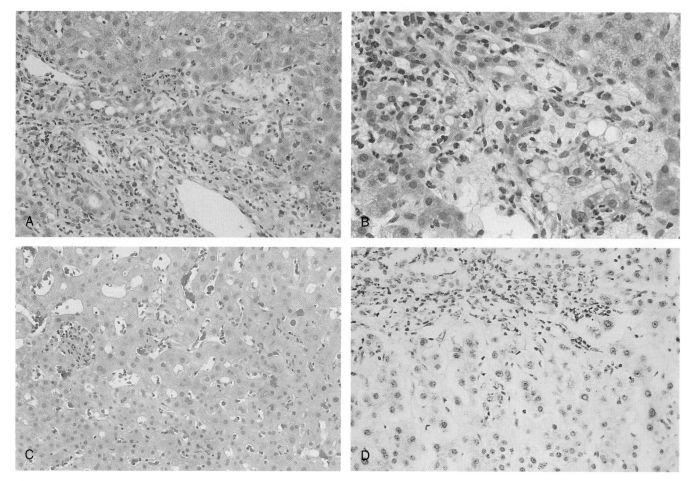

Fig. 15.25 Chlorpromazine-induced chronic cholestasis. All figures from same case. (**A**) Marked portal inflammation (neutrophils, eosinophils) and acute cholangiolitis. H & E. (**B**) Periportal focus of pseudoxanthomatous transformation. H & E. (**C**) Moderate cholestasis and focal necrosis (left). H & E. (**D**) Moderate copper accumulation (red granules) in periportal liver cells. Rhodanine.

tolbutamide, ajmaline and several other drugs listed in Table 15.11.[143-147] Table 15.12 contains a comparison of the features of the drug-induced chronic cholestatic syndrome with those of primary biliary cirrhosis. Duct destruction and portal inflammation are less prominent in the drug-induced syndrome than in primary biliary cirrhosis but may be part of the lesion[88] (Fig. 15.25). Indeed, the syndrome has been called the 'vanishing duct syndrome'.[90]

Biliary sclerosis

Biliary sclerosis is the term that has been applied to the injury produced by therapy of hepatic metastatic carcinoma, with floxuridine infused into the hepatic artery.[150-155] The incidence appears to be high, and the lesion consists of blebs and oedema in the duct epithelial surface and compression and distortion of the duct lumen[155] (Fig. 15.26). Ludwig et al[155] have attributed the

ductal injury to occlusive arterial injury and have labelled the biliary lesion an 'ischaemic cholangiopathy'. On cholangiography, the lesion resembles sclerosing cholangitis. Clinical features include upper abdominal aching, anorexia, weight loss, and jaundice.

Vascular lesions

A number of important vascular lesions can be produced by drugs (Table 15.4).[156] Two involve blockade of efferent blood flow and congestive hepatopathy, leading to necrosis involving zone 3 and, when severe, zone 2. Prolonged occlusion leads to fibrotic bridging between adjacent acini and a picture resembling cardiac cirrhosis. The two occlusive lesions are thrombosis of the hepatic veins (Fig. 15.27) and fibrotic occlusion of the hepatic venules (Fig. 15.28). A third vascular lesion is peliosis hepatis (Fig. 15.29). Additional lesions include sinusoidal dilatation (Fig. 15.30),

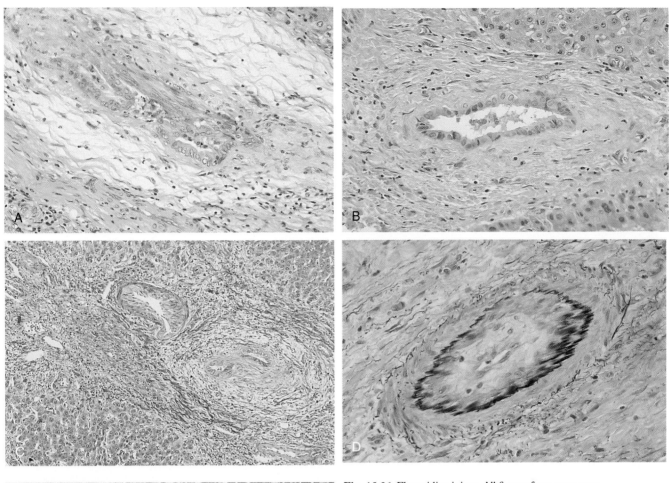

Fig. 15.26 Floxuridine injury. All figures from same case. (**A**) Tangentially-sectioned interlobular bile duct shows degeneration and neutrophilic infiltration. H & E. (**B**) Periductal sclerosis. Note cholestasis in zone 1. H & E. (**C**) Periductal sclerosis, thick-walled artery and occluded vein (left) in portal area. Masson trichrome. (**D**) Hepatic artery branch in portal area shows marked intimal thickening with almost complete occlusion of the lumen, medial hypertrophy and a thickened elastica. Musto. (**E**) Portal vein branch shows old fibrotic occlusion. Masson trichrome.

perisinusoidal fibrosis (Fig. 15.23), and hepatoportal sclerosis (Fig. 15.22).

Hepatic vein thrombotic occlusion

The lesion is the classic cause of the Budd–Chiari syndrome. At least 100 instances have been reported in patients taking oral contraceptives and have been attributed to the thrombogenic effects of contraceptive steroids.[141,157,158] Most of the individuals involved appear to have had overt or latent myeloproliferative disease, but fully a third of the studied cases have not.[157,158] According to Valla et al,[158] the risk of developing hepatic vein thrombosis seems to be more than twice as great in patients taking oral contraceptives as in other women. The incriminability of oral contraceptives as a cause of the Budd–Chiari syndrome, however, remains controversial.[159]

Veno-occlusive disease (VOD)

Injury and occlusion of the efferent hepatic venules has long been known to be produced by pyrrolizidine

Table 15.12 Comparison of primary biliary cirrhosis (PBC) with drug-induced chronic cholestasis (DICC): from Zimmerman (1978)[18]

Characteristics	PBC	DICC
Associated diseases	Sicca syndrome, other 'collagen' disease	Irrelevant
Drug intake	Irrelevant	Phenothiazines Organic arsenicals Tolbutamide ?Other cholestasis-producing drugs
Symptoms		
Pruritus	+	+
Jaundice	– or + (a)	+
Signs		
Skin pigmentations	+	
Jaundice	– or +	+
Xanthomas	+ or –	+ or –
Hepatomegaly	+ or –	+ or –
Splenomegaly	+ or –	+ or –
Biochemical features		
Bilirubin	1–5 mg/dl	1–20 mg/dl
AST/ALT	1–5×	1–5×
Alkaline phosphatase	3–10×	3–10×
Cholesterol	Increased	Increased
ß-globulin	Increased	Increased
IgM	Increased	?
Histological features		
Non-suppurative cholangitis(b)	+	–
Ductopenia	+	+/–
Hepatic granulomas	+	–
Copper in hepatocytes	+	+
Cirrhosis	+ (eventually)	+/–
Prognosis	Variable(c)	Good

(a) Jaundice is usually slight and tends to come relatively late in the course of PBC, while it is early in the course of DICC.
(b) Refers to inflammatory response in portal area
(c) In most instances; outcome is eventually poor when cirrhosis develops.
+ = usually present; – = usually absent; +/– = present but of slight degree

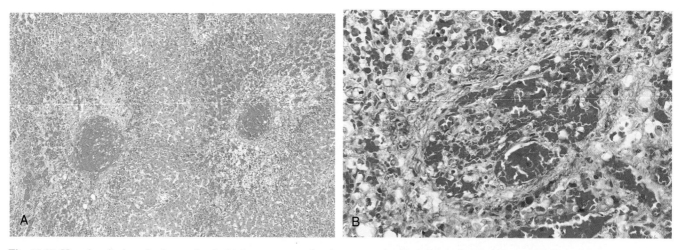

Fig. 15.27 Hepatic vein thrombosis associated with long-term use of oral contraceptive. Both figures from same case. (**A**) Recent thrombi in two terminal hepatic venules with necrosis in zone 3 and marked sinusoidal dilatation and congestion. H & E. (**B**) Thrombosed and recanalized terminal hepatic venule. Masson' trichrome.

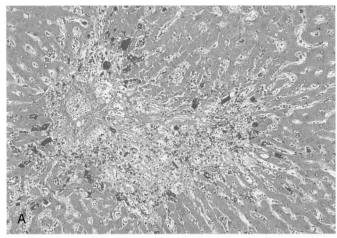

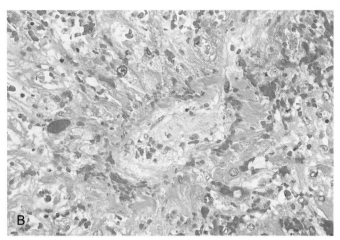

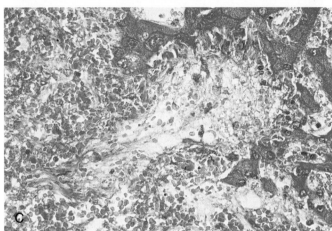

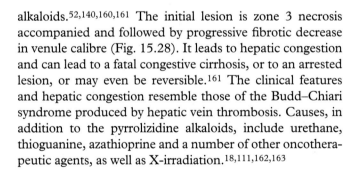

Fig. 15.28 Veno-occlusive disease associated with chemoradiation used for preconditioning prior to bone marrow transplantation. All figures from same case. (**A**) Haemorrhagic necrosis involving zone 3. Terminal hepatic venule (left) shows marked intimal thickening. H & E. (**B**) Wall of terminal hepatic venule is thickened by oedema, and there are numerous extravasated erythrocytes in the intima. H & E. (**C**) Same features shown in (**B**) are present but the lumen of the vein is completely occluded. Masson' trichrome.

alkaloids.[52,140,160,161] The initial lesion is zone 3 necrosis accompanied and followed by progressive fibrotic decrease in venule calibre (Fig. 15.28). It leads to hepatic congestion and can lead to a fatal congestive cirrhosis, or to an arrested lesion, or may even be reversible.[161] The clinical features and hepatic congestion resemble those of the Budd–Chiari syndrome produced by hepatic vein thrombosis. Causes, in addition to the pyrrolizidine alkaloids, include urethane, thioguanine, azathioprine and a number of other oncotherapeutic agents, as well as X-irradiation.[18,111,162,163]

Peliosis hepatis

This lesion consists of large blood-filled cavities (Fig. 15.29). It has long been of interest to pathologists but its clinical significance was recognized only recently.[164–170] The lesion has been produced in experimental animals by administration of lasiocarpine[171] and of phalloidin.[172] Since phalloidin has a special proclivity for injury to membranes[172] its production of peliosis would be consistent with the theory that the lesion reflects 'weakening' of sinusoidal supporting membranes.[172] Necrosis also has been suggested as the initial injury.

Incriminated causes of the lesion in humans include anabolic steroids,[156,167–170] diethylstilboestrol,[166] contraceptive steroids,[173,174] tamoxifen[175] and azathioprine.[176,177] Of practical import is the observation of marked sinusoidal dilatation in livers that show peliosis hepatis, even in sites remote from the lesion.[168] Furthermore, anabolic and contraceptive steroids can lead to sinusoidal dilatation, even when no peliosis has developed.[178] Indeed, a characteristic lesion of prominent dilatation of sinusoids in zone 1 (Fig. 15.30) has been described in patients taking contraceptive steroids.[178,179]

Hepatic neoplasia

Benign tumours

Adenoma, a lesion almost restricted to females in the child-bearing years, was until recently an extremely uncommon tumour.[29] During the past few years, however, many more cases have been encountered, almost all in recipients of contraceptive steroids[27,29,180–182] (see Ch. 16). Perhaps the most convincing evidence for a cause–effect relationship is the reported regression of this tumour following withdrawal of oral contraceptives.[183]

Less convincing is the reported association between the development of ***focal nodular hyperplasia*** and contraceptive steroids;[181] although in some instances contracep-

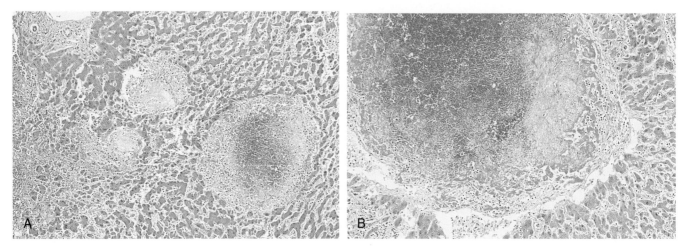

Fig. 15.29 Peliosis hepatis associated with oxymetholone therapy given to patient with aplastic anaemia. Both figures from same case. (**A**) Peliotic cavities are of variable size. H & E. (**B**) Blood in cavity is clotted, with fibrin accumulation at the periphery of the cavity. The cavity has no endothelial lining. H & E.

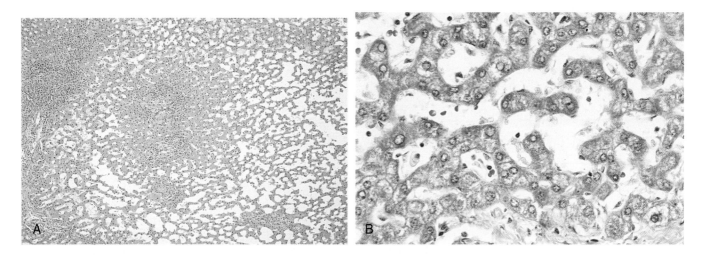

Fig. 15.30 Sinusoidal dilatation associated with long-term use of oral contraceptive. Both figures from same case. (**A**) Note portal area in centre of field. H & E. (**B**) Atrophy of liver plates and striking sinusoidal dilatation. H & E.

tive steroids seem to have had a trophic effect on the growth of focal nodular hyperplasia.[184]

Malignant tumours (see Ch. 16)

Carcinomas, both hepatocellular and cholangiocarcinoma, can be experimentally produced. A large number of chemical and botanical toxins can produce hepatocellular tumours;[185,186] and while most of the cholangiocarcinomas which have been produced are probably variants of hepatocellular carcinoma, true adenocarcinomas have been induced.[185,187–189] In man, Thorotrast has produced hepatocellular and cholangiocellular carcinomas as well as haemangiosarcomas, lesions that may be due to the radioactivity rather than the chemical toxicity of the agent.[190] Epidemiological studies suggest that mycotoxins

as well as synthetic chemicals encountered occupationally may also be carcinogenic in man.[24,25,186,191]

Several medicinal agents have come under suspicion as possible hepatocarcinogens. Development of hepatocellular carcinoma in at least 40 long-term recipients of anabolic steroids has made these agents suspect.[26,28,192] The contraceptive steroids also have been incriminated in the development of hepatocellular carcinoma.[30,31,193] While griseofulvin,[194] and isoniazid[195] are experimental hepatocarcinogens, there is no evidence of their carcinogenicity for man.

Haemangiosarcoma came into sharp focus as a malignant tumour occurring in individuals with occupational exposure to vinyl chloride.[26,196,197] This rare tumour also has developed in vintners with long exposure to inorganic arsenic, in patients with psoriasis treated with arsenicals or

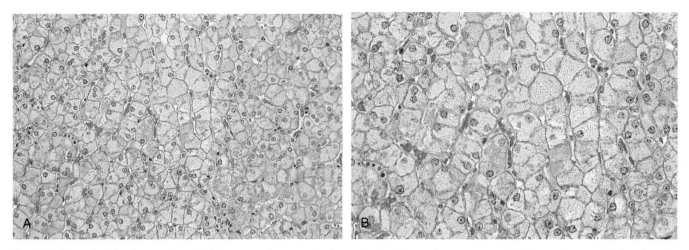

Fig. 15.31 Enzymic induction associated with long-term therapy with phenytoin. Both figures from same case. (**A**) Liver cells are markedly enlarged and have a lightly stained, very finely vesiculated cytoplasm. H & E. (**B**) Higher magnification of induced hepatocytes. Nuclei are located either centrally or eccentrically. H & E.

who had ingested arsenic-contaminated water or had other environmental exposures,[198,199] and in patients who had been injected with Thorotrast.[190,200-204] A case of haemangiosarcoma in a 54-year-old man who had sprayed vineyards with copper sulphate for 35 years raises a possible aetiological relationship of this neoplasm to another heavy metal.[87] Of interest in this context is the occurrence of several cases of haemangiosarcoma in patients with haemochromatosis.[200] Other drugs incriminated rarely as causes of this tumour, include androgenic-anabolic steroids,[205] diethylstilboestrol,[206] and phenelzine.[207]

OTHER DRUG-ASSOCIATED MORPHOLOGICAL FEATURES

Adaptive changes

Ground-glass hepatocytes may develop in long-term therapy with some drugs (Fig. 15.31). This change was first reported by Klinge & Bannasch[208] in patients on long-term therapy with chlorpromazine and barbiturates, and in some patients who had chronic hepatitis, cirrhosis or hepatocellular carcinoma. Other drugs that have been implicated in this change include azathioprine, steroids, resorcin and some analgesics,[209] as well as phenytoin.[210] The change was attributed to a marked, diffuse hyper-trophy of the smooth endoplasmic reticulum (SER) by Klinge & Bannasch,[208] and this has been confirmed in ultrastructural studies.[211-213] It is associated with in-creased activity of microsomal NADPH cytochorme c reductase.[213] Subsequently, the same type of change was found in clinically healthy HBsAg carriers.[214,215] Special stains (aldehyde fuchsin and thionin, and orcein) that have been found to stain the ground-glass hepatocyte

containing HBsAg in the SER, do not stain drug-induced ground-glass cells.[83, 209, 216]

The prognostic significance of the drug-induced ground-glass transformation is not known. Serologically this change is accompanied by elevated levels of γ-glutamyltransferase (GGT)[213] and is believed to account for the hepatomegaly commonly observed in patients on anticonvulsant and other drugs.[212] It is not associated with acute or chronic injury caused by the same drug, and there are no long-term studies of patients with this drug-induced hepatic change. Nevertheless, as noted by several authors, the borderline between adaptation and toxicity remains an uncharted terrain.[211, 217]

A dramatic form of ground-glass change (Fig. 15.32) has been noted in alcoholic patients undergoing aversion therapy.[218-221] At first attributed to disulfiram, it now appears more clearly relatable to cyanamide treatment. The ground-glass cells differ from those described in the foregoing paragraph, in that the cyanamide-associated altered cells contain 'inclusion bodies' that contain glycogen in beta granules, secondary lysosomes, lipid vesicles and residues of degenerate organelles. Furthermore, this lesion can lead to cirrhosis.[222]

Pigment deposits

Several types of pigmentary deposits may follow exposure to exogenous chemicals. These include lipofuscin, haemo-siderin, copper, Thorotrast, gold, titanium and bilirubin.

Lipofuscin, the least significant of these, occurs normally in perivenular hepatocyte lysosomes; it is more prominent in elderly people (Fig. 15.33). It also becomes increased in patients on various long-term medications, such as phena-cetin, *Cascara sagrada* and chlorpromazine,[223] as well as

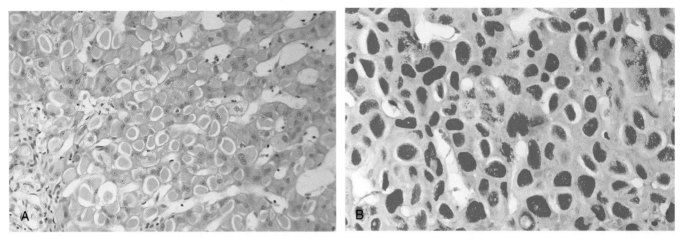

Fig. 15.32 Cyanamide-induced injury. Both figures from same case. (**A**) Periportal liver cells contain large, eosinophilic (ground-glass) inclusions surrounded by an artefactual space. H & E. (**B**) Inclusions are still strongly PAS-positive after diastase digestion.

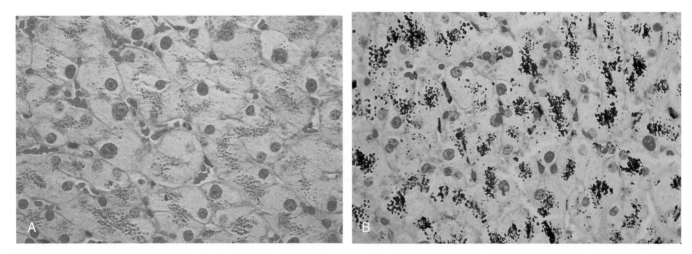

Fig. 15.33 Excess lipofuscin accumulation in liver cells in patient on long-term chlorpromazine therapy. Both figures from same case. (**A**) H & E. (**B**) Pigment accumulation is well demonstrated by the Fontana stain.

anticonvulsant therapy.[212] Ceroid pigment, a lipofuscin, may become more prominent in Kupffer cells following recent necrosis, and increased deposits may follow intravenous infusion of fat emulsions.[224, 225] Tiny black granules (Fig. 15.34) may reflect presence of *gold* as a residue of use of gold compounds for treatment of arthritis,[85] or *titanium* which may be found in the liver of parenteral drug abusers.[226]

Haemosiderin deposits are seen in association with several forms of chemical hepatic injury. In the iron overload associated with alcoholism, haemosiderin is seen in hepatocytes, Kupffer cells and macrophages.[227] Similar deposits are seen in patients with porphyria cutanea tarda associated with alcohol intake[228] or due to chemical (hexachlorobenzene) injury.[229,230] Hepatic haemosiderosis has been reported in patients on long-term haemodialysis who had received parenteral iron[231, 232] (Fig. 15.35).

Copper accumulation, a regular concomitant of primary biliary cirrhosis, may also be seen in drug-induced chronic cholestasis, for example that induced by chlorpromazine,[88] (Fig. 15.25D) and is found in all other forms of prolonged cholestasis. Copper has been demonstrated histochemically in Kupffer cells and within granulomas in patients occupationally exposed to sprayed copper salts.[87]

Thorotrast remained in the livers of patients many years after they had received this radioactive material. It appears as glistening, greyish-brown granules engorging macrophages or lying free in dense fibrous tissue (Fig. 15.36).

Bilirubin is, of course, the pigment most likely to be seen in patients with toxic hepatic injury. In intrahepatic cholestasis it is particularly prominent in canaliculi of zone 3, and may also be seen in Kupffer cells and in hepatocytes (Fig. 15.17).

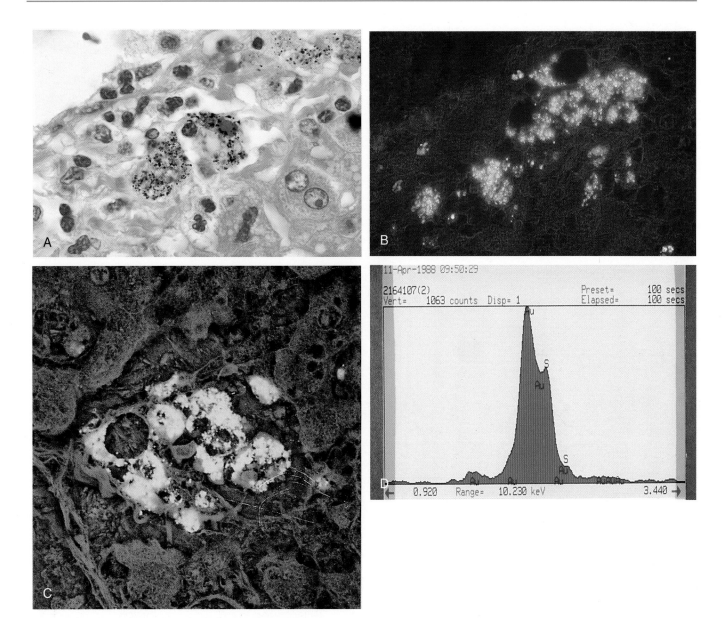

Fig. 15.34 Patient who had received gold therapy for rheumatoid arthritis. All figures from same case. (**A**) Granular, black pigment in Kupffer cells. H & E. (**B**) Pigment granules display a golden birefringence in polarized light. (**C**) The pigment granules are readily identified by scanning electron microscopy using the back scatter technique. ×1500. (**D**) X-ray microanalysis reveals the presence of the elements gold and sulphur in the pigment granules.

BIOCHEMICAL, FUNCTIONAL AND CLINICAL MANIFESTATIONS OF INJURY

The biochemical manifestations of hepatotoxicity reflect the histological patterns of injury (Table 15.13). Toxic necrosis leads to changes in the blood and to clinical features similar to those of acute viral hepatitis. Toxic steatosis leads to qualitatively similar, but quantitatively more modest abnormalities. The histological pattern and

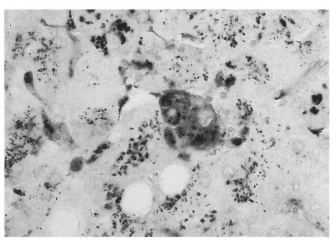

Fig. 15.35 Marked haemosiderosis (reticuloendothelial and hepatocellular) in patient on renal haemodialysis who had received intramuscular iron therapy. Mallory's stain for iron.

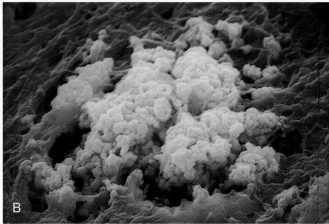

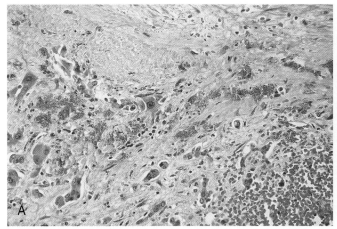

Fig. 15.36 Thorotrast — all figures from same case. (**A**) Coarsely granular deposits of Thorotrast are pink-brown in colour, and are surrounded by dense fibrous tissue. H & E. (**B**) Thorotrast particles are readily identified by scanning electron microscopy. × 3000. (**C**) Element thorium is identified in Thorotrast deposits by X-ray microanalysis.

Table 15.13 Histological types of acute toxic hepatic injury and associated biochemical and clinical aspects

Histological lesion	Biochemical abnormalities in serum[a]			Clinical aspects	Examples[b]
	AST and ALT	Alkaline phosphatase	Cholesterol		
I. Cytotoxic					
Zonal necrosis	10–500×	1–2×	Normal or low	Hepatic and renal failure	Carbon tetrachloride, MSH, P, HALO
Diffuse necrosis	10–200×	1–2×	Normal or low	Severe hepatitis-like disease	INH, methyldopa, HALO
Steatosis	5–20×	1–2×	Normal or low	Resembles fatty liver of pregnancy and Reye's syndrome	Tetracycline
II. Cholestatic					
With portal tract inflammation (hepatocanalicular)	1–10×	3–10×	High	Resembles obstructive jaundice	CPZ, EE
Without portal tract inflammation (canalicular)	1–5×	1–3×	Normal or high	Resembles obstructive jaundice	Anabolic and contraceptive steroids
III. Mixed (mixtures of cytotoxic and cholestatic)	10–100×	1–10×	Normal or high	May resemble hepatitis or obstructive jaundice	PBZ, PAS, sulphonamides

[a] Degree of abnormality indicated as fold increase. AST = aspartate transaminase; ALT = alanine transaminase
[b] PAS = para-aminosalicylic acid; MSH = poisonous mushrooms; P = paracetamol; HALO = halothane; INH = isoniazid; CPZ = chlorpromazine; EE = erythromycin estolate; PBZ = phenylbutazone

biochemical changes of cholestasis mimic those of biliary tract obstruction.

Hepatocellular necrosis produces in the blood high levels of enzymes released from the damaged liver. Most extensively studied, in this regard, are the levels of the transaminases (aminotransferases) which may be increased to values that are 10- to 500-fold the normal; but a number of other enzymes also reflect the change sensitively.[233] In contrast to the logarithmic increase in levels of transaminases, the values for serum alkaline phosphatase, 5'-nucleotidase and leucine aminopeptidase increase no more than one- to three-fold, in response to necrosis.

Depressed levels of plasma coagulation factors are characteristic of hepatic necrosis, and in the usual clinical setting are reflected in the one-stage prothrombin time. Indeed, the most useful clinical clues to severity of necrosis are the prothrombin time and bilirubin levels.[234]

Albumin levels do not change appreciably in the early phase of acute necrosis. Hypoalbuminaemia ensues only late in the clinical course, or in association with subacute or chronic disease. Globulin levels also may stay unchanged although in subacute and chronic drug-induced disease the gamma globulin levels may increase somewhat. Indeed, in drug-induced chronic hepatitis gamma globulin levels may be strikingly increased.[107] Plasma cholesterol levels tend to be low or normal in acute hepatic necrosis.

Microvesicular steatosis leads to less dramatic biochemical evidence of hepatic injury than does acute necrosis. Values for the serum transaminases in tetracycline toxicity increase to 5- to 20-fold the upper limit of normal. Bilirubin levels are only modestly increased. Values for alkaline phosphatase resemble those of hepatic necrosis in their slight degree of increase. Prolonged prothrombin times are characteristic. Hypoglycaemia may be prominent.[18] Macrovesicular steatosis leads to even lesser degrees of abnormality.

Cholestatic injury is manifested clinically by jaundice and itching. The transaminase levels in the two types of cholestasis do not differ appreciably. In hepatocanalicular cholestasis alkaline phosphatase may be increased to three- to ten-fold the normal level and the cholesterol values are increased, whereas in the canalicular type the alkaline phosphatase increases are less than three-fold and the cholesterol level is usually normal.

Toxic porphyria may accompany several forms of hepatic injury. The hepatic steatosis, necrosis and cirrhosis produced in humans[229] and experimental animals[230] by hexachlorobenzene is accompanied by a form of porphyria resembling porphyria cutanea tarda. Most cases of porphyria cutanea tarda, however, are associated with alcoholism and alcoholic liver disease[228,235] or chronic hepatitis C.[235a] Griseofulvin-induced hepatic injury also may be accompanied by a similar defect in porphyrin metabolism.[194]

Some of the clinical manifestations of drug-induced hepatic injury are systemic and extrahepatic. Fever, rash

Table 15.14 Salient features of syndromes of acute toxic hepatic injury from Zimmerman (1978)[18]

	CCl4	Phosphorus	Toxic mushrooms	Paracetamol
Phase I (1st 24 h)				
Diarrhoea	+	+*	–	–
Vomiting		+*	+	+/–
Pain		+	–	–
Haemorrhage	–	+	–	
Shock	–	+		+/–
Phase II (24–72 h)				
Asymptomatic period	–	+	+	+
Jaundice	+	–	–	–
Renal	+/–	+/–	+	–
CNS	–	–	+	–
Phase III (48–72 h)				
Hepatic failure	+	+	+	+
Jaundice	4+	4+	4+	+
Renal failure	+	+	+	+/–
Haemorrhagic phenomena	+	+	+	+
Hepatic lesion				
Steatosis	+	4+	4+	+/–
Necrosis	Zone 3	Zone 1	Zone 3	Zone 3
Mortality	10–20%	30–40%	25%	15%

* Phosphorescent appearance and garlic odour to vomitus and faeces

and eosinophilia may precede or accompany the hepatic injury. Indeed, the pseudomononucleosis syndrome of fever, rash, lymphadenopathy, and lymphocytosis with 'atypical' lymphocytes in the blood is a classic reaction to injury by phenytoin, sulphonamides, dapsone, para-aminosalicylic acid and other drugs.[18,236,237] Renal injury may occur as a result of nephrotoxic metabolites, e.g. methoxyflurane,[238] or as a manifestation of generalized hypersensitivity.[237]

Syndromes of injury produced by a number of known hepatotoxins tend to consist of three phases: (i) immediate severe, neurological or gastrointestinal manifestations; (ii) a period of relative well-being; (iii) the phase of overt hepatic injury that often includes renal failure. This sequence is characteristic of poisoning due to CCl4,[239] phosphorus,[3] hepatotoxic mushrooms[240,241] and, to some degree, of that due to paracetamol[18] (Table 15.14).

ANALYSIS OF HEPATOTOXIC REACTIONS ACCORDING TO CIRCUMSTANCES OF EXPOSURE

OCCUPATIONAL AND DOMESTIC HEPATOTOXINS

A host of agents with hepatotoxic potential have been employed in the munitions, rocketry, plastics, agricultural,

Table 15.15 Partial list of agents likely to be encountered occupationally with indication of hepatic lesion in experimental animals and humans[a]

	Demonstrated in		Lesions
	Experimental animals	Humans	
Beryllium	+	?	Granuloma, necrosis; MZ
Carbon disulphide[b]	+	0	Ballooning, fat; PV
Chlorinated aromatic compounds[d]	+ to ++++	+ to ++++	Necrosis, fat; PV
Chloronitroaromatic compounds[d]	+ to ++++	+ to ++++	Necrosis, fat; PV
Chloronitroparaffins[d]	+++	0	Necrosis; PV or M
Copper	+	+	Granuloma
4'4-Diaminodiphenylmethane[e]	+	+	Cholestasis
Dimethylformamide	+	+	Microvesicular steatosis, necrosis
Dioxan	+	+	Necrosis; PV
Diphenyloxide	+	+	Necrosis; PV
Furans	±	±	Necrosis; PV
Nitroaromatic compounds	+ to ++++	+ to ++++	Necrosis; PV or M
Nitroparaffins			
Nitroethane	++	0	Necrosis
Nitromethane	+	0	Necrosis
1-Nitropropane	+++	0	Necrosis
2-Nitropropane	++	+	Necrosis

[a] References 18, 50, 79
[b] Injury slight unless drug-metabolizing enzymes induced
[c] PV = perivenular (acinar zone 3); M = massive; MZ = midzonal (acinar zone 2)
[d] Brominated and iodinated compounds cause injury similar to that of chorinated ones
[e] Agent of Epping jaundice, reference 247

paint, cosmetic, pharmaceutical and other chemical industries (Table 15.15). Nevertheless, overt, acute hepatic injury is an uncommon consequence of occupational exposure to toxic chemicals.[18]

Hepatotoxins encountered in the home (Table 15.16) include:

1. Some of the industrial toxins, e.g. CCl$_4$, and other chemicals such as phosphorus and copper salts.

2. Ordinarily safe drugs if taken in large overdoses, e.g. paracetamol; others are discussed in the appropriate sections later in this chapter.

3. Mycotoxins and other botanical agents. Poisonous mushrooms are still an important cause of acute hepatic injury in some parts of the world.[6,240-242] Food contaminated with aflatoxins has been implicated in causing acute hepatic disease.[77,243] and, on epidemiological grounds, in the aetiology of hepatocellular carcinoma.[24,25] Consump-

Table 15.16 Hepatotoxic agents to which household exposure is known or potential

Agents	Exposure	Lesion
Chlorinated hydrocarbons	Careless use, accidental, 'solvent sniffing'	Perivenular necrosis (zone 3), steatosis
Phosphorus (yellow)	Suicidal or accidental	Steatosis, periportal necrosis (zone 1)
Toxic chemicals as inadvertent contaminants of food:		
4-4'-Diaminodiphenylmethane	Contaminant of flour ('Epping jaundice')	Cholestatic jaundice
Hexachlorobenzene	Fungistatic added to wheat	Steatosis, necrosis, toxic porphyria
Chlorinated biphenyls	Contaminant of rice (Japan)	Steatosis, necrosis
Toxic drugs	Poisonous overdose (paracetamol)	Perivenular necrosis (zone 3)
Drug abuse	Sniffing of chloroform, trichloroethylene, halothane, glue	Varies with toxic agent; Most often perivenular necrosis (zone 3)
Toxic foods of plant origin:		
Amanita phalloides and related species	Ingested as food in ignorance of toxicity	Perivenular necrosis (zone 3), steatosis
Cycad nut	Ingested as food in ignorance of toxicity	Necrosis, steatosis, cirrhosis, hepatocellular carcinoma
Senecio, Heliotropium, Crotalaria, and other plants that contain pyrrolizidine alkaloids	Ingested as additive to foods, as medicinal decoction, or as abortifacient	Perivenular necrosis (zone 3), veno-occlusive disease, congestive cirrhosis
Nutmeg	Ingested as abortifacient	Steatosis, midzonal necrosis (zone 2)
Mycotoxins		
Aflatoxins	Present mainly in legumes and other foods of vegetable origin when climatic conditions permit	Steatosis, necrosis, cirrhosis, hepatocellular carcinoma
Ochratoxin		
Luteoskyrin		

tion of plants containing pyrrolizidine alkaloids has long been known to cause acute and chronic hepatic disease, and continues to be responsible for epidemics of veno-occlusive disease.[244,245] Ingestion of the cycad nut can cause acute hepatic disease[246] and has the potential for causing chronic liver disease including carcinoma.[23]

4. Food containing preservatives, or accidentally or carelessly contaminated with toxic chemicals. Epping jaundice,[247] an epidemic of cholestatic jaundice caused by the use of flour contaminated by methylene dianiline,[248] by a bakery in Epping, England, was an example of hepatic injury acquired in the home. The possible synthesis in the gastrointestinal tract of hepatotoxic and hepatocarcino-genic nitrosamines from ingested nitrites and secondary amines has been the subject of speculation.[249]

5. Exposure to insecticides including a number of chlorinated aromatic hydrocarbons is widespread by way of foodstuffs, occupational exposure and, at times, accidental or suicidal ingestion. Long-term storage in human tissues of DDT and other insecticides and their metabolites has been demonstrated.[250] Nevertheless, there is no significant evidence of hepatic injury form sustained occupational exposure to the chlorinated insecticides. Accidental ingestion of large amounts of DDT (approximately 6 g[251]) and of paraquat (approximately 20 g),[252] however, has led to rare instances of zone 3 hepatic necrosis. Paraquat poisoning also can lead to cholestasis.[35,89,252] The early injury is zone 3 necrosis; the later injury is cholestasis. The clinical relevance of the known ability of DDT and related compounds to induce the drug-metabolizing enzyme system and so affect hepatotoxic exposure is open to speculation.[43]

The usual circumstances of exposure and the character of the injury produced by household hepatotoxins are summarized in Table 15.16. The toxicity of several of these agents, however, warrants description in more detail.

Carbon tetrachloride poisoning

Instances of CCl_4 intoxication still occur, but are now rare.[2] Most victims are alcoholics since alcoholism enhances susceptibility to this hepatotoxin and leads to increased carelessness with its use. Inhalation of the agent, usually during careless domestic use, or accidental ingestion of the toxin during a state of alcoholic intoxication has been the usual mode of exposure.[239,253] There is little evidence to support an early view that poisoning by inhalation produces mainly renal injury and that poisoning by ingestion leads mainly to hepatic injury.[15]

The clinical syndrome consists of hepatic failure regularly accompanied by renal failure. Indeed, CCl_4 poisoning may rarely lead to renal failure with little or no evidence of hepatic injury. Prior to the appearance of hepatic injury there are usually neurological and gastrointestinal manifestations and a variable degree of vascular collapse.[237,239,253]

The main histological abnormalities are in the liver and kidney, but there are also changes in the lung, heart, pancreas and brain. The liver shows necrosis and some steatosis in acinar zone 3 (Fig. 15.3). The degree of steatosis is variable, presumably reflecting, at least in part, the effects of the usually associated alcoholism. Prominent ballooning may precede the necrosis. Renal abnormalities include necrosis and fatty change of the tubules.[254] The lungs of fatal cases show oedema, an alveolar pseudomembrane, and thickened, fibrotic alveolar walls with epithelial proliferation. These changes may reflect renal failure rather than the pulmonary toxicity of CCl_4.[255] Myocardial degeneration also may be a complication of renal failure or of its treatment, or may reflect a toxic effect of CCl_4 on the myocardium. Pancreatitis is a frequent finding.[254] The mortality rate in CCl_4 poisoning ranged from 10–25%,[18] prior to the use of extracorporeal dialysis for renal failure, and may be lowered further by treatment with acetyl-cysteine and hyperbaric oxygen.[256]

Other chloroalkanes, e.g. trichloroethylene, may produce a similar syndrome and histological changes.[254,257] The relative toxicity and likelihood of producing these changes depends on the energy of the carbon–halogen bond of the respective compound and the relative ease of formation of the active metabolite.[256–258,259]

Mushroom and phosphorus poisoning

A somewhat similar clinical syndrome results from poisoning by the hepatotoxic mushroom Amanita phalloides and related species, and by phosphorus. The mortality rate of mushroom poisoning has been above 25%[8,242,260] and that of phosphorus poisoning has been in excess of 50%.[3]

Mushroom poisoning presents as severe diarrhoea followed by amelioration and subsequently by severe hepatic and renal failure.[242,260] The liver shows very prominent steatosis and zone 3 necrosis (Fig. 15.5).

Phosphorus poisoning is characterized by more severe gastrointestinal symptoms and shock than is CCl_4 poisoning, and by phosphorescence and garlic-like odour of excreta and vomitus. The fully-developed clinical picture is that of fulminant hepatic and renal failure. Histologically, the liver may show only or mainly steatosis, at first in the periportal zones and then throughout the acini. Necrosis may, however, be present and is also predominantly periportal in distribution.[5]

Toxic epidemic syndrome is a multisystem illness that appeared in Spain in 1981 and was attributed to illegally sold cooking oil that had been adulterated with aniline-denatured rapeseed oil.[261–263] Approximately 50 000 to 100 000 people consumed the poisoned oil, of whom 18 000 required medical treatment and 350 died.[262] Almost a quarter of the patients treated at one medical facility had biochemical or, less often, clinical evidence of hepatic involvement, but the majority were asymptomatic.[261,262]

The histopathological changes were those of a cholestatic hepatitis that resembled chlorpromazine-induced liver injury.[262] Of 24 patients studied by Solis-Herruzo et al[262] 11 had bile-duct degenerative and inflammatory lesions, in addition to cholestasis and necro-inflammatory changes.

MEDICINAL AGENTS

There is an interesting and useful relationship between the pharmacological category of a drug and the type of hepatic injury that it can produce. General anaesthetics, many of the drugs used to treat rheumatic and musculoskeletal disease, antidepressants and anticonvulsants produce cytotoxic injury. Most neuroleptic drugs, and some antithyroid and antidiabetic agents, produce cholestatic injury. Other antithyroid and antidiabetic agents lead to cytotoxic injury. Anabolic and contraceptive steroids also produce cholestasis, albeit of a somewhat different category from the tranquillizers. The diversity of drugs employed in cardiovascular and microbial disease precludes such generalizations.[18,264]

Anaesthetic drugs (Table 15.17)

Volatile anaesthetics that injure the liver produce the cytotoxic type of injury. None leads to cholestasis. Among the anaesthetics there are agents that behave as intrinsic hepatotoxins, others that produce hepatic injury as idiosyncratic reactions, and a third group that has rarely been incriminated as the cause of hepatic injury. Intrinsic hepatotoxins include $CHCl_3$, trichlorethylene, vinyl ether and tribromoethanol. All can produce hepatic necrosis in experimental animals. None of this group are used as anaesthetics today and, accordingly, their toxicity is largely of historical and toxicological interest. The toxicity of trichlorethylene, however, remains relevant, since it has caused hepatic injury as a drug of abuse[257] and as an occupational hazard.[265] Furthermore, the similarity of the zone 3 necrosis produced by halothane, methoxyflurane, and enflurane to that produced by the known hepatotoxic anaesthetics warrants emphasis. These multi-halogenated hydrocarbons, widely used during the past 25 years, have generally had a safe record. Nevertheless, agents in this group, particularly halothane, have been incriminated in many cases of hepatic injury.[266–276]

Halothane

There is today no doubt that halothane-induced hepatic injury is a real phenomenon, albeit of low incidence.[268, 270, 274–277] There have been dissenters,[278] and the issue has been somewhat controversial.[279–284] The incidence of hepatic injury is uncertain. Overall, a figure of one in 2 500 has been offered.[274] Prevalence is greater after multiple exposures than after a single one. Indeed, the figure exceeds 1% in women treated for carcinoma of the cervix with repeated radium implantation under halothane anaesthesia.[285–287] In other settings the incidence is as low as 1 in 10 000 individuals on first exposure and 1 in 1000 in those previously exposed.[18] Despite the low incidence, the widespread and extensive use of halothane and the severity of halothane-induced injury made it an important cause of acute hepatic failure[14,18] until other haloalkanes with lower incidence of hepatic injury began to be employed in its place.

Susceptibility to hepatic injury appears to be somewhat greater in females, to be enhanced by advancing age and obesity, and to be low in children.[275] Over three-quarters of patients have had multiple exposures.[267,268] Many of the patients had had fever with or without eosinophilia after the previous exposure to halothane.[266,270,288–291] The clinical syndrome in more than half of the reported cases includes features that appear to reflect hypersensitivity followed or accompanied by manifestations of severe hepatic disease.[267,268,270,271,288–291] The onset of illness is earlier (average 3 days) in patients who have had prior exposure to halothane than in those who develop hepatic damage after the first exposure (average 6 days).[267,268,270,288–291] Fatal cases are characterized by progressively deepening jaundice, haemorrhagic phenomena, ascites and coma.

The hepatic injury is cytotoxic, consisting of necrosis and slight steatosis. There are some differences in the literature regarding the type of necrosis. Massive necrosis, zonal necrosis, or diffuse hepatitis-like degeneration and necrosis have each been reported.[18] It is our view that zone 3 necrosis, resembling that of CCl_4 as described by Morgenstern et al[291] and Peters et al,[53] is the most charac-

Table 15.17 Hepatotoxic potential of general anaesthetics

Hepatotoxicity for man	Agents[a]	Lesion[b] Steatosis	Necrosis
I. Intrinsic hepatotoxins	Chloroform	+	PV
	Trichlorethylene	+	PV
	Vinyl ether	–	PV
	Tribromoethylalcohol	–	PV
II. Agents hepatotoxic only as idiosyncratic reactions	Halothane	–	PV, M
	Methoxyflurane	–	PV, M, D
	Fluroxene	–	PV, M, D
	Enflurane	–	PV, M, D
	Isoflurane	?[c]	?[c]
III. Agents that seem virtually free of potential for significant hepatic injury in man	Cyclopropane	–	–
	Ether	–	–
	Nitrous oxide	–	–

[a] Distinction between weaker hepatotoxins in group 1 and agents in group II may be quite arbitrary

[b] PV = perivenular (acinar zone 3); M = massive; D = diffuse and hepatitis-like; + = variable and usually slight

[c] Likelihood of injury has been controversial, but several cases now reported (see text)

istic lesion, particularly in patients whose prior exposure was recent.[55] Even in cases which are described as massive necrosis, there is often a remnant of residual tissue in the periportal zone, suggesting that the lesion is severe zonal necrosis rather than massive necrosis. Uncommonly, we have seen instances of periportal necrosis.[55]

Sections obtained by biopsy in mildly or moderately severe illness, however, may reveal diffuse acidophilic degeneration, sinusoidal ('free') acidophilic bodies and mononuclear infiltration, changes that are said to be indistinguishable from those of viral hepatitis.[270] Even in moderately severe injury, however, biopsy sections usually show zonal injury.[53,55] Furthermore, the sharp demarcation of the areas of necrosis in halothane injury is an infrequent feature of fatal cases of viral hepatitis. In general, inflammatory infiltration is much less prominent in halothane-induced injury than in viral hepatitis,[19,55] although the liver from some patients shows a prominent, eosinophilic inflammatory response. Dordal et al[292] and Shah & Brandt[293] have described granulomatous inflammation.

The prognosis of recognized cases has been grave with estimates of 14–70% mortality.[18,266,268,274] Milder involvement, however, probably goes unrecognized. Cirrhosis has been reported to follow repeated occupational (anaesthetist) exposure.[294] Thomas[295] has attributed one case of chronic active hepatitis to halothane-induced injury, an attribution not substantiated by any other reports.

The mechanism of injury, at least in part, appears to involve an immunological response to halothane or a metabolite.[270,274,296] The importance of multiple exposures, the prevalence of fever and eosinophilia, the demonstration of sensitivity to planned or inadvertent exposure, reports of eosinophilic aggregates in the liver and serological studies all support this view.[18,270,289,290,296,297] The zonal necrosis of halothane toxicity, however, resembles the lesion of intrinsic toxins such as CCl$_4$ and not that of apparent hypersensitivity-dependent hepatic injury.[53,297] This raises the possibility that a toxic metabolite formed in zone 3 hepatocytes might contribute to the hepatic injury,[297,298] and there is some experimental evidence to support this view.[275,276,298] Recent studies[296] suggest that the metabolite of halothane produced by oxidative metabolism reacts with hepatocyte components to produce a neoantigen that provokes immunological responses leading to hepatic necrosis; while the metabolite of reductive metabolism is a free radical leading to hepatic injury.

Other anaesthetics

Methoxyflurane. This agent may also produce hepatic necrosis resembling that following exposure to halothane.[296] The syndrome is similar to that observed in halothane-induced injury, differing only in the propensity for methoxyflurane to produce renal injury, characterized by a long-persistent defect in concentrating capacity. The necrosis

of methoxyflurance jaundice is also usually in zone 3, although it may be massive.[53] The renal lesion associated with methoxyflurane apparently results from the toxic effects on the renal tubule of fluoride liberated from the methoxyflurane.[299]

Enflurane. This agent, which was developed shortly after halothane, also has led to a number of instances of hepatic injury similar to that of halothane.[273,300–303] The usual lesion is necrosis involving zone 3, and clinical and biochemical features resemble those of halothane injury.[273]

Isoflurane. Injury due to this agent is even more rare than that due to enflurane, but convincing cases have been reported.[304–307] These reports suggest that isoflurane-induced hepatic injury is a real, though rare, entity.[307]

Fluroxene. This anaesthetic, which saw limited use, caused zone 3 necrosis.[54,308] Enzyme induction was found to enhance markedly the necrogenic effects of the agent in humans[54] and in animals.[309]

Cyclopropane and ether. These agents are essentially non-hepatotoxic anaesthetics that have been employed extensively. In our opinion, there is no convincing evidence that they produce hepatic injury in humans.

Psychotropic and anticonvulsant drugs
(Table 15.18)

There is a striking and useful correlation between the form of injury and the therapeutic category of the drugs in this group. Chlorpromazine and other neuroleptics produce mainly cholestatic injury.[18,264,310–313] Antidepressant hydrazines and most anticonvulsants cause cytotoxic injury, although phenobarbital and carbamazepine cause either cholestatic or cytotoxic injury.[18,264,312] The tricyclic antidepressants cause injury that appears to be more variable in character, both hepatocellular and cholestatic injury having been reported.[18,312] The hepatic injury associated with psychotropic agents is summarized in Table 15.18.

Neuroleptic drugs

Chlorpromazine. Jaundice occurs in approximately 1% of all patients who receive this drug.[18,237] A period of 1–5 weeks of drug administration precedes the development of jaundice in 90% of cases.[237] Re-administration of small doses leads to prompt recurrence of hepatic dysfunction or jaundice in approximately half of the patients.[313]

The hepatic injury is primarily cholestatic, of the hepatocanalicular type. Severe itching is common. Liver biopsy in most patients reveals prominent cholestasis with only mild hepatocyte degeneration and necrosis, and occasional sinusoidal acidophilic bodies.[15,19,88,237] The inflammatory response is mainly in the portal area, is usually rich in eosinophils, and is prominent only early in the course of the illness.[19] A small proportion of patients develop hepatic necrosis and high transaminase levels, as well as prominent

Table 15.18 Hepatic injury produced by psychotropic drugs*

Drug	Type of injury[a]	Drug	Type of injury[a]
I. Neuroleptics		II. Antidepresants	
A. Phenothiazines		A. Monoamine oxidase inhibitors[e]	
Chlorpromazine (Thorazine)		Hydrazines	
Carphenazine (Proketazine)		Iproniazid (Marsilid)	
Fluphenazine (Prolixin)		Isocarboxid (Marplan)	
Laevopromazine (Veratril)		Nialamide (Niamid)	
Mepazine (Pacatal)	Ch or M	Phenelzine (Nardil)	H-Cell
Perhenazine (Trilafon)		Pheniprazine (Catron)	
Prochlorperazine (Compazine)		Phenoxypropazine (Drazine)	
Promazine (Sparine)[b]		Privaloylbenzylhydrazine (Tersavid)	
Promethazine (Phenergan)[c]		Mebanazine (Actomal)	
Thioridazine (Mellaril)			
Triflupromazine (Vesprin)			
B. Thioxanthenes[d]		B. Non-hydrazines	
Chlorprothixene (Tractan)		Tranylcypromine (Parnate)[d]	H-Cell
Chlorpenthixol (Sordinol)	Ch or M		
Thiothixene (Navene)			
C. Butyrophenones		C. Tricyclic antidepressants	
Haloperidol (Haldol)	Ch or M	Amitryptiline (Elavil)	
		Desipramine (Pertofran)	
		Doxepin (Sinequan)	Ch or H-Cell
		Imipramine (Tofranil)	
		Nortriptyline (Aventyl)	
D. Anxiolytics		D. Other antidepressants[d]	
Benzodiazepines[d]		Femoxitin	H-Cell
Alprazolam (Xanex)		Mianserine (Tolvin)	Ch
Chlordiazepoxide (Librium)[f]		Nomifensine (Merital)	H-Cell
Diazepam (Valium)	Ch or M		
Flurazepam (Dalmane)			
Triazolam (Halcion)			

[a] Ch = cholestatic injury—consists mainly of bilirubin casts in canaliculi, usually with portal inflammatory infiltrate and with or without mild parenchymal injury; H-Cell = hepatocellular injury-consists mainly of necrosis with or without inflammation; M = mixed. See Table 15.13 for biochemical features.
[b] No reports of injury according to review of Rees[310] and very few to our knowledge
[c] No cases of hepatic injury reported
[d] Too few cases for clear picture
[e] Use of all in this group, except isocarboxazid and phenelzine, abandoned
[f] Rare instances of hepatocellular injury in recipients of chlordiazepoxide plus other drugs
* Trade names included because of multiplicity of drugs with similar names and roles

cholestasis and high alkaline phosphatase levels (mixed jaundice).[237,314]

The prognosis of chlorpromazine jaundice is generally good. Two-thirds of the patients recover within 8 weeks. Most of the remainder require 2–12 months to return to normal.[237] There have been a number of reported instances of a prolonged cholestatic syndrome, with clinical and biochemical (marked hypercholesterolaemia, xanthomatosis) and, in some patients, even histological features that have resembled those of primary biliary cirrhosis.[88,143–146,315] Similar chronic cholestasis has been produced by prochlorperazine[88,147] and haloperidol.[316]

The clinical features of chlorpromazine-induced jaundice and the prompt recurrence of hepatic abnormality in many of those given a challenge dose suggest that hypersensitivity is responsible for the hepatic injury.[237,313] The suggestion that the mechanism also involves an adverse effect of the drugs on the liver which, when potentiated by drug hypersensitivity, can lead to frank jaundice, has been cited in an earlier section of this chapter.

Other neuroleptic drugs. Most other neuroleptics also lead to cholestatic injury (Table 15.18)[18,264] Exceptions are *loxapine*[317] and *molindone*,[318] which have been incriminated in hepatocellular injury.

Antidepressants

Iproniazid and other hydrazine derivatives. Amine oxidase inhibitors that are hydrazine derivatives can produce hepatic injury in susceptible individuals,[15,18,237] and their use has been largely abandoned. Iproniazid was the earliest of these drugs and it was estimated by Rosenblum et al[319] to produce jaundice in approximately 1% of recipients. The clinical, biochemical and histological features indicated hepatocellular injury. The mortality rate was about 15%.[15,18,51,319]

The liver showed extensive, diffuse parenchymal degeneration and necrosis; in some cases, bilirubin casts were prominent.[15,18,51,319] In some instances there was predominant necrosis in acinar zone 3. Where massive necrosis developed, the lesion resembled that of fatal viral hepatitis.[51] The inflammatory response was usually sparse. The suggestion of Rosenblum et al[319] that the mechanism for the hepatic injury was the production of hepatotoxic metabolites of iproniazid found support in the experimental studies of Mitchell & Jollow.[43] Presumably the responsible metabolites are formed or accumulate in greater amounts in susceptible persons. The hepatic injury produced by other antidepressant hydrazides is similar to that of iproniazid.

Other antidepressants. Of the non-hydrazine antidepressants, *tranylcypromine* has produced a hepatocellular jaundice similar to the hydrazines,[320] but that induced by the tricyclic group may apparently be cholestatic or cytotoxic.[18,106,312,321] Instances of hepatocellular injury due to *zimelidine*[322] and *nomifensine*[323,324] have been reported recently. Injury due to other antidepressants is shown in Table 15.18.

Anticonvulsants

Several anticonvulsant agents have led to toxic hepatitis (Table 15.19). The frequent use of multiple drugs in patients whose convulsions are difficult to control, however, complicates incrimination of individual drugs. Nevertheless, the role of a number of them in producing hepatic injury and the character of the injury has become quite clear.

Phenytoin. The incidence of jaundice in recipients of phenytoin (Dilantin®, diphenylhydantoin-DPH) appears to be low.[18] The drug, however, is very widely used; during the half century of its use, many instances of hepatic injury have been reported. The mortality rate of the full-blown syndrome of generalized hypersensitivity and jaundice appears to be approximately 30%.[8,325-339] The hepatic damage is predominantly cytotoxic;[18,210] although cholestasis may be prominent[325] and warrants designation of the injury as mixed hepatocellular.[18]

Table 15.19 Hepatic injury produced by anticonvulsant drugs

Drug	Type of injury[a]
Carbamazepine (Tegretol)[b]	H-Cell, Ch, M
Mephenytoin (Mesantoin)	H-Cell, M
Paramethadione (Paradione)	H-Cell, M
Phenacemide (Phenurone)	H-Cell, M
Phenytoin (Dilantin)	H-Cell, M
Phenobarbital	H-Cel or Ch
Trimethadione (Tridione)	H-Cell, M
Valproic acid (Depakene)	H-Cell

(a) See footnote (a) Table 15.18. H-Cell = hepatocellular; M = mixed
(b) Can lead to chronic cholestasis

Less dramatically overt hepatic injury may also be caused by phenytoin. Abnormal levels of serum aminotransferases have been recorded in about 20% of patients taking the drug.[340] Granulomatous and granulomatoid inflammation has been described.[84,85,210,331,332]

The liver shows diffuse degeneration, multifocal or even massive necrosis, and multiple acidophilic bodies accompanied by a rich inflammatory response.[210,236,326-332] The latter often includes clusters of eosinophils or lymphocytes, and at times focal aggregates of hyperplastic Kupffer cells having a granulomatoid appearance.[210] The hepatic lesion — with lymphocyte 'beading' in sinusoids, granulomatoid changes and frequent hepatocyte mitoses — may resemble that of infectious mononucleosis (Fig. 15.14).[210,236,334] Indeed, in some instances, severe generalized hypersensitivity, rather than hepatic failure per se, appears to be responsible for the devastating clinical syndrome. Almost all patients develop a generalized rash that may become exfoliative.[333,338,339] In addition, periarteritis nodosa,[335] curious pseudolymphomatous lymph node changes[336] and bone marrow injury[337] may accompany the liver damage.

The symptoms, signs and laboratory features offer strong clinical support for the view that the hepatic injury is a manifestation of drug hypersensitivity.[18,327,328] Indeed, the 'pseudomononucleosis' syndrome of lymphadenopathy, lymphocytosis and circulating atypical lymphocytes resembles serum sickness.[18,336]

Phenacemide led to injury similar to that of phenytoin in an incidence as high as 2% of patients, and its use was abandoned.[18] Similar injury also has been associated with reactions to *mephenytoin, trimethadione, thiohydantoin* and *5-phenyl-5 thienylhydantoin*.[8,332]

Carbamazepine has led to several forms of hepatic injury. Among the estimated 250 cases of overt hepatic injury attributed to this drug,[341] cholestatic and hepatocellular injury as well as hepatic granulomas have all been reported.[342-351] Cholestatic injury may fail to subside for many months or may even lead to chronic cholestasis with disappearance of intrahepatic bile ducts.[350]

The morphological changes have been hepatocellular in about 25% of cases, cholestatic in about the same proportion of cases, and mixed in the others. A few of the hepatocellular cases have shown massive necrosis, the others have shown lesser degrees of necrosis. Some of the cholestatic cases have shown prominent cholangitis and, as cited above, chronic cholestasis with disappearance of bile ducts has been recorded.[350]

Valproic acid has led to severe hepatic injury in a number of patients.[48,49,110,351-359] At least 100 fatal cases and 25 recovered ones have been reported. The liver has shown microvesicular steatosis, necrosis, or both, as well as cirrhosis in some instances (Fig. 15.37).[48] The microvesicular steatosis seems clearly ascribable to the valproic acid, since a similar lesion can be produced in experimental animals by the agent,[360-363] but the role of

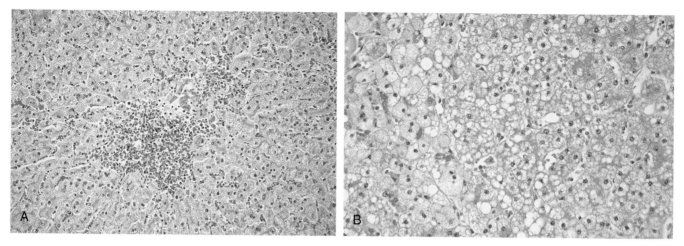

Fig. 15.37 Valproate-associated injury. (**A**) Zone 3 necrosis. Preserved liver cells show microvesicular steatosis. H & E. (**B**) Higher magnification of steatosis in case illustrated in (**A**).

valproic acid, and other drugs taken concurrently, in the production of the necrosis is not clear.[48] The syndrome develops after 3–6 months of therapy; it is characterized by somnolence, hyperammonaemia, coma and coagulopathy.

Anti-inflammatory agents and other drugs used in musculoskeletal disease (Table 15.20)

A number of the non-steroidal anti-inflammatory agents (NSAIDs) and other drugs employed in the treatment of rheumatic disease, gout and musculoskeletal disease have been reported to cause hepatic injury.[18,264, 364–371] Indeed, the past decade has seen a sharp focus on the hepatic injury induced by the NSAIDs, largely generated by the dramatic hepatic injury noted in patients taking benoxaprofen (Oroflex®) as well as by the large number of new NSAIDs that have entered clinical use or are undergoing clinical testing.[366] The hepatic injury induced by agents in this group is not uniform with regard to character or mechanism of its production. Some of the drugs produce cytotoxic injury, others lead to cholestasis (Table 15.21).

Cinchophen, once used to treat rheumatic disease and gout, fell into disuse half a century ago.[99,371] Nevertheless, it remains of interest as the first agent reported to produce idiosyncratic hepatic injury and as the prototype of drug-induced hepatocellular jaundice.[18] Indeed, reports of cinchophen-associated hepatic injury continue to appear.[372] The reported mortality was high, approaching 50%.[99,370] Fatal cases showed acute or subacute hepatic necrosis.[99] In those with a prolonged course the liver was described as showing 'toxic cirrhosis'.[98]

Glafenine, an NSAID with chemical similarity to cinchophen, produces similar hepatic injury.[373–375] It has led to acute hepatic injury as well as to chronic hepatitis.[372] It also has recently been withdrawn from use.[375]

Table 15.20 Hepatic injury produced by non-steroidal anti-inflammatory drugs and other agents used to treat rheumatic and myotonic disease

	Type of injury[a]	References
Allopurinol[f]	H-Cell or Ch	445–451
Benoxaprofen[c]	Ch	401–403
Chlorzoxazone	H-Cell	457
Cinchophen[c]	H-Cell	18, 371, 372
Clometacine[e]	H-Cell	393–396
Colchicine[d]	H-Cell	18
Dantrolene	H-Cell[e]	455, 456
Diclofenac	H-Cell	387–392
Diflunisal	Ch	431, 432
Etodolac	H-Cell	365, 409
Fenbufen	H-Cell	406, 407
Fenclozic acid[b]	H-Cell	264, 365
Fenoprofen[b]	AT	365, 367
Glafenine	H-Cell	373–375
Gold preparations	Chol or H-Cell	434–438
Ibufenac[c]	H-Cell	383, 384
Ibuprofen	H-Cell	385, 386
Indomethacin	H-Cell	379–382
Naproxen[f]	Ch or H-Cell	404, 405
Oxphenbutazone[f]	H-Cell or Ch	18
Paracetamol	H-Cell	9–11, 18
Penicillamine	H-Cell	440–442
Phenylbutazone[f]	H-Cell or Ch	376–378
Piroxicam[b]	H-Cell or Ch	414–418
Pirprofen	H-Cell	411–413
Probenecid[g]	H-Cell	443
Salicylates	H-Cell	419–426
Seatone	Granulomas	433
Sulindac	Ch or H-Cell	397–400
Tolmetin[b]	H-Cell	367
Zoxazolamine	H-Cell	452–454

[a] See footnote Table 15.18, H-Cell = hepatocellular; Ch = cholestatic; AT = abnormal transaminase levels
[b] Too few cases reported for clear picture
[c] Largely or completely withdrawn from clinical use
[d] Hepatic injury observed mainly in experimental animals
[e] Can also cause chronic active hepatitis
[f] Can cause granulomas
[g] So rare as to suggest that the reported cases may have been coincidental rather than caused by the drug

Table 15.21 Various forms of injury[a] caused by non-steroidal anti-inflammatory agents

	PAR[b]	PBZ[b]	CINC[b]	ASP[b]	BEN[b]	SU[b]
Form of injury[a]						
Hepatocellular	+	+	+	+	−	(+)
Cholestatic	−	(+)	−	−	+	+
Granulomas	−	+	−	−	−	−
Mechanism						
Intrinsic toxicity	+(c)	(+)(c)	−	+	−	−
Idiosyncrasy						
Hypersensitivity	−	+	−	−		+
Metabolic	(e)	(+)	+	+(b)	+(d)	−
Dose-dependent	+(c)	+(c)		+	+(d)	

(a) + = typical injury; (+) = less characteristic injury
(b) PAR = paracetamol (acetaminophen); PBZ = phenylbutazone; CINC = cinochopen; ASP = aspirin; BEN = benoxaprofen; SU = sulindac
(c) Causes necrosis in large overdose
(d) Susceptibility also age-related
(e) Susceptibility enhanced by cytochrome P-450 induction or glutathione depletion or both
(f) Susceptibility enhanced by active rheumatic disease

Phenylbutazone. Jaundice has occurred in 0.25% of recipients.[376] The mechanism appears to be hypersensitivity.[377] The injury is cytotoxic in at least two-thirds of the patients. In these patients the liver shows parenchymal necrosis, and the jaundice is hepatocellular.[18,377] However, instances of cholestatic jaundice due to phenylbutazone also occur.[377,378] Some of these have shown granulomas, especially in the portal areas. *Oxyphenbutazone* apparently produces similar injury.

Indomethacin has been reported to produce relatively few instances of jaundice. The injury is usually hepatocellular. Necrosis may be zonal or massive and may be accompanied by microvesicular steatosis.[379–382] The incidence appears to be very low.

Ibufenac, which was withdrawn from use, produced elevated transaminase levels in about 30% and jaundice in about 5% of recipients.[383,384] The jaundice was hepatocellular. Transaminase levels were high. The liver showed necrosis and there were instances of fatal liver disease. A closely related drug, *ibuprofen,* appears to have a much lower incidence of hepatic injury, but cases of hepatocellular damage have been reported.[385,386] A case of fatal injury with microvesicular steatosis has been reported.[386]

Diclofenac, a recently introduced and widely used NSAID, has been incriminated in at least 60 reported instances of hepatic injury.[387–392] We have studied 180 cases reported to the Food and Drug Administration.[392] Almost all have had clinical and biochemical evidence of hepatocellular injury, and histologically there was focal necrosis. In some cases a lesion resembling chronic hepatitis has been recorded.[387,392]

Clometacine, which has been used mainly in France, has led to a number of cases of acute or chronic hepatocellular injury.[393–396] The cases of chronic injury resembled autoimmune chronic active hepatitis[391,394,395] and have led to cirrhosis in some instances.[396]

Sulindac has been incriminated in more than 100 instances of hepatic injury, most cholestatic but some hepatocellular.[397–400] Circumstances and associated clinical features suggest the mechanism to have been hypersensitivity.

Benoxaprofen was withdrawn from clinical use in the USA and UK after it was found to lead to a number of instances of a fatal syndrome characterized by cholestatic jaundice (Fig. 15.38) and renal failure.[401–403] The fatal outcome was curious since cholestatic jaundice rarely leads to death. Accordingly, Prescott et al have suggested that impaired hepatic and renal excretion might have combined to produce lethal blood levels.[403]

Naproxen has led to instances of hepatocellular injury including cases of massive necrosis, and also to cases of cholestatic and mixed jaundice.[404,405]

Fenbufen,[406,407] *fentiazac,*[408] *etodolac*[409] and *feprazone*[410] have each been incriminated in instances of hepatic injury, mainly hepatocellular.

Pirprofen has been involved in at least 14 published cases of hepatocellular injury, 4 fatal.[411–413] Most of the patients were female and over 60 years of age. The lesion is usually non-zonal necrosis, accompanied in some cases by microvesicular steatosis.

Piroxicam also has led to instances of hepatocellular injury, some fatal,[414–416] as well as to cases of cholestasis.[417] It also has been implicated in cases of pancreatitis.[418]

Salicylates, long considered to be free of potential for producing hepatic injury, have recently been found to lead to hepatic degeneration and focal necrosis when blood levels are high. Aspirin levels above 15 mg/dl can lead to high transaminase levels, hyperbilirubinaemia and biopsy evidence of parenchymal injury.[419–428] These aspirin levels in the serum are achieved with the full dosage employed to treat rheumatic fever, acute rheumatoid arthritis, and systemic lupus erythematosus (SLE). The phenomenon appears to depend on the salicylate moiety since it has

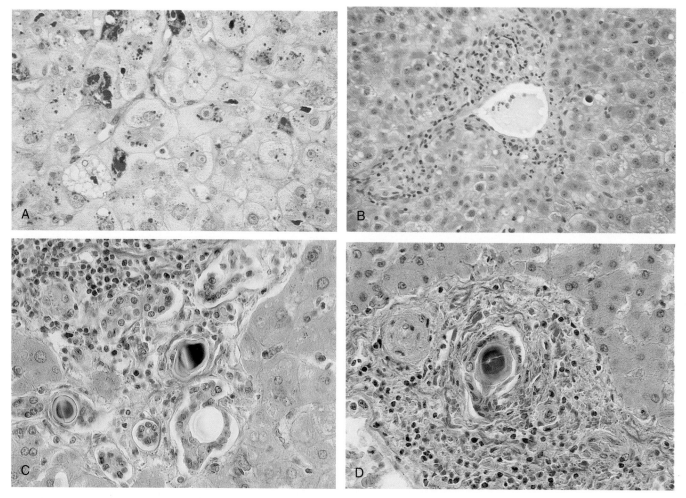

Fig. 15.38 Hepatic injury due to benoxaprofen. (**A**) Perivenular cholestasis with numerous bile plugs: there is marked swelling of hepatocytes with some cytoplasmic vacuolation; there are mild reactive inflammatory changes with some ceroid-laden macrophages. PAS–diastase (**B**) Same case as cholestasis was panacinar; note bile plugs in cholangioles and a mild cholangiolitis. H & E. (**C**) and (**D**) Autopsy liver in a further case showing inspissated bile plugs in cholangioles and bile ducts. van Gieson.

been observed with aspirin, choline salicylate and sodium salicylate.[419] Histologically the liver has shown focal necrosis and inflammation. Patients with active juvenile rheumatoid arthritis and active SLE seem particularly vulnerable to aspirin-induced injury, but patients with inactive disease and normal subjects also are susceptible.[420,421] Hypoalbuminaemia appears to enhance susceptibility.[426]

During the past few years attention has focused on the possible role of salicylates in provoking Reye's syndrome in children with acute viral illness.[427-430] An increasingly voluminous literature attests to the widespread acceptance of the association although there has also been scepticism.[430] Nevertheless, the similarity of the lesion of aspirin poisoning to that of Reye's syndrome[76] and the suggestive, albeit challenged[430], evidence support the likelihood of this association.

Diflunisal, a difluorophenyl derivative of salicylate, has been associated with hepatic injury.[431,432] At least one instance of cholestatic[431] and three of mixed hepatocellular[432] jaundice have been reported.

Gold compounds have led to a number of instances of hepatic injury.[434-438] Both cholestatic and hepatocellular injury has been reported, cholestatic more frequently. Fatalities have been reported among the cases of hepatocellular injury, but the prognosis among the cholestatic cases has been good. Some of the reported cases have appeared to reflect immunological idiosyncrasy (hypersensivity); others, especially those with hepatocellular injury, may reflect metabolic idiosyncrasy.[18] In rare instances, prolonged treatment with a gold preparation may lead to accumulation of the metal within lysosomes and ultimate rupture of the lysosomes with resulting hepatic necrosis.[438]

Penicillamine has been reported to lead to at least 20 instances of cholestatic jaundice. Accompanying circumstances have suggested the mechanism to be hypersensitivity.[439-442]

Probenecid, to our knowledge, has produced jaundice with hepatic necrosis in only one case.[443] The rarity of the lesion, despite the wide use of the drug, suggests that even this episode may have been a coincidence.

Allopurinol has now been incriminated in many instances of hepatic abnormality. These include minor hepatic dysfunction,[444] hepatic granulomas,[445–447] cholestasis[447] and some cases of hepatic necrosis.[448–451] The instances of necrosis have been in association with manifestations of systemic hypersensitivity phenomena.

Zoxazolamine, briefly in use as a muscle relaxant several decades ago, produced severe hepatic necrosis in recipients, and this led to its abandonment.[452–454]

Dantrolene, which was introduced for the treatment of severe muscle spasm associated with grave neurological disease, also can produce cytotoxic hepatic injury. Both acute and subacute hepatic necrosis have been reported. The subacute lesion has resembled chronic active hepatitis, while the acute lesion has resembled that produced by cinchophen, iproniazid and zoxazolamine. Overt hepatic injury, which occurs in about 0.5% of recipients, tends to spare children below the age of 10 and adults taking daily doses below 200 mg. It usually does not appear until at least six weeks after starting the drug.[455,456]

Chlorzoxazone, a muscle relaxant structurally similar to dantrolene, has produced cases of severe hepatic necrosis.[457]

Agents employed in the treatment of endocrine disease

A number of hormones and their derivatives and other agents used in endocrine disease produce hepatic dysfunction and jaundice (Table 15.22). These include the thiourea derivatives, some of the oral hypoglycaemic agents, the C-17 alkylated anabolic steroids and the oral contraceptive agents and several other agents that can play endocrine or 'quasi-endocrine' roles.[18]

Thiourea derivatives

There appear to be differences between the types of injury produced by different derivatives of thiourea.[8,264] The instances of jaundice induced by *thiourea, methimazole, carbimazole* and *methylthiouracil* appear to have been cholestatic (hepatocanalicular or mixed hepatocanalicular).[18,264] Those reported in recipients of *propylthiouracil* appear to have been hepatocellular.[18,264,458–461] Several have had features of chronic active hepatitis. Mehimazole and carbimazole tend to produce cholestasis.[462–465] The association of rash, fever, eosinophilia, and neutropenia with hepatic injury suggests that the mechanism for the hepatotoxicity of the thiourea derivatives has been hypersensitivity to the respective drug.[18]

Table 15.22 Hepatic injury produced by hormonal derivatives and other agents used in endocrine diseases.

	Type of injury*	Other lesions
Steroids and associated agents		
Anabolic-Androgen (C-17)	Ch-Can	See Table 15.23
Oral contraceptives	Ch-Can	
Tamoxifen	Ch-Can	Peliosis hepatis
Danazol	Ch-Can	Carcinoma
Glucocorticoids		Steatosis
Oral hypoglycaemics		
Acetohexamide	H-Cell-M	
Azepinamide	H-Cell-M	
Carbutamide	H-Cell-M	
Chlorpropamide	Ch-H-Can	
Glibenclamide	Ch-H-Can	
Metahexamide	H-Cell-M	
Tolazemide	Ch-H-Can	Chronic cholestasis
Tolbutamide	Ch-H-Can	Chronic cholestasis
Antithyroid drugs		
Carbimazole	Ch-H-Can	
Methimazole	Ch-H-Can	
Thiouracil	Ch-H-Can	
Propylthiouracil	H-Cell	Chronic hepatitis

*Ch-Can = cholestasis, canalicular type; Ch-H-Can = cholestasis, hepatocanalicular type; H-Cell = hepatocellular; H-Cell-M = mixed hepatocellular injury (see footnote (a) Table 15.18)

Oral hypoglycaemic drugs

Hepatic injury has occurred in 0.5–1% of recipients of carbutamide, chlorpropamide, or metahexamide.[18] The incidence of jaundice among patients taking acetohexamide appears to be lower.[18,264,466–468] Tolbutamide, despite its extremely wide use, has been incriminated in only a few instances of jaundice.[469] The jaundice of chlorpropamide has been cholestatic (hepatocanalicular); that of metahexamide, acetohexamide, and carbutamide appears to have been mixed hepatocellular.[18,237,466–468] The few reported examples of tolbutamide jaundice have appeared to be cholestatic.[18] Gregory et al[469] have described a case of prolonged jaundice with features resembling those of primary biliary cirrhosis and a fatal outcome in a patient taking tolbutamide. We have seen two other instances of chronic intrahepatic cholestasis in patients who had been taking tolbutamide. Sulphonylurea derivatives also can produce granulomas in the absence of other evidence of hepatic injury.[470] Lesions associated with other sulphonylurea derivatives are listed in Table 15.22.

Only isolated instances of hepatic injury have been ascribed to biguanides,[471] and those may have been coincidental. Phenformin, to our knowledge, has not been reported to produce hepatic damage, somewhat surprisingly, since it is structurally related to the hepatotoxic agent synthalin.[472]

Anabolic and contraceptive steroids

The hepatic effects of the C-17 alkylated anabolic and of the oral contraceptive steroids have much in common

Table 15.23 Adverse effects associated with alkylated steroids[a]

	Anabolic	Contraceptives
Acute cholestasis	+	+
Chronic cholestasis	?	?
Budd–Chiari syndrome	–	+
Carcinoma		
Hepatocellular	+	±
Cholangiocellular	±	–
Adenoma	±	+
Nodular regenerative hyperplasia	±	±
Focal nodular hyperplasia	–	?
Peliosis hepatis	+	±
Sinusoidal dilatation[b]	±	+
Lithogenesis	–	±

[a] + = association definite; ± = association possible; = no association
[b] Dilatation associated with contraceptive steroids is in zone 1;
dilatation possibly associated with anabolic steroids is in zone 3

(Table 15.23). Both groups of drugs are intrinsic hepatotoxins capable of producing acute, cholestatic jaundice. Both have led to instances of peliosis hepatitis[165–170] and have been implicated in hepatic tumour production.[26–31,165,173,180–184,192,193] There are differences also. While both have been incriminated in the development of both hepatocellular carcinoma and adenoma, anabolic steroids have been particularly incriminated in hepatocarcinogenesis, and contraceptive steroids have been far more clearly related to the development of hepatocellular adenomas.[28] Furthermore, hepatic vein occlusion and the Budd–Chiari syndrome is apparently related to the thrombogenic effect of the oestrogenic component of the contraceptive preparations.[18,264]

The structure of these agents is important. The presence of an alkyl or ethinyl group on carbon-17 appears to be essential for the production of cholestatic jaundice. Testosterone does not lead to jaundice or impaired hepatic function. Unsaturation of ring A, a characteristic of native oestrogens, appears to enhance the adverse effect of steroids on hepatic function, as may be deduced from the greater potency of the oestrogenic than of the progestogenic component of contraceptive preparations.[473]

The incidence of jaundice in patients who receive anabolic steroids appears to be very low, although hepatic dysfunction occurs in almost all patients who take them in sufficiently large doses. In most of the patients in whom jaundice has developed, the drug had been taken for 1–6 months.[237]

The impression gained from the anabolic steroid phenomenon, that individual susceptibility permits a mildly adverse effect to be translated into the development of jaundice, is even more apparent with respect to the contraceptive steroids. The latter are far more likely to lead to jaundice in women who have a personal or familial history of jaundice of pregnancy.[474–477] This, and the clustering of cases of 'pill jaundice' in Chile[475] and Scandinavia,[173,477] suggest a genetic susceptibility to this type of hepatic injury.[18]

These steroids are cholestatic hepatotoxins,[18] and the jaundice appears to result from selective interference with transport of bile acids across the sinusoidal membrane of the hepatocyte[46] and perhaps of constituents of bile across the canalicular membrane.[44,478] There is evidence that they interfere with both bile-salt-dependent and bile-salt-independent flow.[18] The histological features are those of the cholestatic canalicular type.[237] Death has been reported only in patients who were debilitated or had other disease.[15,237] In other patients, jaundice has subsided, although one case of 'biliary cirrhosis' has been ascribed to methyltestosterone.[479]

Curiously, *stilboestrol* and *diethylstilboestrol* appear to have the potential to produce parenchymal injury. Lesions produced by large doses include necrosis and steatosis,[18] and steatonecrosis with Mallory bodies (non-alcoholic steatohepatitis).[125] Mallory bodies have been induced in the Armenian hamster by diethylstilboestrol.[73]

Hepatocellular carcinoma has been reported in at least 33 recipients of the alkylated anabolic steroids[192] and in at least as many patients who had been taking contraceptive steroids.[26,31,193] In view of the large number of women who have taken contraceptives, and the relatively limited number of patients who have used alkylated anabolic steroids, hepatocarcinogenesis would appear to be more readily attributable to anabolic than to contraceptive steroids.[264] The atypical character of the tumours described in recipients of anabolic steroids, however, led to a questioning of their true carcinomatous nature.[480]

Hepatocellular adenoma seems clearly relatable to the taking of contraceptive steroids. Hundreds of cases have now been recorded.[26,27,29,30,165,180–184,481] Almost all of those in the files of the AFIP have presented since the introduction of 'the pill' and almost all patients with this tumour have been users of it — a far more convincing relationship to the steroid than that of focal nodular hyperplasia.[181] A few instances of nodular regenerative hyperplasia have been attributed to the use of contraceptive or androgenic-anabolic steroids.[482] The histological features of these tumours are considered in chapter 16.

Reports of hepatic haemangiosarcoma in recipients of oestrogenic and androgenic compounds have also appeared.[56,205,206,483] Several instances of intrahepatic cholangiocarcinoma have been reported in patients on androgenic-anabolic steroids.[484,485]

Anti-oestrogens

Tamoxifen, an anti-oestrogen chemically related to stilboestrol, has been reported to lead to cholestatic and mixed jaundice[486,487] and to peliosis hepatis.[175] This agent also has been implicated in development of a 'benign cyst'[488] and marked steatosis.[489]

Clomiphene, an ovulation-inducing agent employed to treat infertility, has been implicated in two instances of tumorigenesis. One involved development of hepatoblastoma in an infant whose mother had received the agent.[490] The other involved development of an adenoma in a woman who had been taking the drug for two years.[491]

Cyclofenil has been implicated in the development of biochemical evidence of hepatic injury in at least 35% of recipients[492–494] and of overt hepatitis in 1% of them.[493]

Antihypophyseal drugs. Danazol, a compound structurally related to the C-17 anabolic steroids, also can produce cholestatic jaundice.[495,496] It also has been implicated in several cases of hepatocellular tumours — both adenomas[497] and carcinomas.[497–499] *Octreotide*, an analogue of somatostatin, has been implicated in a case of hepatocellular injury.[500]

Antimicrobial agents

A number of agents in this category can produce hepatic dysfunction or jaundice. The form of injury and the presumed mechanism are shown in Table 15.24. A few of the agents warrant special comment.

Tetracyclines produce a characteristic microvesicular steatosis, resembling the fatty liver of pregnancy or of Reye's syndrome.[18,78,501] Hepatocytes contain many small sudanophilic droplets. There is little or no necrosis and little cholestasis. Initially described as an adverse reaction to chlortetracycline,[502, 503] it also has followed administration of oxytetracycline and tetracycline[501] and, presumably, could result from any tetracycline derivative that shares the antimicrobial properties of the group and reaches the hepatocyte in sufficiently high concentration. An instance of hepatic steatosis attributed to minocycline hydrochloride, a semi-synthetic tetracycline, has been reported to differ

Table 15.24 Hepatic injury produced by antimicrobial agents

Agent	Type of injury[a]	Agent	Type of injury
Antibiotics		*Antimetazoal and antiprotozoal agents*	
Chloramphenicol	H-Cell, M	Antimonials	Steatosis
Cephalosporins	Ch	Amodiaquine	H-Cell
Clindamycin	H-Cell	Hycanthone	H-Cell
Erythromycins[b]		Mepacrine[g]	H-Cell
Penicillins[c]		Niclofan	Ch
G	Ch	Thiabendazole	Ch[e]
Amoxicillin	AT		
Ampicillin	H-Cell		
Carbenicillin	AT		
Oxacillin	Ch		
Cloxacillin	Ch		
Augmentin[d]	Ch	*Antituberculosis*	
Tetracyclines	Steatosis	Cycloserine	AT
		Ethionamide	H-Cell
		Isoniazid	H-Cell
Synthetic drugs		p-Aminosalicylate	H-Cell
Arsenicals, organic	Ch[e]	Pyrazinamide	H-Cell
Nitrofurantoin	H-Cell,Ch, CAH	Rifampicin	H-Cell[i]
Sulphonamides	H-Cell-M, CAH	Thiosemicarbazone	H-Cell
Sulphones	H-Cell		
Sulphomethoxazole–trimethoprim	Ch, H-Cell	*Antiviral agents*	
		Cytarabine	J
Antifungal agents		Idoxuridine	M
Amphotericin[f]	H-Cell	Vidarabine	H-Cell
5-Fluorocytosine[g]	Ch	Xenalamine	CH
Griseofulvin[h]	Ch	Zidovudine	Ch, H-Cell
Hydroxystilbamidine	H-Cell		
Ketoconazole	H-Cell		
Pentamidine[g]	H-Cell		

[a] See footnote (a) Table 15.18. Ch = cholestatic; H-Cell = hepatocellular; M = mixed type; J = jaundice, details not clear; CAH = chronic active hepatitis; AT = abnormal transaminase levels
[b] All erythromycins except base
[c] Natural penicillin rarely leads to hepatic injury, semisynthetic ones are more likely to do so
[d] Trade name for amoxicillin–clavulanic acid combination
[e] Can lead to chronic cholestasis–PBC like
[f] Hardly any convincing cases
[g] Too few cases for clear picture
[h] Causes necrosis, steatosis, carcinoma, and Mallory bodies in mice
[i] Dose-related dysfunction leading to hyperbilirubinaemia

from that due to tetracycline, in that it was predominantly macrovesicular.[504] The microvesicular steatosis of tetracycline can be reproduced in experimental animals.[505]

The clinically significant syndrome of severe fatty liver with hepatic failure occurs in patients who have received the drug intravenously in a dose of 1.5 g/day or more, particularly if the recipient is in the last trimester of pregnancy or has renal disease.[501] While pregnancy appears to enhance susceptibility to tetracycline-induced hepatic injury,[501,506] non-pregnant females and males are also susceptible.[78,502,503] The clinical manifestations include nausea, vomiting and abdominal pain, possibly related to the frequently associated pancreatitis. Jaundice is rarely intense. Most of the reported patients have died.[18,501,506] Less severe cases probably go unrecognized or unrecorded. The mechanism for the liver damage is clearly that of intrinsic hepatotoxicity. The lesion appears to be mainly the result of inhibition of transport of lipid from the liver and perhaps impaired mitochondrial oxidation of fatty acids.[38, 505]

Erythromycin estolate was for many years considered to be the only erythromycin derivative which produced jaundice.[18,507–511] It is now clear that *erythromycin ethylsuccinate,*[512–515] *erythromycin propionate,*[516–518] perhaps *erythromycin stearate*[518] or even *erythromycin base*[519] can produce the same syndrome and lesion. Jaundice occurs in about 1–2% of adults taking erythromycin estolate but very rarely in children taking the drug.[509] The jaundice is hepatocanalicular with high values for alkaline phosphatase and moderate elevated transaminase values.[18] Liver biopsy usually shows only bile casts and prominent portal inflammatory infiltration, usually rich in eosinophils.[514] However, hepatic necrosis occurs in some patients,[510,514,518] and *erythromycin lactobionate*, administered intravenously, has been incriminated in an instance of severe hepatic necrosis.[520]

The blood and tissue eosinophilia, fever and rash that accompany the hepatic injury have led to the inference that it is a manifestation of hypersensitivity.[18] The high incidence of hepatic dysfunction in patients taking erythromycin estolate[508] and the demonstration that it is damaging to suspensions of hepatocytes in vitro[521] and the ex-vivo perfused liver,[522] suggest that intrinsic hepatotoxicity of the agent may contribute to the hepatic injury.[18]

Chloramphenicol jaundice has been reported in a number of recipients of this agent. The scanty data available suggest that both hepatic parenchymal necrosis and cholestasis can occur. The mechanism for the apparent hepatotoxicity is unclear.[18]

Triacetyloleandomycin (troleandomycin) produced jaundice in 4% and hepatic dysfunction in over 50% of one group of patients who had taken 2 g daily for two or more weeks.[523] Characteristically, the injury due to this drug is mixed, with both cytotoxic and cholestatic features, the latter predominating.[523] Triacetyloleadomycin or a metabolite appears to be a mild intrinsic hepatotoxin. Metabolic differences between different individuals presumably determine the extent of hepatic injury.[523] Patients taking this drug and oral contraceptives appear more likely to develop jaundice than those taking either preparation alone.[524,525]

Novobiocin, now little used, can produce unconjugated hyperbilirubinaemia, apparently by blockade of conjugation.[526] Accordingly, it should be categorized as a mild intrinsic hepatotoxin. Rare instances of hepatic necrosis due to idiosyncrasy have been described.[527,528]

Penicillin commonly leads to generalized hypersensitivity, but rarely to hepatic injury.[529,530] Among the huge number of patients who have been given penicillin very few instances of liver damage have been reported.[531–537] Several semisynthetic derivatives (Table 15.24), however, seem to produce jaundice or biochemical evidence of hepatic injury more commonly.[538–559] *Cloxacillin, dicloxacillin* and *floxicillin* have led to multiple instances of cholestasis.[553–559] The combination of the drug, amoxicillin–clavulanate (*Augmentin*), has led to a number of instances of cholestatic injury.[560,561]

Organic arsenicals. 'Intrahepatic obstructive' jaundice in patients given *arsphenamine* was first described by Hanger & Gutman.[562] Their careful description of the first clearly recognized cases of cholestatic jaundice apparently owing to the drug allergy is a milestone in the history of drug-induced hepatic disease. Based on the occurence of fever and eosinophilia, they ascribed the syndrome to drug hypersensitivity and distinguished it from the hepatic parenchymal lesion (zonal or massive necrosis) produced by very large doses of arsenicals and from the needle-transmitted hepatitis that plagued venereal disease clinics before the days of disposable needles. The pattern of biochemical abnormality closely simulated that of obstructive jaundice. The alkaline phosphatase levels were increased more than fourfold and measures of parenchymal injury (flocculation tests) were normal or only mildly deranged. Hypercholesterolaemia was common. The livers showed cholestasis and a variably prominent portal inflammatory infiltration. A syndrome resembling that of primary biliary cirrhosis has been reported to follow arsenical jaundice.[142,563]

Sulphonamides have been incriminated in several hundred instances of hepatic injury. Many have shown hepatic necrosis and hepatocellular jaundice, although instances of cholestatic jaundice have been described. The hepatic damage caused by these agents appears to be mixed hepatocellular, and the mechanism involves hypersensitivity.[564]

The sulphamethoxazole–trimethoprim combination has led to a number of instances of jaundice.[530] Both cholestatic and hepatocellular injury have been reported, in some cases accompanied by pancreatitis.[530,565] While the clinical inference has led to implication of the sulphonamide component as responsible for the injury,[564] there is evidence that the trimethoprim can contribute.[566] The hepatic injury attributed to sulphasalazine is thought to be related to its content of sulphapyridine.[567] Injury due to other sulphonamide-containing preparations is shown in Table 15.24.

Sulphones, long used in the treatment of leprosy, appear to produce hepatic injury more often than do the sulphonamides. The incidence has been reported to be about 5% in recipients of the prototypic compound, 4,4'-diaminodiphenylsulphone (dapsone). Jaundice appears to be mixed hepatocellular. The mechanism for the hepatic injury is not clear; it is presumably hypersensitivity.[568]

Nitrofurantoin. Most cases of hepatic injury have been cholestatic, but hepatocellular forms also have been observed in recipients of this drug.[569] The drug appears to have led to a number of instances of chronic active hepatitis,[107,569–572] and to granulomatous hepatitis.[571]

Antituberculous drugs

Clarification of the aetiological role of a particular agent in this group as the cause of hepatic injury has been complicated by the frequent use of several drugs in combination. Nevertheless, observations recorded from the period when para-aminosalicylic acid (PAS) was employed alone or with streptomycin, and the recent practice of treating 'tuberculin converters' with isoniazid (INH) alone, has permitted some deductions regarding the ability of each of these agents to produce hepatic injury.[18] Streptomycin and dihydrostreptomycin appear to be free of hepatotoxic potential, but PAS can cause liver damage. Ethambutal leads to very rare instances of cholestatic jaundice.[572] Rifampin also has been implicated in cases of hepatic injury. It appears to potentiate the ability of INH to produce hepatic injury and vice versa (see below). By far the most important member of this group with regard to hepatotoxicity is INH. Similar injury is caused by its congeners, pyrazinamide and ethionamide.[18]

Para-aminosalicylic acid. Hepatic injury is part of a generalized hypersensitivity which occurs in 0.3–5% of patients taking the drug. The reaction appears after 1–5 weeks of taking PAS; it includes fever, rash, eosinophilia, lymphadenopathy, and often atypical circulating lymphocytes ('pseudomononucleosis'). Approximately 25% of patients with this generalized hypersensitivity develop jaundice and biochemical evidence of hepatic injury. The biochemical and morphological evidence of both parenchymal injury and prominent cholestasis seen in the liver warrant designation of the jaundice as mixed hepatocellular.[237] The histological changes include prominent inflammation accompanying the diffuse degeneration, necrosis and cholestasis.[237] Necrosis may be massive in fatal cases. In some non-fatal cases, there may be striking periportal necrosis. While the decreased use of PAS has

decreased the immediate relevance of its hepatotoxic effects, the syndrome of hepatic injury is an important and classic one and warrants description.

Isoniazid apparently showed only a slight potential for producing hepatic injury during almost two decades of its clinical use.[95] Despite the huge number of recipients of INH, only a few instances of jaundice had been attributed to it prior to 1972, and these were usually in patients who also had been taking other drugs. In that year, however, Garibaldi et al[573] reported 19 instances of hepatocellular injury, most of them accompanied by jaundice, out of 2321 patients taking INH for chemoprophylaxis. These authors also cited a number of other previously unreported instances of INH hepatotoxicity described to them by other physicians. Since then, other reports have appeared.[94,95] The frequency of jaundice among recipients of INH approaches 1%. The incidence is very low under the age of 20, and rises to greater than 2% in patients over 50.[95] The clinical features and experimental data support the view that metabolic idiosyncrasy leading to toxic metabolites is responsible for the injury.[47]

Examination of liver biopsies has revealed diffuse degeneration and necrosis, and fatal cases have shown massive necrosis.[94,95,573] In a few patients biopsy has shown changes consistent with chronic active hepatitis.[95] The fatality rate is in excess of 10% of icteric cases.[94,95,573]

Minor elevations (less than threefold) of serum transaminases may occur in 10–20% of patients during the first two months of INH therapy, yet in most of these the abnormality does not progress or may even subside despite continued administration of the drug.[574,575] Such patients show minor histological abnormalities on biopsy.[574]

Rifampin. A number of patients have developed jaundice while taking rifampin and INH, or rifampin alone. Several reports suggest that rifampin and INH together may be more hepatotoxic than either alone.[576,577] This view seems to be supported by the report of Hugues and his colleagues[578] who found that rats developed hepatic necrosis when given rifampin and INH together, but not when given either drug alone.

Hepatic injury due to rifampin appears during the first month of therapy,[579] in contrast to INH jaundice, most cases (85%) of which present 2–12 months after starting treatment.[95] Rifampin-induced injury is mainly hepatocellular, although cholestasis may be present. Degeneration and necrosis are characteristic and tend to be more marked in zone 3 than elsewhere. The inflammatory response appears to be more prominent than that of INH injury.[579] Some reports[580] suggest that the prognosis is guarded, with a high case fatality rate, while others[579] suggest that the disease is relatively mild.

Presumably unrelated to this hepatic injury is the ability of rifampin to produce unconjugated hyperbilirubinaemia and impaired BSP excretion in experimental animals and patients. Apparently the drug competes with other substances cleared by the liver for excretion into bile or uptake from sinusoidal blood by the hepatocyte.[581]

Antifungal agents

Griseofulvin, a known experimental hepatotoxin, produces hepatic necrosis, hepatocellular carcinoma and toxic porphyria in mice.[582-584] Denk et al[72] have described inclusions identical to alcoholic hyalin in mice given griseofulvin and have employed the model to study the lesion. Humans have developed porphyrinuria, and those with acute intermittent porphyria in remission may experience a relapse while taking the drug.[585,586] We are aware of only two reported cases of jaundice, both cholestatic, due to the drug.[587,588] Other vague reference to liver damage in humans has appeared.[589]

Ketoconazole, an antifungal drug introduced several years ago, has been reported to lead to more than 100 instances of hepatocellular injury and a much smaller number of cases of apparent cholestatic injury.[590-592] The incidence of jaundice appears to be low. Based on apparent usage, it has been estimated to range from 0.01%-0.1%.[591,592] Minor elevations of aspartate transaminase levels occur in about 10% of recipients.[592] *Fluconazole* can lead to a 15-20% incidence of elevated transaminase levels.[593]

Flucytosine is converted to 5-fluorouracil, a transformation on which its antifungal activity depends. Data on the hepatic effects of this drug are scanty; it appears to lead to transient elevations of serum transaminases in 10% of recipients[594] and has been incriminated in the causation of hepatic necrosis.[595]

Amphotericin B appears to be a very rare cause of hepatic injury.[18] At least two reported cases have been attributed to the drug, one convincingly proved by withdrawal and readministration.[596, 597] Both had hepatocellular injury.

Antiviral agent

Information on the hepatotoxicity of agents in this group is limited. *Idoxuridine* has been reported to produce cholestatic jaundice,[598, 599] as well as instances of serum aspartate transaminase levels elevated to a degree that suggests hepatocellular injury.[600] *Xenelamine* has led to instances of cholestatic jaundice,[601,602] and *cytosine arabinoside* has led to jaundice of uncertain type.[603,604] *Zidovudine* has been incriminated in an instance of cholestatic jaundice,[605] one of hepatocellular injury[606] and in several instances of elevated transaminase levels.[607] *Didanosine* (ddi, Videx) leads to a high incidence of elevated transaminase levels[608] and has been incriminated in at least one instance of hepatic failure accompanied by microvesicular steatosis.[609]

Antiprotozoan and antihelminthic agents

Most of the agents employed to treat malaria, amoebiasis and other protozoan diseases have had little overt hepatotoxic effect.[18] *Amodiaquine*, an antimalarial, has led to a number of instances of severe hepatitis, several fatal.[610] Pentamidine used for the treatment of *Pneumocystis carinii* infection has led to a 30% incidence of elevated transaminase levels.[611] Other antiprotozoan agents reported to produce hepatic injury are listed in Table 15.24.

Chlorinated hydrocarbons and organic antimonials, long used as antihelminthics, are known to cause hepatic injury. *Hycanthone*, used for the treatment of schistosomiasis, has also been found to produce hepatocellular injury and, in some cases, fatal necrosis.[612] *Thiobendazole* has produced intrahepatic cholestasis, in some instances progressing to a syndrome resembling primary biliary cirrhosis.[613,614] *Niclofolan* has been incriminated in causing cholestatic jaundice.[615] *Piperazine* has been reported to cause acute hepatocellular injury.[616] *Albendazole*[617] and *mebendazole*[618] also have been reported to produce hepatic injury.

Drugs used in cardiovascular disease

A number of the drugs which are employed in treatment of cardiac disease, hypertension and atherosclerosis can produce hepatic injury (Table 15.25). A few warrant special comment.

Phenindione, an anticoagulant, has led to well over 100 instances of generalized hypersensitivity. About 10% of these were accompanied by jaundice, which had both cholestatic and hepatocellular features.[237] The approximately 10% case fatality rate was mainly due to generalized hypersensitivity rather than to liver failure.[619] *Warfarin* also has been incriminated in instances of cholestatic injury.[620]

Quinidine. A number of cases of hepatic injury due to quinidine have been reported.[621-623] In the reported patients the syndrome has been ushered in with fever within 6-12 days of initiation of treatment. In most cases, readministration of a single dose of quinidine has led to prompt recurrence of fever and to elevated transaminase levels. Hepatic injury is hepatocellular with degeneration and focal necrosis. Liver biopsy has shown granulomas in several patients.

Procainamide may rarely cause hepatic injury. We are aware of only 5 reported cases[624-628] and of 3 unpublished ones. In these patients the injury appeared to be mixed hepatocellular. *Aprindin*, an anti-arrhythmic agent with local anaesthetic properties similar to those of procainamide, has been reported to cause hepatic injury with both cytotoxic and cholestatic features.[629,630]

Amiodarone, also an anti-arrhythmic, can produce a lesion resembling alcoholic liver disease with steatosis and Mallory bodies (Fig. 15.11). Accompanying these changes there is also phospholipidosis[68-71] (Fig. 15.13a). Other anti-

Table 15.25 Hepatic injury produced by various agents used to treat cardiovascular disease

Agent	Type of injury[a]	Agent	Type of injury[a]
Anti-anginal		*Beta blockers*	
Benziodarone	H-Cell	Acebutalol	H-Cell
Coralgil[j]	H-Cell[b]	Atenolol	Ch
Perhexiline	H-Cell[b]	Labetalol	H-Cell
Nitroglycerine	AT	Metoprolol	H-Cell
		Propanolol	H-Cell
Anti-arrhythmics			
Ajmaline[f]	Ch	*Calcium blockers*	
Aprindine	H-Cell, M	Bepridil	H-Cell
Disopyramide	Ch, M	Diltiazem	H-Cell
Encainide	H-Cell	Nifedipine	H-Cell, Ch, M[b,c,d]
Flecainide	AT	Nicardipine	H-Cell
Mexiletine	H-Cell	Verapamil	H-Cell
Procainamide	H-Cell, M[c]		
Propafenone	Ch	*Diuretics*	
Quinidine	H-Cell[e]	Chlorthalidone	Ch
Tocainide	H-Cell	Frusemide	H-Cell[e]
		Quinethazone	Ch
		Thiazides	Ch
		Ticrynafen	H-Cell[d]
Antithrombotics		*Lipid-lowering*	
Acenocoumarol	H-Cell, M	Cholestyramine	AT
Dipyridamole	H-Cell	Clofibrate	Ch
Heparin	AT	Fenofibrate	Ch, M
Phenindione	Ch	Gemfibrozil	AT
Phenoprocoumon	H-Cell, Ch	Lovastatin	H-Cell
Sulphinpyrazole	O	Nicotinic acid	H-Cell
Streptokinase	AT[h]	Plethoryl	H-Cell
Ticlopidene	H-Cell, Ch, M		
Warfarin	Ch[g,h]		
Antihypertensive		*Miscellaneous*	
Captopril	Ch, M, H-Cell	Nafronyl	H-Cell
Dihydralazine	H-Cell[c]	Papaverine	H-Cell[d]
Enalapril	M	Pentoxyfyllene	H-Cell[i]
Hydralazine	H-Cell[c]	Pyridinol carbamate	H-Cell
Methyldopa	H-Cell[c,d]	Suloctidyl	H-Cell

(a) See footnote (a) in Table 15.18. Ch = cholestatic; H-Cell = hepatocellular; M = mixed; AT = abnormal transaminase levels
(b) Lesions may include Mallory bodies, phospholipidosis or both, and may lead to cirrhosis
(c) Also lead to hepatic granulomas
(d) Can lead to chronic active hepatitis
(e) In experimental animals
(f) Includes congeners: prajmaline, detajmium; all three can lead to chronic cholestatic syndrome resembling primary biliary cirrhosis
(g) Also led to microvesicular steatosis in large doses
(h) Also has led to rupture of the liver
(i) None published
(j) Trade name for 4'4-diethylaminoethoxyhexoestrol, a Japanese drug no longer in use

arrhythmic agents that produce hepatic injury include *disopyramide*, which leads to cholestatic or mixed injury,[631] and ajmaline.

Ajmaline, an alkaloid derived from the root of *Rauwolfia serpentina*, is closely related to quinidine in structure and has found similar clinical applications. This drug and several derivatives have been incriminated in a number of instances of jaundice.[632-635] In most of these patients, the jaundice has been cholestatic with high levels of alkaline phosphatase, modestly elevated transaminase values, and evidence of cholestasis on biopsy. A number of cases have become chronic, and bile-duct injury, with a syndrome resembling primary biliary cirrhosis, has been reported as a complication of ajmaline therapy.[635]

Hydralazine has been reported to lead to acinar zone 3 necrosis[636,637] and also to a cholangitic and granulomatous reaction.[638]

Methyldopa. During almost two decades of widespread clinical use this drug has led to hepatic injury in at least 80 reported cases.[639] Presumably, there are many unreported cases. The available data suggest that the incidence of overt hepatic disease is well under 1% but that trivial injury reflected by biochemical abnormalities and apparent hepatic dysfunction is more frequent.

The hepatic disease has been acute in 85% of recorded cases and chronic in the remainder. The predominant acute injury has been hepatocellular and has resembled that of acute viral hepatitis.[639,640] There has usually been a prodromal period of anorexia, malaise, and fever, followed in a few days by frank jaundice. Values for aspartate transaminase in most patients have ranged up to 3000 iu/l; and those for alanine transaminase have been at least as high. Levels of serum alkaline phosphatase have been elevated in almost all patients, but in 90% of them have been less than three times the normal.

Coombs-positive haemolytic anaemia occurs in 3% of patients with hepatic injury, a figure similar to the overall incidence in recipients of methyldopa. Lupus erythematosus (LE) cells may be demonstrable, and serum antinuclear and anti-smooth muscle antibodies may be transiently present.[639] The majority of recipients of the drug who develop acute hepatocellular injury, however, have not shown these autoimmune serological markers. Blood eosinophilia has also been rare.

The histological changes resemble those of acute viral hepatitis. Ballooning degeneration, 'free' acidophilic bodies and areas of necrosis are characteristic. The inflammatory response tends to be concentrated in the portal and periportal zones. It consists mainly of lymphocytes and other mononuclear cells with some neutrophils. Tissue eosinophilia is uncommon. Prominence of plasma cells is also not characteristic of the acute form of injury but, as described below, is seen in the patients with the chronic active hepatitis form of damage. Bridging necrosis extending between portal areas (peri-acinar) and from portal to central areas was prominent among the patients of Maddrey & Boitnott,[97] and several reported patients have had severe subacute hepatic necrosis.[97,639–641] The prognosis of the acute form of hepatocellular injury approximates that of other forms of drug-induced hepatocellular damage. Approximately 10% of the reported patients with acute hepatic injury have died.[639,640] In non-fatal cases, recovery is usually prompt after discontinuation of the drug, and jaundice is gone by 3–8 weeks.

A chronic syndrome, which in all regards resembles that of the autoimmune type of chronic active hepatitis (CAH), has been attributed to methyldopa.[17,101,639–641] Biopsy has revealed confluent areas of parenchymal necrosis and collapse, condensation of reticulin, and an intense inflammatory response in the portal and periportal areas. The inflammatory cells have consisted of lymphocytes, plasma cells, and varying numbers of eosinophils. Biopsy specimens from some patients have shown fibrous septum formation; several have had the pattern of frank macronodular cirrhosis in a setting of chronic necro-inflammatory disease.[103] The clinical features, like those of other forms of CAH, have been a mixture of acute and chronic hepatic disease. Some patients had already developed clinical evidence of cirrhosis when first recognized to have hepatic disease. Others have presented with apparently acute hepatocellular injury, only to have the biopsy reveal CAH.[639]

The calcium channel blockers *nifedipine, diltiazem* and *verapamil* have been incriminated in instances of hepatic injury (Table 15.25), both hepatocellular and cholestatic.[642–645] Each has been incriminated in cases of hepatocellular injury. Nifedipine and diltiazem have been reported to produce Mallory bodies.[71] Diltiazem has been reported to lead to granulomas.[644]

Captopril and *enalapril* have led to both cholestatic and hepatocellular jaundice, more commonly cholestatic.[646,647] The congener, *lisinopril*, has led to hepatocellular jaundice.[648]

Several *beta blockers* have been incriminated in hepatic injury. These include *lobetalol*, which has led to at least 11 reported cases of hepatocellular jaundice, 4 fatal,[649] *acebutalol* which also led to hepatocellular jaundice,[650] and *atenolol* which has been reported to lead to cholestasis.[651]

Clofibrate, used to treat hypercholesterolaemia, appears to have little important adverse effect on the liver. It leads to mild and transient increases in aminotransferases and to impaired hepatic excretory function.[18] It has been reported to lead to cholestatic injury[652] and to hepatic granulomas.[653]

Fenofibrate has been reported to lead to instances of cholestasis[654] and of chronic hepatitis.[108] While clofibrate and its congeners lead to peroxisome proliferation and carcinoma in experimental animals, there is no evidence that either of these occurs in man.

Nicotinic acid and its derivatives, also employed to treat hypercholesterolaemia, have caused hepatic dysfunction in about one-third and jaundice in 3–5% of long-term recipients.[655] The long-acting preparation appears to be particularly prone to cause the injury. The demonstration of parenchymal degeneration and necrosis on biopsy, and the high serum levels of alanine transaminase, indicate the jaundice to have been hepatocellular; massive necrosis has been reported.[656,657] Employment of huge doses of nicotinic acid to treat psychiatric disease has led to several instances of jaundice with features of both hepatocellular injury and cholestasis.[658,659]

Several inhibitors of hydroxymethylglutaryl CoA (HMGCoA) reductase, *lovastatin* and *simvastatin*, can produce dose-dependent hepatotoxic injury in experimental animals, but in the doses used in humans to treat hypercholesterolaemia they produce hepatic injury rarely. The incidence of transaminase elevation appears to be less than 5%. Rare cases of heptocellular[660,661] and of cholestatic[662] injury have been reported.

Diuretic drugs

Rare instances of jaundice, apparently hepatocanalicular, have been observed in patients taking thiazide diuretics. *Quinethazone, ethacrynic acid, chlorthalidone,* and *frusemide* have been reported to lead to instances of jaundice, perhaps due to hypersensitivity.[15,663] Mitchell & Jollow,[43] however, have shown that large doses of frusemide lead to acinar zone 2 necrosis in rats. Their studies demonstrated clearly that the injury was caused by a metabolite of the drug. A recent experimental, light microscopic and ultrastructural study of frusemide injury in mice revealed zone 3 necrosis, and suggested an important role for the plasma membrane in the development of hepatic damage.[664] Reports of injury in man are very rare.

Ticrynafen is a uricosuric diuretic that led to severe acute hepatocellular injury and to instances of chronic hepatitis and cirrhosis. Indeed, it remained in clinical use in the USA for less than one year.[665]

Other drugs involved in treatment of cardiac disease are listed in Table 15.25.

Antineoplastic and immunosuppressive agents

The number of candidate oncotherapeutic agents studied in experimental animals and tested in patients is far too great, and the data regarding the possible adverse effects of many of them on the liver are far too scant, to permit systematic analysis of the hepatotoxicity of cancer chemotherapy. However, the effects of a number of these agents are listed in Table 15.26.

While the forms of hepatic injury produced by agents in this category are similar to those produced by other drugs, there are several forms of injury particularly characteristic of some oncotherapeutic and immunosuppressive agents. Steatosis is a characteristic lesion of a number of them.[111] Veno-occlusive disease (VOD), the dramatic lesion characteristically resulting from pyrrolizidine alkaloids (Fig. 15.28), is produced by several cancer chemotherapy agents singly and in various combinations.[111,666–670] Some antineoplastic drugs appear to spare the liver or to produce hepatic injury rarely as the result of host idiosyncrasy.[670]

Antimetabolites and related agents

Some antimetabolites, selective enzyme poisons and antibiotics are intrinsic hepatotoxins with a dose-related ability to produce liver damage. In this category are methotrexate (MTX), some antipyrimidine and antipurine compounds, asparaginase and a number of antineoplastic antibiotics.

Methotrexate. Shortly after its introduction 40 years ago for the treatment of leukaemia, hints that it might be hepatotoxic appeared.[137] Subsequently, even more convincing evidence of the hepatotoxicity of this agent came from its use for the treatment of psoriasis. By now there have been many reports of psoriatic patients treated with methotrexate who developed cirrhosis, fibrosis or fatty liver.[671–681] The likelihood of liver damage seems directly related to duration of therapy and inversely related to the length of the interval between doses.[672,673] Daily small doses are more likely to lead to liver damage than are larger doses at weekly intervals.[673–675] The role of cofactors such as age, obesity and alcoholism has been especially stressed in the studies of Nyfors & Poulsen.[675] Indeed, it has become increasingly clear that significant hepatic injury

Table 15.26 Hepatic injury produced by oncotherapeutic agents

Drug	Type of injury[a]	Other lesions
Aclarubicin	AT	
Actinomycin D[b]	H-Cell	Steatosis, VOD
Aminoglutethamide	Ch	
Amsacrin[c]	H-Cell/Ch	Steatosis
Anabolic steroids	Ch	Peliosis hepatis
Asparaginase	H-Cell[d]	
Azathioprine[e,f]	H-Cell-M	VOD; peliosis hepatis
Bleomycin	H-Cell[d]	Steatosis
Busulfan	Ch	VOD; peliosis hepatis
Carmustine	H-Cell	Steatosis
Chlorambucil	H-Cell	
Chloropurine	H-Cell	
Cisplatin	H-Cell	Steatosis
Cyclosporin	Ch	
Cytoxan	H-Cell	
Cytarabine	H-Cell	VOD
Dacarbazine	H-Cell	VOD
Daunorubicin	H-Cell[b]	VOD
Dichloromethotrexate	H-Cell	
Diethylstilboestrol[d]	H-Cell	
Doxorubicin	H-Cell	VOD
Oestrogens (steroid)	Ch	Possibly VOD; peliosis hepatis
Etoposide	H-Cell	
Floxuridine[k]	H-Cell-M	VOD
Homoharringtonine	AT	
Hydrazines	H-Cell	Steatosis
Hydroxyprogesterone	Ch	
Hydroxyurea	H-Cell	Peliosis hepatis
Indicine-N oxide	H-Cell	VOD
Interferons	AT	
Interleukin-2[j]	Ch	Steatosis
Lomustine	—	—
Mechlorethamine	—	—
Medroxyprogesterone	Ch	
Melphalan	AT	
Mercaptopurine	H-Cell-M	
Methotrexate[g]	H-Cell	Steatosis
Mithramycin	H-Cell	
Mitomycin	H-Cell	Steatosis; VOD
Mitoxantrone	AT	
Monomethylformamide	H-Cell	
Procarbazine	H-Cell[h]	
Semustine	AT	
Streptozotocin	H-Cell	Steatosis
Tamoxifen	Ch	Peliosis hepatis
Teniposide	H-Cell	
Thioguanine	H-Cell	
Thiotepa[i]	H-Cell	Steatosis
Triethylmelamine	—	—
Uracil mustard	—	—
Urethane	H-Cell	
Vinca alkaloids	H-Cell[b]	VOD

(a) See footnote (a) in Table 15.18. H-Cell = hepatocellular; Ch = cholestatic; H-Cell/Ch = either; AT = elevated transaminase levels; PL = phospholipidosis; VOD = veno-occlusive disease
(b) Only when given with other agents or radiotherapy
(c) Cholestasis is the more characteristic lesion
(d) Minor component of lesion
(e) Can cause chronic cholestasis
(f) Can cause chronic active hepatitis
(g) In large parenteral doses
(h) Rare
(i) Zone 1 injury resembling white phosphorus poisoning
(j) Pattern of injury is consistently cholestatic. Histological changes show more variation
(k) Characteristic injury is sclerosing cholangitis when drug is administered by pump infusion into hepatic artery

is uncommon in the non-drinking, non-obese, non-diabetic patient.[681]

The biochemical changes produced are extremely mild and may be misleading in relation to the hepatic damage. Histological changes include steatosis, ballooning degeneration and necrosis of hepatocytes, fibrosis and ultimately cirrhosis (Fig. 15.24). Portal inflammation is usually moderate and consists of lymphocytes, macrophages and neutrophils. Hepatocyte nuclei are usually hyperchromatic, pleomorphic and vacuolated (Fig. 15.24C).

Increasingly, methotrexate has been employed in the treatment of rheumatoid arthritis. Thus far, relatively little hepatic injury has been noted, apparently less than that recorded in treated psoriatic patients. Series of arthritic patients monitored for injury have revealed only steatosis and some fibrosis,[682-686] although individual instances of severe hepatic disease have been recorded,[687,688] including cirrhosis.[126]

Prevention of injury in patients with psoriasis or arthritis treated with methotrexate requires adherence to a few principles. Exclusion of patients who take alcohol regularly or who are obese diabetics, use of small doses of the drug and administration of the drug no more frequently than weekly, minimizes the likelihood of hepatic injury.[673,680,681] Monitoring for injury requires liver biopsy, since biochemical or other non-invasive methods are insufficiently sensitive.[676-678] Recommended frequency of monitoring has been based on cumulative dose, with varying figures of 1.5–2.0 g,[680] 2–4 g,[689] and 4 g[678] recommended for the interval between biopsies. Treatment of neoplastic disease with large doses of MTX can lead to acute injury, even necrosis,[690,691] but the incidence is low.[692] Cirrhosis is even less likely to be a problem, since prolonged therapy is not usual.

Antipyrimidines. Azauridine and *azacytidine* are pyrimidine antagonists that have been shown to produce steatosis and necrosis in experimental animals.[693-695] Cytosine arabinoside (cytarabine) produces hepatocellular injury which is apparently mild.[696] 5-Fluorouracil[696] can produce hepatic injury when given intravenously but not orally.[697]

Floxuridine given by 'pump-infusion' via the hepatic artery for treatment of colonic carcinoma metastatic to the liver has led to a high incidence of sclerosing cholangitis[150-155] (Fig. 15.26). The blebbing necrosis, inflammation and distortion of the biliary tree has been called an 'ischaemic cholangiopathy' since it appears to result from injury to branches of the hepatic artery[155] (Fig. 15.26D).

Antipurines. Azaserine is a glutamine antagonist which inhibits purine synthesis. It produces steatosis as well as some liver-cell necrosis.[698,699]

6-Mercaptopurine, an agent which may also be used as an immunosuppressant, may produce hepatic injury, with jaundice in 6–40% of recipients.[700-702] While cholestasis is prominent in some patients, the predominant injury is hepatocellular, and fatal hepatic necrosis has occurred.

Possible potentiation of the hepatotoxicity of mercaptopurine by doxorubicin has been suggested by Minow et al[703] because of the frequency and severity of hepatic injury when these two drugs are in combination for the treatment of refractory leukaemia.[703,704] *6-Chloropurine* has led to similar hepatic injury.[700] *Thioguanine* has been reported to cause jaundice[705] and veno-occlusive disease.[163]

Azathioprine, a derivative of mercaptopurine used mainly as an immunosuppressant, has led to a few reported instances of cholestatic injury.[706-709] It has also been incriminated in a number of instances of hepatocellular injury,[710-716] and the lesion has been characterized as mixed.[717] This drug also can lead to striking sinusoidal dilatation,[718] peliosis hepatis,[176] and VOD.[719-721]

Frentizole, an antipurine used as an immunosuppressant, leads to a high incidence of elevated transaminase levels and to hepatocellular jaundice.[722,723] Pentostatin, an antileukaemia agent, also leads to hepatocellular injury.[723] Hepatic injury due to other purines and pyrimidines is shown in Table 15.26.

L-Asparaginase (colaspase), although an enzyme, behaves like an antimetabolite. It catalyses the deamination of asparagine, depriving the neoplastic cell of this amino acid, and blocking protein synthesis. Presumably, the steatosis which asparaginase produces in 60–90% of recipients[723-726] depends on the same mechanism, although some authors have attributed the hepatic injury to a contaminant of the enzyme.[726]

Antibiotics

Some antineoplastic antibiotics produce necrosis, while others cause steatosis, presumably by mechanisms related to their antineoplastic effects.[18] Nevertheless, some potent cytostatic agents (actinomycin D, cycloheximide, daunorubicin) cause necrosis of bone marrow and intestinal mucosa, but not hepatic lesions. The potentiation of the hepatic injury of 6-mercaptopurine by Adriamycin (doxorubicin), however, has been noted previously.[703,727] Similarly, severe liver toxicity may follow the administration of actinomycin D after nephrectomy and irradiation for Wilms' tumour.[728] Adverse effects of other oncotherapeutic antibiotics are shown in Table 15.26.

Alkaloids

Vinca alkaloids. Vincristine and vinblastine differ from each other somewhat in their toxic side effects, but both lead to little or no hepatic injury in man or in experimental animals. One early report[729] drew attention to the small areas of hepatic necrosis observed at autopsy in patients who had been treated with vincristine. Al Saghir & Hawkins[730] observed transient serum enzyme elevations in a patient on vincristine therapy. We are aware of two patients who developed an acute necrosis of the small intrahepatic bile ducts while under treatment with vinblastine and vincristine, respectively. It is of interest that a similar lesion has been reported in a patient who had been taking vincristine and several other agents. The lesion was ascribed by the authors to a 'graft-versus-host' reaction.[731] Coupled with radiation, these agents can apparently lead to necrosis.[732]

Emetine, used mainly for the treatment of amoebic abscess, has intermittently been tried as an anticancer agent, but without success. It is an extremely powerful inducer of hepatic steatosis in experimental animals,[735] but hepatic injury has not been recognized in man during its long years of use as an anti-amoebic drug.

Alkylating agents

Four groups of alkylating agents have been utilized in the treatment of neoplastic diseases (Table 15.26). As nearly as can be ascertained from the available literature,[733,734] the *ethylenimine* derivatives have not been incriminated in the production of liver damage.[111] Among the *nitrogen mustards*, the prototypic mechlorethamine and melphalan also seem free of responsibility for hepatic injury, although several other members of the groups have been incriminated in the production of liver damage.[111] *Chlorambucil* has been incriminated in several instances of hepatocellular jaundice. Cholestatic jaundice has been attributed[736] to an alkyl sulphonate (*busulfan*). The most convincing evidence for some hepatotoxic potential applies to the nitrosoureas.

Other antitumour agents

Urethane, formerly used to treat leukaemia and multiple myeloma, is a known hepatotoxin and hepatocarcinogen.[49,111,737,738] It has produced perivenular necrosis and fibrosis in association with injury to the efferent hepatic veins and venules. The histological changes and syndrome resemble the veno-occlusive disease of pyrrolizidine toxicity.[739] *4'4-Diaminodiphenylamine* (known as M&B 938) was tested for therapeutic value in multiple myeloma a quarter of a century ago and found to produce cholestatic jaundice.[739] Other agents incriminated in hepatic injury are listed in Table 15.26.

Miscellaneous drugs (Table 15.27)

The number of other drugs that have been implicated in hepatic injury is too large for inclusion. Some are listed in Table 15.27. A few warrant special comment.

Drugs used in gastrointestinal disease

Histamine (H₂) receptor antagonists. The widely used agents cimetidine and ranitidine appear to have a very low incidence of hepatic injury. Mildly elevated transaminase levels have been noted in a small proportion of patients taking cimetidine[740] or ranitidine.[741] Each of these drugs appears to have been incriminated in an estimated 15–25 cases of clinically evident hepatic injury.[742–756] Both hepatocellular and cholestatic injury have been recorded. Several closely related compounds have appeared to be more likely to produce hepatocellular injury and have been abandoned.[757,758] Other H₂ receptor antagonists in clinical use appear not to have been implicated in hepatic injury.

Cimetidine and, to a lesser extent, ranitidine can inhibit cytochrome P-450.[758] Indeed, the potent inhibition of P-450 involves particularly the isoform involved in paracetamol metabolism. Accordingly, cimetidine can inhibit the metabolism and hepatotoxicity of paracetamol in experimental animals.[759] This effect has not yet been shown to be of benefit in humans.

Omeprazole, also used to treat peptic ulcer, is not an H² receptor antagonist. It is an inhibitor of gastric mucosal ATPase.[760] This drug induces cytochrome P-450 (especially P-450IA1) an effect that might modify response to other hepatotoxic agents.[760]

Oxyphenisatin. This agent had been in use as a component of laxative preparations for many years, when it was first recognized as a cause of hepatic disease.[761–765] Within 3–4 years more than 100 cases had been identified. About two-thirds of these presented with chronic hepatitis, while the remainder apparently had acute disease.[18,762–764]

The majority of patients were women, perhaps because of their greater use of laxatives. Those with acute liver damage presented with anorexia, fatigue and jaundice, often accompanied by slight upper abdominal distress.[765] A similar presentation also was found in some patients with chronic liver damage, although most presented with an insidious onset.[102,764] Chronic liver injury seemed to develop particularly in patients who continued taking oxyphenisatin after jaundice had appeared and been ignored, or where the relationship to the drug had been overlooked.[8,102] Serological features, typical for lupoid hepatitis, including LE cells, antinuclear and anti-smooth muscle antibodies, were observed in a number of patients with the chronic syndrome.[18,102,764]

The histological changes in oxyphenisatin-induced disease ranged from those typical for acute hepatitis, through changes classic for CAH, to frank cirrhosis.[18,102,764] Patients with the acute syndrome showed diffuse hepatocellular necrosis, acidophilic bodies, acinar disarray, Kupffer cell prominence and inflammation, mainly portal.[5,764] The pattern somewhat resembled that of acute viral hepatitis, although cholestasis and steatosis appeared to be more prominent in oxyphenisatin jaundice. Ultrastructural differences have been cited.[15] Patients with the syndrome of CAH might show subacute hepatic necrosis.[102]

More often the changes were those classic for CAH with piecemeal necrosis, portal and periportal inflammation which included plasma cells and lymphocytes, 'rosette'

Table 15.27 Hepatic injury produced by miscellaneous drugs

	Type of injury[a]	References
Analgesics		
Paracetamol[a]	PV necrosis	9–11, 776
Propoxyphene	Ch	18
Cholecystographic dyes		
Bunamidoyl	[d]	18
Iopanic acid	[d]	18
Iodipamid	[d]	18
Cimetidine	Ch or H-Cell	740, 742–749
Cocaine	H-Cell	80, 778–782
Disulfiram	H-Cell-M	218–222, 786–789
Essential oils		
Apiol[a,e]	Steatosis	18
Myristicin[a,e]	Steatosis	18
Pennyroyal[a,e]	Steatosis	18
Etretinate	H-Cell[f]	794–799
Heavy metal antagonists		
BAL[a,e]	Steatosis	18
Penicillamine	Ch	18
Iodide ion (povidone–iodine)	PV necrosis	18
Lergotrile mesylate	H-Cell	18
Levodopa[b]	H-Cell (?)	18
Methyl methacrylate	Steatosis	18
Oxyphenisatin	H-Cell	18
Phenazopyridine	H-Cell	18
Pyridine	H-Cell	18
Quinine	Granulomas	18, 264
Ranitidine	H-Cell or Ch	741, 750–755
Sulphasalazine[c]	H-Cell-M	766–771
Streptokinase	AT	559
Tannic acid[a]	H-Cell	18
Total parenteral nutrition	Ch, fibrosis, cirrhosis	814
Trimethobenzamide[b,c]	H-Cell-M	18
Tripellannamine[b,c]	Ch	18
Thorotrast	CA, SA, fibrosis, cirrhosis[g]	18
Vitamin A[e]	PV degeneration, necrosis, fibrosis	790–793
X-Irradiation[h]	MZ necrosis, venous injury	18

* See footnote (a) in Table 15.18. Ch = cholestatic injury; H-Cell = hepatocellular; M = mixed; PV = perivenous, acinar zone 3; MZ = midzonal acinar zone 2

[a] Toxic in overdose and in therapeutic doses in unusually susceptible individuals

[b] So rare as to suggest that the reported cases may have been coincidental rather than caused by the drug

[c] Too few cases for clear picture

[d] Interferes with bilirubin clearance by competition for uptake

[e] Hepatic injury observed mainly in experimental animals

[f] Can also cause chronic active hepatitis syndrome

[g] Can lead to angiosarcoma, hepatocellular carcinoma and cholangiocarcinoma

[h] Causes perivenous fibrosis

formation and periportal architectural distortion.[15,18,764] A number of patients had frank cirrhosis.[15,102]

The prognosis in most patients with acute injury was quite good. Withdrawal of the drug usually led to prompt improvement, although instances of progression of disease even after stopping the drug were described.[18] Even patients with chronic disease usually improved after the drug was stopped, but might continue to show active disease.[764] Cirrhosis once established, however, presumably remained.

Use of oxyphenisatin has been largely abandoned. However, the drug remains of interest as having led to the first, and to the most, cases of drug-induced chronic active hepatitis.

Sulphasalazine. This combination of sulphapyridine and 5-aminosalicylate has been implicated in at least 25 published instances of hepatic injury. Injury has been more frequently hepatocellular than cholestatic, although either may occur.[766–773] In about 10% of instances, the hepatic injury is severe enough to lead to massive necrosis and death. The necrosis is non-zonal, similar to that of other forms of sulphonamide-associated injury. Granulomatous hepatitis also has been reported.[771]

5-Aminosalicylate. Reactions to sulphasalazine had been assumed to be due to the sulphonamide component. However, there are recent reports of injury due to 5-aminosalicylate.[772,773]

Analgesics and drugs of abuse

Paracetamol. This mild analgesic has virtually no side effects when taken in the usual therapeutic doses. It produces severe hepatic necrosis when large doses are ingested, usually in attempted suicide.[9–11,774–777] Doses taken in these suicidal attempts have ranged from 7 g to more than 70 g. Biochemical features of importance include striking elevation of transaminase levels, hypoprothrombin-aemia and, in severe injury, lactic acid acidosis.[9,774–777] Transaminase levels range from a 50- to 500-fold increase. Histological changes in the liver consist of perivenular (zone 3) necrosis and sinusoidal congestion, at times accompanied by microvesicular steatosis.

The studies of Mitchell & Jollow[43] demonstrated that a metabolite of the drug leads to the necrosis, apparently as a consequence of the covalent binding of the metabolite to tissue macromolecules. Necrosis occurs only when the quantity of drug taken yields amounts of metabolite that exceed the binding capacity of tissue glutathione.

The prognosis is similar to that of acute hepatic necrosis induced by other drugs. Approximately 10% of all patients who have taken an overdose and 25% of those who develop hepatic injury have developed hepatic failure. The ultimate prognosis seems to correlate with peak levels of unmetabolized drug as measured between 4–15 hours after ingestion.[775]

While the vast majority of instances of paracetamol-induced hepatic necrosis appear to have resulted from large suicidal overdose of the drug, a number of instances of hepatic injury have been the result of therapeutic misadventures involving doses in the therapeutic range.[776,777] For the most part these have involved alcoholic patients, in whom the inducing effect of alcohol on the cytochrome P-450 was held responsible for increased production of hepatotoxic metabolite. Depletion of glutathione secondary to alcoholism is also considered to play a role.

Aspirin. Effects of this NSAID on the liver, when employed for prolonged therapy of rheumatic disease, are discussed elsewhere in this chapter. Single doses used for analgesia do not lead to hepatic injury. Only in the setting of evolving viral infection have single doses of aspirin appeared to provoke hepatic disease — namely Reye's syndrome.

Propoxyphene. This widely used analgesic has been incriminated in rare instances of hepatic injury. Several cases of cholestatic injury have now been recorded.[18]

Cocaine. Long known to produce serious systemic, cardiac and neurological injury, this agent of abuse has now been shown to produce hepatic injury in experimental animals[778–780] and man.[780–783] In mice, cocaine leads to dose- and time-dependent toxicity manifest by elevated transaminase levels and by necrosis and steatosis.[778–780] The necrosis has been described as zonal, but the zone involved has varied, apparently, according to strain of mouse and status of the P-450 system.[778–780] In man, the reported cases have shown coagulative necrosis involving zone 3, zone 2 or the entire acinus and microvesicular steatosis.[80,781–783]

The mechanism of injury appears to involve intrinsic hepatotoxicity for mice, apparently implemented by a toxic, oxidative metabolite of cocaine.[778–780] Presumably,

a similar mechanism applies to injury in man but distinction of the effects of shock and anoxia from those of the drug has been difficult. Nevertheless, whereas the zone 3 necrosis might be ascribed to hypoxia, the microvesicular steatosis is presumably cocaine-induced. Induction of cytochrome P-450 appears to enhance cocaine hepatotoxicity.[780] Particularly relevant is the enhancement of hepatotoxic effects by ethanol, presumably through induction of P-450 2E1.[784]

Other drugs of abuse. Inhalation of chloroform, trichloroethylene and related compounds can lead to zone 3 necrosis and/or steatosis.[18] 'Glue sniffing' and inhalation of other euphorogenic intoxicating agents also may lead to hepatic disease. Nevertheless, these agents may contain non-hepatotoxic (e.g. acetone) or only mildly toxic agents (e.g. toluene) and lead to little or no hepatic injury. The adverse effects of opiates on the liver of the drug abuser are, in great part, obscured by other effects of the associated life style on the liver (hepatitis, alcoholism). Nevertheless, no important hepatotoxic effects can be ascribed to the opiates.[18]

Amphetamines have long been suspected to cause hepatic injury when taken as a form of drug abuse, but evidence for the effects is scant.[18] However, use of 3,4 methylenidioxymethamphetamine ('ecstasy') has recently been reported to cause hepatic injury. Both cholestatic and hepatocellular injury was seen among the 7 cases reported from a single institution.[785]

Disulfiram and cyanamide. These drugs, both of which have been employed in 'aversion therapy' of alcoholism, have each led to different forms of hepatic injury. Disulfiram (Antabuse) has been incriminated in at least 30 reported instances of hepatic injury.[18,786–789] The injury has been mainly hepatocellular, in some instances leading to fulminant hepatic failure. *Cyanamide* can lead to a dramatic form of ground-glass change resembling Lafora bodies (Fig. 15.32A), a lesion that can lead to cirrhosis.[218–222]

Vitamin A and related drugs

Vitamin A toxicity. Although hepatic injury from acute vitamin A poisoning is said to have been known for more than a century,[790,791] vitamin A associated chronic hepatic injury has come into focus only during the past quarter of a century. More than 100 cases of chronic hepatic disease have now been reported.[133,791–793] There are undoubtedly many more. Indeed, 41 cases were recently reported from a single centre.[791]

Excessive doses of this vitamin, continued for months or years, can lead to chronic hepatic disease. The systemic manifestations of the poisoning include headache, anorexia, weight loss, fatiguability, pollar, pruritus, dry skin and loss of body hair. The clinical evidence of hepatic disease is hepatomegaly and splenomegaly, at times accompanied by ascites. Jaundice is uncommon but may occur.[791,792]

Tissue changes may include zone 3 fibrosis, veno-occlusive disease and striking prominence of perisinusoidal cells[133,791,792] (Fig. 15.23). Portal hypertension may be the result of the hepatoportal sclerosis that is characteristic of vitamin A toxicity or of frank cirrhosis. In the excellent study of 41 patients with vitamin A hepatotoxicity by Geubel et al,[790] there was cirrhosis in 59%, chronic hepatitis in 34%, microvesicular steatosis in 21%, sinusoidal fibrosis in 14% and peliosis hepatis in 3%. Critical histological features of vitamin A toxicity are the prominence of perisinusoidal cells (fat-storing cells) and their fluorescence. The sinusoidal changes and frank peliosis have drawn special attention.[793]

Chronic intoxication has resulted from the intake of doses as small as the recommended daily dose continued for years, to doses as high as 20 times the approved dose that may lead to hepatic injury in a few months.

Etretinate. A number of patients receiving the aromatic retinoid derivative of vitamin A, etretinate, in the treatment of psoriasis have developed liver abnormalities including elevations of transaminases, cholestatic reactions, periportal fibrosis, chronic active hepatitis and even cirrhosis.[794–799] That hypersensitivity may be the mechanism for the injury in some cases is suggested by associated eosinophilia and fever in those cases.[796] Reappearance of etretinate-induced liver injury upon challenge also has been demonstrated.[797] *Acitretin*, a metabolite of etretinate, also has been reported to cause severe hepatic injury that progressed to cirrhosis.[799]

Radiation injury

Radiation. The delivery of 3000–6000 rads to the upper abdomen leads to a lesion and syndrome termed 'radiation hepatitis'.[800–802] Clinical features consist of ascites, hepatomegaly, splenomegaly, slight jaundice and, in some patients, abdominal pain. These manifestations appear within 2–6 weeks of a course of radiation therapy. Histological features include sinusoidal congestion and necrosis or atrophy of hepatocytes in zone 3 and internal proliferation or fibrotic occlusion of terminal hepatic veins. These changes are accompanied by periportal fibrosis, periductal fibrosis and phlebosclerosis. The historical and clinical features of radiation injury veno-occlusive disease resemble those of the VOD induced by pyrrolizidine alkaloids.[162]

Thorotrast. This colloidal preparation of thorium dioxide was employed as a parenterally administered contrast agent during the second quarter of this century. It was abandoned by 1955 as late, devastating sequelae of its use became apparent.[190] A large number of reports have appeared describing tumours of the liver and, less frequently, of other organs, as well as lympho- and myeloproliferative syndromes and non-neoplastic lesions of the liver.[18,190,803–811] The Thorotrast-induced lesion that has drawn the most attention is haemangiosarcoma,[190,200–204,805] but cholangiocarcinoma and hepatocellular carcinomas have been attributed to Thorotrast with almost equal frequency.[806–811] Hepatic leiomyosarcoma has also been reported.[812] A number of instances of more than one tumour type in the same patient have been described. (Thorotrast-associated tumours are discussed in Ch 16).

Non-malignant hepatic lesions attributed to Thorotrast include periportal fibrosis, veno-occlusive lesions and cirrhosis.[190] The fibrosis is particularly marked in the subcapsular region. An additional lesion of note is peliosis hepatis, which may be fatal.[813]

The distinctive marker of Thorotrast-induced disease is the presence of particles of Thorotrast free or in macrophages, often in clusters. The particulate, grey-brown, refractile particles are approximately $10\,\mu m$ in diameter (Fig. 15.36). They are illuminated by phase contrast, and shown by microradiography[809] and energy dispersive X-ray analysis, and clearly defined by scanning electron microscopy.[814]

The injury is attributed to the radiation. Thorium dioxide has a biological half-life of about 400 years and a far longer physical half-life. Emitted radiation consists predominantly (90%) of alpha particles but also includes beta and gamma radiation. Despite the interval of almost four decades since use of Thorotrast was largely abandoned, reports of Thorotrast-induced disease continue to appear.

Tacrine

This drug, which has been under study for the treatment of Alzheimer's disease, has hepatotoxic potential. In the doses employed, it has been found to lead to a 40–50% incidence of elevated transaminase levels, about half of which have been more than threefold the normal.[815–817]

Lergotrile masilate

This dopaminergic ergot derivative with apparent therapeutic promise in Parkinson's disease was abandoned because of a 50% incidence of abnormal ALT levels.[18]

Other drugs worthy of mention as the cause of hepatic injury are listed in Table 15.27.

REFERENCES

1. Phillips M J, Poucell S, Patterson J, Valencia P. The liver. An atlas and text of ultrastructural pathology. New York: Raven Press, 1987
2. Ruprah M, Mant T G K, Flanagan R J. Acute carbon tetrachloride poisoning in 19 patients: Implications for diagnosis and treatment. Lancet 1985; i: 1027–1029
3. Diaz-Rivera R S, Collazo P J, Pons E R, Torregrosa M V. Acute phosphorus poisoning in man, a study of 56 cases. Medicine 1950; 29: 269–298
4. Rodriguez-Iturbe B. Acute yellow-phosphorous poisoning. N Engl J Med 1971; 284: 157
5. Salfelder K, Doehnert H R, Doehnert G, Sauerteg K, Deliscano T R, Fabrega S E. Fatal phosphorous poisoning. A study of forty-five autopsy cases. Beitr Pathol 1972; 147: 321–340

6. Benhamou J-P. Drug-induced hepatitis: Clinical aspects. In: Fillastre J P, ed. Hepatotoxicity of drugs. Rouen: Université de Rouen, 1985: pp 22–30

7. Florsheim G L. Toxins and intoxications from the toadstool Amanita phalloides. Trends Pharmacol Sci 1983; 4: 263–266

8. Editorial. Death-cap poisoning. Lancet 1972; i: 1320–1321

9. Clarke R, Borirakchanyavat V, Davidson A R, Thompson R P H, Widdop B, Goulding R, Williams R. Hepatic damage and death from overdose of paracetamol. Lancet 1973; i: 66–70

10. Hamlyn A N, Douglas A P, James O. The spectrum of paracetamol (acetaminophen) overdose: Clinical and epidemiological studies. Postgrad Med J 1978; 5: 400–404

11. Prescott L F. Paracetamol overdose. Drugs 1983; 25: 290–298

12. Bjorneboe M, Iversen O, Olsen S. Infective hepatitis and toxic jaundice in a municipal hospital during a five-year period. Acta Med Scand 1967; 182: 491–501

13. Koff R S, Gardner P, Harinasuta U, Pihl C O. Profile of hyperbilirubinemia in three hospital populations. Clin Res 1970; 18: 680–681

14. Trey C, Lipworth L, Chalmer T, Davidson C S, Gottlieb L S, Popper H, Saunders S J. Fulminant hepatic failure. Presumable contribution of halothane: N Engl J Med 1968; 279: 798–801

15. Klatskin G. Toxic and drug-induced hepatitis. In: Schiff L, ed. Diseases of the liver, 4th edn. Philadelphia: J B Lippincott, 1975: pp 604–710

16. Schaffner F, Raisfeld I H. Drugs and the liver: A review of metabolism and adverse reactions. Adv Intern Med 1969; 15: 221–259

17. Maddrey W C, Boitnott J K. Drug-induced chronic liver disease. Gastroenterology 1977; 72: 1348–1353

18. Zimmerman H J. Hepatotoxicity: the adverse effects of drugs and other chemicals in the liver. New York: Appleton Century Crofts, 1978

19. Scheuer P J. Liver biopsy interpretation, 3rd edn. Baltimore: Williams & Wilkins, 1980: pp 88–101

20. Popper H, Thomas L B. Alterations of liver and spleen among workers exposed to vinyl chloride. Ann NY Acad Sci 1975; 246: 172–194

21. Tomatis L. The IARC program in the evaluation of carcinogenic risk of chemicals to man. Ann NY Acad Sci 1976; 271: 396–409

22. Kraybill H R. The toxicology and epidemiology of natural hepatotoxin exposure. Isr J Med Sci 1974; 10: 416–425

23. Magee P N. Liver carcinogens in the human environment. In: Liver cancer, IARC Scientific Publication 1. Lyon: International Agency for Research on Cancer, 1971: pp 110–120

24. Wogan G N. Aflatoxins and their relationship to hepatocellular carcinoma. In: Okuda K, Peters R L, eds. Hepatocellular carcinoma. New York: John Wiley, 1976: pp 25–41

25. Wogan G N. Aflatoxins as risk factors for hepatocellular carcinoma in humans. Cancer Res 1992; 52 (suppl): 2114s–2118s

26. Ishak K G. Hepatic neoplasms associated with contraceptive and anabolic steroids. In: Lingeman C H, ed. Carcinogenic hormones. Berlin: Springer-Verlag, 1979: pp 73–128

27. Mays E T, Christofferson W. Hepatic tumors induced by sex steroids. Semin Liv Dis 1984; 4: 147–157

28. Ishak K G, Zimmerman H J. Hepatotoxic effects of the anabolic androgenic steroids. Semin Liv Dis 1987; 7: 230–236

29. Edmondson H A, Henderson B, Benton B. Liver cell adenomas associated with use of oral contraceptives. N Engl J Med 1976; 294: 470–472

30. Henderson B E, Preston-Marin S, Edmondson H A, Peters R L, Pike M C. Hepatocellular carcinoma and oral contraceptives. Br J Cancer 1983; 48: 437–440

31. Neuberger J, Williams R. Halothane anesthesia and liver damage. Br Med J 1984; 289: 1136–1139

32. Popper H. Drug-induced hepatic injury. In: Gall E A, Mostofi F K, eds. The liver: Baltimore: Williams & Wilkins, 1973: pp 182–198

33. Sherlock S. Drugs and the liver. In: Diseases of the liver and biliary system, 6th edn. Oxford: Blackwell Scientific Publications, 1991: pp 295–322

34. Himsworth H P. Lectures on the liver and its disease. Cambridge, Massachusetts: Harvard University Press, 1947

35. Mullick F G, Ishak K G, Mahabir R, Stromeyer F W. Hepatic injury associated with paraquat toxicity in humans. Liver 1981; 1: 209–221

36. Farber E. Biochemical pathology. Annu Rev Pharm 1971; 11: 71–96

37. Farber E. The pathology of transcription and translation. New York: Marcel Dekker, 1972

38. Schenker S, Breen K J, Heimberg M. Pathogenesis of tetracycline induced fatty liver. In: Gerok W, Sickinger K, eds. Drugs and the liver. Stuttgart: F K Schattauer-Verlag, 1972: pp 269–280

39. Lieber C S. Alcohol-induced hepatotoxicity. In: Meeks R G, Harrison S D, Brill R J, eds. Hepatotoxology. Boca Raton: CRC Press, 1991: pp 481–523

40. Videla L, Bernstein H, Israel Y. Increased oxidative capacity in the liver following ethanol administration. In: Khanna J M, Israel Y, Kalant H, eds. Alcoholic liver pathology. Toronto: Addiction Research Foundation, 1975: pp 311–340

41. Farber E. Some fundamental aspects of liver injury. In: Khanna J M, Israel Y, Kalant H, eds. Alcoholic liver pathology. Toronto: Addiction Research Foundation, 1975: pp 289–303

42. Farber J L, El-Mofty S K. The biochemical pathology of liver cell necrosis. Am J Pathol 1975; 81: 237–250

43. Mitchell J R, Jollow D J. Metabolic activation of drugs to toxic substances. Gastroenterology 1975; 68: 392–410

44. Arias I M. Effects of a plant acid (icterogenic) and certain anabolic steroids on the hepatic metabolism of bilirubin and sulfobromophthalein (BSP). Ann NY Acad Sci 1963; 104: 1014–1025

45. Zimmerman H J, Lewis J H. Drug-induced cholestasis. Med Toxicol 1987; 2: 112–160

46. Reichen J, Simon F. Mechanisms of cholestasis. Int Rev Exper Pathol 1984; 26: 232–274

47. Mitchell J R, Zimmerman H J, Ishak K G, Thorgeirsson U P, Timbrell J A, Snodgrass W R, Nelson S D. Isoniazid liver injury. Clinical spectrum, pathology and probable pathogenesis. Ann Intern Med 1976; 84: 181–192

48. Zimmerman H J, Ishak K G. Valproate-induced hepatic injury. Analysis of 23 fatal cases. Hepatology 1982; 2: 591–597

49. Eadie M J, Hooper W D, Dickinson R G. Valproate-associated hepatotoxicity and its biochemical mechanism. Med Toxicol 1988; 3: 85–106

50. Rouiller C. Experimental toxic injury of the liver. In: Rouiller C, ed. The liver, vol II. New York: Academic Press, 1964: pp 335–476

51. Popper H, Rubin E, Gardiol D, Schaffner F, Paronetto F. Drug-induced liver disease. Arch Intern Med 1965; 115: 128–136

52. McLean E K. The toxic actions of pyrrolizidine (Senecio) alkaloids. Pharmacol Rev 1970; 22: 429–483

53. Peters R L, Edmondson H A, Reynolds T B, Meister J C, Curphey T J. Hepatic necrosis associated with halothane anesthesia. Am J Med 1967; 47: 748–764

54. Reynolds E S, Brown B R, Vandam L D. Massive hepatic necrosis after fluoroxene anesthesia — case of drug interaction? N Engl J Med 1972; 86: 530–531

55. Benjamin S, Goodman Z D, Ishak K G, Zimmerman H J, Irey N S. The histopathology of halothane-induced hepatic injury: A comparison of biopsy and autopsy cases. Hepatology 1985; 5: 1163–1170

56. Rees K R, Tarlow M J. The hepatotoxic action of allyl formate. Biochem J 1985; 104: 757–761

57. Mitchell J R, Potter W Z, Hinson J A, Snodgreass W R, Timbrell J A, Gillette J R. Toxic drug reactions. In: Eichler O, Farah A, Hecken H, Welsch AD, eds. Handbook of experimental pharmacology; new series, vol 28/3, Berlin: Springer-Verlag, 1975: pp 382–419

58. Slater T F. Necrogenic action of carbon tetrachloride in the rat: A speculative mechanism based on activation. Nature 1966; 209: 36–40

59. Reed W D, Christie B, Krishna G, Mitchell J R, Moskowitz J, Brodie B B. Bromobenzene metabolism and hepatic necrosis. Pharmacology 1971; 6: 41–55

60. Mitchell J R, Jollow D J, Potter W Z. Acetaminophen induced hepatic necrosis. I. Role of drug metabolism. J Pharmacol Exp Ther 1973; 187: 185–194

61. Belinsky S A, Matsumura T, Kauffman F C, Thurman R G. Rates of allyl alcohol metabolism in periportal and pericentral regions of the liver lobule. Mol Pharmacol 1984; 25: 158–164

62. Decker K, Keppler D. Galactosamine induced liver injury. Prog Liver Dis 1972; 4: 183–199

63. Kerr J F R, Wyllie A H, Currie A R. Apoptosis: a basic biologic phenomenon with wide ranging implications in tissue kinetus. Br J Cancer 1972; 26: 239–257

64. Rabin L. The morphologic spectrum of alcoholic liver disease. In: Seeff L B, Lewis J H, eds. Current perspective in hepatology. New York: Plenum Medical 1989: pp 123–139

65. Paliard P, Vitrey D, Fournier G, Belhadjali J, Patricot L, Berger F. Perhexiline maleate-induced hepatitis. Digestion 1978; 17: 419–427

66. Poupon R, Rosensztajn L, Prudhomme de Saint-Maur P, Lageron A, Gombeau T, Darnis F. Perhexiline maleate-associated hepatic injury: Prevalence and characteristics. Digestion 1980; 20: 145–150

67. Forbes G B, Rake M D, Taylor D J E. Liver damage due to perhexiline maleate. J Clin Pathol 1979; 32: 1282–1285

68. Poucell S, Ireton J, Valencia-Mayoral P et al. Amiodarone-associated phospholipidosis and fibrosis of the liver: Light, immunohistochemical and electron microscopic studies. Gastroenterology 1984; 86: 926–936

69. Babany G, Dhumeaux D. L'amiodarone hepatotoxique? Gastroenterol Clin Biol 1985; 505–507

70. Lewis J H, Ranard R C, Caruso A et al. Amiodarone hepatotoxicity: Prevalence and clinopathologic correlations among 104 patients. Hepatology 1989; 9: 679–685

71. Babany G, Uzzan F, Larrey D et al. Alcoholic-like liver lesions induced by nifedipine. J Hepatol 1989; 9: 252–255

72. Denk H, Gschnait F, Wolff K. Hepatocellular hyaline (Mallory bodies) in long term griseofulvin-treated mice. A new experimental model for the study of hyaline formation. Lab Invest 1975; 32: 773–776

73. Coe J E, Ishak K G, Ross M J. Diethylstilbestrol-induced jaundice in the Chinese and Armenian hamster. Hepatology 1983; 3: 489–496

74. Hoyumpa A M Jr, Green H L, Dunn G B, Schenker S. Fatty liver: Biochemical and clinical considerations. Am J Dig Dis 1975; 20: 1142–1170

75. Peters R L, Edmondson H A, Mikkelsen W, Tatter D. Tetracycline induced fatty liver in non-pregnant patients. Am J Surg 1967; 113: 622–632

76. Uchida T, Kao H, Quispe-Sjogren M, Peters R L. Alcoholic foamy degeneration—A pattern of acute alcoholic injury of the liver. Gastroenterology 1983; 8: 683–692

77. Starko K M, Mullick F G. Hepatic and cerebral pathology findings in children with fatal salicylate intoxication: Further evidence for a causal relation between salicylate and Reye's syndrome. Lancet 1983; i: 326–329

78. Bourgeois C, Olson L, Comer D et al. Encephalopathy and fatty degeneration of the viscera: A clinicopathologic analysis of 40 cases. Am J Clin Pathol 1971; 56: 571–588

79. Redlich C A, West A B, Fleming L, True L D, Cullen M R, Riely C A. Clinical and pathological characteristics of hepatotoxicity associated with occupational exposure to dimethylformamide. Gastroenterology 1990; 99: 748–757

80. Wanless I R, Dore S, Gopinath N et al. Histopathology of cocaine hepatotoxicity. Report of four patients. Gastroenterology 1990; 98: 497–501

81. Shikata T, Oda T, Naito C, Kanotaka T, Suzuki H. Phospholipid fatty liver: A proposal of a new concept and its electron microscopical study. Acta Pathol Jpn 1970; 20: 467–486

82. Lullmann H, Lullman-Rauch R, Wasserman O. Drug-induced phospholipidosis. CRC Crit Rev Toxicol 1975; 4: 185–218

83. Ishak K G. Light microscopic morphology of viral hepatitis. Am J Clin Pathol 1976; 65: 787–827

84. McMaster K R, Hennigar G R. Drug-induced granulomatous hepatitis. Lab Invest 1981; 44: 61–73

85. Ishak K G, Zimmerman H J. Drug-induced and toxic granulomatous hepatitis. Bailliere's Clin Gastroenterol 1988; 2: 463–480

86. Stoeckle J D, Hardy H L, Weber A L. Chronic beryllium disease. Long-term follow-up of sixty cases and selective review of the literature. Am J Med 1986; 46: 545–561

87. Pimentel J C, Menezes A P. Liver granulomas containing copper in vineyard sprayer's lung. A new etiology of hepatic granulomatosis. Am Rev Respir Dis 1975; 111: 189–195

88. Ishak K G, Irey N S. Hepatic injury associated with the phenothiazines: Clinicopathologic and follow-up study of 36 patients. Arch Pathol 1972; 93: 283–304

89. Matsumoto T, Matsumori H, Kuwabara N, Fukuda Y, Ariwa R. A histopathological study of the liver in paraquat poisoning. An analysis of fourteen autopsy cases with emphasis on bile duct injury. Acta Pathol Jpn 1980; 30: 859–870

90. DeGott C, Feldmann G, Larrey D et al. Drug-induced prolonged cholestasis in adults: A histological semiquantitative study demonstrating ductopenia. Hepatology 1992; 15: 244–251

91. Boyer J L, Klatskin G. Pattern of necrosis in acute viral hepatitis. Prognostic value of bridging (subacute hepatic necrosis). N Engl J Med 1970; 283: 1063–1071

92. Miller J, Rutherford H. Discussion on atrophy of the liver. Br Med J 1920; 2: 581

93. Bridge J C, Swanston C, Lane R E, Davie T B. Discussion on trinitrotoluene poisoning. Proc Royal Soc Med 1942; 35: 553–560

94. Maddrey W C, Boitnott J K. Isoniazid hepatitis. Ann Intern Med 1973; 79: 1–12

95. Black M, Mitchell J R, Zimmerman H J, Ishak K G, Epler G R. Isoniazid-associated hepatitis in 114 patients. Gastroenterology 1975; 69: 289–302

96. Schweitzer I L, Peters R L. Acute submassive hepatic necrosis due to methyldopa: A case demonstrating possible initiation of chronic liver disease. Gastroenterology 1974; 66: 1203–1211

97. Maddrey W C, Boitnott J K. Severe hepatitis from methyldopa. Gastroenterology 1975; 68: 351–360

98. Weir J F, Comfort M W. Toxic cirrhosis caused by cinchophen. Arch Intern Med 1933; 52: 685–724

99. Palmer W L, Woodall P S, Wang K C. Cinchophen and toxic necrosis of the liver: A survey of the problem. Trans Am Assoc Physicians 1936; 51: 381–393

100. Shalev O, Mosseri M, Ariel I, Stalikowicz R. Methyldopa-induced immune hemolytic anemia and chronic active hepatitis. Arch Intern Med 1983; 143: 592–593

101. Goldstein G B, Lam K C, Mistilis S P. Drug-induced active chronic hepatitis. Am J Dig Dis 1973; 18: 177–184

102. Reynolds T B. Laxative liver disease. In: Gerok W, Sickinger K, eds. Drugs and the liver. Stuttgart: F K Schattauer-Verlag, 1975: pp 319–325

103. Tonder M, Nordoy A, Elgio K. Sulfonamide-induced chronic liver disease. Scand J Gastroenterol 1974; 9: 93–96

104. Wright R. Drug-induced chronic hepatitis. Springer Semin Immunopathol 1980; 3: 331–338

105. Seeff L B. Drug-induced chronic liver disease with emphasis on chronic active hepatitis. Semin Liv Dis 1981; 1: 104–115

106. Pessayre D, Larrey D. Acute and chronic drug-induced hepatitis. Bailliere's Clin Gastroenterol 188; 2: 385–422

107. Sharp J R, Ishak K G, Zimmerman H J. Chronic active hepatitis and severe hepatic necrosis associated with nitrofurantoin. Ann Intern Med 1980; 92: 14–19

108. Homberg J C, Abuaf N, Helmi-Khalil S et al. Drug-induced hepatitis associated with anticytoplasmic organelle antibodies. Hepatology 1985; 5: 722–727

109. Poupon R, Longchal C, Darnis F. Hepatie chronique associee a la prise prolongee de papaverine. Gastroenterol Clin Biol 1978; 2: 305–308

110. Zimmerman H J. Lesions of drug-induced liver disease and valproate toxicity. In: Levy R H, Penry J K, eds. Idiosyncratic reactions to valproate: clinical risk patterns and mechanisms of toxicity. New York: Raven Press, 1991: pp 31–45

111. Zimmerman H J. Hepatotoxic effect of oncotherapeutic agents. Prog Liver Dis 1986; 8: 621–642

112. Lewis D, Wainwright H C, Kew H C, Zwi S, Isaacson C. Liver damage associated with perhexiline maleate. Gut 1979; 20: 186–189

113. Shaikh N A, Downer E, Butany J. Amiodarone — an inhibitor of phospholipase activity: A comparative study of the inhibiting activity of amiodarone, chloroquine and chlorpromazine. Mol Cell Biochem 1987; 76: 163–172

114. Hostetler K Y, Giordano J R, Hoyumpa A M Jr, Jellison E J. In vitro inhibition of lysosomal phospholipase A of rat lung by amiodarone and desethylamiodarone. Biochem Bioph Acta 1988; 959: 316–321

115. Shepherd N A, Dawson A M, Crocker P R, Levison D A. Granular cells — a pathological and analytical study. J Clin Pathol 1987; 40: 418–423

116. Simon J B, Manley P N, Brien J F, Armstrong P N. Amiodarone hepatotoxicity simulating alcoholic liver disease. N Engl J Med 1984; 311: 167–172

117. Lim P K, Trewby P N, Storey G C, Holt D W. Neuropathy and fatal hepatitis in a patient receiving amiodarone. Br Med J 1984; 288: 1638–1639

118. Dake M, Madison J M, Montgomery C K, Shellito J E, Hinchcliffe W S, Winkler M L, Bainton D F. Electron microscopic demonstration of lysosomal inclusion bodies in lung, liver, lymph nodes and blood leukocytes of patients with amiodarone pulmonary toxicity. Am J Med 1985; 78: 506–512

119. Pessayre D, Bichara M, Feldmann G, Degott C, Patet F, Benhamou J P. Perhexiline maleate-induced cirrhosis. Gastroenterology 1979; 76: 170–177

120. Babany G, Mallat A, Zafrani E S, Saint-Marc Girardin M F, Carcone B, Dhumeaux D. Chronic liver disease after low daily doses of amiodarone. Report of three cases. J Hepatol 1986; 3: 228–232

121. Rinder H M, Love J C, Wexler R. Amiodarone hepatotoxicity (letter). N Engl J Med 1986; 314: 318–319

122. Lewis J H, Mullick F G, Ishak K G et al. Histopathological analysis of suspected amiodarone hepatotoxicity. Hum Pathol 1990; 21: 59–67

123. McGovern B, Garan H, Kelly E, Ruskin J N. Adverse reactions during treatment with amiodarone hydrochloride. Br Med J 1983; 287: 175–180

124. Pieterse A S, Rowland R, Dunn D. Perhexiline maleate induced cirrhosis. Pathology 1983; 15: 201–203

125. Seki K, Minami Y, Nishikawa M, Kowata S, Miyoshi S, Imai Y, Tarui S. "Nonalcoholic steatohepatitis" induced by massive doses of synthetic estrogen. Gastroenterol Jpn 1983; 18: 197–203

126. Gilbert S C, Klintman G, Menter A, Silverman A. Methotrexate induced cirrhosis requiring liver transplantation in three patients with psoriasis. Arch Intern Med 1990; 150: 889–891

127. Zachariae H, Kragballe K, Sogaard H. Methotrexate induced liver cirrhosis. Br J Dermatol 1980; 102: 407–412

128. Mikkelsen W P, Edmondson H A, Peters R L, Redeker A G, Reynolds T B. Extra and intrahepatic portal hypertension without cirrhosis. (Hepatoportal sclerosis). Ann Surg 1965; 162: 602–620

129. Zeegen R, Stansfeld A G, Dawson A M, Hunt A H. Prolonged survival after portal decompression of patients with non-cirrhotic intrahepatic portal hypertension. Gut 1970; 11: 610–617

130. Neale G, Azzopardi J G. Chronic arsenical poisoning and noncirrhotic portal hypertension — A case for diagnosis. Br Med J 1971; 4: 725–730

131. Pimentel J C, Menezes A P. Liver disease in vineyard sprayers. Gastroenterology 1977; 72: 275–283

132. Edmundson H A, Peters R L, Reynolds T B, Kuzuma OT. Sclerosing hyaline necrosis of the liver in the chronic alcoholic. Ann Intern Med 1963; 59: 646–673

133. Russell R M, Boyer J L, Bagheri S A, Hruban Z. Hepatic injury from chronic vitaminosis A resulting in portal hypertension and ascites. N Engl J Med 1974; 291: 435–440

134. Shepherd P, Harrison D J, Idiopathic portal hypertension associated with cytotoxic drugs. J Clin Pathol 1990.; 43: 206–210

135. Snover D C, Weisdorf S, Bloomer J, McGlaye P, Weisdorf D. Nodular regenerative hyperplasia of the liver following bone marrow transplantation. Hepatology 1989; 9: 443–448

136. Colsky J, Greenspan E M, Warren T N. Hepatic fibrosis in children with acute leukemia after therapy with folic acid antagonists. Arch Pathol 1955; 59: 198–206

137. Hutter R V, Shipkey F H, Tan C T, Murphy M L, Chowdhury M. Hepatic fibrosis in children with acute leukemia: A complication of therapy. Cancer 1960; 13: 288–307

138. Cameron G R, Karunaratne W A E. Carbon tetrachloride cirrhosis in relation to liver regeneration. J Path Bact 1936; 42: 1–21

139. Brodsky I, Johnson H, Killman S A, Cronkite E P. Fibrosis of central and hepatic veins and perisinusoidal spaces of the liver following prolonged administration of urethane. Am J Med 1961; 30: 976–980

140. Brooks S E H, Miller C G, McKenzie K, Audretsch J J, Bras G, Acute veno-occlusive disease of the liver. Arch Pathol 1970; 89: 507–520

141. Lewis J H, Tice H, Zimmerman H J. Budd-Chiari syndrome associated with oral contraceptive steroids. Review of treatment of 47 cases. Dig Dis Sci 1983; 28: 673–683

142. Haubrich W S, Sancetta S M, Spontaneous recovery from hepatobiliary disease with xanthomatosis. Gastroenterology 1954; 26: 658–665

143. Myers J D, Olson R E, Lewis J H, Moran T J. Xanthomatous biliary cirrhosis following chlorpromazine with observations indicating overproduction of cholesterol, hypoprathrombinemia and the development of portal hypertension. Trans Ass Am Physic 1957; 70: 243–261

144. Kohn N N, Myerson R M. Xanthomatous biliary cirrhosis following chlorpromazine. Am J Med 1961; 31: 665–670

145. Walker C O, Combes B. Biliary cirrhosis induced by chlorpromazine. Gastroenterology 1966; 51: 631–640

146. Hurt P, Wegmann T. Protracted Largactil jaundice deepening into primary biliary cirrhosis. Acta Hepatol Splenol 1961; 8: 87–95

147. Lok A S, Ng I O. Prochlorperazine-induced chronic cholestasis J Hepatol 1988; 6: 369–373

148. Weir J F. Cirrhosis associated with chronic inorganic arsenical poisoning. Proc Staff Meet Mayo Clin 1930; 5: 173–175

149. Franklin M, Bean W B, Hardin R C. Fowler's solution as an etiologic agent in cirrhosis. Am J Med Sci 1950; 219: 589–596

150. Hohn D, Rayner A A, Economou J S, Ignoffo R J, Lewis B J, Stagg R J. Toxicities and complications of implanted pump hepatic arterial and intravenous floxuridine infusion. Cancer 1986; 57: 465–470

151. Bolton J S, Bowen J C. Biliary sclerosis associated with hepatic artery infusion of floxuridine. Surgery 1986; 99: 119–122

152. Botet J F, Watson R C, Kemeny N, Daly J M, Yeh S. Cholangitis complicating intraarterial chemotherapy in liver metastasis. Radiology 1985; 156: 335–337

153. Anderson S D, Holley H C, Berland L L, Van Dyke J A, Stanley R J. Causes of jaundice during hepatic artery infusion chemotherapy. Radiology 1986; 161: 439–442

154. Doria M I, Shepard K V, Levin B, Riddell R H. Liver pathology following hepatic arterial infusion chemotherapy. Cancer 1986; 58: 855–861

155. Ludwig J, Kim C H, Wiesner R H, Krom R A, Floxuridine-induced sclerosing cholangitis: An ischemic cholangiopathy? Hepatology 1989; 9: 215–218

156. Zafrani E S, Pinaudeau Y, Dhumeaux D. Drug-induced vascular lesions of the liver. Arch Intern Med 1983; 143: 495–502

157. Valla D, Le M G, Poynard T, Zucman N, Rueff B, Benhamou J P. Risk of hepatic vein thrombosis in relation to recent use of oral contraceptives. A case control study. Gastroenterology 1986; 90: 807–811

158. Valla D, Casadevall N, Lacombe C et al. Primary myeloproloferative disorder and hepatic vein thrombosis in 20 patients with Budd-Chiari syndrome. Ann Intern Med 1985; 103: 329–334

159. Maddrey W C, Hepatic vein thrombosis (Budd-Chiari syndrome): Possible association with the use of oral contraceptives. Semin Liv Dis 1987; 7: 32–39

160. Stuart K L, Bras G. Veno-occlusive disease of the liver. Q J Med 1957; 26: 291–315

161. Bras G, Brandt K H. Vascular disorders. In: MacSween R N M, Anthony P P, Scheuer P J, eds. Pathology of the liver, 2nd edn. Edinburgh: Churchill Livingstone, 1987: pp 478–502

162. Reed G B Jr, Cox A J Jr. The human liver after radiation injury. A form of veno-occlusive disease. Am J Pathol 1966; 48: 597–611

163. Griner P F, E l Badawi A, Packman C H. Veno-occlusive disease after chemotherapy of acute leukemia. Report of two cases. Ann Intern Med 1976; 85: 578–582

164. Yanoff M, Rawson A J. Peliosis hepatis. An anatomic study with demonstration of two varieties. Arch Pathol 1964; 77: 159–165

165. McGiven A R. Peliosis hepatis. Case report and review of pathogenesis. J Pathol 1970; 101: 283–285

166. Puppala A R, Ro J A. Possible association between peliosis hepatis and diethylstilboestrol. Report of two cases. Postgrad Med 1979; 65: 277–281

167. Delage C, Lagace R. La peliose hepatiquee: Role etiologique possible des medicaments. L'Union Med Canada 1974; 102: 1888–1893

168. Bagheri S A, Boyer J L, Peliosis hepatis associated with androgenic-anabolic steroid therapy: A severe form of hepatic injury. Ann Intern Med 1974; 81: 610–618

169. Nadell J, Kosek J. Peliosis hepatis. Twelve cases associated with oral androgen therapy. Arch Pathol Lab Med 1977; 101: 405–410

170. Taxy J B. Peliosis: A morphologic curiosity becomes an iatrogenic problem. Hum Pathol; 1978; 9: 331–340

171. Allen J R, Carstens L A. Monocrotaline-induced Budd-Chiari syndrome in monkeys. Am J Dig Dis 1970; 16: 111–121

172. Tuchweber B, Kovacs K, Khandekar J D, Gorg B D. Peliosis-like changes induced by phalloidin in rat liver. A light and electron microscopic study. J Med (Basel) 1973; 4: 327–345

173. Sherlock S. Progress report. Hepatic adenomas and oral contraceptives. Gut 1975; 16: 753–756

174. Schonberg L A. Peliosis hepatic and oral contraceptives. J Reprod Med 1983; 27: 753–756

175. Loomus G N, Aneja P, Bota R A, A case of peliosis hepatis in association with tamoxifen therapy. Am J Clin Pathol 1983; 80: 881–883

176. Degott C, Rueff B, Kreis H et al. Peliosis hepatis in recipients of renal transplants. Gut 1978; 19: 748–753

177. McDonald G B, Tirumali N. Intestinal and liver toxicity of neoplastic drugs. West J Med 1984; 140: 250–259

178. Poulsen H, Winkler K. Liver disease with periportal sinusoidal dilatation. Digestion 1973; 8: 441–442

179. Molleken K. Liver biopsy finding after intake of oral contraceptives. Zentrabl Allg Pathol 1979; 123: 195–201

180. Baum J K, Holtz F, Bockstein J J, Klein E W. Possible association between benign hepatomas and oral contraceptives. Lancet 1973; ii: 926–929

181. Ishak K G, Rabin L. Benign tumors of the liver. Med Clin N Am 1975; 59: 995–1013

182. Klatskin G. Hepatic tumors: Possible relationship to use of oral contraceptives. Gastroenterology 1977; 73: 386–394

183. Edmondson H A, Reynolds T B, Henderson B, Benton B. Regression of liver cell adenomas associated with oral contraceptives. Ann Intern Med 1977; 86: 180–182

184. Ishak K G. Hepatic lesions caused by anabolic and contraceptive steroids. Sem Liver Dis 1981; 1: 116–128

185. Butler W H. Pathology of liver cancer in experimental animals. In: Liver Cancer. IARC Scientific Publication 1. Lyon: WHO International Agency for Research in Cancer, 1971: pp 30–41

186. Miller E K, Miller J A. Hepatocarcinogenesis by chemicals. Progr Liver Dis 1976; 5: 699–711

187. Sternberg S S, Popper H, Oser B L, Oser M. Gall bladder and bile duct adenocarcinomas in dogs after long term feeding of aramite. Cancer 1960; 13: 780–789

188. Tilak T B. Induction of cholangiocarcinoma following treatment of a rhesus monkey with aflatoxin. F Cosm Toxicol 1975; 13: 247–249

189. Reddy K P, Buschmann R J, Chomet B. Cholangiocarcinomas induced by feeding 3'-methyl-4-dimethylaminoazobenzene to rats. Am J Pathol 1977; 87: 189–204

190. Selinger M, Koff R S. Thorotrast and the liver: A reminder. Gastroenterology 1975; 68: 799–803

191. Farber E. On the pathogenesis of experimental hepatocellular carcinoma. In: Okuda K, Peters R L, eds. Hepatocellular carcinoma. New York: John Wiley, 1976: pp 3–24

192. Westaby D, Williams R. Androgen and anabolic steroid-related liver tumors. In: Davis M, Tredger J M, Williams R, eds. Drug reactions and the liver. New York: Pitman 1981: pp 284–289

193. Forman D, Vincent T J, Doll R. Cancer of the liver and the use of oral contraceptives. Br Med J 1986; 292: 1357–1361

194. Hurst P, Paget G E, Protoporphyria, cirrhosis and hepatomata in livers of mice given griseofulvin. Br J Dermatol 1963; 75: 105–112

195. Rosenkrantz H S, Carr H S. Hydrazine antidepressants and isoniazid: Potential carcinogen. Lancet 1971; 1: 1354–1355

196. Heath C W Jr, Falk H, Creech J L Jr. Characteristics of cases of angiosarcoma of the liver among vinyl chloride workers in the United States. Ann NY Acad Sci 1975; 246: 231–236

197. Mark I, Delmore F, Creech J L Jr et al. Clinical and morphologic features of hepatic angiosarcoma in vinyl chloride workers. Cancer 1976; 37: 149–163

198. Falk H, Caldwell G G, Ishak K G, Thomas L B, Popper H. Arsenic-related angiosarcoma. Am J Indust Med 1981; 2: 43–50

199. Kasper M L, Schoenfield L, Strom R L, Theologides A. Hepatic angiosarcoma and bronchoalveolar carcinoma induced by Fowler's solution. JAMA 1984; 252: 3407–3408

200. Ishak K G. Mesenchymal tumors of the liver. In: Okuda K, Peters R L, eds. Hepatocellular carcinoma. New York: John Wiley, 1976: pp 247–307

201. De Motta C L, Da Silva Horta J, Taveres M H. Prospective epidemiological study of Thorotrast exposed patients in Portugal. Environ Res 1979; 18: 152–153

202. Baxter P J, Langlands A O, Anthony P P, MacSween R N M, Scheuer P J. Angiosarcoma of the liver: A marker tumour for the late effects of Thorotrast in Great Britain. Br J Cancer 1980; 41: 446–453

203. Falk H, Herbert J, Crowley S, Ishak K G, Thomas L B, Popper H, Caldwell G G. Epidemiology of hepatic angiosarcoma in the United States: 1964–1974. Envir Hlth Persp 1981; 41: 107–113

204. Yamada S, Hosoda S, Tateno H, Kido C, Takahashi S. Survey of Thorotrast-associated liver cancers in Japan. J Nat Cancer Inst 1983; 70: 31–35

205. Falk H, Thomas L B, Popper H, Ishak K G. Hepatic angiosarcoma associated with androgenic-anabolic steroids. Lancet 1979; ii: 1120–1123

206. Hoch-Ligeti C. Angiosarcoma of the liver associated with diethylstilbestrol. JAMA 1978; 240: 1510–1511

207. Daneshmend T K, Scott G L, Bradfield J W B. Angiosarcoma of liver associated with phenelzine. Br Med J 1979; 1: 1679

208. Klinge O, Bannasch P. Zur Vermehrung des glatten endoplasmatischen Retikulum in Hepatocyten Menschlicher Leberpunktate. Verhandl Dtsch Gesell Pathol 1968; 52: 568–573

209. Winckler K, Junge U, Creutzfeldt W. Ground-glass hepatocytes in unselected liver biopsies. Ultrastructure and relationship to hepatitis B surface antigen. Scand J Gastroenterol 1976; 11: 167–170

210. Mullick F G, Ishak K G. Hepatic injury associated with diphenylhydantoin therapy: A clinicopathologic study of 20 cases. Am J Clin Pathol 1980; 74: 442–452

211. Jezequel A M, Orlandi F. Fine morphology of the human liver as a tool in clinical pharmacology. In: Orlandi F, Jezequel A M, eds. Liver and drugs. London: Academic Press, 1972: pp 145–192

212. Jezequel A M, Librari M L, Mosca P, Novelli G, Lorenzini I, Orlandi F. Changes induced in human liver by long-term anticonvulsant therapy. Functional and ultrastructural data. Liver 1984; 4: 307–317

213. Pamperl H, Gardner W, Fridrich L, Pointner H, Denk H. Influence of long-term anticonvulsant treatment on liver ultrastructure in man. Liver 1984; 4: 294–300

214. Hadziyannis S, Gerber M A, Vissoulis C, Popper H. Cytoplasmic hepatitis B antigen in "ground glass" hepatocytes of carriers. Arch Pathol 1973; 96: 327–330

215. Klinge O, Kaboth U, Winckler K. Feingewebliche Befunde an der Leber Klinisch gesunder Australia-Antigen-(HB-Ag-) Trager. Virchows Arch (A) 1973; 361: 359–368

216. Shikata T, Uzawa T, Yoshiwara N, Akatsuka T, Yamazahi S. Staining methods of Australia antigen in paraffin section— detection of cytoplasmic inclusion bodies. Jpn J Exper Med 1974; 44: 25–36

217. Feinman L, Rubin E, Lieber C S. Adaptation of the liver to drugs. In: Orlandi F, Jezequel A M, eds. Liver and drugs. London: Academic Press, 1972: pp 41–83

218. Vazquez J J, Pardo-Mindan J. Liver cell injury (bodies similar to Lafora's) in alcoholics treated with disulfiram (Antabuse). Histopathology 1979; 3: 377–384

219. Vazquez J J, Pervera S. Cyanamide-induced liver injury in alcoholics. Lancet 1980; i: 361–362

220. Vazquez J J, Guillen F J, Zozaya Lahoz M. Cyanamide-induced liver injury. A predictable lesion. Liver 1983:3: 225–231

221. Thomsen P, Reincke V. Ground glass inclusions in liver cells in an alcoholic treated with cyanamide (Dipsan). Liver 1981; 1: 67–73

222. Vazquez J J. Ground-glass hepatocytes: light and electron microscopy. Characterization of the different types. Histopathology 1990; 5: 379–386

223. Ishak K G. The liver. In: Riddell R H, ed. Pathology of drug-induced and toxic diseases. New York: Churchill Livingstone, 1982: pp 457–513

224. Koga Y, Swanson V L, Hays D M. Hepatic "intravenous fat pigment" in infants and children receiving lipid emulsion. J Pediatr Surg 1976; 10: 641–648

225. Passwell J H, David R, Katznelson D, Cohen B E. Pigment deposition in the reticuloendothelial system after fat emulsion infusion. Arch Dis Child 1976; 51: 366–368

226. Coelho Filbo J C, Morreua R A, Crocker P R, Levison D A. Identification of titanium pigment in drug addicts' tissues. Histopathology 1991; 19: 190–192

227. Bothwell T H, Bradlow M B. Siderosis in the Bantu: A combined histopathological and chemical study. Arch Pathol 1960; 70: 279–292

228. Lundvall O. Alcohol and porphyria cutanea tarda. In: Engel A, Larsson T, eds. Alcoholic cirrhosis and other toxic hepatopathies Stockholm: Nordiska Bokhandelns Forlag, 1970: pp 356–372

229. Schmid R. Cutaneous porphyria in Turkey. N Engl J Med 1960; 263: 397–398

230. Ockner R K, Schmid R. Acquired porphyria in man and rat due to hexachlorobenzene intoxication. Nature 1961; 189: 499–502

231. Ali M, Fayemi Riglusi R, Frasuno J, Marsen T, Malcolm D. Hemosiderosis in hemodialysis patients: An autopsy study of 50 cases. JAMA 1980; 244:343–345

232. Kothari T, Swamy A P, Lee J C K, Mangla J C, Cestero R V M. Hepatic hemosiderosis in maintenance hemodialysis (MHD) patients. Dig Dis Sci 1980; 25: 363–368

233. Zimmerman H J, Seeff L B. Enzymes in hepatic disease. In: Coodley E L, ed. Diagnostic enzymology. Philadelphia: Lea & Febiger, 1970: pp 1–38

234. Zimmerman H J. Hepatic failure. In: Gall E A, Mostofi F K, eds. The liver. Baltimore: Williams & Wilkins, 1973: pp 384–405

235. Meyer U A, Maxwell J D. Human and experimental porphyria: Relationship of defects in heme biosynthesis to drug idiosyncrasy. In: Gerok W, Sickinger K, eds. Drugs and the liver. Stuttgart Schattauer-Verlag, 1975: pp 201–207

235a. Fargiori S, Piperno A, Cappellini M D et al Hepatitis C virus and porphyria cutanea tarda: evidence of a strong association. Hepatology 1992; 16: 1322–1326

236. Harinasuta U, Zimmerman H J. Diphenylhydantoin sodium hepatitis. JAMA 1968; 203: 1015–1018

237. Zimmerman H J. Clinical and laboratory manifestations of hepatotoxicity. Ann NY Acad Sci 1963; 104: 954–987

238. Elkington S G, Goffinet J A, Conn H O. Renal and hepatic injury associated with methoxyflurane anesthesia. Ann Intern Med 1968; 69: 1229–1236

239. Jennings R B. Fatal fulminant acute carbon tetrachloride poisoning. AMA Arch Pathol 1955; 59: 269–284

240. Rueff B, Benhamou J-P. Acute hepatic necrosis and fulminant hepatic failure. Gut 1973; 14: 805–815

241. Litten W. The most poisonous mushrooms. Sci Am 1975; 232: 91–101

242. Floersheim G L. Treatment of human amatoxin mushroom poisoning. Myths and advances in therapy. Med Toxicol 1987; 2: 1–9

243. Krishnamachari K A V R, Bhat R V, Nagarajan V, Tilak T B G. Hepatitis due to aflatoxicosis. An outbreak in western India. Lancet 1975; i: 1061–1063

244. Mohabbat O, Srivastava R N, Sediq G G, Merzad A A, Aram G N. An outbreak of hepatic veno-occlusive diseases in north-western Afghanistan. Lancet 1976; ii: 269–271

245. Tandon B N, Randon R K, Tandon H D, Narndranathan M, Joshi Y K. An epidemic of veno-occlusive disease of liver in central India. Lancet 1976; ii: 271–272

246. Fukunishi R. Acute hepatic lesions induced by cycasin. Acta Pathol Jpn 1973; 23: 639–646

247. Kopelman H, Scheuer P J, Williams R. The liver lesion of the Epping jaundice. Q J Med 1966; 35: 553–564

248. McGill D B, Motto J D. An industrial outbreak of toxic hepatitis due to methylenedianiline. N Engl J Med 1974; 291: 278–282

249. Lijinsky W, Greenblatt M. Carcinogen dimethylnitrosamine produced in vitro from nitrite and aminopyrine. Nature (New Biology) 1972; 236: 177–178

250. Bick M. Chlorinated hydrocarbon residues in human body fat. Med J Aust 1967; 1: 1127–1130

251. Smith N J. Death following accidental ingestion of DDT. JAMA 1948; 136: 469–471

252. Bullivant C M. Accidental poisoning by paraquat: Report of two cases in man. Br Med J 1966; 1: 1272–1273

253. Hardin B L Jr. Carbon tetrachloride poisoning — a review. Ind Med Surg 1954; 23: 93–105

254. Von Oettingen W F. The halogenated hydrocarbons of industrial and toxicological importance. Amsterdam: Elsevier 1964

255. Umiker W, Pearce J. Nature and genesis of pulmonary alterations in carbon tetrachloride poisoning. Arch Pathol 1953; 55: 203–217

256. Williams A T, Burk R F. Carbon tetrachloride hepatotoxicity: An example of tree radical mediated injury. Sem Liver Dis 1990; 10: 279–284

257. Baerg R D, Kimberg D V. Centrilobular hepatic necrosis and acute renal failure in 'solvent sniffers.' Ann Intern Med 1970; 73: 713–720

258. Slater T F. Free radical mechanisms in tissue injury. Bristol: JW Arrowsmith, 1972: pp 118–163

259. Recknagel R O, Glende E A Jr. Carbon tetrachloride hepatotoxicity: An example of lethal cleavage. CRC Crit Rev Tox 1973; 2: 263–297

260. Harrison D C, Paaso B T. Amanita phalloides poisoning. West J Med 1983; 138: 731–732

261. Kilbourne E, Rigau-Perez J G, Heath C W, Zach M M, Flak H, Martin-Macros M, De Carlos A. Clinical epidemiology of toxic oil syndrome. Manifestation of a new illness. N Engl J Med 1983; 309: 1408–1414

262. Solis Herruzo J A, Castellano G, Colina F, Morillas J D, Munoz-Yague M T, Coca M D C, Jelavic D. Hepatic injury in the toxic epidemic syndrome caused by ingestion of adulterated cooking oil. Hepatology 1984; 4: 131–139

263. Diaz de Rojas F, Castro G M, Abaitua B I et al. Hepatic injury in the toxic oil syndrome. Hepatology 1985; 5: 166–174

264. Zimmerman H J, Maddrey W M. Toxic and drug induced hepatitis. In: Schiff L, Schiff E R, eds. Disease of the liver. Philadelphia: Lippincott 1987: pp 591–667

265. Little D M, Wetstone H J. Anesthesia and the liver. Anesthesiology 1964; 25: 815–853

266. Little D M. Effects of halothane on liver function. In: Greene N M, ed. Clinical anesthesia: Halothane. Philadelphia: F A Davis, 1968: pp 85–137

267. Gottlieb L S, Trey C. The effects of fluorinated anesthetics on the liver and kidneys. Annu Rev Med 1974; 25: 411–429

268. Inman W H W, Mushin W M. Jaundice after repeated exposure to halothane: An analysis of reports to the Committee on Safety of Medicine. Br Med J 1974; 1: 5–10

269. Joshi P H, Conn H O. The syndrome of methoxyflurane-associated hepatitis. Ann Intern Med 1974; 80: 395–401

270. Klatskin G, Smith D P. Halothane-induced hepatitis. In: Gerok W, Sickinger K, eds. Drugs and the liver. Stuttgart: F K Schattaure-Verlag, 1975: pp 289–296

271. Moult P, Sherlock S. Halothane-related hepatitis. Q J Med 1975; 44: 99–114

272. Bottinger L E, Dalen E, Hallen B. Halothane-induced liver damage: An analysis of the material reported to the Swedish Adverse Drug Reaction Committee 1966–1973. Acta Anaesth Scand 1976; 20: 40–46

273. Lewis J H, Zimmerman H J, Ishak K G, Mullick F G. Enflurane hepatotoxicity: A clinicopathologic study of 24 cases. Ann Intern Med 1983; 98: 984–992

274. Carney F M, Van Dyke R A. Halothane hepatitis: A critical review. Anesth Analg, Current Researches 1972; 51: 135–160

275. Cousins M J, Plummer J L, Hall P. Toxicity of volatile anaesthetic agents. Can Anaesth Soc J 1985; 32: S52–S55

276. Brown B R, Gandolfi A J. Adverse effects of volatile anaesthetics. Br J Anaesth 1984; 59: 14–23

277. Stock J G, Strunin L. Unexplained hepatitis following halothane. Anesthesiology 1985; 63: 424–439

278. Simpson B R, Strunin L, Walton B. Evidence for halothane hepatotoxicity is equivocal. In: Ingelfinger F J, Relman A S, Finland M, eds. Controversy in internal medicine. Philadelphia: WB Saunders, 1974: p 580

279. Schaffner F. Halothane hepatitis. In: Ingelfinger F, Ebert P, Finland M, Relman A, eds. Controversy in internal medicine II. Philadelphia: WB Saunders, 1974: pp 565–584

280. Peters R L. Halothane hepatitis (Letter). Lancet 1978; ii: 790–791

281. Strunin L. Halothane hepatitis. Lancet 1978; 2: 790

282. Fee J P, Black G W, Dundee J W, McIlroy P D, Black F H, Doggart J R. Halothane and anicteric hepatitis (Letter). Lancet 1980; i: 361

283. Watts G T. Halothane and anicteric hepatitis. (Letter). Lancet 1980; i: 361

284. Venning G R. Does halothane cause hepatic necrosis? Br Med J 1983; 286: 1216

285. Hughes M, Powell L W. Recurrent hepatitis in patients receiving multiple halothane anesthetics for radium treatment of carcinoma of the cervix uteri. Gastroenterology 1970; 58: 790–797

286. Davis P, Holdsworth C D. Jaundice after multiple halothane anesthetics administered during the treatment of carcinoma of the uterus. Gut 1973; 14: 566–568

287. Trowell J, Peto R, Smith A C. Controlled trial of repeated halothane anesthetics in patients with carcinoma of the uterus. Lancet 1975; i: 821–823

288. Klion F M, Schaffner F, Popper H. Hepatitis after exposure to halothane. Ann Intern Med 1969; 71: 467–477

289. Sherlock S. Progress report. Halothane hepatitis. Gut 1971; 12: 324–329

290. Reed W D, Williams R. Halothane hepatitis as seen by the physician. Br J Anesth 1972; 44: 935–940

291. Morgenstern L, Sacks H J, Marmer M J. Postoperative jaundice associated with halothane anesthesia. Surg Gyn Obst 1965; 121: 728–732

292. Dordal E, Galgov S, Orlando R A, Platz C, Fatal halothane hepatitis with transient granulomas. N Engl J Med 1970; 283: 357–359

293. Shah I A, Brandt H. Halothane-associated granulomatous hepatitis. Digestion 1983; 28: 245–249

294. Klatskin G, Kimberg D V. Recurrent hepatitis attributable to halothane sensitization in an anesthetist. N Engl J Med 1969; 280: 515–522

295. Thomas F B. Chronic aggressive hepatitis induced by halothane. Ann Intern Med 1974; 81: 487–489

296. Neuberger J, Kenna J G. Halothane hepatitis: A model of immune mediated drug hepatotoxicity. Clin Sci 1987; 72: 263–270

297. Zimmerman H J. The spectrum of hepatotoxicity. Persp Biol Med 1968; 12: 135–161

298. Reynolds E S, Moslen M T. Liver injury following halothane anesthesia in phenobarbital-pretreated rats. Biochem Pharmacol 1974; 23: 189–195

299. Mazze R I, Cousins M J. Renal toxicity of anesthetics: With specific reference to the nephrotoxicity of methoxyflurane. Can Anaesth Soc J 1973; 20: 64–80

300. Masone R J, Goldfarb J P, Manzione N C, Biempica L. Enflurane hepatitis. J Clin Gastroenterol 1982; 4: 541–545

301. Sigurdson J, Hreidarsson A B, Thjodlerfasson B. "Enflurane hepatitis". A report of a case with a previous history of halothane hepatitis. Acta Anaesthesiol Scand 1985; 29: 495–496

302. Paull J D, Fortune D W. Hepatotoxicity and death following two enflurane anesthetics. Anaesthesia 1987; 42: 1191–1196

303. Foutch P G, Ferguson D R, Tuthill R J. Enflurane-induced hepatitis with prominent cholestasis. Cleve Clin J Med 1987; 54: 210–213

304. D'eramo C, Ghinelli F, Zucolli P. Dano epatico ed anestetici alognato; esperienza clinica preliminare. Acta Bio-Med Ateneo Parmensen 1985; 56: 155–160

305. Brunt E M, White H, Marsh J W, Holtmann B, Peters M S. Fulminant hepatic failure after repeated exposure to isoflurane anesthesia: A case report. Hepatology 1991; 13: 1017–1021

306. Stoelting R K, Blitt C D, Cohen P J, Merin R G. Hepatic dysfunction after isoflurane anesthesia. Anesth Annlg 1987; 66: 147–153

307. Zimmerman H J. Even isoflurane (editorial). Hepatology 1991; 13: 1251–1253

308. Harris J A, Cromwell T H. Jaundice following fluroxene anaesthesia. Anesthesiology 1972; 37: 462–463

309. Harrison G G, Smith J S. Massive lethal hepatic necrosis in rats anesthetized with fluroxene after microsomal enzyme induction. Anesthesiology 1973; 39: 619–625

310. Rees L. Drugs used in the treatment of psychiatric disease. Abst Wld Med 1966; 39: 129–141

311. Teller D N. Phenothiazines and butyrophenones in relation to neurochemistry and pharmacology. In: Denbar H C B, ed. Psychopharmacological treatment: theory and practice. New York: Marcel Dekker, 1975; pp 28–42

312. Zimmerman H J. Update of hepatotoxicity due to classes of drugs in common clinical use: Nonsteroidal drugs, anti-inflammatory drugs, antibiotics, antihypertensives and cardiac and psychotropic agents. Sem Liver Dis 1990; 10: 322–338

313. Hollister L E. Allergy to chlorpromazine manifested by jaundice. Am J Med 1957; 23: 870–879

314. Zelman S. Liver cell necrosis in chlorpromazine jaundice. Am J Med 1959; 27: 708–729

315. Levine R A, Briggs G W, Lowell D M. Chronic chlorpromazine cholangiolitic hepatitis: Report of a case with immunofluorescent studies. Gastroenterology 1966; 50: 665–670

316. Dincsoy H P, Saelinger D A. Haloperidol-induced chronic cholestatic liver disease. Gastroenterology 1982; 83: 694–700

317. FDA ADR Highlights August 14, 1980

318. Bhatia S C, Banta L E, Erlich D W. Molindone and hepatotoxicity. Drug Intell Clin Pharm 1985; 19: 744–746

319. Rosenblum L E, Korn R J, Zimmerman H J. Hepatocellular jaundice as a complication of iproniazid therapy. Arch Intern Med 1960; 105: 583–593

320. Brandt C, Hoffbauer F W. Liver injury associated with tranylcypromine therapy. JAMA 1964; 188: 752–753

321. Short M H, Burns J M, Harris M E. Cholestatic jaundice during imipramine therapy. JAMA 1968; 206: 1791–1792

322. Somerville J M, McLaren E H. Severe headache and disturbed liver function during treatment with Zimelidine. Br Med J 1982; 285: 1009–1010

323. Brandes J W, Korst H A, Littman K P. Gelbsucht nach Nomifensin Med Welt 1980; 31: 1607–1608

324. Vaz F G, Singh R, Nurussaman M. Hepatitis induced by nomifensine. Br Med J 1984; 289: 1268

325. Martin W, Rickers J. Cholestatische Hepatose nach Diphenylhydantoin. Wien Klin Wochenschr 1972; 84: 41–45

326. Dhar G J, Pierach C A, Ahamed P N, Howard R B. Diphenylhydantoin-induced hepatic necrosis. Postgrad Med 1974; 56: 128–134

327. Haruda F. Phenytoin hypersensitivity: Thirty eight cases. Neurology 1979; 29: 1480–1485

328. Aaron J S, Bank S, Ackert G. Diphenylhydantoin-induced hepatotoxicity. Am J Gastroenter 1985; 80: 200–202

329. Parker W A, Shearer C A. Phenytoin hepatotoxicity: a case report and review. Neurology 1979; 29: 175

330. Lee T J, Carney C N, Lapid J, Higgins T, Fallon H J. Diphenylhydantoin-induced hepatic necrosis. A case study. Gastroenterology 1976; 70: 422–424

331. Cook I F, Shilkin K B, Reed W D. Phenytoin induced granulomatous hepatitis. Aust NZ J Med 1981; 11: 539–541

332. Gram L, Bentssen R D. Hepatic toxicity of antiepileptic drugs: A review. Acta Neurol Scand (suppl) 1983; 97: 81–90

333. Gropper A L. Diphenylhydantoin sensitivity: Report of a fatal case with hepatitis and exfoliative dermatitis. N Engl J Med 1956; 254: 522–524

334. Brown M, Schubert T. Phenytoin hypersensitivity, hepatitis and mononucleosis syndrome. J Clin Gastroenterol 1986; 8: 469–477

335. Van Wyk J J, Hoffman C R. Periarteritis nodosa. A case of fatal exfoliative dermatitis resulting from "dilantin sodium" sensitization. Arch Intern Med 1948; 81: 605–611

336. Gams R A, Neal J A, Conrad E G. Hydantoin-induced pseudo-lymphoma. Ann Intern Med 1968; 69: 557–568

337. Easton J D. Potential hazards of hydantoin use. Ann Intern Med 1972; 77: 998–999

338. Sheretz E F, Jegasothy B V, Lazarus G S. Phenytoin hypersensitivity reaction presenting with toxic epidermal necrolysis and severe hepatitis. Report of a patient treated with corticosteroid pulse therapy. J Am Acad Dermatol 1985; 12: 1783

339. Tomsick R S. The phenytoin syndrome. Cutis 1983; 32: 535–538

340. Andreasen P B, Lyngbye J, Trolle E. Abnormalities in liver function tests during long-term diphenylhydantion therapy in epileptic outpatient. Acta Med Scand 1973; 194: 261–264

341. Hadzie N, Portmann B, Davies E T, Mowat A P, Mieli-Vergani G. Acute liver failure induced by carbamazepine. Arch Dis Child 1990; 65: 315–317

342. Fellows W K. A case of aplastic anemia and pancytopenia with tegretol therapy. Headache 1969; 9: 92–95

343. Zucker P, Daum F, Cohen M I. Fatal carbamazepine hepatitis. J Pediatr 1977; 91: 667–668

344. Bertram P D, Taylor R J. Carbamazepine hepatotoxicity: Clinical and histopathological features. Am J Gastroenterol 1980; 74: 78–83

345. Levy M, Goodman M W, Van Dyne B J, Sumner H W. Granulomatous hepatitis secondary to carbamazepine. Ann Intern Med 1981; 95: 64–65

346. Rigau Canaardo J, Bruguera M, Sese J, Morlans G. Hepatite aigue cholestatique due a la carbamazepine. Gastroenterol Clin Biol 1984; 8: 769–770

347. Williams S J, Ruppin D C, Grierson J M, Farrell G C. Carbamazepine hepatitis: The clinicopathological spectrum. J Gastroenterol Hepatol 1986; 1: 159–163

348. Larrey D, Hadengue A, Pessayre D. Carbamazepine-induced acute cholangitis. Dig Dis Sci 1987; 32: 554–557

349. Hopen G, Nesthus I, Laerum O D. Fatal carbamazepine-associated hepatitis. Report of two cases. Acta Med Scand 1981; 210: 333–335

350. Forbes G M, Jeffrey G P, Shilkin K B, Reed W D. Carbamazepine hepatotoxicity: Another case of the vanishing bile duct syndrome. Gastroenterology 1992; 102: 1385–1388

351. Jeavons P M. Hepatotoxicity of antiepileptic drugs. In: Oxley J, Jauz O, Meinardi H, eds. Chronic toxicity of antiepileptic drugs. New York: Raven Press, 1982: pp 601–610

352. Powell-Jackson P R, Tredger J M, Williams R. Hepatotoxicity to sodium valproate. A review. Gut 1984; 25: 673–681

353. Dreifuss F E, Santilli N, Langer D H et al. Valproic acid hepatic fatalities: A retrospective review. Neurology 1987; 37: 379–385

354. Colletti R B, Trainer T D, Krawisz B R. Reversible valproate fulminant hepatic failure. J Pediatr Gastroenterol Nutr 1986; 5: 990–994

355. Scheffner D, Konig S, Rauterberg-Ruland I et al. Fatal liver failure in 16 children with valproate therapy. Epilepsia 1988; 29: 530

356. Zafrani E S, Bertelot P. Sodium valproate in the induction of unusual hepatotoxicity. Hepatology 1982; 2: 648–649

357. Jeavons P M. Non-dose-related side effects of valproate. Epilepsia 1984: 25: s50–s55

358. Keene D L, Humphrey P, Carpenter B, Fletcher J P. Valproic acid producing a Reye-like syndrome. Can J Neurol Sci 1982; 9: 435–437

359. Young R S, Bergman A, Gang D L, Richardson E P. Fatal Reye-like syndrome associated with valproic acid. Ann Neurol 1980; 7: 389

360. Lewis J H, Zimmerman H J, Garrett C T, Rosenburg E. Valproate-induced hepatic steatogenesis in rats. Hepatology 1982; 2: 870–873

361. Kesterson J W, Granneman G R, Machinist J M. The hepatotoxicity of valproic acid and its metabolites in rats. I. Toxicology, biochemical and histopathologic studies. Hepatology 1984; 4: 1143–1152

362. Granneman G R, Wang S I, Kesterson J W, Machinist J M. The hepatotoxicity of valproic acid and its metabolites in rats. II. Intermediary and valproic acid metabolism. Hepatology 1984; 4: 1153–1158

363. Sugimoto T, Woo M, Nishida N et al. Hepatotoxicity in rat following administration of valproic acid. Epilepsia 1987; 28: 142–146

364. Lewis J H. Hepatic toxicity of nonsteroidal anti-inflammatory drugs. Clin Pharm 1984; 3: 128–138

365. Koff R S. Liver disease induced by nonsteroidal anti-inflammatory drugs. In: Borda I T, Koff R S eds. NSAIDS: a profile of adverse effects. St. Louis: Mosley 1992: pp 133–146

366. Paulus H E. Arthritis Advisory Committee meeting. Arthritis Rheum 1982; 25: 595–596

367. Katz L M, Love P Y. NSAIDs and the liver. In: Famely J A, Paulus H E, eds. Therapeutic applications of NSAIDS: Subpopulations and new formulations. New York: Marcel Dekker, 1992: pp 247–263

368. Rabinovitz M, Van Thiel D H. Hepatotoxicity of nonsteroidal anti-inflammatory drugs. Am J Gastroenterol 1992; 87: 1696–1704

369. Cuthbert M F. Adverse reactions to non-steroidal anti-inflammatory drugs. Curr Med Res Opin 1974; 2: 600–610

370. Offerhaus L. Nonsteroidal anti-inflammatory drugs in the treatment of rheumatic disorders: Pitfalls and problems with the present plethora. Neth J Med 1983; 26: 173–175

371. Hueper W E. Cinchophen (Atophan): A critical review. Medicine 1948; 27: 43–103

372. Cutr'in P, Priesto C, Nietopol E, Batella Eiras A. Toxic hepatitis from cinchophen. Report of 3 cases. Med Clin (Barc) 1991; 97: 104–106

373. Stricker B H, Blok A P, Bronkhorst F B. Glafenine-associated hepatic injury: Analysis of 38 cases and review of the literature. Liver 1986; 6: 63–72

374. Ypma R T J M, Festen J J M. Hepatotoxicity of glafenine (Letter). Lancet 1978; ii: 480–481

375. Anon. Withdrawal of glafenine. Lancet 1992; 339: 357

376. Kuzell W C, Schaffarzick R E, Naugler W E, Gaudin G, Mankle E A. Phenylbutazone: Further clinical evaluation. Arch Intern Med 1953; 92: 646–661

377. Benjamin S, Ishak K G, Zimmerman H J, Grushka A. Phenylbutazone liver injury: A clinical-pathologic survey of 23 cases and review of the literature. Hepatology 1981; 1: 255–263

378. Ishak K G, Kirchner J P, Dhar J K. Granulomas and cholestatic-hepatocellular injury associated with phenylbutazone. Report of two cases. Am J Dig Dis 1977; 22: 611–617

379. Fenech F F, Bannister W H, Grech J L. Hepatitis with biliverdinaemia in association with indomethacin therapy. Br Med J 1967; 3: 155–156

380. Kelsey W M, Scharyj M. Fatal hepatitis probably due to indomethacin. JAMA 1967; 199: 586–587

381. Opolon P, Cartron P, Chicot D, Carole J. Application due test de transformation lymphoblastique (TTL) au diagnostic de certaines hepatites medicamenteuses. Presse Med 1969; 77: 2041–2044

382. DeKraker-Sangster M, Bronkhorst F B, Brandt K H, Boersma J W. Massive hepatocellular necrosis after administration of indomethacin in combination with aminophenazone. Med Tijdschr Geneeskd 1981; 125: 1828–1831

383. Thompson M, Stephenson P, Percy J S. Ibufenac in the treatment of arthritis. Ann Rheum Dis 1964; 23: 397–404

384. Hart F D, Boardman P L. Ibufenac (4-isobutylphenyl acetic acid). Ann Rheum Dis 1965; 24: 61–65

385. Stempel D A, Miller J J. Lymphopenia and hepatic toxicity with ibuprofen. J Pediatr 1977; 90: 657–658

386. Bravo J F, Jacobson M P, Mertens B F. Fatty liver and pleural effusion with ibuprofen therapy. Ann Intern Med 1977; 87: 200–201

387. Iveson T J, Ryley N A, Kelly P M A, Trowell J M, McGee J O, Chapman R W. Diclofenac associated hepatitis. J Hepatol 1990; 10: 85–89

388. Breen E G, McNicholl J, Cosgrove E, McCabe J, Steven F M. Fatal hepatitis associated with diclofenac. Gut 1986; 27: 1390–1393

389. Helfgott S M, Sandberg-Cook J, Zakim D, Nestler J. Diclofenac-associated hepatotoxicity. Beth Israel Hospital. JAMA 1990; 264: 2660–2662

390. Ouellette G S, Slitsky B E, Gates J A, Lagarde S, West A B. Reversible hepatitis associated with diclofenac. J Clin Gastroenterol 1991; 13: 205–210

391. Purcell P, Henry D, Melville G. Diclofenac hepatitis. Gut 1991; 32: 1381–1385

392. Banks T, Zimmerman H J, Harter J, Ishak K G. Diclofenac-associated hepatic injury analysis of 181 cases. (In press)

393. Spreux A, Larousse C. Hepatites survenant au cours d'un traitement par la clomentacine. Therapie 1981; 36: 293–297

394. Metreau J M, Andre C, Zafrani E S et al. Hepatites chroniques actives associees a des anticorps anti-DNA natif: Frequence de l'etiologie medicamenteuse. Gastroenterol Clin Biol 1984; 8: 833–837

395. Chagnon J P, Barge J. Hepatite chronique active a la clometacine et antigene HLA B8. Gastroenterol Clin Biol 1983; 7: 556

396. Meyer C, Chassagnon C. Un nouveau cas mortel de cirrhose du a la clometacine. J Med Lyon 1984; 251: 339

397. Park G D, Spector R, Headstream T, Goldberg M. Serious adverse reactions associated with sulindac. Arch Intern Med 1982; 142: 1292–1294

398. Wood L J, Mundo F, Searle J, Powell L W. Sulindac hepatotoxicity: Effects of acute and chronic exposure. Aust NZ J Med 1985; 15: 397–401

399. Whittaker S J, Amar J N, Wanless I R, Heathcote J. Sulindac hepatotoxicity. Gut 1982; 23: 875–877

400. Terazi E, Harter J G, Zimmerman H J, Ishak K G, Eaton R. Sulindac-associated hepatic injury. Analysis of 91 cases reported to the FDA. Gastroenterology 1993; 104: 569–574

401. Taggert H M, Allerdice J M. Fatal cholestatic jaundice in elderly patients taking benoxaprofen. (Letter). Br Med J 1982; 284: 1372

402. Goudie B M, Birnie G F, Watkinson G, MacSween R N M, Kissen L H, Cunningham N E. Jaundice associated with the use of benoxaprofen. Lancet 1982; i: 959

403. Prescott L P, Leslie P J, Padfield P. Side effects of benoxaprofen. Br Med J 1982; 284: 1783

404. Law I P, Knight H. Jaundice associated with naproxen (Letter). N Engl J Med 1976; 295: 1201

405. Victorino R M M, Silveira J C B, Baptista A, de Moura M C. Jaundice associated with naproxen. Postgrad Med J 1980; 56: 368–370

406. Crossley R J. Side effects and safety data for fenbufen. Am J Med 1983; 75: 84–90

407. Becker A, Hoffmeister R T. Fenbufen, a new non-steroidal anti-inflammatory agent in rheumatoid arthritis, its efficiency and toxicity. J Int Med Res 1980; 8: 333–338

408. Bunde B, Deckers Y, Dequeker J. Fentiazac in rheumatoid arthritis. Comparison with sulindac and long-term tolerance. Curr Med Res Opin 1983; 8: 310–314

409. Ryder S, Salom I, Jacob G. Etodolac (ULTRADOL). The safety profile of a new structurally nonsteroidal anti-inflammatory drug. Curr Ther Res 1983; 33: 948

410. Wiggins J, Scott D L. Hepatic injury following feprazone therapy. Rheumatol Rehab 1981; 20: 44–45

411. Danan G, Trunet P, Bernuau J et al. Pirprofen-induced fulminant hepatitis. Gastroenterology 1985; 89: 210–213

412. De Herder W W, Scherder P, Purnode A et al. Pirprofen-associated hepatic injury. J Hepatol 1987; 4: 127–132

413. Geneve J, Hayat-Bonan B, Labbe G et al. Inhibition of mitochondrial b-oxidation of fatty acids by pirprofen. Role in microvesicular steatosis due to this nonsteroidal anti-inflammatory drug. J Pharmacol Exp Ther 1987; 242: 1133–1137

414. Lee S M, O'Brien C J, Williams R, Whitaker S, Gould S R. Subacute hepatic necrosis induced by piroxicam. Br Med J 1986; 293: 540–541

415. Planas R, Leon R D, Quer J C, Barranco C, Bruguera M, Gassull M A. Fatal submassive necrosis of the liver associated with piroxicam. Am J Gastroenterol 1990; 85: 468–470

416. Bismuth H, Samuel D, Gugenheim J et al. Emergency liver transplantation for fulminant hepatitis. Ann Intern Med 1987; 107: 337–341

417. Hepps K S, Maliha G M, Estrada R, Goodgame R W. Severe cholestatic jaundice associated with piroxicam. Gastroenterology 1991; 101: 1737–1740

418. Haye O. Piroxicam and pancreatitis (letter). Ann Intern Med 1986; 104: 895

419. Zimmerman H J. Effects of aspirin and acetaminophen on the liver. Arch Intern Med 1981; 141: 333–342

420. Seaman W E, Ishak K G, Plotz P H. Aspirin-induced hepatotoxicity in patients with systemic lupus erythematosus. Ann Intern Med 1974; 80: 1–8

421. Seaman W E, Ploitz P H. Effect of aspirin on liver tests in patients with rheumatoid arthritis or systemic lupus erythematosus and in normal volunteers. Arthritis Rheum 1974; 19: 155–160

422. Russell A S, Sturge R A, Smith M A. Serum transaminases during salicylate therapy. Br Med J 1971; 2: 428–429

423. Rich R R, Johnson J S. Salicylate hepatotoxicity in patients with juvenile rheumatoid arthritis. Arthr Rheum 1973; 16: 1–9

424. Bernstein B H, Singsen B H, King K K, Hanson V. Aspirin-induced hepatotoxicity and its effect on juvenile rheumatoid arthritis. Am J Dis Child 1977; 131: 659–663

425. Schaller J G. Chronic salicylate administration in juvenile rheumatoid arthritis: Aspirin hepatotoxicity and its clinical significance. Pediatrics 1978; 62: 916–925

426. Gitlin N. Salicylate hepatotoxicity: The potential role of hypoalbuminemia. J Clin Gastroenterol 1980; 2: 281–285

427. Hurwitz E S, Barrett M J, Bregman D et al. Public Health service study of Reye's syndrome and medications. Report of the main study. JAMA 1987; 257: 1905–1911

428. White J M. Reye's syndrome and salicylates. JAMA 1987; 258: 3117

429. Arrowsmith J B, Kennedy D L, Kuritsky J N, Faich G A. National patterns of aspirin use and Reye syndrome reporting US 1980–1985. Pediatrics 1987; 79: 858–863

430. Daniels S R, Greenberg R S, Ibrahim M A. Scientific uncertainties in the studies of salicylate use and Reye's syndrome. JAMA 1983; 249: 1311–1316

431. Warren J S. Diflunisal-induced cholestatic jaundice. Br Med J 1978; 2: 736–737

432. Cook D J, Achong M R, Murphy F R. Three cases of diflunisal hypersensitivity. Can Med Assoc J 1988; 138: 1029–1030

433. Ahern M J, Milazzo S E, Dymock R. Granulomatous hepatitis and seatone. Med J Austr 1980; 2: 151–152

434. Schenker S, Olson K N, Dunn D, Breen K J, Combes B. Intrahepatic cholestasis due to therapy of rheumatoid arthritis. Gastroenterology 1973; 64: 622–624

435. Favreau M, Tannenbaum H, Lough J. Hepatic toxicity associated with gold therapy. Ann Intern Med 1977; 87: 717–719

436. Pessayre D, Feldman G, Degott C et al. Gold salt-induced cholestasis. Digestion 1979; 19: 56–64

437. Watkins P B, Schade R, Mills A S, Carithers R L Jr, Van Thiel D H. Fatal hepatic necrosis associated with parenteral gold therapy. Dig Dis Sci 1988; 33: 1025–1029

438. Fleischner G M, Morecki I, Manaichi T, Hayaski H, Sternlieb I. Light and electron microscopical study of a case of gold salt induced hepatotoxicity. Hepatology 1991; 14: 422–425

439. Wildhirt E. Therapie chronische Leberkrankheiten Mit D-Penicillamin. Munch Med Wochen 1974; 116: 217–220

440. McLeod B D, Kinsella T D. Cholestasis associated with D-

penicillamine for rheumatoid arthritis. Can Med Assoc J 1979; 120: 965–966

441. Devogelaer J P, Huaux J P, Choche E, Rahier J, Nagant de Deuxchaisnes C. A case of cholestatic hepatitis associated with D-penicillamine therapy for rheumatoid arthritis. Int J Clin Pharmacol Res 1985; 5: 35–38

442. Gefel D, Harats N, Lijovetsky G, Eliakim M. Cholestatic jaundice associated with D-penicillamine therapy. Scand J Rheumatol 1985; 14: 303–306

443. Reynolds E S, Schlant R C, Gonick H C, Dammin G J. Fatal massive necrosis of the liver as a manifestation of hypersensitivity to probenecid. N Engl J Med 1957; 256: 592–596

444. Gutman A B. The past four decades of progress in the knowledge of gout, with an assessment of the present status. Arthritis Rheum 1973; 16: 431–445

445. Esperitu C R, Alaln J, Glueckauf L G, Lubin J. Allopurinol-induced granulomatous hepatitis. Am J Dig Dis 1976; 21: 804–806

446. Simmons F, Feldman B, Gerety D. Granulomatous hepatitis in a patient receiving allopurinol. Gastroenterology 1972; 62: 101–104

447. Chawla S K, Patel H D, Parrino G R, Soterakis J, Lopresti P A, D'Angelo W A. Allopurinol hepatotoxicity. Arthritis Rheum 1977; 20: 1546–1549

448. Al-Kawas F H, Seeff L B, Berendson R A, Zimmerman H J, Ishak K G. Allopurinol hepatotoxicity. Report of two cases and review of the literature. Ann Intern Med 1981; 95: 588–590

449. Boyer T D, Sun N, Reynolds T B. Allopurinol hypersensitivity and liver damage. West J Med 1977; 126: 143–147

450. Butler R C, Shah S M, Gurnow W A, Texter E C. Massive hepatic necrosis in a patient receiving allopurinol. JAMA 1977; 237: 473–474

451. Hande K R, Noone K R, Stone W J. Severe allopurinol toxicity: Description and guidelines for prevention in patients with renal insufficiency. Am J Med 1984; 76: 47–56

452. Jasper H. Jaundice in a patient receiving zoxazolamine (Flexin). Am J Gastroenterol 1960; 34: 419–421

453. Carr H J J Jr, Knauer F. Death due to hepatic necrosis in a patient receiving zoxazolamine. N Engl J Med 1961; 264: 977–980

454. Lubell D L. Fatal hepatic necrosis associated with zoxazolamine therapy. NY St J Med 1962; 62: 3807–3810

455. Utili R, Boitnott J, Zimmerman H J. Dantrolene-associated hepatic injury. Incidence and character. Gastroenterology 1977; 72: 610–616

456. Chan C H. Dantrolene sodium and hepatic injury. Neurology 1990; 40: 1427–1432

457. Powers B J, Cattau E L, Zimmerman H J. Chlorzoxazone hepatotoxic reactions. Arch Intern Med 1986; 146: 1183–1186

458. Bloch C A, Jenski L J, Balistreri W F, Dolan L M. Propylthiouracil-associated hepatitis. Arch Intern Med 1985; 145: 2129–2130

459. Fedotin M S, Lefer L G. Liver disease caused by propylthiouracil. Arch Intern Med 1975; 135: 319–321

460. Mihas A A, Holley P, Koff R S, Hirschowitz B I. Fulminant hepatitis and lymphocyte sensitization due to propylthiouracil. Gastroenterology 1976; 70: 770–774

461. Limaye A, Ruffolo P R. Propylthiouracil-induced fatal hepatic necrosis. Am J Gastroenterol 1987; 82: 152–154

462. Wheeler D C, Ayres J G H, Skinner C. Carbamazole-induced jaundice. J R Soc Med 1985; 78: 75–78

463. Vitug A C, Goldman J M. Hepatotoxicity from antithyroid drugs. Hormone Res 1985; 21: 229–234

464. Schmidt G, Boersch G, Mueller K M, Wegener M. Methimazole associated cholestatic liver injury: Case report and brief literature review. Hepatogastroenterology 1986; 33: 244–246

465. Wildert E. Toxische choelstatische hepatore durch thimazol un Carbamaol. Dtsch Med Wochenschr 1982; 107: 1531–1533

466. Balodimos M C, Graham C A, Marble A, Krall L P. Acetohexamide in the therapy of diabetes mellitus. Metabolism 1968; 17: 669–680

467. Council on Drugs. An oral hypoglycemic agent: Acetohexamide (Dymelor). JAMA 1965; 191: 127–128

468. Goldstein M J, Rothenberg A J. Jaundice in a patient receiving acetohexamide. N Engl J Med 1966; 275: 97–99

469. Gregory D H, Zaki G F, Sarosi G A, Carey J B. Chronic cholestasis following prolonged tolbutamide administration. Arch Pathol 1967; 84: 194–201

470. Bloodworth J M B Jr. Morphologic changes associated with sulfonylurea therapy. Metabolism 1963; 12: 287–301

471. Smetana H F. The histopathology of drug-induced liver disease. Ann NY Acad Sci 1963; 104: 821–846

472. Creutzfeld W, Soling H O. Oral treatment of diabetes (a clinical and experimental review), translated by C Gless. Berlin: Springer-Verlag, 1961

473. Urban E, Frank B W, Kern F Jr. Liver dysfunction with mestranol but not with norethynodrel in a patient with enovid-induced jaundice. Ann Intern Med 1968; 68: 598–602

474. Holzbach R T, Sanders J H. Recurrent intrahepatic cholestasis of pregnancy: Observations on pathogenesis. JAMA 1965; 193: 542–544

475. Orellana-Alcalde J M, Dominguez J P. Jaundice and oral contraceptive drugs. Lancet 1966; ii: 1278–1280

476. Metreau J M, Dhumeaux D, Bethelot P. Oral contraceptives and the liver. Digestion 1972; 7: 318–335

477. Eisalo A, Jarvinen P A, Luukkainen T. Hepatic impairment during the intake of contraceptive pills. Clinical trial with post-menopausal women. Br Med J 1964; 2: 426–427

478. Wheeler H O. Secretion of bile. In: Schiff L, ed. Diseases of the liver, 4th edn. Philadelphia: J B Lippincott, 1975: pp 87–110

479. Glober G A, Wilkerson J A. Biliary cirrhosis following the administration of methyltestosterone. JAMA 1968; 204: 170–173

480. Anthony P P. Hepatoma associated with androgenic steroids. Lancet 1975; i: 685–686

481. Stubblefield P G. Oral contraceptives and neoplasia. J Reprod Med 1984; 29: 524–529

482. Stromeyer F W, Ishak K G. Nodular transformation (nodular 'regenerative' hyperplasia) of the liver: A clinicopathologic study of 30 cases. Human Pathol 1981; 12: 60–71

483. Ham J M, Pirola R C, Crouch R I. Hemangioendothelial sarcoma of the liver associated with long-term estrogen therapy in man. Dig Dis Sci 1980; 25: 879–883

484. Stromeyer F W, Smith D H, Ishak K G. Anabolic steroid therapy and intrahepatic cholangiocarcinoma. Cancer 1979; 43: 440–443

485. Turani H, Levy J, Zevin D, Kessler E. Hepatic lesions in patients on anabolic androgenic therapy. Isr J Med Sci 1983; 19: 332–337

486. Agrawal B L, Zelkowitz L. Bone "flare", hypercalcemia and jaundice after tamoxifen therapy. Arch Intern Med 1981; 141: 1240

487. Blackburn A M, Amiel S A, Millis R R, Rubens R D. Tamoxifen and liver damage. Br Med J 1984; 289: 288

488. Nand S, Gordon L I, Brestan E, Harris C, Brandt T. Benign hepatic cyst in patient on antiestrogen therapy for metastatic breast cancer. Cancer 1982; 50: 1882–1883

489. Noguchi M, Taniya T, Tajiri K et al. Fatal hyperlipaemia in a case of metastatic breast cancer treated by tamoxifen. Br J Surg 1987; 74: 586–587

490. Melamed I, Bujanover Y, Hammer J, Spirer Z. Hepatoblastoma in an infant born to a mother after hormonal treatment for sterility. N Engl J Med 1982; 307: 820

491. Carrasco D, Barrachina M, Prieto M, Berenguer J. Clomiphene citrate and liver-cell adenoma. N Engl J Med 1984; 310: 1120–1121

492. Hogh B, Stenhammar L. Cyclotenin in childhood scleroderma. Acta Dermatol Venereol 1983; 63: 445–446

493. Olsson R, Tyllstrom J, Zettergren L. Hepatic reactions to cyclifenil. Gut 1983; 24: 260–263

494. Bouvet B, Rocas P, Paliard P, Brette R, Trepo C. Hepatite ague du au cyclofenil (Ondoyne). A propos de deux cas. Gastroenterol Clin Biol 1985; 9: 941–943

495. Boue F, Coffin B, Delfrasissy J F. Danazol and cholestatic hepatitis. Ann Intern Med 1986; 105: 139–140

496. Ohsawa T, Iwashito S. Hepatitis associated with danazol (letter). Drug Intell Clin Pharm 1986; 20: 889

497. Kahn H, Manzarbeitia C, Theise N, Schwartz M, Miller C, Swan N T. Danazol-induced hepatocellular adenomas. A case report and review of the literature. Arch Pathol Lab Med 1991; 115: 1054–1057

498. Buamah P K. An apparent danazol-induced primary hepatocellular carcinoma. J Surg Oncol 1985; 28: 114–116

499. Fermand J P, Levy Y, Bouscary D, D'Agay M F, Clot P, Frija J, Brouet J C. Danazol-induced hepatocellular adenoma. Am J Med 1990; 88: 529–530

500. Arosio M, Bazzoni N, Ambrosi B, Faglia G. Acute hepatitis after treatment of acromegaly with octreotide (letter). Lancet 1988; 2: 1498

501. Davis J. Liver damage due to tetracycline and its relationship to pregnancy. In: Meyler L, Peck H M, eds. Drug-induced diseases. Amsterdam: Excerpta Medica, 1968: pp 103–110

502. Lepper M H, Wolfe C K, Zimmerman H J, Caldwell E R, Spies H W, Dowling H F. Effect of large doses of aureomycin on human liver. Arch Intern Med 1951; 88: 27–283

503. Lepper M H, Zimmerman H J, Caldwell E R Jr, Carroll G, Spies H W, Wolfe C K, Dowling H F. Effect of large doses of aureomycin, terramycin, and chloramphenicol on livers of mice and dogs. Arch Intern Med 1951; 88: 284–295

504. Burette A, Finet C, Prigogine T, DeRoy G, Deltenre M. Acute hepatic injury associated with minocycline. Ann Intern Med 1984; 44: 1491–1492

505. Breen K, Schenker S, Heimberg M. The effect of tetracycline on the hepatic secretion of triglyceride. Biochem Acta 1972; 270: 74–80

506. Kunelis C T, Peters J L, Edmondson H A. Fatty liver of pregnancy and its relationship to tetracycline therapy. Am J Med 1965; 38: 359–377

507. Robinson M M. Demonstration by "challenge" of hepatic dysfunction associated with proprionyl erythromycin ester lauryl sulfate. Antibiot Chemother 1962; 12: 147–151

508. Ticktin H E, Robinson M D. Effects of some antimicrobial agents on the liver. Ann NY Acad Sci 1963; 104: 1080–1092

509. Braun P. Hepatotoxicity of erythromycin. J Infect Dis 1969: 300–306

510. Havens W P Jr. Cholestatic jaundice in patients treated with erythromycin estolate. JAMA 1962; 180: 30–32

511. Viteri A L, Green J F Jr, Dyck W P. Erythromycin ethylsuccinate-induced cholestasis. Gastroenterology 1979; 76: 1007–1008

512. Diehl A M, Latham P, Boitnott J K, Mann J, Maddrey W C. Cholestatic hepatitis from erythromycin ethlysuccinate. Am J Med 1984; 76: 931–934

513. Sullivan D, Csuka M E, Blanchard B. Erythromycin ethylsuccinate hepatotoxicity. JAMA 1980; 243: 1074

514. Zafrani E S, Ishak K G, Rudzki C. Cholestatic and hepatocellular injury associated with erythromycin esters: Report of nine cases. Am J Dig Dis 1979; 24: 385–396

515. Pesayre D, Marie C, Benhamou J-P. Hepatite due au propionate d'erythromycine. Arch Fr Mal App Dis 1976; 65: 405–408

516. Ortuno J A, Olasso V, Berenquez J. Hepatitis colestasica par propionato de eritromicin. Med Clin (Barc) 1984; 82: 912

517. Paliard P, Stremsdoerfer N, Meindrot H. Hepatite aigue aux esters d'erythromycine (propionate et ethylsuccinate). Gastronterol Clin Biol 1983; 17: 100–101

518. Hosker J P, Jewell D P. Transient, selective factor X deficiency and acute liver failure following chest infection treated with erythromycin. Br Postgrad Med J 1983; 59: 514–515

519. Inman W H, Rawson N S. Erythromycin estolate and jaundice. Br Med J 1983; 286: 1954–1955

520. Ghoulson C F, Warren G H. Fulminant hepatic failure associated with intravenous erythromycin lactobionate. Arch Intern Med 1990; 150: 215–216

521. Zimmerman H J, Kendler J, Libber S, Lukacs L. Hepatocyte suspensions as a model for demonstration of drug hepatotoxicity. Biochem Pharmacol 1974; 23: 2187–2189

522. Kendler J, Anuras S, Laborda O, Zimmerman H J. Perfusion of the isolated rat liver with erythromycin estolate and other derivatives. Proc Soc Exp Bio Med 1972; 139: 1272–1275

523. Ticktin H E, Zimmerman H J. Hepatic dysfunction and jaundice in patients receiving triacetyloleandomycin. N Engl J Med 1962; 267: 964–968

524. Haber I, Hubens H. Cholestatic jaundice after triacetyloeandomycin and oral contraceptives. The diagnostic value of gamma glutamyl transpeptidase. Acta Gastroenterol Belg 1980; 43: 475–482

525. Miguet J P, Vintton D, Pessayre D. Jaundice from troleandomycin and oral contraceptives (letter). Ann Intern Med 1980; 92: 434

526. Hargreaves T, Lathe G H. Inhibitory aspects of bile secretion. Nature 1963; 200: 1172–1176

527. Bridges R A, Berendes H, Good R A. Serious reactions to novobiocin. J Pediatrics 1957; 50: 579–585

528. Perisco L. L'ittero da novobiocina. Policlinico (Prat) 1966; 73: 1607–1614

529. Davies G E, Holmes H E. Drug-induced immunological effects on the liver. Br J Anaesth 1973; 44: 941–945

530. Zimmerman H J, Lewis J H. Hepatic toxicity of antimicrobial agents. In: Root R K, Sande M A, eds. New dimensions of antimicrobial therapy. New York: Livingstone, 1984: pp 153–202

531. Felder S L, Felder L. Unusual reaction to penicillin. JAMA 1950; 143: 361–362

532. Girard J P, Haenni B, Bergoz R, Kapanaci Y, Cruchand A. Lupoid hepatitis following administration of penicillin: Case report and immunological studies. Helv Med Acta 1967; 34: 23–25

533. Goldstein L I, Ishak K G. Hepatic injury associated with penicillin therapy. Arch Pathol 1974; 98: 114–117

534. Murphy E S, Mireles M. Shock, liver necrosis and death after penicillin injection. Arch Pathol 1962; 73: 355–362

535. Rabinovitch J, Snitkof M C. Acute exfoliative dermatitis and death following penicillin-therapy. JAMA 1948; 138: 496–498

536. Valdiva-Barriga V, Feldman A, Orellana J. Generalized Hypersensitivity with hepatitis and jaundice following the use of penicillin and streptomycin. Gastroenterology 1963; 45: 114–117

537. Waugh D. Myocarditis, arteritis and focal hepatic, splenic and renal granulomas apparently due to penicillin sensitivity. Am J Pathol 1952; 28: 437–447

538. Ross S, Lovrien E W, Zaremba E A, Bourgeois L, Puig J R. Alpha-aminobenzyl penicillin — new broad spectrum antibiotic: Preliminary clinical and laboratory observations. JAMA 1962; 182: 238–242

539. Freedman M A. Oxacillin-apparent hematologic and hepatic toxicity. Rocky Mt Med J 1965; 62: 34–36

540. Ten-Pas A, Quinn E L. Cholestatic hepatitis following the administration of sodium oxacillin. JAMA 1965; 191: 674–675

541. Walker S H, Standiford W E. The treatment of infants with oxacillin sodium. Am J Dis Child 1967; 114: 64

542. Silverblatt F, Turck M. Laboratory and clinical evaluation of carbenicillin (carboxybenzyl penicillin). In: Hobby G L, ed. Antimicrobial agents and chemotherapy. 1968. Baltimore: Williams & Wilkins, 1969: pp 279–285

543. Boxerbaum B, Doershuk C P, Pittman S, Mathews L W. Efficacy and tolerance of carbenicillin in patients with cystic fibrosis. In: Hobby G L, ed. Antimicrobial agents and chemotherapy. 1968. Baltimore: Williams & Wilkins, 1969: pp 292–295

544. Neu H C, Swarz H. Carbenicillin: Clinical and laboratory experience with a parenterally administered penicillin for treatment of pseudomonas infections. Ann Intern Med 1969; 71: 903–911

545. Fowle A S E, Zorab P A. Esch. coli endocarditis successfully treated with oral trimethoprim and sulfamethoxazole. Br Heart J 1970; 32: 127–129

546. Bodey G P, Whitecar J P Jr, Middleman E, Rodriguez V. Carbenicillin therapy for pseudomonas infections. JAMA 1971; 218: 62–66

547. Knirsch A K, Gralla E J. Abnormal serum transaminase levels after parenteral ampicillin and carbenicillin administration. N Engl J Med 1970; 282: 1081–1084

548. Kosmidis J, Williams J D, Andrews J, Goodall J A D, Geddes A M. Amoxicillin — pharmacology, bacteriology and clinical studies. Br J Clin Pract 1972; 26: 341–346

549. Dismukes W E. Oxacillin-induced hepatic dysfunction. JAMA 1973; 226: 861–863

550. McArthur J E, Dyment P G. Stevens-Johnson syndrome with hepatitis following therapy with ampicillin and cephalexin. NZ Med J 1975; 81: 390–392

551. Wilson F M, Belamaric J, Lauter C B, Lerner A M. Anicteric

carbenicillin hepatitis: Eight episodes in four patients. JAMA 1975; 232: 818–821

552. Cavanzo F J, Garcia C F, Botera R C. Chronic cholestasis paucity of bile ducts, red cell aplasia and the Stevens-Johnson syndrome. Gastroenterology 1990; 99: 854–856

553. Enat R, Pollack S. Ben-Arieh Y, Livini E, Barzilai D. Cholestatic jaundice caused by cloxacillin macrophage inhibition factor test in prevention rechallenge with hepatotoxins drugs. Br Med J 1980; 1: 982–983

554. Kleinman M S, Presberg J E. Cholestatic hepatitis after dicloxacillin-sodium therapy. J Clin Gastroenterol 1986; 8: 77–78

555. Victorino R M, Maria V A, Correoa A P, de Moura C. Floxacillin-induced cholestatic hepatitis with evidence of lymphocyte sensitization. Arch Intern Med 1987; 147: 987–989

556. Tauris P, Jorgensen N F, Petersen C M, Albertson K. Prolonged severe cholestasis induced by oxacillin derivatives. A report of two cases. Acta Med Scand 1985; 217: 567–569

557. Deboever G. Cholestatic jaundice due to derivation of oxacillin (letter). Am J Gastroenterol 1987; 82: 483

558. Bengtsson F, Floren C H, Hagerstrand I. Flucloxacillin-induced cholestatic liver damage. Scand J Infect Dis 1985; 17: 125–128

559. Stricker B H C, Spoelstra P. Drug-induced liver injury. Amersterdam: Elsevier, 1985: pp 45–76

560. Reddy K R, Brillant P, Schiff E R. Amoxicillin-clavulanate potassium-associated cholestasis. Gastroenterology 1989; 96: 1135–1141

561. Dowsett J F, Gillow T, Haggerty A. Amoxycillin/clavulanic acid (Augmentin) induced intrahepatic cholestasis. Dig Dis Sciences 1989; 34: 1290–1293

562. Hanger F M Jr, Gutman A B. Postarsphenamine jaundice apparently due to obstruction of intrahepatic biliary tract. JAMA 1940; 115: 263–271

563. Stolzer B L, Miller C, White W A Jr, Zukerfrod M. Post-arsenical obstructive jaundice complicated by xanthomathosis and diabetes mellitus. Am J Med 1950; 9: 124–132

564. Dujvone C A, Chan C H, Zimmerman H J. Sulfonamide hepatic injury. Review of the literature and report of a case due to sulfamethoxazone. N Engl J Med 1967; 277: 785–788

565. Alberti-Flor J J, Hernandez M E, Ferrer J P, Howell S, Jeffers L. Fulminant liver failure and pancreatitis associated with the use of sulfamethoxazole-trimethoprim. Am J Gastroenterology 1989; 84: 1577–1579

566. Tanner A R. Hepatic cholestasis induced by trimethoprim. Br Med J 1986; 293: 1072–1073

567. Fich A, Schwartz J, Braverman D, Zifroni A, Rochmilewitz D. Sulfasalazine hepatotoxicity. Am J Gastroenterol 1984; 79: 401–402

568. Johnson D A, Cattau E L, Kuritsky J N, Zimmerman H J. Liver involvement in the sulfone syndrome. Arch Intern Med 1986; 146: 875–877

569. Goldstein L I, Ishak K G, Burns W. Hepatic injury associated with nitrofurantoin therapy. Am J Dig Dis 1974; 19: 987–998

570. Selroos O, Edgar J. Lupus-like syndrome associated with pulmonary reaction to nitrofurantoin. Report of three cases. Acta Med Scand 1975; 197: 125–129

571. Sippel P J, Agger W A. Nitrofurantoin-induced granulomatous hepatitis. Urology 1981; 18: 177–178

572. Gulliford M, Mackay A D, Prowse K. Cholestatic jaundice caused by ethambutol. Br Med J 1986; 292: 866–867

573. Garibaldi R A, Drusin R E, Ferebee S H, Gregg M B. Isoniazid-associated hepatitis: report of an outbreak. Am Rev Respir Dis 1972; 106: 357–365

574. Scharer L, Smith J P. Serum transaminase elevations and other hepatic abnormalities in patients receiving isoniazid. Ann Intern Med 1969; 71: 1113–1120

575. Mitchell J R, Thorgeissson U P, Black M et al. Increased incidence of isoniazid hepatitis in rapid acetylators. 1 Possible relation to hydrazine metabolites. Clin Pharmacol Ther 1975; 18: 70–79

576. Kochman S, Bureau G, Dubois De Montreynaud J M D. A propos de 5 cas d'icteres a la rifampicine (I). Presse Med 1971; 79: 524

577. Pessayre D. Present views on isoniazid and isoniazid-rifampin hepatitis. Aggressologie 1982; 23: 13–15

578. Hugues F C, Marche C, Marche J. Effects hepatobiliares de l'association rifamipicine-isoniazide. Therapie 1969; 24: 899

579. Scheuer P J, Summerfield J A, Lal S, Sherlock S. Rifampicin hepatitis. A clinical and histological study. Lancet 1974; i: 421–425

580. Lesobre R, Ruffino J, Treyssier L, Achard F, Brefort G. Les icteres au cours du traitement par la rifamipicine. Rev Tubercul Pneumolog 1969; 33: 393–403

581. Cohn H D. Clinical studies with new rifampicin derivative. J Clin Pharmacol J N Drgs 1969; 9: 118–125

582. Matillia A, Molland E A. A light and electron microscope study of the liver in case of erythro-hepatic protoporphyria and griseofulvin-induced porphyria in mice. J Clin Pathol 1974; 27: 698–709

583. Barich L L, Schwarz J, Barich D J, Horowitz M G. Toxic liver damage in mice after prolonged intake of elevated doses of griseofulvin. Antibiot Chemother 1961; 11: 566–571

584. Hurst E W, Paget G E. Protoporphyria, cirrhosis and hepatomata in livers of mice given griseofulvin. Br J Dermatol 1963; 75: 105–112

585. Berman A, Franklin R L. Precipitation of acute intermittent porphyria by griseofulvin therapy. JAMA 1968; 188: 466

586. Redeker A G, Sterling R E, Bronow R S. Effect of griseofulvin in acute intermittent porphyria. JAMA 1964; 188: 466–468

587. Chiprut R O, Viteri A, Jamroz C, Dyck W P. Intrahepatic cholestasis after griseofulvin administration. Gastroenterology 1967; 70: 1141–1143

588. Breinstrup H, Sogaard-Anderson J. Cholestasis: Intrahepatic after griseofulvin behandling. Ugeskrift for Laeger 1966; 128: 145–146

589. Simon N, Berko G, Polay A, Kocsis G. Der Einflus der Griseofulvin-Therapie auf die Leberfunktion und den Porphyrin-Stoffwechsel. Arch Dermatol Forsch 1971; 241: 148–155

590. Lewis J H, Zimmerman H J, Benson G D, Ishak K G. Hepatic injury associated with ketoconazole therapy. Gastroenterology 1984; 86: 503–513

591. Stricker B H, Block A P, Bronkhorst F B, Van Parys G E, Desmet V J. Ketoconazole-associated hepatic injury. A clinicopathological study of 55 cases. J Hepatol 1986; 3: 399–406

592. Lake-Bakaar G, Scheuer P J, Sherlock S. Hepatic reactions associated with ketoconazole in the United Kingdom. Br Med J 1987; 294: 419–422

593. Ikemoto H. Clinical study of fluconazole for treatment of deep mycoses. Diag Microbiol Infect Dis (suppl 4) 1989; 12: 239S–247S

594. Medical Letter on Drugs and Therapeutics. Annotation. Flucytosine (Ancobon): A new antifungal drug. Med Lett Drugs Ther 1972; 14: 29

595. Record C O, Skinner J M, Sleight P, Speller D C B. Candida endocarditis treated with 5-fluorocytosine. Br Med J 1971; 1: 262–264

596. Carnecchia B M, Kurtzke J F. Fatal toxic reaction to amphotericin B in cryptococcal meningo-encephalitis. Ann Intern Med 1960; 53: 1027–1036

597. Miller M A. Reversible hepatotoxicity related to amphotericin B. Can Med Ass J 1984; 131: 1245–1247

598. Dayan A D. Lewis P D. Idoxuridine and jaundice. Lancet 1969; ii: 1073

599. Silk B R, Roome A P C H. Herpes simplex encephalitis treated with intravenous idoxuridine. Lancet 1970; i: 411–412

600. Breeden C J, Hall T C, Tyler H R. Herpes simplex encephalitis treated with systemic 5-iodo-2'-deoxyuridine. Ann Intern Med 1966; 65: 1050–1056

601. Hecht Y, Levy V G, Agnolucci M T, Caroli J. Hepatites cholostatiques dues a la xenalamine. Arch Fr Mal App Dig 1965; 54: 615–636

602. Herbeuval R, Rauber G, Dornier R. Hepatite cholostatique a la xenalamine. Therapie 1966; 21: 781–786

603. Traggis D G, Dohliwitz A, Das L, Jaffe N, Maloney W C, Hall T C. Cytosine arabinoside in acute leukemia of childhood. Cancer 1971; 28: 815–818

604. Hryniuk W, Foerster J, Shojania M, Chow A. Cytarabine for herpes virus infections. JAMA 1972; 219: 715–718

605. Dubin G, Braffman M N. Zidovudine-induced hepatotoxicity. Ann Intern Med 1989; 110: 85–86

606. Gradon J D, Chapnick E K, Sepkowitz D V. Zidovudine hepatitis. J Intern Med 1992; 23: 317–318

607. Melamed A J, Muller R J, Gold J W, Campbell S W, Kleinberg M L, Armstrong P. Possible zidovudine-induced hepatotoxicity. JAMA 1987; 258: 2063

608. Lambert J S, Seidlin M, Reichman R C et al. 2'3'-Dideoxyinosine (ddI) in patients with the acquired immunodeficiency syndrome or AIDS-related complex. N Engl J Med 1990; 322: 1333–1340

609. Lai K K, Gang D L, Zawacki J K, Cooley T P. Fulminant hepatic failure associated with 2,3'dideoxyuridine (ddI). Ann Intern Med 1991; 115: 283–284

610. Larry D, Castot A, Pessayre D. Amodiaquine-induced hepatitis. A report of seven cases. Ann Intern Med 1986; 104: 801–803

611. Wharton J M, Coleman D L, Wofsy C B et al. Trimethoprim-sulfamethoxazole or pentamidine for Pneumocystis carinii pneumonia in the acquired immunodeficiency syndrome. Ann Intern Med 1986; 105: 37–44

612. Farid Z, Smith J H, Bassily S, Sparks H A. Hepatotoxicity after treatment of schistosomiasis with hycanthone. Br Med J 1972; 2: 88–89

613. Jalota R, Freston J A. Severe intrahepatic cholestasis due to thiobendazole. Am J Trop Med Hyg 1974; 23: 676–678

614. Rex D, Lumeng L, Eble J, Rex L. Intrahepatic cholestasis and sicca complex after thiabendazole. Gastroenterology 1983; 85: 718–721

615. Reshev R, Lok A, Sherlock S. Cholestatic jaundice in fascioliasis treated with niclofolan. Br Med J 1982; 285: 1243–1244

616. Hamlyn A N, Morris J S, Sarkany I, Sherlock S. Piperazine hepatitis. Gastroenterology 1976; 70: 1144–1147

617. Jagota S C. Jaundice due to albendazole. Indian J Gastroenterol 1989; 8: 58

618. Jung U, Mahr W. Mebendazole hepatitis. Z Gastroenterol 1983; 21: 736–741

619. Perkins J. Phenindione jaundice. Lancet 1962; i: 125–127

620. Adler E, Benjamin S B, Zimmerman H J. Cholestatic hepatic injury related to warfarin exposure. Arch Intern Med 1986; 146: 1837–1839

621. Geltner D, Chajeck T, Rubinger D, Levij I S. Quinidine hypersensitivity and liver involvement. A survey of 32 patients. Gastroenterology 1976; 70: 650–652

622. Koch M J, Seeff L B, Crumley C E, Rabin L, Burns W A. Quinidine hepatotoxicity: A report of a case and review of the literature. Gastroenterology 1976; 70: 1136–1140

623. Chajek T. Letter. Quinidine and granulomatous hepatitis. Ann Intern Med 1975; 82: 282

624. King J A, Blount R E Jr. An unexpected reaction to procainamide. JAMA 1963; 186; 603–604

625. Farber H I. Fever, vomiting and liver dysfunction with procainamide therapy. Postgrad Med 1974; 56: 155–156

626. Rotmensch H H, Yust I, Siegman-Igra Y, Liron M, Ilie B, Vardinon N. Granulomatous hepatitis: A hypersensitivity response to procainamide. Ann Intern Med 1978; 89: 646–647

627. Berg P A, Brattig N. Role of immune mechanism in drug-induced diseases. In: Davis M, Tredger J M, Williams R, eds. Drug reactions and the liver. London: Pitman Medical, 1981: pp 105–107

628. Worman H J, Ip J H, Winters S L, Tepper D C, Igomes A J. Hypersensitivity reaction associated with acute hepatic dysfunction following a single intravenous dose of procainamide. J Intern Med 1992; 232: 361–363

629. Brandes J W, Schmitz-Moormann P, Lehmann F G, Martini G A. Gelbusucht nach Aprindin. Eine hepatitisahnliche Arneimittelschadfingung. Dtsch Med Wochenschr 1976; 101: 111–113

630. Herlong H F, Reid P R, Boitnott J K, Maddrey W C. Aprindine hepatitis. Ann Intern Med 1978; 89: 359–361

631. Meinertz T, Langer K H, Kasper W, Just H. Disopyramide-induced intrahepatic cholestasis. Lancet 1977; ii: 828–829

632. Dolle W. Intrahepatische chollestasee durch Ajmaline. Med Klin 1962; 57: 1648–1650

633. Buscher H P, Talke H P, Rademacher J P, Gessner U, Oelhert W, Gerok W. Intrahepatische Cholestase durch N-Propyl-Ajmalin. Deutsche Medizinische Wochenschrift 1976; 101: 699–703

634. Beerman B, Ericsson J L E, Hellstrom K, Wengle B, Werner B. Transient cholestasis during treatment with ajmaline and chronic xanthomatous cholestasis after administration of ajmaline, methyltestosterone and ethinylestradiol. Acta Med Scand 1971; 1900: 241–250

635. Larrey D, Pessayre D, Duhamel G et al. Prolonged cholestasis after ajmaline-induced acute hepatitis. J Hepatol 1986; 2: 81–87

636. Bartoli E, Massarolli G, Solinas A, Faedda R, Chiandusi L. Acute hepatitis with bridging necrosis due to hydralazine intake. Arch Intern Med 1979; 130: 698–699

637. Itoh S, Ichinoe A, Tsukada Y, Itoh Y. Hydralazine-induced hepatitis. Hepatogastroenterology 1981; 28: 13–16

638. Myers J L, Augur N A. Hydralazine-induced cholangitis. Gastroenterology 1984; 87: 1185–1188

639. Rodman J S, Deutsch D J, Gutman S I. Methyldopa hepatitis. A report of six cases and review of the literature. Am J Med 1976; 60: 941–948

640. Toghill P J, Smith P G, Benton P, Brown R C, Matthews H L. Methyldopa liver damage. Br Med J 1974; 3: 545–548

641. Williams E R, Khan M A. Liver damage in patients on methyldopa. J Ther Clin Res 1967; 1: 5–9

642. Shaw D R, Misan G H, Johnson R D. Nifedipine hepatitis. Aust NZ J Med 1987; 17: 447–448

643. Hare D L, Horowitz J D. Verapamil hepatotoxicity: A hypersensitivity reaction. Am Heart J 1986; 111: 610–611

644. Sarachek N S. Diltiazem and granulomatosis hepatitis. Gastroenterology 1985; 5: 1260–1262

645. Beaugrand M, Denis J, Callard P. Tous les inhibiteurs caliques preventils entrainer des lesions d'hepatite alcoolique (HA)? Gastroenterol Clin Biol 1987; 11: 76

646. Rahmat J, Gelfand R L, Gelfand M, Winchester J F, Schreiner G E, Zimmerman H J. Captopril-associated cholestatic jaundice. Ann Intern Med 1985; 102: 56–63

647. Rosellini S R, Costa P L, Gaudio M, Saragoni A, Miglio F. Hepatic injury related to enalapril. Gastroenterology 1989; 97: 810

648. Larrey O, Babany G, Benan J et al. Fulminant hepatitis after lisinopril. Gastroenterology 1990; 99: 1832–1833

649. Clark J A, Zimmerman H J, Tanner L A. Labetalol hepatotoxicity. Ann Intern Med 1990; 113: 210–213

650. Tanner L A, Bosco L A, Zimmerman H J. Hepatotoxicity after acebutolol therapy. Ann Intern Med 1989; 111: 33–34

651. Schwartz M S. Atenolol-associated cholestasis. Am J Gastroenterol 1989; 184: 1084–1088

652. Valdes M, Jacobs W H. Intrahepatic cholestasis following the use of atromid-s. Am J Gastroenterol 1976; 66: 69

653. Pierce E H, Chesler D L. Possible association of granulomatous hepatitis with clofibrate therapy. N Engl J Med 1978; 299: 314

654. Massen H, Furet Y. Hepatitie au fenofibrate. Cahiers d'Anesthesiol 1986; 34: 249–250

655. Christensen N A, Anchor R W P, Berge K G, Mason H L. Nicotinic acid treatment of hypercholesterolemia. JAMA 1961; 177: 546–550

656. Clementz G L, Holmes A W. Nicotinic acid-induced fulminant hepatic failure. J Clin Gastroenterol 1987; 9: 582–584

657. Mullin G E, Greenson J K, Mitchell M C. Fulminant hepatic failure after ingestion of sustained release nicotinic acid. Ann Intern Med 1989; 111: 253–255

658. Winter S L, Boyer J L. Hepatic toxicity from large doses of vitamin B (Nicotinamide). N Engl J Med 1973; 289: 1180–1182

659. Einstein N, Baker A, Galper J, Wolfe H. Jaundice due to nicotinic acid therapy. Am J Dig Dis 1975; 20: 282–286

660. Raveh D, Arnon R, Israeli A, Eisenberg S. Lovastatin-induced hepatitis. Isr J Med Sci 1992; 28: 101–102

661. Feydy P, Bogomoltz W V. A case of hepatitis caused by simvastatin (letter). Gastroenterol Clin Biol 1991; 15: 94–95

662. Ballare M, Campanin M, Catania E, Bordin G, Zaccala G,

Monteverde A. Acute cholestatic hepatitis during simvastatin administration. Recent Prog Med 1991; 82: 233–235

663. Dargie H J, Dollery C T. Adverse reactions to diuretic drugs. In: Meyler's Side effects of drugs, vol 8. Amsterdam: Excerpta Medica, 1975: pp 483–501

664. Walker R M, McElligott T F. Furosemide induced hepatotoxicity. J Pathol 1981; 135: 301–314

665. Zimmerman H J, Lewis J H, Ishak K G, Maddrey W C. Ticrynafen-associated hepatic injury: Analysis of 340 cases. Hepatology 1984; 4: 315–323

666. Weitz H, Gokel J M, Loeschke K et al. Veno-occlusive disease of the liver in patients receiving immunosuppressive therapy. Virchows Arch 1982; 395: 245–256

667. Asbury R F, Rosenthal S N, Descalzi M E, Ratcliffe R L, Arsenead J C. Hepatic veno-occlusive disease due to DTIC. Cancer 1980; 45: 2670–2674

668. Rollins B J. Hepatic veno-occlusive disease. Am J Med 1986; 81: 297–306

669. Greenstone M A, David P M, Mikhailidis D P, Scheuer P J. Hepatic vascular lesions associated with dacarbazine treatment. Br Med J 1981; 282: 1744–1745

670. Schein P S, Winokur S H. Immunosuppressive and cytotoxic chemotherapy: Long-term complications. Ann Intern Med 1975; 82: 84–95

671. Almeyda J, Barnardo D, Baker H. Drug reactions XV. Methotrexate, psoriasis and the liver. Br J Dermatol 1971; 85: 302–305

672. Dahl M G C, Gregory M M, Scheuer P J. Liver damage due to methotrexate in patients with psoriasis. Br Med J 1971; 1: 625–630

673. Dahl M G C, Gregory M M, Scheuer P J. Methotrexate hepatotoxicity in psoriasis — comparison of different dose regimens. Br Med J 1972; 1: 654–656

674. Millward-Sadler G H, Ryan T J. Methotrexate induced liver disease in psoriasis. Br J Dermatol 1974; 90: 661–667

675. Nyfors A, Pouslen H. Liver biopsies from psoriasis related to methotrexate. Acta Pathol Microbiol Scand 1976; 84: 253–261

676. Podurgiel B J, McGill D B, Ludwig J, Taylor W F, Muller S A. Liver injury associated with methotrexate therapy for psoriasis. Mayo Clinic Proc 1973; 48: 787–792

677. Roenigk H R Jr, Bergfeld W F, St Jacques R, Owens F J, Hawk W A. Hepatotoxicity of methotrexate in the treatment of psoriasis. Arch Dermatol 1971; 103: 250–261

678. Roenigk H R Jr. Methotrexate and liver biopsies. Is it really necessary? Arch Intern Med 1990; 150: 773–774

679. Weinstein C, Roenigk H R, Maibach H, Cosmides J, Halprin K, Millard M. Psoriasis – liver methotrexate interactions. Arch Dermatol 1970; 108: 36–42

680. Lewis J H, Schiff E R. Methotrexate-induced chronic liver injuries. Guidelines for detection and prevention. The AGC Committee on FDA-related matters. Am J Gastroenterol 1988; 83: 1337–1345

681. Kaplan M M. Methotrexate treatment of chronic cholestatic liver disease: Friend or foe. Q J Med 1989; 72: 757–761

682. Kremer J M, Lee R G, Tolman K G. Liver histology in patients with rheumatoid arthritis undergoing long term treatment with methotrexate. Arthritis Rheum 1989; 132: 121–127

683. Brick J E, Moreland L W, Al-Kawas F, Chang W W, Layne R D, DiBartolomeo A G. Prospective analysis of liver biopsies before and after methotrexate therapy in rheumatoid patients. Semin Arthritis Rheum 1989; 19: 31–44

684. Rau R, Karger T, Herborn G, Frenzel H. Liver biopsy findings on patients with rheumatoid arthritis undergoing long term treatment with methotrexate. J Rheumatol 1989; 14: 489–493

685. Kevat S, Ahern M, Hall P. Hepatotoxicity of methotrexate in rheumatic diseases. Med Toxicol 1988; 3: 197–208

686. Shergy W J, Polisson R P, Caldwell D S, Rice J R. Methotrexate-associated hepatotoxicity: Retrospective analysis of 210 patients with rheumatoid arthritis. Am J Med 1988; 85: 771–774

687. Kujala G A, Shamma's J M, Chang W L, Brick J E. Hepatitis with bridging fibrosis and reversible hepatic insufficiency in a woman with rheumatoid arthritis taking methotrexate. Arthritis Rheum 1990; 33: 1037–1041

688. Hopwood D, Nyfors A. Liver ultrastructure in psoriatics related to methotrexate therapy. I. A prospective study of findings in

hepatocytes from 24 patients before and after methotrexate treatment. Acta Pathol Microbiol Scand 1977; 85: 787–800

689. Nyfors A. Liver biopsies from psoriatics related to methotrexate therapy. 3. Finding in post-methotrexate liver biopsies from 160 psoriatics. Acta Pathol Microbiol Scand Sect A 1977; 85: 511–518

690. McInstosh S, Davidson D L, O'Brien R T, Pearson H A. Methotrexate hepatotoxicity in children with leukemia. J Pediatr 1977; 90: 1019–1021

691. Hersh E M, Wong V G, Henderson E S, Freireich E J. Hepatotoxic effects of methotrexate. Cancer 1966; 19: 600–606

692. Locasciulli A, Mura R, Fraschini D et al. High dose methotrexate administration and acute liver damage in children treated for acute lymphoblastic leukemia. A prospective study. Haematologica 1992; 77: 49–53

693. Jiricka Z, Smetana K, Janku I, Elis J, Novotny J. Studies on 6-azauridine and 6-azacytidine. I Toxicity studies of 6-azauridine and 6-azacytidine in mice. Biochem Pharmacol 1965; 14: 1517–1523

694. Bellet R E, Mastrangelo M J, Engstrom P F, Causter R P. Hepatotoxicity of 5-azacytidine. A clinical and pathologic study. Neoplasma 1973; 20: 303–309

695. Bellet R E, Mastrangelo M J, Engstrom P F, Strawitz J G, Weiss V, Yarbor J W. Clinical trial with subcutaneously administered 5-azacytidine. Cancer-chemotherapy 1974; 58: 217–222

696. Ganesan T S, Barnett M J, Amos R J, Piall E M, Aherne G W, Man A, Lister T A. Cytosine arabinoside in the management of recurrent leukemia. Hematol Oncol 1987; 5: 65–69

697. Bateman J R, Pugh R P, Cassidey F R, Marshall G J, Irwin L E. 5-Florouracil given once weekly: Comparison of intravenous and oral administration. Cancer 1971; 78: 907–913

698. Sternberg S S, Phillips F S. Azaserine: Pathological and pharmacological studies. Cancer 1957; 10: 889–901

699. Hruban Z, Swift H, Slesers R. Effect of azaserine on the fine structure of the liver and pancreatic acinar cells. Cancer Research 1965; 25: 708–723

700. Ellison R H, Karnofsky D A, Burchenal J H. Clinical evaluation of 6-chloropurine in leukemia of adults. Blood 1958; 13: 705–724

701. Einhorn M, Davidsohn I D. Hepatotoxicity of mercaptopurine. JAMA 1964; 188: 802–806

702. Shorey J, Schenker S, Suki W N, Combes B. Hepatotoxicity of mercaptopurine. Arch Intern Med 1968; 122: 54–58

703. Minow R A, Stern M H, Casey J H, Rodriguez V, Luna M. Clinicopathological correlation of liver damage in patients treated with 6-mercaptopurine and adriamycin. Cancer 1976; 38: 1524–1528

704. Rodriguez V, Bodey G P, McCredie K B, Freireich E J, Monow R A, Casey J H, Luna M. Combination 6-mercaptopurine-adriamycin in refractory adult acute leukemia. Clin Pharm Therapeutics 1975; 18: 462–466

705. Council on Drugs. Evaluation of two antineoplastic agents. JAMA 1967; 200: 619–620

706. Sparberg M, Simon N, Del Greco F. Intrahepatic cholestatis due to azathioprine. Gastroenterology 1969; 57: 439–441

707. Drinkard J P, Stanley T M, Dornfeld L, Austin R C, Barnett E V, Pearson C M. Azathioprine and prednisone in the treatment of adults with lupus nephritis. Clinical, histological, and immunological changes with therapy. Medicine 1970; 49: 411–432

708. Greaves M W, Dawber R. Azathioprine in psoriasis. Br Med J 1970; 2: 237–238

709. Haas J, Patzold U, Stamm T. Intrahepatische Cholestasein eine allergische Reaktion bei Azothioprin-Therapie. Dtsch Med Wochenschr 1978; 103: 1576–1577

710. Torisu M, Yokoyama T, Amemiya H et al. Immunosuppression, liver injury, and hepatitis in renal, hepatic and cardiac homograft recipients: with particular reference to the Australian Antigen. Ann Surg 1971; 174: 620–637

711. Malekzadeh M H, Grushkin C M, Wright H T, Fine R N. Hepatic dysfunction after renal transplantation in children. J Pediatr 1972; 81: 279–285

712. Zarday A, Veith F J, Gliedman M L, Soberman R. Irreversible liver damage after azathioprine. JAMA 1972; 222: 690–691

713. Briggs W A, Lazarus M, Birtch A G, Constantine L H, Hager E B, Merrill J P. Hepatitis affecting hemodialysis and transplant patients. Arch Intern Med 1973; 132: 21–28

714. Millard P R, Herbertson B M, Evans D B, Calne R Y. Azathioprine hepatotoxicity in renal transplantation. Transplantation 1973; 16: 527–529

715. Ireland P, Rashid A, von Lichtenberg F, Cavallo T, Merrill J P. Liver disease in kidney transplant patients receiving azathioprine. Arch Intern Med 1973; 132: 29–37

716. Ware A J, Luby J P, Eigenbrodt E H, Long D L, Hull A R. Spectrum of liver disease in renal transplant recipients. Gastroenterology 1975; 68: 755–764

717. DePinho R O, Goldberg C S, Lefkowitch J H. Azathioprine and the liver. Evidence favoring idiosyncratic mixed cholestatic-hepatocellular injury in humans. Gastroenterology 1984; 86: 162–165

718. Gerlag P G, Lobatto S, Driessen W M et al. Hepatic sinusoidal dilation with portal hypertension during azathioprine treatment after kidney transplantation. J Hepatol 1986; 1: 339–348

719. Adler M, Delhaye M, Deprez C et al. Hepatic vascular disease after kidney transplantation. Report of two cases and review of the literature. Nephrol Dial Transplant 1987; 2: 183–188

720. Weitz H, Gokel J M, Possinger K, Loeschke K, Possinger K, Eder M. Veno-occlusive disease of the liver in patients receiving immunosuppressive therapy. Virchows Arch (A) 1982; 395: 245–256

721. Marubbio A T, Denielson B. Hepatic veno-occlusive disease in a renal transplant patient receiving azathioprine. Gastroenterology 1975; 69: 739–743

722. Sabharwal U K, Vaughan J H, Kaplan R A, Robinson C A, Curd J G. Frentizole therapy in systemic lupus erythematosus. Arthritis Rheum 1980; 23: 1376–1380

723. Sznol M, Ohnuma T, Holland J F. Hepatic toxicity of drugs used for hematologic neoplasms. Semin Liver Dis 1987; 7: 237–256

724. Gross M A, Speer R J, Hill J M. Hepatic lipidosis associated with L-asparaginase treatment. Proc Soc Exp Biol Med 1969; 130: 733–736

725. Grundman E, Oettgen H, eds. Experimental and clinical effects of L-asparaginase. Berlin: Springer-Verlag, 1970

726. Haskell C M, Canellos G P, Leventhal B G, Carbone P P, Block J B, Serpick A A, Selawry O S. L-asparaginase. Therapeutic and toxic effects in patients with neoplastic disease. N Engl J Med 1969; 281: 1028–1034

727. Aviles A, Herreta J, Ramos E, Ambriz R, Aguirre J, Pizzuto J. Hepatic injury during doxorubicin therapy. Arch Pathol Lab Med 1984; 108: 912–913

728. McVeagh P, Ekert H. Hepatotoxicity of chemotherapy following nephrectomy and radiation therapy for right-sided Wilms' tumor. J Pediatr 1975; 87: 627–628

729. Costa G, Hreshchyshyn M M, Holland J F. Initial clinical studies with vincristine. Cancer Chemo Rpts 1963; 24: 39–44

730. Al Saghir N S, Hawkins K A. Hepatotoxicity following vincristine therapy. Cancer 1984; 54: 2006–2008

731. Ford J M, Lucey J J, Cullen M H, Tobias J S, Lister T A. Fatal graft-versus-host disease following transfusions of granulocytes from normal donors. Lancet 1976; ii: 1167–1169

732. Hansen M M, Ranek L, Walbom S, Nissen N I. Fatal hepatitis following irradiation and vincristine. Acta Med Scand 1982; 212: 171–174

733. Perry M C. Hepatotoxicity of chemotherapeutic agents. Semin Oncol 1982; 9: 65–74

734. McDonald G B, Tirumali N. Intestinal and liver toxicity of neoplastic drugs. West J Med 1984; 140: 250–259

735. Dianzani M U. Toxic liver injury by protein synthesis inhibitors. Prog Liver Dis 1976; 5: 232–245

736. Underwood J C E, Shahani R T, Blackburn E K. Jaundice after treatment of leukaemia with busulfan. Br Med J 1971; 1: 556–557

737. Choudari Kommineni V R, Greenblatt M, Vesselinovitch S D, Mihailovich N. Urethane carcinogenesis in rats. Importance of age and dose. J Nat Cancer Inst 1970; 45: 687–696

738. Weiss D L, De Los Santos R. Urethane-induced hepatic failure in man. Am J Med 1960; 28: 476–481

739. Denman A M, Ward H W C. Jaundice during treatment of myelomatosis with M and B 938. Br Med J 1960; 1: 482–483

740. Capurso L, Monte P R D, Mazzeo F, Menardo G, Morettini A, Saggioro A, Tafner G. Comparison of cimetidine 800 mg once daily and 400 mg twice daily in acute duodenal ulceration. Br Med J 1984; 289: 1418–1420

741. Zantac (Ranitidine hydrochloride) In: Product Information section. Physicians Desk Reference, 1991, p 1041

742. Zuchner H. Cholestatische hepatose unter cimetidine. Deutsche Medizine Wochenschrift 1977; 102: 1788–1789

743. Lilly J R, Hitch D C, Javitt N B. Cimetidine cholestatic jaundice in children. J Surg Res 1978; 24: 384–387

744. Khalsa J H. Cimetidine (Tagamet®)-associated cholestatic jaundice. ADR Highlights. No 83–10, 1983

745. Villeneuve J P, Warner H A. Cimetidine hepatitis. Gastroenterology 1979; 77: 143–144

746. Ruiz del Arbol L, Mureira V, Moreno A. Bridging hepatic necrosis associated with cimetidine. Am J Gastroenterol 1980; 74: 267

747. Lorenzini I, Jezequel A M, Orlandi F. Cimetidine-induced hepatitis: Electron microscopic observation and clinical pattern of liver injury. Dig Dis Sci 1981; 26: 275–280

748. Boyd P T, Lepre F, Dickey J D. Chronic active hepatitis associated with cimetidine. Br Med J 1989; 298: 324–325

749. Schwartz J T, Gyorkey F, Graham D Y. Cimetidine hepatitis. J Clin Gastroenterol 1986; 8: 681–686

750. Barr G D, Piper D W. Possible ranitidine hepatitis. Med J Austr 1981; 2: 421

751. Souza-Lima M A. Hepatitis associated with ranitidine. Ann Intern Med 1984; 101: 207–208

752. Black M, Scott Jr W E, Kanter R. Possible ranitidine hepatotoxicity. Ann Intern Med 1984; 101: 208–209

753. Cleator I. Adverse effects of ranitidine therapy. Can Med Assoc J 1983; 129: 405

754. Lauritsen K, Havelund T, Rask-Madsen J, Fenger C. Ranitidine and hepatotoxicity (letter). Lancet 1984; ii: 1471

755. Hiesse C, Cantarovich M, Santelli E et al. Ranitidine hepatotoxicity in renal transplant patients (letter). Lancet 1985; i: 1280

756. Farup P G. Zaltidine: An effective but hepatotoxic H2 receptor antagonist. Scand J Gastroenterol 1988; 23: 655–658

757. Zimmerman H J, Jacob L, Bassan H, Gillespie J, Lukacs L, Abernathy C O. Effects of H2 blocking agents on hepatocytes in vitro: Correlation with potential for causing hepatic disease in patients. Proc Soc Exp Biol Med 1986; 182: 511–514

758. Speeg K V Jr, Patwardhan R V, Avant G R, Mitchell M C, Schenker S. Inhibition of microsomal drug metabolism by histamine H_2 receptor antagonist studied in vivo and in vitro in rodents. Gastroenterology 1982; 82: 89–96

759. Mitchell M C, Schenker S, Speeg K V. Selective inhibition of acetaminophen oxidation and toxicity by cimetidine and other histamine H_2 receptor antagonists in vivo and in vitro in the rat and in man. J Clin Invest 1984; 74: 383–391

760. Diaz D, Fabre I, Daujat M, Saint-Aubert B et al. Omeprazole is an arylhydrocarbon-like inducer of human hepatic cytochrome P450. Gastroenterology 1990; 99: 737–747

761. Editorial. Below the belt. Lancet 1971; ii: 253

762. Reynolds T B, Lapin A C, Peters R L, Yamahiro H S. Puzzling jaundice due to laxative ingestion. JAMA 1970; 211: 86–90

763. Reynolds T B, Peters R L, Yamada S. Chronic active and lupoid hepatitis caused by a laxative oxyphenisatin. N Engl J Med 1971; 285: 813

764. Dietrichson O, Juhl E, Nielsen J O, Oxlund J J, Christoffersen P. The incidence of oxyphenisatin-induced liver damage in chronic non-alcoholic liver disease. A control investigation. Scand J Gastroenterol 1974; 9: 473–478

765. Australian Drug Evaluation Committee. Withdrawal of oxyphenisatin acetate, diacetoxydiphenolisatin and triacetyldiphenolisatin from the Australian market. Med J Aust 1972; 1: 1051–1053

766. Taffet L S, Kiron M D. Sulfasalazine adverse effects and desensitization. Dig Dis Sci 1983; 28: 833–842

767. Boyer D L, Li B U, Fyda J N, Friedman R A. Sulfasaclazione-induced hepatotoxicity in children with inflammatory bowel disease. J Pediatr Gastroenterol Nutr 1989; 8: 528–532

768. Larcan A, Lambert H, Janot C, Perarnaud J, Delorme F, Tibbek F. Hepatite mortelle au cours d'un traitement per sulfasalazine. Therapie 1982; 37: 315–319

769. Ribe J, Benkov K J, Thung S N, Shen S C, LeLeioka N S. Fatal massive hepatic necrosis: A probable hypersensitivity reaction to sulfasalizine. Am J Gastroenterol 1986; 81: 205–208

770. Gulley M, Mirza A, Kelly C. Hepatotoxicity of salicylazolpyridine. A case report and review of the literature. Am J Gastroenterol 1979; 72: 561–564

771. Namias A, Bhalotra R, Donowitz M. Reversible sulfasalazine-induced granulomatous hepatitis. J Clin Gastroenterol 1981; 3: 193–198

772. Turunen U, Eloman I, Antila V J et al. Mesalalazine tolerance in patients with inflammatory bowel disease and previous intolerance in patients or allergy to sulfasalazine or sulphonamides. Scand J Gastroenterol 1987; 22: 798–802

773. Burke D A, Manning A P, Williamson J M, Axon A T. Adverse reactions to sulphasalazine and 5-amino salicylic acid in the same patient. Aliments Pharmacol Ther 1987; 1: 201–208

774. Portmann B, Talbot I C, Day D W et al. Histopathological changes in the liver following a paracetamol overdose: correlation with clinical and biochemical parameters. J Pathol 1975; 117: 179–181

775. Rumack B H, Peterson R G. Acetaminophen overdosage: Incidence, diagnosis, and management in 416 patients. Pediatrics 1978; 62: 898–903

776. Black M. Acetaminophen hepatotoxicity. Annu Rev Med 1984; 35: 577–593

777. Seeff L B, Cuccherini B A, Zimmerman H J, Adler E, Benjamin S B. Acetaminophen hepatotoxicity in alcoholics—a therapeutic misadventure. Ann Intern Med 1986; 104: 399–404

778. Kloss M W, Rosen G M, Rauckman E J. Cocaine-mediated hepatotoxicity. A critical review. Biochem Pharm 1984; 33: 169–173

779. Mallat A, Dhumeaux D. Cocaine and the liver. J Hepatol 1991; 12: 272–278

780. Kanel G C, Cassidy W, Shuster L, Reynolds T B. Cocaine-induced liver cell injury: comparison of morphological features in man and in experimental models. Hepatology 1990; 11: 646–651

781. Perino L E, Warren G H, Levine J S. Cocaine-induced hepatotoxicity in humans. Gastroenterology 1987; 93: 176–180

782. Wanless I R, Dore S, Gopinath N et al. Histopathology of cocaine hepatotoxicity. Report of four patients. Gastroenterology 1990; 98: 497–501

783. Silva M O, Roth D, Reddy K R, Fernandez J A, Albores-Saavedra J, Schiff E R. Hepatic dysfunction accompanying acute cocaine intoxication. J Hepatol 1991; 12: 312–315

784. Smith A C, Freeman R W, Harbison R D. Ethanol enhancement of cocaine-induced hepatotoxicity. Biochem Pharm 1981; 30: 453–458

785. Henry J A, Jeffreys K J, Dawling S. Toxicity and deaths from 3,4-methylenedioxymethamphetamine ("ecstasy"). Lancet 1992; 340: 384–387

786. Eisen H J, Ginsberg A L. Disulfiram-hepatotoxicity. Ann Intern Med 1975; 83: 673–674

787. Kristensen M E. Toxic hepatitis induced by disulfiram in a nonalcoholic. Acta Med Scand 1981; 209: 335–336

788. Nassberger L. Disulfiram-induced hepatitis—a report of a case and review of the literature. Postgrad Med J 1984; 60: 639–641

789. Berlin R G. Disulfirm hepatotoxicity. A consideration of its mechanism and clinical spectrum. Alcohol Alcoholism 1989; 24: 241–245

790. Geubel A P, De Galocsy C, Alves N, Rahier J, Dive C. Liver damage caused by therapeutic vitamin A administration: estimate of dose-related toxicity in 41 cases. Gastroenterology 1991; 100: 1701–1079

791. Hathcock J N, Hattan D G, Jenkins M Y, McDonald J T. Evaluation of vitamin A toxicity. Am J Clin Nutr 1990; 52: 183–202

792. Inkeles S B, Connor W E, Illingworth D R. Hepatic and dermatologic manifestation of chronic hypervitaminosis A in adults. Report of two cases. Am J Med 1986; 80: 491–496

793. Zafrani E S, Bernuau D, Feldmann G. Peliosis-like ultrastructural changes in the hepatic sinusoids in human chronic hypervitaminosis A. Hum Pathol 1984; 15: 1166–1170

794. Camuto P, Shupack J, Orbuch P, Tobias H, Sidhu G, Feiner H. Long-term effects of etretinate on the liver in psoriasis. Am J Surg Path 1987; 11: 30–37

795. Khouri M R, Saul S H, Dlugosz A A, Soloway R D. Hepatocanalicular injury associated with vitamin A derivative etretinate, an idiosyncratic hypersensitivity reaction. Dig Dis Sci 1987; 32: 1207–1211

796. Weiss V, West D P, Ackerman R, Robinson L A. Hepatotoxic reactions in a patient treated with etretinate therapy. Arch Dermatol 1984; 120: 104–106

797. Weiss V, Layden T, Spinowitz A, Buys C M, Nemchausky B A, West D P, Emmons K M. Chronic active hepatitis associated with etretinate therapy. Br J Dermatol 1985; 112: 591–597

798. Kamm M A, Davies D J, Breen K J. Acute hepatitis due to etretinate. J Gastroenterol Hepatol 1988; 3: 663–666

799. Halioua B, Saurat J H. Risk: benefit ratio in the treatment of psoriasis with systemic retinoids. Br J Dermatol 1990; 122 (suppl 36): 135–150

800. Ingold J A, Reed G B, Kaplan H S, Bagshaw M A. Radiation hepatitis. Am J Roentgen 1965; 93: 200–208

801. Lansing A M, Davis W M, Brizel H E. Radiation hepatitis. Arch Surg 1968; 96: 878–882

802. Lewin K, Mills R R. Human radiation hepatitis. A morphologic study with emphasis on the late changes. Arch Pathol 1973; 96: 21–26

803. Horta J, Da Motta C, Taveres M H. Thorium dioxide effects in man. Epidemiological, clinical and pathogical studies (Experience in Portugal). Environ Res 1974; 8: 131–134

804. Batlifora H A. Thorotrast and tumors of the liver. In: Okuda K, Peters R L, eds. Hepatocellular carcinoma. New York: John Wiley, 1976: pp 247–307

805. Falk H, Herbert J, Crowley S. Epidemiology of hepatic angiosarcoma in the United States: 1964–1974. Environ Hlth Persp 1981; 41: 107–113

806. Rubel L R, Ishak K G. Thorotrast associated cholangiocarcinoma. Cancer 1982; 50: 1408–1415

807. Khan A A. Thorotrast-associated liver cancer. Am J Gastroenterol 1985; 80: 699–703

808. Marant R, Rultner J R. Late complications of Thorotrast. Experiences from Zurich. Schweitz Med Wochensche 1987; 117: 952–957

809. Levy D W, Rindsberg S, Friedman A C et al. Thorotrast-induced hepatosplenic neoplasia: C T identification. Am J Roentgenol 1986; 146: 997–1004

810. Ito Y, Kojiro M, Nakashima T, Mori T. Pathomorphologic characteristics of 102 cases of thorotrast-related hepatocellular carcinoma, cholangiocarcinoma and hepatic angiosarcoma. Cancer 1988; 62: 1153–1162

811. Andersson M, Storm H H. Cancer incidence among Danish Thorotrast-exposed patients. J Natl Cancer Inst 1992; 84: 1318–1325

812. Shurbaji M S, Olson L J, Kuhajda P. Thorotrast-associated hepatic leiomyosarcoma and cholangiocarcinoma. Hum Pathol 1987; 18: 524–526

813. Okuda K, Omata M, Itoh Y, Ikezaki H, Nakashima T. Peliosis hepatis as a late and fatal complication of Thorotrast liver disease: Report of five cases. Liver 1981; 1: 110–122

814. Ishak K G. Applications of scanning electron microscopy to the study of liver disease. Prog Liv Dis 1986; 8: 1–31

815. O'Brien J T, Eagger S, Levy R. Effects of tetrahydroaminoacridine on liver function in patients with Alzheimer's disease. Age Ageing 1991; 129–131

816. Molloy D W, Guyatt G H, Wilson D B, Duke R, Ress L, Singer J. Effect of tetrahydroaminoacridine on cognition, function and behavior in Alzheimer's disease. Can Med Assoc J 1991; 144: 29–34

817. Davis K, Thal L J, Gamzu E R et al. A double-blind placebo-controlled multicenter study of tacrine for Alzheimer's disease. N Engl J Med 1992; 327: 1253–1259

16

Tumours and tumour-like lesions of the liver and biliary tract

P. P. Anthony (with a contribution by P. Bannasch)

Benign epithelial tumours
    Liver-cell (hepatocellular) adenoma
    Bile-duct adenoma
    Bile-duct cystadenoma
    Biliary papillomatosis

Liver-cell (hepatocellular) carcinoma
    Epidemiology
    Aetiology
    The role of cirrhosis
    Precancerous changes in the human liver
    Clinical presentation, radiological investigation and
        laboratory findings
    Paraneoplastic syndromes
    α-Fetoprotein
    Pathology

Hepatoblastoma

Bile-duct carcinoma (cholangiocarcinoma)
    Epidemiology, aetiology and pathogenesis
    Types of bile-duct carcinoma
    Microscopic appearances
    Differential diagnosis and special techniques
    Spread and prognosis

Bile-duct cystadenocarcinoma

Mixed liver-cell and bile-duct carcinomas and other malignant epithelial tumours

Benign non-epithelial tumours
    Haemangioma
    Infantile haemangioendothelioma
    Lymphangioma
    Angiomyolipoma
    Other rare benign soft tissue tumours

Malignant non-epithelial tumours
    Angiosarcoma
    Malignant epithelioid haemangioendothelioma

    Undifferentiated (embryonal) sarcoma
    Rhabdomyosarcoma
    Other primary sarcomas
    Primary lymphoma of the liver

Rare primary tumours

Metastatic tumours

Tumour-like lesions
    Cysts
    Focal nodular hyperplasia
    Nodular regenerative hyperplasia
    Mesenchymal hamartoma
    Biliary hamartoma (von Meyenburg complex)
    Inflammatory pseudotumour
    Miscellaneous tumour-like lesions

Experimental liver tumours (*P. Bannasch*)

Aetiology: exogenous and endogenous factors
    Chemical agents
    Physical factors
    Hepadnaviruses
    Genetic events

Stages of neoplastic development

Sequential cellular changes during neoplastic development

Liver tumours continue to attract an interest that seems to be out of proportion to their numerical importance, at least in the Western world, where liver-cell or hepatocellular carcinoma is uncommon. There are several reasons for this: (i) carcinogenesis in the liver has been the most intensively studied experimental model for many years and, understandably, the stimulus is there to look for the equivalent findings in man; (ii) the number of people affected in Africa and South-East Asia is huge, hence there is moral obligation to take notice; (iii) in the whole field of clinically relevant cancer research, it is perhaps in this area where the most exciting advances have been made. Suffice to mention but a few of these: the discovery of α-fetoprotein as a tumour marker, the role of the hepatitis B and C viruses and of aflatoxin as major aetiological agents, and recent molecular biological and genetic studies on viral DNA integration, the X protein transgene and p53 mutation. More is yet to come.

It must be appreciated that many different tumours arise in the liver in addition to hepatocellular and cholangiocarcinomas and that these, though individually rare, represent a significant number even in Europe and North America. Moreover, some are treatable and indeed curable. The old term 'hepatoma' is still used from time to time: it has no precise clinical or pathological meaning and should be discarded for ever. Table 16.1 is based on a revised classification of liver tumours by an expert group of histopathologists originally sponsored by the World Health Organization and now by the Armed Forces Institute of Pathology.[1] This is an abbreviated list but it serves to indicate the multiplicity of tumour types encountered at this site. Tissue diagnosis remains mandatory, despite advances in laboratory and imaging techniques.

Our knowledge of the worldwide distribution of tumours is based on data derived from cancer registries in many parts of the world. These have been published in successive volumes of the series *Cancer Incidence in Five Continents*, the latest of which appeared in 1987.[2] Tumours are registered under their International Classification of Diseases (ICD) code number. This combined all hepatobiliary tumours under a single heading until 1968 when it separated them into 'neoplasms of the liver' and 'neoplasms of the gallbladder and extrahepatic bile ducts'. However, the 1977 revision still had not made the important distinction between hepatocellular and intrahepatic bile-duct carcinomas. The latest classification of tumours (ICD-O), which appeared in 1990, has now remedied this defect.[3]

Accurate registration of the major types of liver cancer is essential. It is evident from numerous population-based and hospital centre studies that the marked geographical variability in incidence is due to just one tumour type, namely hepatocellular carcinoma, which predominates in tropical Africa and South-East Asia. Intrahepatic bile-duct carcinoma is the next commonest. It occurs with much the same frequency everywhere, except in South-East Asia where its high incidence is associated with liver fluke infestation. Other tumour types are all rare but some have interesting and, from the public health point of view, important aetiological associations.

The outlook for malignant hepatobiliary tumours is, in general, poor. In 1974, Waterhouse published data on survival from all types of cancer based on the Birmingham Cancer Registry.[4] Primary liver tumours made up rather less than 0.5% of all cancers and the 5-year survival was nil for hepatocellular carcinoma and only 1.5% for bile-duct carcinoma. The figures collected by the Cancer Research Campaign from England and Wales in 1982 by Toms[5] were similar for all types of liver cancer: 2% for males and 3% for females. In this survey, however, much better results were recorded in patients under 45: 12% and 14% respectively. This may reflect, first of all, the better prognosis of certain types of tumour such as fibrolamellar carcinoma or epithelioid haemangioendothelioma in adolescents and young adults and of hepatoblastoma in children. Steady advances have since been made in patient selection, surgical techniques and chemotherapy.[6–8]

How large is the problem? The American Cancer Society estimated 11 600 new cases of liver and biliary tract carcinomas per year throughout the 1980s, with a death rate of 9300 annually.[9] Figures for the United Kingdom and most of Europe are similar pro rata but elsewhere, particularly in Africa and South-East Asia, they are much higher: an estimated number of 1 000 000 deaths annually from hepatocellular carcinoma alone.[10]

Table 16.1 An abbreviated classification of primary tumours of the liver

	Benign	Malignant
Epithelial tumours	Liver-cell adenoma Bile-duct adenoma Bile-duct cystadenoma Biliary papillomatosis	Liver-cell (hepatocellular) carcinoma Bile-duct carcinoma (cholangiocarcinoma) Bile-duct cystadenocarcinoma Combined and mixed carcinomas Hepatoblastoma
Non-epithelial tumours	Haemangioma Angiomyolipoma Other benign tumours	Haemangiosarcoma Epithelioid haemangioendothelioma Embryonal sarcoma Rhabdomyosarcoma Other sarcomas, lymphomas, germ cell tumours
Tumour-like lesions	Cysts Focal nodular hyperplasia Nodular regenerative hyperplasia Mesenchymal hamartoma Peliosis Inflammatory pseudotumour	

The epidemiology, aetiological associations and pathology of liver tumours have been described in many textbooks, atlases and proceedings of symposia.[1,11-16]

BENIGN EPITHELIAL TUMOURS

LIVER-CELL (HEPATOCELLULAR) ADENOMA

This is much the most important benign tumour of the liver, and its association with oral contraceptive steroid usage is well established. Our attention to this was first drawn by a report in 1973[17] which followed closely another report on hepatocellular carcinoma in patients on androgenic/anabolic steroids.[18] It soon became evident that the type of tumour induced by both female and male synthetic gonadal steroids is the same[19] and genuine malignancy in either situation is rare. All the compounds incriminated so far, whether they be male or female hormones, have been 17-alkyl (α-ethinyl) substituted derivatives of the basic steroid structure. Liver-cell adenoma unrelated to synthetic gonadal steroids is extremely rare.

Aetiology

A number of anecdotal reports in the 1970s were eventually followed by convincing case-control studies and other epidemiological evidence to show that liver-cell adenoma was indeed related to the use of oral contraceptive steroids.[20-29] These data and the hepatotoxicity and carcinogenicity of the agents have been comprehensively reviewed in recent years.[30-32] A registry of cases was set up in the United States, and the clinical and pathological features have been described in detail.[22,26]

The development of liver-cell adenoma in a woman taking oral contraceptive steroids relates to dose, duration of usage and increasing age, usually over 30 years. The relative risk has been estimated as 25 and 500, after 9 and 7 years of drug use, respectively, in two studies in the United States.[20,25] These large discrepancies are probably due to differences in case selection, methodology and other confounding factors.[31,32] Similar studies from Europe[27] produced much lower figures. The number of cases in the United Kingdom is not known but is likely to be low, and there has been much greater concern with genital cancers, particularly of the cervix.[33] In any case, the absolute risk is very small given the rarity of liver-cell adenoma in the general population. The estimated annual incidence in the United States has been put at 3.4 per 100 000 oral contraceptive users or 288 cases per year[25] and is probably falling. Mestranol was at first thought to carry a greater risk than ethinyloestradiol (the two most commonly used compounds) until it was realized that the difference could be explained by a change-over from the one to the other in the late 1960s and the subsequent reduction in the dosage used. The earlier introduction of hormonal contraceptive methods, the much greater number of women at risk, and the larger doses of drugs used initially all go towards explaining the comparatively higher incidence of liver-cell adenoma in the United States than in Europe and elsewhere, where this form of contraception was adopted later and on a smaller scale. There is no evidence that the progestogen component of combined preparations carries any risk, nor that smoking or alcohol adds significantly to it.[30-32] Low dose oral contraceptives in current use seem to carry little or no risk of tumour development.[33a]

Liver-cell tumours also occur in adult men and women treated with androgenic/anabolic steroids for impotence or as part of a sex change regime, and in children of either sex treated with the same drugs for Fanconi's syndrome, refractory anaemias and bone marrow aplasia. The most commonly incriminated drugs have been methyltestosterone, oxymetholone and norethandrolone.[18,34-39] A fatal case of rupture of a hepatic tumour, thought to be a liver-cell adenoma with possible malignant transformation, has been reported in an athlete/body-builder who was taking anabolic steroids.[40] In a similar case, a liver tumour which had ruptured but was not resected, later regressed after discontinuation of self-medication.[40a] In another rare instance, liver-cell adenoma and focal nodular hyperplasia were attributed to high endogenous sex steroids, both androgens and oestrogens.[41]

The hepatic side effects of female and male synthetic gonadal steroids include cholestatic jaundice, sinusoidal dilatation, Budd-Chiari syndrome and gallstone formation for the former, and cholestatic jaundice and peliosis hepatis for the latter.[23,30-32,35,39] These are seldom seen in combination with tumours except for peliosis hepatis, which may be quite extensive in liver-cell adenoma due to androgenic/anabolic steroids.[34,35,39] Most gonadal steroid-related liver tumours do not produce α-fetoprotein and they do not metastasize, despite a frequently equivocal microscopic appearance that suggests malignancy. Instances of spontaneous regression after discontinuation of either type of drug are rare[42-44] and so are reports of progression and/or malignant change[45-51] (see also pp 16.12-16.13).

Other, much less frequent aetiological agents and associations include clomiphene,[52] danazol,[53-55] norethisterone,[56] glycogen storage disease type Ia,[57,58] familial diabetes mellitus[59] and Klinefelter syndrome.[60] An increasing number of 'spontaneous' cases in both sexes and at any age, including childhood, are also being reported in which no cause could be found.[61-63] Finally, a unique primary placental liver-cell adenoma has also been described.[64]

Clinical presentation

Most patients present with acute abdominal pain which almost invariably is due to haemorrhage into the tumour; the risk of rupture into the peritoneal cavity is high. In two large surgical series, this occurred in half of the cases.[46,48]

There were no deaths in these series, both from specialist units, but surveys of case reports and registry data reveal a mortality of 20%.[22,26–28,31] Other patients complain of episodic abdominal pain or discomfort, and liver-cell adenomas are seldom discovered incidentally. Tumours larger than 10 cm are at risk of rupture and they should be removed for this reason alone.[46,48] This risk may be particularly high at the time of menstruation[20] and during pregnancy[65,66] when oestrogen levels are low. Increased nuclear and cytosolic oestrogen receptors have been reported in liver-cell adenomas; such receptors were absent in the tumour of a patient who had been taking tamoxifen.[67] These differences in binding capacity suggest a potential for hormone responsiveness in liver-cell adenoma.

Pathology

The macroscopic and microscopic appearances are reasonably characteristic; confusion with focal nodular hyperplasia and mesenchymal hamartoma should no longer arise.[11–13,16,22,26,28,68–70] The simultaneous occurrence of liver-cell adenoma and focal nodular hyperplasia has been observed from time to time but the two are probably unrelated.[28,29,68–71] The term mesenchymal hamartoma is now reserved to designate a tumour-like lesion of the liver in childhood which arises as a result of ductal plate maldevelopment.

Liver-cell adenomas arise anywhere in an otherwise normal liver. They are commonly solitary and seldom multiple, when they may number 2–6. Occasionally they may be pedunculated. Rare instances of 'liver cell adenomatosis' have been recorded with nodules described as 'more than ten' or 'numerous' and often small.[72–74] It is unclear whether this represents a distinct entity but there is no relationship to the sex of the patient or to synthetic gonadal steroids and other agents. In most cases of liver-cell adenoma, the tumour is seen as a bulging mass with dilated blood vessels running over its surface and it may be large, measuring up to 30 cm and weighing 3000g. On sectioning, it is well demarcated, usually spherical and is seldom encapsulated. The colour varies from yellow to tan, the consistency is soft or friable, and areas of necrosis or haemorrhage are frequently present. All tumours are highly vascular and those associated with androgenic/anabolic steroids may also show peliosis. Areas of scarring indicate previous episodes of infarction.

The histological hallmark of liver-cell adenoma is that it consists solely of liver cells which are arranged in plates that are two to three cells thick and never more (Fig. 16.1). These are separated by inconspicuous, slit-like sinusoids lined by endothelium. Mitoses are absent or few. The normal reticulin pattern is well preserved (Fig. 16.2). Despite earlier reports, Kupffer cells are present in liver-cell adenomas, albeit in variable numbers,[75] and, when active, they may be demonstrated by PAS–diastase or

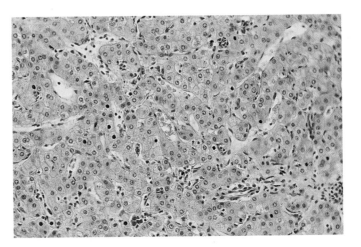

Fig. 16.1 Liver-cell adenoma arranged in plates that are two to three cells thick. These are separated by sinusoids. The patient was an adolescent, and scanty foci of extramedullary haemopoiesis are present. H & E.

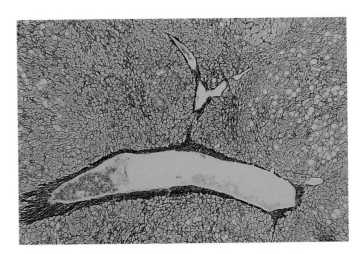

Fig. 16.2 The normal reticulin pattern is well preserved throughout; note the large blood vessels and patchy fatty change. Reticulin – Van Gieson.

Perls' stains (Fig. 16.3). Tumour cells are generally larger than normal hepatocytes, their nuclei are uniform and the cytoplasm is either pale and eosinophilic or almost clear, due to excess glycogen or fat. Bile ducts are absent in any shape or form but bile may present as droplets in the cytoplasm or as plugs in distended canaliculi. Large tortuous arteries and dilated, thin-walled veins are seen which may contain thrombi. Hyaline globules that are usually PAS–diastase-positive and consist of α_1-antitrypsin are occasionally seen. They are not related to oral contraceptive steroid use as was once thought.[76] Other, rare, features include appearances resembling alcoholic hepatitis with fatty change, polymorphs and Mallory bodies,[77] and giant cell granulomas which may be quite numerous.[74,78] Foci of extramedullary haemopoiesis may be seen in tumours of children or adolescents. Finally, liver-cell dysplasia, sometimes extensive, may be present.

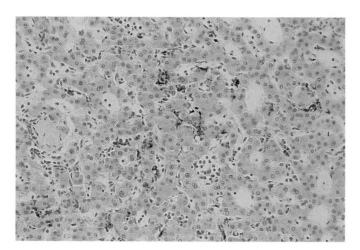

Fig. 16.3 Haemosiderin-laden Kupffer cells near an area of old haemorrhage. Perls' stain.

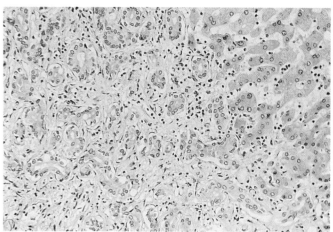

Fig. 16.4 Bile-duct adenoma made up of small ducts set in a fibrous stroma; normal liver is seen on the right. H & E.

Differential diagnosis

The main difficulty lies in the distinction between liver-cell adenoma and well-differentiated liver-cell carcinoma, and this may at times be impossible on histological grounds alone. Liver-cell plates more than three cells thick, acinar structures, decreased nuclear:cytoplasmic ratio, prominent nucleoli, mitoses, cytoplasmic basophilia, loss of the reticulin pattern, absence of Kupffer cells, presence of vascular invasion and of stainable α-fetoprotein, all indicate carcinoma. However, none of these features can be relied upon with certainty as some may rarely be seen in liver-cell adenoma and others are commonly absent in well-differentiated liver-cell carcinoma. The most helpful, perhaps, are the thickness of liver-cell plates (e.g. more or less than three cells), the amount of reticulin (normal or deficient) and vascular invasion (present or absent). The usefulness of special techniques is discussed on pages 16.26–16.28. It should be noted that male sex, cirrhosis and chronic hepatitis B virus infection strongly indicate that a liver-cell tumour, no matter how well differentiated, is in fact malignant. Conversely, female sex and a history of oral contraceptive use support the diagnosis of liver-cell adenoma. Some situations present exceptional difficulties, e.g. tumours associated with metabolic disorders (glycogen storage disease type Ia, hereditary tyrosinaemia) in which both liver-cell adenoma and carcinoma develop in the course of time.

BILE-DUCT ADENOMA

Earlier synonyms for this tumour included 'benign cholangioma' and 'cholangioadenoma'. It is always discovered incidentally, e.g. at laparotomy, when it may be mistaken for a metastasis on frozen section. Bile-duct adenoma is considered rare but, in one study, it was found in 26 of 95 livers sliced finely and serially at autopsy.[79] The tumour is usually solitary, white and fibrous, and measures up to 2 cm in size. The histological appearances are consistent:[80,81] a maze of small ducts which are lined by a single layer of cuboidal cells that may secrete mucin (Fig. 16.4). The immunophenotype of these structures is similar to that of interlobular bile ducts but there is no communication between them, and bile is not seen in the lumens. The stroma is fibrous and it may be cellular or hyalinized; it typically contains lymphocytes. There is no capsule, and normal portal tracts may be included in the lesion. Two examples have been reported that contained clusters of endocrine cells resembling carcinoid tumour.[82] Rarely, large or 'atypical' examples may be seen, with papillary or cribriform patterns and cysts, but no authentic example of malignant change is known. The term 'biliary adenofibroma' has recently been applied to a 7 cm solitary lesion with worrying histological features.[82a]

BILE-DUCT CYSTADENOMA

This tumour is rare but not unique to the liver, in that cystadenomas of similar appearance also occur in the pancreas and, quite commonly, in the ovary. Some 100 cases have been reported in the liver but only half of these were acceptable on review.[82,84] The majority occur in women, with a peak incidence in the fifth decade. Patients present with pain or discomfort, a palpable mass or, less commonly, jaundice, rupture or infection. Bile-duct cystadenomas grow slowly, frequently to a large size, and may become malignant. Surgical resection is invariably indicated and is usually curative.[85]

Bile-duct cystadenoma differs from other, usually congenital, cysts in being multilocular. The contents are clear to cloudy, mucinous or gelatinous fluid or jelly, the colour of which is yellow to brown but may be frankly haemorrhagic and rarely purulent. The inner surface of the locules may be smooth, trabeculated or show small sessile projections.

Histologically, a *mucinous* type is commonest.[83,84] It is lined by columnar, cuboidal or flattened, mucus-secreting epithelium which is generally single layered but may show small papillary structures or cystic invaginations. A basement membrane separates the lining from the underlying stroma which varies in thickness and may be relatively acellular and hyaline or highly cellular and compacted, resembling ovarian stroma (Fig. 16.5). The latter feature has been referred to as 'mesenchymal' and is only seen in women.[84] Elevated serum CA 19–9 levels were demonstrated in two cases.[85a] In another study of five cases, immunocytochemistry and electron microscopy suggested that these tumours arise from ectopic embryonal tissues destined to form the adult gall bladder.[85b] The septa between cysts often show secondary changes: foamy or pigmented macrophages, cholesterol clefts, fibrosis, scarring and sometimes calcification. Foci of cellular atypia, particularly nuclear enlargement and hyperchromasia, multilayering or solid epithelial masses indicate 'borderline' change; capsular invasion signifies malignancy. A much less common *serous* type is becoming increasingly recognized.[1] This consists of numerous small locules lined by a single layer of cuboidal cells with a clear cytoplasm that is rich in glycogen. A *papillary cystic tumour* has also been reported.[86] These latter two varieties are similar to tumours seen in the pancreas.[87] Bile-duct cystadenoma has been reported in an oral contraceptive steroid user; tumour tissue had a high oestrogen receptor content.[88]

Biliary cystadenomas do not communicate with the biliary tree but rare examples may indent, or even project into, major hepatic ducts.[84] This may result in cholangitis.[88a]

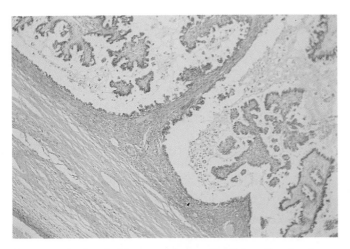

Fig. 16.5 Multilocular biliary cystadenoma lined by papillary fronds which display cytological atypia ('borderline' change). Note the narrow layer of compacted, cellular stroma. H & E.

BILIARY PAPILLOMATOSIS

This condition is rare but over 50 cases have now been reported.[89–93] Patients usually present in middle to old age, and men outnumber women by 2 to 1. Multiple papillomas are present in the intra- and extrahepatic bile ducts, including the common bile duct. The gallbladder and the major pancreatic ducts may also be involved. The lumens of these structures contain soft, friable, papillary excrescences which are composed of mucus-secreting columnar epithelial cells supported by thin fibrovascular stalks. Paneth cells and neuroendocrine elements may be demonstrable. Variable degrees of structural and cytological atypia and foci of invasion may be seen. The condition is relentlessly progressive with episodes of obstructive jaundice, sepsis and haemobilia; patients die from these complications even in the absence of malignant transformation. Curettage and drainage may relieve symptoms for a time but cure can probably only be achieved by total hepatectomy and liver transplantation. Occasional cases have been associated with ulcerative colitis, Caroli's disease and polyposis coli.[89–93] Cases of solitary villous adenoma of the common bile duct, causing obstructive jaundice, have also been reported.[93a,b]

LIVER-CELL (HEPATOCELLULAR) CARCINOMA

This tumour shows a remarkable geographical variability in incidence which has attracted the attention of epidemiologists since the middle of the century. It soon became evident that racial and genetic factors were of little, if any, importance and incidence rates were found to be closely related to environmental factors — the prevalence of chronic hepatitis B virus infection in particular.

EPIDEMIOLOGY

The longstanding failure of coding liver tumours by specific histogenetic type has already been alluded to in the introduction to this chapter. It must also be appreciated that the data collected by cancer registries in many countries, especially those with the highest incidence rates, are unlikely to be complete and must represent underestimates. Despite these difficulties, a reasonably accurate tabulation can be built up, aided by nationwide or regional surveys and reports from centres with a specialist interest in case finding, prevention and treatment. These have been regularly summarized and updated over the years.[10,94–102] and the following is a brief summary of the data accumulated during the last ten years.

Liver-cell carcinoma is one of the most common internal malignancies worldwide, with an annual occurrence of at least 1 000 000 new cases. In rank order, it is the seventh most common malignant tumour in males and the ninth in females. Mortality is nearly the same, as the overwhelming majority die in a few weeks or, at most, months. Thus the death toll is considerable.[10,98,99,102]

The geographical distribution is highly uneven and, in broad terms, countries may be divided into three groups: those with low, intermediate and high incidence rates (Table 16.2). The highest rates of all are obtained in South-East Asia and tropical Africa where, in countries such as Mozambique, frequencies have been estimated to be up to 150/100 000/year. In these areas, the tumour is the commonest or next commonest in the list of all cancers. The lowest rates are found in Western countries, South America and the Indian subcontinent. Intermediate rates prevail in Japan, the Middle East and the Mediterranean area.[10,94,96,99–102]

Whites, wherever they live, have a low incidence, even in Africa or South-East Asia where hepatocellular carcinoma is rampant in the native population. It has been suggested, and is probably true, that they are protected by maintaining the lifestyle and environment of their home countries. This applies even after several generations of 'expatriate' living as in East, Central and South Africa. The same is not true for Indians who settled in Singapore or Hong Kong since the end of the last century: their incidence rates are roughly double those observed in their home country. Chinese are at a high risk, whether they live in Shanghai, Singapore, Hong Kong or anywhere else. The probable reason is that most of them are first or second generation immigrants; after that, tumour incidence decreases slowly as it does also amongst Koreans and Japanese in California or Hawaii. The black population of the United States, West Indies and Brazil shows an incidence rate that is only marginally above that of whites, amongst whom they have lived since the beginning of the slave trade in the 17th century. Much of this variation in incidence rates in migrating populations can be explained by differences in hepatitis B virus carrier rates which they closely reflect.[10,97,99,101,102]

Lesser variations in tumour incidence have been observed in racially homogeneous countries such as Greece, Spain or Italy and in African countries like Kenya or Swaziland. In the former, this may be explained by differences in hepatitis B virus carriage, consumption of alcohol and smoking; in the latter, it may be related to variable levels of exposure to aflatoxins.[94–96] Higher than average European rates have also been reported in Switzerland, a highly industrialized country. This calls attention to the potential role of chemicals, also suspected in China, where high mortality rates from liver-cell carcinoma have been recorded in coastal and riverside areas with stagnant, polluted water supplies. Moving from a rural to an urban environment can be associated with an increase in risk as, apparently, in Norway and Poland, or with a decrease, as in South Africa.[10,99,100,102] Environmental changes again, are responsible: exposure to hepatotoxic agents and improved living standards, respectively.

Constant risk factors in all parts of the world are male sex, age and cirrhosis.[10,95,97,101,102] Males predominate over females particularly in high incidence areas, though the ratio may be exaggerated by incomplete registration of women. The mean age of patients is greater in low and intermediate than in high incidence areas, and Africans develop the tumour earlier in life than Asians. Cirrhosis, from whatever cause, appears to be a precancerous condition.

Emphasis in recent years has shifted from descriptive epidemiological studies to the identification of specific aetiological agents. It is unlikely that liver-cell carcinoma has a single cause and, in all probability, this tumour develops in a multifactorial and multistep manner that converges through mechanisms that may be shared by several agents.[101,103–107]

As regards the reported increase in the incidence of the disease in Western countries in particular, this is probably an artefact, due to 'diagnostic drift' caused by the greater availability and increased sophistication of specialist medical facilities.[108]

AETIOLOGY

The inter-relationships between tumour, virus, chemicals, hormones, alcohol, nutrition, and presence or absence of cirrhosis are complex.[101,103–107] The following is an account of current views and recent observations concerning each. Molecular biological techniques are likely to revolutionize this field, in which much of our knowledge is still based on circumstantial evidence.[109]

Table 16.2 The relative frequency of liver-cell carcinoma in the world, expressed as a number of cases/100 000 population/year

High (20–150)	Intermediate (5–20)	Low (less than 5)
East, West and Central Africa (blacks)	South-East Asia and South Africa (Indians)	North, West and Central Europe
South-East China	Japan	North and South America
Taiwan	Middle East	Australia
Korea	India, Pakistan	North and South Africa (Arabs, whites)
Thailand	South and East Europe	Central Asia
Vietnam	Central America	
Burma	Alaska	
Hong Kong		
Singapore		
Oceania		

Age and sex

The incidence of hepatocellular carcinoma increases with age in all populations but there is a tendency for it to fall off in the elderly.[10,94, 96, 99,102,110] In general, the age peak is inversely related to the frequency of the tumour, patients being the youngest in high and the oldest in low incidence areas. In Mozambique, 50% are less than 30 years old and the frequency of the tumour amongst them is 500 times higher than in the same age group in Western countries; the difference then falls to 15-fold in the elderly.[2] Marked age differences are also seen between whites and South-East Asians in California and whites and blacks in South Africa, whilst immigrants from India to South-East Asia, from Japan to Hawaii and from the Eastern Mediterranean area to Europe, Australia and the United States fall in between. Liver-cell carcinoma also occurs in childhood. This is most commonly seen in high incidence areas where it is associated with the acquisition of chronic hepatitis B virus infection early in life. In Western countries, congenital abnormalities and various inborn errors of metabolism account for some cases, and others are fibrolamellar carcinomas, a special subtype with a known predilection for the young.[111]

A male to female predominance is observed everywhere and ranges from 4:1 in low to 8:1 in high incidence areas.[10,94,96,99,102] The same is true in rats and mice, in which experimental liver tumours are more easily induced in males than in females.[112–114] Moreover, orchidectomy reduces the carcinogenic effect of chemicals in male rodents to the level found in females; implantation of stilboestrol or oestradiol pellets has a similar though not quite as marked effect.[114]

The observations in humans and findings in experimental animals suggest that sex hormones and/or receptors for them may play a role in the development of liver-cell carcinoma. Much work has been done recently in this area but the results are far from clear.[114a] The presence of androgen receptors in the normal liver has been both denied[115] and confirmed.[116,117] However, both groups of authors demonstrated these receptors in hepatocellular carcinomas and the suggestion has been made that this tumour is androgen dependent.[118] Liver-cell tumours associated with androgenic/anabolic steroids may regress after withdrawal of the drug,[39,51] as indeed do those induced by oral contraceptive steroids.[42–44] Androgen and oestrogen receptors in the cytosol and nuclei of normal and cancerous liver cells have been quantitated.[119] Androgen receptors were elevated in most tumours; results for oestrogen receptors were variable but tended to be of the same or a lower level. Androgen receptors in both normal and malignant liver cells specifically bind androgens,[120] and androgen receptor messenger RNAs have been demonstrated in both.[121] Oestrogen and progesterone receptors have also been reported in both liver-cell adenomas and carcinomas[122,123] and their levels correlated with that of androgen receptors:[124] the titre was highest for androgen, intermediate for oestrogen and lowest for progesterone receptors.

It is highly unlikely that sex steroids are carcinogenic by themselves but they may act as promoters of abnormal growth.[116,118,125,126] Recent therapeutic trials introducing several compounds that interfere with hormone action and receptors, such as tamoxifen and cytoproterone, have shown variable and disappointing results[125,127] though, in one study, there was some beneficial effect with prolonged survival.[127a] A search for others is continuing. A simple explanation for the higher frequency of liver-cell carcinoma amongst males has also been offered: they more often smoke and drink alcohol and suffer from cirrhosis more commonly.[128] However, it has been demonstrated that the risk of liver-cell carcinoma in cirrhosis is related to DNA synthesis rate in the liver and this is higher in men than in women.[128a]

Genetics, congenital anomalies and metabolic disorders

A genetic predisposition to cirrhosis and liver cancer has been produced in highly inbred strains of mice[129] but we have no evidence of this occurring in man. However, there are numerous rare examples of liver-cell carcinoma complicating diseases that are genetic, congenital or metabolic in origin and, in some instances, the tumour develops early in life.

MHC and blood group antigens

Analysis of major histocompatibility complex (MHC) antigens in 102 patients and 208 controls in South Africa failed to show a link with either hepatitis B virus infection or hepatocellular carcinoma.[130] The distribution of MHC and blood group antigens was also found to be the same in patients with the tumour and healthy controls in China.[131]

Family clusters

Five recent reports have documented 100 cases of liver-cell carcinoma in children aged 8 months to 16 years[132–137] which involved seven families for up to three generations.[134,136] Chronic hepatitis B virus infection was demonstrated in 95 cases and was invariably associated with both vertical (from mother to child) and horizontal (among siblings) transmission of the virus. Most cases occurred in boys, some were associated with cirrhosis and the tumour was rapidly progressive in all. It is not known whether additional environmental factors could have hastened tumour development but all reports have emphasized the need for early vaccination of children against the hepatitis B virus when the infection is clustered in families.

Congenital anomalies and syndromes

A growing number of inherited conditions are being catalogued in which hepatocellular carcinoma occurred on occasion.[111] Three cases have been reported in familial polyposis of the colon,[138-140] 6 in Alagille's syndrome,[141-143a] and 3 in ataxia-telangiectasia,[144] Others included hereditary haemorrhagic telangiectasia,[145] Byler-type familial cholestatic cirrhosis[146,147] as well as neonatal hepatitis/biliary atresia, congenital hepatic fibrosis, neurofibromatosis, Soto's syndrome, situs inversus and the fetal alcohol syndrome.[111,137] Some of these may have been due purely to chance.

Inborn errors of metabolism

The chronic form of hereditary tyrosinaemia (type I) carries the greatest risk of malignancy in this group of disorders. In one study, 16 of 43 patients developed liver-cell carcinoma despite dietary control.[148] The sequence of events is progression from micro- to macronodular cirrhosis, liver-cell dysplasia, elevated serum α-fetoprotein levels and, finally, hepatocellular carcinoma.[149,150] It is now recommended that hepatectomy and liver transplantation be carried out by two years of age.[149] The liver tumours that develop in type I glycogen storage disease are usually adenomas[57,58] but carcinoma has been described.[151] There are persistent reports of an association between liver-cell carcinoma and the hepatic types of porphyria, both acute intermittent and cutanea tarda,[152,153] in which the relative risk of malignancy has been calculated as 61-fold in a study of 245 patients.[154]

α_1-Antitrypsin (α_1AT) deficiency (see Ch. 4)

α_1-Antitrypsin is an inhibitor of serine proteinases which include trypsin, chymotrypsin and leucocyte elastase. It is synthesized in liver cells and then secreted into the blood stream. This process is under genetic control, for which up to 75 allelic variants are known. These are termed Pi (protease inhibitor) genes and are named after the electrophoretic or other properties of their protein product. PiZ is the variant associated with subnormal serum levels of α_1AT: 10–15% in PiZZ homozygotes and 50–60% in PiZS, M, F, etc. heterozygotes. The enzyme is normally produced in liver cells in α_1AT deficiency but it is not secreted. This leads to accumulation of PAS-positive, diastase-resistant globules that consist of α_1AT.

α_1AT deficiency is associated with neonatal jaundice and cirrhosis in early childhood and with pulmonary emphysema and cirrhosis in adult life. These and other aspects have been comprehensively reviewed[155-157] but many unanswered questions remain. Why is it, for example, that only 10–15% of PiZZ individuals develop any form of liver disease whilst Pi–(null) subjects, who do not produce

α_1AT at all, have normal livers but die early in life from emphysema? Many reports have both suggested[158,159] and refuted[160,161] an association between α_1AT deficiency and liver-cell carcinoma in both PiZ hetero- and homozygous individuals and in both low and high incidence areas for the tumour.[155-157] Most of the evidence in support for an association has come from Scandinavia, and the last word for the moment rests with Eriksson et al[162] who re-examined their data on all autopsies performed in the city of Malmö, Sweden, from 1963 to 1982. They concluded that there was a strong relationship between α_1AT deficiency and both cirrhosis and primary liver cancer. However, when the data were stratified for sex, these associations were statistically significant only for males. They suggested the possibility of additional exogenous factors such as alcohol or occupational toxins.

Other puzzling facets include the well-documented observations that α_1AT globules can be found in liver tumour cells, both of adenomas[76] and carcinomas,[163,164] in patients who do not have the PiZ gene and are not deficient in the enzyme. The simultaneous presence of α_1AT deficiency, copper storage and Mallory bodies has also been reported in 3 patients with hepatocellular carcinoma for no reason that could be ascertained.[165] The suggestion has been put forward that the inability to discharge α_1AT by the liver cells of PiZ carriers or by liver carcinoma cells may have a promoting effect on tumour growth by allowing proteases to destroy contact inhibition amongst transformed liver cells.[155,157]

Iron overload (see Ch. 5)

Genetic haemochromatosis is an autosomal recessive disorder that is associated with HLA-A3, B7 and B14 MHC antigens and a putative defect on the short arm of chromosome 6. It commonly affects males and results in cirrhosis of the liver. The risk of hepatocellular carcinoma is high and was found to be the cause of death in 22% of patients in a study covering 50 years from 1917 to 1968.[166] Mortality has decreased in recent years, and only 16 to 163 patients died of tumour in another study of patients diagnosed between 1959 and 1983.[167] The relative risk, however, was still 219-fold over the general population. All these patients were males and had cirrhosis though 11 of them no longer had an iron overload. In a 7-year follow-up study of 93 haemochromatosis patients, 7 developed hepatocellular carcinoma; again, all were male and had cirrhosis.[167a] Malignancy is rare in females or in the pre-cirrhotic phase of the disease.[168,168a] It has been suggested that iron itself may exert a carcinogenic effect through the production of free radicals or in association with alcohol or hepatitis B virus infection but there is no firm evidence for this.[169] It seems that the relationship is between male sex, cirrhosis and cancer and not between iron and cancer.[170] Proliferative, and often dysplastic iron-free foci of liver cells are present in the majority of cases before hepatocellular carcinoma develops.[168a] Non-hereditary iron overload syndromes have also been described, especially in Africans amongst whom liver-cell carcinoma is highly prevalent. Iron is ingested from home-made beer brewed in steel drums but it is no longer thought to be causally related to the tumour for which other aetiologies, namely hepatitis B virus infection and aflatoxins, are much more likely.

Copper storage

Large amounts of copper accumulate in Wilson's disease, another autosomal recessive condition that tends to affect males and results in cirrhosis. Ten patients with liver-cell carcinoma are on record, all of whom had cirrhosis of long duration, and 8 were male.[171] Hepatocellular carcinoma may also complicate primary biliary cirrhosis, another condition in which copper accumulates in the liver: 16 cases are on record[172,173] of whom 6 were males, a surprisingly high proportion in a disease that affects mainly females.

Membranous obstruction of the inferior vena cava

Reports have appeared from South Africa,[174] Japan[175] and occasionally elsewhere[176] of an association between abnormalities of the inferior vena cava and hepatocellular carcinoma. The exact incidence of the lesion is difficult to assess because it is seldom sought and is easily overlooked. Two types of occlusion have been described: a high membranous one where the vein joins the right atrium, and a fibrous occlusion of variable length below this level. The lesion has been regarded as congenital in nature due to malformation of the Eustachian valve[174] or as acquired due to mechanical injury, infection and thrombosis.[175] Whatever its aetiology, the obstruction is longstanding as the liver shows changes of chronic passive congestion. In South Africa, 20% of all cases with liver-cell carcinoma had the lesion at autopsy and 47.5% of patients with radiologically demonstrated caval obstruction during life subsequently developed carcinoma.[174]

Host–tumour interactions

Klein[177] speaks of tumour development as a play with many different *dramatis personae*. The main character, the villain, is the cancer cell which tries to evade or overcome the defensive responses of the host. These are mainly immunological and are directed against cell surface antigens; T and B cells, the complement system, natural killer cells and macrophages may all play a part. The various components of the response are not necessarily defensive and some actually facilitate growth.[178] In animals, tumours induced by a virus evoke a response that is the same against all tumours induced by the virus; the response to

tumours induced by chemicals is specific to individuals and not to the agents. In man, many examples have been recorded of spontaneous regression of in-situ and invasive cancers, disappearance of the primary tumour in the presence of metastases, unexpected survival and sudden precipitous growth. All these phenomena imply a defensive response or a failure of it, but many studies that have evaluated host immunity have been inconclusive and attempts made at immunotherapy, in most instances, have been fruitless.[179] As regards liver tumours, almost nothing is known about control by the host[180] and there is no evidence for any genetic or acquired alteration in immune responses to have a role in their development. The question is not whether immune responses can control neoplasia but why they so commonly fail to do so.

Nutrition

Malnutrition is common in most areas with a high incidence of liver-cell carcinoma but so are hepatitis B virus infection and exposure to hepatotoxic agents. Existing knowledge on diet and cancer indicates that it is over-nourishment, rather than lack of calories or deficiency of protein, that promotes tumour development.[181] Epidemiological studies indicate a relationship between high dietary fat, cholesterol and obesity and carcinomas of the breast and endometrium in women, carcinoma of the prostate in men, and carcinomas of the colon and pancreas in both sexes. Other, specific tumour-enhancing effects have been attributed to deficiencies of vitamins A, C and E and of the trace element selenium. Disturbance of immune defence mechanisms also occurs in protein deficiency, which is common in the tropics and in chronic liver disease of alcoholics in Western countries, but its role is in doubt. In one study from Japan, inadequate and unbalanced nutritional intake were commoner in patients with cirrhosis and hepatocellular carcinoma than in the general population but it was unclear whether this was a cause and effect relationship.[182] Prolonged parenteral nutrition in infancy may be complicated by cholestasis, liver fibrosis and cirrhosis; cases of liver-cell carcinoma are on record that occurred in infants at 6 and 26 months of age.[183,184]

Parasites

There is no evidence for a causative role for any of the large number of protozoa and helminths that affect man. Some, notably *Schistosoma mansoni* and *japonicum*, produce a fibrogenic response to eggs deposited in the liver and this is the most important cause of portal hypertension in sub-Saharan Africa, Brazil and South-East Asia.[185] Earlier suggestions that hepatic schistosomiasis may lead to neoplasia have not received support. Patients who develop hepatocellular carcinoma are found to have cirrhosis associated with serological markers of chronic hepatitis B virus infection. In Africa, a rapidly growing tumour may be confused with an amoebic abscess but there is no connection between the two. Malaria, trypanosomiasis and leishmaniasis may affect the immune system of the host, and indeed the peculiar geographical distribution of Burkitt's lymphoma and nasopharyngeal carcinoma have been attributed to the immunosuppressive effect of chronic malaria infection. However, there is no evidence for a role in liver-cell carcinoma, which is not linked epidemiologically to any of these infections.

Naturally occurring carcinogens

The term refers to a vast array of substances that have been found in drinking water, foodstuffs, native remedies and the like.[10,14,94-96,99-101,104,186] Most are only suspected to be carcinogens and few have been studied in any detail (Table 16.3). Interest in these agents seems to have waned in recent years, with the exception of mycotoxins which merit separate consideration.

Pyrrolizidine alkaloids are proven hepatotoxins. They are found in species of *Senecio*, *Crotalaria* and *Heliotropium* plants. The four listed in Table 16.3 are credited with the ability to induce tumours in the liver of rodents after conversion by the mixed-function oxidase system. Male rats and those on a low lipotrope diet are particularly susceptible. In man, acute poisoning from drinking herbal teas may result in acute liver failure whilst chronic ingestion leads to veno-occlusive disease as observed in Jamaica, India and Afghanistan. *Comfrey*, widely used in Western countries as a green vegetable, tea or animal fodder, is carcinogenic to rats but there are no reports of a similar effect in man. Cycads are palm-like plants which grow in many tropical countries and their seeds or roots are used as food in times of drought and famine. They contain β-glycosides generally known as *cycasins*. The active principle, methylazoxymethanol, is similar to dimethylnitrosamine. Cycasins readily produce liver tumours in many animals

Table 16.3 Naturally occurring carcinogens

Pyrrolizidine alkaloids:
    isatidine
    lasiocarpine
    monocrotaline
    retrorsin
Comfrey
Cycasins:
    methylazoxymethanol
Safrole
Tannic acid
Nitrosamines and nitrosamides
Mycotoxins:
    aflatoxins
    sterigmatocystin
    luteoskyrin
    cyclochlorotine

and are potentially hazardous to man. However, they are water-soluble and are removed by prolonged soaking during preparation of the plant prior to ingestion. *Safrole* occurs in many essential oils, formerly used as medicines and flavouring agents. It produces liver tumours in rodents and its use is no longer permitted. *Tannic acid* is a powerful liver carcinogen in rats. It is present in tea, coffee, beer and wine but there is no evidence to link it to liver-cell carcinoma in man.

N-nitroso compounds, such as *nitrosamines and nitrosamides*, should not be regarded simply as experimental laboratory agents that produce liver tumours in fish, rodents and mammals. Human exposure may occur in two ways, through ingestion of pre-formed compounds or simultaneous ingestion of nitrate and nitrosatable substances.[187] Pre-formed nitrosamines are found in many common foodstuffs like cheese, fish and meat products but generally in minute quantities. Higher levels have, however, been associated with specific processing conditions, e.g. frying. Formation of *N*-nitroso compounds from nitrite and secondary amines in the human stomach has also been demonstrated. A potential carcinogenic hazard thus exists to liver, stomach and bowel but its seriousness has not been determined.

Mycotoxins

The term applies to a large number of toxic metabolites produced by fungi some of which, notably aflatoxins, are carcinogenic to animals and may represent a hazard to populations in certain parts of the world.

Aflatoxins

Interest in fungi as causative agents of liver disease was stimulated by the outbreak of a mysterious disease which affected turkeys, ducklings and farm animals in the 1960s. This was soon traced to groundnut meal contaminated with the mould *Aspergillus flavus*. A number of closely related substances, known as aflatoxins, were isolated and found to be metabolic products of this fungus. Aflatoxins B1, B2, G1 and G2 are so designated because of their blue or yellow-green autofluorescence; of the four, B1 is the most potent. They can be measured in foodstuffs, and further derivatives such as P1 and M1 can be detected in the serum and body fluids. Their chemistry, mode of action and toxicity have been well studied and extensively reviewed.[10,94-96,99-101,188-190]

Aflatoxins have been found in peanut, soya bean, corn, rice, wheat, barley and cotton seed. Hot, humid climatic conditions and prolonged storage encourage the growth of fungi and lead to high levels of contamination. *Aspergillus flavus* is, in fact, the commonest cause of food spoilage in the tropics.

The effects of aflatoxins in animals vary from acute liver necrosis to dysplasia and the development of liver-cell carcinoma. The rat is the most susceptible species. The carcinogenic effect is dose dependent and it is more readily evident in males and young animals. Aflatoxins also produce liver tumours in the ferret, marmoset, tree shrew, duck and trout; of all species tested, only the mouse is resistant.

The risk of dietary exposure to aflatoxins and a high incidence of hepatocellular carcinoma coexist in many parts of Africa and South-East Asia[191–194] but a lack of association is also on record.[195] There are considerable difficulties in evaluating this relationship. Food samples from stores and markets may show a high level of contamination but this is reduced after selection by housewives and subsequent cooking; current levels of exposure are not necessarily relevant to past rates of tumour incidence; data on the latter may be incomplete and the time lag between ingestion and neoplasia in individuals is bound to vary. A recent large-scale follow-up study in Shanghai, comparing patients who developed liver-cell carcinoma with up to 10 controls who remained healthy, showed a strong relationship between exposure to aflatoxins and risk of tumour.[196] The method used was urinary assay for aflatoxin B1, its derivatives P1 and M1, and DNA-adduct AFB1-N^7-Gua, which are regarded as reliable indicators of recent exposure. A retrospective study of urinary aflatoxin metabolite levels and background rates of hepatocellular carcinoma in Taiwan also showed a strong correlation that was independent of other risk factors.[196a] Assays for serum albumin adducts to aflatoxin are also available now and may assess dietary intake in the longer term. A study using one such assay demonstrated a high prevalence of aflatoxin–albumin adducts in sera of pregnant women and in cord blood samples of their offspring at delivery in the Gambia.[197] The conclusion drawn was that in-utero exposure occurs in Africa and may account for the early onset of liver-cell carcinoma for which this geographical area is so well known. Associated risk factors include alcohol, smoking and, most of all, chronic hepatitis virus B infection[193,194,196] but, even allowing for these, exposure to aflatoxins remains a strong and independent predictor of malignancy.[191]

The most interesting observations that have come to light recently are those concerning the tumour suppressor gene p53. Mutations are commonly found in cancers at many sites and often lead to synthesis of a faulty protein that has lost its normal growth regulatory function.[198] A selective guanine to thymine (G to T) transversion at codon 249 occurs specifically in some hepatocellular carcinomas and is the same as that caused by exposure to aflatoxin B1. Two reports, from China[199] and South Africa,[200] demonstrated this mutational 'hotspot' in up to half of cases. In a subsequent report of results on 167 tumour samples from 14 countries, G to T transversion at codon 249 was found in 12 of 72 from Africa and South-East Asia and in none of 95 from North America, Europe, the Middle East and Japan.[201] Within Africa the mutation was more frequent in Mozambique (a high risk area) than in Transkei (a low risk area). Multiple mutations of the p53 gene have been demonstrated in a small proportion of cases of hepatocellular carcinoma in Britain,[201a,b] the United States,[201c–g] Japan,[201h–j] and other countries. Some of these were associated with loss of heterozygosity on a number of chromosomes and a few had evidence of hepatitis B or C virus infection. It has been suggested that accumulation of changes in multiple tumour suppressor genes, including p53, are involved in the progression of liver cancer.

Other mycotoxins[186,188,189–191]

These include *sterigmatocystin*, which is also produced by *Aspergillus* species and is similar to aflatoxins, but the dose required to produce tumours in the rat is much higher and a survey of foodstuffs in South Africa failed to indicate that it was a health hazard. *Luteoskyrin* and *cyclochlorotine* are metabolites of *Penicillium islandicum* which is frequently found in spoiled rice and grain in Japan, Ethiopia and South Africa. A carcinogenic effect has been demonstrated in rodents but there is no evidence of a risk to man.

Synthetic chemicals and occupational hazards

Hundreds of chemicals — some purely experimental, others industrial — can produce liver damage and tumours in rodents when administered in large amounts or can be shown to have a mutagenic effect in test systems such as the one devised by Ames[94–96,104,186–188] Indeed, both rodent toxicity assays and the Ames test have been used on a large scale and for many years to identify carcinogens in, and eliminate them from, foodstuffs, cosmetics, cleaning agents, pharmaceuticals, pesticides and a myriad of other man-made products. The chemicals which have caused most concern are nitrites, hydrocarbons, solvents, organochlorine pesticides, primary metals and polychlorinated biphenyls.[94–96,186] However, convincing epidemiological evidence is lacking for a carcinogenic role in most instances. A lively controversy on the subject has been provoked recently by Ames himself, following the publication of a series of review articles on carcinogens and human health in the journal *Science*; this has been summarized[202] and the main points are as follows.

Tumours are thought to arise from damage to nuclear DNA in cells which then escape normal repair mechanisms and undergo permanent mutation. An essential prerequisite for this change is mitosis, which 'fixes' the abnormality in the cell line. Ames contends that tumours that develop after the administration of artificially high doses of chemicals to rats and mice represent false positive results for carcinogenicity because, at such toxic levels, they produce a chronic mitogenic response. The same might also be said about mutagenicity assays which involve rapidly dividing bacteria. In low doses and often trace amounts, the same chemicals do not stimulate mitosis in man and therefore no harm results. In other words, Ames has questioned the fundamental assumption that an extrapolation from high dose to low dose effect is ever justified. He has suggested that the most important environmental agents are those whose chief effect is to cause chronic division of cells; these include tobacco smoke, alcohol, chronic virus infection, steroids and prolonged low dose ingestion of natural compounds such as aflatoxins. The argument does not invalidate acute animal experiments as valuable tools for the study of changes that accompany neoplastic development but it does raise the question of 'Which causes of cancer matter in the real world?'[202]

Studies aimed at specific occupational hazards have also produced inconclusive results. A large-scale case–control study in New Jersey, USA, showed weak odds ratios for male farm labourers, wine makers, bartenders, dry cleaners and petrol station attendants and for female cleaning service workers; hepatitis and cirrhosis could not be evaluated.[203] In a similar study from Alabama, USA,[204] no positive association was found between liver-cell carcinoma and any particular occupation, industry or chemical exposure, whilst in yet another, from New York,[205] positive associations were found with employment in household work, cleaning, food and beverage services and transport: cirrhosis was an additional factor in all of them. The one industrial agent that may rarely cause hepatocellular carcinoma is vinyl chloride monomer;[206] this is discussed, along with Thorotrast and arsenic, under angiosarcoma of the liver (p 16.39–16.40).

Iatrogenic agents: drugs and radiation

The aetiological role of oral contraceptive and androgenic/anabolic steroids in liver-cell adenoma is beyond doubt (p. 16.3).

As regards usage of oral contraceptive steroids, a number of reports of malignant change in liver-cell adenoma or de novo liver-cell carcinoma have appeared, usually after many years of exposure to the drug.[45,47,50,207,208] In a study of 126 cases of liver-cell carcinoma in women during the period 1970–1975 in the United States,[209] it was found that 39 had used an oral contraceptive, 26 had not, and the history was not known in 61. In users, the peak incidence occurred in the age group 26–35 years whilst in non-users the tumour was commoner in those aged over 35; the age distribution fell between users and non-users in those with an unknown history. A report from the United Kingdom in 1980[207] documented 3 liver-cell adenomas and 7 hepatocellular carcinomas; 8 in all had used oral contraceptive steroids for 5 years or longer. Attention was drawn to the importance of tumour subtype in a study of 128 cases of liver-cell carcinoma in women between 1953 and 1980.[210] There were 48 patients under the age of 40, and 13 of these had used the drug. However, the majority of tumours in young women and in those who had been on the pill were fibrolamellar carcinomas which have a known predilection for young people of both sexes. The conclusion reached was that the association was between a particular type of liver cancer and age, and that the use of oral contraceptive steroids was incidental. Further studies, however, both from the United States[211,212] and the United Kingdom,[213] showed a significantly greater usage of the drug in women with liver-cell carcinoma and a rise in mortality rates from the tumour in young women from the late 1970s. Two groups of investigators from the United Kingdom[214,215] have calculated the relative risk of liver-cell carcinoma in oral contraceptive users as 7.2 and 20.1 after 8 years or more on the drug and yet another study from the United States put the risk at 5.5-fold after 5 years of use.[216] The association between liver-cell carcinoma and oral contraceptive steroid usage now seems certain in areas of low incidence for the tumour but the absolute, as opposed to the relative, risk is small and the tumour remains rare.[217] There is no evidence that oral contraceptives increase the risk in high tumour incidence areas where hepatitis B virus infection is endemic.[218,219]

The number of liver tumours associated with androgenic/anabolic steroids is small. These have been regarded as carcinomas on account of their histological appearance but they seldom produce α-fetoprotein and do not metastasize; most are therefore liver-cell adenomas and not carcinomas.[19,34–36,51,220] They have been seen in two groups of patients: in children with Fanconi's syndrome and other refractory anaemias, and in adults with sexual problems — impotence, hypogonadism and female-to-male transsexualism. Peliosis may develop in these tumours.[35,36,39] Two cases, allegedly malignant, have been reported in athletes/body-builders on anabolic steroids over long periods.[40,221]

Amongst a variety of drugs, single anecdotal case reports have incriminated methotrexate, danazol and tamoxifen[222] and, more recently, cytoproterone acetate.[223] Tamoxifen is undoubtedly capable of inducing liver cancer in rats.[223a,b]

Ionizing radiation, which includes radioactivity and X-rays, has been held to be carcinogenic to the liver.[224] In animals, tumour induction depends on age and sex, dose of radiation and survival time, mitotic agents such as carbon tetrachloride or partial hepatectomy, state of nutrition and other, poorly understood factors. In man, therapeutic doses lead to cell death and any carcinogenic effect can only operate at low doses and before repair can take place. Once again, this necessitates a mitotic agent as cell turnover in the normal liver is low. One radioactive agent, however, that undoubtedly causes liver tumours is Thorotrast (thorium dioxide). These are usually angiosarcomas and bile-duct carcinomas but a few cases of liver-cell carcinoma are on record.[225-228] Thorotrast, once introduced into the body, emits low-dose alpha radiation for the duration of the life of the individual. On the other hand, the one-dose radiation suffered by survivors of the atomic bombs dropped on Hiroshima and Nagasaki did not lead to an increase in liver tumours.[229]

Alcohol, tobacco and other cofactors

A history of chronic alcohol abuse is frequently found in patients with hepatocellular carcinoma, particularly in low incidence areas where hepatitis B virus infection is uncommon.[10,94-104] Alcohol has also been incriminated in the genesis of carcinomas at other sites, notably the mouth, larynx and oesophagus, where the evidence for an aetiological role is much stronger.[230-232] Alcohol may, however, act as a co-carcinogen with other agents, notably hepatitis B virus infection, aflatoxins and smoking, in addition to its general role as a cirrhosis-inducing agent.

Alcohol, by itself, has never been demonstrated to have a carcinogenic effect in experimental animals. Problems also remain with the different effects of the amount, rate and route of administration.[232,233] Alcohol is a powerful inducer of the microsomal cytochrome *P*-450 biotransformation system which is responsible for the metabolic activation and inactivation of diverse chemical carcinogens. The latter include aflatoxins, and a synergistic effect has been demonstrated in a case–control study in the Philippines.[234] Individuals consuming more than both 24 g alcohol and 4 µg of aflatoxin B_1 per day had a 35-fold increase in relative risk of liver-cell carcinoma, whereas the risk was halved by similar aflatoxin exposure but little or no alcohol consumption. Cytochrome *P*-450 is also highly inducible by smoking and excessive tobacco use has been found to be a significant risk factor, either alone or in combination with alcohol and chronic hepatitis B virus infection.[235-240] Other effects of alcohol that may have a role in liver carcinogenesis include inhibition of DNA repair, enhancement of integration of genetic material from the hepatitis B virus, formation of adducts with acetaldehyde, altered steroid metabolism and an immunosuppressive effect.[233-235] The greatest interest, perhaps, has been generated by reports of a higher than expected prevalence of chronic hepatitis B virus infection amongst alcoholics, either in a serologically demonstrable, replicative or as a seronegative, integrated form. The evidence for the former seems reasonably convincing[235-239] but it is of variable strength and the methodology employed in some studies has been questioned. In any event, the greatest odds ratios are associated with hepatitis B virus infection, and those for alcohol or smoking are much less.[240a] Earlier reports that hepatitis B virus DNA exists in an integrated form in the genome of liver-cell carcinoma cells in the majority of alcoholic cirrhotic patients without serological evidence of infection[241] have

not been substantiated by others[242] and the matter remains controversial; more sensitive techniques, such as the polymerase chain reaction, may clarify the situation.[243] Recently, an association of alcohol with hepatitis C virus infection alone[244] or with hepatitis B virus as well[245] has also been demonstrated in patients with hepatocellular carcinoma. One thing is certain about the role, if any, of alcohol: continued consumption is not necessary for the development of liver-cell carcinoma once cirrhosis is established and the risk actually increases with time after cessation of drinking.[246] The overall life-time risk, culled from many studies,[10,94-104] seems to be around 15%.

Another curious facet arises from the observation that Mallory bodies occur in liver-cell carcinoma cells of alcoholic and non-alcoholic patients alike[247,248] as indeed they do also in liver-cell adenomas.[77] This points to some sort of a link in the pathogenesis of alcoholic liver disease and of liver cancer but it could equally represent a secondary disturbance in intermediate filament metabolism.

Hepatitis B virus

The virology, mode of transmission and natural history of infections with the hepatitis viruses A, B, C, D and E (HAV, HBV, HCV, HDV, and HEV) are discussed in Chapter 6. An encounter with HAV and HEV does not lead to chronic liver disease and HDV requires the presence of HBV in the liver either simultaneously (coinfection) or previously (superinfection). Both HBV and HCV may become established as a carrier state and lead to chronic hepatitis, cirrhosis and liver-cell carcinoma. HBV is the more important of the two and will be discussed first; our knowledge of diseases associated with HCV is still evolving.

Generally speaking, detection of HBV surface antigen (HBsAg) and core antibody (anti-HBc) indicate active infection, and the presence of 'e' antigen (HBeAg) a high level of replication. The level of these markers in the blood declines later in the course of chronic infection when HBV becomes integrated in the nuclei of liver cells. The risk of malignancy probably relates both to the replicative phase, through continuing liver-cell damage due to chronic hepatitis and cirrhosis, and to the integrated state when oncogenic events may occur. HBV is transmissible to the chimpanzee but no tumour has yet developed in this animal. On the other hand, HBV-like viruses cause hepatitis, cirrhosis and liver-cell carcinoma in woodchucks, squirrels and ducks: these are collectively known as the hepadna (hepatitis DNA) viruses.

The complex relationships between HBV and hepatocellular carcinoma are best discussed under separate headings. Some aspects, namely the influences of age and sex and cofactors such as alcohol, aflatoxins and smoking, have been covered in the preceding sections; the role of cirrhosis will be further analysed below. Table 16.4 lists the main lines of evidence that link HBV with liver-cell

Table 16.4 The main points of evidence for an aetiological association between the hepatitis B virus (HBV) and liver-cell carcinoma (LCC)

HBV carrier rate matches incidence of LCC
Strength of relationship in case–control studies
Prospective studies and follow-up
Greater risk of malignancy in cirrhosis due to HBV
Liver-cell dysplasia, LCC and HBV
Presence of integrated HBV DNA in LCC
Production of HBV antigens by LCC cell lines in culture
Molecular biological studies
HBV-like viruses in animals with LCC

carcinoma based on hundreds of original articles and many reviews.[10,94–107,249–261a,b]

Geographical distribution of hepatitis B virus carrier state

Areas where chronic HBV infection is common include most parts of Africa below the Saharan desert belt, South-East Asia, China and Oceania; the virus is uncommon in Western Europe, North America and Australia; an intermediate prevalence is seen in Japan, India, the Middle East and Mediterranean countries.[10,15,94,96,99,100,102,249–251,257,259] Indeed, maps and tabulations have been constructed that show almost identical frequencies of HBV carriage rates and incidence of liver-cell carcinoma.[94,96,98–100,102,249–251,253] Greenland Eskimos seem to be an exception: a 10% population infection rate is not matched by a 2.3/100 000/year tumour incidence.[262] The same does not apply to Alaskan Eskimos but they also show unusual features, namely an association of hepatocellular carcinoma with chronic hepatitis rather than cirrhosis.[263]

Variations in tumour incidence within a country or region generally relate to differences in HBsAg carriage rate.[264,265] Pockets of high frequency for both HBV infection and liver-cell carcinoma are found in areas where neither is common and are confined to population subsets, e.g. Oriental immigrants in the United States and elsewhere, Mozambican Shangaans who go to work in the mines of South Africa and, generally, in recently arrived communities from high incidence areas anywhere.[10,15,94,96,98–100] Interesting studies have also been carried out on those who had seen military service in the tropics during World War II. British ex-servicemen showed an elevated rate of HBV infection, cirrhosis and hepatocellular carcinoma[266] but US veterans did not.[267,267a] Thus, the geographical association of the virus with cancer is almost, but not quite, universal.

It is generally agreed that a particularly high risk of acquisition of the chronic HBV carrier state and of the subsequent development of liver-cell carcinoma is associated with infection at or near birth or in childhood.[10,94,96,98–100,250–253] The risk is further increased in families.[132–136] Perinatal and childhood transmission are well recognized in South-East Asia and in tropical Africa. Among those infected at birth, the likelihood of becoming a carrier is approximately 95%, which may be explained by the immaturity of the immune system in the newborn. The risk falls to around 40% in those infected in childhood. In both instances, the mother rather than the father is the source of infection, directly or through siblings. Significantly, she is likely to be positive not only for HBsAg and anti-HBc but also for HBeAg, i.e. to be a highly replicative, infectious source of the virus. In adults, the risk of the carrier state after an encounter with HBV is 10% or less.[250–253]

Case–control studies

Numerous reports from many countries have uniformly and conclusively shown a much higher frequency of hepatitis B virus markers in patients with hepatocellular carcinoma than in controls, whether these were healthy blood donors, office workers, villagers, or hospital patients with other types of cancer or other forms of liver disease. This holds true even after allowing for varying carrier rates in different populations.[10,94,96,98–100,250–253] Thus, in tropical Africa and South-East Asia where the background infection rate may be 10–20%, patients with liver-cell carcinoma are positive for HBsAg and/or HBcAg in 70–95% of cases; in Western countries the figures are less than 1% and 20–25% respectively but the strength of the association is just as strong. Single-centre studies from Europe, North America and South Africa, dealing with patients from a variety of ethnic origins, have also shown appropriately low and high infection rates in whites and in blacks or Orientals, whilst those from the Eastern Mediterranean, Middle East or India were in an intermediate position, with liver-cell cancer rates to match.

Prospective studies and follow up

Long-term follow-up studies have been of the greatest interest. In Taiwan, a total of 22 707 male Chinese government employees were followed up for a mean of 4.7, 6.2 and 8.9 years for the purposes of three successive reports.[252,259,268] They were chosen because of their high HBV carrier rate and high incidence of hepatocellular carcinoma; all had life insurance policies provided by the State; an accurate record of causes of illness and death was kept in all cases. Of the total enrolled between 1975 and 1978, 3454 (15.2%) were HBsAg positive, 2248 (9.9%) were anti-HBc positive, 15 570 (68.6%) were anti-HBs positive and 1272 (5.6%) were negative for all three HBV markers. By 31 December 1986, 202 000 man-years of follow up were available for evaluation. The results were striking: 152 of 161 cases of liver-cell carcinoma developed in HBsAg carriers and 9 in those positive for anti-HBc, 7 of whom were also positive for anti-HBs. No case occurred in individuals who were negative for all three HBV markers on enrolment. HBsAg emerged as the most significant predictor of liver-cell carcinoma from this study with a relative death risk of 98.4, whilst the figure for mortality from cirrhosis was 24; these figures exceed the relative lung cancer risk in heavy smokers, for example. Large-scale prospective studies are difficult, time-consuming and expensive, but limited undertakings in Japan, England and Wales and the United States have also provided evidence in support of a high life-time risk of cirrhosis and liver-cell carcinoma in individuals chronically infected with HBV.[96,98–100,252,254–257,259–261]

Subtypes

The relationship of HBsAg subtypes (a, d, y, r and w) to risk of developing hepatocellular carcinoma was also studied but no evidence has come to light of an 'oncogenic strain'; moreover, expression of these subtypes may differ among normal hepatocytes and tumour cells in the same individual, an observation that has no explanation at present.[269]

Hepatitis D virus (delta agent)

Earlier studies of cases of liver-cell carcinoma with or without cirrhosis suggested that HDV infection was as common as or less common than in patients with chronic hepatitis or cirrhosis without the tumour and that the presence of this virus was related to its geographical distribution in different populations.[270–272] The obligatory symbiosis of HDV with HBV makes evaluation of its role difficult but more recent evidence indicates that HDV infection imposes an additional burden on the already damaged liver. Patients with liver-cell carcinoma and both HBV and HDV infection are younger than those with HBV but without HDV; this has been attributed to the fact that cirrhosis develops at an earlier age in the former group.[273,274] In chronic woodchuck hepatitis virus and HDV infection, liver-cell carcinoma also develops much earlier than in animals with woodchuck hepatitis virus infection alone.[275] Severe necro-inflammatory liver disease associated with florid replication of both viruses may represent an additional promoting effect in both man and the woodchuck.

Integration of hepatitis B virus in the liver

During the replicative phase of the infection, HBV antigens (HBsAg, HBcAg and HBeAg) are readily identifiable in the non-tumorous liver of 'healthy' carriers and patients with cirrhosis and hepatocellular carcinoma by immunohistochemical means, but they are not found in tumour cells.[276] Nevertheless, a human liver cancer cell line grown in culture has been shown to produce HBsAg[277] and transplantation of tumour tissue into nude mice has resulted in the production of all three major antigens as well as HBV DNA polymerase;[278] moreover, a liver-cell carcinoma line transfected with cloned viral DNA was shown to pro-

duce free Dane particles, i.e. the complete virion.[279] Clearly, HBV cannot be visualized in tumour cells in a replicative form but it can be demonstrated, once integrated, by molecular biological techniques.

Oncogenic viruses, whether they be DNA viruses or RNA retroviruses, integrate into the genome of the cell which then undergoes malignant transformation. HBV is a small double-stranded DNA virus with genes that encode for HBsAg, HBcAg, HBeAg, DNA polymerase and the X protein. Replication requires reverse transcription, and integration can occur, both being features of the life cycle of known animal oncogenic viruses.[280] Numerous studies have been carried out during the last decade on the presence, mode and patterns of integration of HBV in liver cells prior to, or after, the development of liver-cell carcinoma in patients who did or did not have serological evidence of infection; the results have been complex and, at times, conflicting.[243,254–258,260,261,281–285] Some of the discrepancies at least may represent technical problems such as the efficiency of hybridization, or the choice of particular restriction enzymes; artefacts, due to contamination, are difficult to eliminate in polymerase chain reaction assays in particular. Integration of HBV DNA precedes the development of hepatocellular carcinoma and it occurs in the majority of tumours from both HBsAg positive and negative patients but more commonly after replication of the virus has declined or ceased and the patient has become seronegative. A preferential site for HBV insertion has not been identified so far and integration appears to be multiple and random. In a few instances, viral DNA sequences have been found within or near cellular proto-oncogenes but these seem to be exceptional, and probably chance events. Integrated sequences may also show deletions and rearrangements or be split into fragments. HBV DNA may not be found in the genome of liver cells from a minority of HBV-infected patients, which indicates that integration is not an obligatory oncogenic event. Moreover, HBV does not possess a gene that resembles any known oncogene.

The smallest HBV genomic open reading frame encodes for a protein of 154 amino acids known as the X protein. When integrated, this is capable of activating cellular genes at a distance, a phenomenon known as 'transactivation'. The X gene of HBV and the *tat* gene of HTLV-1 (human T-cell leukaemia virus-1) are positioned identically with respect to their genomic organization. The *tat* gene is probably essential for the transforming effect of HTLV-1, and the X gene may play a similar role; it has, indeed, been shown to influence the expression of cellular proto-oncogenes C-*fos* and C-*myc*.[283,285,286] Hepatitis B X gene is expressed in hepatocellular carcinoma tissue and it activates protein kinase C, a mediator of cell transformation by various tumour-promoting agents.[286a,b]

Molecular biological techniques have also enabled studies to be carried out on the clonality of hepatocellular carcinomas. Several investigators have found that, using HBV DNA as a genetic marker, identical patterns of integration were present in multifocal liver-cell carcinomas and in primary tumours and their metastases. This established their origin from a single clone of cells in which HBV integration had occurred before malignant transformation.[287,288] However, different patterns of integration have also been demonstrated in one case where two nodules of hepatocellular carcinoma in the same liver appeared to be of independent derivation.[289]

Hepadnaviruses in animals

Liver-cell carcinoma has been observed in several mammalian and avian species in association with chronic infection by HBV-like hepadnaviruses. These include the woodchuck hepatitis virus (WHV) of *Marmota monax*, the ground squirrel hepatitis virus (GSHV) of *Spermophilus beecheyi* and the duck hepatitis virus (DHV) of *Anas domesticus*.[14,96,254,282,290] Other hepadnaviruses have been described in tree squirrels, stink snakes, kangaroos and probably other birds and mammals but these are not associated with hepatocellular carcinoma. WHV may be directly oncogenic: all woodchucks infected at birth in the laboratory become carriers and develop liver-cell carcinoma within 36 months. Infected adult animals tend to revert to anti-WHV serological status and seldom become carriers or develop tumours. The sequence of events in carrier woodchucks has been thoroughly studied.[14,291,292] It shows a continuum from normal liver to hyperplastic nodules and liver-cell dysplasia and finally overt hepatocellular carcinoma. The rest of the liver shows chronic hepatitis and extramedullary haemopoiesis but not cirrhosis. WHV is present in both replicative and integrated forms throughout.[293] The changes in ground squirrels and ducks have been less well studied but are probably similar.

Prevention through vaccination

The ultimate proof of the causative role of HBV in liver-cell carcinoma is yet to come. Effective immunization against the virus in populations with a high incidence of the tumour must result in a substantial decline. Unfortunately, poor health care resources do not allow for mass immunization in countries that would benefit most. Safe and effective vaccines, either plasma-derived or yeast recombinant, are available but still expensive. Strategies aim at vaccinating infants and young children in South-East Asia and Africa and high risk groups in Europe, North America and elsewhere.[294] In Taiwan a nationwide immunization programme was introduced in 1984 and led to a fall in HBsAg carrier rate amongst children from 10% to 2%.[295] A more recent report documented a 100% protective efficacy rate in neonates.[295a] In the Gambia, a limited field trial proved to be 97% effective in preventing

chronic infection.[296] However, the existing reservoir of carriers is estimated to be 300 million and elimination of the virus from them is impossible: millions are destined to die for decades to come.

Hepatitis C virus

It has long been recognized that a past history of post-transfusion hepatitis, in the absence of HBV markers, was a risk factor for hepatocellular carcinoma, especially in Western countries. This was attributed to 'non A, non B' hepatitis which also occurred in sporadic and epidemic forms.[297] The riddle was finally solved when molecular cloning techniques had led to the development of serological tests for the detection of HCV.[298] These are still being refined and no doubt some earlier results will have to be revised. From 1989 onwards, a large number of case-control studies have been published to show evidence of an association between chronic HCV infection and both cirrhosis and liver-cell carcinoma from Spain,[299] Italy,[300-302] Japan,[303,304] South Africa[305] and the United States.[306,307] The situation at present is reminiscent of the 1970s when similar studies poured forth to establish the link of HBV with hepatocellular carcinoma. Much is yet to be learnt about HCV, e.g. whether it also exists in an integrated form like HBV or whether its effect, like that of HDV, is exerted through an additional necro-inflammatory burden on the liver. Recent epidemiological surveys indicate that HCV seropositivity in hepatocellular carcinoma is substantial in many countries.[307a,b] A method for the detection of HCV RNA by the polymerase chain reaction has been developed and it demonstrated its presence in both liver and tumour tissue.[307c]

THE ROLE OF CIRRHOSIS

It is evident from the foregoing that almost any form of chronic liver disease that leads to cirrhosis may be complicated by liver-cell carcinoma; therefore cirrhosis, from whatever cause, is in itself a precancerous condition. Considerable variations exist, however, between areas with a low or high incidence of the tumour that may reflect on aetiology, duration of cirrhosis and its morphology.[10,14,98,101,102,104,254-256,308-310,310a] The main differences are summarized in Table 16.5 from data collected from many parts of the world.

In low incidence areas for hepatocellular carcinoma, such as Europe and North America, cirrhosis is common, usually alcoholic in origin, and carries a relatively low risk of tumour development. In this setting, cirrhosis is micronodular initially but becomes macronodular with prolonged survival, and the risk of malignancy persists even after cessation of drinking.[246] The majority of patients die of cirrhosis rather than cancer. Male preponderance is moderate and patients are middle-aged or elderly. HBV infection

Table 16.5 Clinicopathological patterns of liver-cell carcinoma and cirrhosis

	Europe and America	Africa and South-East Asia
Incidence of liver-cell carcinoma	Low	High
Age and sex of patients	Middle to old age, male	Young to middle age, male
Incidence of cirrhosis	Common	Uncommon (?)
Aetiology of cirrhosis	Alcoholic	Hepatitis B virus, aflatoxins
Duration of cirrhosis	Long	Short (?)
Morphology of cirrhosis	Micronodular	Macronodular
Liver-cell carcinoma arising in cirrhosis	80–90%	60–70%
Cirrhosis terminating in liver-cell carcinoma	5–15%	40–50%
Relative proportion of liver-cell carcinoma and cirrhosis	Cirrhosis outnumbers liver-cell carcinoma	True incidence of cirrhosis unknown but probably less than liver-cell carcinoma

seems to carry a relatively minor role. Cirrhosis precedes tumour and the typical presentation of liver-cell carcinoma is an abrupt and rapid deterioration of the condition of a cirrhotic patient.[14,104,255,309,310]

In high tumour incidence areas of tropical Africa and South-East Asia, the prevalence of cirrhosis is poorly documented and may be, by itself, relatively uncommon. Alcoholism is rare and most cases of hepatocellular carcinoma are related to chronic HBV infection acquired early in life. The characteristic presentation is acute and is not preceded by previous signs or symptoms of liver disease. Nevertheless, 'silent cirrhosis' is still found in the majority of cases, though not quite in such high proportion as in low incidence areas. The morphological pattern of cirrhosis is macronodular and usually of the so-called incomplete septal type. The life-time risk of cirrhosis terminating in liver-cell carcinoma is high. Male predominance is more marked than it is in low incidence areas and patients are often young, in their 30s or 40s, particularly in Africa.[14,104,256,309,310]

Many explanations, and permutations thereof, have been put forward regarding the role of cirrhosis in the pathogenesis of hepatocellular carcinoma: clearly, the former is neither an essential prerequisite nor is the latter an inevitable consequence. One explanation is that the two simply share a common cause; this does not explain the variability of the risk of malignancy associated with particular aetiologies — low in the case of alcohol and high in chronic HBV infection, for example. Another is that neoplasia is an inevitable consequence of hyperplasia that is inherent in the cirrhotic process; this cannot be true as most patients with any form of chronic liver disease do not develop the tumour even after many years. The third, most plausible, explanation is that cirrhosis increases the susceptibility of the liver to malignant change, the magnitude of which depends on additional factors which include all those discussed in the preceding section. This certainly best fits the epidemiological evidence and is also compatible with experimental studies. Neoplastic development in the liver is seen as a multi-step process that is triggered by a variety of events.[14,101,103–107,309–311] The normal liver is mitotically inactive but, when stimulated to divide, it

becomes exquisitely sensitive to carcinogenesis.[312] Sustained and rapid proliferation of liver cells occurs in man in a variety of conditions that end in cirrhosis. This prevents the repair of any damage to DNA by viruses or chemicals and the abnormality is then 'fixed' and transmitted to the progeny, giving rise to an altered cell line. The 'right' combination of sites of damage that result in neoplastic transformation is an improbable and rare event, hence it takes time for the tumour to develop. In this light, cirrhosis may be seen as a promoter of neoplastic transformation after initiation by a variety of agents. From many studies, HBV-associated cirrhosis has emerged as the one most likely to be complicated by liver-cell carcinoma.[98,101,102,254–256,309,313–315]

The tumour also occurs in the absence of cirrhosis in a small, but significant, proportion of cases.[316–318] In high incidence areas, most relate to chronic HBV infection and may occur in childhood. In low incidence areas they form a heterogenous group but HBV, synthetic gonadal steroids and, possibly, chemicals are causative factors. The fibrolamellar subtype of liver-cell carcinoma is exceptional in that it is not associated with any of these aetiologies, and arises in normal livers and equally in both sexes.

PRECANCEROUS CHANGES IN THE HUMAN LIVER

The multi-step development of hepatocellular carcinoma in laboratory animals, its relevance to man and the interplay with viruses have already been alluded to[14,101,103–107,319,320] and are discussed in the second part of this chapter (see p. 681). Morphologically, the abnormal hepatocyte populations that precede the development of overt, metastasizing cancer may appear as hyperplastic areas, clear cell, acidophilic or basophilic cell foci, 'tigroid' cells, oval cells, megalocytosis and so forth; the gradual loss of adult liver-cell enzymes and the appearance of fetal enzymes are well documented: the roles of proto-oncogenes or tumour suppressor genes are being explored. Ethical considerations prohibit the study of the sequence of events in man and we still have comparatively little knowledge of what precedes the development of malignancy in the human liver. Two lesions, however, adenomatous hyperplasia and liver-cell dysplasia, have received the most attention.

Adenomatous hyperplasia

Regenerative liver nodules in cirrhosis are an integral part of the process but may occasionally grow to a large size and appear tumour-like. A number of terms have been applied to these lesions: 'hepatocellular pseudotumour', 'macroregenerative nodule', 'adenomatous hyperplasia' or 'adenomatous hyperplastic nodule' and 'dysplastic nodule',[321] of which 'adenomatous hyperplasia' is the most frequently used.

No satisfactory definition exists of what should be referred to as adenomatous hyperplasia in terms of size; reported examples have ranged from 1 to 15 cm, but most measured 2–3 cm.[321] They are readily detected by modern imaging methods and usually in individuals who are being screened for hepatocellular carcinoma. They have been reported to be larger and/or more numerous in the presence of the tumour,[322,323] to contain 'nodules in nodules',[324,325] to show changes variously described as 'atypical', 'dysplastic' or 'early malignant',[323,326–328] and to undergo malignant transformation over time as evidenced by doubling in volume and changes in imaging characteristics.[329] Almost all recent studies have been published from Japan but the existence of large nodules in cirrhosis has been recognized for a long time in Europe and the United States, albeit considered to be a rare occurrence.

Adenomatous hyperplastic nodules may be partly or completely surrounded by a fibrous rim and typically bulge on their cut surface. The surrounding liver tissue may appear compressed. There are no internal septa or a central scar as in focal nodular hyperplasia and no necrosis or haemorrhage as in liver-cell adenoma or, indeed, carcinoma. The rest of the liver always shows cirrhosis — alcoholic, HBV-related or both — from which one or more of these lesions stand out by their size and sometimes lighter colour. In a 'typical' case, the lesion consists of normal-appearing hepatocytes arranged in plates one or two cells thick; areas of fatty change, basophilia and disordered or uneven growth may be seen; nuclear atypia is absent.[321] In cases described as 'atypical', 'dysplastic' or 'early malignant' further changes are observed. These include nodules in nodules, nuclear enlargement, prominent nucleoli, increased nucleo-cytoplasmic ratio, 'proliferation centres', liver-cell dysplasia, clear cell or fatty change, increased basophilia, acinar structures and trabecular growth into areas of fibrosis.[323–330] (Fig. 16.6). Various authors have described the same appearances with different interpretations as to whether they were precancerous, early malignant or overtly cancerous, and the criteria are open to interpretation. Several groups have attempted to refine criteria for morphological assessment.[330a–c]

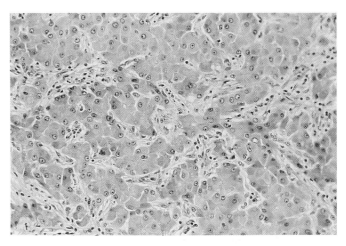

Fig. 16.6 'Atypical adenomatous hyperplasia' displaying irregular trabecular growth, variable cytoplasmic granularity and conspicuous nucleoli in small areas of a 3 cm large cirrhotic nodule. H & E.

Further evidence has been sought from special studies utilizing a variety of techniques. Resistance to iron accumulation is well known as a phenotypic marker of preneoplasia and neoplasia during experimental carcinogenesis in rodents overloaded with iron and it also occurs in cirrhotic patients with haemochromatosis when they develop liver-cell carcinoma. Studies carried out on large numbers of adenomatous macroregenerative nodules have shown both decreased[331] and increased[332] content of iron when compared with the rest of the cirrhotic liver. Iron-free foci have been described as 'borderline lesions' or 'malignant;[331–333] and could be identified by magnetic resonance imaging in vitro.[333] Mallory body clustering in cells showing cellular atypia and resistance to iron has also been reported.[334] In one case, two nodules of atypical adenomatous hyperplasia, one of which contained a small focus of 'overt hepatocellular carcinoma', showed the same restriction pattern of integrated HBV DNA, indicating a common clonal origin.[335] However, in another single case report, absence of HBV integration was found in nodules of adenomatous hyperplasia and dysplasia.[336] Hyperplastic nodules were also studied in alcoholic cirrhosis and it was found that they appeared following reduction or cessation of drinking; the conclusion was that consumption of alcohol actually inhibits liver-cell proliferation.[337] Cytophotometric DNA analysis of 'ordinary' and 'atypical' adenomatous hyperplastic nodules and foci of 'apparent hepatocellular carcinoma' produced somewhat overlapping diploid, hyperploid and aneuploid patterns.[338] A phenotypic analysis showed increasing expression of A, B, and H blood group antigens, *Ulex europaeus* agglutinin 1 and factor VIII-related antigen on the sinusoidal endothelium from normal liver through cirrhosis to adenomatous hyperplasia and liver-cell carcinoma,[339] whilst ultrastructural studies showed loss of sieve plates in carcinoma, some capillarization in adenomatous hyperplasia and occasional large gaps in fetal liver.[340] A study utilizing proliferating cell nuclear antigen showed an increase in activity from cirrhotic nodules through adenomatous hyperplasia to liver-cell carcinoma, suggesting a stepwise progression.[341] Further reports, along the same lines, continue to emphasize the pre-cancerous nature of nodular lesions in the liver.[341a-e] Japanese workers have produced a considerable body of evidence to incriminate adenomatous hyperplasia in the pathogenesis of liver-cell carcinoma with recent support from the United States.[330a,b]

Liver-cell dysplasia

The term was introduced some 20 years ago and refers to the presence of large, abnormal cells with bizarre, hyperchromatic and occasionally multiple nuclei, which occur in groups or sometimes occupy whole cirrhotic nodules.[342-344] The appearances are quite striking (Fig. 16.7) and there has been no disagreement on the characteristics of liver-cell dysplasia, only about its nature, i.e. whether it is a regenerative, degenerative or precancerous change. In the original study of 552 African patients,[342] liver-cell dysplasia was found in 2 of 200 (1%) patients with normal livers, in 3 of 43 (6.9%) patients with normal livers bearing liver-cell carcinoma, in 35 of 175 (19.3%) patients with cirrhosis and in 80 of 124 (64.5%) patients with cirrhosis and liver-cell carcinoma. On average, cirrhotic patients without dysplasia were 10 years younger than those with carcinoma. There was a strong relationship between liver-cell dysplasia, male sex, macronodular cirrhosis and HBsAg carriage. From this circumstantial evidence it was concluded that liver-cell dysplasia was a precancerous change. Similar studies followed from many parts of the world to confirm these findings — Italy, Hungary, Thailand, Hong Kong and some from Japan; others from Japan and South Africa disputed the suggestion, though they accepted the associa-

tion with chronic HBV infection.[345,346] A recent study from South Africa[347] recorded opposite conclusions to two earlier reports from that country. A difference in the prevalence of liver-cell dysplasia was found in 160 patients with liver-cell carcinoma, 75.6% in HBsAg–positive individuals versus 29.4% in those negative for this marker. There was also a significant relationship with macronodular cirrhosis, domicile (rural rather than urban), younger age and evidence of ongoing viral replication, e.g. serum HBeAg and/or tissue HBcAg positivity. Careful monitoring of HBsAg–positive patients with liver-cell dysplasia was recommended. Follow-up studies from Italy reached similar conclusions: liver-cell dysplasia was found to be associated with an increased risk of malignancy during a mean observation period of 32 months.[348,349] Liver-cell dysplasia has also been documented in patients with a history of 'non A, non B' hepatitis and cirrhosis[350] and in liver-cell adenomas associated with oral contraceptive steroids;[351,352] in both instances, it was held to be a precancerous change. Doubts have persisted in Japan where liver-cell dysplasia was divided into large and small cell types,[353] the former corresponding to the original description and the latter characterized by a high nucleo–cytoplasmic ratio, basophilia and a tendency to form small round foci. Electron microscopy suggested large dysplastic cells to be regenerative and small dysplastic cells to be precancerous. An alternative interpretation might be that the latter are hyperplastic, as in cirrhotic and adenomatous nodules. However, the association of large cell dysplasia with HBV, in free or integrated forms, has been confirmed in Japan also.[354,355]

As with adenomatous hyperplasia, attention has turned to studies utilizing special techniques. An enzyme histochemical study in cirrhotic patients showed that neither dysplastic liver cells nor HBsAg positive hepatocytes showed patterns of deviation similar to those seen in liver-cell carcinoma.[356] Immunocytochemical studies failed to show differences in expression of HBV antigens, α-fetoprotein, carcinoembryonic antigen, α_1-antitrypsin and ferritin between normal and dysplastic liver cells.[357-359] Morphometric analyses of nuclear parameters such as shape, size, symmetry, nucleo–cytoplasmic or nucleolo–nuclear ratios have both supported (from Italy)[359,360] and refuted (from Japan)[361] the precancerous nature of liver-cell dysplasia. Flow cytometric studies of nuclear DNA content produced similarly discrepant results form the same areas.[362-363] A recent study, once again, reaffirmed that liver-cell dysplasia is a morphological entity that is associated with DNA aneuploidy.[363a] In a study from the United States, HBsAg positive liver cells were found to exhibit both dysplastic and hyperplastic changes.[364] In cirrhosis, a small number of cells were found to show expression of α-fetoprotein messenger RNA but these were morphologically indistinguishable from surrounding hepatocytes.[365] In another study, it was demonstrated in cells that were morphologically dysplastic.[366]

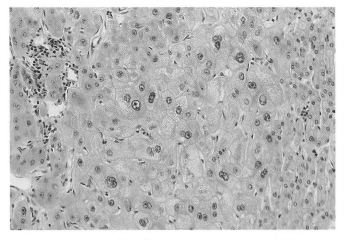

Fig. 16.7 A group of dysplastic liver cells in the middle, with normal liver cells on either side. H & E.

Expression of *ras*, *myc*, *fos* and other oncogenes may also prove to be an indicator of preneoplasia.[367,368] Recently, the claim has been made that high numbers of silver staining nucleolar organiser regions (AgNORs) in hepatocytes in chronic liver disease are indicative of an increased risk of malignancy.[368a] These changes, however, are not associated with morphological abnormalities.

In summary, the precancerous nature of both adenomatous hyperplasia and liver-cell dysplasia remains controversial, workers from Japan favouring the former and others, notably from Italy, Africa and the Far East, the latter as the more likely candidate. Sufficient evidence exists, however, in the case of both for close follow up of patients, with serial estimation of serum α-fetoprotein and ultrasound or magnetic resonance imaging of the liver.[321,345,369]

CLINICAL PRESENTATION, RADIOLOGICAL INVESTIGATION AND LABORATORY FINDINGS

Liver-cell carcinoma produces no symptoms or signs pathognomonic of its presence, and diagnosis is late except in those 'early' cases detected by screening. The tumour is often large and/or multifocal. The mode of presentation in high and low incidence areas is different.[370-372] In Western countries, patients are usually middle-aged or elderly, have had cirrhosis for years, and the onset of malignancy is heralded by the sudden and otherwise unexplained deterioration of their clinical condition. The commonest complaints are pain in the right upper quadrant and weight loss. An arterial bruit and/or hepatic friction rub may be heard over the liver in a quarter or so of cases. Fever is sometimes prominent. Hepatic decompensation develops rapidly with jaundice, ascites and encephalopathy. In tropical Africa, patients are often young adults and cirrhosis is first discovered at the same time as the tumour after a fulminating course that mimicks liver abscess. In South-East Asia, Japan and other, intermediate incidence areas, clinical presentation is somewhere in between the above. Rupture of the tumour and intraperitoneal haemorrhage, often massive and fatal, occurs fairly commonly in Africa[373] and the Far East[374,375] and much less frequently elsewhere. There is also a risk of haemorrhage from ruptured oesophageal varices which may develop in the absence of cirrhosis, owing to tumour growth into the hepatic or portal veins.[373-375] An uncommon but striking presenting feature is obstructive jaundice due to involvement of the main hepatic or common bile ducts; some of these patients may also manifest haemobilia.[376,376a] Presentation with metastases is rare but it may occasionally occur at odd sites: stomach,[376b] ovary[377] and bone.[378] Various staging methods, including one based on the TNM system, have been devised in order to provide guidance to treatment.[379] These and other clinical aspects are covered in detail in surgical textbooks[6-8] and reviews.[370-372]

Radiological imaging techniques have progressed considerably and, in specialist centres, almost to the exclusion of a need for tissue diagnosis.[380] The most routinely employed methods are ultrasonography and computer-assisted tomography which are both non-invasive and highly accurate; magnetic resonance imaging is increasingly preferred but not yet widely available. Angiography is not free of risk but it adds considerably to the pre-operative evaluation of resectability.

Conventional biochemical tests are of limited value but the combination of a high serum alkaline phosphatase level with a normal or only slightly raised bilirubin is highly suggestive of a tumour in the appropriate clinical setting. A bewildering variety of enzyme and other biological markers, present in the serum, have been offered for diagnostic use.[370-372,381,382] These include a specific γ-glutamyltransferase,[383] fucosyltransferase,[384] α-L-fucosidase,[385,386a] des-γ-carboxy prothrombin (PIVKA-II)[387-389a] and ferritin.[390] Others include tumour-specific alkaline phosphatase, transcobalamine, tissue polypeptide antigen, α₁-antitrypsin and C-reactive protein. These and other substances are normally produced by fetal or adult liver cells or may result from the interruption of normal metabolic pathways in carcinoma cells.[391]

PARANEOPLASTIC SYNDROMES

A number of paraneoplastic manifestations occur in patients with hepatocellular carcinoma, some of which are clinically manifest, whilst others are detected only by laboratory tests.[370-372,381,382]

Hypoglycaemia is seen in about one-quarter or so of cases in South-East Asia but much less commonly elsewhere. It takes two distinct forms. In one, it develops during the last few weeks of life and is similar to that observed in the terminal stage of many malignancies; it is possibly due to uptake of glucose and other nutrients by rapidly growing masses of tumour. In the other, it occurs early in the clinical course of the disease and is severe and unresponsive to treatment; this may be due to ectopic secretion of substances with an insulin-like activity, such as insulin growth factor II (IGF II).[392] *Hypercalcaemia* may develop with both liver-cell and bile-duct carcinoma but it is relatively rare; ectopic parathormone production, prostaglandins and osteoclast activating factor are possible explanations but none has been convincingly demonstrated. *Erythrocytosis* occurs in up to 10% of cases and it has been attributed to an erythropoietin-like substance, demonstrable in the serum but not in tumour tissue, though malignant liver cells grown in culture have been shown to produce it. Synthesis of cholesterol by liver carcinoma cells appears to be autonomous and *hypercholesterolaemia* is relatively common. *Sexual changes* may occasionally occur. These include gynaecomastia, feminization and isosexual precocity. Raised serum levels of chorionic gonadotropin, placental lactogen and testosterone have been found in a few patients.

Various *rare syndromes and manifestations* include secondary porphyria, especially cutanea tarda, carcinoid syndrome, dysfibrinogenaemia, hypertrophic pulmonary osteoarthropathy, hypertension, hyperthyroidism, polyneuropathy and skin rashes. Neurotensin and a vitamin B_{12}-binding protein are markers of the fibrolamellar variant of liver-cell carcinoma and are discussed under that heading.

α-FETOPROTEIN (AFP)

This is the most thoroughly characterized carcinofetal gene product and its usefulness in the diagnosis of hepatic and testicular tumours as well as in the detection of neural tube defects is well established. AFP is the major fetal globulin during early gestation. The chemistry, physiology and usefulness of AFP have been extensively reviewed.[381,382,391,393] It is produced mainly by liver cells with a contribution from gastrointestinal mucosa and the yolk sac. The peak concentration in the blood of the fetus is reached at around weeks 12–14 of gestation and thereafter falls off quite rapidly. The level of AFP after birth decreases gradually to the normal adult range of 10–20 ng/ml within a few weeks or months and in all cases by the end of the first year of life. During normal development, production of AFP is gradually switched to that of albumin in the same way as adult haemoglobin replaces fetal haemoglobin. Prolonged elevations are seen in neonatal hepatitis, ataxia–telangiectasia and tyrosinaemia. The serum AFP level is increased in pregnant women during the second trimester and is much higher in those carrying an abnormal fetus with anencephaly, rachischisis and spina bifida; the level is still more elevated in the amniotic fluid. The possible biological roles of AFP are an immunosuppressive effect which may help to maintain the fetus as an allograft, and a growth promoting potential which is called for to aid regeneration after liver injury.

Sensitive radioimmunoassay has replaced immunodiffusion and countercurrent immunoelectrophoresis for the measurement of AFP and it detects a level of less than 1 ng/ml. Modest rises above 20 ng/ml and up to 200–400 ng/ml occur in acute and chronic hepatitis, toxic injury, trauma to the liver and partial hepatectomy; occasionally, higher levels have been recorded. The rise is often related to transaminase activity and is transient or episodic, occurring during periods of liver-cell damage and regeneration. A steady increase in cirrhosis, especially when related to HBV infection, indicates the development of liver-cell carcinoma: AFP estimation and imaging by ultrasound constitute the best form of screening for those at risk.[321,345,369] It appears, however, that an increase in the serum level to over 400–500 ng/ml does not occur until the tumour has reached a size of 2–3 cm. Thereafter, the level stabilizes in the individual patient, no matter how large the tumour may grow, and shows little fluctuation. Several investigations have both suggested and refuted a relationship between high levels of AFP and young age, HBV carriage and poor tumour differentiation. In a minority of cases, 5–10% in high and 15–20% in low tumour incidence areas, a diagnostic rise above 400–500 ng/ml is not seen at any stage; indeed, the level may remain within normal limits.

High serum levels of AFP are seen in patients with hepatoblastoma and yolk sac tumours of the testis or ovary, which are easily distinguished from liver-cell carcinoma on other grounds. It must be noted, however, that rare cases of AFP positive carcinoma have been recorded at other sites, notably the stomach (particularly those described as 'hepatoid'),[394,395a] gallbladder,[396,396a] papilla of Vater,[397] rectum,[398] pancreas (pancreatoblastoma and acinar carcinoma),[399,399a] lung,[400] kidney,[401,402] endometrium[403] and ovary.[404,404a] In most such cases, however, serum AFP levels have been fairly low or AFP could only be demonstrated in tumour tissue.

The usefulness of AFP for the diagnosis of hepatocellular carcinoma may be improved by its degree of fucosylation[405,405a] and lectin binding,[406,406a] which may make it more 'liver specific'. Finally, tumour tissue expression and hypomethylation of AFP messenger RNA have been found to correlate with young age, HBsAg seropositivity, serum level of AFP, tumour size, poor histological grade and length of survival.[406b]

PATHOLOGY

The macroscopic and microscopic appearances of liver-cell carcinoma have been described in detail over the years; criteria for diagnosis and nomenclature have been clarified; special subtypes with a better prognosis have been recognized.[1,11–16,373,407–409] A major landmark was the classification proposed by the WHO, first in 1978 and now revised.[1] This recognized the histological patterns and cytological features as separate but equally important. Additions and modifications are still being made and the interest in special techniques, especially immunocytochemistry, is reflected in an ever-growing number of publications. It must be admitted, however, that the morphological features, with few exceptions, have little epidemiological, biological or clinical significance.

Macroscopic appearances

Liver-cell carcinoma forms soft, haemorrhagic, occasionally bile-stained nodules and masses with a tendency to necrosis. The macroscopic classification of Eggel, devised at the turn of the century, was subsequently adopted by most workers. This distinguished three forms: (i) the

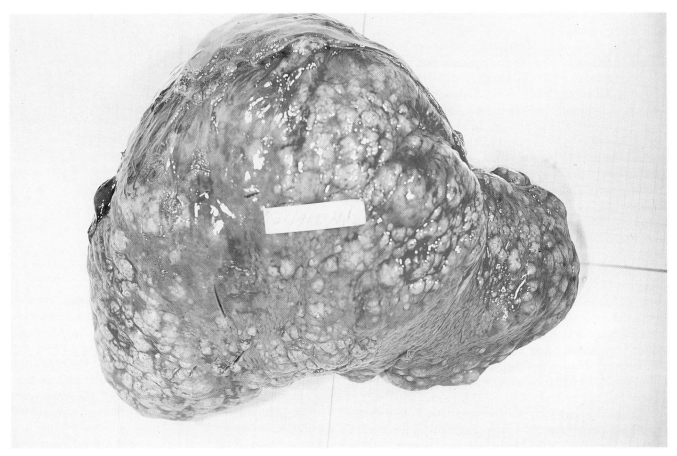

Fig. 16.8 Masses and nodules of hepatocellular carcinoma replace most of the liver at autopsy.

multinodular, in which more or less rounded and sharply demarcated nodules of tumour are scattered throughout the liver; (ii) the massive, in which a solitary mass replaces most or all of the right or left lobe of the liver with small 'satellite' nodules elsewhere; and (iii) the diffuse, in which numerous small tumours seem to replace the entire liver. In advanced cases at autopsy, a combination of these patterns is often seen with a large mass surrounded by smaller but still sizeable nodules and obvious intravascular spread (Fig. 16.8). The macroscopic diagnosis is often easy in the case of multinodular or massive tumours but it may be difficult in the diffuse variety when small tumour nodules are hardly distinguishable from cirrhotic nodules (Fig. 16.9).

Recently, more detailed classifications have been proposed that relate gross morphology to mode of growth, vascular spread and metastasis. A collaborative study of autopsy material from Japan, the United States and South Africa[410] defined three patterns: (i) expanding (further subdivided into cirrhotomimetic, pseudoadenomatous and sclerosing variants), (ii) spreading (with cirrhotomimetic and infiltrative variants), and (iii) multifocal (composed of several small tumours at multiple sites in the liver). An 'indeterminate type' was that in which classification was not possible due to necrosis or haemorrhage, and others presented a combination of patterns. The same classifica-

tion has been reproduced in the Armed Forces Institute of Pathology monograph on liver tumours.[12] Further modifications[11,409,411] have divided liver-cell carcinomas into infiltrative or expansive, single or multinodular, and mixed types with further observations on encapsulation, intrahepatic venous spread and special subtypes such as pedunculated or 'small'. Not all would agree that such

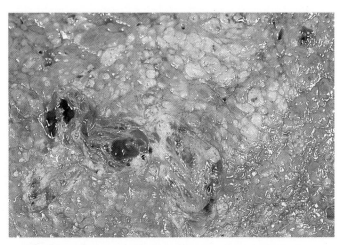

Fig. 16.9 Cut surface of cirrhotic liver with numerous yellow-green tumour nodules that are difficult to distinguish; note vascular invasion.

detailed categorizations are easily reproducible or necessarily meaningful.

The intrahepatic vascular changes have been extensively studied, using post-mortem angiography and injection of coloured gelatins.[11,409] Liver-cell carcinomas have an arterial blood supply but both the hepatic and portal veins proliferate alongside and cavernous structures develop in collaterals.[412,413] Consequently, intra- and extrahepatic spread can take place in all directions: commonly to all parts of the liver,[414] hepatic veins, inferior vena cava and right atrium[415] and the portal system; rarely, spread may involve gastric and oesophageal varices.[416,417] This propensity of hepatocellular carcinoma for local intravascular spread has been noted for many years but distant metastases may not occur until quite late.[373] It is, however, a major factor in the development of spontaneous rupture that follows from widespread thrombotic occlusion and infarction.[373–375] It is also responsible for variceal haemorrhage in the absence of cirrhosis which may rarely be seen. Direct extension of the tumour into the main hepatic or common bile ducts may also be seen macroscopically and, indeed, the patients may have presented with large duct obstruction.[11,376,376a,409] Finally, direct spread to stomach and/or duodenum may occur with bleeding due to luminal ulcers.[376b,418]

The significance of capsule formation has been debated and it has been interpreted as a passive result of mechanical compression[419] or as an active defence reaction against growth of the tumour.[420]

Microscopic features

The majority of liver-cell carcinomas conform to a fairly monotonous pattern but, in a minority, the appearances are quite variable and confusion with bile-duct carcinoma and metastatic tumours may arise. It must be remembered that the main characteristic of hepatocellular carcinoma is its resemblance to the normal liver, both in its plate-like growth and in its cytology, and this is usually evident in at least part of the tumour. A positive diagnosis must rest on the identification of this basic pattern and, in its absence, only a tentative opinion should be expressed, subject to confirmation by evidence of AFP production, or else a further opinion should be sought.

The most widely adopted classification of liver-cell carcinoma is that proposed by the WHO[1] and this, with or without added variants, has been used or adopted by others over the years.[11–16,373,407–409,421]

The following histological patterns may be seen:

Trabecular, plate-like or sinusoidal. This is the basic structure from which all others derive (Fig. 16.10). In two-dimensional sections, tumour cells appear to grow as cords but are, in reality, plates which vary in thickness from two to many cells. They are separated by sinusoids lined by flat endothelial cells. Kupffer cells are absent or

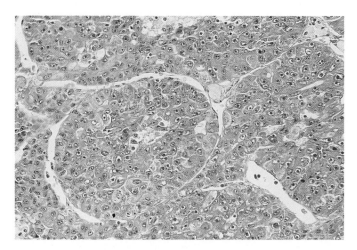

Fig. 16.10 The usual appearance of liver-cell carcinoma: trabeculae or plates of varying thickness are separated only by sinusoids. H & E.

reduced in number.[422,423] Sometimes, large cavernous blood spaces form, communicating either with arteries or veins as demonstrated by angiography; these are often associated with intrahepatic vascular spread.[11,410,412,413] A few collagen fibres may be demonstrated in Disse's space surrounding the sinusoids, as well as a basement membrane, i.e. they become 'capillarized'. Similarly, a basement membrane may also be visualized by anti-laminin and anti-collagen antibodies.[423,424] There is usually little or no fibrous stroma, unless scarring has followed infarction or septa have developed between nodules.

Pseudoglandular, adenoid or acinar.[425] This pattern may result from central degeneration and breakdown of otherwise solid trabeculae. The content of these gland-like spaces is at first made up of cellular debris, macrophages and exudate (Fig. 16.11), which are then absorbed and replaced by homogeneous, colloid-like material, the whole resembling thyroid follicles (Fig. 16.12). This material may stain with PAS diastase and be mistaken for mucin, but it

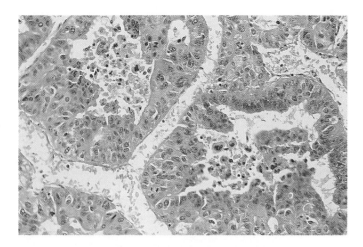

Fig. 16.11 The origin of a pseudoglandular pattern most frequently lies in central breakdown of thick trabeculae of tumour cells. H & E.

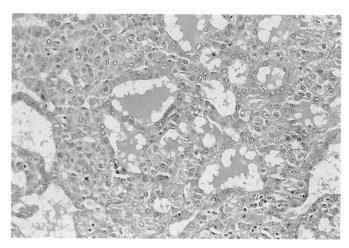

Fig. 16.12 Eosinophilic proteinaceous fluid fills gland-like spaces amongst poorly formed trabeculae. H & E.

is mainly fibrin and this can be shown by appropriate trichrome methods or immunocytochemistry. Fronds and papillae formed by tumour cells may also be seen and at times are prominent to the extent of being marcoscopically visible. Rarely, the lumens contain foamy macrophages and/or cholesterol crystals. A glandular pattern can also result from dilatation of canaliculi between tumour cells. These may contain bile which is often abnormal in appearance, being granular and varying in colour from yellow to dark brown. Finally, longitudinal splits may develop in cords of tumour cells, imparting a small duct-like appearance once referred to as 'cholangiolocellular', but the term is now obsolete.

Compact, solid or scirrhous. With few exceptions, such appearances are the result of compression artefact, scarring or chemo/radiotherapy (Fig. 16.13) or else the tumour is not of liver-cell origin. The term 'sclerosing hepatic carcinoma' has been applied to a group of tumours associated with hypercalcaemia: on close examination, they were a heterogeneous group, some being of liver-cell and others of bile-duct or mixed origin. The age and sex distribution and metastatic pattern of a large series of 30 cases was closer to bile-duct than to liver-cell carcinoma, none was HBsAg positive and only two tumours produced AFP.[426]

The following cytological features are important:

Hepatic or ***liver-like.*** This appearance is the commonest (Figs 16.10–16.13). Tumour cells are polygonal, with vesicular nuclei and prominent nucleoli. The degree of nuclear hyperchromasia and pleomorphism varies with the degree of differentiation, as does the nucleo–cytoplasmic ratio. The cytoplasm is finely granular and is often more basophilic than that of normal or of benign adenomatous liver cells. Bile canaliculi may be seen on high power magnification and can be readily demonstrated by polyclonal anti-carcinoembryonic antigen (CEA) antibody or electron microscopy.

Pleomorphic cells, often huge and possessing multiple bizarre nuclei (Fig. 16.14), are seldom numerous but at times occupy large areas and form solid masses; in some instances, the trabecular or plate-like growth pattern is genuinely lost.

Clear cells. These can be predominant but are usually still arranged in plates, and confusion with renal cell carcinoma should not arise (Fig. 16.15). The clarity of the cytoplasm is most often due to large amounts of glycogen but it may be due to water or fat. It has been suggested that clear cell carcinoma constitutes an entity, further characterized by an association with hypoglycaemia and a less aggressive course, particularly in Oriental patients.[11,409] Rare instances have also been reported in Caucasians, and sudden death, from a catastrophically low level of blood glucose, has been recorded.[427] However, clear cell areas are often seen in 'ordinary' liver-cell carcinomas and their significance is doubtful.

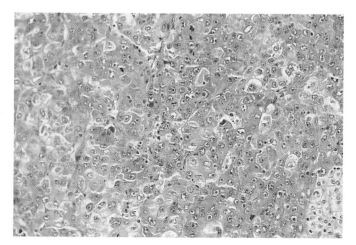

Fig. 16.13 Liver-cell carcinoma with thick trabeculae compressed into a compact mass; however, the sinusoids are still distinguishable and could be demonstrated by appropriate endothelial markers. H & E.

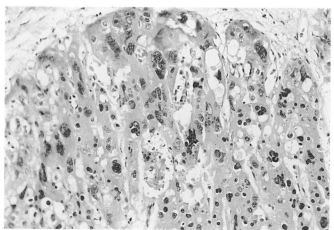

Fig. 16.14 Pleomorphic liver-cell carcinoma with hyperchromatic, giant or multiple nuclei; a vague trabecular arrangement is still evident. H & E.

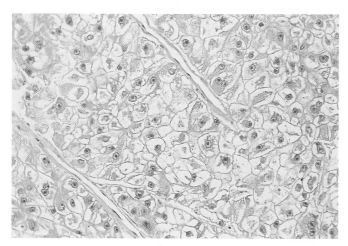

Fig. 16.15 The clear cell variant of hepatocellular carcinoma: the clarity of the cytoplasm could be shown by the PAS method to be due to excess glycogen. H & E.

An *oncocyte-like* appearance is characteristic of the fibro-lamellar variant of liver-cell carcinoma but such cells may be seen in small numbers in otherwise 'ordinary' tumours; they contain numerous mitochondria. *Spindle, carcinoid-like, giant, strap-like* and *rhabdoid* cell types have been noted[11,12,409] but it is debatable whether tumours that are predominantly of such an appearance are of liver-cell origin.

A number of **intracellular inclusions** may be seen, the nature of which can readily be identified by immuno-cytochemistry or electron microscopy.

Globular hyaline bodies have been reported in up to 15% of hepatocellular carcinomas (Fig. 16.16a). They may be intra- or extracellular and of varying size, are often acidophilic or weakly PAS positive, and stain orange to red with most trichrome stains. They can usually be shown to be composed of α_1-antitrypsin, albumin, fibrinogen, ferritin or some other 'export' protein of liver cells. Similar hyaline inclusions can also be seen in other tumours. Typical *Mallory bodies* (Fig. 16.16b) are rarely seen but may be numerous and seem to be specific for liver-cell carcinoma.

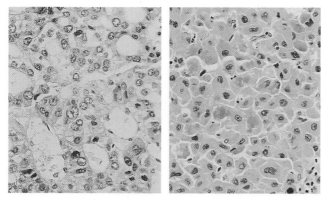

Fig. 16.16 Cytoplasmic inclusions in liver-cell carcinoma: (a) acidophilic globules on the left (trichrome), and (b) Mallory bodies on the right, H & E.

They presumably represent a disturbance in intermediate filament metabolism by the tumour cell and are not necessarily related to an alcoholic aetiology or the presence of cirrhosis.[247,248,428] *Pale bodies* are round to ovoid, clear or lightly eosinophilic and may contain albumin or fibrinogen. *Ground glass inclusions* may contain HBsAg and represent non-neoplastic liver cells entrapped in the tumour or else consist of liver proteins, especially fibrinogen, in dilated cisterns of the endoplasmic reticulum.[429] A large amount of *Dubin–Johnson-like pigment* in tumour cells, imparting a black colour to the macroscopic specimen, has also been described.[430] Many other deopsits and inclusions can be identified ultrastructurally: giant lysosomes, myelin figures, megamitochondria, abnormal accumulations of glycogen and all sorts of degenerative products.[431] Liver carcinoma cells may also show *eosinophilic intranuclear inclusions* which are due to complex infolding of the nuclear membrane and the apparent incorporation of part of the cytoplasm into the nucleus.

Other, rare features are the presence of epithelioid and giant cell granulomas[432] and foci of extramedullary haemopoiesis, especially in younger individuals.[11,409]

Grading

Many years ago, Edmondson & Steiner devised a system which divided hepatocellular carcinoma into four grades, from I to IV, on the basis of histological differentiation.[433] Grade I is the best differentiated and consists of small liver-like tumour cells arranged in thin trabeculae. The cells of grade II tumours are larger, with abnormal nuclei and eosinophilic cytoplasm; glandular structures may be seen. Giant tumour cells are more numerous in grade III tumours. The cells of grade IV tumours are the least well-differentiated with intensely hyperchromatic nuclei, little cytoplasm and loss of a trabecular pattern. Most liver-cell carcinomas are grade II or III. Difficulties arise at both ends of the scale. Grade I carcinomas may be difficult to distinguish from liver-cell adenomas and atypical hyperplastic nodules, and grade IV carcinomas from other anaplastic tumours. Histological grade has been correlated with gross morphology, metastases, laboratory parameters, enzyme histochemistry and AFP production, but the effect on prognosis is small and probably negligible.[1,11, 12,16,373,407–411,434]

The usefulness of special staining techniques

Most cases of liver-cell carcinoma can be diagnosed readily in sections stained with haematoxylin and eosin. *Silver impregnation* helps to outline the sinusoids but the reticulin pattern so demonstrated is always deficient when compared with normal or cirrhotic liver and is never as complete as it is in liver-cell adenoma (Fig. 16.17). The *periodic acid–Schiff (PAS)* method shows the presence of finely stippled glycogen in the cytoplasm; large amounts may be present

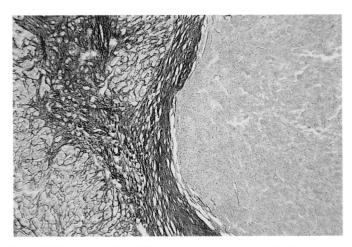

Fig. 16.17 A large nodule of liver-cell carcinoma on the right is devoid of reticulin, in contrast to cirrhotic liver on the left. Reticulin stain.

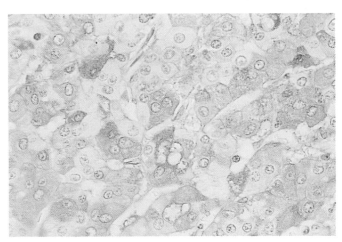

Fig. 16.18 Liver-cell carcinoma stained for cytoplasmic albumin; similar results may be obtained for fibrinogen, α₁-antitrypsin and other 'export' proteins. Immunoperoxidase.

in clear cell tumours. Epithelial mucin is not found in liver-cell carcinoma and its presence indicates bile-duct or some other adenocarcinoma, e.g. metastasis. Therefore, any PAS-positive, diastase-resistant material must be verified by other means such as staining with mucicarmine since α_1-antitrypsin globules and fibrinogen are also PAS positive. *Trichrome* methods are useful for demonstrating cytoplasmic inclusions and fibrinogen. *Iron* and *lipofuscin* are not seen in liver-cell carcinoma cells.

Enzyme histochemistry requires fresh tumour tissue, preferably snap-frozen. In general, the activities of *'adult' liver enzymes* (e.g. adenosine triphosphatase, glucose-6-phosphatase) decrease whilst those of *'fetal' enzymes* (e.g. γ-glutamyltransferase) increase as they do during experimental hepatic carcinogenesis.[346] A positive bile canalicular staining for *alkaline phosphatase* has been claimed to distinguish benign liver tumours from hepatocellular carcinoma and hepatoblastoma, in which this enzyme is absent or greatly reduced.[434] Expression of glutathione S-transferases has also been shown to be different in liver-cell and bile-duct carcinomas.[435]

The role of **immunocytochemistry** has been extensively reviewed.[346,381,408] The demonstration of normal 'export' proteins (Fig. 16.18) such as *albumin, fibrinogen, α₁-antitrypsin and chymotrypsin, ferritin, C-reactive protein* and *metallothionein* is useful in identifying the tumour as being of liver-cell origin.[346,381,408,436,437] Major histocompatibility complex (MHC) antigens are not expressed by normal liver cells but both Class 1 and 2 antigens are present on most liver carcinoma cells.[438] Patterns of *ABH* and *Lewis* antigen expression and tumour markers CA 19-9 and CA 50 have been suggested as being helpful in the differential diagnosis of liver-cell from bile-duct carcinoma.[439,440] Similar claims have been made also for *tissue polypeptide antigen*.[408] *Ulex europaeus lectin, collagen type IV, fibronectin* and *laminin* have also been studied and found to relate to tumour differentiation and degree of capillariza-

tion of sinusoids.[441,442] A strong expression of *transferrin receptor* has been found in hepatocellular carcinoma and hepatoblastoma but not in benign liver tumorus or hyperplastic nodules.[443] Normal adult liver cells contain *cytokeratins* Nos 8 and 18 as defined in Moll's catalogue, whereas bile-duct and gallbladder epithelial cells contain Nos 7, 8, 18 and 19. Metastatic carcinomas express sets of cytokeratins that derive from their primary sites of origin but these often overlap. Initial studies have suggested that monoclonal antibodies against individual cytokeratins might help to distinguish between liver-cell and bile-duct carcinoma and at least some metastatic carcinomas, e.g. from the colon and rectum.[444–446] It was later found, however, that expression of cytokeratins may change when malignancy develops. In particular, liver-cell carcinoma cells can express cytokeratins normally found in bile-duct epithelial cells, as indeed do fetal liver cells, embryonal-type cells in hepatoblastoma, and adult liver cells in chronic cholestatic conditions and focal nodular hyperplasia.[447,448] These findings indicate a common cell of origin not only for normal liver and bile-duct cells but also for their malignant counterparts; the existence of such a stem cell, however, remains to be proven.

The specificity of *AFP* is high but, unfortunately, its sensitivity is low in tumour tissue. It can only be demonstrated in about one-quarter of adult liver-cell carcinomas and, even then, its expression is often patchy and weak.[408,436,437] This is in contrast to its strong positive staining in fetal liver cells and in most hepatoblastomas. The reasons are not clear but tumour size below 3 cm, a lack of association with HBV, female sex, good differentiation and low serum levels have all been suggested. In a recent study it was found that AFP-positive cells were present in 9 of 10 liver-cell carcinomas with serum levels exceeding 5000 ng/ml but were absent in all 17 tumours with levels below this figure; there was also a relationship between positive AFP staining and poor degrees of differ-

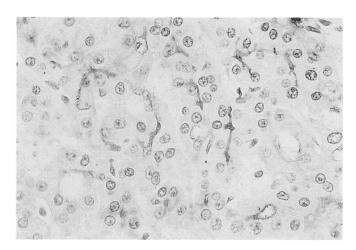

Fig. 16.19 Polyclonal antibody against CEA demonstrates numerous bile canaliculi. Immunoperoxidase.

entiation.[436] *Carcinoembryonic antigen* (CEA) is widely distributed in tissues derived from the endoderm and it is almost always demonstrable in bile-duct carcinomas, in mixed liver-cell/bile-duct carcinomas and in some fibrolamellar carcinomas, but not in pure liver-cell carcinomas if monoclonal antibodies are used.[436,437] However, most liver-cell carcinomas show a characteristic bile canalicular staining pattern when polyclonal antisera, unabsorbed by biliary glycoproteins, are applied[449,449a] and this is diagnostically useful (Fig. 16.19). The reason is that CEA belongs to a family of glycoproteins that are found on the luminal surface of biliary epithelial cells, and antisera raised against the group as a whole cross-react readily with its individual members. Occasionally, both α and β subunits of *human chorionic gonadotrophin* (HCG) are demonstrable in a few cells of hepatocellular carcinoma but their presence is commoner in hepatoblas-

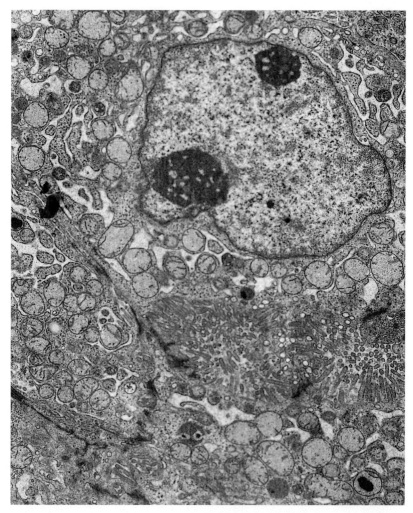

Fig. 16.20 An obliquely cut bile canaliculus, rich in microvilli, is seen in the lower half of the field. Surrounding neoplastic liver cells show many mitochondria. The nucleus in the top half of the field contains two large, abnormal nucleoli. x 4800. Courtesy of Prof K Lapis, Budapest.

toma.[408,436,437] Positivity for markers indicating a 'neuro-endocrine' differentiation has also been reported.[450]

Several *oncogenes*, notably *N-ras* and *C-myc*, have been identified in liver-cell carcinoma but their interest is theoretical rather than practical.[451,452] *Ras* oncogene p21 product was found to be absent in normal liver tissue but was expressed in cirrhotic nodules (macronodular more than micronodular), in all cases with liver-cell dysplasia, in all but one with adenomatous hyperplasia, and in most liver-cell carcinomas.[453] Abnormal forms of p53 have also been found in liver-cell carcinoma cell lines[454] and in tumour tissue.[452] Both p21 and p53 products were associated with chronic HBV infection.[453,455] Recently, molecular biological techniques have also been used to demonstrate *AFP messenger RNA* in preneoplastic cells in cirrhosis, in liver-cell carcinoma and in hepatoblastoma.[366,456] Tissue expression and hypomethylation of the AFP gene have been found to correlate with greater aggressiveness of hepatocellular carcinoma and shorter survival of patients.[406b] (see page 16.22)

Ki67 is a nuclear protein expressed by cells during the proliferative cycle. It has been suggested that a numerical score based on the number of positive cells is useful in the distinction between liver-cell adenoma and carcinoma.[457] A similar claim has been made for the quantitative argyrophil technique which detects nucleolar organizer region associated proteins — the *AgNOR* count[458] but this has not been confirmed by others.[459] Monoclonal antibodies against *DNA polymerase alpha*[460] and *proliferating cell nuclear antigen* (PCNA/cyclin)[461a-c] have both been used successfully to detect liver cells in the mitotic cycle in hepatitis, cirrhosis and liver-cell carcinoma. *Flow cytometry* is an excellent tool for the demonstration of ploidy. A number of studies have suggested a relationship between aneuploidy and high AFP levels and short survival,[462-465] but others could not confirm these results.[466] *Morphometric analyses* have found changes in mean cell size, nuclear size, shape and texture and nucleo–cytoplasmic ratio to be useful in the differential diagnosis between benign and malignant liver lesions.[467-469a,b]

The increasing popularity of immunocytochemistry, its wide availability and ready applicability to routinely processed material have resulted in a virtual neglect of *electron microscopy* in the diagnosis of liver-cell tumours other than for the elucidation of the structure of cytoplasmic inclusion bodies and the like. The ultrastructural features have been well described and are still useful,[11,470,471] especially for the demonstration of numerous cytoplasmic organelles, intercellular canaliculi and bile which are pathognomonic of liver-cell carcinoma (Fig. 16.20).

Fine needle aspiration cytology

Aspiration cytology for the primary diagnosis of tumours in the liver has been advocated by those with sufficient experience.[472-476] Key cytological features of malignancy are pleomorphic polygonal cells, a raised nucleo–cytoplasmic ratio, trabecular fragments, sinusoidal blood vessels, intracytoplasmic bile droplets and Mallory-type or hyaline inclusions (Fig. 16.21a,b). In most reported series, false positive diagnoses were rare but false negatives rather common. Results improve with centrifuging needle washings and embedding tissue fragments.[476a,b] The spring-loaded, high speed 'Biopty TM' gun has also been used with success.[477] The most useful immunocytochemical technique for the diagnosis of liver-cell carcinoma seems to be staining of bile canaliculi by polyclonal anti-CEA sera.[478,479] It should be noted that intraperitoneal spread of liver-cell carcinoma is rare and malignant cells are seldom present in ascitic fluid.

The differential diagnosis of liver-cell carcinoma

The main problems arise in the distinction of well and poorly differentiated liver-cell carcinomas from liver-cell

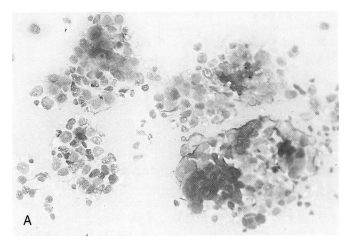

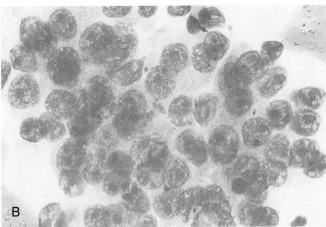

Fig. 16.21 (a) Liver-cell carcinoma: cohesive trabecular fragments of polygonal tumour cells. Romanowsky. Courtesy of Dr E Hudson, London. (b) Liver-cell carcinoma: prominent nucleoli and bile droplets in the centre. Romanowsky. Courtesy of Dr E Hudson, London

adenomas and from other poorly differentiated tumours, respectively. Special stains, immunocytochemistry and, in some cases, electron microscopy, as outlined above, are all helpful. The distinction between liver-cell adenoma and well-differentiated carcinoma has been discussed on page 16.5. In the case of equivocal or poorly differentiated tumours, the demonstration of mucin secretion and of CEA by a monoclonal antibody indicates bile-duct or other metastatic adenocarcinoma, but it cannot distinguish between them. Mixed liver-cell and bile-duct carcinomas and tumours with a sarcomatous component are rare and will be discussed on page 16.37. Difficulties may be experienced when tumour cells appear to grow in continuity with liver cells as if in transition from benign to malignant. Such a replacing or infiltrative pattern is, in fact, commoner in metastatic carcinoma, especially from the breast (Fig. 16.22). Special types of tumour, in which a likely primary source outside the liver can be established or strongly suggested, include oat cell carcinoma of the lung, renal cell carcinoma, melanoma, carcinoid and islet cell tumours, carcinomas of the prostate and thyroid, teratoma and lymphoma. Tumours of liver-like but odd appearance may represent primary carcinoid tumour, epithelioid leiomyoma or peripheral neuroectodermal tumour. None of these, if closely examined, shows the hallmark of liver-cell carcinoma which is a plate-like growth of cells separated by vascular sinusoids.

Spread and prognosis

The characteristic tendency of hepatocellular carcinoma for intravascular spread and the involvement of major hepatic veins and of the portal vein have already been discussed on page 16.20, together with the much less common direct spread into the hepatic and common bile ducts. The tumour seldom breaches Glisson's capsule and growth into adjacent structures or the omentum, through the diaphragm or the abdominal wall, is rarely seen.

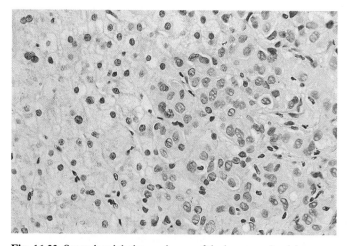

Fig. 16.22 Secondary lobular carcinoma of the breast on the right replacing normal liver-cell cords on the left. H & E.

Dissemination throughout the peritoneal cavity is least common of all. At autopsy, metastases are present in 40–60% of cases.[11,12,410,480,481] These are more commonly lymphatic to nodes in the porta hepatis, around the pancreas and the coeliac axis. Haematogenous spread occurs less often and most of all to the lungs; other sites include adrenal, stomach, heart, pancreas, kidney, spleen, ovary[377] and bone.[378] The routes and sites of metastasis may also be influenced by coexistent cirrhosis, e.g. via collaterals, as opposed to absence of cirrhosis when spread most commonly occurs via the hepatic veins to the lungs.

Treatment modalities have included surgical resection, hepatic arterial embolization, injection of alcohol, radiation, systemic and local chemotherapy, and hepatectomy followed by transplantation.[6,7,13,15,261,282,482–485] Their discussion is outside the scope of this account; suffice it to say that the results are poor and most patients die within 2–6 weeks of presentation from liver failure, haemorrhage and infections. Better results and even cure have been obtained with small 'early' tumours, less than 3–5 cm in diameter, and in special subtypes such as fibrolamellar or pedunculated carcinomas.

A small number of well-documented cases of spontaneous regression have been reported;[486–489] the reasons or mechanisms are unknown.

Special subtypes of liver-cell carcinoma

These deserve consideration as their natural history is different.

Fibrolamellar carcinoma

This is probably the only genuine subtype in that it differs in almost all aspects from 'ordinary' liver-cell carcinoma yet it is of liver-cell origin and it is malignant. It has been described under a variety of names in the past: 'eosinophilic hepatocellular carcinoma with fibrous stroma',[490] 'polygonal cell type hepatocellular carcinoma with fibrous stroma',[491] 'fibrolamellar oncocytic hepatoma'[492] and 'fibrolamellar carcinoma of the liver';[493] the last of these terms is now firmly established.[494]

In Western countries fibrolamellar carcinoma may constitute up to 5% of cases but the proportion rises to 15–40% in children and adolescents. Over 90% occur under 25 years of age and less than 5% over the age of 50 but, rarely, cases have been reported in patients aged 70–85 years.[494–496] Females are affected slightly more commonly than males. Patients present with abdominal pain, malaise and weight loss. A mass is readily palpable and is frequently large. Jaundice is rare. Serum AFP is seldom raised, less than 10% of patients show evidence of HBV infection and they do not have cirrhosis.[490–497] An abnormal transcobalamin-1 protein, that binds vitamin B_{12},[498] and neurotensin[499] may be found in the serum but neither of these findings have been widely confirmed. In rare cases, elevated levels of CEA[500] and hypercalcaemia[499] have also been reported. Fibrolamellar carcinomas are usually solitary and often large, the average weight being around 1000g. Two-thirds of reported cases have arisen in the left lobe of the liver. The surgical resectability rate is high. Multiple tumours may still be curable by hepatectomy and transplantation. The 5-year survival rate recorded in three large series was around 50% and progress is slow even when the tumour has not been completely eradicated.[495,496,501] In fatal cases, metastases are most commonly seen in regional lymph nodes and the lungs, and seldom elsewhere.

Macroscopically, the tumour is well defined and may show a lobular arrangement with interconnecting fibrous septa or a central, stellate scar. Smaller satellite nodules may be seen adjacent to the tumour mass. The distinctive histological features include both parenchymal and stromal components (Figs 16.23 and 16.24). Tumour cells are

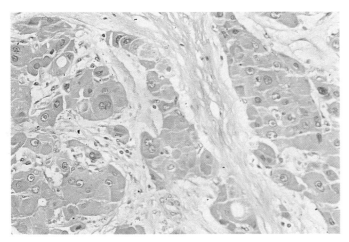

Fig. 16.23 Fibrolamellar carcinoma: large polygonal tumour cells with granular eosinophilic cytoplasm are separated by abundant fibrous stroma. H & E.

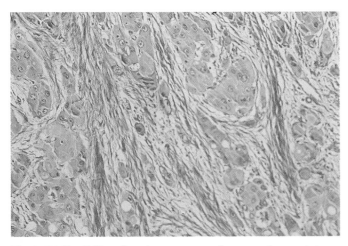

Fig. 16.24 Parallel lamellae of coarse, ropy collagen are characteristic. Van Gieson.

large, eosinophilic and polygonal, with vesicular nuclei and prominent, usually single, nucleoli. The conspicuous granularity of the cytoplasm is due to the presence of numerous mitochondria. Cytoplasmic globules and 'pale bodies' most commonly represent α_1-antitrypsin and fibrinogen, respectively; other secretory products include albumin, ferritin and C reactive protein.[502] AFP is seldom demonstrable but polyclonal antisera to CEA outline bile canaliculi and, occasionally, true bile ductular differentiation is present with production of mucin.[503] Tumour cells may contain bile droplets, copper and copper-associated protein.[500] An enzyme histochemical study indicated a highly differentiated liver-cell pattern but it also recorded production of CEA, serotonin and the presence of neurosecretory granules.[504] Fibrolamellar carcinomas express both 'hepatic' (Nos 8,18) and 'biliary' (Nos 7,19) cytokeratins.[505] An abundant fibrous stroma is characteristic and is a *sine qua non* requirement for diagnosis. It is arranged in distinct parallel lamellae around nests, cords and sheets of tumour cells and it is rich in fibronectin.[506] This fibrous incarceration of the tumour has been held to be responsible for its slow growth and favourable prognosis in contrast to 'ordinary' liver-cell carcinoma which has a rich vascular stroma.[507] Ultrastructural descriptions have accompanied many of the reports of this tumour.[492,508-510] The main findings are intra- and extracytoplasmic lumens, bile canaliculi, numerous mitochondria, granular and filamentous inclusions, Mallory bodies and large peroxisomes.

Fibrolamellar carcinoma is not always 'pure' in that it may contain areas of liver-cell carcinoma and vice versa, as well as a bile-duct carcinomatous component: it is not known whether survival differs in patients with such mixed tumours. Positive staining for markers of 'neuroendocrine' differentiation have led to suggestions that fibrolamellar carcinoma is a 'primary carcinoid' of the liver[450] or that it arises from focal nodular hyperplasia on account of its macroscopic resemblance to it, i.e. nodularity and central scarring;[511] neither proposition has found much support. These uncertainties of histogenesis are mirrored by an almost complete absence of any aetiologies. Recorded associations with primary sclerosing cholangitis, Fanconi's syndrome and others remain anecdotal, and integrated HBV-DNA sequences have been found in only one case.[512]

Pedunculated liver-cell carcinoma

This tumour does not greatly differ from 'ordinary' hepatocellular carcinoma as regards age and sex distribution, association with cirrhosis and chronic HBV infection, production of AFP and microscopic appearances. Some 40 cases are on record.[513-514,515a] Its good prognosis may relate to a relative separation from the main mass of the liver which acts as a mechanical impediment to spread. This also contributes to surgical resectability despite a large size: the recorded average weight is over 1 kg. Most such tumours are attached to the undersurface of the right lobe of the liver near the anterior edge. Accessory lobes are most commonly found at this site and it is likely that pedunculated liver-cell carcinomas arise in them. Rarely, liver-cell adenoma and focal nodular hyperplasia may be found in the same location and be also pedunculated.

Minute, small or encapsulated liver-cell carcinoma

Most cases have been reported from South-East Asia, especially Japan.[11,408,410] Definitions vary but do not refer just to size or encapsulation. All hepatocellular carcinomas must start small and some may acquire a capsule, but tumours reported under this term appear to be biologically distinctive.[516–521] The main characteristics are a small size (variously recorded as 2–5 cm), slow growth, encapsulation by fibrous tissue, an almost invariable association with cirrhosis, low prevalence of HBV infection and serum levels of AFP usually below the level of 500 ng/ml. The histological features do not differ from those of 'ordinary' liver-cell carcinoma except that these tumours are usually well differentiated. Apart from the small size, the prognosis is best if encapsulation is complete and when there is no capsular or vascular invasion (Fig. 16.25). Five-year survival rates have been reported as ranging from 100% for tumours with the best prognostic features, to 25% for those with multinodularity, breach of the capsule and portal vein invasion.[522–524] These reports suggest that there may be an early, subclinical, slow-growing phase in some liver-cell carcinomas of cirrhotic patients in which cure by surgery is possible. It is unclear, however, why this phenomenon is confined to South-East Asia and, particularly, to Japan.

HEPATOBLASTOMA

This tumour has been comprehensively described in

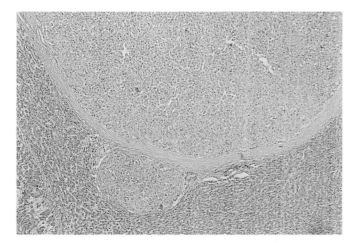

Fig. 16.25 Small, encapsulated hepatocellular carcinoma with a nodular extension into adjacent liver. H & E.

textbooks[1,12,16,525,526] and classic reviews of large numbers of cases.[110,527–531] It accounts for only 0.2–5.8% of malignancies in childhood but for 25–45% of primary hepatic tumours and for 50–62% of those that are malignant. The incidence is the same in all parts of the world and is about one-third that of neuroblastoma and one-sixth that of nephroblastoma. The vast majority, 83–92%, occur under 5 years of age and 66% in the first 2 years of life. Rarely, it may be present at birth. Adolescents or young adults are seldom affected but a few cases have been recorded up to middle life and even in old age.[532] Males are twice as commonly affected as females but the frequency is near equal in older children. One-third of patients with hepatoblastoma have some form of congenital anomaly, syndrome or other childhood tumour.[111,525,526] These include hemihypertrophy, cleft palate, talipes, cardiac and renal malformations, diaphragmatic hernia, Beckwith–Wiedemann and Down syndromes, and nephroblastoma. Some 30 cases of an association of this tumour with familial colonic polyposis have been reported up to 1992, and it is now considered to be part of this syndrome.[533,534] Two cases occurred in the same family.[535] Simultaneous hepatoblastoma in twins has also been encountered.[536] Anecdotal case reports have attempted to link hepatoblastoma to maternal oral contraceptive use but this has been refuted by a large case–control study which also excluded alcohol, smoking and HBV infection, but pointed to the possible role of parental occupational exposure to metals, solvents and pigments.[537]

The usual presentation is failure to thrive, loss of weight and a rapidly enlarging upper abdominal mass. Fewer, vomiting and diarrhoea are less common and jaundice is rare. The serum AFP level is almost invariably high. Virilization is seen in a small minority of cases, due to production of chorionic gonadotropin (HCG) by the tumour.[538–540] Increased excretion of cystathionine in the urine occurs in about one-half of cases. Hypercholesterolaemia has been associated with a poor prognosis. These paraneoplastic phenomena occur independently of one another.

Hepatoblastoma usually forms a single mass and is often large when first detected, up to 25 cm, and may weigh over 1 kg. The tumour has a variegated appearance, according to the proportion of its histological components, i.e. brown to green, fibrous or calcified, and often shows areas of necrosis, cystic change and haemorrhage. Vascularity is usually prominent, a thin capsule may be present and the rest of the liver is normal.

Most hepatoblastomas fall into the epithelial or mixed epithelial and mesenchymal categories;[527,528] rare variants are anaplastic small cell,[528] macrotrabecular,[529] teratoid[541] and mucoid.[542] The epithelial component may be of several types, the presence of two or more of which is required for the diagnosis, which is further enhanced by the presence of osteoid (Fig. 16.26). *Fetal-type cells* are

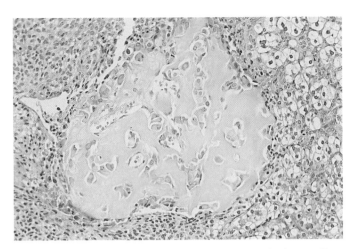

Fig. 16.26 Hepatoblastoma showing granular and clear fetal-type cells and an island of osteoid in the centre. H & E.

polygonal and relatively large, almost the size of normal liver cells. They have round to oval nuclei, single nucleoli and the cytoplasm may be granular or clear, depending on the amount of glycogen and fat. These cells are generally organized into irregular plates with bile canaliculi and sinusoids. Extramedullary haemopoiesis is commonly seen. *Embryonal-type cells* are small, elongated or fusiform and darkly staining. They have hyperchromatic nuclei and little cytoplasm. They may be arranged in rosettes, cords or ribbons. *Anaplastic small cells* grow in sheets and are indistinguishable from neuroblastoma and other primitive tumours of childhood. Some anaplastic tumours have a *mucoid stroma*. The *macrotrabecular* component resembles adult liver-cell carcinoma. Intestinal-type *glandular elements* and areas of *squamous metaplasia*, often highly keratinized, may also be seen. The mesenchymal component characteristically consists of *osteoid* and undifferentiated spindle-celled mesenchyme. Other elements, namely cartilage, striated muscle and neural tissue, are rarely seen but have led to descriptions of *teratoid hepatoblastoma*.[541] Combined hepatoblastoma and yolk sac tumour[542a] and a melanin-containing hepatoblastoma with endocrine differentia-tion[542b] have been reported.

Immunocytochemical studies have demonstrated AFP, HCG, CEA, epithelial membrane antigen, both hepatic (Nos 8, 18) and biliary (Nos 7, 19) cytokeratins, vimentin, α_1-antitrypsin, ferritin, S100 protein, chromogranin A and neurone-specific enolase in a varying proportion of cases.[531,538,540,543–545] AFP is readily demonstrable in fetal and embryonal types of cell, HCG in giant cells and vimentin in anaplastic cells; cells embedded in osteoid express cytokeratins. Ultrastructural studies have shown simple cytoplasmic organelles, few mitochondria, bile canaliculi with microvilli, dilated endoplasmic reticulum and fibrillar or amorphous inclusions.[525,526,543]

Surgical resection is the primary treatment, preceded by accurate staging and chemo/radiotherapy. Operative mortality is high, around 25%, but results are improving,

with long-term survival of 15–35% being recorded in large series.[111,525,526,530,531] Poor prognostic indicators are age under one year, large size, involvement of vital structures and predominance of small anaplastic cells or adult liver-cell carcinoma-like macrotrabeculae: the former are associated with a uniformly fatal outcome and the latter are resistant to chemotherapy. The most notable feature of tumours after treatment is the extensive presence of osteoid.[545a]

BILE-DUCT CARCINOMA (CHOLANGIOCARCINOMA)

Bile-duct carcinoma is much less common worldwide than liver-cell carcinoma but it is more evenly distributed and represents a greater problem in Western countries. Improvements in surgical techniques and treatment results are currently of the greatest interest and little progress has been made in recent years in our understanding of the disease. Bile-duct carcinoma is a disease of older individuals and it affects both sexes equally. There is no association with cirrhosis. The highest incidence is seen in South-East Asia where liver fluke infestation is common. There are three main forms — intrahepatic, hilar and extrahepatic — which differ in clinical presentation, course and, to some extent, aetiology.

EPIDEMIOLOGY, AETIOLOGY AND PATHOGENESIS

The inaccuracies contained in the system of registration of liver tumours based on the International Classification of Diseases of the WHO have already been discussed on page 16.2. Despite this, much reliable information is available from studies in specific areas of the world.[12,16,373,546–553] The highest incidence rates of intrahepatic bile-duct carcinoma are recorded in South-East Asia, particularly Hong Kong, Canton and Thailand, where it represents an additional cancer burden to liver-cell carcinoma. However, the latter still predominates in males.[546,547,549,551]

Intrahepatic bile-duct carcinoma in South-East Asia is linked to infestation with liver flukes: *Clonorchis sinensis* in Hong Kong and Canton (Fig. 16.27) and *Opisthorchis viverrini* in Thailand.[546,547,549,551a] Millions of people are affected in swampy lowlands, around canals and in river deltas. The habit of eating raw or under-cooked fish is clearly responsible. The life cycle of liver flukes requires poor environmental conditions with human waste discharged into water, snails as intermediate hosts and penetration of free-living cercariae into the flesh of fish, where they encyst as metacercariae. When ingested in a viable state by man, these hatch in the duodenum and juvenile flukes settle in the liver where they mature and lay eggs. These, in turn, are excreted in bile to leave the body on defaeca-

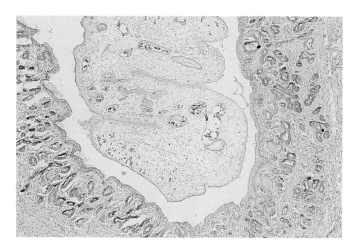

Fig. 16.27 A gravid female Clonorchis fluke lies in the lumen of a bile duct which shows adenomatous proliferation of its lining. H & E.

tion and the cycle is endlessly repeated. Infestation is acquired early in life and increases in intensity to middle and old age.[546,547,549] The majority of individuals with light to moderate parasite load are symptomless but those with heavy infestation present with cholangitis, liver abscess or carcinoma. Changes seen prior to the development of malignancy are hyperplasia of the bile-duct epithelium, adenomatous proliferation of glands and an increase in mucus-secreting goblet cells (Fig. 16.27); ulceration and squamous metaplasia are uncommon.[546] The presence of flukes may not, in itself, be sufficient and a study carried out in Thailand suggested endogenous nitrosamines, derived from substances in the diet, to have a co-carcinogenic effect.[554] No such synergism could be demonstrated for chronic HBV infection or aflatoxins.[555] Other parasites that settle in the liver, notably *Schistosoma mansoni* and *japonicum* and *Fasciola hepatica*, are not associated with neoplasia.[548]

An association between *hepatolithiasis* and intrahepatic bile-duct carcinoma has been reported mainly from Japan[556,557] and Taiwan.[558,588a] The development of the tumour may be preceded by dysplasia of the ductal epithelium.[559,559a] *Congenital anomalies of the biliary tree*, with or without infection or stones, also represent an increased risk of malignancy. These include cystic dilatation of the bile ducts or Caroli's disease,[560,561] solitary or multiple cysts, including choledochal cyst of the common bile duct,[562-564] and multiple biliary microhamartomas or von Meyenburg complexes.[565] The risk of malignant change in choledochal cysts is high and, for this reason alone, they should always be removed as soon as they are discovered. Several reports, mainly from Japan, have also linked anomalies of the union between the pancreatic and common bile ducts with an increased risk of carcinoma of the gallbladder, the biliary tree and the pancreas.[566,567] Tumours associated with stones, cysts and anomalies may be partly or wholly squamous.

Intra- and extrahepatic bile-duct and gallbladder carcinoma represent a rare but significant complication of long-standing *ulcerative colitis*, commonly preceded by sclerosing cholangitis and epithelial dysplasia.[568-571a] A study from Egypt suggested an association with the typhoid carrier state.[572] Use of the radiological contrast medium *thorium dioxide* (Thorotrast) led to the development of liver tumours in many patients; initially these were mainly haemangiosarcomas but, in recent years, bile-duct and liver-cell carcinomas have predominated.[226-228,573] Smoking, alcohol consumption and oral contraceptive steroids have also been suggested as possible aetiological agents.[574,575] Finally, an association of bile-duct carcinoma has been shown with familial polyposis coli and hereditary non-polyposis colorectal carcinoma.[576] *Ras* gene mutations, similar to those observed in large bowel carcinomas, were found in intrahepatic bile-duct carcinomas.[577]

TYPES OF BILE-DUCT CARCINOMA

The clinical course of bile-duct carcinomas varies according to site, i.e. whether they arise within the liver, near the hilum or from the extrahepatic ducts. Their pathology is relatively simple: nearly all are mucus-secreting adenocarcinomas.[578-580]

Intrahepatic or peripheral bile-duct carcinoma (cholangiocarcinoma)

The above synonyms are usually applied to tumours that arise from ducts proximal to (i.e. above) the hilum of the liver.[12,16,373,548,550,552] This intrahepatic location is the commonest in all parts of the world and is invariably found in cases associated with liver flukes, hepatolithiasis, congenital anomalies, microhamartomas and Thorotrast.

Most patients present in the fifth or sixth decade of life and the sex distribution is about equal. Common symptoms are abdominal pain, weight loss and weakness; jaundice and ascites are rare. Early diagnosis, except by chance, is almost impossible and many tumours are in an advanced stage when first recognized. A mass, which is often palpable, is readily visualized by modern imaging techniques and is characteristically avascular on angiography. Laboratory investigations are not particularly helpful but the level of AFP is usually in the normal range and that of CEA is raised.

The gross appearance is a grey-white, tough, scirrhous type of growth which is often solitary but may be multinodular or a combination of both. Sclerosis is particularly marked in the centre and, in some cases, extensive calcification may be present. Finger-like extensions around the main mass represent spread along portal lymphatic channels. Involvement of blood vessels and growth into major bile ducts are rarely seen. The prognosis is poor due to lack of symptoms, late presentation and limited resectability; few patients survive longer than a year. In a small minority, the tumour grows slowly, may reach a huge size and even calcify. Results have improved recently, with advances in surgical techniques.[6,7,548,550,581a] Metastatic spread is common and it occurs first to regional lymph nodes followed by the lungs and many distant sites. Peritoneal carcinomatosis is also frequent in the terminal stage. Death is usually due to widespread dissemination of the tumour, cachexia and liver failure.

Hilar adenocarcinoma (Klatskin tumour)

This term refers to a carcinoma arising from the main hepatic duct or one of its lobar branches in the hilum of the liver (Fig. 16.28). Klatskin[582] recognized three main types as seen at laparotomy: a smal fibrous nodule, segmental stenosis or a papillary growth. Series of cases have subsequently been published but this type of bile-duct carcinoma is relatively rare.[583–585] Males are more commonly affected than females and the peak age is around the sixth decade. The tumour may be associated with ulcerative colitis and, rarely, with past exposure to Thorotrast. Patients present with slow, relentless, obstructive jaundice associated with pruritus which mimicks primary biliary cirrhosis, but mitochondrial antibodies are absent in the serum. The characteristic gross appearance is a large, green liver with collapse of the gallbladder and the extrahepatic bile ducts. The tumour is not easily visualized and may be missed. When seen, it most commonly presents as an ill-defined structure. A frozen

section for diagnosis may be difficult to interpret as the tumour is submerged in abundant fibrosis stroma where it appears as scanty clumps, strands or tubules which are often well differentiated. It is recommended that the surgeon takes a nearby lymph node along with the biopsy as metastasis is frequently present even in the absence of enlargement. Hilar adenocarcinoma grows slowly and prolonged survival is possible even in unresectable cases, provided that some form of biliary drainage can be established.[585a]

Carcinoma of the extrahepatic bile ducts

This tumour may arise anywhere between the confluence of the hepatic and cystic ducts and the ampulla of Vater. About one-half are found in the common hepatic, cystic and upper common bile ducts, one-quarter in the middle and one-tenth in the lower common bile duct; the rest are multiple or diffuse tumours.[552,581,586–590a] Published series often include carcinomas of the gallbladder and, indeed, this organ may also be involved in a small minority of cases as well as the pancreas. In general, the prognosis is worse for carcinomas of the proximal, than for the distal, segments of the extrahepatic biliary tree.

The age range is similar to that for carcinomas of the intrahepatic biliary tree and of the gallbladder and shows a peak in the seventh decade. Males are more commonly affected than females. Most patients present with obstructive jaundice, and some with ascending cholangitis or haemobilia. Pain, weight loss and a palpable mass are features of

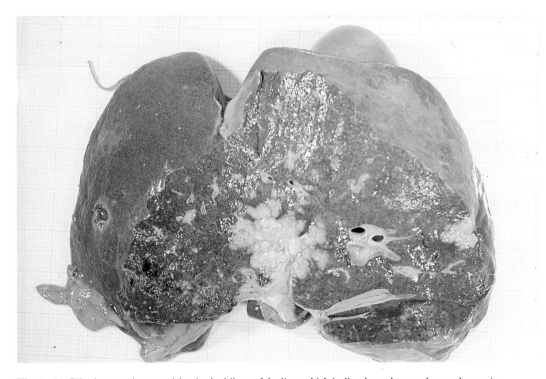

Fig. 16.28 Bile-duct carcinoma arising in the hilum of the liver which is discoloured green due to obstruction.

advanced disease. At laparotomy, extrahepatic bile-duct carcinoma may appear as a polyp, a stricture or a diffuse thickening. The latter may be difficult to distinguish from primary sclerosing cholangitis and a frozen section is often required for diagnosis.

Known associations include congenital malformations, particularly choledochal cyst, malunion between the main pancreatic and common bile ducts, and ulcerative colitis.

MICROSCOPIC APPEARANCES

Whether the tumour is intra- or extrahepatic, the usual finding is an adenocarcinoma.[1,12,16,550,552,578,580,582,583] The commonest histological apperance is a well to moderately differentiated *tubular* adenocarcinoma set in abundant fibrous stroma (Fig. 16.29). PAS–diastase-resistant or mucicarmine-positive mucus is readily demonstrable in glandular lumens that are lined by small cuboidal cells with round nuclei and small nucleoli. Occasionally, tumour cells are large, columbar or pleomorphic. They may also grow in *cord-like* or *papillary* patterns, but cysts of any size are seldom formed. Rarely, intraheptic bile-duct carcinoma may be *mucinous* with large amounts of extracellular mucus in which clumps of tumour cells appear to float freely or be of *signet-ring cell* type or *solid and acinar* with closely set fine glandular lumens. A *sarcomatous* spindle cell component may rarely be present.[590b] Bile, produced by liver cells nearby, may be entrapped at the margins of the tumour: it is always extracellular. Bile-duct hyperplasia, atypical hyperplasia and carcinoma in situ are demonstrable in the majority of resection or autopsy specimens away from the main tumour mass.[578,591,592] A three-dimensional reconstruction technique based on 1 mm slides of liver has demonstrated a wide zone of dysplasia around the main mass.[593] This clearly has therapeutic implications as the margin of excision needs to be wide if curative surgery is intended: it unfortunately also explains why this is seldom achieved. In the extrahepatic biliary tree, better differentiated tubular or papillary tumours predominate.[552,588,594–596] They may be entirely intraluminal or mural or a combination of both.[597] Metaplasia, dysplasia and adenoma may be found in the vicinity, and these have been suggested to be precursor lesions.

DIFFERENTIAL DIAGNOSIS AND SPECIAL TECHNIQUES

Both intra- and extrahepatic bile-duct carcinomas may be so well differentiated that difficulties arise in the distinction from inflammatory and reactive bile-duct proliferations.[321] In the intrahepatic location, this is particularly so when obstruction, cholangitis or hepatolithiasis are present, with or without malformation of the bile-duct system.[598] Morphological features in favour of malignancy are nuclear enlargement and pleomorphism, prominent nucleoli, increased nucleo–cytoplasmic ratio and cribriform or back-to-back glandular patterns.[550,578,599] Expression of intracytoplasmic, rather than luminal, CEA is also a marker of malignancy.[595,598,599] Even more difficult, and usually impossible, is the distinction between a primary intrahepatic bile-duct and a metastatic adenocarcinoma, unless carcinoma in situ or perineural invasion can be demonstrated in the vicinity. Bile-duct carcinoma may, occasionally, grow in a liver-like trabecular pattern but the intervening stroma is fibrous and not sinusoidal (Fig. 16.30).

The immunocytochemistry of primary malignant epithelial tumours of the liver has been discussed on pages 16.26–16.28. Bile-duct carcinomas readily express biliary-type cytokeratins Nos 7 and 19, monospecific CEA, EMA, blood group antigens and carbohydrate antigen CA 19-9. These are helpful in the distinction from

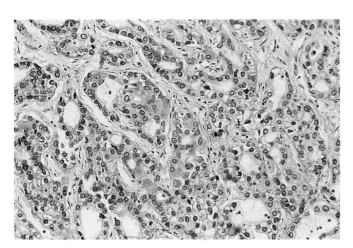

Fig. 16.29 The periphery of an intrahepatic bile-duct carcinoma (cholangiocarcinoma); note entrapped normal liver cells in the centre. H & E.

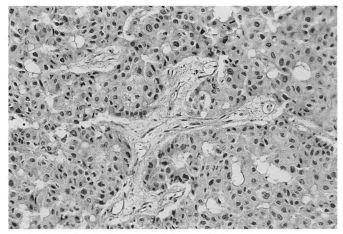

Fig. 16.30 Bile-duct carcinoma growing in thick liver-like cords; the intervening stroma, however, is fibrous. Both mucin secretion and intracytoplasmic CEA could be demonstrated. H & E.

liver-cell carcinoma but not from most metastatic adeno-carcinomas, i.e. those from stomach, pancreas or large bowel, with sufficient certainty. Biliary epithelial cells express amylase but liver-cells don't. This difference is retained in carcinomas that arise from them and can be useful in differential diagnosis.[599a] Electron microscopy, even on formalin-fixed and paraffin-embedded tissue, may be used to demonstrate glandular characteristics: lack of organelles, presence of tonofilaments and a basal lamina[11,470,471] (Fig. 16.31). Expression of *C-myc*, *C-ras* and *C-erb*B2 oncogenes relate to tumour differentiation but are not otherwise useful for diagnosis.[600] The same applies also to the expression of glycoconjugates.[601] Neuroendocrine differentiation, using a variety of markers, has been related to a particularly poor prognosis.[602] Finally, endoscopic brush cytology has been found to be an effective means in the diagnosis of extrahepatic bile-duct carcinoma.[603]

SPREAD AND PROGNOSIS

The prognosis of bile-duct carcinomas, whether intra- or extrahepatic, is dismal. Most patients deteriorate steadily and die in a few months. The outlook for hilar and extrahepatic tumours is improving slowly, due to new surgical techniques rather than to other modalities, e.g. radio- or chemotherapy, which are largely ineffective.[6,7,580,583-587,589] Metastases develop in nearly all cases and are always found in regional lymph nodes. Blood-borne spread occurs later and to the lungs in particular; other sites include bone, adrenals, kidneys, spleen and pancreas. Both direct involvement of adjacent structures and peritoneal carcinomatosis are common in the terminal stages. Patients with unrelieved obstruction of the major hepatic or common bile ducts die from complications, e.g. liver failure or sepsis, before metastases have developed.

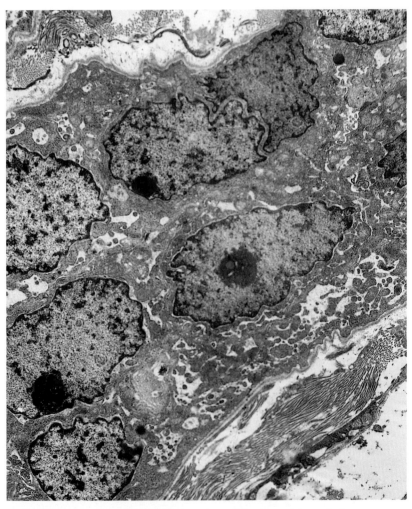

Fig. 16.31 A poorly formed, cord-like structure of bile-duct carcinoma is shown, surrounded by a thin, pale basal membrane and parallel bundles of collagen. × 6500. Courtesy of Prof K Lapis, Budapest

BILE-DUCT CYSTADENOCARCINOMA

This tumour has quite a good prognosis and it is to be distinguished from squamous and adenocarcinomas complicating developmental cysts, which are aggressive. It is the malignant counterpart of bile-duct cystadenoma, which has been discussed on pages 16.5–16.6, and is even less common.[83,84,603a] It is usually recognized histologically on examination of a resected cystic tumour specimen. Signs of malignancy are nuclear pleomorphism, mitoses, multilayering of the epithelial lining and, most important of all, presence of capsular invasion. The majority occur in middle-aged women and cause no symptoms until quite large. Local or metastatic spread is rare and, with few exceptions, the tumour is usually amenable to surgery.[604] Unusual examples have been reported, one with partial liver-cell differentiation,[605] another with extensive oncocytic change[605a] and another arising from the common hepatic duct outside the liver.[606]

MIXED LIVER-CELL AND BILE-DUCT CARCINOMAS AND OTHER MALIGNANT EPITHELIAL TUMOURS

Sell & Dunsford[607] proposed from studies of experimental hepatic carcinogenesis that liver-cell and bile-duct carcinomas arise from a pluripotent stem cell, but tumours of *mixed liver-cell and bile-duct differentiation* are seldom seen in man. In a series of 24 cases, 4 were 'collision' tumours, 12 appeared to be 'transitional' and 8 were fibrolamellar carcinomas with a mucus-secreting component.[503] In general, poorly differentiated or featureless tumours should not be labelled 'hepatobiliary' or 'mixed', nor should they be put into this category purely on immunophenotypic characteristics that may overlap. In the WHO classification[1] such tumours are listed as 'undifferentiated carcinoma' not otherwise specified. *Adenosquamous* and *squamous carcinomas* usually arise in hepatolithiasis, cysts and congenital anomalies of bile ducts[608–610] and rarely in otherwise normal livers.[611] An increasing number of liver-cell or bile-duct carcinomas with *sarcomatous transformation* are being reported, usually of a spindle cell appearance[612–614] and, rarely, with rhabdomyoblastic[615] or giant cell differentiation.[616] Occasionally, carcinomas of liver-cell or bile-duct origin may coexist with leiomyo- or other sarcomas as separate tumours in the same patient. *Mucoepidermoid carcinoma* of salivary gland type may arise from both intra- and extrahepatic bile ducts.[617] α-fetoprotein producing *hepatoid carcinoma of the ovary*, without a germ cell component, i.e. distinct from *hepatoid yolk sac tumour*, is well described[404] but the possibility of metastasis from liver-cell carcinoma to the ovary must always be considered.[377] Similar hepatoid tumours rarely occur in the stomach,[394–395a] gallbladder,[396,396a] intestines,[397,398] pancreas,[399] lung,[400] kidney[401,402] and endometrium;[403] at these latter sites, the evidence rests more on production of AFP by the tumour than a histological resemblance to liver-cell carcinoma. Primary *carcinoid tumours* of the liver,[618] but much more commonly of the bile ducts,[619–623] have long been recognized. They are curiously 'silent' though endocrine products such as somatostatin, pancreatic polypeptide and an unknown hypoglycaemic agent have been identified in them. Their slow growth, resectability and potential for cure make recognition important. *Small-cell neuroendocrine (oat-cell) carcinoma* has also been described.[624] Recently, 6 cases of *hepatic gastrinoma* have been reported.[624a] Finally, an *ectopic liver-cell carcinoma*, arising in the abdominal cavity, has been encountered.[625]

BENIGN NON-EPITHELIAL TUMOURS

The commonest benign soft tissue tumour is haemangioma; angiomyolipoma, which is rare, can cause diagnostic difficulty; the rest are incidental curiosities.

HAEMANGIOMA

This is the commonest benign tumour of the liver.[70] It occurs in both sexes and at all ages. Most never produce symptoms and are discovered incidentally at autopsy; only occasionally do they become large enough to be clinically important. The reported incidence varies widely from 0.4 to 20%, the highest figure being the result of a thorough prospective search.[79] Cavernous haemangioma, sclerosing haemangioma, solitary fibrous nodule and various other synonyms have been used to describe different stages in the development and involution of these lesions.

Haemangiomas are usually solitary, less than 5 cm in size and appear as well-delineated, flat, subcapsular lesions of red-blue colour that may partially collapse on sectioning. Others show varying degrees of fibrosis, calcification and contraction that may mimic umbilication and be mistaken for a metastasis. Least commonly, they may be pedunculated. Microscopically, they consist of cavernous vascular spaces lined by flattened endothelium with fibrous septa, thrombosis, phleboliths, scarring and calcification in varying proportions (Fig. 16.32a,b). Small haemangiomas may become entirely fibrous[626] and stains, such as van Gieson–elastic, may be needed to identify thick-walled vessels buried in a hyaline mass. Haemangiomas that measure 10 cm or more are often referred to as 'giant'. Patients may present with abdominal pain or discomfort and a palpable mass. Rare complications include rupture, thrombocytopenia and consumptive coagulopathy.[627] Most haemangiomas, however, remain stable and tend to involute; the advice, generally, is that they need be resected only if symptoms are severe.[628–630] The role of sex hormones in causing enlargement during pregnancy or recurrence as a result of steroid medication remain

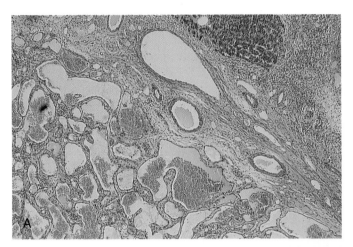

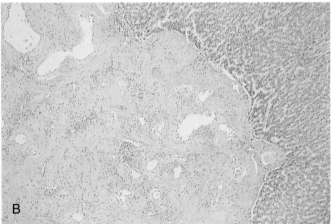

Fig. 16.32 (A) Cavernous haemangioma of the liver made up of large, thick-walled blood vessels. H & E (B) A completely sclerosed example, appearing as a 'solitary fibrous nodule'. H & E.

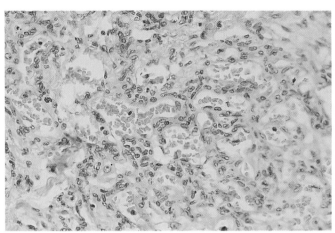

Fig. 16.33 Infantile haemangioendothelioma; an intricate maze of vascular channels is lined by endothelial cells which show nuclear atypia and multilayering. H & E.

disputed.[631] A differential diagnostic problem seldom arises but it includes peliosis, angiosarcoma and hereditary haemorrhagic telangiectasia.

Diffuse systemic haemangiomatosis is a rare disease of adults with involvement of multiple organs including the liver.[632]

INFANTILE HAEMANGIOENDOTHELIOMA

This is the commonest mesenchymal tumour of the liver in infancy.[70] Large published series indicate that nearly all cases are diagnosed during the first six months of life.[628,633–635] Females outnumber males by 2 to 1. Hepatomegaly or a mass, failure to thrive and high output cardiac failure, due to arteriovenous shunting through the tumour, are the presenting features. The natural history is variable but up to two-thirds of symptomatic patients may die. Rupture, thrombocytopenia and hypofibrinogenaemia are rare. Cutaneous haemangiomas are often present.

The tumour is seldom solitary and is usually multinodular or diffuse, spongy and red-brown with variable degrees of scarring. The microscopic appearances were classified into

two types but these frequently coexist.[633] Type 1, the most common pattern, is represented by numerous intercommunicating vascular channels lined by a single layer of endothelial cells. Large cavernous spaces may form and thrombosis and infarction are common. Extramedullary haemopoiesis is a frequent finding. Small bile ducts are present throughout. Type 2 is characterized by nuclear atypia, multilayering and papillary projections of the endothelial lining (Fig. 16.33); solid masses may form and mitoses are present. Some come to resemble angiosarcoma as seen in adults but do not metastasize, although similar tumours may be present simultaneously in spleen, lungs and bone.

Congestive cardiac failure requires vigorous medical treatment but, if the child can be supported without recourse to surgery, the tumour tends to regress gradually over a matter of months. Treatment modalities include steroids, chemo/radiotherapy, embolization or ligation of the hepatic artery and resection. In the latest series,[635] 17 of 20 patients were alive and well 6 months to 14 years after diagnosis.

LYMPHANGIOMA

Hepatic lymphangiomas occur as solitary or, more commonly, multiple masses composed of dilated lymphatic channels containing proteinaceous fluid or blood; indeed, in some patients haemangiomas are also present.[636–638a] Multiple organs and tissues, including the spleen, kidneys, lungs, gastrointestinal tract and skeleton, are usually involved, especially in children.

ANGIOMYOLIPOMA

Tumours of the liver composed of vessels, smooth muscle, fat and haemopoietic tissue occur in various combinations.[321,639] Adults of either sex are usually affected and

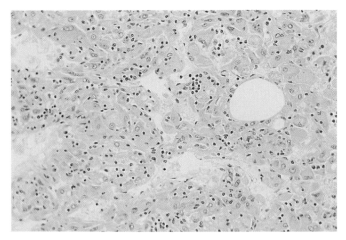

Fig. 16.34 Angiomyolipoma with few fat cells, poorly formed vessels and numerous spindle and polygonal smooth muscle cells of epithelioid appearance. H & E.

most angiomyolipomas are discovered incidentally unless large (up to 20 cm), when they cause symptoms. Some patients have tuberous sclerosis.[640] The unusual histological appearances may cause diagnostic difficulty[640a], especially in the leiomyomatous element which may be either spindle or epithelioid and liver-like (Fig. 16.34). Electron microscopy[641] and immunocytochemistry[642] readily identify the various components of this tumour. Reactivity with the HMB-45 antibody, a melanocytic marker, has been described.[642a]

OTHER RARE BENIGN SOFT TISSUE TUMOURS

These include pure lipoma,[643] myelolipoma,[644] leiomyoma,[645] chondroma,[645a] schwannoma,[645b] localized fibrous mesothelioma,[646] adrenal rest tumour[647] and benign teratoma.[12,70,648] Only a handful of these are on record but granular cell tumours have been reported quite frequently: a recent review has documented 45 examples in 43 patients.[649] They invariably arise from the extrahepatic bile ducts, usually in younger individuals and more commonly in females and American negroes. A variety of unusual soft tissue tumours are often found in the liver in patients with tuberous sclerosis.[650,650a,b]

MALIGNANT NON-EPITHELIAL TUMOURS

Sarcomas of the liver are uncommon when compared with carcinomas but some, notably angiosarcoma, have attracted considerable interest.

ANGIOSARCOMA

This is the commonest sarcoma arising in the liver.[12,651,652] The peak age incidence is in the sixth and seventh decades of life and the male to female ratio is 3:1. A survey covering Great Britain identified only 35 cases during a

15-year period;[653] a similar study from the United States[654] showed an annual incidence of 0.14–0.25 per million. Somewhat higher figures have been reported from Portugal,[225,655] Germany[227] and Japan.[226,228,656]

The commonest aetiological agent is thorium dioxide (Thorotrast), a radiological contrast medium which was much in use from the late 1920s to the mid-1950s. Thorium is radioactive with a biological half-life of approximately 400 years. 70% of the injected dose is taken up by the liver, 20% by the spleen and 10% by the bone marrow; almost none of it is eliminated thereafter. In the mid-1970s some 50–100 000 people were estimated to be still at risk and the incubation period is long: 15–25 years.[657] Particles of Thorotrast are readily visualized as coarse, dirty brown, slightly refractile granules (Fig. 16.35) which are radio-opaque and show short dotted-line tracks of α radiation on autoradiography. In recent years, an increasing number of bile-duct carcinomas[226,228,573] and liver-cell carcinomas[226,228] have been reported as well as peliosis.[658] Multiple different tumours in the same patient have also been documented.[651]

The increased incidence of angiosarcoma of the liver in workers exposed to vinyl chloride monomer (VCM) during the manufacture of polyvinyl chloride (PVC) created much concern in the 1970s but as levels of exposure were quickly brought down, the peak incidence has now passed.[651,659,660] Again, the latent period is 20 years or so and new cases are still expected to occur till the end of the century.[661] In the 1950s, workers would enter the autoclaves in which VCM had been polymerized to PVC to clean them manually, releasing trapped gaseous VCM which led to high exposure levels of 250–10 000 ppm. The gas is mildly narcotic and acute toxicity is manifested by progressive loss of consciousness; chronic effects include scleroderma, Raynaud's phenomenon, acro-osteolysis, portal hypertension and, finally, angiosarcoma. Safety measures were introduced in the 1970s and the statutory limit of exposure is now 10 ppm.

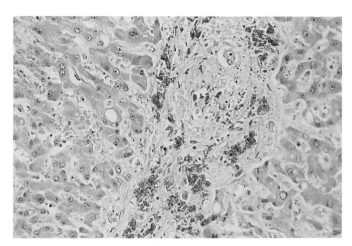

Fig. 16.35 Granular, dirty brown deposits of Thorotrast in a fibrous portal tract. H & E.

Cases of liver-cell carcinoma[206] and of leukaemia and lymphoma[662] are also on record.

Chronic arsenic intoxication has been known for many years to produce angiosarcoma of the liver, both as an occupational hazard amongst vintners and as an iatrogenic effect in patients taking Fowler's solution.[651] Other, rare aetiologies include oral contraceptives and androgenic/anabolic steroids, stilboestrol, phenelzine, radiation and copper sulphate spray.[651] An increased incidence of hepatic angiosarcoma has also been reported among Egyptian farmers exposed to pesticides.[663] However, the cause remains unknown in the majority of cases.

The liver changes that precede the development of angiosarcoma have been well studied both in experimental animals and in man and are remarkably similar, regardless of aetiology. They consist of liver-cell hyperplasia, sinusoidal dilatation, endothelial cell enlargement, nuclear pleomorphism and hyperchromasia, excess reticulin and portal and subcapsular fibrosis.[664-668] Clinically, portal hypertension may be evident at this stage. Indocyanine green clearance test has been recommended as a sensitive indicator of liver damage in VCM workers.[668] Plain films of the abdomen in Thorotrast-related cases show opacification of liver and spleen. Abdominal pain, hepatomegaly, jaundice, gastrointestinal or intraperitoneal haemorrhage, anaemia, thrombocytopenia and disseminated intravascular coagulation indicate that the tumour has developed, and patients die within six months of diagnosis.[651]

At autopsy, angiosarcoma appears as ill-defined, spongy, haemorrhagic nodules that involve the whole of the liver. Metastases are seen in lymph nodes, spleen, lungs, bone and adrenals in about one-fifth of cases. The most characteristic histological pattern is a scaffold-like or tectorial growth on the surface of liver-cell plates (Fig. 16.36) which later atrophy and disappear. Large, cavernous spaces may form with papillary projections into their lumens. Solid cellular masses are seen rarely. The tumour cells are elongated with pleomorphic, hyperchromatic and occasionally multiple nuclei and scanty cytoplasm. Extramedullary haemopoiesis and phagocytosis of red cells may be seen. A coarse reticulin pattern is characteristic. Nearby hepatic and portal vein radicles are often infiltrated and necrosis and haemorrhage are common. The differential diagnosis includes haemorrhagic liver-cell carcinoma, vascular leiomyosarcoma and diffuse metastatic growth in sinusoids, but it is greatly facilitated by positive immunostaining with endothelial markers such as factor VIII-related antigen or von Willebrand factor and Q BEND/10 and by binding of *Ulex europaeus* lectin.[669]

MALIGNANT EPITHELIOID HAEMANGIOENDOTHELIOMA

This tumour was originally described in skin, bone and lung. In the liver, it was regarded as a sclerotic form of bile-duct carcinoma until recently;[670] since then, many more have been reported.[408,651,652,671-675] The age range is from the second to the eighth decades of life, with an average around 50 years, and females predominate over males in a ratio of 2:1. Oral contraceptive steroids have been suggested as possible causative agents in younger women.[671,674] Presentation is usually vague, with malaise, weight loss and upper abdominal discomfort; jaundice, rupture and a Budd–Chiari-like syndrome are rare. Hepatomegaly or a palpable mass are readily felt, the tumour is hypovascular and calcification may be seen on X-ray.

The liver shows multiple, tough, fibrous masses. Microscopically, a characteristic zoning phenomenon may be seen.[673] On the periphery, tumour cells infiltrate sinusoids and vessels, often in clumps. They are large, pleomorphic and 'epithelioid' in appearance (Fig. 16.37). They replace

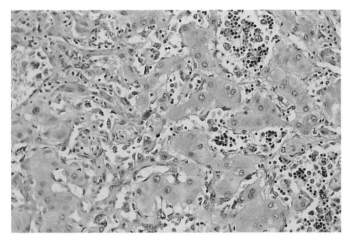

Fig. 16.36 Angiosarcoma of the liver showing an intrasinusoidal 'scaffolding' growth pattern on the surface of surviving liver-cell plates; note foci of extramedullary haemopoiesis. H & E.

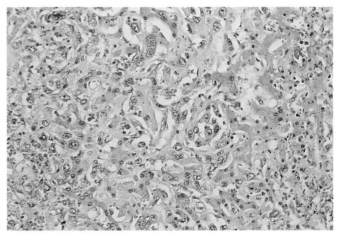

Fig. 16.37 Malignant epithelioid haemangioendothelioma: cords and groups of bizarre tumour cells of an epithelioid appearance diffusely infiltrate the liver. H & E.

liver-cell plates towards the centre and appear as cords and tube-like structures. The centre itself is fibrous, hyaline and often calcified and contains only scanty tumour cells that are elongated or stellate in shape. Cords and clumps of tumour display large vacuoles which may contain red cells and are, in fact, intracytoplasmic vascular lumens (Fig. 16.38). Two types of large vessel involvement may be seen: tongue-like projections of tumour cells in a myxohyaline stroma (Fig. 16.39) and complete fibrous occlusion with few cells. The endothelial nature of tumour cells is readily demonstrated by immunocytochemistry.[669,670,672,673] Electron microscopy shows Weibel–Palade bodies, pinocytotic vesicles and a basal lamina; abundant cytoplasmic filaments may be present which may stain for cytokeratins.

The prognosis is unpredictable but much better than for angiosarcoma: 12 of 17 patients, of whom only 3 had any form of treatment, were alive on an average of 9.8 years of follow up; on the other hand, 6 of 8 who died did so within 2 years.[670] Hepatectomy and liver transplantation have been successfully carried out in an increasing number of cases.[672,674]

UNDIFFERENTIATED (EMBRYONAL, MESENCHYMAL) SARCOMA

The original description of this tumour fifteen years ago[676] has since been further elaborated but not improved upon.[1,12,651,677 – 682] It is the third commonest malignant liver tumour in children after hepatoblastoma and infantile haemangioendothelioma, but is much less common than either and it represents only 6% of all hepatic tumours in childhood.[111] The majority of patients are between 6 and 10 years of age and the sex incidence is about equal. Rare cases have been reported in adults. Abdominal swelling and weight loss are the usual presenting features. Rarely, the tumour invades the inferior vena cava and grows into the heart, when cardiac murmurs and dyspnoea may develop. Laboratory tests are of little help. Imaging methods demonstrate a large, hypodense and avascular mass. The majority arise in the right lobe of the liver.

The majority of tumours are soft and globular and the cut surface is variegated, solid and cystic, glistening or gelatinous, and may show haemorrhage and necrosis. A thin pseudocapsule is usually present. Microscopically, tumour cells are spindle-shaped, stellate or pleomorphic; loosely arranged but compact areas, with a more uniform and rounded morphology, may be seen (Fig. 16.40) as well as fibroblast or smooth muscle-like fascicles and bundles. Cystic fluid-filled spaces of degeneration are common. An abundant acid mucopolysaccharide matrix is characteristic. Extramedullary haemopoiesis is seen in about one-half of cases. Two further special features are PAS-positive diastase-resistant globules and benign-

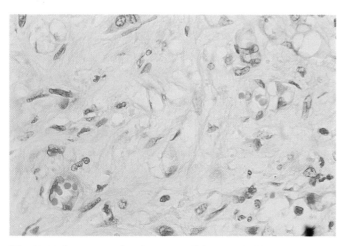

Fig. 16.38 Scanty vacuolated tumour cells in myxohyaline stroma; red cells are visible in some of the primitive vascular lumens. H & E.

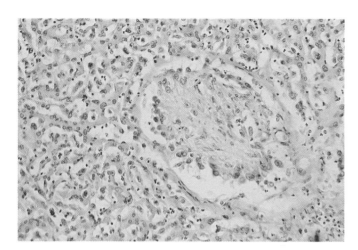

Fig. 16.39 A tongue-like intravascular growth of tumour with a fibrous core. H & E.

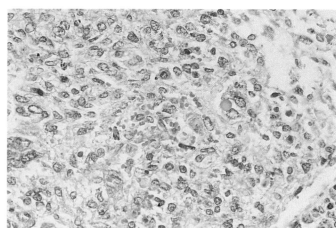

Fig. 16.40 A cellular area in embryonal sarcoma containing numerous acidophilic, extra- and intracellular inclusions of varying size near the centre. H & E.

appearing bile ducts that may be dilated. Immuno-cytochemical and ultrastructural investigations have shown evidence of widely divergent differentiation into both soft tissue and epithelial phenotypes,[651,677–682] probably from a primitive stem cell.

Prognosis has been hopeless until recently, but with aggressive therapy combining excision, chemotherapy and radiation, 5-year survival approaches 15%.[651,678,679,682,683]

RHABDOMYOSARCOMA (SARCOMA BOTRYOIDES)

This tumour is similar to those occurring elsewhere in the body and commonly affects children less than 5 years of age, but it has occasionally been reported in adults.[12,111,651] Patients present with intermittent obstructive jaundice, fever and weight loss. The tumour arises from major bile ducts in or near the porta hepatis, where it forms gelatinous grape-like masses that project into the lumen. These are covered by biliary epithelium. A dense 'cambium' layer of dark, round to oval tumour cells lies immediately beneath the surface (Fig. 16.41). Elsewhere, spindle cells are arranged in a loose myxoid stroma. Mitoses are numerous. Giant and strap-like cells are rare and cross-striations are seldom seen. Immunocytochemistry demonstrates actin, myosin or myoglobin, and thick and thin myofilaments, with recognizable Z bands, are seen by electron microscopy. Prognosis and treatment results are similar to those of undifferentiated embryonal sarcoma.[683]

OTHER PRIMARY SARCOMAS

Most types of sarcoma have been recorded as primary tumours in the liver.[12,651] They usually occur in middle and old age, in either sex, and present late. Progress may be slow but the prognosis is poor as complete excision of

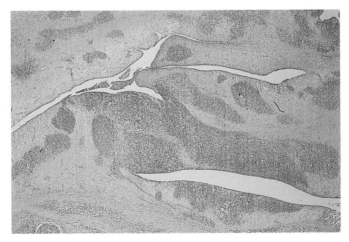

Fig. 16.41 Rhabdomyosarcoma forming polypoid masses in the lumen of a large bile duct; note dense 'cambium' layer. H & E.

large, advanced tumours is seldom possible. *Leiomyosarcoma* may arise from the ligamentum teres and the portal and hepatic veins: the prognosis worsens in this order.[684–686] Other reported malignant soft tissue tumours are *fibrosarcoma*,[687–689] *malignant fibrous histiocytoma*,[690–692] *liposarcoma*,[693] *osteosarcoma*,[694] *osteoclastoma*,[695] *malignant haemangiopericytoma*[696] and sarcomas with divergent lines of differentiation and/or epithelial elements that have been described under terms such as *malignant mesenchymoma* or *malignant mixed tumour*.[697–699] Personal experience includes others, as well as varying mixtures of both liver-cell and bile-duct carcinomas with sarcomas. The possibility of metastases must always be borne in mind.

PRIMARY LYMPHOMA OF THE LIVER

All types of Hodgkin's and non-Hodgkin's lymphoma, leukaemia, as well as histiocytosis and mastocytosis may secondarily involve the liver.[700] An increasing number of primary lymphomas have recently been described and their recognition is important as the outcome is favourable.[701–704b] The tumour occurs over a wide age range with peaks in childhood and adolescence and in middle to old age. Males predominate over females in a ratio of 4:1. Patients present with pain, hepatomegaly or a mass. 'B' symptoms (fever, weight loss) occur in about one-half of cases. A small number have been associated with autoimmune disorders, chronic hepatitis, cirrhosis, HBV infection and AIDS.[703,704] Most tumours form solitary or multiple masses but some are diffuse. Histologically, they are all non-Hodgkin's lymphomas, usually described as 'high grade'. Few cases have been characterized fully but they may be of B or T cell lineage.[703,704] Misdiagnosis — as metastatic carcinoma, chronic hepatitis or inflammatory pseudotumour — is common. The destructive nature of a lymphoid infiltrate is an important clue to diagnosis (Fig. 16.42). The best prognostic indicator is surgical resectability but multi-agent chemotherapy and/or radiation have produced worthwhile results.

RARE PRIMARY TUMOURS

These include occasional examples of primary choriocarcinoma,[12,705,706] endodermal sinus (yolk sac) tumour,[12,707–709a] rhabdoid tumour,[12,710–712] malignant melanoma of bile ducts[12,713] and adrenal or pancreatic rest tumours.[12,714,715]

METASTATIC TUMOURS

The liver is a common site for metastasis from many primary sites, particularly lung, breast and the gastrointestinal tract.[12] Most secondary carcinomas are difficult to assign to their origin but immunocytochemistry is helpful for some — gonads, prostate, thyroid, for example.

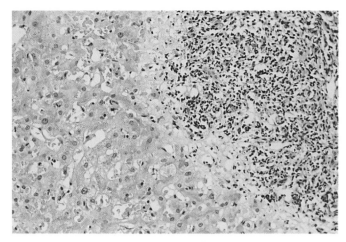

Fig. 16.42 Primary lymphoma of the liver showing a peculiar lytic zone of necrosis between the tumour on the right and the normal liver on the left. H & E.

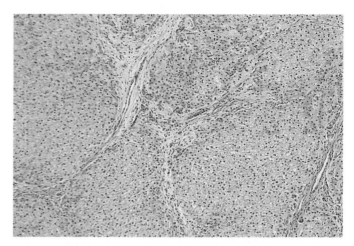

Fig. 16.43 Focal nodal hyperplasia consists of liver nodules which are separated by fibrous septa. Bile ducts, sometimes numerous, are always present at the interface between liver nodules and septa. Trichrome.

Twenty-five cases of *carcinomatous cirrhosis* with jaundice, ascites and bleeding oesophageal varices have been reported, most due to diffuse infiltration of the liver by metastatic breast carcinoma.[716] Patients may also present with obstructive jaundice due to metastatic infiltration of the common bile duct.[717] Tumours may be missed by a biopsy needle but a triad of histological features has been claimed to be helpful; this consists of proliferating bile ducts, leucocytes and focal sinusoidal dilatation.[718]

TUMOUR-LIKE LESIONS

A variety of such lesions occur and it is important to distinguish them from true tumours.[1,12,70]

CYSTS

Multiple intrahepatic cysts occur in polycystic disease, congenital hepatic fibrosis and in Caroli's disease; an extreme example is choledochal cyst (see Chs 3 and 11). Solitary, non-neoplastic, non-parasitic cysts are rare and probably also developmental in origin. They are unilocular and their epithelial lining may be flattened, cuboidal, or squamous. *Ciliated hepatic foregut cyst* has been reported and is thought to arise from embryonic foregut, differentiated towards bronchial structures.[719]

FOCAL NODULAR HYPERPLASIA

This lesion occurs in both sexes and at all ages but most commonly in young adult women.[1,12,70,720–722a] The majority are discovered incidentally and only 15% or so cause symptoms, usually awareness of a mass or upper abdominal pain. Rupture and haemoperitoneum are rare.

Focal nodular hyperplasia is usually solitary, less than 5 cm in size and typically forms a well-circumscribed fibrous globular mass. It tends to bulge on its cut surface and

displays multiple yellow-brown nodules of liver parenchyma separated by fibrous septa. Histologically, it resembles cirrhosis (Fig. 16.43) except that the lesion is focal and the rest of the liver is normal. A central stellate scar is often seen and may contain thick-walled vessels. A mild to moderate lymphocytic infiltrate is present in the septa. The nodules consist of normal liver cells arranged in plates two to three cells thick. They may contain increased amounts of glycogen or fat, show cholestasis with feathery change, bile in the form of intracytoplasmic droplets or canalicular plugs, copper storage and Mallory bodies.[723] Numerous proliferating bile ductules are seen around the liver-cell nodules. Immunocytochemical studies have shown that they arise from the latter by metaplasia.[724]

Lesions of focal nodular hyperplasia may occasionally be large, up to 15 cm, and weigh as much as 700 g, be pedunculated or multiple and be associated with liver-cell adenoma. Whether or not this condition is related to oral contraceptive use has been hotly debated for years but, on the whole, the evidence is against it.[26–32,725,726] Gonadal steroids and pregnancy may, however, increase the vascularity of the lesion and predispose it to rupture. It has been suggested that focal nodular hyperplasia is essentially a vascular malformation with arteriovenous anastomoses and localized overgrowth of all liver constituents.[725,726] A syndromatic form has been reported with intracranial vascular malformations, meningioma and astrocytoma.[727]

Focal nodular hyperplasia is readily distinguished from liver-cell adenoma by its multinodularity, the presence of septa and proliferating bile ductules, and from mesenchymal hamartoma by the lack of immature connective tissue elements. Most patients are treated conservatively and surgery is only necessary for those with symptoms.[722]

NODULAR REGENERATIVE HYPERPLASIA

This condition has been described under a variety of names

— nodular transformation, non-cirrhotic nodulation, adenomatosis and others — but the current term is now universally accepted.[1,12,70] It has been reported in patients of all ages and in both sexes equally.

Nodular regenerative hyperplasia occurs in association with a bewildering number and variety of diseases which include rheumatoid arthritis, Felty's syndrome, scleroderma, systemic lupus erythematosus, CRST syndrome, polyarteritis nodosa, subacute bacterial endocarditis, diabetes, myeloproliferative disorders, lymphomas, after steroid and/or cytotoxic therapy and in recipients of bone marrow and kidney transplants; the list is still growing.[728–734] Common to most of these disorders is some sort of vascular or circulatory abnormality; Wanless[732] has suggested that nodular regenerative hyperplasia is a secondary and non-specific tissue adaptation to heterogeneous distribution of total hepatic blood flow from any cause. Suggestions that it represents a preneoplastic change have been largely discounted.[70] The condition does not always involve the entire liver and may be accentuated near the porta hepatis ('partial nodular transformation').[735]

Nodular regenerative hyperplasia may be an incidental finding, a cause of non-cirrhotic portal hypertension or, occasionally, a source of intraperitoneal haemorrhage. Diagnosis by needle biopsy is difficult and most cases have been recognized only at laparotomy or autopsy. The liver is divided into fine nodules which are 0.1–1.0 cm in size; rarely, some measure up to 10 cm and look like a tumour. Microscopically, the nodules are formed by liver cells, distorting but not effacing the normal architecture; their expansile nature is best appreciated in reticulin preparations. The liver-cell plates are two or more cells thick. The intervening liver parenchyma is atrophic but fibrous septa do not form. The overall appearance is one of pure liver-cell nodularity, enlarging and distorting acini or lobules but not replacing them, and normal portal structures remain evenly distributed. Obliterative vascular changes, involving all types of vessel in the liver, may be seen.[732] The only diagnostic difficulty is the distinction of large nodules from liver-cell adenomas but, be they solitary or multiple, the rest of the liver is normal around adenomas.

MESENCHYMAL HAMARTOMA

This lesion most probably represents a localized abnormality of ductal plate development that precedes birth, and it is related to polycystic disease, congenital hepatic fibrosis and biliary hamartoma.[736] Mesenchymal hamartoma occurs almost exclusively in young children, the average age being 15 months, and it is twice as common in males.[70,737,738] Rarely, it has been reported in adolescents and young adults.[739] Most patients present with progressive abdominal enlargement and imaging techniques show a cystic mass. This is usually large, weighing over 1 kg, smooth-surfaced, soft and fluctuant. Multiple cystic spaces

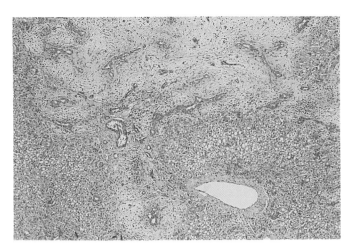

Fig. 16.44 Mesenchymal hamartoma consists of haphazardly arranged liver parenchyma, loose mesenchyme and branching bile ducts. H & E.

contain thin fluid or semi-solid gelatinous material. The solid areas in between may be white and fibrous, yellow and myxoid or brown and liver-like. Microscopically, a haphazard and variable admixture of tissues is seen, from which the liver is normally made up (Fig. 16.44). The predominant component is mesenchymal and consists of loose, oedematous connective tissue rich in acid mucopolysaccharides with dilated lymphatics, vessels and fluid-filled spaces. Numerous, tortuous bile ducts and liver-cell nodules are scattered about randomly or attempt to form ductal plates. Branch-like or nodular extensions are often seen around the main mass. Extramedullary haemopoiesis is commonly present. The prominent mesenchymal component readily distinguishes this lesion from focal nodular hyperplasia and liver-cell adenoma. Surgical excision is curative, recurrence has not been reported and malignant transformation does not occur.

BILIARY HAMARTOMA (VON MEYENBURG COMPLEX)

This lesion is sometimes confused with bile-duct adenoma but it is a malformation, usually multiple and throughout the liver, that is part of the spectrum of fibropolycystic diseases of the liver due to ductal plate malformation.[70,736,740] Biliary hamartomas are incidental findings at laparotomy or autopsy and, being small (less than 0.5 cm) they may be included in a needle biopsy. They consist of small, irregular ducts, sometimes dilated, that are embedded in a fibrous stroma (Fig. 16.45). They may contain proteinaceous or bile-stained fluid but they do not communicate with the biliary system. It has been alleged that bile-duct carcinomas may arise in them.[565]

INFLAMMATORY PSEUDOTUMOUR

About 50 cases have been reported, 18 of them in three series from England,[741] Japan,[742] and China[742a] the rest as

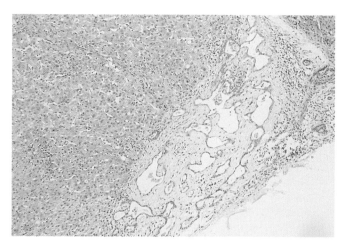

Fig. 16.45 Von Meyenburg complex (biliary hamartoma) at the edge of a needle biopsy of the liver. H & E.

single case reports from many parts of the world. Synonyms include 'pseudolymphoma', 'histiocytoma' and 'plasma cell granuloma' and the lesion has long been known to occur in the lung, orbit and many other sites.[742b] Most patients are young and there is a striking male predominance. The presenting symptoms, in order of frequency, are intermittent fever, abdominal pain, vomiting, diarrhoea and jaundice. A history of travel to tropical destinations or an association with gallstones and stenosis of the common bile duct have been recorded in a few cases. Leucocytosis, a raised ESR and polyclonal hyperglobulinaemia have been observed in approximately one-half of patients. Macroscopically, the lesion is tumour-like, may be solitary or multiple, and measures up to 25 cm. Microscopically, inflammatory pseudotumour shows a mixture of chronic inflammatory cells in which polyclonal plasma cells predominate (Fig. 16.46); other cell types include macrophages, eosinophils and fibroblasts. Sclerosis, with a

whorled or lamellar pattern, is characteristic. Rarely, obliterative endophlebitis and giant cell granulomas may be seen in or outside the lesion. The differential diagnosis includes lymphoma and malignant fibrous histiocytoma; the most helpful feature is the presence of polyclonal plasma cells. The lesion is clearly inflammatory and possibly infective but no causative organism has ever been demonstrated, except in one recently reported case in which culture obtained intraoperatively from the lesion grew *Klebsiella pneumoniae*.[743] Recovery is the rule, but persistent biliary problems and portal hypertension have been recorded when the lesion involved structures near the porta hepatis.

MISCELLANEOUS TUMOUR-LIKE LESIONS

These include those due to infections, i.e. pyogenic and amoebic abscesses, echinococcal cyst, tuberculoma and syphilitic gumma. *Solitary necrotic* or *fibrous nodule*.[744–747a] despite its name, may be multiple. Moreover, the two lesions are different. Nodules with a necrotic centre are due to larval infestation[744,747a] (Fig. 16.47), whilst a densely fibrotic nodule is likely to be a sclerosed haemangioma[745] (Fig. 16.32b). Bearing these features in mind, the two should be readily distinguished.[746] *Pseudolipoma* represents attachment of omental or pericolic fat lobules to the liver[748,749] or ectopia.[750] *Focal fatty change* forming a tumour-like mass is mainly seen in alcoholics.[751] *Compensatory lobar hyperplasia* may follow occlusion of portal vein branches or of major bile ducts.[752] *Endometriosis*[753] and *ectopic hepatic pregnancy*[754] have both been recorded. The commonest pseudotumour of the extrahepatic biliary tree is *adenomyoma*.[755] Branching glandular structures are seen in a stroma of hyperplastic smooth muscle cells; the lumens may contain mucus, bile or stones. Peliosis hepatis is discussed in Chapter 14.

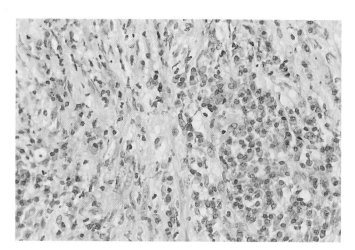

Fig. 16.46 Pools of polyclonal plasma cells are the hallmark of inflammatory pseudotumour. H & E.

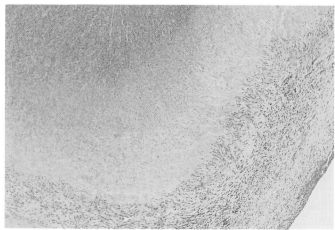

Fig. 16.47 'Solitary necrotic nodule' of the liver with a border of granulation tissue. Larval remains could be demonstrated on serial sectioning. H & E.

EXPERIMENTAL LIVER TUMOURS
P. Bannasch

Nearly all types of primary liver tumour known from human pathology have been produced by various oncogenic agents in different animal species, particularly in small rodents.[756-759] Hepatocellular neoplasms are the commonest and have therefore attracted the greatest attention.[759-761] For a long time, studies on chemically induced liver carcinogenesis predominated.[757,762-764] More recently, however, several animal models of hepatocarcinogenesis associated with hepadnavirus infection have been developed and investigated in detail.[759,765,766] In addition, during the past few years different strains of transgenic mice have been described, which are prone to develop a high incidence of liver tumours and provide an excellent tool for studying the molecular basis of carcinogenesis.[767-769]

A large number of chemicals, some physical agents, and hepadnaviruses have been identified as carcinogens in the liver of various animal species, but as yet only a few of these agents have been accepted as human hepatocarcinogens. Although this discrepancy may indicate a gap in knowledge, our understanding of neoplastic development in the liver has been considerably improved by the systematic analysis of experimental animal models. This holds especially true for a better comprehension of the mechanisms of interaction of the aetiological agents with their target cells, and for a deeper insight into the successive molecular and cellular events that lead step by step to liver neoplasia.

AETIOLOGY: EXOGENOUS AND ENDOGENOUS FACTORS

As a rule, neoplastic development is the result of a complex interaction between exogenous (oncogenic) agents and various endogenous factors which are determined by the genetic disposition of each individual. During the past two decades, particular attention has been given to the elucidation of genetic factors in oncogenesis.[770-775] A variety of genetic changes ranging from point mutations to gross chromosomal aberrations, which may result in the distortion of either gene expression or the biochemical function of genes, have been discovered in human and experimental tumours, including hepatocellular carcinomas. The majority of genes affected are involved in cell proliferation and differentiation under physiological conditions, but have operationally been called proto-oncogenes or tumour suppressor genes. Both the activation of proto-oncogenes and the inactivation of tumour suppressor genes are considered among the rate limiting changes that are responsible for the stepwise development of neoplasia. Thus, both exogenous and endogenous factors have to be taken into account if we are to understand the pathogenesis of liver tumours.

CHEMICAL AGENTS

A large number of compounds, representing many classes of chemicals, act as hepatocarcinogens in laboratory animals, especially in small rodents.[763,775-777] Although there are only a few chemicals for which epidemiological studies provided sufficient evidence of hepatocarcinogenicity in man, it is remarkable that the two most important compounds known hitherto, namely aflatoxin B_1 (a naturally occurring fungal metabolite) and vinyl chloride monomer (an industrial carcinogen) were first identified as hepatocarcinogens in rodents. It is likewise noteworthy that these two chemicals do not only act on the same target tissue but also on the same type of target cell in rodents and man. In both species, aflatoxin B_1 is involved in the development of hepatocellular carcinomas,[777] while vinyl chloride monomer mainly induces liver angiosarcomas originating from the sinusoidal endothelial cells.[778] Another example of striking interspecies similarity is the increased incidence of hepatocellular tumours, predominantly adenomas, and peliosis hepatis in rats treated with different steroids and the increased risk in women using combined oral contraceptives of the development of hepatocellular adenomas, which also occur in men and women treated with anabolic/androgenic steroids, the latter frequently associated with peliosis hepatis.[776] These observations may indicate that the long list of other chemicals which occur in the human environment and induce liver neoplasms in rodents should be seriously considered as risk factors in man, even if no convincing epidemiological data are available at present. This list includes such diverse compounds as nitrosamines, aromatic amines, organochlorine pesticides, polychlorinated biphenyls, phthalates, and hypolipidaemic drugs.[763,775,776,779] It is true, however, that many factors, like the dose and rate of administration of the chemical, the age, sex and genetic background of the animal, the state of nutrition and hormonal balance, and the intrinsic or compound-related rate of cell proliferation, may strongly influence the carcinogenic effect and, hence, complicate the extrapolation of data from animals to man.

The majority of chemicals, both man-made and naturally occurring, are themselves inert (procarcinogens) and require metabolic activation (frequently via an intermediate called proximate carcinogen) to an active agent (ultimate carcinogen). The enzymes that carry out metabolic conversion are members of the 'mixed function oxygenase' system located in the endoplasmic reticulum of the cell. This is a complex of several enzymes, notably P-450, which require NADPH and oxygen. They can carry out several reactions including aromatic ring oxidation, aliphatic hydroxylation, oxidative demethylation, and N-hydroxylation on a great variety of organic compounds. For example, aflatoxin B_1

and vinyl chloride monomer are subject to activation through epoxydation, whilst 2-acetylaminofluorene requires *N*-hydroxylation to an *N*–OH derivative as a first step to become effective. The liver is by far the most active and versatile organ in the metabolism of carcinogens generally, but its capacity can be manipulated experimentally either to activate or to detoxify potential carcinogens, and the ultimate fate of a chemical depends largely on a balance between these two processes. Once an ultimate carcinogen is formed in the liver, it acts as an 'electrophilic reactant' which is a positively charged molecule that reacts avidly with sites of electron density in many cellular constituents. Damage to nuclear DNA is considered the most important early event, but alterations in mitochondrial DNA, in RNA, and in soluble or structural proteins, have also been described.

In addition to electrophilic chemicals that react with DNA and are consequently classified as 'DNA-reactive' or 'genotoxic', a number of 'non-genotoxic' compounds have been identified which apparently do not interact with DNA but, nevertheless, produce liver neoplasms in rodents.[761,775,780] The close correlation between mutagenicity in short-term assays and rodent carcinogenicity, which was emphasized in the 1970s by many authors favouring an essential role of DNA damage in the initiation of carcinogenesis, does not hold true for hepatocarcinogens, for which virtually no correlation could be demonstrated between mutagenicity and carcinogenicity. Non-genotoxic hepatocarcinogens may act as weak but also as strong carcinogens in rodent liver; they comprise compounds such as phenobarbital, methapyriline, chloroform, 1,4-dichlorobenzene, and a diverse group of chemicals including hypolipidaemic drugs (e.g. clofibrate, ciprofibrate), phthalate ester plasticizers, and herbicides, that have in common the ability to increase the number of peroxisomes in hepatocytes ('peroxisome proliferators'). A variety of mechanisms of action have been proposed for non-genotoxic hepatocarcinogens.[757,761,775,780] These chemicals might, for example, elicit cellular processes leading to generation of reactive species such as an activated oxygen or hydrogen peroxide, which could in turn exert genotoxicity. A stimulation of cell proliferation increasing the risk of 'spontaneous' mutations or causing preferential growth of preneoplastic cells might be another mechanism. However, there is no conclusive evidence for these hypothetical mechanisms. Moreover, genotoxic compounds may likewise promote the growth of preneoplastic cells. Consequently, an unequivocal separation of initiating and promoting effects in hepatocarcinogenesis remains elusive.[781]

In any case, cell proliferation is considered to play an important part in the different stages of chemical carcinogenesis.[762,764,782,783] In many animal experiments, it has been shown that the carcinogenic effect of chemicals can be increased considerably by a preceding partial hepatectomy. The mechanism of this enhancing effect is not entirely clear, but it is generally assumed that alterations in DNA, brought about by the carcinogen or occurring spontaneously, are 'fixed' and, hence, become persistent during cell replication. An alternative explanation is that a reduction in liver mass results in a higher dose of the carcinogen per unit of liver. However, both interpretations fail to explain the finding that an enhancing effect of partial hepatectomy on hepatocarcinogenesis was still demonstrable when the carcinogen was given 3–10 weeks after the operation — when both liver mass and cell replication should have returned to the normal state.[784]

PHYSICAL FACTORS

All physical agents that can be held responsible for neoplasia in the liver exert ionizing radiation.[785] Long-term studies of populations exposed to thermonuclear explosions in Hiroshima and Nagasaki have not shown an increased incidence of liver tumours,[786] though mice, when similarly exposed experimentally, did show a high incidence.[787] Both hepatocellular and cholangiocellular neoplasms have also been induced in rats by local X-irradiation[779] and by the intravenous administration of the alpha emitter thorium dioxide (Thorotrast) which, in addition, produced haemangiosarcomas.[788] Thorotrast was used in medical practice between 1930 and 1955 to improve contrast in X-ray examinations. The injected thorium dioxide particles accumulated in different cell types, especially macrophages, or were deposited in the connective tissue of various organs, particularly the liver. Thorotrast has been shown to cause a significant number of malignant epithelial and vascular liver tumours in man.[789] Recent experimental studies in rats receiving zirconium dioxide, an analogue of thorium dioxide not emitting alpha particles, revealed that the liver tumours induced by Thorotrast were due to ionizing radiation and not to mechanical irritation by the colloidal particles.[790]

Like chemical carcinogenesis, radiation carcinogenesis depends on several factors: age and sex of the animal, dose of radiation, the proliferative state of liver cells and post-radiation survival time, in addition to poorly understood nutritional and genetic factors.[791] Development of intrahepatic vascular changes, similar to veno-occlusive disease or chronic Budd–Chiari syndrome, is often seen after radiation in experimental animals as well as occasionally in man.[792,793] Previous partial hepatectomy produces an increased incidence of radiation-induced liver tumours.[794]

HEPADNAVIRUSES

The hepadnaviruses represent a family of closely related DNA viruses which, besides hepatitis B virus (HBV) of man, include woodchuck hepatitis virus (WHV), ground squirrel hepatitis virus (GSHV), duck hepatitis virus (DHV), and heron hepatitis B virus (HHBV).[759–761,765,766] These viruses share close genomic, structural, antigenic and biological similarities such as narrow host range, a significant tropism for hepatocytes, and frequent development of persistent infections associated with chronic hepatitis. From the different animal models of hepadnavirus infection, persistent WHV infection shows the most consistent association with hepatocellular carcinoma and has been studied most thoroughly.[761,795,796]

Though hepadnaviruses contain a DNA genome, they multiply by reverse transcription like RNA retroviruses in animals, some of which are oncogenic. One of the first events following penetration and uncoating of hepadnaviruses in hepatocytes is conversion of the viral DNA, which represents a partly double-stranded circular molecule, into a covalently closed, completely double-stranded molecule. The completed circular DNA molecule accumulates in the nucleus and is believed to serve as a template for the synthesis of viral RNAs, including pre-genomic RNAs and RNAs encoding viral proteins. The pre-genomic RNAs are packed into particles with viral core proteins in the cytoplasm and trigger a complicated process of reverse transcription, eventually leading to virions that are secreted with a partly double-stranded circular DNA molecule, as before. Persistent WHV infection develops more readily in neonatal than in adult woodchucks. The chronic infection is usually characterized by a mild lymphocytic infiltrate in the portal tracts, single cell necrosis in the parenchyma, slight proliferation of sinusoidal endothelial cells and sometimes also bile ductular (oval) cells. Scattered 'ground glass' hepatocytes are present, expressing large amounts of surface antigen like the respective cells in the human liver of chronic HBV carriers.

In woodchucks, integration of hepadnaviral DNA into the host genome is uncommon in the early stages of persistent infection[796] and is mostly detected at advanced stages, particularly in hepatocellular carcinomas. Integration is found at random positions, and nearly all integrations cloned from precancerous liver or hepatocellular carcinoma tissues contained viral DNA lacking some portions of viral coding sequences due to deletion. In several cases WHV integrations occurred within and adjacent to the woodchuck c-*myc* and N-*myc* genes. Whether the integrations in these genes were sufficient to initiate hepatocarcinogenesis or functioned to promote tumour progression remains obscure. In any case, WHV, just like HBV, is only one possible factor in the sequence of successive events leading to liver neoplasms. An interaction of hepadnavirus infection with chemical carcinogens, especially the aflatoxins, has frequently been postulated to be responsible for hepatocarcinogenesis. However, intraperitoneal or oral administration of aflatoxin B_1 to ducks chronically infected with DHV failed to demonstrate any interactive effect of the virus in this species.[777] Whereas aflatoxin B_1 alone significantly increased the incidence of hepatocellular carcinomas, neither persistent DHV infection alone nor DHV infection plus aflatoxin B_1 revealed an oncogenic potential of this hepadnavirus under the experimental conditions chosen. In woodchucks, it has been demonstrated that persistent WHV infection may induce enzyme systems in the hepatic parenchyma, which catalyse the metabolism of several chemical carcinogens including aflatoxin B_1 and may, thus, contribute to the initiation and progression of hepatocarcinogenesis.[797]

GENETIC EVENTS

DNA modifications. The electrophilic intermediates produced by the metabolic activation of many chemical carcinogens result in the formation of complex spectra of DNA adducts, involving binding to various nucleophilic sites in the four bases as well as the phosphate backbone.[798,799] The formation and possible persistence of DNA adducts depend on many factors, including the distribution, metabolic activation and detoxification of the chemical carcinogen, and the proliferation and repair capacity of the target cell. Although DNA modifications are regarded as a critical event in the initiation of hepatocarcinogenesis, the ever-increasing number of chemicals which induce hepatocellular neoplasms in rodents, but do not appear to interact with DNA, suggests alternative mechanisms of action.[764,780]

The regulation of gene expression and cellular differentiation are associated with changes in DNA methylation, and these have also been proposed as an essential step in carcinogenesis.[800] Whereas a number of authors reported DNA hypomethylation in chemical hepatocarcinogenesis,[801,802] others found that the hepatocarcinogen methapyriline leads to an increase in deoxycytosine methylation.[803] Prolonged feeding of diets that are deficient in sources of transferable methyl groups, such as choline and methionine, has been shown to induce a high incidence of hepatocellular carcinomas without added carcinogens.[802,804]

Oncogenes. Oncogenes were first detected in acutely transforming retroviruses which, in addition to viral genes (*gag, pol, env*) encoding the nucleocapsid, the reverse transcriptase, and the envelope, contain one or more genes that are responsible for their ability to induce neoplastic transformation.[770-772,775] More than 20 viral oncogenes have been isolated from animal tumours. They are identified by three-letter codes after the virus or the tumour from which they were first derived. Well-known examples are *src* (Rous sarcoma virus gene), *ras* (murine sarcoma virus gene), *myc* (avian myelocytomatosis virus gene), and *abl* (Abelson murine leukaemia virus gene). Genes homologous to the retroviral oncogens were subsequently found in normal cells of the natural hosts, as well as in other organisms, by techniques of molecular hybridization. It is assumed that the retroviral oncogenes (*v-onc*) were originally picked up by the respective viruses from the cellular genes now called proto-oncogenes (c-*onc*). The viral oncogenes differ from the proto-oncogenes by point mutations or deletions which are considered to entail their transforming activity. Additional cellular oncogenes, without known retroviral counterparts, have been detected by transfection of tumour-DNA to 'immortalized' cultured mouse fibroblasts (NIH 3T3 cell line), which readily take up foreign DNA and undergo transformation after integration of the transfected oncogenes into their genome.

A variety of oncogene products have been described and grouped into five main classes, namely:

1. growth factors (e.g. c-*sis*),
2. plasma membrane-bound receptors (e.g. c-*erb* B),
3. signal-transducing proteins associated with the internal side of the plasma membrane (e.g. tyrosine-specific protein kinases of the *src*-family and GTP-binding proteins of the *ras*-family),
4. cytoplasmic protein kinases (e.g. c-*raf*), and
5. nuclear proteins, most of which represent transcription factors or subunits of these transcription factors (e.g. c-*myb*, c-*jun*, c-*fos*, c-*myc*).[774]

Activation of proto-oncogenes by point mutations, amplifications or rearrangements, resulting in inappropriate gene function and/or expression, has been considered to play an important role during the development of murine hepatocellular tumours.[805-808] Activation of *ras* oncogenes, particularly H-*ras*, has indeed been observed in the majority of hepatocellular adenomas and carcinomas which occurred either spontaneously in B6C3F1 and C3H mice, or were induced in these murine strains by various chemicals such as *N*-hydroxy-2-acetylaminofluorene, vinyl carbamate, and *N*-nitrosodiethylamine. However, *ras* gene activation rarely occurs during rat hepatocarcinogenesis, except in tumours induced by aflatoxin B$_1$.[809,810] The observation that *ras* oncogenes are frequently activated in liver tumours in mouse strains which are highly susceptible to heaptocarcinogens suggests that *ras* activation and/or propensity for clonal expansion of *ras*-containing initiated cells are factors related to susceptibility to hepatocarcinogens.[806,807,811] Several authors proposed that H-*ras* activation may be involved in the pathogenesis of liver tumours in susceptible but not in resistant strains of mice. However, recent comparative studies in three inbred strains and their F$_1$-hybrids revealed that H-*ras* activation frequency does not determine susceptibility to hepatocarcinogens, since a relatively high frequency of H-*ras* mutations was observed in two resistant strains and low frequency was found in the susceptible strain. Pasquinelli and colleagues[812] reported that in HBV transgenic mice, which are prone to develop a high incidence of hepatocellular adenomas and carcinomas, multiple proto-oncogenes (including H-, K- and N-*ras*, N- and c-*myc*, *fos*, *abl*, *sis*, *fms*, *fes*, *erb*-A, *erb*-B, *mos*, *myb*, *raf* and *src*) remained structurally and functionally intact during hepatocarcinogenesis. Persistent hepatocyte nodules produced in rats by the Solt and Farber procedure showed a pattern of expression of mRNA involving 10 cell-cycle-related genes which included c-*fos*, c-*myc*, c-H-*ras* and c-K-*ras*. This was expected on the basis of the degree of cell proliferation which had earlier been shown to lead to cell-cycle-specific activation of a number of proto-oncogenes.[813]

WHV DNA has been shown to be frequently integrated into an N-*myc* gene in hepatocellular carcinomas in woodchucks.[814] The integration occurred in a unique woodchuck N-*myc*-2 cDNA gene (retroposon) and led to its transcriptional activation. WHV integration into c-*myc*, resulting in enhanced expression of this gene in hepatocellular carcinomas, has also been observed in woodchucks.[815,816]

Tumour suppressor genes. The loss of inactivation of 'tumour suppressor genes' or 'anti-oncogenes' has been regarded as an alternative genetic pathway of oncogenesis. Two well-characterized tumour suppressor genes, *p53* and *Rh* (retinoblastoma gene), have recently been studied during hepatocarcinogenesis in HBV transgenic mice.[812] Molecular genetic analysis demonstrated that these two loci were structurally normal and produced normal levels of mRNA. The structural integrity of *p53* in this transgenic mouse model is of particular interest since a high incidence of *p53* point mutations in codon 249 has been described by several authors in human hepatocellular carcinomas in areas with a high level of exposure to aflatoxins,[817-819] whereas *p53* mutations were rarely found in patients exposed to low levels of dietary aflatoxin intake and seemed to occur at late stages of hepatocarcinogenesis in these cases.[819-821]

Transgenes. Gene transfer into the germ line of small mammals such as mice can be achieved by microinjecting a few hundred copies of a gene of interest into the pronucleus of a recently fertilized egg.[822,823] The embryos are then transferred into the oviducts of pseudopregnant females and allowed to develop to term. The resulting progeny carry the extra genes (transgenes) as stable chromosomal integrants and these are inherited in a Mendelian fashion through subsequent generations. In the resulting 'transgenic mice' the transgenes are expressed at both the RNA and protein product level, providing an excellent tool to study a variety of activated genes, including those involved in oncogenesis, in the context of living organisms. Several transgenic mouse models of hepatocarcinogenesis have been developed using different transgenes such as the simian virus 40 large tumour antigen (SV40T-antigen), oncogenic mutants of c-H-*ras* or c-*myc*, the HBV large surface antigen or the *HBx* gene.[767-769,824] The transgenes have been expressed in the liver under the control of tissue-specific promoters like metallothionein, major urinary protein, albumin, and α$_1$-antitrypsin. The findings in transgenic mouse models confirm the concept that hepatocarcinogenesis is a multi-step process in which different oncoproteins may cooperate with one another. The sequence of cellular changes observed during hepatocarcinogenesis in transgenic mice shows striking similarities to that previously described in various models of chemically induced liver carcinogenesis.[769,781]

STAGES OF NEOPLASTIC DEVELOPMENT

Histological and cytological abnormalities preceding invasive neoplasia have long been recognized by pathologists and have been classed as benign or imperfect neoplasia or as precancerous, premalignant or preneoplastic lesions.[825] A multi-stage evolution of neoplasia has also been inferred from the statistical analysis of epidemiological studies in man.[775] The non-linear increase with age in the incidence of cancer suggests that more than one transition is required for the genesis of a neoplasm and, for different types of tumour, the number of stages has been estimated to vary between two and seven. The multi-stage concept of neoplastic development has been particularly advanced by the finding of a variety of genetic changes related to oncogenes and tumour suppressor genes in a large number of malignant and in some benign neoplastic or hyperplastic lesions.[770,771,773,774] In addition to the genetic alterations, epigenetic changes such as DNA hypomethylation have been found in some stages of neoplastic development.

A preferred order of the genetic and epigenetic alterations has been observed during the development of certain tumour types, such as colorectal carcinoma.[826] However, none of these has been found to be restricted to a particular stage of carcinogenesis as defined by histopathological criteria. It has, therefore, been assumed that progressive accumulation rather than a specific sequence of genetic and epigenetic events is responsible for carcinogenesis. This concept precludes a separation of different stages of neoplastic development on the basis of defined genetic and epigenetic alterations. Moreover, once invasive malignancy has developed, it is difficult, if not impossible, to prove retrospectively that a particular genetic change was causal rather than concomitant. Farber & Rubin,[827] summarizing observations in different experimental systems, particularly in chemical hepatocarcinogenesis in rodents, recently challenged the concept of cancer as a genetic disease and postulated that neoplastic development results from adaptive responses to environmental perturbations. Adaptive cellular responses have previously been suggested to play a crucial role during neoplastic transformation of hepatocytes but were regarded as a consequence of genetically or epigenetically fixed aberrations of the intermediate metabolism induced by carcinogens.[828]

The idea that carcinogenesis is a multi-stage process comprising initiation, promotion and progression had originally been inferred from experiments in which two- or three-stage protocols were used to induce tumours of the

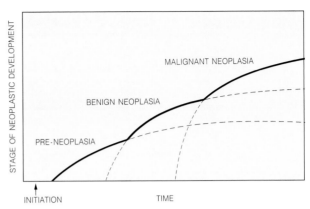

Fig. 16.48 Schematic diagram of the stages of neoplastic development as defined by phenotypic cellular changes.

skin, liver or other tissues.[775] However, an unequivocal explanation of these operationally defined stages has not been reached by this experimental approach. The more recent discovery of characteristic sequential cellular changes during neoplastic development in different organs, especially in the liver, has opened a new approach for the distinction of stages of carcinogenesis, which can now be defined by biological rather than operational criteria.[764] Preneoplasia is represented by phenotypically altered cell populations which have no obvious neoplastic nature but which indicate an increased risk for the development of both benign and malignant tumours. As a rule, preneoplasia and benign neoplasia represent successive stages in a biological continuum leading from the normal to the malignant state (Fig. 16.48). However, some findings suggest that malignant neoplasia may also arise directly from preneoplastic lesions without going through a benign intermediate stage. Another exception to the rule is that some specific types of epithelial neoplasm, such as cystic cholangiomas, are benign end-stages which do not progress to malignancy. There is no doubt that focal preneoplastic lesions frequently persist over long lag periods without giving rise to overt neoplasia, but this should not detract from their significance as early indicators of neoplastic development. This property is being increasingly used for the identification of carcinogenic agents in laboratory animals[781,829] and should also be useful in the early detection and secondary prevention of neoplasia in man.

SEQUENTIAL CELLULAR CHANGES DURING NEOPLASTIC DEVELOPMENT

The liver contains four main target cells for oncogenic agents, namely, the hepatocytes, the bile ductular epithelial, the sinusoidal endothelial and the perisinusoidal cells. In animal experiments all of these cell types may undergo neoplastic transformation and give rise to tumours (Fig. 16.49), the malignant forms of which have been classified as hepatocellular carcinomas, cholangiocarcin-

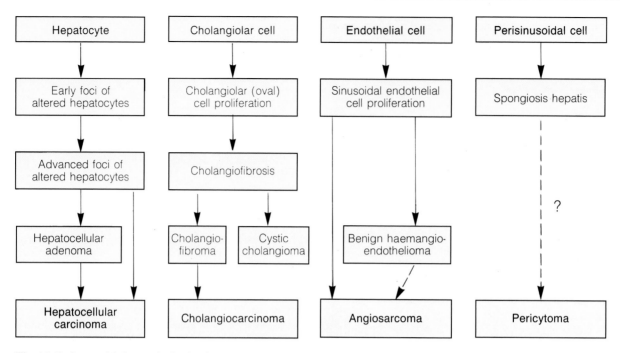

Fig. 16.49 Sequential changes in the development of epithelial and mesenchymal liver tumours.

omas, angiosarcomas and pericytomas.[830] Sequential cellular changes have been observed during the development of most of these neoplasms. Frequently, however, a number of preneoplastic, neoplastic and altered non-neoplastic cellular phenotypes develop concomitantly in the same liver and may show various combinations. It is, thus, not surprising that there is an ongoing debate on the significance of these altered cell populations in neoplastic development.[758,781,831–834] There are two main points at issue: (i) the role of cell damage, cirrhosis and regenerative hyperplasia in hepatocarcinogenesis, and (ii) the possible existence of a pluripotent liver stem cell which might be identical with, or closely related to the so-called oval cells, and be capable of giving rise to different types of liver tumours.

The frequent association between liver cirrhosis and hepatocellular carcinoma dominated the discussion on the pathogenesis of this tumour for more than a hundred years, although it had been known for a long time that it may also occur in the absence of cirrhosis.[835] A number of experiments in rats have clearly shown that toxic liver-cell damage depends on dose and duration of treatment with the chemical.[830] Fibrosis and cirrhosis appear in addition to hepatocellular carcinoma only after continuous administration of high doses which induce severe parenchymal necrosis, predominantly in zone 3 of the liver acinus. After application of low doses that do not produce significant liver-cell necrosis, hepatocellular neoplasms develop independently of fibrosis and cirrhosis. While there seems to be no direct causal relationship between cirrhosis and liver-cell carcinoma, cirrhosis could certainly modify the

action of oncogenic agents on the liver parenchyma (e.g. by leading to increased DNA synthesis and regenerative hyperplasia).

As to the ongoing debate on a possible stem cell of the liver and its relationship to oval cells and liver tumours, we refer to several recent reviews[832–834] (see also Ch.1). Whereas the existence of a liver stem cell remains to be demonstrated, proliferation of oval cells, which most probably originate from bile ductular (cholangiolar) cells, is indeed a frequent event following pronounced parenchymal damage induced by hepatocarcinogenic chemicals, radiation or viruses. However, the postulated transition from oval cells to hepatocytes and their tumours is questionable.[758, 836–838]

The most important argument against a crucial role of oval cells in the development of hepatocellular neoplasms is that, with scarcely necrogenic low doses of chemical carcinogens, hepatocellular adenomas and carcinomas not only develop without accompanying fibrosis and cirrhosis but also without any preceding oval cell proliferation. When appreciable necrotic changes of the parenchyma are produced, reactive oval cell proliferation often occurs and may persist, leading to cholangiocellular but not to hepatocellular neoplasms after long lag periods. In addition, a large number of experiments in a broad spectrum of various species provided convincing evidence that hepatocellular carcinomas induced by chemicals, radiation or viruses originate from preneoplastic foci of altered hepatocytes which apparently derive form differentiated hepatocytes.[761,781,831,839] Although there is circumstantial evidence for occasional transdifferentiation (metaplasia) of hepatocytes into cells resembling bile ductular epithelia in adenoid hepatocellular carcinomas, it appears to be appropriate to follow the sequence of cellular changes during carcinogenesis separately for each major cell type of the liver.

Hepatocytes. Characteristic changes in the biochemical and morphological phenotype of hepatocytes emerge in various species, including primates, long before hepatocellular adenomas and carcinomas become manifest.[758,781,829,831] The abnormal hepatocytes that precede benign and malignant neoplasms usually form foci which are perfectly integrated into the normal liver parenchyma (Fig. 16.50). These foci of altered hepatocytes have been observed in different species, especially in small rodents, after administration of both 'genotoxic' and 'non-genotoxic' chemical carcinogens, in rats after exposure to ionizing radiation, in woodchucks chronically infected with hepadnaviruses, in several transgenic mouse models of hepatocarcinogenesis, and in humans bearing hepatocellular carcinoma or suffering from cirrhosis. Foci of altered hepatocytes may also occur 'spontaneously' in aged animals. Under extreme experimental conditions, such as strongly hepatotoxic dosing regimens or repeated administration of high doses of several carcinogens, the majority of the focal lesions may disappear after cessation of treatment. However, this poorly understood reversion-linked phenotypic instability does not occur after continuous or short-term administration of lower doses of carcinogens which induce persistent, even life-long, lesions without any indication of reversibility.

A multitude of metabolic and morphological alterations have been found in preneoplastic hepatic foci.[762,782, 828,840–846] However, for the separation of stages of neoplastic development, phenotypic cellular changes connected with a shift in carbohydrate metabolism are of particular interest.[761,828] There is compelling evidence that a specific sequence of cellular changes predominates during hepatocarcinogenesis. This sequence leads from clear and acidophilic cell foci storing glycogen in excess, through intermediate and mixed cell formations composing 'late' foci and adenomas, to the glycogen-poor but ribosome-rich (basophilic) cell populations prevailing in hepatocellular carcinomas (Fig. 16.50). The progression of these changes is associated with an ever-increasing rate of cell proliferation. The complete sequence may be induced by a single dose of a potent chemical carcinogen such as *N*-nitrosomorpholine, which indicates that the transition from early to late phenotypic cellular changes is an autogenous process which does not require repeated interaction of the carcinogenic agent with the target cells. Some types of preneoplastic hepatic foci are apparently not integrated into the sequence outlined but may either result from phenotypic modulations of the predominant sequence, or represent intermediate stages in alternative cell lineages leading to hepatic neoplasms.

Cytochemical and microbiochemical studies in rodents revealed that the excessive storage of glycogen (glycogenosis) in preneoplastic hepatocytes is related to a disturbance in glycogen breakdown (Fig. 16.51a–c), most probably as a consequence of alterations in superordiante metabolic regulations such as a disorder in signal transduction at the plasma membrane.[781,847] At the same time, there is a gradual increase in the activities of the key enzyme of the pentose phosphate pathway, glucose-6-phosphate dehydrogenase (Fig. 16.51d), and of the glycolytic enzyme pyruvate kinase. It has been shown that the enhanced activity of glucose-6-phosphate dehydrogenase correlates with an accumulation of the enzyme protein due to overexpression of the coding gene as demonstrated by in-situ hybridization. These findings indicate the beginning of a metabolic shift in the glycogenotic hepatocytes towards alternative metabolic pathways. The enhanced activity of the key enzyme of the pentose phosphate pathway (which provides precursors for nucleic acid synthesis) is closely related to the increased cell proliferation in preneoplastic and neoplastic hepatic lesions.

Additional metabolic changes occur when glycogen storage foci give rise to mixed or basophilic cell foci, adenomas and carcinomas. Thus, the activities of the glycolytic enzymes hexokinase and glyceraldehyde-3-

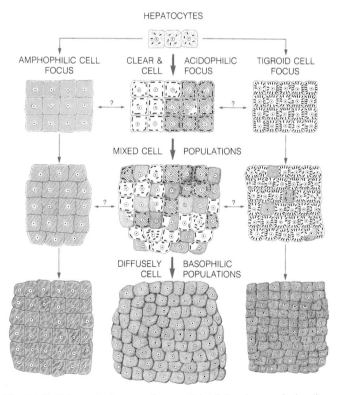

Fig. 16.50 Schematic diagram of sequential cellular changes during the development of hepatocellular neoplasms in rodent liver. In addition to the predominant sequence (centre), two alternative sequences have been established (left and right) which may either occur independently or represent phenotypic modulations of the main sequence.

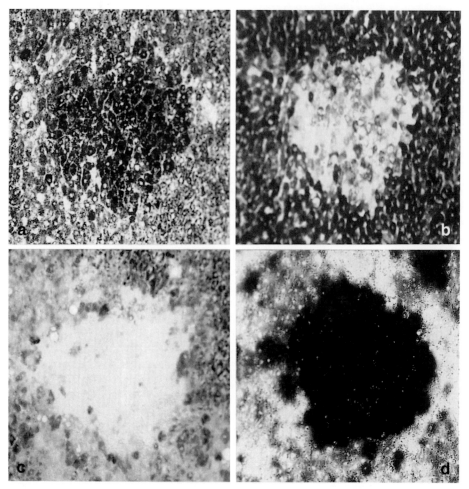

Fig. 16.51 (a–d) Serial sections through glycogenotic focus of hepatocytes induced in rat liver with *N*-nitrosomorpholine. (a) Demonstration of glycogen by the PAS reaction. (b) Decreased activity of glucose-6-phosphatase (lead salt method). (c) Decreased activity of glycogen phosphorylase (iodine staining of newly synthesized glycogen). (d) Increased activity of glucose-6-phosphate dehydrogenase (tetrazolium salt method). Illustrations kindly supplied by R Grobholz, German Cancer Research Center, Heidelberg.

phosphate dehydrogenase and the glycogen-degrading α-glucosidase increase, while the activities of glucokinase and pyruvate kinase decrease, and the glycogen gradually disappears. These findings suggest that the molecular changes underlying excessive storage of glycogen eventually result in a channelling of glucose via a sustained cascade of intermediate steps towards alternative pathways of carbohydrate metabolism, such as the pentose phosphate pathway and glycolysis. The hypothesis that glycogenosis indicates a metabolic aberration which triggers a cascade of events eventually leading to hepatocellular neoplasms is supported by the ever-increasing number of clinical case reports of hepatocellular adenomas and carcinomas in patients who suffer from inborn glycogen storage disease type I.[758] Whether the recently reported reactivation of insulin-like growth factor II, which has been observed in different animal models of hepatocarcinogenesis during late stages of neoplastic development[846,848] and in human hepatocellular carcinomas,[849] is related to the metabolic

shift in carbohydrate metabolism just described is an intriguing question which remains to be answered. Observations that suggest an ordered pattern of metabolic changes during hepatocarcinogenesis have also been described for a number of enzymes involved in drug metabolism, such as various cytochrome *P*-450 isoenzymes and epoxide hydrolase.[846]

Cholangiolar (oval) cells. The neoplastic transformation of bile-duct epithelium follows a complex sequence (Fig. 16.49) usually starting with a proliferation of cells which derive from the ducts of Hering (cholangioles) and are often called 'oval cells'.[758,836,838,850] Severe parenchymal necrosis — as, for example, produced by sublethal doses of chemical carcinogens — appears to be a prerequisite for the early reactive proliferation of cholangiolar cells. The majority of these cells die but those that survive undergo 'intestinal metaplasia' or 'cholangiolar mucopolysaccharidosis' and form mucous cholangiofibrotic lesions (Fig. 16.52) which have been shown to represent

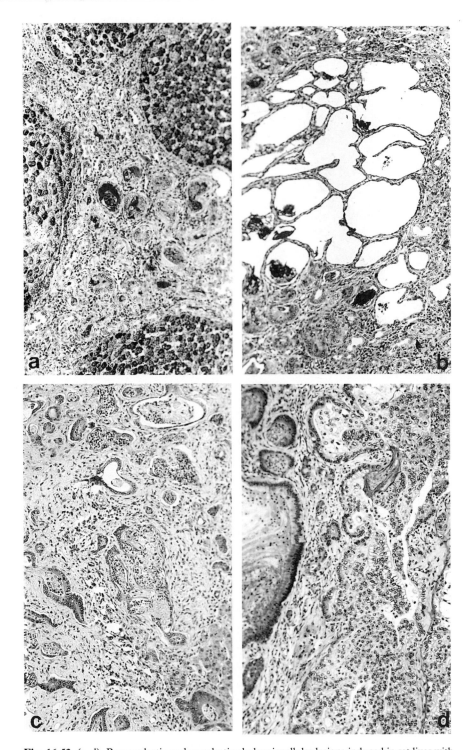

Fig. 16.52 (a–d) Preneoplastic and neoplastic cholangiocellular lesions induced in rat liver with *N*-nitrosomorpholine. (a) Cholangiofibrosis, PAS. (b) Benign cystic cholangioma, PAS. (c) Cholangiofibroma, H & E. (d) Cholangiocarcinoma. Note transition from component rich in mucous substances (to the left) into mucus-free carcinoma. Alcian blue. From Bannasch & Zerban[830]

an intermediate stage in the development of benign and malignant cholangiocellular neoplasms. In the cholangio-fibrotic lesions many ductular cells exhibit a conversion into goblet cells which store and secrete abundant mucous substances. This mucus production seems to be specific for carcinogen-induced cholangiolar proliferation and may represent a phenomenon analogous to hepatocellular glycogenosis. In line with this assumption it has been

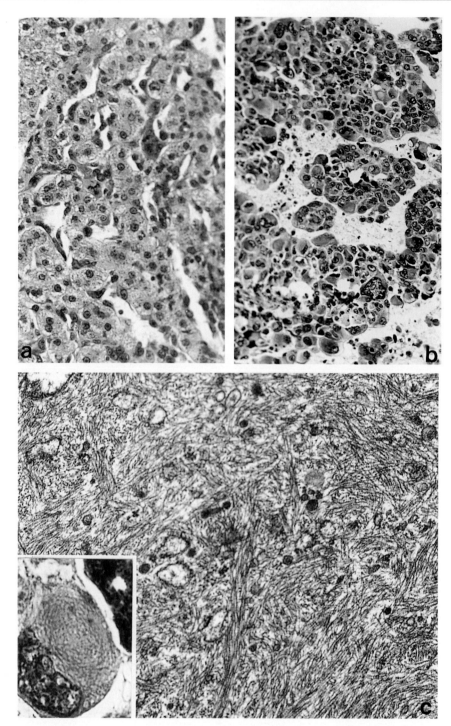

Fig. 16.53 (a–c) Early and advanced neoplastic changes of sinusoidal endothelial cells induced in rat liver with *N*-nitrosomorpholine. (a) Proliferation of atypical endothelial cells along the sinusoids, H & E. (b) Angiosarcoma, H & E. (c) Electron microscope demonstration of accumulation of intermediate filaments of the vimentin type in angiosarcoma cell. Uranyl acetate and lead nitrate, × 36 000. Inset: Vimentin storage in cell as seen under the light microscope. H & E. From Bannasch & Zerban[830]

demonstrated by histochemical assays that cholangiolar mucopolysaccharidosis shares many enzymatic alterations with hepatic glycogenosis.[836,838] According to Chou & Gibson,[851] an accumulation of mucopolysaccharides may also play an important role in the development of human cholangiocarcinomas. They have shown that bile ductular proliferation and excessive mucus secretion occur in individuals chronically infested with liver flukes. In rat liver,

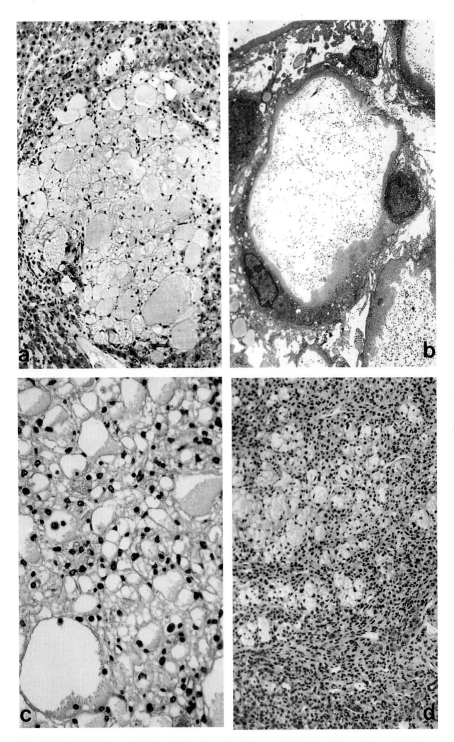

Fig. 16.54 (a–d) Spongiosis hepatis (a–c) and pericytoma (d) induced in rat liver with *N*-nitrosomorpholine. (a) Spongiosis hepatis as seen under the light microscope. H & E. (b) Portion of spongiosis hepatis as seen under the electron microscope. Uranyl acetate and lead nitrate, × 1760. (c) Spongiosis hepatis showing considerable cell proliferation, H & E. (d) Pericytoma, H & E. From Bannasch & Zerban[830]

two types of tumour may develop from the cholangio-fibrotic lesions (Fig. 16.52b and c): (i) benign cystic chol-angioma, the formation of which is accompanied by a marked change in the epithelial phenotype from cylin-drical to flat cells no longer secreting mucus, and (ii) cho-langiofibroma, which is characterized by a particularly pronounced production of collagen fibres and mucous substances.[758] As a rule, cholangiofibroma does not metastasize, but it is a potentially malignant tumour which may progress to a cholangiocarcinoma (Fig. 16.52d). Again, the excessive production of mucus gradually disappears during this process. In rats, not only short-term administration of high doses but also long-term application of low doses of chemical hepatocarcinogens can lead to bile-duct proliferation, benign cystic cholangioma and, perhaps, also cholangiocarcinoma, without producing cholangiofibrosis as an early stage.

Endothelial cells. The sequential cellular changes that occur during the genesis of angiosarcomas in rodents and man show many similarities.[756,758,778] The endothelial cells may give rise to three types of vascular lesions after treatment with chemical carcinogens, namely sinusoidal peliosis hepatis, benign angioma, and angiosarcoma (Fig. 16.53a and b). Sinusoidal peliosis is a benign lesion characterized by an irregular focal dilatation of the sinuses. The lining endothelial cells may show some minor alterations such as nuclear enlargement. In *Mastomys* species all transitions from peliosis to unequivocal angiosarcoma can be observed after single or two-fold intraperitoneal injections of *N*-nitrosodiethylamine.[843] Anabolic/androgenic steroids, which have been related to liver-cell adenomas and peliosis hepatis in man, may induce this lesion in rats too. Transitions from benign angioma to angiosarcoma may occur in nitrosamine-treated rodents but this is the exception rather than the rule. The majority of angiosarcomas originate from highly atypical endothelial cells without an obvious benign precursor stage. The atypical endothelial cells accumulate excessive amounts of a cytoskeletal filament protein called vimentin (Fig. 16.53c).

Perisinusoidal cells. The perisinusoidal cells are also possible targets of oncogenic agents as demonstrated especially for chemical carcinogens in rodents and fish.[758,852] They have only been clearly identified during the past two decades and have variously been called Ito cells, lipocytes, or fat-storing cells.[853] These cells are located between the endothelial cells and the hepatocytes and have been shown to be involved in the metabolism of vitamin A and in the production of collagen, as well as in the secretion of hepatocyte growth factor and transforming growth factor β.[853,854] In rats and fish treated with different chemical carcinogens the perisinusoidal cells are considered to be the site of origin of a cyst-like multilocular lesion (Fig. 16.54a and b) designated as 'spongiosis hepatis'.[758, 852] The lobules of spongiosis are not filled with blood but with glycosaminoglycans as demonstrated histochemically. There is circumstantial evidence for the rare progression of spongiosis hepatis to malignant mesenchymal tumours classified as pericytomas, after very long lag periods (Fig. 16.54c and d). The accumulation of glycosaminoglycans in spongiotic lesions ceases during transformation into pericytomas. Whereas no counterpart of spongiosis hepatis has as yet been described in man, human hepatic pericytomas have rarely been observed.

REFERENCES

1. Ishak K G, Anthony P P, Sobin L H. Histological typing of tumours of the liver. World Health Organization International Histological Classification of Tumours, 2nd edn. Berlin: Springer-Verlag, 1994 (in press)
2. Muir C, Waterhouse J, Mack T, Dowell J, Whelan S, eds. Cancer incidence in five continents. Vol V. Lyon: International Agency for Research on Cancer, 1987
3. World Health Organization International Classification of Diseases for Oncology (ICD-O). Geneva: World Health Organization, 1990
4. Waterhouse JAH. Cancer handbook of epidemiology and prognosis. Edinburgh: Churchill Livingstone, 1974
5. Toms J R. Trends in cancer survival in Great Britain. London: Cancer Research Campaign, 1982
6. Blumgart L H, ed. Surgery of the liver and biliary tract. Edinburgh: Churchill Livingstone, 1988
7. McDermott W V, ed. Surgery of the liver. Boston: Blackwell, 1988
8. Schweizer P, ed. Hepatobiliary surgery in childhood. Stuttgart: Schattauer, 1991
9. Lefkowitch J H. The epidemiology and morphology of primary malignant liver tumors. Surg Clin North Am 1981; 61: 169–181
10. Rustgi V K. Epidemiology of hepatocellular carcinoma. Gastroenterol Clin North Am 1987; 16: 545–551
11. Nakashima T, Kojiro M. Hepatocellular carcinoma. An atlas of its pathology. Tokyo: Springer-Verlag, 1987
12. Craig J R, Peters R L, Edmondson H A. Tumors of the liver and intrahepatic bile ducts. Atlas of tumor pathology, 2nd series, fascicle 26. Washington DC: Armed Forces Institute of Pathology, 1989
13. Okuda K, Ishak K G, eds. Neoplasms of the liver. Tokyo: Springer-Verlag, 1988
14. Bannasch P, Keppler D, Weber G, eds. Liver cell carcinoma. Falk Symposium 51. Dordrecht: Kluwer, 1989
15. Tabor E, Di Bisceglie A M, Purcell R H. Etiology, pathology and treatment of hepatocellular carcinoma in North America. Advances in Applied Biotechnology Series, Vol 13. Houston: Gulf Publishing, 1991
16. Anthony P P. Tumours of the hepatobiliary system. In: Fletcher C D M, ed. Diagnostic histopathology of tumours. Edinburgh: Churchill Livingstone, 1994 (in press)
17. Baum J K, Holtz F, Bookstein J J, Klein E W. Possible association between benign hepatomas and oral contraceptives. Lancet 1973; ii: 926–929
18. Johnson F L, Feagler J R, Lerner K G. Association of androgenic–anabolic steroid therapy with development of hepatocellular carcinoma. Lancet 1972; ii: 1273–1276
19. Anthony P P. Hepatoma associated with androgenic steroids. Lancet 1975; i: 685–686
20. Edmondson H A, Henderson B, Benton B. Liver cell adenomas associated with use of oral contraceptives. N Engl J Med 1976; 294: 470–472
21. Nissen E D, Kent D R, Nissen S E. Etiologic factors in the pathogenesis of liver tumors associated with oral contraceptives. Am J Obstet Gynecol 1976; 127: 61–66
22. Christopherson W M, Mays E T. Liver tumors and contraceptive steroids: experience with the first hundred registry patients. J Natl Cancer Inst 1977; 58: 167–171
23. Klatskin G. Hepatic tumors: possible relationship to use of oral contraceptives. Gastroenterology 1977; 73: 386–394
24. Vana J, Murphy G P, Aronoff B L, Baker H W. Primary liver tumors and oral contraceptives. JAMA 1977; 238: 2154–2158
25. Rooks J B, Ory H W, Ishak K G et al. Epidemiology of hepatocellular adenoma. The role of oral contraceptive use. JAMA 1979; 242: 644–648
26. Christopherson W M, Mays E T, Barrows G H. Liver tumors in young women: a clinical pathologic study of 201 cases in the Louisville Registry. In: Fenoglio C M, Wolff M, eds. Progress in surgical pathology, vol II. New York: Masson, 1980: pp 187–205

27. Mettlin C, Natarajan N. Studies of the role of oral contraceptive use in the etiology of benign and malignant liver tumors. J Surg Oncol 1981; 18: 73–85

28. Valla D, Benhamou J-P. Liver diseases related to oral contraceptives. Dig Dis 1988; 6: 76–86

29. Shortell C K, Schwartz S I. Hepatic adenoma and focal nodular hyperplasia. Surg Gynecol Obstet 1991; 173: 426–431

30. Gregoire A T, Blye R P, eds. Contraceptive steroids. Pharmacology and safety. New York: Plenum Press, 1986

31. Huggins G R, Zucker P K. Oral contraceptives and neoplasia: 1987 update. Fertil Steril 1987; 47: 733–761

32. Prentice R L, Thomas D B. On the epidemiology of oral contraceptives and disease. In: Klein G, Weinhouse S, eds. Advances in cancer research, vol 49. Orlando: Academic Press, 1987: pp 285–401

33. Beral V, Hannaford P, Kay C. Oral contraceptive use and malignancies of the genital tract. Lancet 1988; ii: 1331–1335

33a. Lindgren A, Olsson R. Liver damage from low-dose oral contraceptives. J Intern Med 1993; 234: 287–292

34. Paradinas F, Bull T B, Westaby D, Murray-Lyon I M. The development of peliosis hepatis and liver tumours during long-term methyltestosterone therapy: a light and electron microscopical study. Histopathology 1977; 1: 225–246

35. Ishak K G. Hepatic lesions caused by anabolic and contraceptive steroids. Semin Liver Dis 1981; 1: 116–128

36. Westaby D, Portmann B, Williams R. Androgen related primary tumours in non-Fanconi patients. Cancer 1983; 51: 1947–1952

37. Chandra R S, Kapur S P, Kelleher J, Luban N, Patterson K. Benign hepatocellular tumors in the young. Arch Pathol Lab Med 1984; 108: 168–171

38. Carrasco D, Prieto M, Pallardó L et al. Multiple hepatic adenomas after long-term therapy with testosterone enanthate — review of the literature. J Hepatol 1985; 1: 573–578

39. Ishak K G, Zimmerman H J. Hepatotoxic effects of the anabolic/androgenic steroids. Semin Liver Dis 1987; 7: 230–236

40. Creagh T M, Rubin A, Evans D J. Hepatic tumour induced by anabolic steroids in an athlete. J Clin Pathol 1988; 41: 441–443

40a. Klava A, Super P, Aldridge M, Horner J, Guillou P. Body builder's liver. J Roy Soc Med 1994; 87: 43–44

41. Grangé J-D, Guéchot J, Legendre C, Giboudeau J, Darnis F, Poupon R. Liver adenoma and focal nodular hyperplasia in a man with high endogenous sex steroids. Gastroenterology 1987; 93: 1409–1413

42. Edmondson H A, Reynolds T B, Henderson B, Benton B. Regression of liver cell adenomas associated with oral contraceptives. Ann Intern Med 1977; 86: 180–182

43. Steinbrecher U P, Lisbona R, Huang S N, Mishkin S. Complete regression of hepatocellular adenoma after withdrawal of oral contraceptives. Dig Dis Sci 1981; 26: 1045–1050

44. Bühler H, Pirovino M, Akovbiantz A et al. Regression of liver cell adenoma. A follow up study of three consecutive patients after discontinuation of oral contraceptive use. Gastroenterology 1982; 82: 775–782

45. Tesluk H, Lawrie J. Hepatocellular adenoma. Its transformation to carcinoma in a user of oral contraceptives. Arch Pathol Lab Med 1981; 105: 296–299

46. Kerlin P, Davis G L, McGill D B, Weiland L H, Adson M A, Sheedy P F. Hepatic adenoma and focal nodular hyperplasia: clinical, pathologic and radiologic features. Gastroenterology 1983; 84: 994–1002

47. Gordon S C, Reddy K R, Livingstone A S, Jeffers L J, Schiff E R. Resolution of a contraceptive-steroid induced hepatic adenoma with subsequent evolution into hepatocellular carcinoma. Ann Intern Med 1986; 105: 547–549

48. Leese T, Farges O, Bismuth H. Liver cell adenomas. Ann Surg 1988; 208: 558–564

49. Marks W H, Thompson N, Appleman H. Failure of hepatic adenoma (HCA) to regress after discontinuance of oral contraceptives. Ann Surg 1988; 208: 190–195

50. Gyorffy E J, Bredfeldt J E, Black W C. Transformation of hepatic cell adenoma to hepatocellular carcinoma due to oral contraceptive use. Ann Intern Med 1989; 110: 489–490

51. See K L, See M, Gluud C. Liver pathology associated with the use of anabolic-androgenic steroids. Liver 1992; 12: 73–79

52. Carrasco D, Barrachina M, Prieto M, Berenguer J. Clomiphene citrate and liver cell adenoma. N Engl J Med 1984; 310: 1120–1121

53. Middleton C, McCaughan G W, Painter D M, Stephen M S, Beale M, Fraser I. Danazol and hepatic neoplasia: a case report. Aust NZ J Med 1989; 19: 733–735

54. Fermand J P, Levy Y, Bouscary D et al. Danazol-induced hepatocellular adenoma. Am J Med 1990; 88: 529–530

55. Kahn H, Manzarbeitia C, Theise N, Schwartz M, Miller C, Thung S N. Danazol-induced hepatocellular adenomas. Arch Pathol Lab Med 1991; 115: 1054–1057

56. Kalra P A, Guthrie J A, Dibble J B, Turney J H, Brownjohn A M. Hepatic adenomas induced by norethisterone in patients receiving renal dialysis. Br Med J 1987; 294: 808

57. Coire C I, Quizilbash A H, Castelli M F. Hepatic adenomata in type la glycogen storage disease. Arch Pathol Lab Med 1987; 111: 166–169

58. Poe R, Snover D C. Adenomas in glycogen storage disease Type I. Am J Surg Pathol 1988; 12: 477–483

59. Foster J H, Donahue T A, Berman M M. Familial liver-cell adenomas and diabetes mellitus. N Engl J Med 1978; 299: 239–241

60. Beuers U, Richter W O, Ritter M M, Wiebecke B, Schwandt P. Klinefelter syndrome and liver adenoma. J Clin Gastroenterol 1991; 13: 214–216

61. Wheeler D, Edmondson H A, Reynolds T B. Spontaneous liver cell adenoma in children. Am J Clin Pathol 1986; 85: 6–12

62. Kogure K, Nagamachi Y, Sasamoto K, Ogawa T. Liver cell adenoma: a case report and a review of 30 cases reported in Japan. J Gastroenterol Hepatol 1987; 2: 325–331

63. Pulpeiro J R, Orduna M, Jimenez J, Gallego M S, Millan J M. Primary hepatocellular adenoma in men. J Clin Ultrasound 1989; 17: 269–274

64. Chen K T K, Ma C K, Kassel S H. Hepatocellular adenoma of the placenta. Am J Surg Pathol 1986; 10: 436–440

65. Estebe J-P, Malledant Y, Guillon Y-M et al. Rupture spontanée d'un adénome du foie pendant la grossesse. J Chir 1988; 125: 654–656

66. Tsang V, Halliday A W, Collier N, Benjamin I S, Blumgart L H. Hepatic cell adenoma: spontaneous rupture during pregnancy. Dig Surg 1989; 6: 86–87

67. Porter L E, Elm M S, Van Thiel D H, Eagon P K. Hepatic estrogen receptor in human liver disease. Gastroenterology 1987; 92: 735–745

68. Nime F, Pickren J W, Vana J. The histology of liver tumors in oral contraceptive users observed during a national survey by the American College of Surgeons Commission on Cancer. Cancer 1979; 44: 1481–1489

69. Mays E T, Christopherson W. Hepatic tumors induced by sex steroids. Semin Liv Dis 1984; 4: 147–157

70. Goodman Z D. Benign tumors of the liver. In: Okuda K, Ishak K G, eds. Neoplasms of the liver. Berlin: Springer-Verlag, 1988: pp 105–125

71. Goldfarb S. Sex hormones and hepatic neoplasia. Cancer Res 1976; 36: 2584–2588

72. Chen K T K, Bocian J J. Multiple hepatic adenomas. Arch Pathol Lab Med 1983; 107: 274–275

73. Flejou J F, Barge J, Menu Y et al. Liver adenomatosis: an entity distinct from liver adenoma? Gastroenterology 1985; 89: 1132–1138

74. Le Bail B, Jouhanole H, Deugnier Y et al. Liver adenomatosis in two patients on long-term oral contraceptives. Am J Surg Pathol 1992; 16: 982–987

75. Goodman Z D, Mikel U V, Lubbers P R, Ros P R, Langloss J M, Ishak K G. Kupffer cells in hepatocellular adenomas. Am J Surg Pathol 1987; 11: 191–196

76. Palmer P E, Christopherson W M, Wolfe J H. Alpha-1-antitrypsin, a protein marker in oral contraceptive-associated hepatic tumors. Am J Clin Pathol 1979; 68: 736–739

77. Heffelfinger S, Irani D R, Finegold M J. 'Alcoholic hepatitis' in a hepatic adenoma. Hum Pathol 1987; 18: 751–754

78. Malatjalian D A, Graham C H. Liver adenoma with granulomas. Arch Pathol Lab Med 1982; 106: 244–246

79. Karhunen P J. Benign hepatic tumours and tumour-like conditions in men. J Clin Pathol 1986; 39: 183–188

80. Govindarajan S, Peters R L. The bile duct adenoma. Arch Pathol Lab Med 1984; 108: 922–924

81. Allaire G S, Rabin L, Ishak K G, Sesterhenn I A. Bile duct adenoma: a study of 152 cases. Am J Surg Pathol 1988; 12: 708–715

82. O'Hara J B, McCue P A, Miettinen M. Bile duct adenomas with endocrine component. Am J Surg Pathol 1992; 16: 21–25

82a. Tsui W M S, Loo K T, Chow L T C, Tse C C H. Biliary adenofibroma. A heretofore unrecognized benign biliary tumor of the liver. Am J Surg Pathol 1993; 17: 186–192

83. Ishak K G, Willis G W, Cummins S D, Bullock A A. Biliary cystadenoma and cystadenocarcinoma. Cancer 1977; 39: 322–338

84. Wheeler D A, Edmondson H A. Cystadenoma with mesenchymal stroma (CMS) in the liver and bile ducts. Cancer 1985; 56: 1434–1445

85. Lewis W D, Jenkins R L, Rossi R L et al. Surgical treatment of biliary cystadenoma. Arch Surg 1988; 123: 563–568

85a. Thomas J A, Scriven M W, Puntis M C A, Jasani B, Williams G T. Elevated serum CA 19–9 levels in hepatobiliary cystadenoma with mesenchymal stroma. Cancer 1992; 70: 1841–1846

85b. Subramony C, Herrera G A, Turbat-Herrera E A. Hepatobiliary cystadenoma. Arch Pathol Lab Med 1993; 117: 1036–1042

86. Kim Y I, Kim S T, Lee G K, Choi B I. Papillary cystic tumor of the liver. Cancer 1990; 65: 2740–2746

87. Bogomoletz W V. Cystic tumours of the exocrine pancreas. In: Anthony P P, MacSween R N M, eds. Recent advances in histopathology, No. 15. Edinburgh: Churchill Livingstone, 1992: pp 141–155

88. Suyama Y, Horie Y, Suou T et al. Oral contraceptives and intrahepatic biliary cystadenoma having an increased level of estrogen receptor. Hepato-gastroenterol 1988; 35: 171–174

88a. Wang Y-J, Lee S-D, Lai K-H, Wang S S, Lo K-J. Primary biliary cystic tumors of the liver. Am J Gastroenterol 1993; 88: 559–603

89. Okulski E G, Dolin B J, Kandawalla N M. Intrahepatic biliary papillomatosis. Arch Pathol Lab Med 1979; 103: 647–649

90. Mercadier M, Bodard M, Fingerhut A, Chigot J P. Papillomatosis of the intrahepatic bile ducts. World J Surg 1984; 8: 30–35

91. Padfield C J H, Ansell I D, Furness P N. Mucinous biliary papillomatosis: a tumour in need of wider recognition. Histopathology 1988; 13: 687–694

92. Bottger T, Sorger K, Jenny E, Junginger T. Progressive papillomatosis of the intrahepatic and extrahepatic bile ducts. Acta Chir Scand 1989; 155: 125–129

93. Hubens G, Delvaux G, Willems G, Bourgain C, Klöppel G. Papillomatosis of the intra- and extrahepatic bile ducts with involvement of the pancreatic duct. Hepato-gastroenterol 1991; 38: 413–418

93a. Buckley J G, Salimi Z. Villous adenoma of the common bile duct. Abdom Imaging 1993; 18: 245–246

93b. Hanafy M, McDonald P. Villous adenoma of the common bile duct. J Roy Soc Med 1993; 86: 603–604

94. Munoz N, Linsell A. Epidemiology of primary liver cancer. In: Correa P, Haenszel W, eds. Epidemiology of cancer in the digestive tract. The Hague: Nijhoff, 1982: pp 161–195

95. Okuda K, MacKay I. Hepatocellular carcinoma. UICC Technical Report Series vol 74. no 17. Geneva: UICC, 1982

96. Linsell A. Primary liver cancer: epidemiology and etiology. In: Wanebo H J, ed. Hepatic and biliary cancer. New York: Dekker, 1986: pp 3–15

97. Okuda K. Primary liver cancer. Dig Dis Sci 1986; 31(9) suppl: 1335–1465

98. Omata M. Current perspectives on hepatocellular carcinoma in Oriental and African countries compared to developed Western countries. Dig Dis 1987; 5: 97–115

99. Munoz N, Bosch X. Epidemiology of hepatocellular carcinoma. In: Okuda K, Ishak K G, eds. Neoplasms of the liver. Berlin: Springer-Verlag, 1988: pp 3–19

100. Bosch F X, Munoz N. Epidemiology of hepatocellular carcinoma. In: Bannasch P, Keppler D, Weber G, eds. Liver cell carcinoma. Falk Symposium No 51. Dordrecht: Kluwer, 1989: pp 3–14

101. Lau JY-N, Lai C-L. Hepatocarcinogenesis. Trop Gastroenterol 1990; 11: 9–24

102. Simonetti R G, Camma C, Fiorello F, Politi F, d'Amico G, Pagliaro L. Hepatocellular carcinoma. A worldwide problem and the major risk factors. Dig Dis Sci 1991; 36: 962–972

103. Harris C C, Sun T. Multifactorial etiology of human liver cancer. Carcinogenesis 1984; 5: 697–701

104. Farber E, ed. Experimental, epidemiological and clinical aspects of liver carcinogenesis. Cancer Surveys 1986; 5: 695–819

105. Farber E, Sarma D S R. Hepatocarcinogenesis: a dynamic cellular perspective. Lab Invest 1987; 56: 4–22

106. Popper H. Viral versus chemical carcinogenesis. J Hepatol 1988; 6: 229–238

107. Kaldor J M, Bosch F X. Multistage theory of carcinogenesis: the epidemiological evidence for liver cancer. Bull Cancer 1990; 77: 515–519

108. Andersen I B, Sørensen T I A, Prener A. Increase in incidence of disease due to diagnostic drift: primary liver cancer in Denmark, 1943–85. Br Med J 1991; 302: 437–440

109. Okuda K. Hepatocellular carcinoma: recent progress. Hepatology 1992; 15: 948–963

110. Stevens R G, Merkle E J, Lustbader E D. Age and cohort effects in primary liver cancer. Int J Cancer 1984; 33: 453–458

111. Weinberg A G, Finegold M J. Primary hepatic tumors in childhood. Hum Pathol 1983; 14: 512–537

112. Butler W H, Newberne P M. Mouse hepatic neoplasia. Amsterdam: Elsevier, 1975

113. Newberne P M, Butler W D. Rat hepatic neoplasia. Cambridge: MIT Press, 1978

114. Grasso P. Experimental liver tumours in animals. In: Williams R, Johnson P J, eds. Liver tumours. Baillière's Clinical Gastroenterology 1987; 1: 183–305

114a. Nagasue N, Kohno H. Hepatocellular carcinoma and sex hormones. HPB Surgery 1992; 6: 1–6

115. Iqbal M J, Wilkinson M L, Johnson P J, Williams R. Sex steroid proteins in foetal, adult and malignant human liver tissue. Br J Cancer 1983; 48: 791–796

116. Eagon P K, Porter L E, Francavilla A, Di Leo A, Van Thiel D H. Estrogen and androgen receptors in liver: their role in liver disease and regeneration. Semin Liv Dis 1985; 5: 59–69

117. Nagasue N, Ito A, Yukaya H, Ogawa Y. Androgen receptors in hepatocellular carcinoma and surrounding parenchyma. Gastroenterology 1985; 89: 643–647

118. Ohnishi S, Murakami T, Moriyama T, Mitamura K, Imawari M. Androgen and estrogen receptors in hepatocellular carcinoma and in the surrounding non-cancerous liver tissue. Hepatology 1986; 3: 440–443

119. Eagon P K, Francavilla A, Di Leo A et al. Quantitation of estrogen and androgen receptors in hepatocellular carcinoma and adjacent normal human liver. Dig Dis Sci 1991; 36: 1303–1308

120. Nagasue N, Kohno H, Chang Y, Hayashi T, Nakamura T. Specificity of androgen receptors of hepatocellular carcinoma and liver in humans. Hepato-gastroenterol 1990; 37: 474–479

120. Nakagama H, Gunji T, Ohnishi S et al. Expression of androgen receptor mRNA in human hepatocellular carcinomas and hepatoma cell lines. Hepatology 1991; 14: 99–102

121. Carbone A, Vecchio F M. Presence of cytoplasmic progesterone receptors in hepatic adenomas. Am J Clin Pathol 1986; 85: 325–329

123. Nagasue N, Ito A, Yukaya H, Ogawa Y. Estrogen receptors in hepatocellular carcinoma. Cancer 1986; 57: 87–91

124. Nagasue N, Kohno H, Yamanoi A, Kimoto T, Chang Y-C, Nakamura T. Progesterone receptor in hepatocellular carcinoma: correlation with androgen and estrogen receptors. Cancer 1991; 67: 2501–2503

125. Carr B I, Van Thiel D H. Hormonal manipulation of human hepatocellular carcinoma. J Hepatol 1990; 11: 287–289

126. Porter L E, Van Thiel D H, Eagon P K. Estrogens and progestins as tumour inducers. Semin Liv Dis 1987; 7: 24–31

127. d'Arville C N, Johnson P J. Growth factors, endocrine aspects and hormonal treatment in hepatocellular carcinoma — an overview. J Steroid Biochem Mol Biol 1990; 37: 1007–1012

127a. Farinati F, De Maria N, Fornasiero A et al. Prospective controlled trial with antiestrogen drug Tamoxifen in patients with unresectable hepatocellular carcinoma. Dig Dis Sci 1992; 37: 659–662

128. Lai C-L, Gregory P B, Wu P-C, Lok ASF, Wong K-P, Ng MMT. Hepatocellular carcinoma in Chinese males and females: possible causes for the male predominance. Cancer 1987; 60: 1107–1110

128a. Tarao K, Ohkawa S, Shimizu A et al. The male preponderance in incidence of hepatocellular carcinoma in cirrhotic patients may depend on the higher DNA synthetic activity of cirrhotic tissue in men. Cancer 1993; 72: 369–374

129. Heston W E, Development and utilization of inbred strains of mice for cancer research. In: Mammalian genetics and cancer. (The Jackson Laboratory Fiftieth Anniversary Symposium.) New York: Liss, 1981: pp 279–298

130. Kew M C, Gear A J, Baumgarten I, Dusheiko G M, Maier G. Histocompatibility antigens in patients with hepatocellular carcinoma and their relationship to chronic hepatitis B virus infection in these patients. Gastroenterology 1979; 77: 537–539

131. Chan S H, Simons M J, Oon C J. HLA antigens in Chinese patients with hepatocellular carcinoma. J Natl Cancer Inst 1980; 65: 21–23

132. Hsu H-C, Wu N-Z, Chang M-H, Su I-J, Chen D S. Childhood hepatocellular carcinoma develops exclusively in hepatitis B surface antigen carriers in three decades in Taiwan. J Hepatol 1987; 5: 260–267

133. Wu T C, Tong M J, Hwang B, Lee S-D, Hu M M. Primary hepatocellular carcinoma and hepatitis B infection during childhood. Hepatology 1987; 7: 46–48

134. Leuschner I, Harms D, Schmidt D. The association of hepatocellular carcinoma in childhood with hepatitis B virus infection. Cancer 1988; 62: 2363–2369

135. Lok A S F, Lai C-L. Factors determining the development of hepatocellular carcinoma in hepatitis B surface antigen carriers. Cancer 1988; 61: 1287–1291

136. Cheah P L, Looi L-M, Lim H-P, Yap S-F. Childhood primary hepatocellular carcinoma and hepatitis B virus infection. Cancer 1990; 65: 174–176

137. McGoldrick J P, Boston V E, Glasgow J F T. Hepatocellular carcinoma associated with congenital macronodular cirrhosis in a neonate. J Pediatr Surg 1986; 21: 177–179

138. Weinberger J M, Cohen Z, Berk T. Polyposis coli preceded by hepatocellular carcinoma. Dis Colon Rectum 1981; 24: 296–300

139. Zeze F, Ohsato K, Mitani H, Ohkuma R, Koide O. Hepatocellular carcinoma associated with familial polyposis of the colon. Dis Colon Rectum 1983; 26: 465–468

140. Laferla G, Kaye S B, Crean G P. Hepatocellular and gastric carcinoma associated with familial polyposis coli. J Surg Oncol 1988; 38: 19–21

141. Kaufman S S, Wood P, Shaw B W, Markin R S, Gridelli B, Vanderhoof J A. Hepatocarcinoma in a child with the Alagille syndrome. Am J Dis Child 1987; 141: 698–700

142. Rabinovitz M, Imperial J C, Schade R R, Van Thiel D H. Hepatocellular carcinoma in Alagille's syndrome: a family study. J Pediatr Gastroenterol Nutr 1989; 8: 26–30

143. Le Bail B, Bioulac-Sage P, Arnoux R, Perissat J, Saric J, Balabaud C. Late recurrence of a hepatocellular carcinoma in a patient with incomplete Alagille syndrome. Gastroenterology 1990; 99: 1514–1516

143a. Keeffe E B, Pinson C W, Ragsdale J, Zonana J. Hepatocellular carcinoma in arteriohepatic dysplasia. Am J Gastroenterol 1993; 88: 1446–1448

144. Weinstein S, Scottalini A G, Loo S Y T, Caldwell P C, Bhagavan N V. Ataxia telangiectasia with hepatocellular carcinoma in a 15 year old girl and studies of her kindred. Arch Pathol Lab Med 1985; 109: 1000–1004

145. Jameson C F. Primary hepatocellular carcinoma in hereditary haemorrhagic telangiectasia. Histopathology 1989; 15: 550–552

146. Barrett-Dahma B. Hepatoma in familial cholestatic cirrhosis in childhood; its occurrence in twin brothers. Arch Pathol Lab Med 1979; 103: 30–33

147. Ugarte N, Gonzalez-Crussi F. Hepatoma in siblings with progressive familial cholestatic cirrhosis of childhood. Am J Clin Pathol 1981; 76: 172–177

148. Weinberg A G, Mize C E, Worthan H G. The occurrence of hepatoma in the chronic form of hereditary tyrosinaemia. J Pediatr 1976; 88: 434–438

149. Dehner L P, Snover D C, Sharp H L, Ascher N, Nakhleh R, Day D L. Hereditary tyrosinaemia type 1 (chronic form). Hum Pathol 1989; 20: 149–158

150. Manowski Z, Silver M M, Roberts E A, Supesina R A, Phillips M J. Liver cell dysplasia and early liver transplantation in hereditary tyrosinaemia. Mod Pathol 1990; 3: 694–701

151. Conti J A, Kemeny N. Type Ia glycogenosis associated with hepatocellular carcinoma. Cancer 1992; 69: 1320–1322

152. Lithner F, Wetterberg L. Hepatocellular carcinoma in patients with acute intermittent porphyria. Acta Med Scand 1984; 215: 271–274

153. Slersema P D, ten Kate F J W, Mulder P G H, Wilson J H P. Hepatocellular carcinoma in porphyria cutanea tarda: frequency and factors related to its occurrence. Liver 1992; 12: 56–61

154. Kauppinen R, Mustajoki P. Acute hepatic porphyria and hepatocellular carcinoma. Br J Cancer 1988; 57: 117–120

155. Sharp H L. Alpha-1-antitrypsin: an ignored protein in understanding liver disease. Semin Liv Dis 1982; 2: 314–328

156. Crystal R G. Alpha-1-antitrypsin deficiency, emphysema and liver disease. J Clin Invest 1990; 85: 1343–1352

157. Schwarzenberg S J, Sharp H L. Pathogenesis of α_1-antitrypsin deficiency — associated liver disease. J Pediatr Gastroenterol Nutr 1990; 10: 5–12

158. Eriksson S, Hägerstrand I. Cirrhosis and malignant hepatoma in α_1-antitrypsin deficiency. Acta Med Scand 1974; 195: 451–458

159. Larsson C. Natural history and life expectancy in severe alpha-1-antitrypsin deficiency, PiZ. Acta Med Scand 1978; 204: 345–351

160. Govindarajan S, Ashcavai M, Peters R L. Alpha-1-antitrypsin phenotypes in hepatocellular carcinoma. Hepatology 1981; 1: 628–631

161. Cohen C, Berson S D, Budgeon R B. Alpha-1-antitrypsin deficiency in Southern African hepatocellular carcinoma patients, an immunoperoxidase and histochemical study. Cancer 1982; 49: 2537–2540

162. Eriksson S, Carlson J, Velez R. Risk of cirrhosis and primary liver cancer in alpha-1-antitrypsin deficiency. N Engl J Med 1986; 314: 736–739

163. Palmer P E, Wolfe H J. Alpha-1-antitrypsin deposition in primary hepatic carcinoma. Arch Pathol Lab Med 1976; 100: 232–236

164. Reintoft I, Hägerstrand I E. Demonstration of alpha-1-antitrypsin in hepatomas. Arch Pathol Lab Med 1979; 103: 495–498

165. Rubel L R, Ishak K G, Benjamin S B, Knuff T E. Alpha-1-antitrypsin deficiency and hepatocellular carcinoma. Arch Pathol Lab Med 1982; 106: 678–681

166. Purtilo D T, Gottlieb L S. Cirrhosis and hepatoma occurring at Boston City Hospital (1917–1968). Cancer 1973; 32: 458–462

167. Niederau C, Fischer R, Sonnenberg A, Stremmel W, Trampisch H J, Strohmeyer G. Survival and causes of death in cirrhotic and in non-cirrhotic patients with primary haemochromatosis. N Engl J Med 1985; 313: 1256–1262

167a. Adams P C. Hepatocellular carcinoma in hereditary hemochromatosis. Can J Gastroenterol 1993; 7: 37–41

168. Fellows I W, Stewart M, Jeffcoate W J, Smith P G. Hepatocellular carcinoma in primary haemochromatosis in the absence of cirrhosis. Gut 1988; 29: 1603–1606

168a. Deugnier Y, Guyader D, Crantock L et al. Primary liver cancer in genetic hemochromatosis: a clinical, pathological and pathogenetic study of 54 cases. Gastroenterology 1993; 104: 228–234

169. Deugnier Y, Battistelli D, Jouanolle H et al. Hepatitis B virus infection markers in genetic haemochromatosis. J Hepatol 1991; 13: 286–290

170. MacSween R N M, Scott A R. Hepatic cirrhosis: a clinico-pathological review of 520 cases. J Clin Pathol 1973; 26: 936–942

171. Polio J, Enriquez R E, Chow A, Wood W M, Atterbury C E. Hepatocellular carcinoma in Wilson's disease. J Clin Gastroenterol 1989; 11: 220–224

172. Melia W H, Johnson P J, Neuberger J, Zaman S, Portmann B C, Williams R. Hepatocellular carcinoma in primary biliary cirrhosis. Gastroenterology 1984; 87: 660–663

173. Nakanuma Y, Terada T, Doishita K, Miwa A. Hepatocellular carcinoma in primary biliary cirrhosis: an autopsy study. Hepatology 1990; 11: 1010–1016

174. Simpson I W. Membranous obstruction of the inferior vena cava and hepatocellular carcinoma in South Africa. Gastroenterology 1982; 82: 171–178

175. Okuda K. Membranous obstruction of the inferior vena cava: etiology and relation to hepatocellular carcinoma. Gastroenterology 1982; 82: 376–379

176. Hautekeete M L, Brenard R, Hadengue A et al. Membranous obstruction of the inferior vena cava and hepatocellular carcinoma in a Caribbean patient. J Clin Gastroenterol 1990; 12: 214–217

177. Klein G. Immune and non-immune control of neoplastic development: contrasting effects of host and tumor evolution. Cancer 1980; 45: 2486–2499

178. Lachmann P J. Tumour immunology: a review. J Roy Soc Med 1984; 77: 1023–1029

179. Baker H W. Biologic control of cancer. Arch Surg 1986; 121: 1237–1241

180. Paroli M, Perrone A, Bonavita M S, Barnaba V. Immunology of hepatocellular carcinoma. Ital J Gastroenterol 1991; 23: 494–497

181. Willett W C, MacMahon B. Diet and cancer — an overview. N Engl J Med 1984; 310: 633–638, 697–703

182. Munehisha T, Nakata K, Muro T et al. Nutritional study in the area with high incidence of liver cirrhosis and hepatocellular carcinoma in Japan. Jpn J Gastroenterol 1983; 80: 828–836

183. Vileisis R A, Sorensen K, Gonzalez-Crussi F, Hunt C E. Liver malignancy after parenteral nutrition. J Pediatr 1982; 100: 88–90

184. Patterson K, Kapur S P, Chandra R S. Hepatocellular carcinoma in a non-cirrhotic infant after prolonged parenteral nutrition. J Pediatr 1985; 106: 797–800

185. De Cock K M. Hepatosplenic schistosomiasis: a clinical review. Gut 1986; 27: 734–745

186. IARC Monographs on the evaluation of carcinogenic risks to humans. Vols 1–50 1972–1992 and Suppl 2, 5–8 1980–1990. Geneva: World Health Organization

187. Magee P N, Montesano R, Pruessman R. N-nitroso compounds and related carcinogens. American Cancer Society Monographs 1976; 173: 491–625

188. Wogan G N. Aflatoxins and their relationship to hepatocellular carcinoma. In: Okuda K, Peters R L, eds. Hepatocellular carcinoma. New York: Wiley, 1976: pp 25–41

189. Linsell C A. Liver cell cancer — intervention studies. J Cancer Res Clin Oncol 1981; 99: 51–56

190. Berry C L. The pathology of mycotoxins. J Pathol 1988; 154: 301–311

191. Wogan G N. Aflatoxins as risk factors for hepatocellular carcinoma in humans. Cancer Res 1992; 52 (suppl): 2114S–2118S

192. Yaobin W, Lizun L, Benfa Y et al. Relationship between geographical distribution of liver cancer and climate — aflatoxin B1 in China. Sci Sin 1983; 26: 1166–1175

193. Van Rensburg S J, Cook-Mozaffari P, Van Schalkwyk D J, Van Der Watt J J, Vincent T J, Purchase I F. Hepatocellular carcinoma and dietary aflatoxin in Mozambique and Transkei. Br J Cancer 1985; 51: 713–726

194. Peers F, Bosch X, Kaldor J, Linsell A, Pluijmen M. Aflatoxin exposure, hepatitis B virus infection and liver cancer in Swaziland. Int J Cancer 1987; 39: 545–553

195. Campbell T C, Chen J, Lin C, Li J, Parpia B. Non association of aflatoxin with primary liver cancer in a cross-sectional ecological survey in the People's Republic of China. Cancer Res 1990; 50: 6682–6893

196. Ross R K, Yuan J-M, Yu M C et al. Urinary aflatoxin biomarkers, a risk of hepatocellular carcinoma. Lancet 1992; 339: 943–946

196a. Hatch M C, Chen C-J, Levin B et al. Urinary aflatoxin levels, hepatitis-B virus infection and hepatocellular carcinoma in Taiwan. Int J Cancer 1993; 54: 931–934

197. Wild C P, Rasheed F N, Jawla M F B, Hall A J, Jansen L A M, Montesano R. In-utero exposure to aflatoxin in West Africa. Lancet 1991; 337: 1602

198. Hollstein M, Sidransky D, Vogelstein B, Harris C C. p53 mutations in human cancers. Science 1991; 253: 49–53

199. Hsu I C, Metcalf R A, Suu T, Welsh J A, Wang N J, Harris C C. Mutational hotspot in the p53 gene in human hepatocellular carcinomas. Nature 1991; 350: 427–428

200. Bressac B, Kew M, Wands J, Ozturk M. Selective G to T mutations of p53 gene in hepatocellular carcinoma from Southern Africa. Nature 1991; 350: 429–431

201. Ozturk M and collaborators. p53 mutation in hepatocellular carcinoma after aflatoxin exposure. Lancet 1991; 338: 1356–1359

201a. Challen C, Lunec J, Warren W, Collier J, Bassendine M F. Analysis of the p53 tumor-suppressor gene in hepatocellular carcinomas from Britain. Hepatology 1992; 16: 1362–1366

201b. Collier J D. Carpenter M, Burt A D, Bassendine M F. Expression of mutant p53 protein in hepatocellular carcinoma. Gut 1994; 35: 98–100

201c. Hsia C C, Kleiner D E, Axiotis C A et al. Mutations of p53 gene in hepatocellular carcinoma: roles of hepatitis B virus and aflatoxin contamination in the diet. J Natl Cancer Inst 1992; 83: 1638–1641

201d. Buetow K H, Sheffield V C, Zhu M et al. Low frequency of p53 mutations observed in a diverse collection of primary hepatocellular carcinomas. Proc Natl Acad Sci USA 1992; 89: 9622–9626

201e. Choi S W, Hytiroglou P, Geller S A et al. The expression of p53 antigen in primary malignant epithelial tumors of the liver: an immunohistochemical study. Liver 1993; 13: 172–176

201f. Goldblum J R, Bartos R E, Carr K A, Frank T S. Hepatitis B and alterations of the p53 tumor suppressor gene in hepatocellular carcinoma. Am J Surg Pathol 1993; 17: 1244–1251

201g. Shieh Y S C, Nguyen C, Vocal M V, Chu H-W. Tumor-suppressor p53 gene in hepatitis C and B virus-associated human hepatocellular carcinoma. Int J Cancer 1993; 54: 558–562

201h. Hayashi H, Suglo K, Matsumata T et al. The mutation of codon 249 in the p53 gene is not specific in Japanese hepatocellular carcinoma. Liver 1993; 13: 279–281

201i. Konishi M, Kikuchi-Yanoshita R, Tanaka K et al. Genetic changes and histopathological grades in human hepatocellular carcinomas. Jpn J Cancer Res 1993; 84: 839–899

201j. Nishida N, Fukuda Y, Kokuryu H et al. Role and mutational heterogeneity of the p53 gene in hepatocellular carcinoma. Cancer Res 1993; 53: 368–372

202. Forman D. Editorial. Ames, the Ames test, and the causes of cancer. Br Med J 1991; 303: 428–429

203. Stemhagen A, Slade J, Altmann R, Bill J. Occupational risk factors and liver cancer. Am J Epidemiol 1983; 117: 443–454

204. Austin H, Delzell E, Grufferman S et al. Case-control study of hepatocellular carcinoma, occupational and chemical exposures. J Occup Med 1987; 29: 665–669

205. Fleisher J M. Occupational and non-occupational risk factors in relation to an excess of primary liver cancer observed among residents of Brooklyn, New York. Cancer 1990; 65: 180–185

206. Evans D M, Williams W J, King I T. Angiosarcoma and hepatocellular carcinoma in vinyl chloride workers. Histopathology 1983; 7: 377–388

207. Neuberger J, Portmann B, Nunnerley H B, Laws J W, Davis M, Williams R. Oral contraceptive-associated liver tumours: occurrence of malignancy and difficulties in diagnosis. Lancet 1980; 1: 273–276

208. Hromas R A, Srigley J, Murray J L. Clinical and pathological comparison of young adult women with hepatocellular carcinoma with and without exposure to oral contraceptives. Amer J Gastroenterol 1985; 80: 479–485

209. Vana J, Murphy G P. Primary malignant liver tumors. Association with oral contraceptives. NY State J Med 1979; 79: 321–325

210. Goodman Z D, Ishak K G. Hepatocellular carcinoma in women: probable lack of etiologic association with oral contraceptive steroids. Hepatology 1982; 2: 440–444

211. Henderson B E, Preston-Martin S, Edmondson H A, Peters R L, Pike M C. Hepatocellular carcinoma and oral contraceptives. Br J Cancer 1983; 48: 437–440

212. Palmer J R, Rosenberg L, Kaufmann D W, Warshauer N E, Stolley P, Shapiro S. Oral contraceptive use and liver cancer. Am J Epidemiol 1989; 130: 878–882

213. Forman D, Doll R, Peto R. Trends in mortality from carcinoma of the liver and the use of oral contraceptives. Br J Cancer 1983; 48: 349–354

214. Forman D, Vincent T J, Doll R. Cancer of the liver and the use of oral contraceptives. Br Med J 1986; 292: 1357–1361

215. Neuberger J, Forman D, Doll R, Williams R. Oral contraceptives and hepatocellular carcinoma. Br Med J 1986; 292: 1355–1357

216. Yu M C, Tong M J, Govindarajan S, Henderson B E. Nonviral risk factors for hepatocellular carcinoma in a low risk population, the non-Asians of Los Angeles County, California. J Natl Cancer Inst 1991; 83: 1820–1826

217. Prentice R L. Epidemiologic data on exogenous hormones and hepatocellular carcinoma and selected other cancers. Prev Med 1991; 20: 38–46

218. The WHO Collaborative Study of Neoplasia and Steroid Contraceptives. Combined oral contraceptives and liver cancer. Int J Cancer 1989; 43: 254–259

219. Kew M C, Song E, Mohammed A, Hodkinson J. Contraceptive steroids as a risk factor for hepatocellular carcinoma: a case/control study in South African black women. Hepatology 1990; 11: 298–302

220. Moldvay J, Schaff Z, Lapis K. Hepatocellular carcinoma in Fanconi's anemia treated with androgen and corticosteroid. Zentralbl Pathol 1991; 137: 167–170

221. Overly W L, Dankoff J A, Wang B K, Singh U D. Androgens and hepatocellular carcinoma in an athlete. Ann Intern Med 1984; 100: 158–159

222. Anthony P P. Liver tumours. In: Bircher J, ed. Adverse drug reactions in the differential diagnosis of GI and liver diseases. Baillière's Clinical Gastroenterology, vol 2, no 2. London: Baillière Tindall, 1988: pp 501–522

223. Ohri S K, Gaer J A R, Keane P F. Hepatocellular carcinoma and treatment with cyproterone acetate. Br J Urol 1991; 67: 213

223a. Hirsimäki P, Hirsimäki Y, Nieminen L, Payne B J. Tamoxifen induces hepatocellular carcinoma in rat liver: a 1-year study with two antiestrogens. Arch Toxicol 1993; 67: 49–54

223b. Williams G M, Iatropoulos M J, Djordjevic M V, Kaltenberg O P. The triphenylethylene drug tamoxifen is a strong liver carcinogen in the rat. Carcinogenesis 1993; 14: 315–317

224. Kohn H I, Fry R J M. Radiation carcinogenesis. New Engl J Med 1984; 310: 504–511

225. Horta da Silva J, Cayolla da Motta L, Tavares M H. Thorium dioxide effects in man; epidemiological clinical and pathological studies (experience in Portugal). Env Health Res 1974; 8: 131–159

226. Yamada S, Hosoda S, Tateno H, Kido C, Takahashi S. Survey of thorotrast-associated liver cancers in Japan. J Natl Cancer Inst 1983; 70: 31–35

227. Van Kaick G, Muth H, Kaul A, eds. The German Thorotrast Study. Luxembourg: Commission of the European Communities, 1984

228. Ito Y, Kojiro N, Nakashima T, Mori T. Pathomorphologic characteristics of 102 cases of Thorotrast-related hepatocellular carcinoma, cholangiocarcinoma and hepatic angiosarcoma. Cancer 1988; 62: 1153–1162

229. Schreiber W H, Kato H, Robertson J D. Primary carcinoma of the liver in Hiroshima and Nagasaki, Japan. Cancer 1970; 26: 69–75

230. MacSween R N M. Alcohol and cancer. Br Med Bull 1982; 38: 31–33

231. Bassendine M F. Alcohol — a major risk factor for hepatocellular carcinoma? J Hepatol 1986; 2: 513–519

232. Lieber C S, Garro A, Leo N A, Mak K M, Worner T. Alcohol and cancer. Hepatology 1986; 6: 1005–1019

233. Naccarato R, Farinati F. Hepatocellular carcinoma, alcohol and cirrhosis: facts and hypotheses. Dig Dis Sci 1991; 36: 1137–1142

234. Bulatao-Jayme J, Almero E M, Castro C A, Jardeleza T H, Salamat L A. A case–control dietary study of primary liver cancer risk from aflatoxin exposure. Int J Epidemiol 1982; 11: 112–119

235. Austin H, Delzell E, Grufferman S et al. A case–control study of hepatocellular carcinoma and the hepatitis B virus, cigarette smoking and alcohol consumption. Cancer Res 1986; 46: 962–966

236. Trichopoulos D, Day N E, Kaklamani E et al. Hepatitis B virus, tobacco smoking and ethanol consumption in the etiology of hepatocellular carcinoma. Int J Cancer 1987; 39: 45–59

237. Nomura H, Kashiwagi S, Hayashi J et al. An epidemiologic study of effects of alcohol in the liver in hepatitis B surface antigen carriers. Am J Epidemiol 1988; 128: 277–284

238. Yu H, Harris R E, Kabat G C, Wynder E L. Cigarette smoking, alcohol consumption and primary liver cancer: a case–control study in the USA. Int J Cancer 1988; 42: 325–328

239. Tsukuma H, Hiyama T, Oshima A et al. A case–control study of hepatocellular carcinoma in Osaka, Japan. Int J Cancer 1990; 45: 231–236

240. Chen C-J. Liang K-Y, Chang A-S et al. Effects of hepatitis B virus, alcohol drinking, cigarette smoking and familial tendency on hepatocellular carcinoma. Hepatology 1991; 13: 398–406

240a. Tanaka K, Hirohato T, Takeshita S et al. Hepatitis B virus, cigarette smoking and alcohol consumption in the development of hepatocellular carcinoma: a case-control study in Fukuoka, Japan. Int J Cancer 1992; 51: 509–514

241. Bréchot C, Nalpas B, Couroucé A-M et al. Evidence that hepatitis B virus has a role in liver cell carcinoma in alcoholic liver disease. N Engl J Med 1982; 306: 1384–1387

242. Walter E, Blum H E, Meier P et al. Hepatocellular carcinoma in alcoholic liver disease: no evidence for a pathogenetic role of hepatitis B virus infection. Hepatology 1988; 8: 745–748

243. Paterlini P, Bréchot C. The detection of hepatitis B virus (HBV) in HBsAg negative individuals with primary liver cancer. Dig Dis Sci 1991; 36: 1122–1129

244. Shimizu S, Kiyosawa K, Sodeyama T, Tanaka E, Nakano M. High prevalence of antibody to hepatitis C virus in heavy drinkers with chronic liver diseases in Japan. J Gastro-enterol Hepatol 1992; 7: 30–35

245. Nalpas B, Driss F, Pol S et al. Association between HCV and HBV infection in hepatocellular carcinoma and alcoholic liver disease. J Hepatol 1991; 12: 70–74

246. Lee F I. Cirrhosis and hepatoma in alcoholics. Gut 1966; 7: 77–85

247. Nakanuma Y, Ohta G. Is Mallory body formation a preneoplastic change? Cancer 1985; 55: 2400–2404

248. Nakanuma Y, Ohta G. Expression of Mallory bodies in hepatocellular carcinoma in man and its significance. Cancer 1986; 57: 81–86

249. Szmuness W. Hepatocellular carcinoma and the hepatitis B virus: evidence for a causal association. Prog Med Virol 1978; 24: 40–69

250. Maupas P, Melnick J L. Hepatitis B virus and primary hepatocellular carcinoma. Prog Med Virol 1981; 27: 1–202

251. Melnick J L. Hepatitis B virus and liver cancer. In: Phillips L A, ed. Viruses associated with human cancer. New York: Marcel Dekker, 1983: pp 337–367

252. Beasley R P, Hwang L-Y. Epidemiology of hepatocellular carcinoma. In: Vyas G H, Dienstag J L, Hoofnagle J H, eds. Viral hepatitis and liver disease. New York: Grune & Stratton, 1984: pp 209–224

253. Tabor E. Hepatitis B virus and primary hepatocellular carcinoma. In: Gerety R J, ed. Hepatitis B. Orlando: Academic Press, 1985: pp 247–267

254. Bassendine M F. Hepatocellular carcinoma. In: Jewell D P, Mahida Y R, eds. Topics in gastroenterology, no 15. Oxford: Blackwell, 1987: pp 101–114

255. Bassendine M F. Aetiological factors in hepatocellular cancer. In: Williams R, Johnson P J, eds. Liver tumours. Baillière's Clinical Gastroenterology, vol 1, no 1. London: Baillière Tindall, 1987: pp 1–16

256. Bréchot C. Hepatitis B virus and hepatocellular carcinoma. Bull Inst Pasteur 1987; 85: 125–149

257. Shafritz D A. Role of various molecular forms of HBV-DNA in chronic liver disease and primary liver cancer. Hepatology Rapid Literature Review 1987; 17 (6): XI–XVIII

258. Zuckerman A J, Harrison T J. Hepatitis B virus, chronic liver disease and hepatocellular carcinoma. Postgrad Med J 1987; 63 (suppl 2): 13–19

259. Beasley R P. Hepatitis B virus. The major etiology of hepatocellular carcinoma. Cancer 1988; 61: 1942–1956

260. Zuckerman A J, ed. Viral hepatitis. Br Med Bull 1990; 46: 301–564

261. Colombo M. Hepatocellular carcinoma. J Hepatol 1992; 15: 225–236

261a. Chen D-S. Natural history of chronic hepatitis B infection: new light on an old story. J Gastroenterol Hepatol 1993; 8: 470–475

261b. Schirmacher P, Rogler C E, Dienes H P. Current pathogenetic and molecular concepts in viral liver carcinogenesis. Virchows Archiv B Cell Pathol 1993; 63: 71–89

262. Melbye M, Skinhøy P, Nielsen N H et al. Virus-associated cancers in Greenland: frequent hepatitis B virus infection but low primary hepatocellular carcinoma incidence. J Natl Cancer Inst 1984; 73: 1267–1272

263. Popper H, Thung S N, McMahon B J, Lanier A P, Hawkins I, Alberts S R. Evolution of hepatocellular carcinoma associated with chronic hepatitis B virus infection in Alaskan Eskimos. Arch Pathol Lab Med 1988; 112: 498–504

264. Trichopoulos D, Papaevangelou G, Violaki M, Vissoulis C H, Sparos L, Manousos O N. Geographic correlation between mortality from primary hepatic carcinoma and prevalence of hepatitis B surface antigen in Greece. Br J Cancer 1976; 34: 83–87

265. Kaklamani E, Tzonou A, Sparos L, Koumantaki I, Trichopoulos D. Hepatitis B virus and primary liver cancer: relative risk estimation from population correlations. IRCS Med Sci 1983; 11: 707–708

266. Cobden I, Bassendine M F, James O F W. Hepatocellular carcinoma in North-East England: importance of hepatitis B infection and ex-tropical military service. Q J Med 1986; 60: 855–863

267. Seeff L B, Beebe G W, Hoofnagle J H et al. A serologic follow-up of the 1942 epidemic of post-vaccinal hepatitis in the United States Army. N Engl J Med 1987; 316: 965–969

267a. Norman J E, Beebe G W, Hoofnagle J H, Seeff L B. Mortality follow-up of the 1942 epidemic of hepatitis B in the US Army. Hepatology 1993; 18: 790–797

268. Beasley R P, Hwang L-Y, Lin C C, Chien C-S. Hepatocellular carcinoma and hepatitis B virus. A prospective study of 22707 men in Taiwan. Lancet 1981; ii: 1129–1133

269. Nakatsuji Y, Kiyosawa K, Tanaka E et al. Expression of hepatitis B surface antigen subtypes in liver of patients with hepatocellular carcinoma; comparison of subtypes in serum and liver. Liver 1991; 11: 176–184

270. Govindarajan S, Hevia F J, Peters R L. Prevalence of delta antigen/antibody in B-viral-associated hepatocellular carcinoma. Cancer 1984; 53: 1692–1694

271. Kew M C, Dusheiko G M, Hadziyannis S J, Patterson A. Does delta infection play a part in the pathogenesis of hepatitis B virus related hepatocellular carcinoma? Br Med J 1984; 288: 1727

272. Trichopoulos D, Day N E, Tzonou A et al. Delta agent and the etiology of hepatocellular carcinoma. Int J Surg 1987; 39: 283–286

273. Bonino F, Brunetto M R, Negro F, Smedile A, Ponzetto A. Hepatitis delta virus, a model of liver cell pathology. J Hepatol 1991; 13: 260–266

274. Verme G, Brunetto M R, Oliveri F et al. Role of hepatitis delta virus infection in hepatocellular carcinoma. Dig Dis Sci 1991; 36: 1134–1136

275. Schlipkoter V, Ponzetto A, Fuchs K et al. Different outcomes of chronic hepatitis delta virus infection in woodchucks. Liver 1990; 10: 291–301

276. Kawano Y. Localization of hepatitis B surface antigen in hepatocellular carcinoma. Acta Pathol Jpn 1983; 33: 1087–1093

277. Alexander J J, Van der Merwe C F, Saunders R M, McElligott S E, Desmyter J. A comparison between in vitro experiments with a hepatoma cell line and in vivo studies. Hepatology 1982; 2 (Suppl): 92S–96S

278. Matsui T, Takano M, Miyamoto K et al. Nude mice bearing human primary hepatocellular carcinoma that produces hepatitis B surface, core and e antigens, as well as deoxyribonucleic acid polymerase. Gastroenterology 1986; 90: 135–142

279. Tsurimoto T, Fujiyama A, Matsubara K. Stable expression and replication of hepatitis B virus genome in an integrated state in a human hepatoma cell line transfected with the cloned viral DNA. Proc Natl Acad Sci USA 1987; 84: 444–448

280. Tiollais P, Purcell C, Dejean A. The hepatitis B virus. Nature 1985; 317: 489–495

281. Bréchot C, Degos F, Lugassy C et al. Hepatitis B virus DNA in patients with chronic liver disease and negative tests for hepatitis B surface antigen. N Engl J Med 1985; 312: 270–276

282. Dusheiko G M. Hepatocellular carcinoma associated with chronic viral hepatitis. Br Med Bull 1990; 46: 492–511

283. Robinson W S, Klote L, Aoki N. Hepadnaviruses in cirrhotic liver and hepatocellular carcinoma. J Med Virol 1990; 31: 18–32

284. Paterlini P, Gerken G, Nakajima E et al. Polymerase chain reaction to detect hepatitis B virus DNA and RNA sequences in primary liver cancers from patients negative for hepatitis B surface antigen. N Engl J Med 1990; 323: 80–85

285. Pugh J C, Bassendine M F. Molecular biology of hepadnavirus replication. Br Med Bull 1990; 46: 329–353

286. Rogler C E. Recent advances in hepatitis B viruses and hepatocellular carcinoma. Cancer Cell Mon Rev 1990; 2: 366–370

286a. Diamantis I D, McGandy C E, Chen T-J, Liaw Y-F, Gudat F, Bianchi L. Hepatitis B X-gene expression in hepatocellular carcinoma. J Hepatol 1992; 15: 400–403

286b. Kekulé A S, Lauer U, Weiss L, Luber B, Hofschneider P H. Hepatitis B virus transactivator HBX uses a tumour promoter signalling pathway. Nature 1993; 361: 742–745

287. Blum H E, Offensperger W-B, Walter E et al. Hepatocellular carcinoma and hepatitis B virus infection: molecular evidence for monoclonal origin and expansion of malignantly transformed hepatocytes. J Cancer Res Clin Oncol 1987; 113: 466–472

288. Govindarajan S, Craig J R, Valinluck B. Clonal origin of hepatitis B virus-associated hepatocellular carcinoma. Hum Pathol 1988; 19: 403–405

289. Sakamoto M, Hirohashi S, Tsuda H, Shimosato Y, Makuuchi M, Hosoda Y. Multicentric independent development of hepatocellular carcinoma revealed by analysis of hepatitis B virus integration pattern. Am J Surg Pathol 1989; 13: 1064–1067

290. Summers J. Three recently described animal virus models for human hepatitis B virus. Hepatology 1981; 1: 179–183

291. Popper H, Roth L, Purcell R H, Tennant B C, Gerin J L. Hepatocarcinogenicity of the woodchuck hepatitis virus. Proc Natl Acad Sci USA 1987; 84: 866–870

292. Ponzetto A, Forzani B. Animal models of hepatocellular carcinoma: hepadnavirus-induced liver cancer in woodchucks. Ital J Gastroenterol 1991, 23: 491–493

293. Fuchs K, Heberger C, Weimer T, Roggendorf M. Characterization of woodchuck hepatitis virus DNA and RNA in

the hepatocellular carcinomas of woodchucks. Hepatology 1989; 10: 215–220

294. Catterall A P, Murray-Lyon M I. Strategies for hepatitis B immunization. Gut 1992; 33: 576–579

295. Tsen Y-J, Chang M-H, Hsu H-Y, Lee C-Y, Sung J-L, Chen D S. Seroprevalence of hepatitis B virus infection in children in Taipei, 1989: five years after a mass hepatitis B vaccination program. J Med Virol 1991; 34: 96–99

295a. Lo K-J, Lee S-D, Tsai Y-T et al. Hepatitis B vaccine trial in neonates. J Gastroenterol Hepatol 1993; 8: S99–S102

296. Whittle H C, Inskip H, Hall A J, Mendy M, Downes R, Hoare S. Vaccination against hepatitis B and protection against chronic viral carriage in the Gambia. Lancet 1991; 337: 747–750

297. Alter H J. The hepatitis C virus and its relationship to the clinical spectrum of NANB hepatitis. J Gastroenterol Hepatol 1990; Suppl 1: 78–94

298. Choo K L, Kuo G, Weiner A J, Overby L R, Bradley D W, Houghton M. Isolation of a cDNA clone derived from a blood borne non-A non-B viral hepatitis genome. Science 1989; 244: 359–362

299. Bruix J, Barrera J M, Calvet X et al. Prevalence of antibodies to hepatitis C virus in Spanish patients with hepatocellular carcinoma and hepatic cirrhosis. Lancet 1989; ii: 1004–1006

300. Colombo M, Kuo G, Choo Q L et al. Prevalence of antibodies to hepatitis C virus in Italian patients with hepatocellular carcinoma. Lancet 1989; ii: 1006–1008

301. Farinati F, Faginoli S, De Maria N et al. Anti-HCV positive hepatocellular carcinoma in cirrhosis. J Hepatol 1992; 14: 183–187

302. Simonetti R G, Camma C, Fiorello F et al. Hepatitis C virus infection as a risk factor for hepatocellular carcinoma in patients with cirrhosis. Ann Intern Med 1992; 116: 97–102

303. Saito I, Miyamura T, Ohbayashi A et al. Hepatitis C virus infection is associated with the development of hepatocellular carcinoma. Proc Natl Acad Sci USA 1990; 87: 6547–6549

304. Tanaka K, Hirohata T, Koga S et al. Hepatitis C and hepatitis B in the etiology of hepatocellular carcinoma in the Japanese population. Cancer Res 1991; 51: 2842–2847

305. Kew M C, Houghton M, Choo Q L, Kuo G. Hepatitis C virus antibodies in southern African blacks with hepatocellular carcinoma. Lancet 1990; 335: 873–874

306. Hasan F, Jeffers L J, Medina M et al. Hepatitis C-associated hepatocellular carcinoma. Hepatology 1990; 12: 589–591

307. Di Bisceglie A M, Order S E, Klein J L et al. The role of chronic viral hepatitis in hepatocellular carcinoma in the United States. Am J Gastroenterol 1991; 86: 335–338

307a. Esteban R. Epidemiology of hepatitis C virus infection. J Hepatol 1993; 17 (Suppl. 3): S67–S71

307b. Resnick R H, Koff R. Hepatitis C-related hepatocellular carcinoma. Prevalence and significance. Arch Intern Med 1993; 153: 1672–1677

307c. Gerber M A. Relation of hepatitis C virus to hepatocellular carcinoma. J Hepatol 1993; 17 (Suppl. 3): S108–S111

308. Anthony P P, Ishak K G, Nayak N C, Poulsen H E, Scheuer P J, Sobin L H. The morphology of cirrhosis. J Clin Pathol 1978; 31: 395–414

309. Kew M C, Popper H. Relationship between hepatocellular carcinoma and cirrhosis. Semin Liver Dis 1984; 4: 136–146

310. Johnson P J, Williams R. Cirrhosis and the aetiology of hepatocellular carcinoma. J Hepatol 1987; 4: 140–147

310a. Colombo M. Hepatocellular carcinoma in cirrhotics. Semin Liv Dis 1993; 13: 374–383

311. Berman J J. Cell proliferation and the aetiology of hepatocellular carcinoma. J Hepatol 1988; 7: 305

312. Callea F, Brisigotti M, Fabretti G, Sciot R, Van Eyken P, Favret M. Cirrhosis of the liver, a regenerative process. Dig Dis Sci 1991; 36: 1287–1293

313. Tiribelli C, Melato M, Croce L S, Giarelli L, Okuda K, Ohnishi K. Prevalence of hepatocellular carcinoma and relation to cirrhosis: comparison of two different cities in the world: Trieste, Italy and Chiba, Japan. Hepatology 1989; 10: 998–1002

314. Hadengue A, N'Dri N, Benhamou J-P. Relative risk of hepatocellular carcinoma in HBsAg positive vs alcoholic cirrhosis. A cross sectional study. Liver 1990; 10: 147–151

315. Kobayashi K, Unoura M, Tanaka N, Hattori N. A comparison between hepatocellular carcinoma-developing and non-carcinoma-developing patients with cirrhosis over a long follow-up period. Hepato-gastroenterol 1990; 37: 445–448

316. Tabarin A, Bioulac-Sage P, Boussarie L. Hepatocellular carcinoma developed on non-cirrhotic livers. Arch Pathol Lab Med 1987; 111: 174–180

317. Smalley S R, Moertel C G, Hilton J F et al. Hepatoma in the non-cirrhotic liver. Cancer 1988; 62: 1414–1424

318. Kalayci C, Johnson P J, Davies S E, Williams R. Hepatitis B virus related hepatocellular carcinoma in the non-cirrhotic liver. J Hepatol 1991; 12: 54–59

319. Farber E. Hepatocyte proliferation in stepwise development of experimental liver cell cancer. Dig Dis Sci 1991; 36: 973–978

320. Sakamoto M, Hirohashi S, Shimosato Y. Early stages of multistep hepatocarcinogenesis. Hum Pathol 1991; 22: 172–178

321. Crawford J M. Pathologic assessment of liver cell dysplasia and benign liver tumors: differentiation from malignant tumors. Semin Diagn Pathol 1990; 7: 115–128

322. Furuya K, Nakamura M, Yamamoto Y, Togei K, Otsuka H. Macroregenerative nodule of the liver. Cancer 1988; 61: 99–105

323. Wada K, Kondo F, Kondo Y. Large regenerative nodules and dysplastic nodules in cirrhotic livers: a histopathologic study. Hepatology 1988; 8: 1684–1688

324. Arakawa M, Kage M, Sugihara S, Nakashima T, Suenaga M, Okuda K. Emergence of malignant lesions within an adenomatous hyperplastic nodule in a cirrhotic liver. Gastroenterology 1986; 91: 198–208

325. Arakawa M, Sugihara S, Kenmochi K et al. Small mass lesions in cirrhosis: transition from benign adenomatous hyperplasia to hepatocellular carcinoma? J Gastroenterol Hepatol 1986; 1: 3–14

326. Nakanuma Y, Terada T, Terasaki S et al. 'Atypical adenomatous hyperplasia' in liver cirrhosis: low grade hepatocellular carcinoma or borderline lesion? Histopathology 1990; 17: 27–35

327. Ohno Y, Shiga J, Machinami R. A histopathological analysis of five cases of adenomatous hyperplasia containing minute hepatocellular carcinoma. Acta Pathol Jpn 1990; 40: 267–278

328. Sakamoto M, Hirohashi S, Shimosato Y. Early stages of multistep hepatocarcinogenesis: adenomatous hyperplasia and early hepatocellular carcinoma. Hum Pathol 1991; 22: 172–178

329. Takayama T, Makuuchi M, Hirohashi S et al. Malignant transformation of adenomatous hyperplasia to hepatocellular carcinoma. Lancet 1990; 336: 1150–1153

330. Eguchi A, Nakashima O, Okudaira S, Sugihara S, Kojira M. Adenomatous hyperplasia in the vicinity of small hepatocellular carcinoma. Hepatology 1992; 15: 843–848

330a. Ferrell L, Wright T, Lake J, Roberts J, Ascher N. Incidence and idagnostic features of macroregenerative nodules vs. small hepatocellular carcinoma in cirrhotic livers. Hepatology 1992; 16: 1372–1381

330b. Ferrell L D, Crawford J M, Dhillon A P, Scheuer P J, Nakanuma Y. Proposal for standardized criteria for the diagnosis of benign, borderline and malignant hepatocellular lesions arising in chronic advanced liver disease. Am J Surg Pathol 1993; 17: 1113–1123

330c. Nakanuma Y, Terada T, Ueda K, Terasaki S, Nonomura A, Matsui O. Adenomatous hyperplasia of the liver as a precancerous lesion. Liver 1993; 13: 1–9

331. Terada T, Nakanuma Y. Iron negative foci of siderotic macroregenerative nodules in human cirrhotic liver. A marker of incipient neoplastic lesions. Arch Pathol Lab Med 1989; 113: 916–920

332. Terada T, Nakanuma Y. Survey of iron-accumulative macroregenerative nodules in cirrhotic livers. Hepatology 1989; 10: 851–854

333. Terada T, Kadoya M, Nakanuma Y, Matsui O. Iron accumulating adenomatous hyperplastic nodule with malignant

foci in the cirrhotic liver. Histopathologic, quantitative iron and magnetic resonance imaging in vitro studies. Cancer 1990; 65: 1994–2000

334. Terada T, Hoso M, Nakanuma Y. Mallory body clustering in adenomatous hyperplasia in human cirrhotic livers: report of four cases. Hum Pathol 1989; 20: 886–890

335. Tsuda H, Hirohashi S, Shimosato Y, Terada M, Hasegawa H. Clonal origin of atypical adenomatous hyperplasia of the liver and clonal identity with hepatocellular carcinoma. Gastroenterology 1988; 95: 1664–1666

336. Govindarajan S, Conrad A, Lim B, Valinluck B, Kim A M, Schmid P. Study of preneoplastic changes of liver cells by immunohistochemical and molecular hybridization techniques. Arch Pathol Lab Med 1990; 114: 1042–1045

337. Gluud C, Christoffersen P, Eriksen J et al. Influence of ethanol on development of hyperplastic nodules in alcoholic men with micronodular cirrhosis. Gastroenterology 1987; 92: 256–260

338. Hoso M, Nakanuma Y. Cytophotometric DNA analysis of adenomatous hyperplasia in cirrhotic livers. Virchows Arch (A) 1991; 418: 401–404

339. Terada T, Nakanuma Y. Expression of ABH blood group antigens, receptors of Ulex europaeus agglutinin I and factor VIII-related antigen on sinusoidal endothelial cells in adenomatous hyperplasia in human cirrhotis livers. Hum Pathol 1991; 22: 486–493

340. Haratake J, Hisaoka M, Yamamoto O, Horie A. An ultrastructural comparison of sinusoids in hepatocellular carcinoma, adenomatous hyperplasia and fetal liver. Arch Pathol Lab Med 1992; 116: 67–70

341. Matsuno Y, Hirohashi S, Furuya S, Sakamoto M, Mukai K, Shimosato Y. Heterogeneity of proliferative activity in nodule-in-nodule lesions of small hepatocellular carcinoma. Jpn J Cancer Res 1990; 81: 1137–1140

341a. Motohashi I, Okudaira M, Takai T, Kaneko S, Ikeda N. Morphological differences between hepatocellular carcinoma and hepatocellular carcinoma like lesions. Hepatology 1992; 16: 118–126

341b. Terada T, Nakanuma Y. Cell proliferative activity in adenomatous hyperplasia of the liver and small hepatocellular carcinoma. Cancer 1992; 70: 591–598

341c. Orsatti G, Theise N D, Thung S N, Paronetto F. DNA image cytometric analysis of macroregenerative nodules (adenomatous hyperplasia) of the liver: evidence in support of their preneoplastic nature. Hepatology 1993; 17: 621–627

341d. Seki S, Sakaguchi H, Kawakita N et al. Detection of preneoplastic lesions of small hepatocellular carcinoma in cirrhotic livers. J Gastroenterol Hepatol 1993; 8: 582–586

341e. Terada T, Ueda K, Nakanuma Y. Histopathological and morphometric analysis of atypical adenomatous hyperplasia of human cirrhotic livers. Virchows Archiv A Pathol Anat Histopathol 1993; 422: 381–388

342. Anthony P P, Vogel C L, Barker L F. Liver cell dysplasia: a premalignant condition. J Clin Pathol 1973: 26; 217–233

343. Anthony P P. Precursor lesions for liver cancer in humans. Cancer Res 1976; 36: 2579–2582

344. Anthony P P. Precancerous changes in the human liver. J Toxicol Env Health 1979; 5: 301–313

345. Anthony P P. Liver cell dysplasia: what is its significance? Hepatology 1987; 7: 394–396

346. Gerber M A. Recent studies on the developing human hepatocellular carcinoma. Cancer Surveys 1986; 5: 741–763

347. Paterson A C, Kew M C, Dusheiko G M, Isaacson C. Liver cell dysplasia accompanying hepatocellular carcinoma in Southern Africa. J Hepatol 1989; 8: 241–248

348. Borzio M, Bruno S, Roncalli M. Liver cell dysplasia and risk of hepatocellular carcinoma in cirrhosis: a preliminary report. Br Med J 1991; 302: 1312

349. Podda M, Roncalli M, Battezzati P M, Liver cell dysplasia and hepatocellular carcinoma. Ital J Gastroenterol 1992; 24: 39–42

350. Lefkowitch J H, Apfelbaum T F. Liver cell dysplasia and hepatocellular carcinoma in non-A, non-B hepatitis. Arch Pathol Lab Med 1987; 111: 170–173

351. Tao L-C. Oral contraceptive-associated liver cell adenoma and hepatocellular carcinoma. Cancer 1991; 68: 341–347

352. Tao L-C. Are oral contraceptive-associated liver cell adenomas premalignant? Acta Cytol 1991; 36: 338–344

353. Watanabe S, Okita K, Harada T et al. Morphologic studies of the liver cell dysplasia. Cancer 1983; 51: 2197–2205

354. Akagi G, Furuya K, Kanamura A et al. Liver cell dysplasia and hepatitis B surface antigen in liver cirrhosis and hepatocellular carcinoma. Cancer 1984; 54: 315–318

355. Tanaka Y, Esumi M, Shikata T. Frequent integration of hepatitis B virus DNA in non-cancerous liver tissue from hepatocellular carcinoma patients. J Med Virol 1988; 26: 7–14

356. Uchida T, Miyata H, Shikata T. Human hepatocellular carcinoma and putative precancerous disorders. Their enzyme histochemical study. Arch Pathol Lab Med 1981; 105: 180–186

357. Roncalli M, Borzio M, De Biagi G et al. Liver cell dysplasia and hepatocellular carcinoma: a histological and immunohistochemical study. Histopathology 1985; 9: 209–221

358. Roncalli M, Borzio M, De Biagi G et al. Liver cell dysplasia in cirrhosis. A serologic and immunohistochemical study. Cancer 1986; 57: 1515–1521

359. Pollice L, Ricco R, Russo S, Maiorono E, Pagniello G, Delfino-Pesce V. Hepatocellular dysplasia: immunohistochemical and morphometrical evaluation. Appl Pathol 1988; 6: 73–81

360. Roncalli M, Borzio M, Tombesi M W, Ferrari A, Servida E. A morphometric study of liver cell dysplasia. Hum Pathol 1988; 19: 471–474

361. Henmi A, Uchida T, Shikata T. Karyometric analysis of liver cell dysplasia and hepatocellular carcinoma. Cancer 1985; 55: 2594–2599

362. Kagawa K, Deguchi T, Tomimasu H et al. Feulgen DNA cytofluorimetry of the liver cell dysplasia (LCD) in the liver cirrhosis. Jpn J Gastroenterol 1984; 81: 82–91

363. Roncalli M, Borzio M, Brando B, Colloredo G, Servida E. Abnormal DNA content in liver cell dysplasia: a flow cytometric study. Int J Cancer 1989; 44: 204–207

363a. Thomas R M, Bermann J J, Yetter R A, Moore G W, Hutchins G M. Liver cell dysplasia: a DNA aneuploid lesion with distinct morphologic features. Hum Pathol 1992; 23: 496–503

364. Chen M-L, Gerber M A, Thung S N, Thornton J C, Chung W K. Morphometric study of hepatocytes containing hepatitis B surface antigen. Am J Pathol 1984; 114: 217–221

365. Otsuru A, Nagataki S, Koji T, Tamaoki T. Analysis of alpha-feroprotein gene expression in hepatocellular carcinoma and liver cirrhosis by in situ hybridization. Cancer 1988; 62: 1105–1112

366. Di Bisceglie A M, Dusheiko G M, Paterson A C et al. Detection of alpha-fetoprotein messenger RNA in human hepatocellular carcinoma and hepatoblastoma tissue. Br J Cancer 1986; 54: 779–785

367. Haritani H, Esumi M, Uchida T, Shikata T. Oncogene expression in the liver tissue of patients with non-neoplastic liver disease. Cancer 1991; 67: 2594–2598

368. Challen C, Guo K, Collier J D, Cavanagh D, Bassendine M F. Infrequent point mutations in codons 12 and 61 of ras oncogenes in human hepatocellular carcinomas. J Hepatol 1992; 14: 342–346

368a. Derenzini M, Trerè D, Oliveri F et al. Is high AgNOR quantity in hepatocytes associated with increased risk of hepatocellular carcinoma in chronic liver disease? J Clin Pathol 1993; 46: 727–729

369. Regan L S. Screening for hepatocellular carcinoma in high-risk individuals. Arch Intern Med 1989; 149: 1741–1744

370. Vitale G C, Heuser L S, Polk H C. Malignant tumours of the liver. Surg Clin North Am 1986; 66: 723–741

371. Johnson P J. The clinical features and natural history of malignant liver tumours. In: Williams R, Johnson P J, eds. Liver tumours. Baillière's Clinical Gastroenterology, vol 1, no 1. London: Baillière Tindall, 1987: pp 17–34

372. Kassianides C, Kew M C. The clinical manifestations and natural history of hepatocellular carcinoma. Gastroenterol Clin North Am 1987; 16: 553–562

373. Anthony P P. Primary carcinoma of the liver: a study of 282 cases in Ugandan Africans. J Pathol 1973; 110: 37–48

374. Chearani O, Plengvanit U, Asavanich C, Damrongsak D, Sindhvananda K, Boonyapisit S. Spontaneous rupture of primary hepatoma. Cancer 1983; 51: 1532–1536

375. Miyamoto M, Sudo T, Kuyama T. Spontaneous rupture of hepatocellular carcinoma: a review of 172 Japanese cases. Am J Gastroenterol 1991; 86: 67–71

376. Kojiro M, Kawabata K, Kawano Y, Shirai F, Takemoto N, Nakashima T. Hepatocellular carcinoma presenting as intra-bile duct tumor growth. Cancer 1982; 49: 2144–2147

376a. Lai S T, Lam K T, Lee K C. Biliary tract invasion and obstruction by hepatocellular carcinoma: report of five cases. Postgrad Med J 1992; 68: 961–963

376b. De Nardi P, Braga M, Zerbi A et al. Bleeding gastric polyposis-like metastases of hepatocellular carcinoma. Dig Surg 1992; 9: 105–108

377. Young R H, Gersell D J, Clement P B, Scully R E. Hepatocellular carcinoma metastatic to the ovary. Hum Pathol 1992; 23: 574–580

378. Liaw C-C, Ng K-T, Chen T-J, Liaw Y-F. Hepatocellular carcinoma presenting as bone metastasis. Cancer 1989; 64: 1753–1757

379. Manfredi D, Manfredi R, Campioni N et al. A proposed TNM calssification for malignant primary liver tumours. J Surg Oncol 1986; 32: 227–229

380. Ferrucci J T. Liver tumor imaging: current concepts. Am J Roentgenol 1990; 155: 473–484

381. Deugnier Y, Auffret P, Lehry D, Brissot P, Bourel M. Marqueurs biologiques du carcinome hépatocellulaire. Gastroenterol Clin Biol 1987; 11: 648–657

382. Warnes T W, Smith A. Tumour markers in diagnosis and management. In: Williams R, Johnson P J,. eds. Liver tumours. Baillière's Clinical Gastroenterology, vol 1, no 1. London: Baillière Tindall, 1987; pp 63–89

383. Kew M C, Wolf P, Whittaker D, Rowe P. Tumour-associated isoenzymes of gamma-glutamyl transferase in the serum of patients with hepatocellular carcinoma. Br J Cancer 1984; 50: 451–455

384. Hutchinson W L, Du M-Q, Johnson P J, Williams R. Fucosyltransferases: differential plasma and tissue alterations in hepatocellular carcinoma and cirrhosis. Hepatology 1991; 13: 683–688

385. Hutchinson W L, Johnson P J, Du M-Q, Williams R. Serum and tissue α-L-fucosidase activity in the preclinical and clinical stages of hepatocellular carcinoma. Clinical Science 1991; 81: 177–182

386. Marotta F, Chui D H, Safran P, Zhang S C. Serum α-L-fucosidase. A more sensitive marker for hepatocellular carcinoma? Dig Dis Sci 1991; 36: 993–997

386a. Giardina M G, Matarazzo M, Varriale A, Morante R, Napoli A, Martino R. Serum alpha-L-fucosidase. Cancer 1992; 70: 1044–1048

387. Deyashiki Y, Nishioka Y, Takahashi K, Kosaka Y, Suzuki K. Evaluation of des-γ-carboxy prothrombin as a marker protein of hepatocellular carcinoma. Cancer 1989; 64: 2546–2551

388. Nakao A, Virji A, Iwaki Y, Carr B, Iwatsuki S, Starzl E. Abnormal prothrombin (DES-γ carboxy prothrombin) in hepatocellular carcinoma. Hepato-gastroenterol 1991; 38: 450–453

389. Takikawa Y, Suzuki K, Yamazaki K et al. Plasma abnormal prothrombin (PIVKA-II): a new and reliable marker for the detection of hepatocellular carcinoma. J Gastroenterol Hepatol 1992; 7: 1–6

389a. Weitz I C, Liebman H A. Des-γ-carboxy (abnormal) prothrombin and hepatocellular carcinoma: a critical review. Hepatology 1993; 18: 990–997

390. Hann H-W L, Kim C Y, Loudon W T, Blumberg B S. Increased serum ferritin in chronic liver disease: a risk factor for primary hepatocellular carcinoma. Int J Cancer 1989; 43: 376–379

391. Kew M C. Tumour markers of hepatocellular carcinoma. J Gastroenterol Hepatol 1989; 4: 373–384

392. Yonei Y, Tanaka M, Ozawa Y et al. Primary hepatocellular carcinoma with severe hypoglycaemia: involvement of insulin-like growth factors. Liver 1992; 12: 90–93

393. Taketa K. Alpha-fetoprotein: re-evaluation in hepatology. Hepatology 1990; 12: 1420–1432

394. Ishikura H, Kirimoto K, Shamoto M et al. Hepatoid adenocarcinomas of the stomach: an analysis of seven cases. Cancer 1986; 58: 119–126

395. Votte A, Sevestre H, Dupas J-L et al. Adenocarcinome hépatoide de l'estomac. Gastroenterol Clin Biol 1991; 15: 437–440

395a. de Lorimier A, Park F, Aranha G V, Reyes C. Hepatoid carcinoma of the stomach. Cancer 1993; 71: 293–296

396. Hasebe C, Sekiya C, Satoh H et al. A case of α-fetoprotein-producing gallbladder carcinoma. Acta Hepatol Jpn 1984; 25: 1180–1186

396a. Watanabe M, Hori Y, Nojima T et al. Alpha-fetoprotein-producing carcinoma of the gallbladder. Dig Dis Sci 1993; 38: 561–564

397. Gardiner G W, Lajoie G, Keith R. Hepatoid adenocarcinoma of the papilla of Vater. Histopathology 1992; 20: 541–544

398. Nakajima T, Okazaki N, Morinaga S et al. A case of alpha-fetoprotein-producing rectal carcinoma. Jpn J Clin Oncol 1985; 15: 679–685

399. Iseki M, Suzuki T, Koizumi Y et al. Alpha-fetoprotein-producing pancreatoblastoma. Cancer 1986; 57: 1833–1835

399a. Nojima T, Kojima T, Kato H, Sato T, Koito K, Nagashima K. Alpha-fetoprotein-producing acinar cell carcinoma of the pancreas. Hum Pathol 1992; 23: 828–830

400. Ishikura H, Kanda M, Nosaka K, Mizuno K. Hepatoid adenocarcinoma: a distinctive histological subtype of alpha-fetoprotein-producing lung carcinoma. Virchows Archiv (A) 1990; 417: 73–80

401. Morimoto H, Tanigawa N, Inoue H, Muraoka R, Hosokawa Y, Hattori T. Alpha-fetoprotein-producing renal cell carcinoma. Cancer 1988; 61: 84–88

402. Ishikura H, Ishiguro T, Enatsu C et al. Hepatoid adenocarcinoma of the renal pelvis producing alpha-fetoprotein of hepatic type and bile pigment. Cancer 1991; 67: 3051–3056

403. Matsukuma K, Tsukamoto N. α-Fetoprotein producing endometrial adenocarcinoma. Gynec Oncol 1988; 29: 370–377

404. Ishikura H, Scully R E. Hepatoid carcinoma of the ovary. Cancer 1987; 60: 2775–2784

404a. Nogales F F, Concha A, Plata C, Riuz-Avila I. Granulosa cell tumor of the ovary with diffuse true hepatic differentiation simulating stromal luteinization. Am J Surg Pathol 1993; 17: 85–90

405. Aoyagi Y, Suzuki Y, Isemura M et al. The fucosylation index of alpha-fetoprotein and its usefulness in the early diagnosis of hepatocellular carcinoma. Cancer 1988; 61: 769–774

405a. Aoyagi Y, Saitoh A, Suzuki Y et al. Fucosylation index of alpha-fetoprotein, a possible aid in the early recognition of hepatocellular carcinoma in patients with cirrhosis. Hepatology 1993; 17: 50–52

406. Du M-Q, Hutchinson W L, Johnson P J, Williams R. Differential alpha-fetoprotein lectin binding in hepatocellular carcinoma. Cancer 1991; 67: 476–480

406a. Sato Y, Nakata K, Kato Y et al. Early recognition of hepatocellular carcinoma based on altered profiles of alpha-fetoprotein. N Engl J Med 1993; 328: 1802–1806

406b. Peng S-Y, Lai P-L, Chu J-S et al. Expression and hypomethylation of alpha-fetoprotein gene in unicentric and multicentric human hepatocellular carcinomas. Hepatology 1993; 17: 35–41

407. Okuda K, Peters R L. Hepatocellular carcinoma. New York: Wiley, 1976

408. Anthony P P. Liver tumours: an update. In: Anthony P P, MacSween R N M, eds. Recent advances in histopathology, no 14. Edinburgh: Churchill Livingstone, 1989: pp 185–203

409. Kojiro M, Nakashima T. Pathology of hepatocellular carcinoma. In: Okuda K, Ishak K G, eds. Neoplasms of the liver. Berlin: Springer-Verlag, 1988: pp 81–104

410. Okuda K L, Peters R L, Simson I W. Gross anatomic features of hepatocellular carcinoma from three disparate geographical areas. Cancer 1984; 54: 2165–2173

411. Yuki K, Hirohashi S, Sakamoto M, Kanai T, Shimosato Y. Growth and spread of hepatocellular carcinoma. Cancer 1990; 66: 2174–2179

412. Terada T, Hoso M, Nakanuma Y. Development of cavernous vasculatures in livers with hepatocellular carcinoma. An autopsy study. Liver 1989; 9: 172–178

413. Kita K, Hoshima T, Tsuji T. Observation of microvascular casts of human hepatocellular carcinoma by scanning electron microscopy. Gastroenterol Jpn 1991; 26: 319–328

414. Kondo Y, Wada K. Intrahepatic metastasis of hepatocellular carcinoma. Hum Pathol 1991; 22: 125–130

415. Kojiro M, Nakahara H, Sugihara S, Murakami T, Nakashima T, Kawasaki H. Hepatocellular carcinoma with intra-atrial tumor growth. Arch Pathol Lab Med 1984; 108: 989–992

416. Arakawa M, Kage M, Matsumoto S et al. Frequency and significance of tumor thrombi in esophageal varices in hepatocellular carcinoma associated with cirrhosis. Hepatology 1986; 6: 419–422

417. Hiraoka T, Iwai K, Yamashita R, Tada I, Miyauchi Y. Metastases from hepatocellular carcinoma in sclerosed oesophageal varices in cirrhotic patients. Br J Surg 1986; 73: 932

418. Humbert P, Sarmiento J, Boix J et al. Hepatocellular carcinoma presenting with bleeding due to duodenal perforation by the tumor. Endoscopy 1987; 19: 37–38

419. Grigioni W F, D'Errico A, Biagini G et al. The capsule surrounding primary liver tumours: wherefrom its prognostic significance? Int J Cancer 1990; 45: 637–643

420. Torimura T, Ueno T, Inuzuka S, Tanaka M, Abe H, Tanikawa K. Mechanism of fibrous capsule formation surrounding hepatocellular carcinoma. Arch Pathol Lab Med 1991; 115: 365–371

421. Goodman Z D, Ishak K G. Pathology of liver tumors. In: Bottino J C, Opfell R W, Muggia F M, eds. Liver cancer. Boston: Martinus Nijhoff, 1986: pp 3–19

422. Tobe K, Tsuchija T, Fujiwara R. Kupffer cells in well differentiated tissue of hepatocellular carcinoma. Acta Hepatol Jpn 1985; 26: 630–637

423. Tabarin A, Bioulac-Sage P, Boussarie L, Balabaud C, de Mascarel A, Grimaud J A. Hepatocellular carcinoma developed on non-cirrhotic livers. Sinusoids in hepatocellular carcinoma. Arch Pathol Lab Med 1987; 111: 174–180

424. Hanatake J, Scheuer P J. An immunohistochemical and ultrastructural study of the sinusoids of hepatocellular carcinoma. Cancer 1990; 65: 1985–1993

425. Kondo Y, Nakajima T. Pseudoglandular hepatocellular carcinoma. A morphogenetic study. Cancer 1987; 60: 1032–1037

426. Omata M, Peters R L, Tatter D. Sclerosing hepatic carcinoma: relationship to hypercalcaemia. Liver 1981; 1: 33–49

427. Ross J S, Kurian S. Clear cell hepatocellular carcinoma: sudden death from severe hypoglycaemia. Am J Gastroenterol 1985; 80: 188–194

428. Hoso M, Nakanuma Y. Clinicopathological characteristics of hepatocellular carcinoma bearing Mallory bodies: an autopsy study. Liver 1990; 10: 264–268

429. Stromeyer F W, Ishak K G, Gerber M A, Matthew T. Ground-glass cells in hepatocellular carcinoma. Am J Clin Pathol 1980; 74: 254–258

430. Roth J A, Berman E, Befeler D, Johnson F B. A black hepatocellular carcinoma with Dubin–Johnson-like pigment and Mallory bodies. Am J Surg Pathol 1982; 6: 375–382

431. Ichida T. Ultrastructural study of intracytoplasmic deposits in human hepatocellular carcinoma. Gastroenterol Jpn 1983; 18: 560–576

432. Tomimatsu H, Kojiro M, Nakashima T. Epithelioid granulomas associated with hepatocellular carcinoma. Arch Pathol Lab Med 1982; 106: 538–539

433. Edmondson H A, Steiner P E. Primary carcinoma of the liver. A study of 100 cases among 48900 necropsies. Cancer 1954; 7: 462–503

434. Cohen M B, Beckstead J H, Ferrell L D. Yen T S B. Enzyme histochemistry of hepatocellular neoplasms. Am J Surg Pathol 1986; 10: 789–794

435. Hayes P C, May L, Hayes J D, Harrison D J. Glutathione S-transferases in human liver cancer. Gut 1991; 32: 1546–1549

436. Brumm C, Schulze C, Charels K, Morohoshi T, Klöppel G. The significance of alpha-fetoprotein and other tumour markers in differential immunocytochemistry of primary liver tumours. Histopathology 1989; 14: 503–513

437. Hurlimann J, Gardiol D. Immunohistochemistry in the differential diagnosis of liver carcinomas. Am J Surg Pathol 1991; 15: 280–288

438. Sung C-H, Hu C-P, Hsu H-C et al. Expression of Class I and Class II major histocompatibility antigens on human hepatocellular carcinoma. J Clin Invest 1989; 83: 421–429

439. Jovanovic R, Jagirdar J, Thung S N, Paronetto F. Blood-group-related antigen Lewis^x and Lewis^y in the differential diagnosis of cholangiocarcinoma and hepatocellular carcinoma. Arch Pathol Lab Med 1989; 113: 139–142

440. Haglund C, Lindgren J, Roberts P J, Nordling S. Difference in tissue expression of tumour markers CA 19-9 and CA 50 in hepatocellular carcinoma and cholangiocarcinoma. Br J Cancer 1991; 63: 386–389

441. Donato M F, Colombo M, Matarazzo M, Paronetto F. Distribution of basement membrane components in human hepatocellular carcinoma. Cancer 1989; 63: 272–279

442. Terada T, Nakanuma Y. Expression of ABH blood group antigens. Ulex europaeus agglutinin I and type IV collagen in the sinusoids of hepatocellular carcinoma. Arch Pathol Lab Med 1991; 115: 50–55

443. Sciot R, Van Eyken P, Desmet V J. Transferrin receptor expression in benign tumours and in hepatoblastoma of the liver. Histopathology 1990; 16: 59–62

444. Fischer H P, Altmannsberger M, Weber K, Osborn M. Keratin polypeptides in malignant epithelial liver tumours. Am J Pathol 1987; 127: 530–537

445. Johnson D E, Herndier B G, Medeiros L J, Warnke R A, Rouse R V. The diagnostic utility of keratin profiles of hepatocellular carcinoma and cholangiocarcinoma. Am J Surg Pathol 1988; 12: 187–197

446. Lai Y-S, Thung S N, Gerber M A, Chen M-L, Schaffner F. Expression of cytokeratins in normal and diseased livers and in primary liver carcinomas. Arch Pathol Lab Med 1989; 113: 134–138

447. Van Eyken P, Sciot R, Paterson A, Callea F, Kew M C, Desmet V J. Cytokeratin expression in hepatocellular carcinoma. Hum Pathol 1988; 19: 562–568

448. Van Eyken P, Sciot R, Desmet V J. Immunocytochemistry of cytokeratins in primary human liver tumours. 1991; APMIS Suppl 23: 77–85

449. Christensen W N, Boitnott J K, Kuhajda F P. Immunoperoxidase staining as a diagnostic aid for hepatocellular carcinoma. Mod Pathol 1989; 2: 8–12

449a. Ma C K, Zarbo R J, Frierson H F, Lee M W. Comparative immunohistochemical study of primary and metastatic carcinomas of the liver. Am J Clin Pathol 1993; 99: 551–557

450. Wang J, Dhillon A P, Sankey E A, Wightman A K, Lewin J F, Scheuer P J. 'Neuroendocrine' differentiation in primary neoplasms of the liver. J Pathol 1991; 163: 61–67

451. Fausto N, Shank P R. Analysis of proto-oncogene expression during liver regeneration and hepatocarcinogenesis. In: Okuda K, Ishak G, eds. Neoplasms of the liver. Berlin: Springer-Verlag, 1988; pp 57–69

452. Himeno Y, Fukuda Y, Hatanaka M, Imura H. Expression of oncogenes in human liver disease. Liver 1988; 8: 208–212

453. Nonomura A, Ohta G, Hayashi M et al. Immunohistochemical detection of ras oncogene p21 product in liver cirrhosis and hepatocellular carcinoma. Am J Gastroenterol 1987; 82: 512–518

454. Bressac B, Galvin K M, Liang T J, Isselbacher K J, Wands J R, Ozturk M. Abnormal structure and expression of p53 gene in human hepatocellular carcinoma. Proc Natl Acad Sci 1990; 87: 1973–1977

455. Scorsone K A, Zhou Y-Z, Butel J S, Slagle B L. p53 mutations cluster of codon 249 in hepatitis B virus-positive hepatocellular carcinomas from China. Cancer Res 1992; 52: 1635–1638

456. Otsuru A, Nagataki S, Koji T, Tamaoki T. Analysis of alpha-fetoprotein gene expression in hepatocellular carcinoma and liver cirrhosis by in situ hybridization. Cancer 1988; 62: 1105–1112

457. Grigioni W F, D'Errico A, Bacci F et al. Primary liver neoplasms: evaluation of proliferative index using MoAb Ki67. J Pathol 1989; 158: 23–30

458. Crocker J, McGovern J. Nucleolar organiser regions in normal, cirrhotic and carcinomatous livers. J Clin Pathol 1988; 10: 1044–1048

459. Zalatnai A, Lapis K, Fehér I. The nucleolar organizer regions in hyperplastic and tumorous lesions of the human liver. Pathol Res Pract 1993; 189: 536–541

460. Seki S, Sakaguchi H, Kawakita N et al. Identification and fine structure of proliferating hepatocytes in malignant and non-malignant liver diseases by use of a monoclonal antibody against DNA polymerase alpha. Hum Pathol 1990; 21: 1020–1030

461. Kawakita N, Seki S, Sakaguchi H et al. Analysis of proliferating hepatocytes using a monoclonal antibody against proliferating nuclear antigen/cyclin in embedded tissues from various liver diseases fixed in formaldehyde. Am J Pathol 1992; 140: 513–520

461a. Kawakita N, Seki S, Yanai A et al. Immunocytochemical identification of proliferative hepatocytes using monoclonal antibody to proliferating cell nuclear antigen (PCNA/cyclin). Am J Clin Pathol 1992; 97 (Suppl. 1): S14–S20

461b. Ojanguren I, Ariza A, Llatjós M, Castella E, Mate J L, Navas-Palacios J J. Proliferating cell nuclear antigen expression in normal, regenerative and neoplastic liver. Hum Pathol 1993; 24: 905–908

461c. Taniai M, Tomimatsu M, Okuda H, Saito A, Obata H. Immunohistochemical detection of proliferating cell nuclear antigen in hepatocellular carcinoma: relationship to histological grade. J Gastroenterol Hepatol 1993; 8: 420–425

462. Hino A, Onitsuka A, Gotoh M et al. A study on DNA histogram pattern of hepatocellular carcinoma. J Jpn Surg Soc 1988; 89: 871–879

463. Ishizu H. Flow cytometric analysis of the nuclear DNA content of hepatocellular carcinoma. Jpn J Surg 1989; 19: 662–673

464. Chen M-F, Hwang T-L, Tsao K-C, Sun C-F, Chen T-J. Flow cytometric DNA analysis of hepatocellular carcinoma: preliminary report. Surgery 1991; 109: 455–458

465. Fujimoto J, Okamoto E, Yamanaka N, Toyosaka A, Mitsunobu M. Flow cytometric DNA analysis of hepatocellular carcinoma. Cancer 1991; 67: 939–944

466. McEntee G P, Batts K A, Katzmann J A, Ilstrup D M, Nagorney D M. Relationship of nuclear DNA content to clinical and pathologic findings in patients with primary hepatic malignancy. Surgery 1992; 111: 376–379

467. Jagoe R, Sowter C, Dandy S, Slavin G. Morphometric study of liver cell nuclei in hepatomas using an interactive computer technique. Nuclear size and shape. J Clin Pathol 1982; 35: 1057–1062

468. Jagoe R, Sowter C, Slavin G. Shape and texture analysis of liver cell nuclei in hepatomas by computer aided microscopy. J Clin Pathol 1984; 37: 755–762

469. Kondo F, Wada K, Kondo Y. Morphometric analysis of hepatocellular carcinoma. Virchows Arch (A) 1988; 413: 425–430

469a. Deprez C, Vangansbeke D, Fastrez R, Pasteels J-L, Verhest A, Kiss R. Nuclear DNA content, proliferation index, and nuclear size determination in normal and cirrhotic liver, and in benign and malignant primary and metastatic hepatic tumors. Am J Clin Pathol 1993; 99: 558–565

469b. Erler B S, Truong H M, Kim S S, Huh M H, Geller S A, Marchevsky A M. A study of hepatocellular carcinoma using morphometric and densitometric image analysis. Am J Clin Pathol 1993; 100: 151–157

470. Johannessen J V, ed. Electron microscopy in human medicine: the liver, gall bladder and biliary ducts. New York: McGraw-Hill, 1979

471. Phillips M J, Poucell S, Patterson J, Valencia P. The liver: an atlas and text of ultrastructural pathology. New York: Raven Press, 1987

472. Bru C, Maroto A, Bruix J et al. Diagnostic accuracy of fine needle aspiration biopsy in patients with hepatocellular carcinoma. Dig Dis Sci 1989; 34: 1765–1769

473. Glenthoj A, Sehested M, Torp-Pedersen S. Diagnostic reliability of histological and cytological fine needle biopsies from focal liver lesions. Histopathology 1989; 15: 375–383

474. Buscarini L, Fornari F, Bolondi L et al. Ultrasound-guided fine-needle biopsy of focal liver lesions: techniques, diagnostic accuracy and complications. J Hepatol 1990; 11: 344–348

475. Cohen M B, Haber M M, Holly E A, Ahn D K, Bottles K, Stoloff A C. Cytologic criteria to distinguish hepatocellular carcinoma from non-neoplastic liver. Am J Clin Pathol 1991; 95: 125–130

476. Kung I T M, Chan S-K, Fung K-H. Fine needle aspiration in hepatocellular carcinoma. Cancer 1991; 67: 673–680

476a. Zainol H, Sumithran E. Combined cytological and histological diagnosis of hepatocellular carcinoma in ultrasonically guided fine needle biopsy specimens. Histopathology 1993; 22: 581–586

476b. Borzio M, Borzio F, Macchi R et al. The evaluation of fine-needle procedures for the diagnosis of focal liver lesions in cirrhosis. J Hepatol 1994; 20: 117–121

477. Charnley R M, Sheffield J P, Hardcastle J D. Evaluation of a biopsy gun for guided biopsy of impalpable liver lesions using intraoperative ultrasound. HBP Surgery 1990; 3: 265–267

478. Carrozza M J, Calafati S A, Edmonds P R. Immunocytochemical localization of polyclonal carcinoembryonic antigen in hepatocellular carcinomas. Acta Cytol 1991; 35: 221–224

479. Wolber R A, Greene C-A, Dupuis B A. Polyclonal carcinoembryonic antigen staining in the cytologic differential diagnosis of primary and metastatic hepatic malignancies. Acta Cytol 1991; 35: 215–220

480. Lee Y-TM, Geer D A. Primary liver cancer: pattern of metastasis. J Surg Oncol 1987; 36: 26–31

481. Yuki K, Hirohashi S, Sakamoto M, Kanai T, Shimosato Y. Growth and spread of hepatocellular carcinoma. Cancer 1990; 66: 2174–2179

482. Herfarth Ch, Schlag P, Hohenberger P eds. Therapeutic strategies in primary and metastatic liver cancer. Berlin: Springer-Verlag, 1986

483. Dunk A A, Thomas H C. Review: the treatment of hepatocellular carcinoma. Aliment Pharmacol Therap 1988; 2: 187–201

484. Johnson P J, Wilkinson M L, Karani J. Advances in neoplastic disease of the liver and biliary tract. Gut 1991: Suppl: S104–S110

485. Hobbs K E F, Dusheiko G M. Management of hepatocellular carcinoma. J Hepatol 1992; 15: 281–283

486. Suzuki M, Okazaki N, Yoshino M, Yoshida T. Spontaneous regression of a hepatocellular carcinoma. Hepato-gastroenterol 1989; 36: 160–163

487. Ayres R C S, Robertson D A F, Dewbury K C, Millward-Sadler G H, Smith C L. Spontaneous regression of hepatocellular carcinoma. Gut 1990; 31: 722–724

488. Gaffey M J, Joyce J P, Carlson G S, Esteban J M. Spontaneous regression of hepatocellular carcinoma. Cancer 1990; 65: 2779–2783

489. Tocci G, Conte A, Guarascio P, Visco G. Spontaneous regression of hepatocellular carcinoma after massive gastrointestinal haemorrhage. Br Med J 1990; 300: 641–642

490. Peters R L. Pathology of hepatocellular carcinoma. In: Okuda K, Peters R L, eds. Hepatocellular carcinoma. New York: Wiley, 1976; pp 107–168

491. Berman M M, Libbey N P, Foster J H. Hepatocellular carcinoma of polygonal cell type with fibrous stroma — an atypical variant with a favourable prognosis. Cancer 1980; 46: 1448–1455

492. Farhi D C, Shikes R H, Silverberg S G. Ultrastructure of fibrolamellar oncocytic hepatoma. Cancer 1982; 50: 702–709

493. Craig J R, Peters R L, Edmondson H A, Omata M. Fibrolamellar carcinoma of the liver: a tumor of adolescents and young adults with distinctive clinicopathologic features. Cancer 1980; 46: 372–379

494. Rolfes D B. Fibrolamellar carcinoma of the liver. In: Okuda K, Ishak K G, eds. Neoplasms of the liver. Berlin: Springer-Verlag, 1988: pp 138–142

495. Soreide O, Czerniak A, Bradpiece H, Bloom S, Blumgart L. Characteristics of fibrolamellar carcinoma. Am J Surg 1986; 151: 518–523

496. Hodgson H J F. Fibrolamellar cancer of the liver. J Hepatol 1987; 5: 241–247

497. Ruffin M T. Fibrolamellar hepatoma. Am J Gastroenterol 1990; 85: 577–581

498. Paradinas F J, Melia W M, Wilkinson M L et al. High serum vitamin B12 binding capacity as a marker of the fibrolamellar variant of hepatocellular cancer. Br Med J 1982; 285: 840–842

499. Collier N A, Weinbren K, Bloom S R, Hodgson H J F, Blumgart L H. Neurotensin secretion by fibrolamellar carcinoma of the liver. Lancet 1984; i: 538–540

500. Teitelbaum D H, Tuttle S, Carey L C, Clausen K P. Fibrolamellar carcinoma of the liver. Ann Surg 1985; 202; 36–41

501. Starzl T E, Iwatsuki S, Shaw B W, Nalesnik M A, Farhi D C, Van Thiel D H. Treatment of fibrolamellar hepatoma with partial or total hepatectomy and transplantation of the liver. Surg Gynaec Obst 1986; 162: 145–148

502. Berman M A, Burnham J A, Sheahan D G. Fibrolamellar carcinoma of the liver: an immunohistochemical study of nineteen cases and a review of the literature. Hum Pathol 1988; 19: 784–794

503. Goodman Z D, Ishak K G, Langloss J M, Sesterhenn I A, Rabin L, Combined hepatocellular–cholangiocellular carcinoma. Cancer 1985; 55: 124–135

504. Lapis K, Schaff Z S, Kopper L, Karácsonyi S, Ormos J. Das fibrolamelläre Leberkarzinom. Zentralbl Allg Pathol 1990; 136: 135–149

505. Van Eyken P, Sciot R, Brock P et al. Abundant expression of cytokeratin 7 in fibrolamellar carcinoma. Histopathology 1990; 17: 101–107

506. Jagirdar J, Ishak K G, Colombo M, Brambilla C, Paronetto F. Fibronectin patterns in hepatocellular carcinoma and its clinical significance. Cancer 1985; 56: 1643–1648

507. Altmann H W. Some histological remarks on the fibrolamellar carcinoma of the liver. Path Res Pract 1990; 186: 63–69

508. Farhi D C, Shikes R H, Murari P J, Silverberg S G. Hepatocellular carcinomas in young people. Cancer 1983; 52: 1516–1525

509. An T, Ghatak N, Kastner R, Kay S, Lee H M. Hyaline globules and intracellular lumina in a hepatocellular carcinoma. Am J Clin Pathol 1983; 79: 392–396

510. Caballero T, Aneiros J, Lopez-Caballero J, Gomez-Moreles M, Nogales F. Fibrolamellar hepatocellular carcinoma. Histopathology 1985; 9: 445–456

511. Vecchio F M, Fabiano A, Ghirlanda G, Manna R, Massi G Fibrolamellar carcinoma of the liver: the malignant counterpart of focal nodular hyperplasia with oncocytic change. Am J Clin Pathol 1984; 81: 521–526

512. Davison F D, Fagan E A, Portmann B, Williams R. HBV-DNA sequences in tumor and non-tumor tissue in a patient with the fibrolamellar variant of hepatocellular carcinoma. Hepatology 1990; 12: 676–679

513. Horie Y, Katoh S, Yoshida H, Imaoka T, Suou T, Hirayama C. Pedunculated hepatocellular carcinoma. Cancer 1983; 51: 746–751

514. Anthony P P, James K. Pedunculated hepatocellular carcinoma. Is it an entity? Histopathology 1987; 11: 402–414

515. Moritz M W, Shoji M, Sicard G A, Shioda R, DeSchryver K. Surgical therapy in two patients with pedunculated hepatocellular carcinoma. Arch Surg 1988; 123: 772–774

515a. Nishizaki T, Matsumata T, Adachi E, Hayashi H, Sugimachi K. Pedunculated hepatocellular carcinoma and surgical treatment. Br J Cancer 1993; 67: 115–118

516. Tang Z-Y. Subclinical hepatocellular carcinoma. Berlin: Springer-Verlag, 1985

517. Ebara M, Ohto M, Shinagawa T et al. Natural history of minute hepatocellular carcinoma smaller than three centimeters complicating cirrhosis. Gastroenterology 1986; 90: 289–298

518. Watanabe A, Yamamoto H, Ito T, Nagashima H. Diagnosis, treatment and prognosis of small hepatocellular carcinoma. Hepato-gastroenterol 1986; 33: 52–55

519. Kanai T, Hirohashi S, Upton M et al. Pathology of small hepatocellular carcinoma. Cancer 1987; 60: 810–819

520. Nagasue N, Yukaya H, Chang Y C et al. Appriasal of hepatic resection in the treatment of minute hepatocellular carcinoma associated with cirrhosis. Br J Surg 1987; 74: 836–838

521. Lee C-S, Hwang L-Y, Beasley R P, Hsu H-C, Lee H-S, Lin T-Y. Prognostic significance of histologic findings in resected small hepatocellular carcinoma. Acta Chir Scand 1988; 154: 199–203

522. Tang Z-Y, Yu Y-Q, Zhou X-D et al. Surgery of small hepatocellular carcinoma. Cancer 1989; 64: 536–541

523. Lai ECS, Ng IOL, You K T. Hepatic resection for small hepatocellular carcinoma: the Queen Mary Hospital experience. World J Surg 1991; 15: 654–659

524. Dusheiko G M, Hobbs K E F, Dick R, Burroughs A K. Treatment of small hepatocellular carcinoma. Lancet 1992; 340: 285–288

525. Stocker J T, Ishak K G. Hepatoblastoma. In: Okuda K, Ishak K G, eds. Neoplasma of the liver. Berlin: Springer-Verlag, 1988: pp 126–136

526. Stocker J T. Hepatic tumours. In: Balistreri W F, Stocker J T, eds. Paediatric hepatology. New York: Hemisphere 1990: pp 399–488

527. Ishak K G, Glunz P R. Hepatoblastoma and hepatocarcinoma in infancy and childhood. Cancer 1967; 20: 396–422

528. Kasai M, Watanabe I. Histologic classification of liver cell carcinoma in infancy and childhood and its clinical evaluation. Cancer 1970; 25: 551–563

529. Gonzalez-Crussi F, Upton M P, Maurer H S. Hepatoblastoma: attempt at characterization of histologic subtypes. Am J Surg Pathol 1982; 6: 599–612

530. Lack E E, Neave C, Vawter G F. Hepatoblastoma. Am J Surg Pathol 1982; 6: 693–705

531. Schmidt D, Harms D, Lang W. Primary hepatic tumours in childhood. Virchows Archiv (A) 1985; 407: 387–405

532. Altmann H W. Epithelial and mixed hepatoblastoma in the adult. Path Res Pract 1992; 188: 16–26

533. Garber J E, Li F P, Kingston J E et al. Hepatoblastoma and familial adenomatous polyposis. J Natl Cancer Inst 1988; 80: 1626–1628

534. Giardello F M, Offerhaus J A, Krush A J et al. Risk of hepatoblastoma in familial adenomatous polyposis. J Pediatr 1991; 119: 766–768

535. Bernstein I T, Bulow S, Mauritzen K. Hepatoblastoma in two cousins in a family with adenomatous polyposis. Dis Colon Rectum 1992; 35: 373–374

536. Riikonen P, Tuominen L, Seppa A, Perkkio M. Simultaneous hepatoblastoma in identical male twins. Cancer 1990; 66: 2429–2431

537. Buckley J D, Sather H, Ruccione K et al. A case–control study of risk factors for hepatoblastoma. Cancer 1989; 64: 1169–1176

538. Nakagawara A, Ikeda K, Tsuneyoshi M et al. Hepatoblastoma producing both alpha-fetoprotein and human chorionic gonadotropin. Cancer 1985; 56: 1636–1642

539. Heimann A, White P F, Riely C A et al. Hepatoblastoma presenting as isosexual precocity. J Clin Gastroenterol 1987; 9: 105–110

540. Watanabe I, Yamaguchi M, Kasai M. Histologic characteristics of gonadotropin-producing hepatoblastoma: a survey of seven cases from Japan. J Paediatr Surg 1987; 22: 406–411

541. Manivel C, Wick M R, Abenoza P, Dehner L P. Teratoid hepatoblastoma. Cancer 1986; 57: 2168–2174

542. Joshi V V, Kaur P, Ryan B, Saad S, Walters T R. Mucoid anaplastic hepatoblastoma. Cancer 1984; 54: 2035–2039

542a. Cross S S, Variend S. Combined hepatoblastoma and yolk sac tumour of the liver. Cancer 1992; 69: 1323–1326

542b. Ruck P, Kaiserling E. Melanin-containing hepatoblastoma with endocrine differentiation. Cancer 1993; 72: 361–368

543. Abenoza P, Manivel J C, Wick M R, Hagen K, Dehner L P. Hepatoblastoma: an immunohistochemical and ultrastructural study. Hum Pathol 1987; 18: 1025–1035

544. Van Eyken P, Sciot R, Callea F, Ramaekers F, Schaart G, Desmet V J. A cytokeratin immunohistochemical study of hepatoblastoma. Hum Pathol 1990; 21: 302–308

545. Ruck P, Harms D, Kaiserling E. Neuroendocrine differentation in hepatoblastoma. Am J Surg Pathol 1990; 14: 847–855

545a. Saxena R, Leake J L, Shafford E A. Chemotherapy effects on hepatoblastoma. Am J Surg Pathol 1993; 17: 1266–1271

546. Gibson J B, Chan W C. Primary carcinomas of the liver in Hong Kong: some possible aetiological factors. In: Grundmann E. Tulinius H, eds. Current problems in the epidemiology of cancer and lymphomas. Recent results in cancer research, vol 39. Berlin: Springer-Verlag, 1972: pp 107–118

547. Belamaric J. Intrahepatic bile duct carcinoma and *C. sinensis* infection in Hong Kong. Cancer 1973; 31: 468–473

548. Okuda K. Primary liver cancer in Japan. Cancer 1980; 45: 2663–2669

549. Kurathong S, Lerdverasirikul P, Wongpaitoon V et al. *Opisthorchis viverrini* infection and cholangiocarcinoma. Gastroenterology 1985; 89: 151–156

550. Sugihara S, Kojiro M. Pathology of cholangiocarcinoma. In: Okuda K, Ishak K G, eds. Neoplasms of the liver. Berlin: Springer-Verlag, 1988: pp 143–158

551. Srivatanakul P, Sontipong S, Chotiwan P, Parkin D M. Liver cancer in Thailand: temporal and geographic variations. J Gastroenterol Hepatol 1988; 3: 413–420

551a. Haswell-Elkins M R, Satarug S, Elkins D B. *Opisthorchis viverrini* infection in North east Thailand and its relationship to cholangiocarcinoma. J Gastroenterol Hepatal 1992; 7: 538–548

552. Anthony P P. Epidemiology, aetiology and pathology of bile duct tumours. In: Preece P E, Cuschieri A, Rosin R D, eds. Cancer of the bile ducts and pancreas. Philadelphia: Saunders, 1989: pp 1–26

553. Parkin D M, Srivatanakul P, Khlat M et al. Liver cancer in Thailand. I. A case–control study of cholangiocarcinoma. II. A case–control study of hepatocellular carcinoma. Int J Cancer 1991; 48: 323–332

554. Srivanatakul P, Ohshima H, Khlat M et al. *Opisthorchis viverrini* infestation and endogenous nitrosamines as risk factors for cholangiocarcinoma in Thailand. Int J Cancer 1991; 48: 821–825

555. Srivatanakul P, Parkin D M, Jiang Y-Z et al. The role of infection by *Opisthorchis viverrini*, hepatitis B virus and aflatoxin exposure in the etiology of liver cancer in Thailand. Cancer 1991; 68: 2411–2417

556. Koga A, Ichimiya H, Yamaguchi K, Miyazaki K, Nakayama F. Hepatolithiasis associated with cholangiocarcinoma. Cancer 1985; 55: 2826–2829

557. Nakanuma Y, Terada T, Tanaka Y, Ohta G. Are hepatolithiasis and cholangiocarcinoma aetiologically related? Virchows Archiv A 1985; 406: 45–58

558. Chen M-F, Jan Y-Y, Wang C-S, Jeng L-BB, Hwang T-L, Chen S-C. Intrahepatic stones associated with cholangiocarcinoma. Am J Gastroenterol 1989; 84: 391–395

558a. Chen M-F, Jan Y-Y, Wang C-S et al. A reappraisal of cholangiocarcinoma in patients with cholelithiasis. Cancer 1993; 71: 2461–2465

559. Ohta T, Nagakawa T, Ueda N et al. Mucosal dysplasia of the liver and the intraductal variant of peripheral cholangiocarcinoma in hepatolithiasis. Cancer 1991; 68: 2217–2223

559a. Terada T, Nakanuma Y. Cell kinetic analyses and expression of carcinoembryonic antigen, carbohydrate antigen 19-9 and DU-PAN-2 in hyperplastic, preneoplastic and neoplastic lesions of intrahepatic bile ducts in livers with hepatoliths. Virchows Archiv (A) 1992; 420: 327–335

560. Chaduri P K, Chaduri B, Schuler J J, Nyhus L M. Carcinoma associated with congenital cystic dilatation of bile ducts. Arch Surg 1982; 117: 1349–1351

561. Dayton M T, Longmire W P, Tompkins R K. Caroli's disease: a premalignant condition? Am J Surg 1983; 145: 41–47

562. Imamura M, Miyashita T, Tani T, Naito A, Tobe T, Takahashi K. Cholangiocellular carcinoma associated with multiple liver cysts. Am J Gastroenterol 1984; 79: 790–795

563. Rossi R L, Silverman M L, Braasch J W, Munson J L, Remine S G. Carcinomas arising in cystic conditions of the bile ducts. Ann Surg 1987; 205: 377–384

564. Todani T, Watanabe Y, Toki A, Urushihara N. Carcinoma related to choledochal cysts with internal drainage operations. Surg Gynec Obstet 1987; 164: 61–64

565. Burns C D, Kuhns J G, Wiemann T J. Cholangiocarcinoma in association with multiple biliary microhamartomas. Arch Pathol Lab Med 1990; 114; 1287–1289

566. Morohoshi T, Kunimura T, Kanda M et al. Multiple carcinomata associated with anomalous arrangement of the biliary and pancreatic duct system. Acta Pathol Jpn 1990; 40: 755–763

567. Ohta T, Nagakawa T, Ueno K et al. Clinical experience of biliary tract carcinoma associated with anomalous union of the pancreaticobiliary ductal system. Jpn J Surg 1990; 20: 36–43

568. Wee A, Ludwig J, Coffey R J, La Russo N F, Wiesner R H. Hepatobiliary carcinoma associated with primary sclerosing cholangitis and chronic ulcerative colitis. Hum Pathol 1985; 16: 719–726

569. Mir-Madjlessi S H, Farmer R G, Sivak M V. Bile duct carcinoma in patients with ulcerative colitis: relationship to scleroisng cholangitis. Dig Dis Sci 1987; 32; 145–154

570. Haworth A C, Manley P N, Groll A, Pace R. Bile duct carcinoma and biliary tract dysplasia in ulcerative colitis. Arch Pathol Lab Med 1989; 113: 434–436

571. Rosen C B, Nagorney D M, Wiesner R H, Coffey R J, La Russo N F. Cholangiocarcinoma complicating primary sclerosing cholangitis. Ann Surg 1991; 213: 21–25

571a. D'Haens G R, Lashner B A, Hanauer S B. Pericholangitis and sclerosing cholangitis are risk factors for dysplasia and cancer in ulcerative colitis. Am J Gastroenterol 1993; 88: 1174–1178

572. El-Zayadi A, Ghoneim M, Kabil S M, El Tawil A, Selim O. Bile duct carcinoma in Egypt: possible etiological factors. Hepato-gastroenterol 1991; 38: 337–340

573. Rubel L R, Ishak K G. Thorotrast-associated cholangiocarcinoma. Cancer 1982; 50: 1408–1415

574. Yen S, Hsieh C-C, MacMahon B. Extrahepatic bile duct cancer and smoking, beverage consumption, past medical history, and oral-contraceptive use. Cancer 1987; 59: 2112–2116

575. Altaee M Y, Johnson P J, Farrant J M, Williams R. Etiologic and clinical characteristics of peripheral and hilar cholangiocarcinoma. Cancer 1991; 68: 2051–2055

576. Mecklin J P, Järvinen H J, Virolainen M. The association between cholangiocarcinoma and hereditary nonpolyposis colorectal carcinoma. Cancer 1992; 69: 1112–1114

577. Tada M, Omata M, Ohto M. High incidence of *ras* gene mutation in intrahepatic cholangiocarcinoma. Cancer 1992; 69: 1115–1118

578. Weinbren K, Mutum S S. Pathological aspects of cholangiocarcinoma. J Pathol 1983; 139: 217–238

579. Kawarada Y, Mizumoto R. Cholangiocellular carcinoma of the liver. Am J Surg 1984; 147: 354–359

580. Nakajima T, Kondo Y, Miyazaki M, Okui K. A histopathologic study of 102 cases of intrahepatic cholangiocarcinoma. Hum Pathol 1988; 19: 1228–1234

581. Preece P E, Cuschieri A, Rosin R D, eds. Cancer of the bile ducts and pancreas. Philadelphia: Saunders, 1989

581a. Schlinkert R T, Nagorney D M, Van Heerden J A, Adson M A. Intrahepatic cholangiocarcinoma: clinical aspects, pathology and treatment. HPB Surgery 1992; 5: 95–102

582. Klatskin G. Adenocarcinoma of the hepatic duct at its bifurcation within the porta hepatis. Am J Med 1965; 38: 241–256

583. Van Steenbergen W, Van Stapel M J, Geboes K, Ponette E, Fevery J, De Groote J. Carcinoma at the hilus of the liver: clinical, radiological, histological and therapeutic aspects. Neth J Med 1982; 25: 344–353

584. Mizumoto R, Kawarada Y, Suzuki H. Surgical treatment of hilar carcinoma of the bile duct. Surg Gynec Obst 1986; 162; 153–158

585. Lygidakis N J, Van Der Heyde M N, eds. Klatskin tumours. Semin Liver Dis 1990; 10: 85–148

585a. Kimura W, Nagai H, Atomi Y et al. Clinicopathological characteristics of hepatic hilar bile duct carcinoma. Hepato-gastroenterol 1993; 40: 21–27

586. Ligoury C, Canard J M. Tumours of the biliary system. Clin Gasgroenterol 1983; 12: 269–295

587. Anderson J B, Cooper M J, Williamson R C N. Adenocarcinoma of the extrahepatic biliary tree. Ann R Coll Surg Engl 1985; 67: 139–143

588. Frierson H F, Fechner R E. Pathology of malignant neoplasms of the gallbladder and extrahepatic bile ducts. In: Wanebo H J, ed. Hepatic and biliary cancer. New York: Dekker, 1986: pp 281–297

589. Roberts J W. Carcinoma of the extrahepatic bile ducts. Surg Clin North Am 1986; 66: 751–756

590. Gertsch P, Thomas P, Baer H, Lerut J, Zimmermann A, Blumgart L H. Multiple tumors of the biliary tract. Am J Surg 1990; 159: 386–388

590a. Henson D E, Albores-Saavedra J, Corle D. Carcinoma of the extrahepatic ducts. Cancer 1992; 70: 1498–1501

590b. Nakajima T, Tajima Y, Sugano I, Nagao K, Kondo Y, Wada K. Intrahepatic cholangiocarcinoma with sarcomatous change. Cancer 1993; 72: 1872–1877

591. Kurashina M, Kozuka S, Nakasima N, Hirabayasi N, Ho M. Relationship of intrahepatic bile duct hyperplasia to cholangiocellular carcinoma. Cancer 1988; 61; 2469–2474

592. Terada T, Nakanuma Y. Pathological observations of intrahepatic peribiliary glands in 1000 consecutive autopsy livers. Hepatology 1990; 12; 92–97

593. Suzuki M, Takahashi T, Ouchi K, Matsuno S. The development and extension of hepatohilar bile duct cancer. Cancer 1989; 64: 658–666

594. Albores-Saavedra J, Henson D E. Tumors of the gallbladder and extrahepatic bile ducts. Atlas of tumour pathology, 2nd series, Fascicle 22. Washington: Armed Forces Institute of Pathology, 1986

595. Davis R I, Sloan J M, Hood J M, Maxwell P. Carcinoma of the extrahepatic biliary tract: a clinicopathological and immunohistochemical study. Histopathology 1988; 12: 623–631

596. Albores-Saavedra J, Henson D E, Sobin L H. Histological typing of tumours of the gallbladder and extrahepatic bile ducts. World Health Organization International Classification of Tumours, 2nd edn. Berlin: Springer-Verlag, 1991

597. Kozuka S, Tsubone M, Hachisuka K. Evolution of carcinoma in the extrahepatic bile ducts. Cancer 1984; 54: 65–72

598. Ohta G, Nakanuma Y, Terada T. Pathology of hepatolithiasis, cholangitis and cholangiocarcinoma. In: Okuda K, Nakayama F, Wong J, eds. Intrahepatic calculi. New York: Liss, 1984: pp 91–133

599. Nakajima T, Kondo Y. Well differentiated cholangiocarcinoma; diagnostic significance of morphologic and immunohistochemical parameters. Am J Surg Pathol 1989; 13: 569–573

599a. Terada T, Nakanuma Y. An immunohistochemical survey of amylase isoenzymes in cholangiocarcinoma and hepatocellular carcinoma. Arch Pathol Lab Med 1993; 117: 160–162

600. Voravud N, Foster C S, Gilbertson J A, Sikora K, Waxman J. Oncogene expression in cholangiocarcinoma and in normal hepatic development. Hum Pathol 1989; 20: 1163–1168

601. Zhang S, Wu M, Chen H, Zhang X. Expression of glycoconjugates in intrahepatic cholangiocellular carcinoma. Virchows Archiv A 1989; 415; 395–401

602. Hsu W, Deziel D J, Gould V E et al. Neuroendocrine differentiation and prognosis of extrahepatic biliary tract carcinomas. Surgery 1991; 110: 604–611

603. Rabinovitz M, Zajko A B, Hassanein T. Diagnostic value of brush cytology in the diagnosis of bile duct carcinoma. Hepatology 1990; 12: 747–752

603a. Nakajima T, Sugano I, Matsuzaki O et al. Biliary cystadenocarcinoma of the liver. Cancer 1992; 69: 2426–2432

604. Cheung Y K, Chan F L, Leong L L Y, Collins R J, Cheung A. Biliary cystadenoma and cystadenocarcinoma: some unusual features. Clin Radiol 1991; 43: 183–185

605. Tomimatsu M, Okuda H, Saito A, Obata H, Hanyu F, Nakano M. A case of biliary cystadenocarcinoma with morphologic and histochemical features of hepatocytes. Cancer 1989; 64: 1323–1328

605a. Wolf H K, Garcia J A, Bossen E H. Oncocytic differentiation in intrahepatic biliary cystadenocarcinoma. Mod Pathol 1992; 5: 665–668

606. O'Shea J S, Shah D, Cooperman A M. Biliary cystadenocarcinoma of extrahepatic duct origin arising in previously benign cystadenoma. Am J Gastroenterol 1987; 82; 1306–1310

607. Sell S, Dunsford H A. Evidence for the stem cell origin of hepatocellular carcinoma and cholangiocarcinoma. Am J Pathol 1989; 134; 1347–1363

608. Song E, Kew M C, Grieve T, Isaacson C, Myburgh J A. Primary squamous cell carcinoma of the liver occurring in association with hepatolithiasis. Cancer 1984; 53: 542–546

609. Gresham G A, Rue L W. Squamous cell carcinoma of the liver. Hum Pathol 1985; 16: 413–416

610. Pliskin A, Cualing H, Stenger R J. Primary squamous cell carcinoma originating in congenital cysts of the liver. Arch Pathol Lab Med 1992; 116: 105–107

611. Clements D, Newman P, Etherington R, Lawrie B W, Rhodes J. Squamous carcinoma in the liver. Gut 1990; 31: 1333–1334

612. Kakizoe S, Kojiro M, Nakashima T. Hepatocellular carcinoma with sarcomatous change. Cancer 1987; 59: 310–316

613. Nakajima T, Kubosawa H, Kondo Y, Konno A, Iwama S. Combined hepatocellular-cholangiocarcinoma with variable sarcomatous transformation. Am J Clin Pathol 1988; 90: 309–312

614. Haratake J, Horie A. An immunohistochemical study of sarcomatoid liver carcinomas. Cancer 1991; 68: 93–97

615. Kubosawa H, Ishige H, Kondo Y, Konno A, Yamamoto T, Nagao K. Hepatocellular carcinoma with rhabdomyoblastic differentiation. Cancer 1988; 62: 781–786

616. Hood D L, Bauer T W, Leibel S A, MacMahon J T. Hepatic giant cell carcinoma. Am J Clin Pathol 1990; 93: 111–116

617. Koo J, Ho J, Wong J, Ong G B. Mucoepidermoid carcinoma of the bile duct. Ann Surg 1982; 196: 140–148

618. Miura K, Shirasawa H. Primary carcinoid tumor of the liver. Am J Clin Pathol 1988; 89: 561–564

619. Goodman Z D, Albores-Saavedra J, Lundblad D M. Somatostatinoma of the cystic duct. Cancer 1984; 53: 498–502

620. Jutte D L, Bell R H, Penn I, Powers J, Kolinjivadi J. Carcinoid tumor of the biliary system. Dig Dis Sci 1986; 32: 763–769

621. Angeles-Angeles A, Quintanilla-Martinez L, Larriva-Sahd J. Primary carcinoid of the common bile duct. Am J Clin Pathol 1991; 96: 341–344

622. Rugge M, Sonego F, Militello C, Guido M, Ninfo V. Primary carcinoid tumor of the cystic and common bile ducts. Am J Surg Pathol 1992; 16: 802–807

623. Ueyama T, Ding J, Hashimoto H, Tsuyenoshi M, Enjoji M. Carcinoid tumor arising in the wall of a congenital bile duct cyst. Arch Pathol Lab Med 1992; 116: 291–293

624. Van der Wal A C, Van Leeuwen D J, Walford N. Small cell neuroendocrine (oat cell) tumour of the common bile duct. Histopathology 1990; 16: 398–400

624a. Moriura S, Ikeda S, Hirai M et al. Hepatic gastrinoma. Cancer 1993; 72: 1547–1550

625. Kawahara E, Kitamura T, Ueda H et al. Hepatocellular carcinoma arising in the abdominal cavity. Acta Pathol Jpn 1988; 38: 1575–1581

626. Berry C L. Solitary 'necrotic' nodule of the liver: a probable pathogenesis. J Clin Pathol 1985; 38: 1278–1280

627. Shimizu M, Miura J, Itoh H, Saitoh Y. Hepatic giant cavernous hemangioma with microangiopathic hemolytic anaemia and consumption coagulopathy. Am J Gastroenterol 1990; 85: 1411–1413

628. Hobbs KEF. Hepatic haemangiomas. World J Surg 1990; 14: 468–471

629. Gandolfi L, Leo P, Solmi L, Vitelli E, Verros G, Colecchia A. Natural history of hepatic haemangiomas: clinical and ultrasound study. Gut 1991; 32: 677–680

630. Yamagata M, Kanematsu T, Matsumata T, Utsunomiya T, Ikeda Y, Sugimachi K. Management of haemangioma of the liver: comparison of results between surgery and observation. Br J Surg 1991; 78: 1223–1225

631. Conter R L, Longmire W P. Recurrent hepatic hemangiomas. Ann Surg 1988; 207: 115–119
632. Sugimura H, Tange T, Yamaguchi K, Mori W. Systemic haemangiomatosis. Acta Pathol Jpn 1986; 36: 1089–1098
633. Dehner L P, Ishak K G. Vascular tumors of the liver in infants and children. Arch Pathol 1971; 92: 101–111
634. Dachman A H, Lichtenstein J E, Friedman A C, Hartman D S. Infantile hemangioendothelioma of the liver: radiologic pathologic–clinical correlation. Am J Radiol 1983; 140: 1091–1096
635. Stanley P, Geer G D, Miller J H, Gilsauz V, Landing B H, Boechat I M. Infantile hepatic hemangiomas. Cancer 1989; 64: 936–949
636. Van Steenbergen W, Joosten E, Marchall G et al. Hepatic lymphangiomatosis. Gastroenterology 1985; 88: 1968–1972
637. Delamarre J, Lamblin G, Sevestre H et al. Lymphangiome caverneux du foie. Gastroenterol Clin Biol 1990; 14: 576–580
638. Miller C, Mazzaferro V, Makowka L et al. Orthotopic liver transplantation for hepatic lymphangiomatosis. Surgery 1988; 103: 490–495
638a. Haratake J, Koide O, Takeshita H. Hepatic lymphagiomatosis: report of two cases with an immunohistochemical study. Am J Gastroenterol 1992; 87: 906–909
639. Goodman Z D, Ishak K G. Angiomyolipomas of the liver. Am J Surg Pathol 1984; 8: 745–750
640. Robinson J D, Grant E G, Haller J O, Cohen H L. Hepatic angiomyolipomas in tuberous sclerosis. J Ultrasound Med 1989; 8: 575–578
640a. Nonomura A, Mizukami Y, Kadoya M. Angiomyolipoma of the liver: a collective review. J Gastroenterol 1994; 29: 95–105
641. Okada K, Yokoyama S, Nakayama I, Tada I, Kobayashi M. An electron microscopic study of hepatic angiomyolipoma. Acta Pathol Jpn 1989; 39: 743–749
642. Linton P L, Ahn W S, Schwartz M E, Miller C M, Thung S N. Angiomyolipoma of the liver: immunohistochemical study of a case. Liver 1991; 11: 158–161
642a. Tsui W M S, Yuen A K T, Ma K F, Tse C C H. Hepatic angiomyolipomas with a deceptive trabecular pattern and HMB-45 reactivity. Histopathology 1992; 21: 569–573
643. Bruneton J-N, Kerboul P, Drouillard J, Menn Y, Normand F, Santini N. Hepatic lipomas: ultrasound and computed tomographic findings. Gastrointest Radiol 1987; 12: 299–303
644. Nishizaki T, Kanematsu T, Matsumata T, Yasunaga C, Kakizoe S, Sugimachi K. Myelolipoma of the liver. Cancer 1989; 63: 930–934
645. Reinertson T E, Fortune J B, Peters J C, Pagnotta I, Baliut J A. Primary leiomyoma of the liver. Dig Dis Sci 1992; 37: 622–627
645a. Fried R H, Wardzala A, Willson R A, Sinanan M N, Marchioro T L, Haggitt R. Benign cartilaginous tumour (chondroma) of the liver. Gastroenterology 1992; 103: 678–680
645b. Hytiroglou P, Linton P, Klion F, Schwartz M, Miller C, Thung S N. Benign schwannoma of the liver. Arch Pathol Lab Med 1993; 117: 216–218
646. Kottke-Marchant K, Hart W R, Broughan T. Localized fibrous tumour (localized fibrous mesothelioma) of the liver. Cancer 1989; 64: 1096–1102
647. Wallace E Z, Leonidas J-R, Stanek A E, Auramides A. Endocrine studies in a patient with functioning adrenal rest tumour of the liver. Am J Med 1981; 70: 1122–1126
648. Robinson R A, Nelson L. Hepatic teratoma in an anencephalic fetus. Arch Pathol Lab Med 1986; 110: 655–657
649. Eisen R N, Kirby W M, O'Quinn J L. Granular cell tumor of the biliary tree. Am J Surg Pathol 1991; 15: 460–465
650. Grasso S, Manusia M, Sciacca F. Unusual liver lesions in tuberous sclerosis. Arch Pathol Lab Med 1982; 106: 49
650a. Jozwiak S, Pedich M, Rajszys P, Michalowicz R. Incidence of hepatic hamartomas in tuberous sclerosis. Arch Dis Child 1992; 67: 1363–1365
650b. Cheung H, Ambrose R E, Lee P O. Liver hamartomas in tuberous sclerosis. Clin Radiol 1993; 47: 421–423
651. Ishak K G. Malignant mesenchymal tumours of the liver. In:

Okuda K, Ishak K G, eds. Neoplasms of the liver. Berlin: Springer-Verlag, 1988: pp 160–176
652. Zafrani E S. Update on vascular tumours of the liver. J Hepatol 1989; 8: 125–130
653. Baxter P J, Anthony P P, MacSween R N M, Scheuer P J. Angiosarcoma of the liver: annual occurrence and aetiology in Great Britain. Br J Ind Med 1980; 37: 213–221
654. Falk H, Herbert J, Crowley S. Epidemiology of hepatic angiosarcoma in the United States 1964–1975. Environ Health Perspect 1981; 41: 107–113
655. Da Motta C L, Da Silva Horta J, Tavares M H. Prospective epidemiological study of Thorotrast-exposed patients in Portugal. Environ Res 1979; 18: 152–173
656. Kojiro M, Nakashima T, Ito Y, Ikezaki H, Mori T, Kido C. Thorium dioxide-related angiosarcoma of the liver. Arch Pathol Lab Med 1985; 109: 853–857
657. Selinger M, Koff R S. Thorotrast and the liver: a reminder. Gastroenterology 1975; 68: 799–803
658. Okuda K, Omata M, Itoh Y, Ikezaki H, Nakashima T. Peliosis hepatis as a late and fatal complication of thorotrast liver disease. Liver 1981; 1: 110–122
659. Lee F I. Vinyl chloride-induced liver disease. J R Coll Physicians Lond 1982; 16: 226–230
660. Tamburro C H. Relationship of vinyl monomers and liver cancers: angiosarcoma and hepatocellular carcinoma. Semin Liver Dis 1984; 4: 158–169
661. Forman D, Bennett B, Stafford J, Doll R. Exposure to vinyl chloride and angiosarcoma of the liver: a report of the register of cases. Br J Ind Med 1985; 42: 750–753
662. Smulevich V B, Fedotova I V, Filatova V S. Increasing evidence of the rise of cancer in workers exposed to vinyl chloride. Br J Ind Med 1988; 45: 93–97
663. El Zayadi A, Khalil A, El Sammy N, Hamza M R, Selim O. Hepatic angiosarcoma among Egyptian farmers exposed to pesticides. Hepato-gastroenterol 1986; 33: 148–150
664. Thomas L B, Popper H, Berk P D, Selikoff I J, Falk H. Vinyl-chloride-induced liver disease. From idiopathic portal hypertension (Banti's syndrome) to angiosarcomas. N Engl J Med 1975; 292: 17–22
665. Popper H, Thomas L B, Telles N C, Falk H, Selikoff I J. Development of hepatic angiosarcoma induced by vinyl chloride, Thorotrast and arsenic: comparison with cases of unknown etiology. Am J Pathol 1978; 92: 349–376
666. Telles N C, Thomas L B, Popper H, Ishak K G, Falk H. Evolution of Thorotrast-induced hepatic angiosarcomas. Environ Res 1979; 18: 74–78
667. Popper H, Maltoni C, Selikoff I J. Vinyl chloride-induced hepatic lesions in man and rodents. A comparison. Liver 1981; 1: 7–20
668. Tamburro C H, Makk L, Popper H. Early hepatic histologic alterations among chemical (vinyl monomer) workers. Hepatology 1984; 4: 413–418
669. Anthony P P, Ramani P. Endothelial markers in malignant vascular tumours of the liver: superiority of QB-END/10 over von Willebrand factor and Ulex europaeus. J Clin Pathol 1991; 44: 29–32
670. Ishak K G, Sesterhenn I A, Goodman Z D, Rabin L, Stromeyer F W. Epithelioid hemangioendothelioma of the liver: a clinicopathologic and follow-up study of 32 cases. Hum Pathol 1984; 15: 839–852
671. Dean P J, Haggitt R C, O'Hara C J. Malignant epithelioid hemangioma of the liver in young women. Relationship to oral contraceptive use. Am J Surg Pathol 1985; 9: 695–704
672. Scoazec J-Y, Lamy P, Degott C et al. Epithelioid hemangioendothelioma of the liver. Gastroenterology 1988; 94: 1447–1453
673. Dietze O, Davies S E, Williams R, Portmann B. Malignant epithelioid haemangioendothelioma of the liver: a clinicopathological and histochemical study of 12 cases. Histopathology 1989; 15: 225–238
674. Kelleher M B, Iwatsuki S, Sheahan D G. Epithelioid

hemangioendothelioma of the liver. Am J Surg Pathol 1989; 13: 999–1008

675. Scoazec J-Y, Degott C, Reynes M, Benhamou J-P, Feldmann G. Epithelioid hemangioendothelioma of the liver: an ultrastructural study. Hum Pathol 1989; 20: 673–681

676. Stocker J T, Ishak K G. Undifferentiated (embryonal) sarcoma of the liver. Cancer 1978; 42: 336–348

677. Keating S, Taylor G P. Undifferentiated (embryonal) sarcoma of the liver. Hum Pathol 1985; 16: 693–699

678. Leuschner I, Schmidt D, Harms D. Undifferentiated sarcoma of the liver in childhood. Hum Pathol 1990; 21: 68–76

679. Lack E E, Schloo B L, Azumi N, Travis W D, Grier H E, Kozakewich H P W. Undifferentiated (embryonal) sarcoma of the liver. Am J Surg Pathol 1991; 15: 1–16

680. Aoyama C, Hachitanda Y, Sato J K, Said J W, Shimada H. Undifferentiated (embryonal) sarcoma of the liver. Am J Surg Pathol 1991; 15: 615–624

681. Parham D M, Kelly D R, Donnelly W H, Douglass E C. Immunohistochemical and ultrastructural spectrum of hepatic sarcomas in childhood: evidence for a common histogenesis. Mod Pathol 1991; 4: 648–653

682. Walker N I, Horn M J, Strong R W et al. Undifferentiated (embryonal) sarcoma of the liver. Cancer 1992; 69: 52–59

683. Horowitz M E, Etcubanas E, Webber B L et al. Hepatic undifferentiated (embryonal) sarcoma and rhabdomyosarcoma in children. Cancer 1987; 59: 396–402

684. Chen K T K. Hepatic leiomyosarcoma. J Surg Oncol 1983; 24: 325–328

685. Maki H S, Hubert B C, Sajjad S M, Kirchner J P, Kuehner M E. Primary hepatic leiomyosarcoma. Arch Surg 1987; 122: 1193–1196

686. Paraskevopoulos J A, Stephenson T J. Primary leiomyosarcoma of the liver. HPB Surgery 1991; 4: 157–163

687. Bodker A, Boiesen P T. A primary fibrosarcoma of the liver. Hepato-gastroenterol 1981; 28: 218–220

688. Nakahama M, Takanashi R, Yamazaki I, Machinami R. Primary fibrosarcoma of the liver. Acta Pathol Jpn 1989; 39: 814–820

689. Ito Y, Uesaka Y, Takeshita S et al. A case report of primary fibrosarcoma of the liver. Gastroenterol Jpn 1990; 25: 753–757

690. Arends J W, Willebrand D, Blaauw A M M, Bosman F T. Primary malignant fibrous histiocytoma of the liver. Histopathology 1987; 11: 427–432

691. Katsuda S, Kawahara E, Matsui Y, Ohyama S, Nakanishi I. Malignant fibrous histiocytoma of the liver. Amer J Gastroenterol 1988; 83: 1278–1282

692. McGrady B J, Mirakhur M M. Recurrent malignant fibrous histiocytoma of the liver. Histopathology 1992; 21: 290–292

693. Kim Y I, Yu E S, Lee K W, Park E U, Song H G. Dedifferentiated liposarcoma of the liver. Cancer 1987; 60: 2785–2790

694. Hochstetter A R, Hattenschwiler J, Vogt M. Primary osteosarcoma of the liver. Cancer 1987; 60: 2312–2317

695. Horie Y, Hori T, Hiroyama C, Hashimoto K, Yumoto T, Tanikawa K. Osteoclast-like giant cell tumour of the liver. Acta Pathol Jpn 1987; 37: 1327–1335

696. Sano T, Terada T, Hayashi F et al. Malignant hemangiopericytoma of the liver: report of a case. Jpn J Surg 1991; 21: 462–465

697. Kishimoto Y, Hijiya S, Nagasako R. Malignant mixed tumour of the liver in adults. Am J Gastroenterol 1984; 79: 229–235

698. Kawarada Y, Uehara S, Noda M, Yatani R, Mizumoto R. Nonhepatocytic malignant mixed tumor primary in the liver. Cancer 1985; 55: 1790–1798

699. Nakabayashi H, Aiba H, Sakuma S et al. An autopsy case of primary malignant mesenchymoma of the liver with various tissue components. Acta Hepatol Jpn 1985; 26: 369–375

700. Jaffe E S. Malignant lymphomas: pathology of hepatic involvement. Semin Liv Dis 1987; 7: 257–268

701. Osborne B M, Butler J J, Guarda L A. Primary lymphoma of the liver. Cancer 1985; 56: 2902–2910

702. Ryan J, Straus D J, Lange C et al. Primary lymphoma of the liver. Cancer 1988; 61: 370–375

703. Anthony P P, Sarsfield P, Clarke T. Primary lymphoma of the liver: clinical and pathological features of 10 patients. J Clin Pathol 1990; 43: 1007–1013

704. Scoazec J-Y, Degott C, Brousse N et al. Non-Hodgkin's lymphoma presenting as primary tumour of the liver: presentation, diagnosis and outcome in eight patients. Hepatology 1991; 13: 870–875

704a. Ohsawa M, Aozasa K, Horiuchi K et al. Malignant lymphoma of the liver. Dig Dis Sci 1992; 37: 1105–1109

704b. Zafrani E S, Gaulard P. Primary lymphoma of the liver. Liver 1993; 13: 57–61

705. Heaton G E, Matthews T H, Christopherson W M. Malignant trophoblastic tumours with massive hemorrhage presenting as liver primary. Am J Surg Pathol 1986; 10: 342–347

706. Alonso J F, Sáez C, Pérez P, Montano A, Japón M A. Primary pure choriocarcinoma of the liver. Path Res Pract 1992; 188: 375–377

707. Narita T, Moriyama Y, Ito Y. Endodermal sinus (yolk sac) tumour of the liver. J Pathol 1988; 155: 41–48

708. Villaschi S, Balisteri P. Endodermal sinus tumour of the liver. Histopathology 1991; 18: 86–88

709. Wakeley P E, Krummel T M, Johnson D E. Yolk sac tumor of the liver. Mod Pathol 1991; 4: 121–125

709a. Whelan J S, Stebbings W, Owen R A, Calne R, Clark P I. Successful treatment of a primary endodermal sinus tumor of the liver. Cancer 1992; 70: 2260–2262

710. Parham D M, Peiper S C, Robicheaux G, Ribeiro R C, Douglass E C. Malignant rhabdoid tumor of the liver. Arch Pathol Lab Med 1988; 112: 61–64

711. Hunt S J, Anderson W D. Malignant rhabdoid tumor of the liver. Am J Clin Pathol 1990; 94: 645–648

712. Foschini M P, Van Eyken P, Brock P R et al. Malignant rhabdoid tumour of the liver. Histopathology 1992; 20: 157–165

713. Deugnier Y, Turlin B, Lehry D et al. Malignant melanoma of the hepatic and common bile ducts. Arch Pathol Lab Med 1991; 115: 915–917

714. Contreras P, Altieri E, Liberman C et al. Adrenal rest tumour of the liver causing Cushing's syndrome. J Clin Endocrinol Metab 1985; 60: 21–28

715. Wolf H K, Burchette J L, Garcia J A, Michalopoulos G. Exocrine pancreatic tissue in human liver: a metaplastic process? Am J Surg Pathol 1990; 14: 590–595

716. Borja E R, Hori J M, Pugh R P. Metastatic carcinomatosis of the liver mimicking cirrhosis. Cancer 1975; 35: 445–449

717. Engel J J, Trujillo Y, Spellberg M. Metastatic carcinoma of the breast: a cause of obstructive jaundice. Gastroenterology 1980; 78: 132–135

718. Gerber M A, Thung S N, Bodenheimer H C, Kapelman B, Schaffner F. Characteristic histologic triad in liver adjacent to metastatic neoplasm. Liver 1986; 6: 85–88

719. Terada T, Nakanuma Y, Kono N, Ueda K, Kadoya M, Matsui O. Ciliated hepatic foregut cyst. Am J Surg Pathol 1990; 14: 356–363

720. Stocker J T, Ishak K G. Focal nodular hyperplasia of the liver: a study of 21 pediatric cases. Cancer 1981; 48: 336–345

721. Brady M S, Coit D G. Focal nodular hyperplasia of the liver. Surg Gynec Obst 1990; 171: 377–381

722. Pain J A, Gimson A E S, Williams R, Howard E R. Focal nodular hyperplasia of the liver: results of treatment and options in management. Gut 1991; 32: 524–527

722a. Okudaira S. Clinicopathologic study on 23 resected cases of focal nodular hyperplasia. Acta Hepatol Jpn 1993; 34: 621–629

723. Butron Vila M M, Haot J, Desmet V J. Cholestatic features in focal nodular hyperplasia of the liver. Liver 1984; 4: 387–395

724. van Eyken P, Sciot R, Callea F, Desmet V J. A cytokeratin-immunohistochemical study of focal nodular hyperplasia of the liver. Liver 1989; 9: 372–377

725. Wanless I R, Mawdsley C, Adams R. On the pathogenesis of

focal nodular hyperplasia of the liver. Hepatology 1985; 5: 1194–1200

726. Ndimbie O K, Goodman Z D, Chase R L, Ma C K, Lee M W. Hemangiomas with localized nodular proliferation of the liver. A suggestion on the pathogenesis of focal nodular hyperplasia. Am J Surg Pathol 1990; 14: 142–150

727. Goldin R D, Rose D S C. Focal nodular hyperplasia of the liver associated with intracranial vascular malformations. Gut 1990; 31: 554–555

728. Stromeyer F W, Ishak K G. Nodular transformation (nodular 'regenerative' hyperplasia) of the liver. Hum Pathol 1981; 12: 60–71

729. Mones J M, Saldana M J, Albores-Saavedra J. Nodular regenerative hyperplasia of the liver. Arch Pathol Lab Med 1984; 108: 741–743

730. Dachman A H, Ros P R, Goodman Z D, Olmsted W W, Ishak K G. Nodular regenerative hyperplasia of the liver: clinical and radiologic observations. AJR 1987; 148: 717–722

731. Colina F, Alberti N, Solis J A, Martinez-Tello F J. Diffuse nodular regenerative hyperplasia of the liver (DNRH). Liver 1989; 9: 253–265

732. Wanless I R. Micronodular transformation (nodular regenerative hyperplasia) of the liver: a report of 64 cases among 2500 autopsies and a new classification of benign hepatic nodules. Hepatology 1990; 11: 787–797

733. Moran C A, Mullick F G, Ishak K G. Nodular regenerative hyperplasia of the liver in children. Am J Surg Pathol 1991; 15: 449–454

734. Naber A H J, Van Haelst U, Yap S H. Nodular regenerative hyperplasia of the liver: an important cause of portal hypertension in non-cirrhotic patients. J Hepatol 1991; 12: 94–99

735. Wanless I R, Lentz J S, Roberts E A. Partial nodular transformation of the liver in an adult with persistent ductus venosus. Arch Pathol Lab Med 1985; 109: 427–432

736. Desmet V J. Cholangiopathies: past present and future. Semin Liv Dis 1987; 7: 67–76

737. Stocker J T, Ishak K G. Mesenchymal hamartoma of the liver. Pediatr Pathol 1983; 1: 245–267

738. De Maioribus C A, Lally K P, Sim K, Isaacs H, Mahour H. Mesenchymal hamartoma of the liver. Arch Surg 1990; 125: 598–600

739. Gramlich T L, Killough B W, Garvin A J. Mesenchymal hamartoma of the liver: report of a case in a 28-year-old. Hum Pathol 1988; 19: 991–992

740. Summerfield J, Nagafuchi Y, Sherlock S, Codafalch J, Scheuer P J. Hepatobiliary fibropolycystic diseases. J Hepatol 1986; 2: 141–156

741. Anthony P P, Telesinghe P U. Inflammatory pseudotumour of the liver. J Clin Pathol 1986; 39: 761–768

742. Horiuchi R, Uchida T, Kojima T, Shikata T. Inflammatory pseudotumour of the liver. Cancer 1990, 65: 1583–1590

742a. Shek T W H, Ng I O L, Chan K W. Inflammatory pseudotumor of the liver. Am J Surg Pathol 1993; 17: 231–238

742b. Anthony P P. Inflammatory pseudotumour (plasma cell granuloma) of lung, liver and other organs. Histopathology 1993; 23: 501–503

743. Malatjalian D A, Morris J, Bodurtha A. *Klebsiella pneumoniae* from an hepatic inflammatory pseudotumour. Can J Gastroenterol 1992; 6: 84–86

744. Shepherd N A, Lee G. Solitary necrotic nodules of the liver simulating hepatic metastases. J Clin Pathol 1983; 36: 1181–1183

745. Berry C L. Solitary 'necrotic nodule' of the liver: a probable pathogenesis. J Clin Pathol 1985; 38: 1278–1280

746. Matters arising. J Clin Pathol 1990; 43: 348–349

747. Sunderesan M, Lyons B, Akosa A B. 'Solitary' necrotic nodules of the liver: an aetiology re-affirmed. Gut 1991; 32: 1378–1380

747a. Tsui W M S, Yuen R W S, Chow L T C, Tse C C H. Solitary necrotic nodule of the liver: parasitic origin. J Clin Pathol 1992; 45: 975–978

748. Pounder D J. Hepatic pseudolipoma. Pathology 1983; 15: 83–84

749. Karhunen P J. Hepatic pseudolipoma. J Clin Pathol 1985; 38: 877–879

750. Wheeler D A, Edmondson H A, Coelomic fat ectopia in the liver. Arch Pathol Lab Med 1985; 109: 783–785

751. Brawer M K, Austin G E, Lewin K J. Focal fatty change of the liver, a hitherto poorly recognized entity. Gastroenterology 1980; 78: 247–252

752. Hadjis N S, Hemingway A, Carr D, Blumgart L H. Liver lobe disparity consequent upon atrophy. J Hepatol 1986; 3: 285–293

753. Finkel L, Marchevsky A, Cohen B. Endometrial cyst of the liver. Amer J Gastroenterol 1986; 81: 576–578

754. De Almeida Barbosa A, Rodriques de Freitas L A, Mota M A. Primary pregnancy in the liver. Path Res Pract 1991; 187: 329–331

755. Cook D J, Salena B J, Vincic L M. Adenomyoma of the common bile duct. Am J Gastroenterol 1988; 83: 432–434

756. Jones T C, Mohr U, Hunt R D, eds. Monographs on pathology or laboratory animals: Digestive system. Berlin: Springer 1985

757. Roberfroid M B, Preat V, eds. Experimental hepatocarcinogenesis. New York; Plenum, 1988

758. Bannasch P, Zerban H, Tumours of the liver. In: Turusov V S, Mohr U, eds. Pathobiology of tumours in laboratory animals, 2nd edn. Lyon: International Agency for Research on Cancer, 1990: pp 199–240

759. Mason W S, Seeger C, eds. Hepadnaviruses. Curr Top Microbiol Immunol. Berlin: Springer, 1991

760. Okuda K, Ishak K G, eds. Neoplasms of the liver. Berlin: Springer, 1987

761. Bannasch P, Keppler D, Weber G, eds. Liver cell carcinoma. Falk Symposium 51. Dordrecht: Kluwer, 1989

762. Farber E, Sarma D S R. Hepatocarcinogenesis: a dynamic cellular perspective. Lab Invest 1987; 56: 4–22

763. Pitot H C. Hepatic neoplasia: Chemical induction. In: Arias J M, Jakoby W B, Popper H, Schachter D, Shafritz D A, eds. The liver, 2nd edn. Biology and pathobiology. New York; Raven, 1988

764. Bannasch P. Pathobiology of chemical hepatocarcinogenesis: Recent progress and perspectives. Part I. Cytomorphological changes and cell proliferation. Part II. Metabolic and molecular changes. J Gastroent Hepatol 1990; 5: 149–159, 310–320

765. Summers J, Smolec J, Snyder R L. A virus similar to human hepatitis B virus associated with hepatitis and hepatoma in woodchuck. Proc Natl Acad Sci USA 1978; 75: 4533–4537

766. Mason W S, Taylor J M. Experimental systems for the study of hepadnavirus and hepatitis delta virus infections. Hepatology 1989; 9: 635–645

767. Messing A, Chen H Y, Palmiter R D, Brinster R L. Peripheral neuropathies, hepatocellular carcinomas and islet cell adenomas in transgenic mice. Nature 1985; 316: 461–463

768. Chisari F V, Klopchin K, Moriyama T et al Molecular pathogenesis of hepatocellular carcinoma in hepatitis B virus transgenic mice. Cell 1989; 59: 1145–1156

769. Kim C M, Koike K, Saito I, Miyamura T, Jay G. HBx gene of hepatitis B virus induces liver cancer in transgenic mice. Nature 1991; 351: 317–320

770. Bishop J M. Cellular oncogenes and retroviruses. Annu Rev Biochem 1983; 52: 301–315

771. Bishop J M. Molecular themes in oncogenesis. Cell 1991; 64: 235–248

772. Sirica A E, ed. The pathology of neoplasia. New York: Plenum, 1989

773. Stanbridge E J. Human tumor suppressor genes. Ann Rev Genet 1990; 24: 615–657

774. Hunter T. Cooperation between oncogenes. Cell 1991; 64: 249–270

775. Vainio H. Magee P N, McGregor D B, McMichael A J, eds. Mechanisms of carcinogenesis in risk identification. Lyon: International Agency for Research on Cancer, 1992

776. IARC Monograph. Evaluation of the carcinogenic risk of chemicals to humans. Suppl 7 Chemicals, occupational exposures and cultural habits associated with cancer in humans,

vols 1–42. Lyon: International Agency for Research on Cancer, 1987

777. IARC Monograph. Evaluation of the carcinogenic risk of chemicals to humans. Some naturally occurring carcinogens. Lyon: International Agency for Research on Cancer, 1993

778. Popper H, Maltoni C, Selikoff I J, Squire R A, Thomas L B. Comparison of neoplastic hepatic lesions in man and experimental animals. In: Hiatt H H, Watson J D, Winston J A, eds. Origins of human cancer. Book C, Human risk assessment. (Cold Spring Harbor Conference on Cell Proliferation vol 4). Cold Spring Harbor: Cold Spring Harbor Laboratory, 1977: pp 1359–1382

779. Remmer H, Bolt H M, Bannasch P, Popper H, eds. Primary liver tumours. Falk Symposium 24. Lancaster: MTP, 1978

780. Reddy J K, Lalwani N D. Carcinogenesis by hepatic peroxisome proliferators: Evaluation of the risk of hypolipidemic drugs and industrial plasticizers to humans. C R C Crit Rev Toxicol 1983; 12: 1–58

781. Bannasch P, Zerbon H. Predictive value of hepatic preneoplastic lesions as indicators of carcinogenic response. In: Vainio H, Magee P N, McGregor D B, McMichael A J, eds. Mechanisms of carcinogenesis in risk identification. Lyon: International Agency for Research on Cancer, 1992: pp 389–427

782. Rabes H M, Development and growth of early preneoplastic lesions induced in liver by chemical carcinogens. J Cancer Res Clin Oncol 1983; 106: 85–92

783. Rabes H M. Cell proliferation and hepatocarcinogenesis. In: Roberfroid M B, Preat V, eds. Experimental hepatocarcinogenesis. New York: Plenum 1988: pp 121–132

784. Bartsch H, Preat V, Aitio A, Cabral J R P, Roberfroid M B. Partial hepatectomy of rats ten weeks before carcinogen administration can enhance liver carcinogenesis: preliminary observations. Carcinogenesis 1988; 9: 2315–2317

785. Kohn H I, Frey R J M. Radiation carcinogenesis . N Engl J Med 1984; 310: 504–511

786. Schreiber W H, Kato H, Robertson J D. Primary carcinoma of the liver in Hiroshima and Nagasaki. Japan Cancer 1970; 26: 69–75

787. Upton A C, Kimball A W, Furth J, Christenberry K W, Benedict W A. Some delayed effects of atom-bomb radiations in mice. Cancer Res 1960; 20: 1–60

788. Wegener K, Wesch H, Kuttler K, Spiethoff A. Thorotrastosis in humans and animals: pathoanatomical results of the German thorotrast study. In: Taylor D M, Mays C W, Gerger G B, Thomas R G, eds. Risks from radium and thorotrast. BIR Report 1989; 21: 104–107

789. Van Kaick G, Wesch H, Luhrs H et al. The German Thorotrast Study–report on 20 years follow-up. In: Taylor D M, Mays C W, Gerber G B, Thomas R G, eds. Risks from radium and thorotrast. BIR Report 1989; 21: 98–103

790. Spiethoff A, Wesch H, Hover K-H, Wegener K. The combined and separate action of neutron radiation and zirconium dioxide on the liver of rats. Health Phys 1992; 63: 111–118

791. Moore T A, Ferrante W A, Crowson T D. Hepatoma occurring two decades after hepatic irradiation. Gastroenterology 1976; 71: 128–132

792. Lewin K, Mills R R. Human radiation hepatitis. Arch Pathol 1973; 96: 21–26

793. Fajardo L F, Colby T V. Pathogenesis of veno-occlusive liver disease after radiation. Arch Pathol Lab Med 1980; 104: 584–588

794. Dettmer C M, Kramer S, Driscoll D H, Aponte G E. A comparison of chronic effects of irradiation upon the normal, damaged and regenerating rat liver. Radiology 1968; 91: 993–997

795. Popper H, Roth L, Purcell R H, Tennant B C, Gerin J L. Hepatocarcinogenicity of the woodchuck hepatitis virus. Proc Natl Acad Sci USA 1987; 83: 2994–2997

796. Rogler C E, Cellular and molecular mechanisms of hepatocarcinogenesis associated with hepadnavirus infection. Curr Top Microbiol Immunol 1991; 168: 103–140

797. DeFlora S, Hietanen E, Bartsch H et al. Enhanced metabolic activation of chemical hepatocarcinogens in woodchucks

infected with hepatitis B virus. Carcinogenesis 1989; 10: 1099–1106

798. Beland F A, Poirier M C. DNA adducts and carcinogenesis. In: Sirica A E, ed. The pathobiology of neoplasia. New York: Plenum, 1989: pp 57–80

799. Swenberg J A, The role of DNA damage, repair and replication in hepatocarcinogenesis. In: Bannasch P, Keppler D, Weber G, eds. Liver cell carcinoma. Falk Symposium 51. Dordrecht: Kluwer, 1989: pp 261–269

800. Jones P A. DNA methylation and cancer. Cancer Res 1986; 46: 461–466

801. Mikol Y B, Hoover K L, Craesia D, Poirier L A. Hepatocarcinogenesis in rats fed methyl-deficient, amino-acid defined diets. Carcinogenesis 1983; 4: 1619–1629

802. Goshal A K, Farber E. The induction of liver cancer by dietary deficiency of choline methionine without added carcinogens. Carcinogenesis 1984; 5: 1367–1370

803. Hernandez L, Allen P T, Poirier L A, Lijinski W. S-Adenosylmethionine, S-adenosyl-homocysteine and DNA methylation in the liver of rats fed methapyriline and analogs. Carcinogenesis 1989; 10: 557–562

804. Locker J, Reddy T V, Lombardi B. DNA methylation and hepatocarcinogenesis in rats fed a choline-devoid diet Carcinogenesis 1986; 7: 1309–1312

805. Yager J D, Zurlo J. Oncogene activation and expression during carcinogenesis in liver and pancreas. In: Sirica A E, ed. Pathobiology of neoplasia. New York; Plenum, 1989: pp 399–417

806. Buchmann A, Bauer-Hofmann R, Mahr J et al. Mutational activation of the c-Ha-ras gene in liver tumours of different rodent strains: correlation with susceptibility to hepatocarcinogenesis. Proc Natl Acad Sci USA 1991; 88: 911–915

807. Dragani T A, Manenti G, Colombo B M et al. Incidence of H-ras gene mutations in liver tumours of mice genetically susceptible and resistant to hepatocarcinogenesis. Oncogene 1991; 6: 333–338

808. Stanley L A, Devereux T R, Foley J et al. Proto-oncogene activation in liver tumours of hepatocarcinogenesis-resistant strains. Carcinogenesis 1992; 13: 2427–2433

809. McMahon G, Davis E F, Huber L J, Kim Y, Wogan G N. Characterization of c-Ki-ras and N-ras oncogenes in aflatoxin B_1-induced rat liver tumors. Proc Natl Acad Sci USA 1990; 87: 1104–1108

810. Strom S C, Faust J B. Oncogene activation and hepatocarcinogenesis. Pathobiology 1990; 58: 153–167

811. Bauer-Hofmann R, Klimek F, Buchmann A et al. Role of mutations at codon 61 of the c-Ha-ras gene during diethylnitrosamine-induced hepatocarcinogenesis in C3H/He mice. Molecular Carcinogenesis 1992; 6: 60–67

812. Pasquinelli C, Bhavani K, Chisari F V. Multiple oncogenes and tumor suppressor genes are structurally and functionally intact during hepatocarcinogenesis in hepatitis B virus transgenic mice. Cancer Res 1992; 52: 2823–2829

813. Farber E, Chen Z Y, Harris L et al. The biochemical–molecular pathology of the stepwise development of liver cancer: new insights and problems. In: Bannasch P, Keppler D, Weber G, eds. Liver cell cancer. Falk Symposium 51. Dordrecht: Kluwer, 1989

814. Fourel G, Trepo C. Bougueleret L et al. Frequent activation of N-myc genes by hepadnavirus insertion in woodchuck liver tumors. Nature 1990; 347: 294–298

815. Moroy T, Marchio A, Etiemble J et al. Rearrangement and enhanced expression of c-myc in hepatocellular carcinoma of hepatitis virus infected woodchucks. Nature 1986; 324: 276–279

816. Hsu T Y, Moroy T, Etiemble J et al. Activation of c-myc by woodchuck hepatitis infection in hepatocellular carcinoma. Cell 1988; 55: 627–635

817. Bressac B, Kew M, Wands J, Ozturk M. Selective G to T mutations of *p53* gene in hepatocellular carcinoma from southern Africa. Nature 1991; 350: 429–431

818. Hsu I C, Metcalf R A, Sun T et al. Mutational hotspot in the *p53*

gene in human hepatocellular carcinomas. Nature 1991; 350: 427–428

819. Ozturk M et al. *p53* mutation in hepatocellular carcinoma after aflatoxin exposure. Lancet 1991; 338: 1356–1359

820. Kress S, Jahn U R, Buchmann A, Bannasch P, Schwartz M. *p53* mutations in human hepatocellular carcinomas in Germany. Cancer Res 1992; 52: 3220–3223

821. Laurent-Puig P, Flegou J-F, Fabre M et al. Overexpression of *p53*: a rare event in a large series of white patients with hepatocellular carcinoma. Hepatology 1992; 16: 1171–1175

822. Cory S, Adams J M. Transgenic mice and oncogenesis. Am Rev Immunol 1988; 6: 25–48

823. Pattengale P K, Stewart T A, Leder A et al. Animal models of human disease. Pathology and molecular biology of spontaneous neoplasms occurring in transgenic mice carrying and expressing activated cellular oncogenes. Am J Pathol 1989; 135: 39–61

824. Sandgren E P, Quaife C J, Pinkert C A, Palmiter R D, Brinster R L. Oncogene-induced liver neoplasia in transgenic mice. Oncogene 1989; 4: 715–724

825. Foulds L. Neoplastic development, vol 2. New York: Academic Press, 1975

826. Fearon E R, Vogelstein B. A genetic model for colorectal tumorigenesis. Cell 1990; 61: 759–767

827. Farber F, Rubin H. Cellular adaptation in the origin and development of cancer. Cancer Res 1991; 51: 2751–2761

828. Bannasch P, Mayer D, Hacker H J. Hepatocellular glycogenosis and hepatocarcinogenesis. Biochim Biophys Acta 1980; 605: 217–245

829. Ito N, Shirai T, Hasegawa R. Medium-term bioassays for carcinogens. In: Vainio H, Magee P N, McGregor D B, McMichael A J, eds. Mechanisms of carcinogenesis in risk identification. Lyon: International Agency for Research on Cancer. 1992; 353–388

830. Bannasch P, Zerban H. Pathogenesis of primary liver tumors induced by chemicals. Recent Results Cancer Res 1986; 100: 1–15

831. Pitot H C. Altered hepatic foci: their role in murine hepatocarcinogenesis. Annu Rev Pharmacol Toxicol 1990; 30: 465–500

832. Sell S. Is there a liver stem cell? Cancer Res 1990; 50: 3811–3815

833. Aterman K. The stem cells of the liver — a selective review. J Cancer Res Clin Oncol 1992; 118: 87–115

834. Sirica A E, ed. The role of cell types in hepatocarcinogenesis. Boca Raton: CRC, 1992

835. Anthony P P. Precursor lesions for liver cancer in humans. Cancer Res 1976; 36: 2579–2582

836. Steinberg P, Hacker H J, Dienes H P, Oesch F, Bannasch P. Enzyme histochemical and immunohistochemical characterization of oval and parenchymal cells proliferating in livers of rats fed a choline deficient/DL-ethionine-supplemented diet. Carcinogenesis 1991; 12: 225–231

837. Farber E. On cells of origin of liver cell cancer. In: Sirica A E, ed. The role of cell types in hepatocarcinogenesis. Boca Raton: CRC, 1992: pp 1–28

838. Hacker H J, Steinberg P, Toshkov I, Oesch F, Bannasch P. Persistence of the cholangiocellular and hepatocellular lesions observed in rats fed a choline-deficient/DL-ethionine-supplemented diet. Carcinogenesis 1992; 13: 271–276

839. Symposium. Significance of foci of cellular alterations in the rat liver. Toxicol Pathol 1989; 17: 557–735

840. Emmelot P, Scherer E. The first relevant cell stage in rat liver carcinogenesis: a quantitative approach. Biochim Biophys Acta 1980; 605: 247–304

841. Pitot H C, Sirica A E. The stages of initiation and promotion in hepatocarcinogenesis. Biochim Biophys Acta 1980; 605: 191–215

842. Williams G. The pathogenesis of rat liver cancer caused by chemical carcinogens. Biochim Biophys Acta 1980; 605: 167–189

843. Schulte-Hermann R Tumor promotion in the liver. Arch Toxicol 1985; 57: 147–158

844. Moore M A, Kitagawa T. Hepatocarcinogenesis in the rat: the effect of the promoters and carcinogens in vivo and in vitro. Int Rev Cytol 1986; 101: 125–173

845. Sato K. Glutathione *S*-transferases and hepatocarcinogenesis. Jpn J Cancer Res (Gann) 1988; 79: 556–572

846. Schwarz M, Buchmann A, Schulte M et al. Heterogeneity of enzyme-altered foci in rat liver. Toxicol Lett 1989; 49: 297–317

847. Mayer D, Klimek F, Hacker H J. Carbohydrate metabolism in hepatic preneoplasia. In: Bannasch P, Keppler D, Weber G, eds. Liver cell carcinoma. Falk Symposium 51. Dordrecht: Kluwer, 1989: pp 329–345

848. Schirmacher P I, Held W A, Chisari F V et al. Reactivation of insulin-like growth factor II during hepatocarcinogenesis in transgenic mice suggests role in malignant growth. Cancer Res 1992; 52: 2549–2556

849. Cariani E, Laserre C, Seurin D et al. Differential expression of insulin-like growth factor II mRNA in human primary liver cancers, benign liver tumors and liver cirrhosis. Cancer Res 1988; 48: 6844–6849

850. Lenzi R, Liu M H, Tarsetti F et al. Histogenesis of bile duct-like cells proliferating during ethionine hepatocarcinogenesis. Evidence for a biliary nature of oval cells. Lab Invest 1992; 66: 390–402

851. Chou S T, Gibson J B. The histochemistry of biliary mucins and the changes caused by Clonorchis sinensis. J Pathol 1970: 101: 185–197

852. Couch J A. Spongiosis hepatis: chemical induction, pathogenesis, and possible neoplastic fate in a teleost fish model. Toxicol Pathol 1991; 19: 237–250

853. Wake K. Perisinusoidal stellate cells (fat-storing cell, interstitial cells, lipocytes), their related structure in and around the liver sinusoids, and vitamin A-storing cells in extrahepatic organs. Int Rev Cytol 1980; 66: 303–353

854. Michalopoulos G. Liver regeneration and growth factors: old puzzles and new perspectives. Lab Invest 1992; 67: 413–415

17

Liver pathology associated with diseases of other organs

R. N. M. MacSween   A. D. Burt

The preceding chapters have dealt chiefly with the diversity of diseases in which the hepatic involvement has been primary. A group remains in which the primary disease or disease process is predominantly extrahepatic, but in which hepatic dysfunction may develop and sometimes be of clinical and morphological significance. These will be dealt with in turn on a systemic basis, but three morphological entities which represent a response to a variety of causes will be described first. These are:

a. non-specific reactive hepatitis, an ill-defined morphological entity which reflects the general and non-specific response of the liver to a wide variety of systemic processes;

b. hepatic granulomatous conditions, which may arise as part of a generalized granulomatous disease, may be a component of certain primary liver diseases or may also represent a non-specific response to extrahepatic disease; and

c. fatty liver, which may develop in a wide diversity of disorders and which, depending on the aetiology or the presence of associated inflammatory change, may result in both acute and chronic hepatic dysfunction.

NON-SPECIFIC REACTIVE HEPATITIS

This description was first applied by Popper & Schaffner.[1] They succinctly defined a morphological entity which may be widespread within the liver, representing either the residuum of previous inflammatory intrahepatic disease or a response to a variety of extrahepatic disease processes, especially febrile illnesses and inflammation somewhere in the splanchnic bed. The changes may also be localized within the liver, representing a response to a variety of focal liver injuries such as vascular lesions or space-occupying lesions.

There are no specific clinical manifestations and although there may be mild increases in serum transaminase levels there is no specific disturbance of liver function tests. Such symptoms or abnormalities of function as may be present can usually be attributed to the underlying or associated disease.

The morphological features which characterize non-specific reactive hepatitis are outlined below. They may exist in various combinations, and may show varying degrees of severity; the essential feature in making the diagnosis is that, even when the changes are widespread, they still tend to be 'focal'. Thus, only some portal tracts are involved, and the parenchymal changes do not demonstrate a uniform zonal distribution.

Portal tract changes. The medium-sized and smaller portal tracts are affected and there may also be focal periportal inflammation. They contain a variable chronic inflammatory cell infiltrate but an entirely normal portal tract may be seen in the same microscopic field, thus emphasizing the focal nature of these reactive changes. (Fig. 17.1a, b). Lymphocytes usually predominate but ceroid-containing macrophages may also be present and, rarely, a few plasma cells and eosinophils. Neutrophil polymorphs are hardly ever seen. The cellular infiltrate

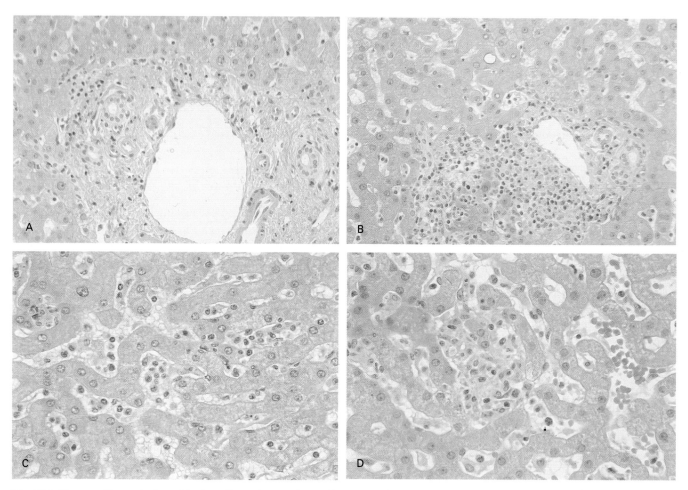

Fig. 17.1 Non-specific reactive hepatitis: these illustrations are from a biopsy taken from a patient with a carcinoma in the ileo-caecal region. (a) Portal tract showing a very light chronic inflammatory cell infiltrate; (b) portal tract showing a mixed lymphocyte and macrophage infiltrate with some periportal spillover; (c) sinusoidal infiltrate of inflammatory cells with reactive Kupffer-cell hyperplasia; (d) granulomatoid aggregate of lymphocytes and macrophages. H & E.

within the portal tract is diffuse. The limiting plate is intact, but where the infiltrate is more intense some irregular spillover into the periportal parenchyma may occur without any liver-cell necrosis. In a few instances, especially in older age groups, well-formed lymphoid follicles may be present.

Parenchymal changes. These comprise foci of liver-cell necrosis and Kupffer-cell prominence. The foci of necrosis may be very small, involving only a few hepatocytes, or may be larger involving several liver-cell plates and producing focal reticulin collapse or condensation. In relation to these foci of liver-cell necrosis, lymphocytes and macrophages accumulate (Fig. 17.1c), and are best demonstrated on a PAS/diastase preparation. The larger foci comprising small macrophage aggregates may be regarded as microgranulomas, although the term granulomatoid reaction is a more accurate description in that epithelioid cells are only poorly developed and giant cells are not seen (Fig. 17.1d). Kupffer-cell hyperplasia occurs near foci of liver-cell necrosis, and in addition generalized Kupffer-cell prominence may be evident, particularly in the perivenular zones. Increased lipofuscin and ceroid pigment deposits are present; there may be irregular focal steatosis and some variation in hepatocyte and nuclear size.

The major differential diagnoses are chronic hepatitis C (HCV) infection and residual viral hepatitis (see Ch. 6). In chronic HCV infection lymphoid follicles, focal hepatocyte necrosis and reactive Kupffer-cell hyperplasia are also seen. In addition, low grade periportal piecemeal necrosis is present and acidophil bodies are evident. In non-specific reactive hepatitis macrophages predominate around intra-acinar foci of liver-cell necrosis. However, in some instances it is not possible to distinguish between the two on the histological features and circulating HCV antibodies should be sought. In residual viral hepatitis there is usually more generalized portal tract involvement, slight portal tract fibrosis with some septum formation may be present, parenchymal changes are predominantly perivenular, some single-cell acidophilic necrosis may be found, and a Prussian blue (Perls') reaction will often show some mild Kupffer-cell siderosis.

SPACE-OCCUPYING LESIONS IN THE LIVER

Tumour deposits and other focal lesions may produce both obstructive and pressure effects and liver biopsies undertaken in the investigation of these may show fairly distinctive features. Non-specific reactive changes are usually present. The portal tracts show some oedema; there is irregularity, sometimes focal, of the limiting plates with a cholangiolitis, comprising prominence of the marginal bile ducts and an infiltrate of neutrophil polymorphs (Fig. 17.2a, b); periductal neutrophils are sometimes conspicuous particularly around the smallest terminal bile ducts and around isolated ducts within the acini

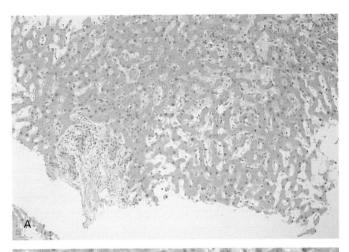

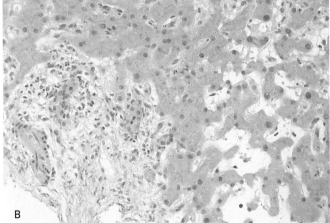

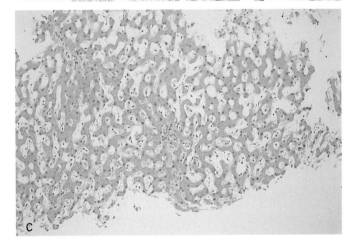

Fig. 17.2 Liver biopsy from a patient suspected of having metastatic tumour. (a) There is some sinusoidal dilatation and the portal tract shows oedema and inflammation which in (b) is associated with an acute cholangiolitis. (c) There is more marked sinusoidal dilatation evident in this area of the biopsy. H & E.

(Fig. 17.2c). The portal tract changes may develop due to local interference with bile flow.[2] In addition, however, sinusoidal dilatation and congestion may occur due to pressure on hepatic venules. The hepatic veins are normal and hepatocytes within zones of dilatation rarely show atrophy. The sinusoidal dilatation is most striking in acinar zone 3 but in some instances the changes are more extensive (Fig. 17.2c).

HEPATIC GRANULOMAS

Granulomas may occur in the liver in a wide variety of disorders, some of which are primary diseases of the liver, but most are part of a generalized disease process. The use of the term *epithelioid cell granuloma* serves to distinguish them from *lipogranulomas*, which are seen in fatty livers, in particular in alcoholic liver disease.[3] The latter comprise loose aggregates of lymphocytes and macrophages, sometimes with a few poorly developed epithelioid cells and rarely one or two multinucleate giant cells (Fig. 17.3a). They occur against a background of hepatic steatosis and lipid material is usually demonstrable around the lesions and within the constituent macrophages.

A number of reports have drawn attention to lipogranulomas which may occur in non-fatty liver and which tend to be more common in portal tracts than in the parenchyma.[4–7] In the parenchyma they are frequently perivenular in distribution and appear as a cluster of variably sized lipid droplets surrounded by a light infiltrate of lymphocytes and macrophages; there is some local increase in fibrous tissue (Fig. 17.3b). Spleen and lymph nodes may also be involved. They appear to be the result of mineral oil deposition and such oils are now widely used in the food industry.[6,7] These lesions are generally of little consequence and are most often seen as incidental findings on liver biopsies or at autopsy. However, Keen et al[8] described two cases in which extensive mineral oil lipogranulomatosis led to venous outflow obstruction.

Bernstein et al[9] drew attention to a peculiar appearance of the hepatic granulomas in Q fever; these show a distinctive ring pattern (Fig. 17.3c) in which fibrin is deposited circumferentially within or at the margin of the granulomas; a central fat vacuole may be present. The association between these so-called fibrin-ring or doughnut granulomas and Q fever has been confirmed.[10,11] It is now apparent, however, that they are not pathognomonic for this disease.[12] Their occurrence in a variety of conditions including Boutonneuse fever,[13] allopurinol hypersensitivity,[14] CMV infection,[15] leishmaniasis,[16] hepatitis A,[17] staphylococcal infection,[18] EBV infection[19] and systemic lupus erythematosus[20] suggests that the granulomas may represent a relatively non-specific but uncommon response to injury.[12,20]

The ensuing account is confined to a discussion of epithelioid cell granulomas. Granulomas may be found in up to 10% of liver biopsies.[21,22] The list of causes of hepatic granulomas (Table 17.1) is a long one and many are rare.[21–37] For the histopathologist few distinguishing morphological features are found in many cases.[2,38,39] In establishing a diagnosis there is a need for a detailed clinical history, appropriate skin testing and careful micro-

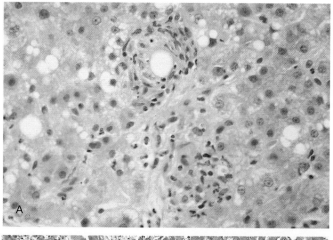

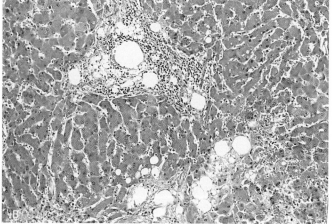

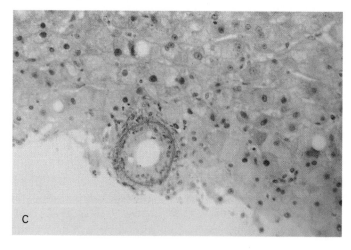

Fig. 17.3 Hepatic granulomas. (a) Lipogranuloma in a fatty liver; the larger one above comprises a central fat globule surrounded by a cuff of inflammatory cells. H & E. (b) Mineral oil granulomas, found incidentally at autopsy, are present both in a portal tract and in the perivenular zone; there is also chronic inflammation of the portal tract, and some increase in fibrous tissue is present around the intra-acinar collection of lipid-laden macrophages. Haematoxylin–phloxine–saffron. Courtesy of Dr I R Wanless. (c) Fibrin ring granuloma from a patient with Q fever; there is a cuff of inflammatory cells in which neutrophils are prominent. MSB. Courtesy of Dr A Sherwood.

Table 17.1 Hepatic granulomas — reported causes

INFECTIOUS DISEASES

Bacterial
- Actinomycosis
- Borrelia (Lyme disease)[24]
- Botryomycosis
- Cat-scratch disease
- Granuloma inguinale
- Listeriosis
- Melioidosis
- Nocardiosis
- Staphylococcal infections[18]
- Syphilis (primary and secondary)
- Tularaemia
- Typhoid
- *Yersinia enterocolitica*[25]

Mycobacterial
- Tuberculosis
- Atypical mycobacteria (e.g. *M. avium intracellulare*)
- BCG immunization and immunotherapy
- Leprosy (lepromatous and tuberculoid)

Rickettsial
- Boutonneuse fever
- Q fever
- *Rickettsia conorii* infection

Chlamydial
- Lymphopathia venereum
- Psittacosis

Fungal
- Aspergillosis
- Blastomycosis (North and South American)
- Candidiasis
- Coccidioidomycosis
- Histoplasmosis
- Mucormycosis
- Paracoccidioidomycosis

Viral
- CMV infection
- EBV — infectious mononucleosis[19]
- Hepatitis A[17]
- HIV infection
- Varicella[26]

Parasitic
- Amoebiasis
- Ancylostomiasis
- Capillariasis
- *Enterobius vermicularis* infection[27]
- Fascioliasis
- Giardiasis
- *Linguatula serrata*[28]
- Opisthorchiasis
- Paragonimiasis
- Pentastomiasis
- Schistosomiasis
- Strongyloidiasis
- Toxocariasis
- Visceral leishmaniasis (kala-azar)

HYPERSENSITIVITY

- Drugs (see Ch. 15, Table 15.8)
- Metals — beryllium, copper, gold

IMMUNOLOGICAL DISEASES

- Chronic granulomatous disease of childhood[29]
- Hypogammaglobulinaemia
- Polymyalgia rheumatica
- Primary biliary cirrhosis
- Rheumatic fever[30]
- Systemic lupus erythematosus
- Vascular diseases
  - allergic granulomatosis
  - necrotizing angiitis in drug abuse[31]
  - polyarteritis nodosa
  - temporal arteritis
- Wegener's granulomatosis

FOREIGN MATERIALS

- Anthracotic pigments
- Barium
- Cement and mica dust
- Mineral oil — radiocontrast media,[5] food additives[6]
- Polyvinyl pyrrolidone
- Silica
- Silicone rubber — renal dialysis tubing[32]
- Starch
- Suture material
- Talc
- Thorotrast

NEOPLASMS

- Extrahepatic malignancy[33]
- Hepatocellular adenoma and liver adenomatosis[34]
- Hodgkin's disease (p. 736)
- Non-Hodgkin's lymphoma (p. 736)

MISCELLANEOUS

- Biliary tract obstruction — bile granulomas
- Chronic inflammatory bowel disease
- Whipple's disease
- Eosinophilic enteritis[35]
- Jejuno-ileal bypass surgery
- Porphyria cutanea tarda[36]
- Psoriasis/hyperuricaemia/gout syndrome[37]
- Sarcoidosis
- Sickle cell anaemia (?)

This table is based on several excellent reviews;[21-23] additional references are given where appropriate. A question mark indicates those conditions in which a coincidental association has not been excluded.

---

biological, serological and biochemical screening. The PAS stain is most useful for defining the number and distribution of granulomas. Involvement of bile ducts with associated ductal damage suggests primary biliary cirrhosis (see Ch. 12); periductal bile granulomas may occur in large duct obstruction but there is an accompanying acute cholangitis.

A non-portal distribution of granulomas is said to be characteristic of tuberculosis;[1] in biopsies caseation is an infrequent feature and alcohol/acid-fast bacilli are demonstrated in less than 10% of proven cases; these findings are much more common in autopsy material. In miliary tuberculosis well-formed giant cell granulomas are infrequent in biopsies and the characteristic features are a marked generalized Kupffer-cell hyperplasia with small macrophage microgranulomas.

Particulate material such as schistosome ova may be seen on routine stains or may be identified on phase-contrast or polarizing microscopy. Serial sectioning may be necessary to show that the lesion is primarily vascular. Special stains are applied when infectious agents are suspected[22,39] and some fungi may be identified by their staining characteristics or by immunohistochemistry.

In Klatskin's survey[21] of over 6000 biopsies, 74% were associated with generalized granulomatous disease, 4% with primary hepatic disease, and in the remaining 22% no definite diagnosis was reached. This failure to establish a cause for hepatic granulomas in 20–25% of patients has been reported by others[40] and in some series the figure has been as high as 50%.[41] Prospective follow-up may result in the aetiology of the granuloma declaring itself in a further 15%.[41,43] However, in some 5–10% of patients no specific diagnosis is reached and they may be regarded as having *idiopathic granulomatous hepatitis*.[38,40,44] Such patients characteristically have a prolonged or recurrent pyrexial illness with weight loss, myalgia, arthralgia and vague abdominal pain.[40] They fail to benefit from a trial of antituberculous drugs[42] but may improve in response to administration of corticosteroids or non-steroidal anti-inflammatory agents; in some patients the condition resolves spontaneously.[45] It should be stressed that the diagnosis of idiopathic granulomatous hepatitis is one of exclusion and should be made only after exhaustive investigation has failed to identify a specific aetiology. The term is in some respects a misnomer, in that there is seldom any significant hepatocellular damage,[40] and it has been suggested that it may represent a form of sarcoidosis confined to the liver.[39]

There is one report of familial granulomatous hepatitis in which two parents and three of their seven children were affected.[46] There is also a report of hepatocellular carcinoma developing in a patient with chronic granulomatous hepatitis;[47] the patient's Kveim test was negative but clinical dyspnoea and the finding of splenic granulomas suggested a diagnosis of sarcoidosis.

SARCOIDOSIS AND THE LIVER

Sarcoidosis, a disease of unknown aetiology,[48] is one of the most common causes of non-caseating hepatic granulomas. The incidence of hepatic involvement in most series ranges from 50 up to 90%,[21,49,50] but Lehmuskallio et al[51] reported a 17% incidence in their series from Scandinavia. The liver follows lymph nodes and lung in frequency of involvement. Klatskin[21] estimated that the affected liver may contain as many as 75 million granulomas but, despite this, the large majority of patients show minimal evidence of clinical or biochemical hepatic dysfunction. In some patients a diagnosis of sarcoidosis has been established on liver biopsy while there was no radiological evidence of pulmonary involvement.[52]

Sarcoid granulomas occur diffusely in the liver but tend to be more frequent in portal tracts or in the periportal area. They consist of a compact aggregate of irregularly arranged large epithelioid cells, sometimes with multinucleated giant cells, and with a surrounding rim of lymphocytes and macrophages; occasional eosinophils may also be present (Fig. 17.4a). The peripheral mantle of lymphocytes is a mixed population of CD4 and CD8 positive cells. There are phenotypic differences between the macrophages in the centre of the lesions which are HLA-DR positive and react with the monoclonal antibody RFD-2, and those in the mantle which are immunoreactive with RFD-1.[53] Schaumann bodies tend to be infrequent in hepatic granulomas of sarcoidosis. Central granular eosinophilic fibrinoid necrosis may occur but caseation is never found. Reticulin fibres are abundant within the granulomas, particularly in older lesions,[38] when a surrounding cuff of fibrous tissue becomes prominent and dense scars taking on some of the staining reactions of amyloid may develop. In the majority of cases resolution is complete, but giant cells may persist for some time in the fibrous scars. A non-specific reactive hepatitis often accompanies the granulomas and may be a prominent feature when there is active clinical disease.[49,50] Damage to bile ducts (Fig. 17.4b) may be seen in some portal tracts, the lesions resembling those seen in primary biliary cirrhosis.

The majority of patients with sarcoidosis and hepatic granulomas have no evidence of liver dysfunction. In some, however, progressive liver disease with portal hypertension, ascites and hepatic encephalopathy ensues.[37,49,49a,54] Maddrey et al,[49] in a review of 300 patients with sarcoidosis, reviewed 20 in whom there was clinical and/or biochemical evidence of liver disease; of these, 10 showed severe functional hepatic impairment with or without portal hypertension. In some progressive portal and parenchymal fibrosis developed. The fibrosis was in part related to the presence of granulomas, but extensive fibrosis unrelated to granulomas also occurred and contributed to the development of cirrhosis. The histological appearances in a similar patient who died of hepatic failure are shown in Figure 17.4c and d. In their recent study of 100 cases of hepatic sarcoidosis Devaney et al[49a] found fibrosis in 21 and cirrhosis in 6.

Portal hypertension may develop in the absence of cirrhosis.[49,55–57] Valla et al[57] described patients with sarcoidosis in whom portal hypertension was the predominant clinical feature. In these 32 patients the portal hypertension was due to a presinusoidal block, the result of a pressure effect by portal tract granulomas, and sometimes with a superimposed sinusoidal block due to fibrosis. Nodular regenerative hyperplasia may contribute in some cases.[49a] Obstruction of hepatic vein branches by sarcoid granulomas is a rare cause of Budd-Chiari syndrome.[58,59]

A chronic prolonged cholestatic syndrome with progression to biliary cirrhosis may rarely occur in sarcoidosis and is more often seen in black people.[60–63] Histologically

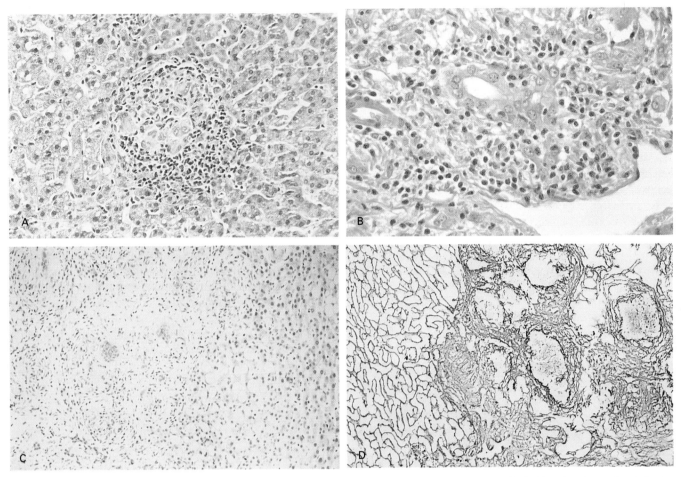

Fig. 17.4 Liver in sarcoidosis. (a) Typical intra-acinar granuloma with a surrounding cuff of lymphocytes. H & E. (b) Portal tract granuloma causing damage to the bile duct. H & E. (c) Diffuse hepatic involvement in sarcoidosis with a confluent aggregate of giant-cell granulomas. H & E. (d) The extensive scarring is shown here on a Gordon & Sweets' reticulin stain.

there is ductopenia which correlates with the amount of fibrosis. Rudzki and his colleagues[60] reviewed 21 such cases and reported five of their own; clinically and biochemically these patients manifested many of the features of primary biliary cirrhosis but anti-mitochondrial antibody was not found and their five additional cases were males. Devaney et al described bile duct lesions similar to primary biliary cirrhosis in 19% of their patient with sarcoidosis and in 13% there were lesions resembling primary sclerosing cholangitis.

Murphy et al[63] emphasized the progressive bile-duct loss which was a feature in their five patients, three of whom were male and all of whom were black. The similarities between sarcoidosis and primary biliary cirrhosis have been reviewed in a number of studies.[63–66] The differential histological diagnosis is discussed in chapter 12. In the 'overlap' patients pulmonary symptoms were the principal initial manifestations with cholestatic liver disease subsequently developing.[65] In general, anti-mitochondrial antibody is not present in sarcoidosis and the Kveim-Siltzbach test is negative in primary biliary cirrhosis. However, there are very rare cases in which both of these

tests are positive[65,67,68] and it remains speculative whether these patients have two co-existing disorders.[66]

FATTY LIVER AND NUTRITIONAL LIVER INJURY

Accumulation of lipid in hepatocytes — *fatty liver* or *steatosis* — is one of the commonest morphological abnormalities in liver biopsy or autopsy material. The presence of fat droplets in occasional hepatocytes is often a non-specific finding of doubtful significance. Minor degrees of steatosis may be considered normal in the ageing liver.[69] The liver has a pivotal role in normal fat metabolism (see Ch. 2) and in this role there are interactions with carbo-hydrate and protein metabolism with involvement of vitamins, hormones and trace elements. Malnutrition may be the cause or may be a contributory factor in certain liver diseases and, conversely, disturbances of nutrition occur in liver disease and are significant factors in the clinical syndromes which accompany hepatic dysfunction. This topic has recently been extensively reviewed.[70,71] In this section, therefore, we propose only to describe some of the morphological changes which comprise fatty liver and which occur both in nutritional disturbances and in a number of other disorders. Some of these are discussed elsewhere in the text, notably metabolic disorders (see Ch. 4) and alcoholic liver disease (see Ch. 8).

The normal human liver contains approximately 5 g lipid per 100 g wet weight, with triglyceride accounting for approximately 20% of this.[72] In severe fatty liver there may be a substantial increase in the size of the liver, lipid then accounting for up to 50% of the wet weight. In autopsy specimens, these livers have a pale yellow greasy appearance (Fig. 17.5a). The colour is due to the presence of excess carotenes and other lipochromes. The mechanisms involved in producing fatty liver are summarized in Table 17.2.[73]

Morphologically, fat accumulates in the liver in two forms:[74] (i) *macrovesicular steatosis*, in which large lipid droplets occupy the cell and displace the nucleus and cytoplasmic organelles to the periphery (Fig. 17.5b); (ii) *microvesicular steatosis*, in which multiple finely dis-persed lipid droplets are present throughout the cell without producing nuclear displacement (Fig. 17.5c, d) and may only be visualized microscopically when fat stains are used on frozen sections. In both forms the fat is present as non-membrane-bound vesicles. Histochemical methods can be used to quantify the lipid in biopsy speci-mens.[75]

Macrovesicular steatosis is seen in many states, including diabetes mellitus, obesity, kwashiorkor, debili-tating illnesses such as chronic inflammatory bowel disease, alcohol-induced liver injury, injury due to other toxins and drugs and in many inherited metabolic disorders. Miscellaneous conditions associated with macrovesicular steatosis include hepatitis C,[76] malaria[77] and immotile cilia syndrome.[78]

The zonal distribution pattern of the fat is variable in the different conditions listed, tending to involve acinar zones 1 and 2 in kwashiorkor and acinar zones 3 and 2 in alcoholic liver disease, but there is no consistent diagnosti-cally helpful pattern.

Focal fatty change was first described in 1980, since

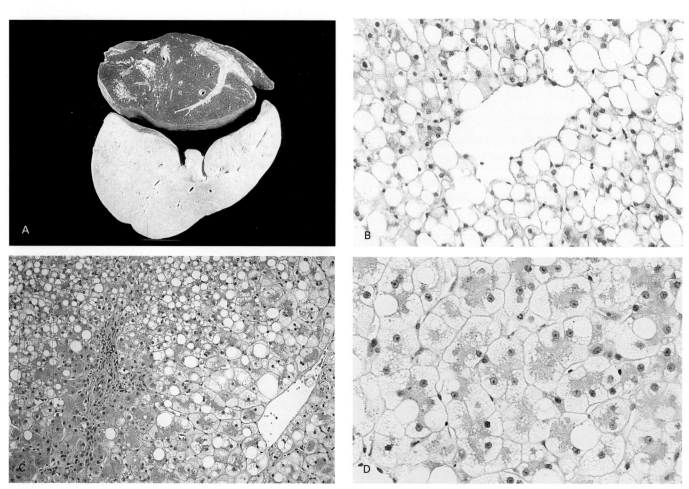

Fig. 17.5 Fatty liver. (a) Gross appearance showing the yellow colour contrasting with a normal liver. (b) Macrovesicular steatosis of acinar zone 3 in an alcoholic patient; there is no fibrosis. Masson's trichrome. (c) Alcoholic foamy degeneration in which both macrovesicular and microvesicular steatosis is present in acinar zones 3 and 2. H & E. (d) Note that the nucleus remains in a central position in the microvesicular pattern, whereas it is displaced when a macrovesicle is present; there is also canalicular and intracellular bilirubinostasis. PAS–diastase.

Table 17.2 Mechanisms which may be involved in causing fatty liver (after Prieto et al[73])

A. Increased triglyceride synthesis
　1. Excessive availability of fatty acids
　　(i) Dietary intake
　　(ii) Adipose tissue, e.g. obesity, diabetes mellitus, corticosteroid therapy
　　(iii) parenteral nutrition
　2. Increased availability of fatty acid precursors
　　(i) Carbohydrate-rich dietary intake
　　(ii) Alcohol
　3. Reduced fatty acid oxidation
　　(i) Mitochondrial dysfunction, e.g. drugs/toxins; Reye's syndrome
　　(ii) Acyl-CoA dehydrogenase deficiency
B. Reduced triglyceride excretion
　1. Reduced apoprotein synthesis
　　(i) Protein malnutrition, e.g. kwashiorkor, gastrointestinal malabsorption
　　(ii) Metabolic diseases (Ch. 4)
　　(iii) Drug/toxin-induced injury, e.g. tetracycline, carbon tetrachloride, alcohol
C. Cryptogenic

when it has become increasingly recognized in that it is picked up by imaging techniques including ultrasound or computed tomography, and may simulate metastatic disease.[79-83] The lesions may be single or multiple, they may sometimes be nodular, and they have occasionally been associated with other hepatic abnormalities such as cirrhosis.[84] The basic acinar architecture of the liver, however, is usually preserved and while some patients have been identified in whom factors predisposing to generalized macrovesicular steatosis were present, the mechanisms leading to a non-homogeneous distribution of fat are not clear although local hypoxia has been postulated to play a role.[83] The lesion must be distinguished from other intrahepatic lipid-rich lesions such as lipoma, angiolipoma, myelolipoma and coelomic fat ectopia.[85-88]

Microvesicular steatosis is the major finding in acute fatty liver of pregnancy (p. 730) and in Reye's syndrome (p. 104), and may also occur in alcoholic foamy degeneration (p. 320) and in drug and toxin-induced liver injury (p. 573). It has also been reported in heatstroke,[89] sudden infant death syndrome,[90] as a consequence of multiple hornet's sting,[91] in hepatitis D infection,[92] in recurrent hepatitis B and D infection in hepatic allografts[93] and in some inherited metabolic disorders (see Ch. 4). In Wolman's disease and cholesteryl ester storage the fat is membrane bound and cholesterol is also present and exhibits birefringence on polarization (p. 174).

In experimental models where steatosis is induced by toxins such as orotic acid[94] and margosa oil,[95] lipid first accumulates as small droplets in the endoplasmic reticulum. Margosa oil, which can cause a Reye's-like syndrome in children, produces mitochondrial injury and glycogen depletion in mice followed by hypertrophy of the endoplasmic reticulum and the development of

microvesicular steatosis.[95] The microvesicular fat globules subsequently coalesce to form large droplets. Such a transition between a microvesicular and a macrovesicular pattern also appears to occur in some forms of human diseases such as alcoholic steatosis and in kwashiorkor.[96,67] Although this suggests that the two morphological types of fatty liver are part of a spectrum, assessment of the predominant form in an individual case is useful in attempting to establish the aetiology of fatty liver. Pure microvesicular steatosis is found in a limited number of disorders but generally has more serious clinical implications than the macrovesicular form.[98]

THE LIVER IN PROTEIN-ENERGY MALNUTRITION

Steatosis is an almost invariable feature of kwashiorkor although it is less frequently encountered in marasmus.[97] The steatosis of kwashiorkor is first seen as small droplets in periportal hepatocytes. These lipid globules later coalesce and the changes progress to involve the entire acinus.[97,99] Following re-feeding, lipid first clears from the perivenular hepatocytes.[97] In the vast majority of cases, the steatosis of kwashiorkor is manifest by asymptomatic hepatomegaly. Biochemical tests of liver function are often normal although occasional cases of severe cholestasis have been described.[100] Histologically, there is little hepatocyte necrosis or inflammation. Mallory body-like material has been described in some cases[97] but a true steatohepatitis does not develop.

It was previously thought that fibrosis and cirrhosis were long-term consequences of the hepatic involvement in kwashiorkor. This concept of so-called nutritional liver disease developed from observations in experimental models, where animals developed cirrhosis when fed nutritionally deficient diets and from epidemiological studies which demonstrated a high incidence of cirrhosis in populations in whom protein-energy malnutrition was a major problem. The concept was further applied to other forms of chronic liver disease and it was at one time suggested that alcoholic cirrhosis might be the result of dietary insufficiency.[101] It is now clear that the observations made in choline- or protein-deficient rats are not relevant to the pathogenesis of human liver disease and that the steatosis of kwashiorkor per se does not lead to cirrhosis.[102] When fibrosis and/or necro-inflammation is present in patients with kwashiorkor it is likely to be related to another factor such as chronic HBV infection.[96]

The pathogenesis of steatosis in kwashiorkor remains controversial. Although aflatoxin ingestion has been considered to be a contributory factor,[103] most evidence suggests that the lipid accumulation results from an imbalance in hepatic carbohydrate, protein and lipid metabolism.[96] Several studies have demonstrated abnormal plasma lipid profiles resulting in an increased delivery of non-esterified fatty acids to hepatocytes.[104] There is also evidence that apolipoprotein deficiency occurs, leading to decreased mobilization of triglycerides from liver cells.[105] Doherty and co-workers[106] have recently shown that hepatocytes in kwashiorkor lack peroxisomes and they have postulated that this may lead to altered beta-oxidation of fat, thereby contributing to the development of steatosis.

Fatty liver is not a feature of the other major form of malnutrition, marasmus. Steatosis, if present, is mild and focal with no particular zonal distribution. The hepatocytes tend to be atrophic and the sinusoids are dilated but there is no intra-acinar inflammation and no fibrosis. Peliosis hepatis has been reported in a patient with marasmus.[107]

NON-ALCOHOLIC STEATOHEPATITIS

A progression from fatty liver to fatty liver hepatitis and eventually cirrhosis was suggested over 30 years ago.[108] In the 1970s the introduction of various gastrointestinal bypass procedures was sometimes accompanied by profound hepatic disturbances and, in some patients, the morphological lesions closely resembled alcoholic hepatitis.[109–111] Similar lesions were then reported in unoperated obese patients,[112] in type II diabetes,[113] and in drug toxicity the topic was reviewed by Schaffner & Thaler.[114] Various terms were applied to this lesion — fatty liver hepatitis, non-alcoholic fatty liver disease, steatonecrosis, pseudo-alcoholic liver disease, alcohol-like hepatitis — but the term non-alcoholic steatohepatitis (NASH) introduced by Ludwig and his colleagues[115] is now widely accepted. The diseases associated with non-alcoholic steatohepatitis are: obesity;[112,116,117] gastroplasty, jejuno-ileal bypass and other surgical procedures for the treatment of morbid obesity;[109,110,118–123] diabetes mellitus, type II (see p. 728); drug-induced injury (see p. 582); total parenteral nutrition; Weber–Christian disease;[123] abetalipoproteinaemia;[124] limb lipodystrophy;[125] and small intestinal diverticulosis.[126] In some patients, however, no recognized associations are present and a diagnosis of non-alcoholic steatohepatitis is made on the basis of the biopsy findings during investigation of mild disturbances in liver function tests and after exclusion of alcohol abuse.[126–133] The histological features (Fig. 17.6) may be indistinguishable from alcoholic hepatitis, but the number of Mallory bodies shows considerable variation in incidence and a periportal distribution of the lesions has been noted in diabetes[134] and in some of the drug-related cases. The lesion tends to be slowly progressive and cirrhosis develops in a proportion of cases.[120,130,131] Hocking and his colleagues found a 29% incidence of progressive liver disease and a 7% incidence of cirrhosis in a follow-up of 100 jejuno-ileal bypass patients.[120] The rate and pattern of progression however vary, depending on the aetiology of the steatohepatitis.[131]

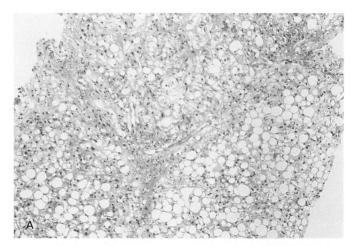

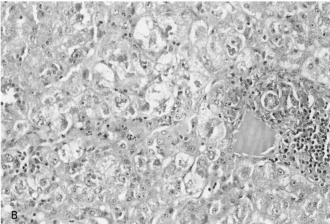

Fig. 17.6 Non-alcoholic steatohepatitis. (a) Following jejuno-ileal bypass; there is macrovesicular steatosis, ballooned hepatocytes some of which contain Mallory bodies, and some irregular fibrosis. H & E. By courtesy of the late Dr R L Peters. (b) In a patient on amiodarone; note the portal tract inflammation and the periportal location of numerous Mallory bodies. By courtesy of Dr N Y Haboubi. H & E.

TOTAL PARENTERAL NUTRITION

Total parenteral nutrition (TPN) by the intravenous route (also referred to as intravenous alimentation) has become an accepted treatment modality over the past 25 years. Peden et al[135] first drew attention to hepatic complications in infants treated with TPN and such complications are now well recognized in both infants and adults. However, it is difficult to define precisely the contribution which TPN might make to liver dysfunction in these patients in that, in many instances, the primary disease for which TPN is indicated and the clinical complications, sepsis for example, which subsequently develop might themselves cause liver injury. The hepatic complications associated with TPN have been reviewed in detail[71,136–139] and, although the same mechanisms may operate in producing some of the liver injuries, the effects in infancy and adults are dissimilar. In both infants and adults biliary sludging, cholelithiasis and acalculous cholecystitis are common and this may result in biliary obstruction.

Hepatic disease in infants. The incidence of TPN-associated cholestasis in infants correlates inversely with the gestational age and birth weight and is also related to the duration of treatment.[139] The diagnosis is one of exclusion, and 'physiological' cholestasis, the numerous other causes of neonatal cholestasis (see Ch. 3) and sepsis have also to be considered.

Morphologically, the changes are not specific and are extremely variable.[135,137–141] Bilirubinostasis affecting liver cells and canaliculi is consistently present and may develop in a matter of days; cholestatic rosettes are frequently observed; bile plugs may also be present in interlobular bile ducts. Steatosis is infrequent. The portal tracts show a variable mixed inflammatory cell infiltrate and, with prolonged therapy, a periportal ductular reaction and progressive fibrosis may lead to a biliary cirrhosis in a few months;[139–142] where treatment is prolonged serial liver biopsy is indicated to assess any liver injury.[143]

The pathogenetic mechanisms involved in TPN-associated cholestasis are not clear.[139,144,145] Physiological immaturity of hepatic excretory function, including bile acid metabolism and transport, the absence of enteral nutrition with disturbances of the normal entero-hepatic circulation, suppression of trophic or secretion-stimulating hormones and the composition of the infusate, including specific unidentified deficiencies, have been variously suggested.

Hepatic disease in adults. Hepatic abnormalities are common following parenteral nutrition in older children and adults but the incidence is difficult to establish and, in most cases, evidence of hepatic dysfunction is transient. High calorie dextrose-based TPN was used initially, whereas lower calorie infusions containing fat are now more common and have been associated with a lower incidence of hepatic dysfunction. However, whereas increases in serum bilirubin are mild and relatively uncommon when compared with that in infants, increases in the serum levels of transaminases, alkaline phosphatase and γ-glutamyltranspeptidase are found in from 20–60% of patients, may develop within 5–20 days of commencing treatment, and may persist in from 15–25% of patients who receive long-term TPN.[136,138,139]

The morphological lesions in the liver (Fig. 17.7) include intrahepatic cholestasis, macrovesicular steatosis, non-alcoholic steatohepatitis, portal and periportal fibrosis.[118,138,139,146–153] Intrahepatic perivenular bilirubinostasis develops after 2–3 weeks on TPN and may be accompanied by periportal inflammation and portal fibrosis which persists after discontinuation of treatment. The macrovesicular steatosis is predominantly periportal and is thought to be due to imbalance in the rate of fat deposition and removal, although carnitine deficiency has been postulated.[154]

Non-alcoholic steatohepatitis may also occur but the true incidence of progression to cirrhosis is not clear.[118,148,155] In Bowyer et al's[148] study of 60 patients treated with long-term TPN, 9 (15%) had persistently abnormal liver function tests; biopsy in 8 of the patients showed steatohepatitis in all of them, with perivenular fibrosis in 3 and nodular regeneration in 1.

THE LIVER IN GASTROINTESTINAL DISEASE

Hepatic involvement in diseases of the gastorintestinal tract is not uncommon, the portal vein affording a means whereby toxins, microorganisms and tumour emboli may gain direct access to the organ. Non-specific reactive hepatitis, intrahepatic sepsis and disseminated intrahepatic metastases result. However, there are also specific hepatobiliary disorders which may accompany chronic inflammatory bowel disease and a few other miscellaneous associations are also outlined below.

CHRONIC INFLAMMATORY BOWEL DISEASE

Liver disease in ulcerative colitis was first reported by Thomas[156] in 1873 who described an enlarged fatty liver in a young male; Lister[157] in 1899 described a patient in whom the ulcerative colitis was accompanied by a diffuse hepatitis. Chapin et al[158] in 1956 first noted that the hepatic lesions in Crohn's disease were similar to those described in ulcerative colitis; with some exceptions, the spectrum of the liver disease in each is essentially similar. Hepatic dysfunction is more frequently associated with colonic involvement and is usually coincident with other extra-intestinal systemic complications.[159] The association between liver dysfunction and chronic inflammatory bowel disease is now well recognized and a number of detailed clinico-pathological reviews have recently been published.[160–163]

The earlier studies describing the hepatic lesions in chronic inflammatory bowel disease[159,160–170] were reviewed by Kern.[171] The classic studies by Mistilis and his colleagues[164,165] drew attention to so-called pericholangitis associated with ulcerative colitis, and they found this liver lesion in 5.4% of 441 ulcerative colitis patients. They emphasized injury to intrahepatic bile ducts as part of this disease entity, which could pursue a chronic course sometimes leading to cirrhosis. In subsequent studies the term pericholangitis became synonymous with the liver involvement in chronic inflammatory bowel disease. The development of endoscopic retrograde cholangiopancreatography (ERCP), however, served to draw attention to those patients in whom there were obliterative lesions in the biliary system, to which the term primary sclerosing cholangitis was applied. It now seems highly unlikely that pericholangitis exists as a disease entity separate from primary sclerosing cholangitis[161,172–174] and histopathologists

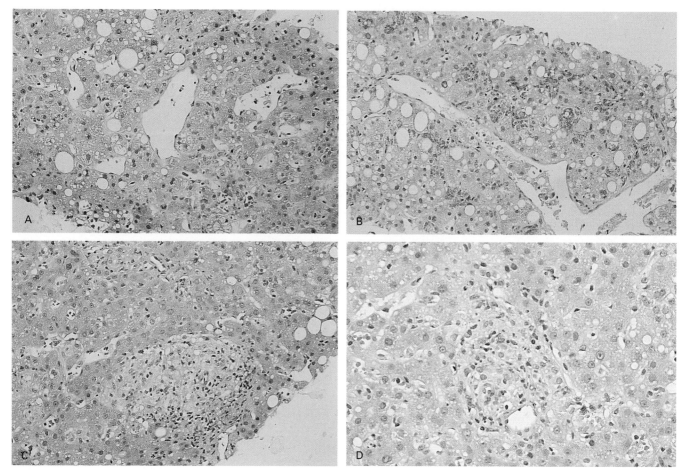

Fig. 17.7 Hepatic changes in a patient with Crohn's disease on total parenteral nutrition. (a) Perivenular macrovesicular and microvesicular steatosis and bilirubinostasis. H & E. (b) Prominent aggregates of ceroid-containing macrophages. PAS–diastase. (c) A granulomatoid aggregate of foamy macrophages with some lymphocytes and plasma cells. H & E. (d) Portal tract inflammation with prominent macrophages, lymphocytes and occasional eosinophils. H & E.

should no longer use the term as a morphological diagnosis.[175,176]

Abnormalities of liver function tests have been reported in approximately 50% of patients with chronic inflammatory bowel disease.[170,177–179] However, the frequency of histologically-proven significant liver disease is considered to be much lower, although there are no prospective studies on patients from the time of first presentation. Estimated frequencies have ranged from 5%[170] to 17%[180] in ulcerative colitis and from 10%[159] to 30%[180] in Crohn's disease. These may be underestimates in that abnormalities of liver function tests do not necessarily correlate with morphological evidence of liver disease. However, if the liver function tests are normal, Broome and his colleagues[181] have reported that less than 3% develop biopsy-proven liver disease on follow-up. In a patient with chronic inflammatory bowel disease and persistently abnormal liver function tests primary sclerosing cholangitis is the most likely diagnosis.

The clinical and pathological features of primary sclerosing cholangitis have been described in chapter 12.

The approximate frequency of the other hepatic lesions which occur in chronic inflammatory bowel disease is summarized in Table 17.3.

Fatty liver

This is the commonest histological abnormality in the liver. It is clinically asymptomatic and hepatomegaly is unusual. It is of a macrovesicular pattern and although its extent seems to be related to the severity of the bowel disease it may persist after colectomy.[167] The development of fatty liver is probably a non-specific manifestation of the accompanying toxaemia, malnutrition and anaemia.

Chronic active hepatitis (CAH)

Prevalence rates up to 10% have previously been reported, but these may have been overestimates due to difficulties in distinguishing between CAH and sclerosing cholangitis. In addition, CAH due to post-transfusional chronic HCV infection was not excluded. An estimate of 1–2% seems

Table 17.3 Liver involvement in chronic inflammatory bowel disease

	Approximate frequency
Fatty liver	50%
Primary sclerosing cholangitis	3–5%
Chronic active hepatitis	1–2%
Cirrhosis	2–5%
Bile duct carcinoma[a]	Risk of tumour increased 10-fold
Gallstones[b]	Increased 5–10 fold
Epithelioid granulomas[c]	5%
Amyloidosis[c]	Rare
Pylephlebitis and pyogenic inflammation	Very rare

[a] Ulcerative colitis only
[b] Crohn's disease only
[c] Probably most common in Crohn's disease

likely for ulcerative colitis, but there is little evidence of an increased incidence in association with Crohn's disease.[161] A diagnosis of CAH should not be made unless the ERCP is normal. The difficulties in establishing the diagnosis have been emphasized by Rabinovitz et al[182] in a report of the simultaneous occurrence of primary sclerosing cholangitis and autoimmune CAH in a patient with ulcerative colitis.

Cirrhosis

The overall prevalence of cirrhosis is about 2–5%.[161,163,177] Edwards & Truelove[183] reported that cirrhosis was present in 2.5% of patients with ulcerative colitis and accounted for 10% of all deaths in a follow-up period of over 20 years. Cirrhosis is 12–50 times commoner in patients with chronic inflammatory bowel disease when compared with controls,[184,185] and is usually associated with extensive disease of the colon. The cirrhosis may develop as a sequel to sclerosing cholangitis where it will be of a micronodular biliary pattern, or as a sequel to CAH (viral or autoimmune) where the pattern will be macronodular. In post-colectomy patients with cirrhosis, bleeding may occur from varices at the ileostomy stoma or at the ileo-rectal anastomosis.[177,186]

Cholangiocarcinoma

This tumour shows a 10–30-fold increase in incidence in patients with ulcerative colitis,[187,188] but in Crohn's disease the association appears to be uncommon.[189] Conversely, in carcinoma of the proximal bile ducts ulcerative colitis was present in 8–10% of patients.[190,191] The clinical and pathological evidence, reviewed by Rosen & Nagomey,[192] suggests that the carcinoma develops as a complication of primary sclerosing cholangitis and, indeed, that primary sclerosing cholangitis may be a premalignant condition in which this tumour develops in 10–15% of cases.[163,192,193] Carcinoma usually develops in patients with longstanding (15 years or more) extensive

and severe ulcerative colitis. On average, the patients are 20 years younger than other patients with cholangiocarcinoma. The tumour may arise some years after total colectomy[187,188] and may involve intra- or extra-hepatic ducts and gallbladder. The differential diagnosis with sclerosing cholangitis is difficult and many tumours are not diagnosed until liver resection at transplantation or at autopsy. The prognosis is dismal, with a mean survival time of approximately 6–18 months.[188,194] Liver transplantation is of limited value and tumours found incidentally at the time of operation may recur in the allograft.[195,196]

Miscellaneous

The hepatic effects of TPN, often instituted in extensive Crohn's disease, have been reviewed on page 722.

Gallstones have a 5–10-fold increased frequency in patients with Crohn's disease of the terminal ileum.[197] This is related to the extent and duration of the ileal disease and the length of bowel which may have to be resected. This complication is thought to be due to bile acid malabsorption[197] and possibly changes in bile acid composition[198] causing cholesterol saturation in the bile. The gallbladder may itself be affected by Crohn's disease.[199]

Amyloidosis of AA type (p. 743) may develop in both ulcerative colitis and Crohn's disease but is more common in Crohn's disease.[200–202] Liver involvement is very uncommon, however.[203] Regression of amyloidosis following colectomy has been reported.[203,204]

Granulomas are found in the liver in approximately 5% of patients, predominantly in Crohn's disease,[159,160,166,185] and may resolve quickly after colectomy.[169,205]

Pylephlebitis and pyogenic abscess of the liver are now rare and avoidable complications[206–208] but may sometimes be the initial presenting feature.[208,209]

Portal vein thrombosis may occur in both ulcerative colitis and Crohn's disease.[158,194] **Budd–Chiari syndrome** has also been reported.[210–212]

MISCELLANEOUS BOWEL DISEASES WITH LIVER INVOLVEMENT

Coeliac disease. Hagander et al[213] found increased serum levels of transaminases and alkaline phosphatase in 39% of 74 adult patients and noted improvement in these indices on a gluten-free diet. Liver biopsy in 13 showed non-specific reactive hepatitis in 5, cirrhosis and/or chronic active hepatitis in 7, and in one case cirrhosis was complicated by a hepatocellular carcinoma. In a retrospective survey of 132 adult patients, abnormalities of liver function tests were found in 47%, 11% having increased alkaline phosphatase levels and 36% increased transaminases.[214] Significant improvement in transaminase levels on a gluten-free diet was seen in 18 of 32 patients studied prospectively; liver biopsies in 37 patients showed non-specific changes in 26, chronic active hepatitis in 5, normal appearances in 5 and primary sclerosing cholangitis in 1 (also accompanied by ulcerative colitis).[214] Mitchison et al[215] noted abnormalities of liver function tests responsive to a gluten-free diet in 3 patients, 1 of whom had steatosis and 2 of whom had non-specific reactive hepatitis.

Lindberg et al[216] reported elevated serum transaminase levels in children with coeliac disease, a finding which they also observed in gastrointestinal allergies and which led them to suggest that the liver dysfunction was non-specific and secondary to mucosal injury. In a retrospective autopsy study of 19 cases of malabsorption Pollock[217] noted that in the 5 patients with a confirmed diagnosis of coeliac disease, 2 had chronic hepatitis, in one of whom cirrhosis and a hepatocellular carcinoma had developed.

Logan et al[218] reported the co-existence of adult coeliac disease in 4 patients with primary biliary cirrhosis, while Hay et al[219] reported primary sclerosing cholangitis in 3 coeliac patients, 2 of whom also had ulcerative colitis.

Whipple's disease may frequently show widespread systemic involvement. the PAS-positive-diastase-resistant foamy macrophages which characterize the intestinal involvement may be found in the liver — Figure 17.8.[220-224] The 'sickle-form' bacilli seen in these macrophages have also been described in Kupffer cells.[225] Non-caseating epithelioid cell granulomas also occur in the liver in Whipple's disease and may precede the onset of intestinal symptoms; these granulomas, however, do not contain bacilli.[226-228]

Eosinophilic gastroenteritis. Hepatic granulomas with a prominent eosinophil infiltrate have been reported in two patients,[35] and in a patient with systemic involvement an intense eosinophilic infiltrate was present in the portal tracts.[229]

THE LIVER IN PANCREATIC DISEASE

EXOCRINE PANCREAS

Cystic fibrosis is discussed in Chapter 4.

Extrahepatic obstruction may occur very rarely as a result of annular pancreas.[230] Jaundice is the initial presenting symptom in 60–70% of patients with carcinoma of the head of pancreas and ampullary region, and eventually develops in 80% of patients.[231] Jaundice, often transient, may develop in 15–75% of patients with acute pancreatitis and may be the result of bile-duct obstruction due to inflammation, or it may result from a common aetiology such as alcohol abuse or gallstones.[232,233] Obstructive jaundice is rare in chronic pancreatitis, but it may occur in an acute exacerbation[233] or from pressure due to a pancreatic pseudocyst.[234] Steatosis, portal tract in-

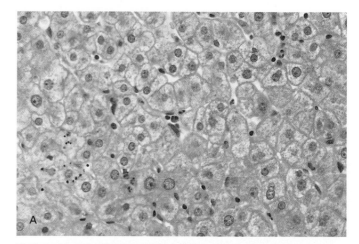

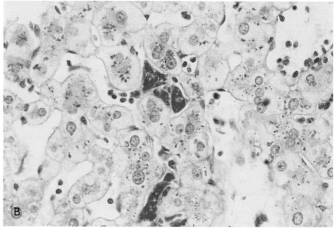

Fig. 17.8 Liver biopsy in a patient with Whipple's disease. (a) There is Kupffer-cell hyperplasia with some large intrasinusoidal cells. H & E. (b) These are strongly PAS-positive. PAS–diastase. Courtesy of Dr Carole D Kooijman.

flammation and fibrosis and cirrhosis are not uncommon associations of chronic pancreatitis, but seem most likely to be due to alcohol abuse or cholelithiasis, common aetiological factors in pancreatitis.

The converse relationships between liver and exocrine pancreas are worth noting. Evidence of acute haemorrhagic pancreatitis has been found in a third of patients with massive liver-cell necrosis[235,236] and may also occur in acute fatty liver of pregnancy.[237]

ENDOCRINE PANCREAS

The liver has a key role in carbohydrate metabolism[238] (see Ch. 2). The possible 'hepatotropic' effects of pancreatic hormones were first investigated by Starzl and his colleagues[239,240] and it is now clear that insulin, glucagon and insulin-like growth factors together with several other hormones and hepatic growth factors, modulate hepatic function in normal circumstances and regulate hepatic regeneration after liver injury (see Ch. 1). Only in diabetes mellitus, however, is there evidence of significant liver disease in association with islet-cell dysfunction.

Diabetes mellitus

Metabolic aspects

The metabolic disturbances which involve the liver have been recently reviewed.[241-243]

In type I diabetes, resulting from insulin lack, the liver contributes to the disturbances in carbohydrate metabolism. The hyperglycaemia results from breakdown of glycogen and over-production of glucose by the liver together with a decreased uptake of glucose from the portal vein blood. The activity of glucose-6-phosphatase is increased with resulting increased glycogenolysis and decreased phosphorylation in the liver. Over-production of glucose also occurs due to a loss of the normal feedback inhibition of gluconeogenesis by plasma glucose levels.[244,245] The uptake of glucose from portal vein blood is considerably reduced[246] and may fall from 60% extraction to as low as 25%.[245] This is the result of low levels of hepatic glucokinase, the enzyme responsible for glucose trapping. The ketoacidosis of severe and prolonged diabetes is due to increased lipolysis, and a release of free fatty acids into the circulation and a failure to inhibit their oxidation in the liver because of the insulin lack, and increased beta-oxidation of the fatty acids.[247,248] Increased levels of glucagon may enhance adipose tissue lipolysis.[249]

In type II diabetes there is altered hepatic responsiveness to insulin. The evidence suggests that, as with fat and muscle tissue, the hepatocyte also acquires insulin resistance by mechanisms which are not yet fully understood.[250] The resistance may be due to a decreased number of insulin receptors[251,252] causing a relative lack of intra-cellular insulin. However, the precise mechanisms involved in the increased hepatic gluconeogenesis which is present in type II diabetes remain uncertain.[253]

Disturbances of lipid metabolism also occur. In type I diabetes, hypertriglyceridaemia results from increased production of VLDL by the liver combined with a decreased peripheral clearance due to a deficiency of lipoprotein lipase.[241,254] In type II diabetes unexplained increased production of VLDL also occurs but lipoprotein lipase levels are normal.

Diabetes mellitus in cirrhosis. Insulin resistance, impaired glucose tolerance and frank diabetes mellitus are common in cirrhosis irrespective of its aetiology. Impaired glucose tolerance is found in about 75% of patients but a diabetic glucose tolerance test is unusual.[238,241,255,256] This glucose intolerance is not fully understood and may be due to hyperinsulinaemia and an acquired insulin resistance,[257-262] and glucose resistance secondary to the liver disease.[263] The hyperinsulinaemia may result from insulin hypersecretion and decreased degradation;[260,261]

the insulin resistance may result from increased insulin antagonists such as glucagon, decreased receptor binding of insulin or a post-receptor defect.[261,262,264-266] However, the mechanisms may be different depending on the aetiology of the cirrhosis.[260]

Clinical aspects

Clinical manifestations of hepatic involvement in diabetes are few. In type I diabetes hepatomegaly occurs when the diabetes is poorly controlled and may be massive, as part of the rare Mauriac's syndrome[267] which occurs in children and is also characterized by retarded growth, obesity, florid facies and hypercholesterolaemia. The hepatomegaly of diabetes is reversible with adequate control and seems primarily to be due to increased glycogen storage.[268,269] Steatosis contributes significantly to the hepatomegaly of type II diabetes. Conventional liver function tests in the well-controlled and uncomplicated diabetic are only minimally abnormal, with some minor elevations of serum alkaline phosphatase and transaminases.

Morphological aspects

The histological changes which occur in the liver have been extensively reviewed.[114,134,255,270,271] Glycogen accumulation is common.[255,269] Glycogenated nuclei, a non-specific feature, may occur in up to 75% of diabetics, especially in type II.[117,271] On electron microscopy the intranuclear glycogen appears in a dispersed form rather than in the rosette form found in the cytoplasm; it may sometimes also be accompanied by an intranuclear glycogen-filled body.[272] The mechanisms of nuclear glycogenation are uncertain, but the appearances are not due to cytoplasmic invagination. Glycogenated nuclei may also occur in the normal liver, in Wilson's disease, sepsis, tuberculosis, biliary tract disease, cirrhosis and autoimmune chronic active hepatitis.[255,270]

Fatty liver of varying degrees of severity is found in 20–80% of diabetics. The incidence is low in type I, probably less than 5%, whereas in type II it is more than 50% and the extent of involvement is related to the degree of accompanying obesity. The fat accumulation in the liver is probably due to an imbalance between the level of synthesis of triglycerides and the ability of the hepatocytes to secrete these in VLDL particles.

The fat may accumulate in any zone of the acinus. In general it is not of clinical significance. However, non-alcoholic steatohepatitis (Fig. 17.9), discussed earlier in the chapter develops in a number of cases.[113,114,134] Nagore & Scheuer[134] in a review of 5451 consecutive liver biopsies noted that 62 (1.13%) were taken from patients with diabetes type II, and in 17 of these the features were of non-alcoholic steatohepatitis. The non-alcoholic steato-

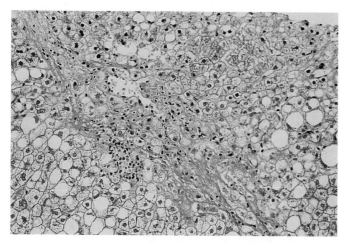

Fig. 17.9 Liver biopsy from a patient with type II diabetes mellitus; there is macrovesicular steatosis with perivenular ballooned hepatocytes, a marked degree of perivenular and pericellular fibrosis and a light, predominantly mononuclear cell infiltrate. Masson's trichrome.

hepatitis may develop several years before the onset of frank diabetes.[272] In a study of 100 liver biopsies from morbidly obese patients it was noted that 36% had features of steatohepatitis and, in addition, that the liver injury, in these patients, correlated in severity with the degree of impaired glucose tolerance.[117] The lesion may sometimes be periportal, and is regarded as pre-cirrhotic although progression may be slow.[131] Collagenization of the space of Disse together with deposition of basement membrane components has been reported in both type I and type II diabetes[273,274] and it was suggested that this lesion might represent liver involvement as part of diabetic microangiopathy.[274]

Cirrhosis is two to three times more frequent in diabetics than in non-diabetics;[255,275] conversely, the frequency of diabetes in cirrhosis shows an increase of similar magnitude as compared with a normal population and, as already mentioned, more than 70% of patients with diabetes have glucose intolerance. Creutzfeldt and his colleagues[255] noted that the diabetes developed before the cirrhosis in 40% of patients, while in 30% the cirrhosis followed the onset of diabetes. There was an increased frequency of hepatitis in early series of diabetics,[276] presumed to be needle-transmitted serum hepatitis and therefore HBV or HCV. It now seems likely that the cirrhosis in diabetes is a sequel to non-alcoholic steatohepatitis. Furthermore, it is to be noted that progression to cirrhosis is not necessarily prevented by control of the diabetes.[114]

Miscellaneous features

There are case reports of liver-cell adenomas,[277] of nodular regenerative hyperplasia,[278] of xanthomatous neuropathy affecting unmyelinated nerve fibres in the hilum and in large portal tracts,[279] and of primary scleros-

ing cholangitis[280] occurring in patients with diabetes. Giant mitochondria, sometimes a feature of alcoholic liver disease, may also occur in diabetes.[281] In one personally studied case prominent giant mitochondria were present in the majority of hepatocytes in a type I diabetic presenting with ketoacidosis and who had gross hepatomegaly.

THE LIVER IN ENDOCRINE DISEASE

Diabetes mellitus has been dealt with in the preceeding section. The effects of gonadal steroids on the liver occur principally in relation to their therapeutic administration, and they have been reviewed elsewhere[243,282–285] and are dealt with in Chapters 15 and 16.

THYROID

The liver is an 'end-organ' in which thyroid hormones modify various hepatocellular synthetic activities and modulate bilirubin and bile acid metabolism; in turn the liver metabolizes these hormones and is the principal site for conversion of T4 to T3. The liver synthesizes the major thyroid-hormone-binding proteins.[286,287] Some thyroid hormones are conjugated as glucuronides and sulphates in the liver, and very small amounts of T3 and T4 are excreted in the bile. Altered thyroid hormone metabolism is found in a variety of acute and chronic liver diseases[286,288,289] and the serum levels of the hormone metabolites may reflect prognosis.[7,290] There is a well-recognized clinical association between autoimmune thyroid disease and primary biliary cirrhosis (see Ch. 12).

Hyperthyroidism. Abnormal liver function tests have been variously reported in from 15–75% of patients with hyperthyroidism.[291,292] Increased serum alkaline phosphatase is the most common abnormality; transaminases and bilirubin may also be increased but this usually resolves when patients become euthyroid. Unexplained clinical jaundice may sometimes develop, and although in early studies on fatal, thyrotoxic crisis cases it was a feature in 20% of patients, in some of these coincidental cardiac failure may have been contributory.[293]

In autopsy studies of patients dying of thyrotoxicosis and its complications, abnormalities were reported in the liver in a significant majority and comprised fatty liver, focal necrosis, venous congestion, parenchymal atrophy and cirrhosis.[294] In biopsy studies, however, only mild non-specific changes were found, comprising mild steatosis, reduced hepatocyte glycogen, cytoplasmic vacuolization, acinar inflammation and Kupffer cell hyperplasia, some nuclear irregularity and hyperchromatism and a minimal increase in portal tract inflammatory cells.[294–297] Ultrastructural studies have shown hypertrophy of the smooth endoplasmic reticulum, mitochondrial enlargement and glycogen depletion.[298]

Hypothyroidism. No constant or specific abnormalities of liver function tests have been reported.[286] There is impaired bile acid synthesis and, experimentally, a reduction in bile flow has been demonstrated due to a reduction in the bile salt-independent component of bile.[299] Increased serum bilirubin levels are common in severe myxoedema, and there is a single case report of cholestasis in association with hypothyroidism.[300]

There are occasional reports of ascites with accumulation of fluid of a high protein content, occurring in the absence of congestive cardiac failure and clearing in response to hormone replacement therapy.[301,302] Baker et al[302] reported concentric thickening of the walls of central veins, perivenular hepatocyte loss and perivenular fibrosis. In the author's experience of a similar case, the liver biopsy failed to show any specific abnormality. Ono & Ishizaki[303] reported a case of nodular regenerative hyperplasia in association with Hashimoto's disease.

In *congenital cretinism*, jaundice due to an unconjugated hyperbilirubinaemia may persist for several weeks, the mechanisms for an apparent failure of hepatocyte uptake being uncertain.[304]

ADRENAL CORTEX

Features of Cushing's syndrome, abdominal striae, facial mooning and acne, may develop in autoimmune hepatitis but without evident adrenal dysfunction.[305] Secondary hyperaldosteronism is a feature of hepatic decompensation (see Ch. 2). Steatosis is a frequent finding in Cushing's syndrome[306] and fatty liver develops after a four-week course of corticosteroid therapy. Fatal fat embolism, of presumed fatty liver origin, has been reported after corticosteroid treatment.[307,308]

Olsson et al[309] reported corticosteroid-responsive elevation of serum transaminases in four patients with Addison's disease; liver biopsy in one showed a lymphocytic infiltrate of the portal tracts. There is a case report of Addison's disease with hypertension and renal and hepatic microthrombosis in the primary antiphospholipid syndrome.[310]

PITUITARY

The interactions between the liver and the pituitary in health and disease have been reviewed in a number of studies.[287,289,311,312] Hepatomegaly is frequently found in acromegaly and is accompanied by increased excretion capacity, the mechanisms for which are uncertain.[313]

MISCELLANEOUS

Orloff reported a syndrome of hyperparathyroidism, cirrhosis and portocaval shunt.[314] Refractory ascites has been reported in POEMS syndrome,[315] in which there is polyneuropathy (P), organomegaly (O), endocrinopathy (E), M (M) protein band and skin (S) changes. In a case of Turner's syndrome, Ulissi & Ricci[316] reported hepatomegaly and the liver showed glandular transformation.

THE LIVER IN PREGNANCY

In the ensuing account the changes which occur in the liver in normal pregnancy and the liver diseases which are peculiar to pregnancy are outlined. In addition, liver disease may develop and complicate pregnancy, and, conversely, established liver diseases may be complicated by pregnancy; for an account of the effects of pregnancy on acute and chronic liver disease the reader is referred to medical and obstetrical texts and to some recent reviews.[317–321]

NORMAL PREGNANCY

In general, the liver functions normally in pregnancy.[322–324] There is no increase in liver size. Although total blood volume and cardiac output are increased by 50%, hepatic blood flow remains unchanged resulting, in the third trimester, in a relative decrease of 25–30% in the proportion of the cardiac output which passes through the liver.[325] Consequently, drugs that are cleared by the liver in a blood-flow-dependent manner have a reduced clearance late in pregnancy.

Conventional liver function tests are altered in the course of pregnancy and the changes are summarized in Table 17.4.[326–328] The crude increase in alkaline phosphatase is in part due to the placental isoenzyme, but the hepatic isoenzyme also increases; the level may remain elevated for four to six weeks post-partum.[328] The serum transaminases, γ-glutamyl transferase, 5-nucleotidase and the prothrombin time remain normal, and in suspected hepatic dysfunction during pregnancy these indices are of most diagnostic help.

Table 17.4 Liver function tests in normal pregnancy

Remain within normal range
    Serum transaminases
    Serum γ-glutamyl transferase
    Serum 5-nucleotidase
    Prothrombin time

Progressive increase
    Serum alkaline phosphatase — × 2–4
    Serum cholesterol — × 2
    Serum fibrinogen — × 1/2
    Bromsulphthalein dye retention — × 5

Progressive decrease
    Serum albumin — × 1/3
    Serum immunoglobulins — slight

Minor change and variable
    Serum bilirubin

Note: all changes maximal at term except for albumin and fibrinogen which change most in the first trimester.

Light microscopic examination of the liver shows minor non-specific changes. These have included cellular and nuclear pleomorphism, increased numbers of binucleate cells, steatosis, increased cellular and nuclear glycogen, mild reactive Kupffer-cell hyperplasia and some lymphocytic infiltration of portal tracts — features which, however, do not constitute a 'liver of pregnancy'. Electron microscopic examination shows features which are considered to be adaptive responses to the hormonal changes; they comprise proliferation of the smooth endoplasmic reticulum, giant mitochondria with increase in crystalline inclusions, and increased numbers of peroxisomes.[329,330]

LIVER DISEASE IN PREGNANCY

Liver disease in pregnancy has been the subject of a number of reviews.[318,319,321,326,327,331] The estimated frequency of jaundice in pregnancy is 1 per 1500 gestations,[326] and it has been subdivided into jaundice in pregnancy and jaundice of pregnancy. *Jaundice in pregnancy* includes any disease which is normally accompanied by icterus, and of these acute viral hepatitis is the most common (40% of all cases of jaundice during pregnancy). Various medical complications in pregnancy (10%) and large-duct obstruction (6%) also contribute significantly.

Jaundice of pregnancy comprises:

(i) recurrent intrahepatic cholestasis (discussed in chapter 11);
(ii) acute fatty liver of pregnancy;
(iii) jaundice in toxaemia of pregnancy;
(iv) a miscellaneous group associated with hyperemesis gravidarum, haemolytic and megaloblastic anaemias of pregnancy, and hydatidiform mole; and an unclassifiable group in which the jaundice is mild and no specific hepatic disease is identified.

Acute fatty liver of pregnancy

This was first defined by Sheehan in 1940,[332] who termed it obstetric acute yellow atrophy; his classic description of the clinical and histological features has not been improved upon. The clinical features are reviewed in a number of papers.[317,333–341] It is a rare disease, but the diagnosis is now being made earlier, suggesting that it may be more common than previously thought.

The large majority of patients are primigravidae, frequently there is a twin pregnancy, the disease occurs at any age in the child-bearing period, and male births are more common than female. Characteristically, it develops in the last 10 weeks and usually in the last 4 weeks of pregnancy. After a mild prodromal illness, severe vomiting and jaundice develop in a few days with rapidly progres-

sive fulminant hepatic failure. Many patients have hypertension and proteinuria suggesting toxaemia of pregnancy, a differential diagnosis which has to be considered.[336,342] Ultrasonography[343] and computed tomography (CT)[344] are useful non-invasive methods of confirming the presence of fatty liver.

Biochemically, the hyperbilirubinaemia is moderate, 100 μmol/l (6 mg/100 ml); there is mild elevation of the transaminases, ~200 iu/l; the prothrombin time is prolonged to 2–4 times normal; hypoglycaemia may be marked and is a contributory factor in the early coma. Serum immunoglobulins are not increased and this contrasts with the findings in acute hepatitis; serum amylase and lipase may be elevated because of an associated pancreatitis.[237] The presence of circulating normoblasts, noted by Sheehan,[345] has been emphasized by Burroughs et al[336] who found them in the blood film in 10 of 11 patients.

The mortality rate for both mother and fetus was as high as 80–85% in earlier series. However, Pockros and his colleagues[338] reported a maternal mortality of 2/18 (11%) and a fetal mortality of 5/20 (25%), an improved survival which they attributed to improved supportive therapy. Early diagnosis and delivery and the occurrence of milder forms of the disease improve the outlook for mother and child.[338,346–348] Liver transplantation has been carried out in two patients.[349,350] In surviving cases there is no report of progression to chronic liver disease and subsequent uncomplicated pregnancy has been reported.[336,348,351–354] There are two case reports of recurrent fatty liver of pregnancy,[355,356] and one case in which intrahepatic cholestasis of pregnancy was later complicated by acute fatty liver of pregnancy.[357]

Macroscopically, the liver is usually smaller than normal and has a distinctive pale yellow colour. Sheehan[332] wrote '...there was a gross fatty change affecting the entire lobule except a sharply defined rim of normal cells around the portal tracts. The affected cells were bloated by a fine foam of tiny white vacuoles throughout the cytoplasm so that they resembled the cells of suprarenal cortex. The nuclei were normal and there was an entire absence of necrobiotic change.' These features are shown in Figure 17.10. In some cases the steatosis may be diffuse without periportal sparing.[336] Canalicular and hepatocellular bilirubinostasis are present. There is Kupffercell hyperplasia, aggregates of ceroid-laden macrophages are conspicuous, and there is usually only a mild, predominantly mononuclear cell infiltrate of the parenchyma and portal tracts, sometimes with a number of eosinophils and occasional plasma cells. Intrasinusoidal fibrin deposits have been reported, occasionally associated with microhaemorrhages.[336]

The reduced liver weight at autopsy despite the presence of steatosis indicates there has been liver-cell loss,[336,358] and morphologically this is best seen with a

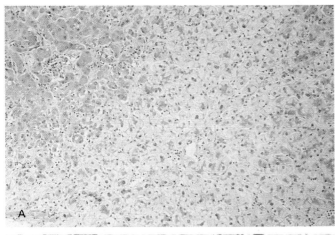

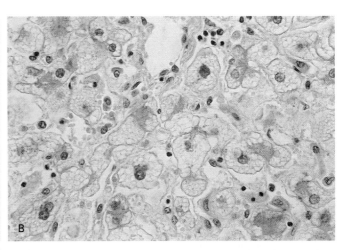

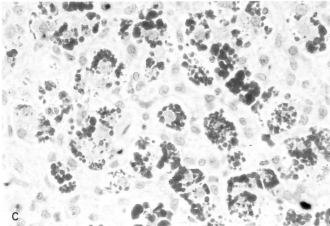

Fig. 17.10 Acute fatty liver of pregnancy (a) Microvesicular steatosis involving acinar zones 2 and 3. H & E. (b) At a higher power note the swollen hepatocytes and the microvesicular fatty accumulation, H & E, shown in (c) with an oil red O stain.

reticulin stain. Joske et al[359] noted mid-zonal necrosis in one case. Serial biopsies in survivors show progressive disappearance of fat from the periportal to the perivenular zone[352] and, in our experience, this happens within days of parturition. Mild steatosis was reported in two of five fetal livers examined.[326]

Ultrastructurally[336,360] the fat is not membrane bound; there is dilatation of the rough endoplasmic reticulum and some cells show cytoplasmic degeneration with autophagic vacuoles; the mitochondria show considerable variation in size and shape (Fig. 17.11).

Extrahepatic complications include gastrointestinal haemorrhage, renal failure, sometimes with fatty infiltration of renal tubules,[361] intravascular haemolysis,[359] pancreatitis and peri-pancreatic bleeding[237,339] and disseminated intravascular coagulation.[338,362] The coagulation defect accounts for many of the complications, and it may be temporarily aggravated by delivery.[338]

The aetiology of acute fatty liver of pregnancy is not known. Sherlock[98] drew attention to the occurrence of microvesicular steatosis in a number of other conditions (for review see Mabie 1992[341]). It is uncertain, however, whether the characteristic liver lesion in these various disorders is the result of a common mechanism, e.g. inhibition of apoprotein synthesis with consequent impaired removal of lipid from the liver, or whether the pathogenesis is different in each. As previously mentioned, some authors have suggested that acute fatty liver of pregnancy is part of the spectrum of pre-eclampsia.[317,339] Minakami et al[363] produced evidence supportive of this, finding microvesicular steatosis in all 41 liver biopsies from cases of pre-eclampsia. However, Ishak and Rolfes[339,342] were of the opinion that there was no similarity between acute fatty liver and the liver changes in pre-eclampsia and eclampsia, a view to which the present authors also subscribe.

The liver in toxaemia of pregnancy

If jaundice occurs in the early stages of toxaemia of pregnancy it is usually haemolytic in type. Haemmerli,[326] in his review of 450 cases of jaundice during pregnancy, attributed 21 to toxaemia, an incidence of just under 5%. The jaundice is usually mild with serum bilirubin levels of less than 100 μmol/l (5.8 mg/dl). Occasional cases may present with severe jaundice.[364,365] The serum alkaline phosphatase is also abnormally elevated and transaminase levels may be in the range of 100–1000 iu/l.

The overall incidence of liver dysfunction in toxaemia is less than 50%.[326] In Barron's[366] experience pre-eclampsia is the commonest cause of hepatic tenderness and disturbed liver function tests in pregnancy, hepatic involvement also being an indicator of severe maternal disease. Liver biopsy has been normal in many jaundiced patients or may show only mild non-specific reactive changes with some hepatocellular pleomorphism.[367] Arias & Marchella-Jimenez[368] reported intrasinusoidal fibrin deposition in all of their series of 12 biopsies, a pattern similar to that which affects renal glomerular capillaries.

In severe and fatal cases the distinctive liver lesion comprises periportal intrasinusoidal fibrin deposition with

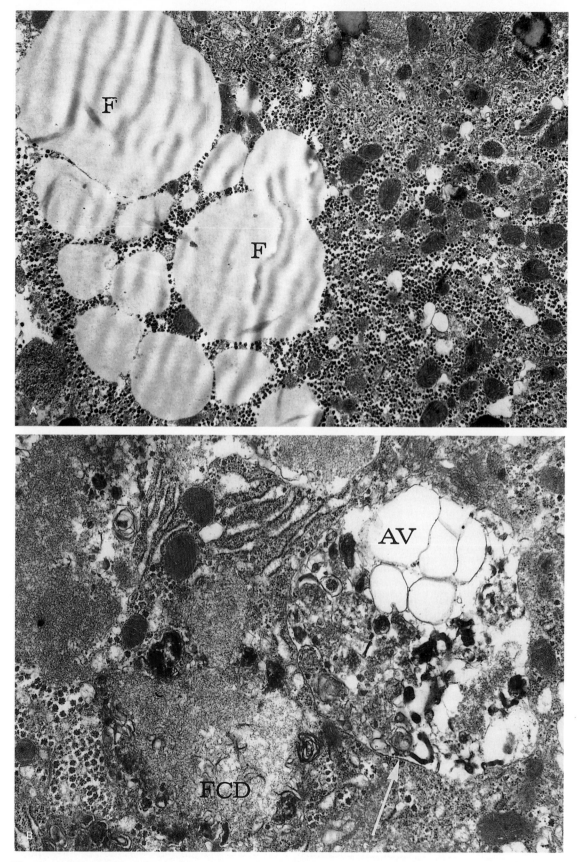

Fig. 17.11 Acute fatty liver of pregnancy. (a) Electron micrograph showing non-membrane-bound fat vacuoles (F) containing slightly osmiophilic material. × 9000. (b) Electron micrograph showing fibrillar material in an area of focal cytoplasmic degeneration (FCD) and a single membrane-bound autophagic vacuole (AV). × 22 500. Reprinted with permission from the article by Burroughs et al[336]

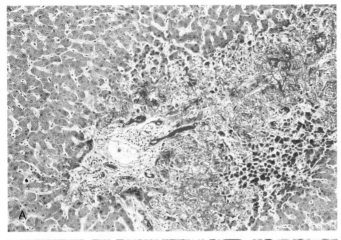

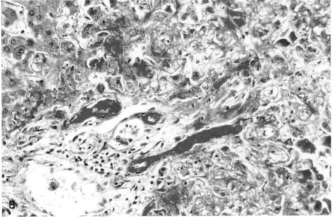

Fig. 17.12 Liver in toxaemia of pregnancy. (a) Area of periportal necrosis with intrasinusoidal fibrin deposition. (b) Hepatic arterioles showing plasmatic vasculosis; intrasinusoidal fibrin deposition is also present. Masson's trichrome.

irregular areas of liver-cell necrosis exciting a minimal inflammatory reaction (Fig. 17.12a). The hepatic arteries and arterioles in the adjacent portal tract show plasmatic vasculosis with seepage of fibrin into and through their walls (Fig. 17.12b). The vascular changes are similar to those occurring in other organs in severe toxaemia and are the result of endothelial cell damage and activation of intravascular coagulation. Sheehan[332] found periportal lesions in 90% of fatal cases, but Antia et al[367] reported them in only 5 of 15 cases.

HELLP syndrome

It is estimated that 2–12% of patients with toxaemia of pregnancy develop the HELLP syndrome which comprises haemolysis (H), elevated liver enzymes (EL) and a low platelet count (LP).[369] It occurs predominantly in multiparous women over 25 years old. Some cases occur a few hours to six days post-partum.[370] Maternal complications include placental abruption, acute renal failure and hepatic rupture, with a maternal mortality rate of 3%.

Recurrence of the syndrome has been reported in only one instance.[371]

There is continuing controversy and confusion as to whether HELLP is a variation of toxaemia of pregnancy or whether it represents a mild form of disseminated intravascular coagulation.[372] The liver biopsy shows features of a non-specific reactive hepatitis with a mild portal tract chronic inflammatory cell infiltrate. However, in some cases periportal or focal parenchymal necrosis with a fibrin exudate has been reported, similar to that described in eclampsia. Intrahepatic haemorrhage and subcapsular haematomas with rupture may occur, and we have seen one case of hepatic infarction.[370]

Miscellaneous liver lesions in pregnancy

Hyperemesis gravidarum. This condition accounted for jaundice in 6% of Haemmerli's cases.[326] When jaundice occurs in hyperemesis gravidarum it is usually mild[373,374] but there may be marked elevation of transaminases.[373] Histological examination of the liver in a small number of cases showed non-specific reactive changes.[332,375,376]

Spontaneous rupture of the liver has now been reported in over 100 cases and there have been recent extended reviews.[377,378] The clinical presentation is usually acute with profound collapse, sometimes out of proportion to the amount of blood in the peritoneal cavity.[379] The rupture is thought to occur from subcapsular haematomas and there may be a history of minor trauma. These haematomas may be found without peritoneal leakage,[380] and they are usually sharply circumscribed. In a case examined by one of the authors, focal intrahepatic haemorrhages were present together with larger areas of haemorrhage immediately subcapsular. The areas of haemorrhage were sharply circumscribed and, within them, periportal areas showed appearances closely resembling those seen in cases of fatal toxaemia.

Spontaneous rupture occurs most commonly in association with toxaemia and in the last trimester of pregnancy. In 15–20% of cases there is no associated hypertension and it sometimes occurs immediately post-partum.

'Liver pregnancy'. A number of extra-uterine pregnancies with placental attachment to the liver are recorded,[381–387] and in one of these the pregnancy went to term but with eventual maternal and fetal death.[383]

THE LIVER IN HAEMATOLOGICAL AND LYMPHORETICULAR DISEASES

Liver involvement in childhood leukaemia, the histiocytoses and the haemophagocytic syndromes is discussed in Chapter 3.

ANAEMIAS

Fatty liver is a frequent accompaniment of anaemia from any cause. In the haemolytic anaemias and in refractory anaemias, secondary iron overload may develop (see Ch. 5). The increased incidence of cholelithiasis in haemolytic syndromes predisposes to biliary obstruction. Morphological changes in *sickle cell anaemia* are common, resulting from a combination of anoxia and impaired sinusoidal blood flow; secondary iron overload is also present.[388-394] Aggregations of red cells and thrombi are prominent in the perivenular zones producing sinusoidal congestion, which in addition, and in contrast to passive venous congestion, may become equally pronounced in all acinar zones. Hepatic vein thrombosis may occur.[395] Crescent-shaped red cells can be readily identified in the sinusoids and in Kupffer cells, which also contain haemosiderin and ceroid pigment (Fig. 17.13). Ultrastructural studies showed collagenization in the space of Disse.[391] In patients dying in sickle cell crisis the liver is enlarged and purplish in colour and, in addition to the severe sinusoidal distension and obstruction, focal liver-cell necrosis may be a prominent feature. Focal nodular hyperplasia, possibly related to local ischaemia, has been reported in children[396] and there is a case report of an hepatic biloma.[397]

Spherocytes in *congenital spherocytosis* and acanthocytes in *abetalipoproteinaemia*[398] may also be recognized within sinusoids on light microscopy.

Hepatic vein, splenic vein and portal vein thrombosis have been reported in patients with *paroxysmal nocturnal haemoglobinuria*.[399,400]

LEUKAEMIAS

Hepatic involvement in acute leukaemia is not usually a significant clinical feature but hepatomegaly and cho-lestasis may occur. In *acute lymphoblastic leukaemia* the infiltrate is usually in the portal tracts whereas both portal tracts and sinusoids are involved in acute myeloid leukaemia. Massive blastic infiltration of the liver producing fulminant liver failure, probably secondary to hepatocellular ischaemia, has been reported in acute leukaemia and also in patients with non-Hodgkin's lymphomas.[401-405]

In *hairy cell leukaemia*, clinical hepatomegaly is present in 30–40% of patients; there may be mild disturbances of liver function tests but infiltration of the liver, both sinusoidal and portal tract, is present in all cases and may produce a characteristic lesion.[406,407] The sinusoidal infiltrate is linear (Fig. 17.14a); there may be peliosis-like lesions, congestion and occasionally granulomas.[408] Nanba et al[409] reported splenic 'pseudo-sinuses' in all of 14 patients and also noted hepatic 'angiomatous lesions' in 3 of 5 liver biopsies. Roquet et al[410] found these angiomatous lesions in 9 of 14 patients. They comprise dilated blood-filled spaces lined by the tumour cells (Fig. 17.14b) and to the walls of which the tumour cells are attached. The lesions are multifocal, may involve portal tracts and

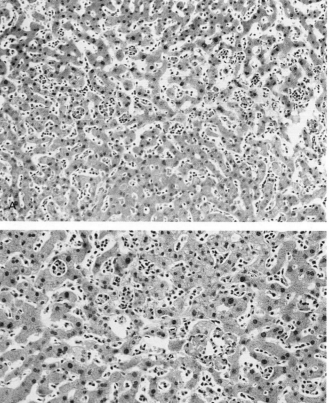

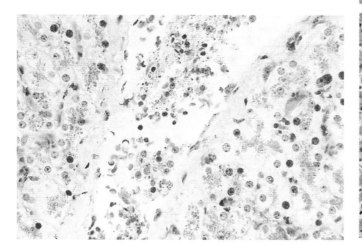

Fig. 17.13 Liver in sickle cell anaemia. Note the sickled red cells in the hepatic vein and congested sinusoids: there is also abundant haemosiderin in perivenular hepatocytes and Kupffer cells. MSB

Fig. 17.14 Liver in hairy cell leukaemia. (a) Sinusoidal dilatation and diffuse intrasinusoidal infiltration by leukaemic cells. (b) Angiomatous lesions comprising congested sinusoids surrounded by a ring of leukaemic cells. H & E. Courtesy of Dr H Tavadia.

sometimes occur in clusters; they resemble haemangiomas or peliosis hepatis. The leukaemic cells have a clear cytoplasm and may be easily overlooked in haematoxylin and eosin-stained sections but are identified by their content of tartrate-resistant acid phosphatase[406,411] or by immunohistochemical methods.[412]

An ultrastructural study of the peliotic lesions demonstrated loss of continuity of sinusoidal lining cells with the hairy cells coming into direct contact with hepatocytes and with extravasation of blood into the space of Disse.[407] These changes resemble those seen in peliosis hepatis[413] and Zafrani and his colleagues suggested that the hairy cells caused endothelial damage.

In *chronic lymphoblastic leukaemias*, liver dysfunction is a late clinical feature and the hepatic infiltrate is predominantly within portal tracts. Nodular regenerative hyperplasia with portal hypertension has been reported.[414] More than 50% of patients with *chronic myeloid leukaemia* have clinical hepatomegaly on presentation and in acute blastic crises sinusoidal infiltration by leukaemic cells is present.

Chronic liver disease, affecting over 65% of children with leukaemias in long-term remission from acute leukaemia, was reported by Locasiulli et al.[415] Some of this was probably drug-related (see Ch. 15), but the authors noted that all of 20 children who had had acute hepatitis developed chronic liver disease. Conversely, there are sporadic reports of a beneficial effect of acute hepatitis in patients with various forms of leukaemia.[416–418]

CHRONIC MYELOPROLIFERATIVE DISORDERS AND MYELODYSPLASTIC SYNDROMES

These myeloproliferating disorders comprise primary polycythaemia (polycythaemia rubra vera), myelofibrosis and essential thrombocythaemia. The hepatic complications in these disorders comprise: (i) Budd–Chiari syndrome; (ii) non-cirrhotic portal hypertension which may develop because of perisinusoidal fibrosis, hepatic infiltration and increased blood flow,[419] nodular regenerative hyperplasia or portal vein thrombosis; (iii) extramedullary haemopoiesis and sinusoidal dilation; (iv) haemosiderosis; and (v) viral and drug-induced hepatitis.

Extramedullary haemopoiesis may be found in the liver, and is usually a feature in over 90% of patients with myelofibrosis.[420–422] Histologically (Fig. 17.15), pleomorphic clumps of erythroid and myeloid precursors together with megakaryocytes are present in the sinusoids and the space of Disse, and portal tract involvement develops as a late feature. In some cases megakaryocytes may be found on their own.[423] The pleomorphism helps to distinguish extramedullary haemopoiesis from the hepatic infiltration in leukaemia, infectious mononucleosis, Felty's syndrome and the tropical splenomegaly syndrome.[423] Extramedullary haemopoiesis is a normal feature in the fetal

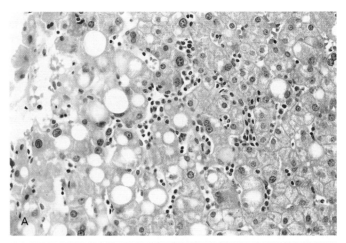

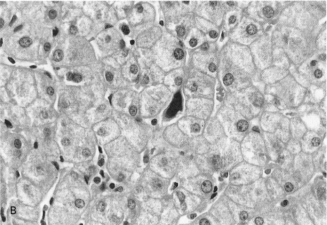

Fig. 17.15 Extramedullary haemopoiesis in the liver. (a) Pleomorphic intrasinusoidal infiltrate and (b) megakaryocyte. H & E.

liver and in the neonatal liver up to 5 weeks of age. It may persist for longer in the presence of neonatal hepatitis or anaemia from any cause. In the adult it may also occur in aplastic anaemia and in a variety of so-called marrow-replacement syndromes including tumour metastases myelomatosis, osteopetrosis and others.

The sinusoidal dilatation found in 50% of patients with myelofibrosis, is thought to be due to obstruction by the extramedullary haemopoiesis.[422] Perisinusoidal fibrosis[424–426] has been attributed to perisinusoidal cell activation by platelet-derived growth factor or other cytokines released by megakaryocytes and activated macrophages.[425,426]

Myelodysplastic syndromes. Haemosiderosis is frequent in the refractory and sideroblastic anaemia categories, and leukaemic infiltration develops when blast transformation occurs.

MYELOMATOSIS

Portal tract and sinusoidal infiltration by extramedullary myeloma deposits is not uncommon[427] and may comprise large focal deposits.[428] In a series of 64 autopsies, hepatic involvement was seen in 40% and in the absence of plasma cell leukaemia.[429]

In *Waldenström's macroglobulinaemia* portal hypertension due to hepatic infiltration by tumour cells[430] and due to nodular regenerative hyperplasia has been reported;[431] macroglobulin deposition in the space of Disse has been observed by the authors, and light chain deposition with peliosis hepatis and nodular regenerative hyperplasia has also been reported in one patient (p. 746).[432]

LYMPHORETICULAR NEOPLASMS

These are subdivided into Hodgkin's disease and non-Hodgkin's lymphoma. The former is always a secondary tumour in the liver but, in addition, a number of hepatic lesions may occur in the absence of hepatic involvement. Primary non-Hodgkin's lymphoma of the liver is discussed in chapter 16. Imaging techniques, in particular CT scanning, and changes in patient management have meant that staging laparotomy with liver biopsy is now less frequently carried out in these diseases.[433,434] Hodgkin's disease has not been reported as primary in the liver.

Hodgkin's disease

Clinical manifestations of hepatic involvement include fever, hepatomegaly and jaundice. Severe cholestatic hepatitis with liver failure and widespread liver involvement by Hodgkin's disease has been reported[435] and occasional patients present with fulminant liver disease.[436]

Liver involvement in Hodgkin's disease is found in about 55% of patients at autopsy.[434] The frequency of diagnostic hepatic lesions on liver biopsy ranges from 5–10% depending on whether percutaneous needle biopsy or wedge biopsy at laparotomy has been examined.[437–439] Deposits in the liver vary considerably in size, in some instances showing a diffuse distribution of uniform small nodules, whilst in others large masses or a combination of these patterns may be present. Hepatic involvement is more common in the lymphocyte depletion and mixed cellularity subtypes and, with the exception of very rare cases,[440,441] has not been found in the absence of splenic involvement.[438,442] Where splenic enlargement was massive, liver involvement was present in 50% of the patients.[434]

Microscopically, the diagnosis is often straightforward, but problems arise in the interpretation of possible early hepatic involvement. Tumour deposits almost invariably involve portal tracts[433] and caution should be exercised in interpreting infiltrates confined to the parenchyma. Non-specific portal tract inflammation — comprising lymphocytes, plasma cells and eosinophils — may frequently be found. Reed–Sternberg cells should be identified before making a definite diagnosis and atypical histiocytes should

be regarded only as suggestive evidence.[439,443] Chronic inflammatory cell infiltration of portal tracts must not be regarded as evidence of liver involvement.[433,444] In our experience mitotic activity within the portal tract infiltration and perivascular 'cushioning' by portal tract lymphoid aggregates should be regarded with suspicion. The bile ducts may be obliterated by the neoplastic cells which may sometimes strikingly surround and extend into the duct epithelium.[435,445] Parenchymal lymphoid aggregates (Fig. 17.16a), sometimes with cytological atypia, may be found in 10% of biopsies from staging laparotomies.[446]

Epithelioid cell granulomas are found in 8–12% of patients.[437,447] They tend to occur in portal tracts, but may also involve the parenchyma and may be diffusely present (Fig. 17.16b–d). Similar granulomas may be found in bone marrow, lymph nodes and in spleen.[448] In some instances they are related to previous lymphangiography,[449] and lipid deposits may be present; in the others the aetiology is uncertain but is possibly related to the altered immunity in patients with Hodgkin's disease.[438,449] They should not be regarded as evidence of organ involvement by Hodgkin's disease, but they have been associated with a better clinical prognosis.[448] In one patient in clinical relapse, caseating hepatic granulomas were found but no causal organism was isolated.[450]

Peliosis hepatis[451] and sinusoidal dilatation (Fig. 17.16e) involving acinar zones 2 and 3[452–454] have been reported in patients who were not receiving androgenic steroids. The frequency of sinusoidal dilatation in these studies ranged from 40–50% and its presence did not correlate with hepatic involvement or with histological type. Bain and his colleagues[453] noted that the sinusoidal dilatation was present concurrently with clinical relapse, while Bruguera et al[454] noted its association with the presence of systemic symptoms.

Clinical jaundice develops in up to 15% of patients with Hodgkin's disease. It may be mild and of a haemolytic nature, may be obstructive and severe when there are extensive hepatic metastases, or may be treatment related.[455] A number of cases of unexplained intrahepatic cholestasis have been reported[455,456] (see Ch. 13) and Lieberman suggested that in 25% of patients the jaundice was unexplained.[455] Hubscher and his colleagues[457] have recently reported three patients with intrahepatic cholestasis in whom liver biopsy showed loss of intrahepatic bile ducts. They suggested that a vanishing bile-duct syndrome was a possible explanation for the intrahepatic cholestasis. We have seen similar cases (Fig. 17.16f). There is a recent report of three patients with primary sclerosing cholangitis in whom Hodgkin's disease developed.[458]

Non-Hodgkin's lymphoma

Macroscopic liver involvement in generalized non-Hodgkin's lymphoma occurs at autopsy with about the

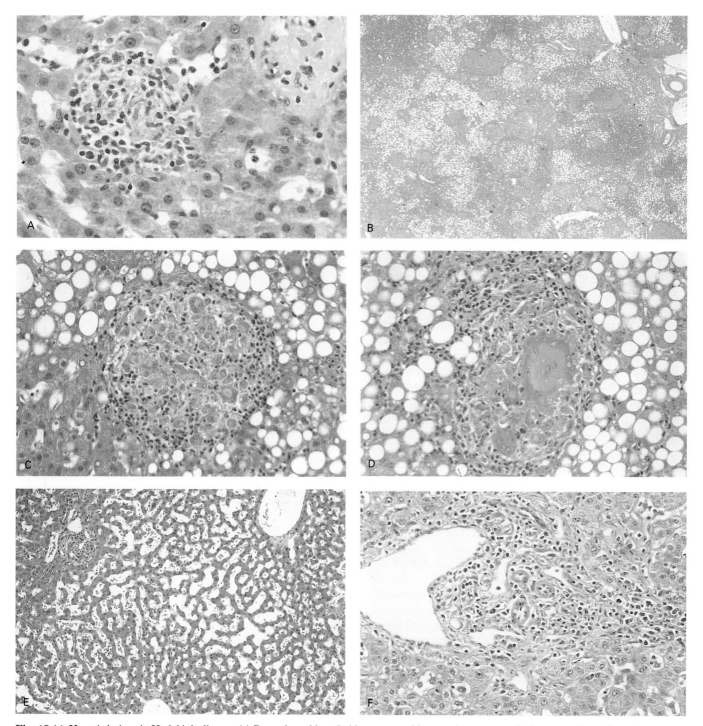

Fig. 17.16 Hepatic lesions in Hodgkin's disease. (a) Parenchymal lymphoid aggregate: this comprises some atypical mononuclear cells and lymphocytes but there are no Reed–Sternberg cells; (b) diffuse granulomatous involvement and fatty liver but with no tumour deposits; these granulomas showed variegated appearances (c and d). (e) Sinusoidal dilatation involving zones 2 and 3. (f) Cholestatic syndrome in a middle-aged male; there is a diffuse chronic inflammatory cell infiltrate of the portal tract in which no bile duct can be identified. H & E.

same frequency as Hodgkin's disease — 52% in the experience of Kim et al.[434] The liver is the organ most commonly involved after lymph nodes, spleen and bone marrow. Liver involvement was found in 15–20% of biopsies undertaken for staging laparotomy[433] and was

almost invariably associated with clinical hepatomegaly and splenic involvement.

The clinico-pathological correlations in the non-Hodgkin's lymphomas are not so well defined as in Hodgkin's disease, largely because of the difficulties arising from the problems of classification. Epithelioid cell granulomas occur in about 10% of ceses and may sometimes be extensive;[459,460] their presence does not indicate hepatic involvement by tumour. Jaundice may occur in the absence of intrahepatic metastases.[461] Patients with concurrent cirrhosis and non-Hodgkin's lymphoma have been reported[462]; in some the cirrhosis was complicated by hepatocellular carcinoma.[463]

B-cell lymphomas. The better differentiated low grade lymphocytic and follicular lymphomas and lymphoid leukaemias tend to produce multiple small nodular deposits, predominantly in portal tracts and sometimes with sinusoidal permeation, whereas the less well differentiated high grade lymphomas produce large irregular deposits which destructively involve both portal tracts and parenchyma. The microscopic features in the liver usually resemble those in involved lymph nodes, although regional and organ diversity in histological appearances is well recognized.[433,439] The differential diagnosis from non-specific inflammation depends on the cytological features, the more extensive, total or near-total involvement of portal tracts, and its tendency to extend beyond the portal tracts and spill over into the periportal parenchyma.[423,434] We have seen lympho-epithelial lesions of the bile ducts in one case. True follicle formation may very occasionally be seen in follicular lymphomas.[439] Immunophenotyping with the demonstration of light chain restriction will establish a diagnosis of malignancy.[464]

In Burkitt's lymphoma, hepatic depostis have been reported in 50–70% of cases,[465,466] sometimes with predominant liver involvement and sometimes with subcapsular involvement only, suggesting direct spread from the peritoneum.

T-cell lymphomas. In peripheral T-cell lymphoma liver involvement is present in about 50% of patients[439] and patients may sometimes present with liver disease.[467] In addition to focal portal tract and parenchymal involvement (Fig. 17.17) there may sometimes be a predominant pattern of intrasinusoidal permeation. In adult T-cell leukaemia the liver infiltrate is usually sinusoidal.[468]

In tropical splenomegaly and non-tropical idiopathic splenomegaly, intrasinusoidal permeation by mononuclear cells is present. The infiltrate in the tropical form is T-cell and there may also be portal fibrosis.[469] In the non-tropical form this pattern of liver involvement was seen in patients who subsequently developed lymphoma.[470] Sandilands et al[471] reported a patient in whom splenomegaly with hepatic sinusoidal lymphocyte infiltration antedated by years a frank leukaemic phase and, at which time, the liver showed a diffuse pattern of perisinusoidal fibrosis. A number of similar cases have now been reported[472,473]: in the case described by Kruskall et al[473] the leukaemia was of T-helper cell type and there was an autoimmune neutropenia.

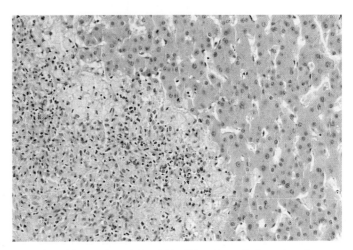

Fig. 17.17 Metastatic peripheral T-cell lymphoma in liver; there is a granulomatoid appearance to the tumour deposit and the hepatocytes at the parenchymal tumour interface show a vacuolated appearance. H & E. Courtesy of Dr R A Burnett.

Hepatic involvement has been reported in *Sezary's syndrome*[474] and in *mycosis fungoides* both in biopsy material and also in 17 of a series of 45 patients examined post-mortem.[475,476] In *angiocentric lymphomas*, focal intrahepatic deposits and intrasinusoidal infiltration may be seen, sometimes accompanied by Kupffer-cell erythrophagocytosis.[439] Liver involvement has also been reported in *angioimmunoblastic lymphademopathy*[439] and there is a case report in which the liver showed nodular regenerative hyperplasia, peliosis hepatic and perisinusoidal fibrosis.[477]

MISCELLANEOUS HAEMATOLOGICAL DISEASES WITH LIVER INVOLVEMENT

Thrombocytopenic purpura

Perisinusoidal fibrosis was reported in 10 patients undergoing splenectomy for thrombocytopenic purpura, in 8 of whom the disease was idiopathic.[478] It was postulated that platelet-derived growth factor and activated macrophages were causal factors in producing the fibrosis, analogous to the similar lesion which has been reported in myelofibrosis.[423–425] Phagocytosis of platelets by Kupffer cells may be seen in autoimmune thrombocytopenia.[479]

Hypereosinophilic syndrome

Chronic active hepatitis has been described in five patients with idiopathic hypereosinophilic syndrome.[480,481] In their patient, Foong et al[481] demonstrated activated eosinophils in a liver biopsy, with deposition of eosinophil major basic protein in areas of hepatocyte injury. Fauci et al[482] noted that 30% of patients with the hypereosinophilic syndrome demonstrated mild hepatomegaly and/or minor distrub-

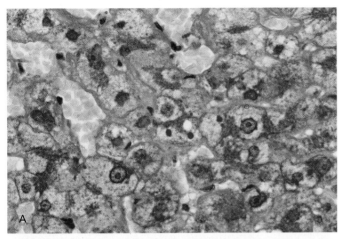

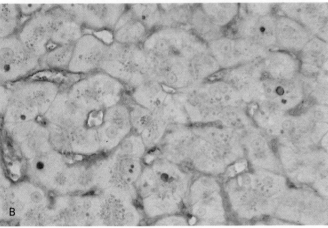

Fig. 17.18 Complement protein accumulation in hepatocytes. (a) Intracytoplasmic globular inclusions showing an intense red staining on a Masson's trichrome. (b) They contain the C4 component of complement and were also weakly positive for C3; there is some perisinusoidal positivity. Immunoperoxidase stain.

ances of liver function tests; sinusoidal congestion, hepatitis and periportal inflammation were present in some cases.

Familial hypofibrinogenaemia/dysfibrinogenaemia

Familial cases of hypofibrinogenaemia have been reported in which hepatocytes contain intracytoplasmic PAS-negative globular inclusions of fibrinogen.[483–485] Similar perivenular globular inclusions have been shown to contain C3 and C4 components of complement[486,487] (Fig. 17.18); these patients had normal serum complement levels. These disorders have now been categorized as endoplasmic reticulum storage diseases (p. 143)

THE LIVER IN THE RHEUMATOID AND CONNECTIVE TISSUE DISEASES

The liver is rarely affected in the collagen diseases.[488,489] With the exception of secondary amyloidosis (type AA), now most commonly seen in rheumatoid

arthritis, evidence for any significant hepatic dysfunction is scant and few specific morphological abnormalities have been described. A generalized necrotizing arteritis may complicate many of the rheumatoid and connective tissue diseases and hepatic involvement may be part of this; nodular regenerative hyperplasia,[431] haematoma[490] and spontaneous hepatic rupture may then develop.[491–493] Many of the therapeutic agents used in the rheumatoid and connective tissue diseases are potentially hepatotoxic and may be responsible for some of the hepatic abnormalities seen in these conditions (see Ch. 15).

RHEUMATOID DISEASES

Rheumatoid arthritis (RA). Based on the evidence provided by the frequency of abnormal liver function tests in RA, in particular raised serum alkaline phosphatase levels, Kendall et al postulated the existence of a 'rheumatoid liver'.[494,495] Increased serum levels of γ-glutamyl-transpeptidase and alkaline phosphatase have been reported in a number of studies, increased levels being found in up to 80% of patients in some series.[496–499] The liver isoenzyme of alkaline phosphatase is predominantly raised.[496] The increases in enzyme levels have been correlated with the clinical activity of RA.[11,13] However, while clinical or scintigraphic evidence of hepatomegaly may be found in 10–20% of patients,[500,501] other clinical signs of chronic liver disease are usually lacking. Liver biopsy and autopsy studies have not revealed any consistent or specific findings, the main abnormalities being non-specific reactive hepatitis, steatosis and minimal portal fibrosis;[502 – 506] chronic active hepatitis and sinusoidal dilatation have occasionally been reported.[507,508] Diseases such as primary biliary cirrhosis or α₁-antitrypsin deficiency may occur coincidentally with RA.[509,510]

Nodular regenerative hyperplasia (Fig. 17.19a) frequently associated with Felty's syndrome, has been reported in a small number of patients with RA[511–513] and its pathogenesis has been associated with rheumatoid vasculitis.[513] Spontaneous rupture of the liver may complicate the vasculitis.[492,493] There is a single case report of rheumatoid nodules in the liver[514] (Fig. 17.19b).

Hepatic fibrosis has been described in RA patients treated with methotrexate.[515] There is evidence of a correlation between the cumulative dose of the drug and increased hepatic collagen, although this relationship has been questioned by Hall et al.[516] In a study by Landas and co-workers, lipogranulomas were found in the livers of 56% of their patients with severe RA.[517] The lesions contained pigment which was shown by spectroscopy to be gold particles, thought to be related to therapy.

Sjögren's syndrome. There is a strong association between the sicca complex and RA. Hepatomegaly and abnormal liver function tests are documented in approximately one quarter of patients with Sjögren's syn-

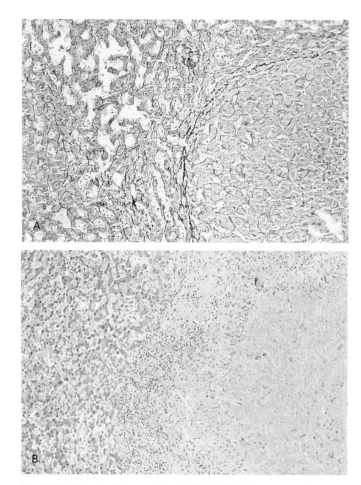

Fig. 17.19 Liver in rheumatoid arthritis. (a) Nodular regenerative hyperplasia in a patient with Felty's syndrome. Gordon & Sweet's reticulin stain. (b) Rheumatoid nodule: this is from the case reported by Smits & Kooijman.[514] Courtesy of Dr Carole D Kooijman.

drome.[500,518] As with RA, there are no consistent changes seen in liver biopsies. In most cases non-specific reactive changes are found.[500] A form of Sjögren's syndrome, which clinically and immunopathologically resembles that associated with rheumatoid arthritis, is seen in patients with primary biliary cirrhosis;[519] clinical symptoms of the sicca complex occur in almost 50% of patients and histological changes diagnostic of Sjögren's syndrome in over 25% — features which suggest that there may be an overlap between the two conditions. Furthermore, an earlier study demonstrated antimitochondrial antibodies in 11% of patients with Sjögren's disease, although this was based on an immunofluorescent test and PBC-specific AMAs were not sought.[500] Montefusco et al[520] reported an association between sclerosing cholangitis, chronic pancreatitis and Sjögren's syndrome.

In *Felty's syndrome*, in which rheumatoid arthritis is accompanied by splenomegaly and neutropenia, mononuclear sinusoidal infiltration may occur[521,522] and the syndrome is frequently complicated by portal hypertension associated with nodular regenerative hyperplasia.[523–526] In

their review of 26 patients with Felty's syndrome and evidence of hepatic dysfunction, Blendis et al[523] reported that 13 had portal hypertension with oesophageal varices, and in 9 of these there was histological evidence of nodular regenerative hyperplasia. On the basis of a further prospective study, Blendis and his colleagues reported that abnormalities of liver architecture may develop in two-thirds of patients with Felty's syndrome and, in at least half of these, nodular regenerative hyperplasia and portal hypertension will be present.[524] The pathogenesis of nodular regenerative hyperplasia in RA and Felty's syndrome is not fully established but recent evidence suggests that rheumatoid vasculitis affecting intrahepatic arterial radicles may play a role[431,513,527] (see also Ch. 15).

Juvenile rheumatoid arthritis (Still's disease). Minor abnormalities of liver function tests have been noted in patients with the febrile systemic type of Still's disease but, in the small number of liver biopsies examined, only non-specific reactive changes were found.[528,529] The hepatic manifestations of the adult onset form of Still's disease (sero-negative arthritis) are similar, with hepatomegaly and raised transaminases being found in a third of patients.[530] However, life-threatening hepatic failure, possibly drug induced, has been noted in three instances with a fatal outcome in one.[530,531]

CONNECTIVE TISSUE DISEASES

Systemic lupus erythematosus (SLE). Dubois et al[532] reported jaundice of a predominantly haemolytic type in 3.8% of 520 patients, and death from hepatic failure of unspecified aetiology in 4% of 249 patients with SLE. Runyon et al,[533] in a retrospective survey of 206 cases, found severe chronic liver disease in 9 (4.4%); these included cirrhosis, chronic active hepatitis and primary biliary cirrhosis. In contrast, Gibson & Myers[534] found no significant liver disease in their series of 81 patients, and in another prospective study, no clinical or biochemical abnormalities of liver function were found in 76% of 260 SLE patients.[535] However, persistent and unexplained increases in serum transaminase levels were found in 15 (8%) patients and, in 12 of these, the enzyme changes matched the SLE activity. This suggests that subclinical liver disease may be a manifestation of SLE in a small minority of patients. In a retrospective reqiew of 1468 cases, Matsumoto and his colleagues[536] noted a history of chronic hepatitis in 36 patients (2.4%), in 8 of whom it was reported to be active; cirrhosis was present in 17 (1.1%).

The commonest histological finding is macrovesicular steatosis;[536] this may in part be due to corticosteroid therapy. Mild periportal inflammation is often present[534] but chronic active hepatitis is rare. Hepatic granulomas have been described in several cases[533] and Murphy et al[20] reported a case in whom the granulomas were of fibrin-ring type; this patient, however, had concomitant cytomegalovirus and staphylococcal infections.

The relationship between 'lupoid' or autoimmune chronic active hepatitis and SLE has been reviewed in detail by Mackay.[537] Although both diseases are characterized by the presence of circulating antinuclear antibodies, the specificities of these antibodies differ. The immunogenetic and pathogenetic mechanisms of CAH and SLE are also dissimilar.[537] Patients in whom both entities are present, such as those described by Runyon et al,[533] probably represent co-existent diseases rather than an 'overlap' syndrome.

Nodular regenerative hyperplasia has been described in SLE.[431,512,536,538] In the autopsy study of Matsumoto et al,[536] 3 of 52 cases of SLE had nodular regenerative hyperplasia suggesting that this may be a relatively common (but clinically silent) complication. The antiphospholipid syndrome, in which there are antiphospholipid antibodies and which is found in a proportion of patients with SLE, is associated with a thrombotic tendency.[539] It has been suggested that by interfering with intrahepatic blood flow, thrombotic occlusion may play a role in the pathogenesis of nodular regenerative hyperplasia in some cases.[540] These antibodies have also been implicated in cases of veno-occlusive disease and Budd-Chiari syndrome occurring in SLE or 'lupus-like' disease.[541,542]

Peliosis hepatis was found in 6 of the cases reported by Matsumoto et al;[536] arteritis, complicated by hepatic infarction in one instance, was a feature in 20% of their patients and might have been of causal significance in the nodular regenerative hyperplasia. Other common findings in their series were sinusoidal congestion and bilirubinostasis which were attributed to the terminal illnesses, rather than SLE per se. Khoury et al[543] also reported hepatic infarction in SLE, and spontaneous rupture of the liver has been reported in 2 patients.[544] There are case reports of primary sclerosing cholangitis[280] and of malacoplakia[545] occurring in patients with SLE. Laxer et al,[546] in reporting 4 cases, suggested that neonatal hepatitis may occur as a complication of neonatal lupus erythematosus with the presence of maternal autoantibodies.

Scleroderma and progressive systemic sclerosis have infrequently been associated with hepatic disease. Bartholomew et al[547] reported liver involvement in 8 of 727 patients with scleroderma, and D'Angelo et al[548] in an autopsy study found cirrhosis in 5 of 57 patients, a lower incidence than in their carefully matched control group. In a study of 4 scleroderma patients with portal hypertension, Morris et al[549] reported that 1 had cirrhosis, 2 had chronic active hepatitis, and in the fourth patient the liver was normal apart from some granulomas. Extrahepatic biliary disease associated with fibrosis of the gallbladder[550] and large duct obstruction due to vasculitis and ulceration[551] have been reported. Primary sclerosing cholangitis associated with systemic sclerosis was reported by Fraile et al.[552]

An association of primary biliary cirrhosis with the CREST syndrome was first suggested by Murray-Lyon et al in 1970[553] and subsequently confirmed in numerous reports (see Ch. 12). Antimitochondrial antibodies are found in up to one quarter of patients with the CREST syndrome although histological changes of primary biliary cirrhosis are present in only 3–4%.[554] Nodular regenerative hyperplasia has been reported in progressive systemic sclerosis[431,512,555] as has hepatic infarction.[556]

Mixed connective tissue disease. This syndrome is characterized by an overlap of the clinical features of SLE, progressive systemic sclerosis and polymyositis and by high titres of antibodies to the ribonucleoprotein fraction of extractable nuclear antigens. In a study of 61 patients, only 4 had clinical evidence of liver disease,[557] and liver biopsy in 1 showed chronic active hepatitis with cirrhosis. A further 3 patients with mixed connective tissue disease and chronic active hepatitis have subsequently been reported.[558,559] Non-specific reactive hepatitis was noted in an autopsy study by Singsen et al[560] of three children with this disease. Budd–Chiari syndrome has been reported in association with mixed connective tissue disease.[561]

MISCELLANEOUS MUSCULOSKELETAL AND MULTI-SYSTEM DISORDERS

Polymyalgia rheumatica. Increased levels of serum alkaline phosphatase are found in over a third of patients and the levels may parallel disease activity.[487,562] Sattar et al[563] reported finding antimitochondrial antibodies in 11 of 36 patients, and primary biliary cirrhosis may co-exist in some cases. Morphological changes in the liver have comprised non-specific reactive hepatitis, steatosis and granulomas; there may sometimes be a moderately intense portal tract inflammation with lymphoid follicles.[564–566] There is an increased frequency of nodular regenerative hyperplasia.[431]

Polymyositis and dermatomyositis. An association between primary biliary cirrhosis and polymyositis has been reported in a small number of cases.[567–569] Unexplained hepatosplenomegaly and minor abnormalities of liver function tests may occur in children with dermatomyositis[570] and there is a case report of a patient with polymyositis of recent onset who was subsequently shown to have a hepatocellular carcinoma.[571]

In Weber–Christian disease, Oram and Cochrane[572] reported severe hepatomegaly due to fatty liver. Inflammation of intrahepatic fat may occur, similar to the panniculitis which characterizes this disease (Fig. 17.20). In a case described by Kimura et al[123] there was steatohepatitis and abundant Mallory bodies were seen. The changes were predominantly in periportal zones; the patient had no other known risk factor for non-alcoholic steatohepatitis.

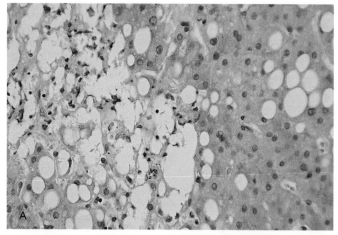

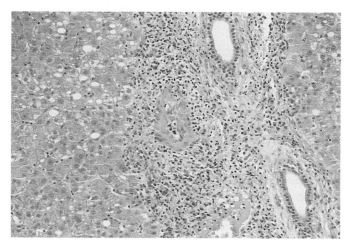

Fig. 17.21 Arteritis in a liver biopsy from a patient with temporal arteritis. H & E. Courtesy of Dr N Y Haboubi.

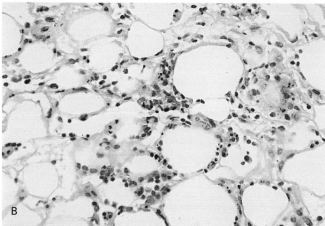

Fig. 17.20 Liver in Weber–Christian disease. (a) There is macrovesicular steatosis and in the accumulation on the left there is inflammation. (b) A mixed mononuclear and neutrophil polymorph infiltrate is present in the inflamed fat. H & E.

Systemic vasculitides. Liver involvement in these disorders is discussed in Chapter 14. The liver may be affected in over 40% of cases of polyarteritis nodosa, producing infarction in many instances.[573] Intrahepatic arterial vasculitis (Fig. 17.21) has also been noted with temporal arteritis.[574] In the vascular subtype of **Behçets' disease**, Budd–Chiari syndrome has been reported.[575,576]

LIVER INVOLVEMENT IN RENAL DISEASE

Hepatic dysfunction is well recognized in patients with chronic renal disease. This is true in patients maintained on haemodialysis and in patients receiving allografts, and in both these groups chronic viral infection is the most common cause of hepatic injury. A number of less common causes of liver dysfunction are also reviewed in this section; the hepatotoxic effects of immunosuppressant therapy in allograft recipients are discussed in chapter 15.

Viral hepatitis

Viral hepatitis is a recognized major complication of haemodialysis. There is no evidence that hepatitis A contributes to the problem.[577,578] In early studies on hepatitis B, serological evidence of infection in haemodialysis patients was found in up to 40%, and chronic HBs antigenaemia was found in 10–15%.[578,579] However, careful screening strategies have resulted in a considerable reduction in these figures and Alter et al[580] reported that whereas the prevalence rate of HBs antigenaemia in haemodialysis units in the USA was 7.8% in 1976, the corresponding figure in 1983 was 0.6%. In both haemodialysis and transplant patients who develop acute hepatitis B the illness is mild[581] and, indeed, in many the acute infection is asymptomatic, although fulminant hepatic failure may occur.[577,582,583] However, acquired HBV infection in these patients is associated with a high risk of chronic infection, a major cause of morbidity and mortality in many transplant centres.[583–590]

The incidence of HBV-associated chronic hepatitis in haemodialysis patients may be as high as 5% and the disease is usually more rapidly progressive, presumably due to the immunosuppressant effects of the patients' azotaemia.[591,592] Similarly, in renal transplant patients histological evidence of more rapidly progressive chronic hepatitis has been found.[588,593,594] It is worth mentioning that in haemodialysis patients only 40–60% have an adequate response to hepatitis B vaccine.[595–597] There is little evidence that persistent HBs antigenaemia jeopardizes the survival of the renal allograft.[579]

The role of HCV in causing liver disease in haemodialysis and transplant patients is currently under intense investigation. There is a high prevalence of HCV antibody in patients maintained on haemodialysis; early studies, using the first generation antibody tests, suggested prevalence rates for HCV infection of 35% in unselected haemodialysis patients[598,599] and 12% in transplant recipients.[600] A recent study from Hong Kong combining RNA and antibody assays reported 25% and 30% positivity rates respectively in a series of 51 patients.[601] In a personal study of 37 transplant patients with biopsy proven liver disease all 3 patients with chronic active hepatitis and 9 of 12 patients with chronic lobular hepatitis were HCV antibody-positive using a second generation RIBA assay.[590]

Cytomegalovirus (CMV) infection is very common in patients being treated for chronic renal disease[577] and acute infection or reactivation may occur in up to 50% of patients undergoing renal transplantation.[602] Clinically, episodes of CMV hepatitis are apparently not modified in these patients. However, the widespread infection in renal transplant recipients makes it difficult to assess a causal role for CMV; absence of histological evidence of infection[590] argues against its having an important role in producing chronic liver dysfunction. Epstein–Barr virus (EBV) and adenovirus infection of the liver in renal patients is relatively rare[577] although more than 80% of allograft recipients harbour EBV in their oropharynx.[603] Herpes simplex (and herpes zoster) seroconversion occurs in a significant proportion of transplant recipients; disseminated infection with hepatic involvement has been reported.[604]

Peliosis hepatis and nodular regenerative hyperplasia

Poliosis hepatis has been reported in two patients on chronic haemodialysis,[605,606] and has also been noted in a number of renal allograft recipients,[607–612] occurring as a complication in 2% of one series of 500 patients.[607] In some cases it was associated with nodular regenerative hyperplasia, a lesion which may also occur on its own in allograft recipients. Allison et al,[590] in reporting nodular regenerative hyperplasia in 5 of 27 transplant patients who had undergone biopsy, estimated that there were 38 previously reported cases in some of whom portal hypertension and hepatic failure had developed.[512,608,610,611–617] Veno-occlusive disease[618–620] and hepatic sinusoidal dilatation, sometimes with portal hypertension,[621] have also been reported in transplant patients.

Nataf et al[622] reported two transplant recipients with *idiopathic portal hypertension* in whose biopsies perisinusoidal fibrosis was present. The aetiology of these vascular complications in the liver remains uncertain. Current evidence suggests that they are related to the use of azathioprine[590,611,621] although sinusoidal endothelial cell disease due to CMV infection has also been postulated.[610]

Miscellaneous liver diseases

Haemosiderosis. Moderate or severe secondary haemosiderosis may develop in patients who receive blood transfusion while on dialysis and may cause hepatic dysfunction after transplantation.[590,623,624] Pahl et al[625] noted haemosiderosis at autopsy in 13 of 78 patients maintained on haemodialysis. Rao & Anderson[624] noted that significant, and sometimes unexplained, haemosiderosis (grade 3 to 4+) was more frequent after renal transplantation and was associated with cirrhosis in a number of patients.

Hepatocellular carcinoma has been reported in a number of patients[626–628] and, of 1436 neoplasms that developed in 1348 patients reported in the Denver Transplant Tumour Registry, 14 were hepatocellular carcinomas.[629]

Intrahepatic haematomas may occur in haemodialysis patients who have developed a bleeding diathesis.[630]

The presence in the liver of silicone particles from dialysis tubing, evoking a *granulomatous reaction* in some cases, has been reported[631–633] and may sometimes lead to scarring.[634] Multiple aluminium-containing epithelioid cell granulomas were found at autopsy in the liver, spleen and lymph nodes of two patients on long-term haemodialysis.[635]

There is a case report of diffuse microscopic hepatic *calcification* in a patient on haemodialysis.[636] In *dialysis-related amyloidosis* (see below), in which β_2-microglobulin is the precursor protein, vascular deposition in the liver has been reported in a very few cases.[637–639]

THE LIVER IN AMYLOIDOSIS AND LIGHT CHAIN DEPOSITION DISEASE

AMYLOIDOSIS

Since the first description by Rokitansky[640] in 1842, amyloid and amyloidosis have continued to intrigue pathologist and clinician alike. Amyloidosis is now classified on the basis of the chemical composition of the amyloid fibrils and their precursor protein.[641–643] Systemic amyloidosis may occur:

1. as *Primary or myeloma-related*:
   a. in association with plasma cell dyscrasias, multiple myeloma, B-cell malignancies and Waldenstrom's disease; the amyloid (A) fibril contains light chain (AL), and the precursor protein is the amino-terminal variable region of kappa or lambda chains, and
   b. in association with heavy chain disease in which the fibril contains heavy chain (AH) and the precursor protein is IgG_1;
2. as *Secondary or reactive* in association with longstanding chronic inflammatory processes, e.g. rheumatoid arthritis and bronchiectasis, Hodgkin's disease, and occasionally non-lymphoid malignancies such as gastric and renal carcinoma and benign tumours including liver-cell adenomas[644]; the fibril is

amyloid A (AA) and the precursor protein, serum AA, is an apolipoprotein which is an acute phase protein (see Ch. 2);

3. in *Heredofamilial forms* which, with the exception of familial Mediterranean fever, are all of autosomal dominant inheritance, show varying geographical or ethnic distribution, affect different organs and whose precursor proteins include various transthyretins;[643] and

4. in patients on *long-term renal dialysis* in which the precursor protein is β_2-microglobulin and where liver involvement is rare.

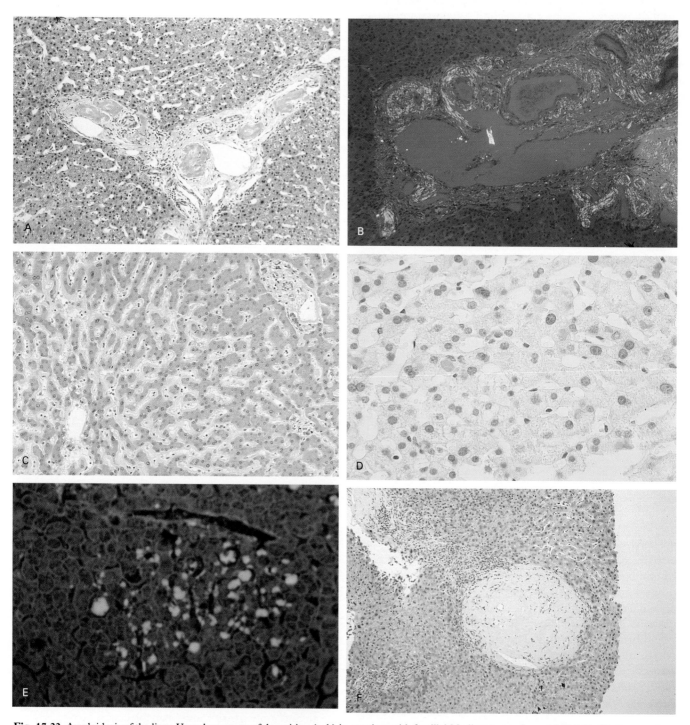

Fig. 17.22 Amyloidosis of the liver. Vascular pattern of deposition (a, b) in a patient with familial Mediterranean fever. (a) H & E. (b) Congo red birefringence. Courtesy of Dr. J. Lough. (c) Linear sinusoidal pattern of deposition, predominantly in acinar zones 2 and 3 and producing compression atrophy of liver-cell plates. H & E . (d, e) Globular sinusoidal pattern. Sirius red and fluorescent microscopy after thioflavine T stain. Courtesy of Dr K G Ishak. (f) Predominantly portal tract deposition. H & E. Courtesy of Dr H Tavadia.

Hepatic involvement in the three major forms of systemic amyloidosis is common.[645-649] Clinical evidence of liver dysfunction is usually not significant.[645,646,648,650,651] Hepatomegaly is present in 20% of patients and may be associated with pain when there is a rapid increase in size;[652] calcification was a feature in one case.[653] Mild jaundice may occur in 5–10% and, rarely, may become severe.[654-656] It may be the presenting feature, however, and this carries a poor prognosis.[655,657,658] The mechanisms of the jaundice are not clear. Portal hypertension may develop[659] and there are case reports of co-existent nodular regenerative hyperplasia[660] and of spontaneous rupture of the liver.[661]

Macroscopically, the liver may be markedly enlarged, weighing up to 9 kg. It is pale, of rubbery consistency and, if amyloid is present in large amounts, it may show the classic waxy lardaceous appearance. Microscopically, the amyloid is demonstrable by conventional stains including Congo red and Sirius red. The AL and AA forms can be distinguished histologically in that pre-treatment with potassium permanganate abolishes the Congo red affinity of the AA fibrils, whereas AL fibrils are resistant to this treatment.[662] In addition, immunohistochemical methods[663] may be applied to show the presence of P component, which has a pentagonal structure, is synthesized by the liver, circulates as serum amyloid P (SAP) and is present in all types of amyloid. There are several patterns of intrahepatic deposition. The amyloid may be deposited in blood vessels — vascular pattern; perisinusoidally in the space of Disse in linear or globular pattern — sinusoidal pattern; in perivascular portal tract fibrous tissue; and in large intrahepatic bile ducts and peribiliary glands.

In the vascular pattern of distribution, hepatic arteries and arterioles are mainly involved (Fig. 17.22a,b) but deposition can also occur in portal veins and, occasionally, in hepatic veins. In the sinusoidal pattern the accumulation is in the space of Disse producing compression atrophy of the liver-cell plates (Fig. 17.22c). A round globular form, 3–40 μm in diameter (Fig. 17.22d,e), may be found involving the space of Disse and portal tracts in patients who are clinically identical to others with amyloidosis;[664,665] some of the globules may be phagocytosed by Kupffer cells. The sinusoidal pattern usually occurs alone, although patients have been noted with coincidental sinusoidal and globular deposition.[647] A pattern of predominantly portal tract deposition (Fig. 17.22f) is sometimes seen (Bruguera—personal observation). Recently, Sasaki and his colleagues[666] noted amyloid deposition (both of AA and AL type) under the lining epithelium of large intrahepatic bile ducts and in the peribiliary glands; they suggested that massive deposition in these sites might cause biliary obstruction.

There may be zonal variation in the amount of amyloid deposited and there is a tendency for the perivenular areas to be less affected.[645] Levine[645] reported one case in which perivenular and periportal deposition occurred without involvement of sinusoids. Accompanying changes may include portal tract fibrosis, portal tract inflammation, and irregularity of the limiting plate with ductular proliferation; cirrhosis has also been recorded.[647]

The distribution pattern in the liver cannot be used to distinguish with certainty between the various forms of systemic amyloidosis.[645,647] Whereas previously it was considered that the vascular pattern was predominant in AL and the sinusoidal pattern in AA, Chopra et al[647] found sinusoidal involvement a consistent feature in the AL form and vascular involvement a consistent feature in the AA form, an observation which was confirmed by Looi & Sumithran.[649] Chopra et al[647] found exclusive parenchymal involvement only in AL and, correspondingly, exclusive vascular involvement only in AA cases.

LIGHT CHAIN DEPOSITION DISEASE

In 1976 Randall and his colleagues[667] first described *non-amyloid light chain disease* in which a plasma cell dyscrasia was associated with tissue deposition of light chains. Presenting with renal failure, their two patients also had hepatic involvement with deposition of light chains in the space of Disse. The disease mainly affects the kidney,[668,669] but skin,[670] pulmonary[671] and vascular involvement[672] have also been reported. Liver involvement is usually incidental, and in only a very few patients has there been significant hepatic dysfunction.[673-679] The clinical manifestations have included hepatomegaly, disturbance of liver function tests and one case of severe unexplained cholestasis.[679]

The striking abnormality in the liver is the deposition of light chains in the space of Disse and in the portal tracts accompanied by sinusoidal dilatation and sometimes peliosis hepatis. These deposits do not contain component P and do not stain with Congo red; they are intensely chromophilic with trichrome stains (Fig. 17.23a) and are PAS-positive diastase-resistant. The light chain nature of the deposits can be confirmed by immunohistochemistry (Fig. 17.23b,c). However, in some cases the deposits have been shown to also contain heavy chains[680,681] and there may also be increased deposition of type I and type IV collagen and of fibronectin.[676,677,679] On electron microscopy the deposits appear as granular non-fibrillar material in the space of Disse and in the pericellular spaces (Fig. 17.23d).

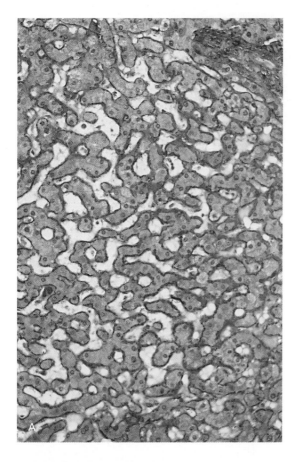

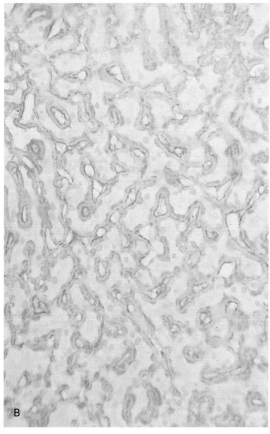

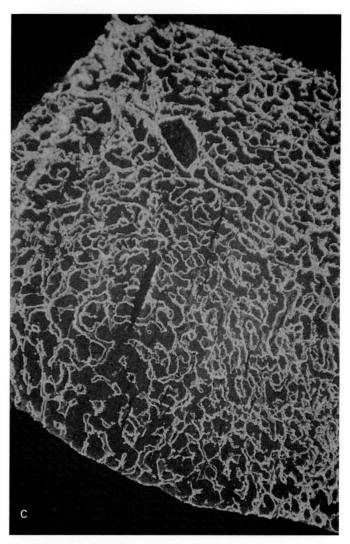

Fig. 17.23 Light chain deposition disease. Perisinusoidal deposition of lambda light chains shown by: (a) Mallory's trichrome stain; (b) Immunoperoxidase staining. (c) Immunofluorescent staining. (d) Electron micrograph showing granular deposits in the space of Disse and also in the intercellular space (double arrows). S = sinusoid lumen. × 4500. Figs (c) and (d) reprinted with permission from the article by Droz et al[676].

There have been a number of recent reports in which light chain deposition and AL amyloid deposits have both been found in the kidney and in the liver.[678,680,682-684] In addition Faa et al[679] noted that at the ultrastructural level, fibrillar material was present in the perisinusoidal deposits in their case of light chain deposition disease. These observations have suggested that light chain deposition disease and amyloidosis of the AL type represent different stages or different patterns of expression in a disease spectrum.

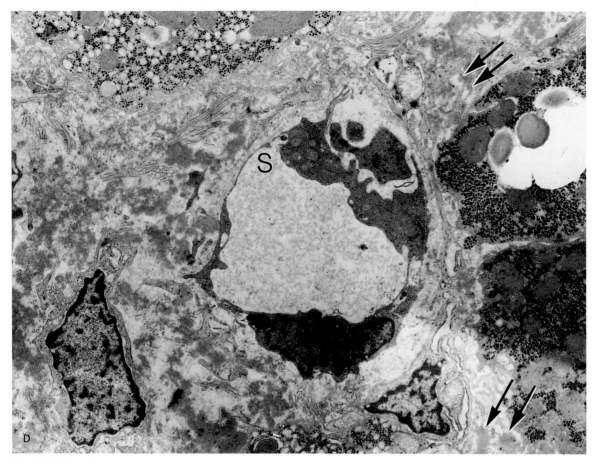

Fig. 17.23 *Contd*

LIVER INVOLVEMENT IN CARDIOVASCULAR DISEASES

Congestive cardiac failure

In prolonged right-sided heart failure the liver is usually enlarged, firm and tender. At autopsy there is a so-called nutmeg pattern on the cut surface in which dark, congested and haemorrhagic perivenular areas alternate with paler zone 2 areas, which may show fatty change, and pale periportal areas.[685] Microscopically, there is venous congestion and sinusoidal congestion in zone 3, compression atrophy of liver-cell plates, and the hepatocytes contain increased amounts of lipofuscin pigment and, occasionally, hyaline globules.[686] With increasing congestion, bridging liver-cell necrosis may link hepatic vein branches[685] and a light inflammatory infiltrate, predominantly neutrophil polymorph, is noted. Perivenular fibrosis develops in the areas of necrosis, and fibrous septa form and extend to link with portal tracts producing the lesion of so-called *cardiac sclerosis* which resembles a micronodular cirrhosis. The basic liver architecture, however, is preserved and a true cardiac cirrhosis rarely, if ever, develops.

Cardiac sclerosis of varying severity is seen in up to 50% of patients with congestive cardiac failure.[685] Nodular regenerative hyperplasia develops in the periportal zones (acinar zone 1) and it is of interest, historically, that this lesion was first described by Steiner[687] in patients with cardiac failure.

Acute circulatory failure

Hepatic injury in acute heart failure and peripheral circulatory shock are thought to be the result of hypoperfusion. They comprise necrosis of hepatocytes initially at the microcirculatory periphery of the acinus, zone 3, but in severe cases there is also involvement of zone 2;[685,688] in some instances zone 2 may be selectively damaged.[689] A similar syndrome, to which the term ischaemic hepatitis has been applied, may develop in many other conditions

Fig. 17.24 Ischaemic hepatitis following myocardial infarction. There is coagulative necrosis involving acinar zones 2 and 3 and with central–central bridging; the hepatocytes in zone 1 show macrovesicular steatosis. H & E.

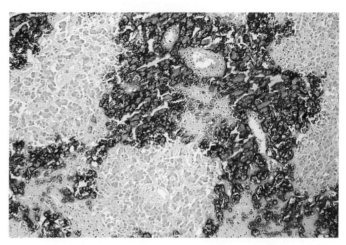

Fig. 17.25 Dystrophic calcification in the autopsy liver of a child aged 6 who had had episodes of ischaemic hepatitis related to surgical treatment of congenital heart disease. H & E. Courtesy of Dr A Howatson.

in which there is systemic hypotension — severe trauma, burns, surgical operation, haemorrhage, pulmonary embolism and peritonitis, for example.[688,690–692] The syndrome may also occur in children.[693] The severity of the liver injury can, in some patients, be related to the degree of hypotension and the duration of the shock state.[694,695] However, in others systemic hypotension may not have been a feature although there was evidence of left ventricular failure.[690]

In ischaemic hepatitis there may be mild jaundice, and there is a dramatic and rapid rise in serum transaminases, with an equally rapid resolution on clinical recovery.[690,692] Fulminant hepatic failure may develop, but this is usually seen when there is acute-on-chronic cardiac failure.[696] Shibayama et al,[697] on the basis of experimental work in rodents, postulated that severe hypotensive episodes caused an increased diffusion of endotoxin from the gastrointestinal tract, with aggravation of the liver injury.

Histologically, there is coagulative necrosis of hepatocytes (Fig. 17.24), sinusoidal congestion and, sometimes, canalicular bilirubinostasis at the periphery of the necrotic areas. Inflammation is minimal and usually comprises neutrophil polymorphs. Loss of liver cells may cause focal collapse with corresponding condensation of the perivenular reticulin framework. With resolution, prominent aggregates of ceroid-containing macrophages are present. Dystrophic calcification may develop[698] (Fig. 17.25).

Hyperpyrexia

Hyperpyrexia of sufficient severity and duration may be fatal. In such patients Gore & Isaacson[699] found an enlarged liver with a mottled appearance. Histologically, the hepatocytes contained small vacuoles, probably micro-

vesicular steatosis, a phenomenon which developed early and was followed approximately 16 hours post-hyperthermia by perivenular necrosis.

Heat stroke

Heat stroke also leads to hepatocellular degeneration with necrosis and congestion in acinar zone 3. Bianchi et al[700] studied two cases of heat stroke; in both patients the blood pressure had at one time dropped to unrecordable levels. Serial liver biopsies were performed. The patients became icteric on the third day and there was a dramatic increase in serum transaminases. At 9 days, the histopathological changes comprised confluent perivenular necrosis, hydropic swelling of hepatocytes, cholestasis, and proliferation of marginal bile ducts with a cholangiolitis. Cholestasis was still present after 4 weeks but there was progressive improvement with complete resolution after 1 year.

Rubel & Ishak[89] studied the liver in the successive stages of fatal exertional heat stroke in 50 young men, most of them military recruits. In those 5 who died 'on the spot' the liver showed microvesicular steatosis, haemosiderosis, congestion, hepatocellular degeneration and extramedullary haemopoiesis. In those who survived up to 8 days microvesicular steatosis was present together with bile stasis (sometimes ductal) and an acute cholangitis and cholangiolitis. The possible mechanisms of the liver injury included, in addition to the hyperthermia, hypoxia (shock, heart failure), coagulopathy, sepsis and endotoxaemia, and in some patients haemolysis. In some cases the hepatic injury due to heat stroke can cause a fatal outcome a week or more after the initial insult; hepatic transplantation may be indicated when progressive clinical decompensation develops.[701]

MISCELLANEOUS LIVER INVOLVEMENT IN OTHER DISEASES

SKIN DISEASES

Liver involvement in mycosis fungoides and Sézary's syndrome has already been noted.

Systemic mastocytosis

Mast cells are very scanty in the normal liver, and although increased numbers are occasionally seen in acute and chronic hepatitis and in cirrhosis[702-704] the numbers present are considerably less than those encountered in mastocytosis.

The terminology of mastocytosis is a little confusing.[705] Systemic mastocytosis may be confined to the skin in 90% of patients — classic urticaria pigmentosa, whereas in 10% of patients other organs, notably bone marrow, spleen, lymph nodes and liver are involved — generalized mastocytosis. There is also a rare malignant mastocytosis in which there is no skin involvement and which follows a rapidly fatal course.

The liver abnormalities in generalized mastocytosis have been reviewed.[706-708] Hepatomegaly is found in 60–80% of patients with liver involvement and mast cell infiltrates, predominantly involving portal tract but also within sinusoids, are present in 40–50% of patients; in only rare cases is the sinusoidal infiltrate predominant; mast cells may also be found within endothelium and subendothelially. Cirrhosis and hepatic fibrosis are found in 4% and 14% of cases respectively. Non-cirrhotic portal hypertension has also been reported,[709-712] accompanied by intractable ascites in some patients.[713,714] The mechanisms of the portal hypertension are uncertain and have been variously attributed to portal fibrosis, perisinusoidal fibrosis and increased splenic blood flow; Bonnet et al[713] noted obstruction of portal and hepatic venules with sinusoidal dilatation and peliosis in their patient.

Lichen planus

Korkij et al,[715] in a retrospective study, found abnormalities of liver function tests in 52% of a series of 73 patients with lichen planus, compared with 36% in 272 control patients with other cutanoeus diseases. Liver biopsy in 8 patients showed 3 cases each of chronic active hepatitis and cirrhosis, the others showing alcoholic hepatitis and metastatic lung carcinoma. In prospective studies Cottoni and colleagues[716] reported associated chronic liver disease in 16 of 62 patients and del Olmo et al,[717] in a study of patients with lichen planus of the mouth, found abnormal liver function tests in 22 of 65 patients with biopsy-proven chronic liver disease in 12 of these. Two cases of hepatocellular carcinoma and lichen planus have been reported.[718]

Other skin disorders

In von Recklinghousen's disease liver complications reported include obstructive jaundice due to a periampullary tumour,[719] a primary neurilemmoma of the liver[720] and hepatic neurofibromas from which a mixed malignant schwannoma and angiosarcoma developed.[721]

Pityriasis rotunda has been shown to be a useful cutaneous marker of hepatocellular carcinoma in South African blacks.[722,723]

Psoriasis. There is no good evidence that psoriasis itself has any specific effects on the liver but the hepatotoxic effects of methotrexate therapy have to be carefully monitored (see Ch. 15). Liver transplantation has been performed in three patients with psoriasis in whom methotrexate-induced cirrhosis developed.[724]

Miscellaneous other associations include reports of acute hepatitis[725] and chronic active hepatitis[726] in patients with **febrile panniculitis**, and of chronic active hepatitis in association with **pyoderma gangrenosum**.[727] Liver involvement may occur in **lipoid proteinosis**, an

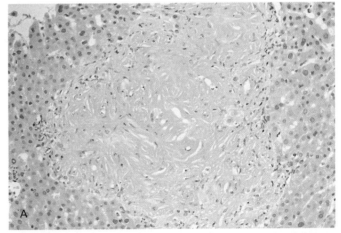

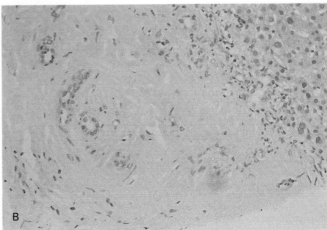

Fig. 17.26 Liver involvement in lipoid proteinosis; (a) Hyalinized matrix glycoprotein deposits have accumulated in the portal tract. H & E. (b) The material is weakly PAS-positive. PAS. Courtesy of Dr Judy Mäkinen.

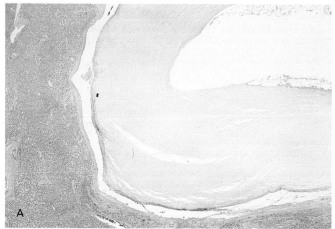

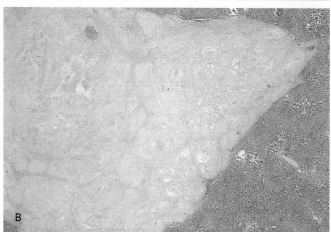

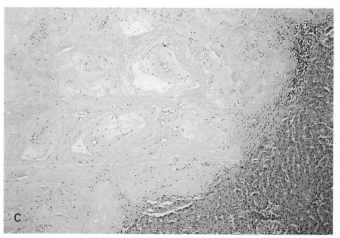

Fig. 17.27 Solitary necrotic nodule of liver. (a) Subcapsular lesion showing an acellular hyalinized outer wall with central loose amorphous material. (b) Intrahepatic nodule which is well circumscribed and which (c) represents a sclerosed haemangioma. H & E.

inherited disorder of collagen metabolism in which hyalinized extracellular matrix glycoproteins are deposited mainly in the skin, oral cavity and larynx.[728,729] The weakly PAS-positive material accumulates in portal tracts (Fig. 17.26) producing compression of the bile ducts.

PNEUMOCONIOSIS

Anthracotic deposits in the liver of coal workers are well recognized[730] and may be found in 10% of cases,[731] correlating with the severity of the patient's pneumoconiosis. Hepatic deposition of other inhaled dust particles may also occur, transport to the liver being effected by circulating macrophages.

NEUROMUSCULAR DISEASES

Nodular regenerative hyperplasia has been reported in a patient with *myasthenia gravis*.[732] In patients with *myotonic dystrophy* elevation of the serum levels of γ-glutamyl-transpeptidase and alkaline phosphatase[733,734] and of serum deoxycholic acid[735] have been reported. Liver biopsy of an affected mother and daughter showed enlargement of perisinusoidal (Ito) cells.[734]

SOLITARY NECROTIC NODULE OF LIVER

Shepherd & Lee[736] described five such lesions comprising a central necrotic core and enclosed by a hyalinized fibrotic capsule containing elastic fibres (Fig. 17.27a). They are usually found incidentally, occurring in the subcapsular region, with occasional deep ones in the liver (Fig. 17.27b, c).[737] They can be mistaken for metastases and represent either effete larval or other parasitic infestation[736,737] or sclerosed haemangiomas.[738]

REFERENCES

1. Popper H, Schaffner F. Liver: structure and function. New York: McGraw-Hill, 1957
2. Gerber M A, Thung S N, Bodenheimer H C Jr, Kapelman B, Schaffner F. Characteristic histological triad in liver adjacent to metastatic neoplasm. Liver 1986; 6: 85–88
3. Christoffersen P, Braendstrup O, Juhl E, Poulsen H. Lipogranulomas in human liver biopsies with fatty change. Acta Pathol Microbiol Scand [A], 1971; 79: 150–158
4. Dincsoy H P, Weesner R E, MacGee J. Lipogranulomas in non-fatty human liver. A mineral oil-induced environmental disease. Am J Clin Pathol 1982; 78: 35–41
5. Cruickshank B, Thomas M J. Mineral oil (follicular) lipidosis: II. Histologic studies of spleen, liver, lymph nodes and bone marrow. Hum Pathol 1984; 15: 731–737
6. Wanless I R, Geddie W R. Mineral oil lipogranulomata in liver and spleen. Arch Pathol Lab Med 1985; 109: 283–286
7. Delladetsima J K, Horn T, Poulsen H. Portal tract lipogranulomas in liver biopsies. Liver 1987; 7: 9–17
8. Keen M E, Engstrand D A, Hafez G R. Hepatic lipogranulomatosis simulating veno-occlusive disease of the liver. Arch Pathol Lab Med 1985; 109: 70–72
9. Bernstein M, Edmondson H A, Barbour B H. The liver lesion in Q-fever. Arch Int Med 1965; 116: 491–498
10. Hofmann C E, Heaton J W. Q fever hepatitis: clinical manifestations and pathological findings. Gastroenterology 1982; 83: 474–479
11. Qizilbash A H. The pathology of Q fever as seen on liver biopsy. Arch Pathol Lab Med 1983; 107: 364–367

12. Marazuela M, Moreno A, Yebra M, Cerezo E, Gomez-Gesto C, Vargas J A. Hepatic fibrin-ring granulomas: a clinicopathologic study of 23 patients. Hum Pathol 1991; 22: 607–613

13. Beorchia S, Rouhier D, Woehrle R et al. Anomalies hépatiques au cours de la fievre boutonneuse méditerranéenne. Ann Gastroenterol Hepatol 1986; 22: 87–90

14. Vanderstigel M, Zafrani E S, Lejonc J L, Schaeffer A, Portos J L. Allopurinol hypersensitivity syndrome as a cause of hepatic fibrin-ring granulomas. Gastroenterology 1985; 90: 188–190

15. Lobdell D H. 'Ring' granulomas in cytomegalovirus hepatitis. Arch Pathol Lab Med 1987; 111: 881–882

16. Moreno A, Marazuela M, Yebra M, Hernandez M, Hellin T, Montalaban C, Vargas J A. Hepatic fibrin-ring granulomas in visceral leishmaniasis. Gastroenterology 1988; 95: 1123–1126

17. Ponz E, Garcia-Pagan J C, Bruguera M, Bruix J, Rodes J. Hepatic fibrin-ring granulomas in a patient with hepatitis A. Gastroenterology 1991; 100: 268–270

18. Font J, Bruguera M, Perez-Villa F, Ingelmo M. Hepatic fibrin-ring granulomas caused by Staphylococcus epidermidis generalized infection. Gastroenterology 1987; 93: 1449–1451

19. Nenert M, Mavier P, Dubuc N, Deforges J, Zafrani E S. Epstein-Barr virus infection and hepatic fibrin-ring granulomas. Hum Pathol 1988; 19: 608–610

20. Murphy E, Griffiths M R, Hunter J A, Burt A D. Fibrin-ring granulomas: a non-specific reaction to liver injury. Histopathology 1991; 19: 91–93

21. Klatskin G. Hepatic granulomata: problems in interpretation. Mount Sinai J Med 1977; 44: 798–812

22. Ishak K G. Granulomas of the liver. In: Ioachim H L, ed. Pathology of granulomas. New York: Raven Press, 1983: pp 307–369

23. Ishak K G. New developments in diagnostic liver pathology. In: Farber E, Phillips M J, Kaufman N, eds. Pathogenesis of liver diseases. Baltimore: Williams & Wilkins 1987: pp 256–262

24. Chavanet P, Dillon D, Lancot J P et al. Granulomatous hepatitis associated with Lyme disease. Lancet 1987; ii: 623–624

25. Stjernberg U, Jilseth C, Ritland S. Granulomatous hepatitis in Yersinia enterocolitica infection. Hepatogastroenterol 1987; 34: 56–57

26. Eshchar J, Reif L, Warou M, Alkan W J. Hepatic lesion in chickenpox: a case report. Gastroenterology 1973; 64: 462–466

27. Mondou E N, Gnepp D R. Hepatic granuloma resulting from Enterobius vermicularis. Am J Clin Pathol 1989; 91: 97–100

28 Mendeloff J. Healed granulomas of the liver due to tongue worm infection. Am J Clin Pathol 1965; 43: 433–437

29 Nakhleh R E, Glock M, Snover D C. Hepatic pathology of chronic granulomatous disease of childhood. Arch Pathol Lab Med 1992; 116: 71–75

30. Kuntz H C, Oellig W P, Thiel H et al. Leber veränderungen bei akuten rheumatischen Fieber. Med Klin 1981; 76: 504–506

31. Citron B P, Halpern M, McCarron M et al. Necrotizing angiitis associated with drug abusers. N Engl J Med 1970; 283: 1003–1011

32. Leong A S Y, Disney A P S, Gove D W. Spallation and migration of silicone from blood-pumping tubing in patients on hemodialysis. N Engl J Med 1982; 306: 135–140

33. Chagnac A, Gal R, Kimche D, Zevin D, Machtey I, Levi J. Liver granulomas: a possible paraneoplastic manifestation of hypernephroma. Am J Gastroenterol 1985; 80: 989–992

34. Le Bail B, Jouhauole H, Deuguier Y et al. Liver adenomatosis with granulomas in two patients on long term oral contraceptives. Am J Surg Pathol 1992; 16: 982–987

35. Everett G D, Mitros F A. Eosinophilic gastroenteritis with hepatic eosinophilic granulomas. Am J Gastroenterol 1980; 74: 519–521

36. Cortes J M, Oliva H, Paradinas F J et al. The pathology of the liver in porphyria cutanea tarda. Histopathology 1980; 4: 471–485

37. Bunim J J, Kimberg D V, Thomas L B, van Scott J, Klatskin G. The syndrome of sarcoidosis, psoriasis and gout. Ann Int Med 1962; 57: 1018–1040

38. Scheuer P J. Hepatic granulomas. Br Med J 1982; 285: 833–834

39. Ferrell L D. Hepatic granulomas: a morphologic approach to diagnosis. Surg Pathol 1990; 3: 87–106

40. Simon H B, Wolff S M. Granulomatous hepatitis and prolonged fever of unknown origin: a study of 13 patients. Medicine 1973; 52: 1–21

41. Sartin J S, Walker R C. Granulomatous hepatitis: a retrospective review of 88 cases at the Mayo Clinic. Mayo Clin Proc 1991; 66: 914–918

42. Cunningham D, Mills P R, Quigley E M M et al. Hepatic granulomas: experience over a 10-year period in the West of Scotland. Q J Med 1982; 202: 162–170

43. Aderka D, Kraus M, Avidor I, Sidi Y, Weinberger A, Pinkhas J. Hodgkin's and non-Hodgkin's lymphomas masquerading as 'idiopathic' liver granulomas. Am J Gastroenterol 1984; 79: 642–644

44. Farrell G C, Powell L W. Chronic granulomatous hepatitis. Austr N Z J Med 1976; 6: 474–478

45. Zoutman D E, Ralph E D, Frei J V. Granulomatous hepatitis and fever of unknown origin. An 11-year experience of 23 cases with three year's follow up. J Clin Gastroenterol 1991; 13: 69–75

46. Mahida Y, Palmer K R, Lovell D, Silk D B A. Familial granulomatous hepatitis: a hitherto unrecognized entity. Am J Gastroenterol 1988; 83: 42–45

47. Melia W M, Calvey H, Portmann B, Williams R. Hepatocellular carcinoma complicating chronic granulomatous hepatitis. J Clin Pathol 1983; 36: 1062–1066

48. James D G, Jones Williams W. Sarcoidosis and other granulomatous disorders. Philadelphia: W B Saunders, 1985

49. Maddrey W C, Johns C J, Boittnott J K, Iber FL. Sarcoidosis and chronic hepatic disease: a clinical and pathologic study of 20 patients. Medicine 1970; 40: 375–395

49a. Devaney K, Goodman Z D, Epstein M S, Zimmerman H J, Ishah K G Hepatic sarcoidosis: clinicopathological features in 100 patients. Am J Surg Pathol 1993; 17: 1272–1280

50 Hercules H de C, Bethlem N M. Value of liver biopsy in sarcoidosis. Arch Pathol Lab Med 1984; 108: 831–834

51 Lehmuskallio E, Hannuksela M, Halme H. The liver in sarcoidosis. Acta Med Scand 1977; 202: 289–293

52. Israel H L, Margolis M L, Rose L J. Hepatic granulomatosis and sarcoidosis. Further observations. Dig Dis Sci 1984; 29: 353–356

53. Mishra B B, Poulter L W, Janossy G, James D G. The distribution of lymphoid and macrophage-like cell subsets of sarcoid and Kveim granulomata: possible mechanism of negative PPD reaction in sarcoidosis. Clin Exp Immunol 1983; 54: 705–715

54. Porter G H. Hepatic sarcoidosis. A cause of portal hypertension and liver failure: review. Arch Int Med 1961; 108: 483–495

55. Le Verger J C, Gosselin M, Laundis B et al. Sarcoidose et hypertension portale: Presentation de 2 cas et revue de la literature. Gastro Clin Biol 1977; 1: 661–669

56. Tekeste H, Latour F, Levitt R E. Portal hypertension complicating sarcoid liver disease: Case report and review of the literature. Am J Gastroenterol 1984; 79: 389–396

57. Valla D, Pessegueiro-Miranda H, Degott C et al. Hepatic sarcoidosis with portal hypertension. A report of seven cases with a review of the literature. Q J Med 1987; 63: 531–544

58. Natalino M R, Goyette R E, Owensby L C, Rubin R N. The Budd–Chiari syndrome in sarcoidosis. JAMA 1978; 239: 2657–2658

59. Russi E W, Bansky G, Pfaltz M, Spinas G, Hammer B, Senning A. Budd-Chiari syndrome in sarcoidosis. Am J Gastroenterol 1986; 81: 71–75

60. Rudzki C, Ishak K G, Zimmerman H J. Chronic intrahepatic cholestasis of sarcoidosis. Am J Med 1975; 59: 373–387

61. Bass N M, Burroughs A K, Scheuer P J, James D G, Sherlock S. Chronic intrahepatic cholestasis due to sarcoidosis. Gut 1982; 23: 417–421

62. Periera-Lima J, Schaffner F. Chronic cholestasis in hepatic sarcoidosis with clinical features resembling primary biliary cirrhosis. Am J Med 1987; 83: 144–148

63. Murphy J R, Sjogren M H, Kikendall J W, Peura D A, Goodman, Z. Small bile duct abnormalities in sarcoidosis. J Clin Gastroenterol 1990; 12: 555–561

64. Stanley N N, Fox R A, Whimster W F, Sherlock S, James D G. Primary biliary cirrhosis or sarcoidosis — or both? N Engl J Med 1972; 287: 1282–1284

65. Fagan E A, Moore-Gillon J C, Turner-Warwick M. Multi-organ granulomas and mitochondrial antibodies. N Engl J Med 1983; 308: 572–575

66. Maddrey W C. Sarcoidosis and primary biliary cirrhosis. Associated disorders? N Engl J Med 1983; 308: 588–590

67. Karlish A J, Thompson R P H, Williams R. A case of sarcoidosis and primary biliary cirrhosis. Lancet 1969; ii: 599

68. Thomas E, Micci D. Chronic intrahepatic cholestasis with granulomas and biliary cirrhosis. Enigmatic diseases and therapeutic dilemma. JAMA 1977; 238: 337–338

69. Findor J, Perez V, Bruch Igartua E, Giovanetti M, Fioravantti N. Structure and ultrastructure of the liver in aged persons. Acta Hepato-Gastroenterol 1973; 20: 200–204

70. Tavill A S, McCullough A J, eds. Nutrition and the liver. Semin in Liver Dis 1991; 11: 265–352

71. Morgan M V. Nutritional aspects of liver and biliary disease. In: McIntyre N, Benhamou J-P, Bircher J, Rizetto M, Rodes J, eds. Oxford textbook of clinical hepatology. Oxford: Oxford University Press, 1991: pp 1339–1388

72. Cairns S R, Peters T J. Biochemical analysis of hepatic lipid in alcoholic and diabetic and control subjects. Clin Sci 1983; 65: 645–652

73. Prieto J, Zozaya J M, Conchillo F. Fatty liver disease and nutritional liver damage. In: Prieto J, Rodes J, Shafritz D A, eds. Hepatobiliary diseases. Berlin: Springer-Verlag, 1991: pp 971–982

74. Popper H. General pathology of the liver: light microscopic aspects serving diagnosis and interpretation. Semin Liver Dis 1986; 6: 175–184

75. Mourelle M, Perez V M, Rojkind M. Lipid quantitation in formalin-fixed liver sections. J Histochem Cytochem 1988; 36: 1471–1474

76. Scheuer P J, Ashrafzadeh P, Sherlock S, Brown D, Dusheiko G M. The pathology of hepatitis C. Hepatology 1992; 15: 567–571

77. Ghisham F K, Myers M G, Younszaik K. Hepatic fatty metamorphosis in latent exoerythrocytic malaria. Am J Gastroenterol 1980; 74: 532–535

78. Paolucci F, Cinti S, Cangiotti A et al. Steatosis associated with immotile cilia syndrome: an unrecognized relationship. J Hepatol 1992; 14: 317–324

79. Brawner M K, Austin G E, Lewin K J. Focal fatty change of the liver: a hitherto poorly recognized entity. Gastroenterology 1980; 78: 247–252

80. Yoshikawa J, Matsui O, Takashima T et al. Fatty change of the liver adjacent to the falciform ligament: CT and sonographic findings in five surgically confirmed cases. Am J Roentgol 1987; 149: 491–494

81. Wang S S, Chiang J H, Tsai Y T et al. Focal hepatic fatty infiltration as a cause of pseudotumors: ultrasonographic patterns and clinical differentiation. J Clin Ultrasound 1990; 18: 401–409

82. Giorgio A, Francica G, Aloisio T et al. Multifocal fatty infiltration of the liver mimicking metastatic disease. Gastroenterol Int 1991; 4: 169–172

83. Grove A, Vyberg B, Vyberg M. Focal fatty change of the liver. A review and a case associated with continuous ambulatory peritoneal dialysis. Virchows Archiv (A) 1991; 419: 69–75

84. Terada T, Nakanuma Y, Hoso M, Saito K, Sasaki M, Nonomura A. Fatty macroregenerative nodule in non-steatotic liver cirrhosis. A morphologic study. Virchows Archiv (A) 1989; 415: 131–136

85. Ishak K G. Mesenchymal tumours of the liver. In: Okuda K, Peters R L, eds. Hepatocellular carcinoma. New York: Wiley, 1976: 247–307

86. Karhunen P J. Hepatic pseudolipoma. J Clin Pathol 1985; 38: 877–879

87. Goodman Z D, Ishak K G. Angiomyolipomas of the liver. Am J Surg Pathol 1984; 8: 745–750

88. Rubin E, Russinovich N A E, Luna R F, Tischler J M A, Wilkerson J A. Myelolipoma of the liver. Cancer 1984; 54: 2043–2046

89. Rubel L R, Ishak K G. The liver in fatal exertional heatstroke. Liver 1983; 3: 249–260

90. Howat A J, Bennett M J, Variend S, Shaw L, Engel P C. Defects of metabolism of fatty acids in the sudden infant death syndrome. Br Med J 1985; 290: 1771–1773

91. Weizman Z, Mussafi H, Ishay J S, Shvil Y, Goitein K, Livini N, Deckelbaum R J. Multiple hornet stings with features of Reye's syndrome. Gastroenterology 1985; 89: 1407–1410

92. Popper H, Thung S N, Gerber M A et al. Histologic studies of severe delta agent infection in Venezuelan Indians. Hepatology 1983; 3: 906–912

93. David E, Rahier J, Pucci A et al. Recurrence of hepatitis D (delta) in liver transplants: histopathological aspects. Gastroenterology 1993; 104: 1122–1128

94. Sabesin S M, Frase S, Ragland J B. Accumulation of nascent lipoproteins in rat hepatic Golgi during induction of fatty liver with orotic acid. Lab Invest 1977; 37: 127–135

95. Sinniah R, Sinniah D, Chia L-S, Baskaran G. Animal model of margosa oil ingestion with Reye-like syndrome. Pathogenesis of microvesicular fatty liver. J Pathol 1989; 159: 255–264

96. Quigley E M, Zetterman R K. Hepatobiliary complications of malabsorption and malnutrition. Semin Liver Dis 1988; 8: 218–228

97. Webber B L, Freiman I. The liver in kwashiorkor. A clinical and electron microscopic study. Arch Pathol 1974; 98: 400–408

98. Sherlock S. Acute fatty liver of pregnancy and the microvesicular fat diseases. Gut 1983; 24: 265–269

99. Praharaj K C, Choudhury U. The liver in kwashiorkor. A clinicohistopathological study. J Ind Med Assoc 1977; 69: 77–80

100. McLean A E N. Hepatic failure in malnutrition. Lancet 1962; ii: 1292–1294

101. Himsworth H P. Lectures on the liver and its diseases, 2nd edn. Oxford: Blackwell, 1950: p 91

102. McLaren D S, Faris R, Zekian B. The liver during recovery from protein-calorie malnutrition. J Trop Med Hyg 1968; 71: 271–281

103. Reid G M. Kwashiorkor. Med Hypotheses 1984; 14: 401–406

104. Truswell A S, Hansen J D L, Watson C E, Wannenburg P. Relation of serum lipids and lipoproteins to fatty liver in kwashiorkor. Am J Clin Nutr 1969; 22: 568–576

105. Sidransky H. Nutritional disturbances of protein metabolism in the liver. Am J Pathol 1976; 84: 649–668

106. Doherty J F, Golden M H N, Brooks S E H. Peroxisomes and the fatty liver of malnutrition: an hypothesis. Am J Clin Nutr 1991; 54: 674–677

107. Simon D M, Krause R, Galambos J T. Peliosis hepatis in a patient with marasmus. Gastroenterology 1988; 95: 805–809

108. Thaler H. Die Fettleber und ihre pathogenetische Beziehung zur Leberzirrhose. Virchows Arch [A] 1962; 335: 180–210

109. Peters R L, Gay T, Reynolds T. Post-jejunoileal-bypass hepatic disease. Its similarity to alcoholic hepatic disease. Am J Clin Pathol 1975; 63: 318

110. Marubbio A T, Buchwald H, Schwartz M Z, Varco R. Hepatic lesions of central pericellular fibrosis in morbid obesity, and after jejunoileal bypass. Am J Clin Pathol 1976; 66: 684–691

111. Galambos J T. Jejunoileal bypass and nutritional liver injury. Arch Pathol Lab Med 1976; 100: 229–231

112. Adler M, Schaffner F. Fatty liver hepatitis and cirrhosis in obese patients. Am J Med 1979; 67: 811–816

113. Falchuk K R, Fiske S C, Haggett R C, Federman M, Trey C. Pericentral hepatic fibrosis and intracellular hyalin in diabetes mellitus. Gastroenterology 1980; 78: 535–541

114. Schaffner F, Thaler H. Nonalcoholic fatty liver disease. In: Popper H, Schaffner F, eds. Progress in liver diseases, vol VIII. New York: Grune & Stratton, 1986: pp 283–298

115. Ludwig J, Viggiano T R, McGill D B et al. Non-alcoholic steatohepatitis: Mayo Clinic experiences with a hitherto unnamed disease. Mayo Clin Proc 1980; 55: 434–438

116. Klain J, Fraser D, Goldstein J et al. Liver histology abnormalities in the morbidly obese. Hepatology 1989; 10: 873–876

117. Silverman J F, O'Brien K F, Long S et al. Liver pathology in morbidly obese patients with and without diabetes. Am J Gastroenterol 1990; 85: 1349–1355

118. Craig R M, Neumann T, Jeejeebhoy K N, Yokoo H. Severe hepatocellular reaction resembling alcoholic hepatitis with cirrhosis after massive small bowel resection and prolonged total parenteral nutrition. Gastroenterology 1980; 79: 131–137

119. Haines N W, Baker A L, Boyer J L. Prognostic indicator of hepatic injury following jejunoileal bypass performed for refractory obesity: a prospective study. Hepatology 1981; 1: 161–167

120. Hocking M P, Duerson M C, O'Leary J P, Woodward E R. Jejunoileal bypass for morbid obesity. Late follow up in 100 cases. N Engl J Med 1983; 308: 995–999
121. Cuellar R E, Tarter R, Hays A, van Thiel D H. The possible occurrence of "alcoholic hepatitis" in a patient with bulimia in the absence of diagnosable alcoholism. Hepatology 1987; 7: 878–883
122. Grimm I S, Schindler W, Haluszka O. Steatohepatitis and fatal hepatic failure after biliopancreatic diversion. Am J Gastroenterol 1992; 87: 775–779
123. Kimura H, Kayo M, Iyo K et al. Alcoholic hyaline (Mallory bodies) in a case of Weber-Christian disease: electron microscopic observations of liver involvement. Gastroenterology 1986; 78: 807–812
124. Partin J S, Partin J C, Schubert W K, McAdams A J. Liver ultrastructure in abetalipoproteinemia: evolution of micronodular cirrhosis. Gastroenterology 1974; 67: 107–118
125. Powell E E, Searle J, Mortimer R. Steatohepatitis associated with limb lipodystrophy. Gastroenterology 1989; 97: 1022–1024
126. Nazim M, Stamp G, Hodgson H J. Non-alcoholic steatohepatitis associated with small intestinal diverticulosis and bacterial overgrowth. Hepato Gastroenterol 1989; 36: 349–351
127. Itoh S, Yougel T, Kawagor K. Comparison between non-alcoholic steatohepatitis and alcoholic hepatitis. Am J Gastroenterol 1987; 82: 650–654
128. Diehl A M, Goodman Z, Ishak K G. Alcohol-like liver disease in non-alcoholics. Gastroenterology 1988; 95: 1056–1062
129. Hay J E, Czaja A J, Rakela J, Ludwig J. The nature of unexplained chronic aminotransferase elevations of a mild to moderate degree in asymptomatic patients. Hepatology 1989; 9: 193–197
130. Lee R G. Non-alcoholic steatohepatitis: a study of 49 patients. Hum Pathol 1989; 20: 594–598
131. Powell E E, Cooksley G E, Hanson R et al. The natural history of nonalcoholic steatohepatitis. A follow-up study of forty-two patients for up to 21 years. Hepatology 1990; 11: 74–80
132. Fletcher L M, Kwoh-Gain I, Powell E E et al. Markers of chronic alcohol ingestion in patients with non-alcoholic steatohepatitis: an aid to diagnosis. Hepatology 1991; 13: 455–459
133. Farahvash M J, Janney C G, Neuschander-Tetri B A, Bacon B R. Non-alcoholic steatohepatitis: an expanded clinical entity. Hepatology 1993; 18: 174A (Abstract)
134. Nagore N, Scheuer P J. The pathology of diabetic hepatitis. J Pathol 1988; 156: 155–160
135. Peden V H, Witzleben C L, Skelton M A. Total parenteral nutrition. J Pediat 1971; 78: 180–181
136. Bower R H. Hepatic complications of parenteral nutrition. Semin Liver Dis 1983; 3: 216–224
137. Baker A L, Rosenberg I H. Hepatic complications of total parenteral nutrition. Am J Med 1987; 82: 489–497
138. Klein S, Nealon W H. Hepatobiliary abnormalities associated with total parenteral nutrition. Semin Liver Dis 1988; 8: 237–246
139. Balistreri W F, Bove K E. Hepatobiliary consequences of parenteral nutrition. In: Popper H, Schaffner F, eds. Progress in liver diseases, vol IX. Philadelphia: W B Saunders, 1990: pp 567–601
140. Cohen C, Olsen M M. Paediatric total parenteral nutrition. Arch Pathol Lab Med 1981; 105: 152–156
141. Body J J, Bleiberg H, Bron D et al. Total parenteral nutrition-induced cholestasis mimicking large bile duct obstruction. Histopathology 1982; 6: 787–792
142. Benjamin D. Hepatobiliary dysfunction in infants and children associated with long-term total parenteral nutrition. A clinicopathologic study. Am J Clin Pathol 1981; 76: 276–283
143. Dahms B B, Halpin T C Jr. Serial liver biopsies in parenteral nutrition-associated cholestasis of early infancy. Gastroenterology 1981; 81: 136–144
144. Whitington P F. Cholestasis associated with total parenteral nutrition in infants. Hepatology 1985; 5: 693–696
145. Roy C C, Belli D C. Hepatobiliary complications associated with TPN: an enigma. J Am Coll Nutr 1985; 4: 651–660
146. Grant J P, Cox C E, Kleinman L M et al. Serum hepatic enzyme and bilirubin elevations during parenteral nutrition. Surg Gyn Obst 1977; 145: 573–580

147. Sheldon G F, Peterson S R, Sanders R. Hepatic dysfunction during hyperalimentation. Arch Surg 1978; 113: 504–508
148. Bowyer B A, Fleming C R, Ludwig J, Petz J, McGill D B. Does long-term home parenteral nutrition in adult patients cause chronic liver disease? JPEN 1985; 9: 11–17
149. Stanko K T, Nathan G, Mendelow H, Adibi S A. Development of hepatic cholestasis and fibrosis in patients with massive loss of intestine supported by prolonged parenteral nutrition. Gastroenterology 1987; 92: 197–202
150. Tulikoura I, Huikuri K. Morphological fatty changes and function of the liver, serum free fatty acids, and triglycerides during parenteral nutrition. Scand J Gastroenterol 1982; 17: 177–185
151. Sax H C, Talamini M A, Brackett K et al. Hepatic steatosis in total parenteral nutrition: failure of fatty infiltration to correlate with abnormal serum hepatic enzyme levels. Surgery 1986; 100: 697–704
152. Wolfe B M, Walker B K, Shaul D B, Wong L, Ruebner B H. Effect of total parenteral nutrition on hepatic histology. Arch Surg 1988; 123: 1084–1090
153. Campos A C, Oler A, Meguid M M, Chen T-Y. Liver biochemical and histological changes with graded amounts of total parenteral nutrition. Arch Surg 1990; 125: 447–450
154. Palombo J D, Schnure F, Bistrian B R et al. Improvement of liver function tests by administration of L-carnitine to a carnitine-deficient patient receiving home parenteral nutrition: A case report. JPEN 1987; 11: 88–92
155. Rabeneck L, Freeman H, Owen D. Death due to TPN-related liver failure. Gastroenterology 1984; 86: 1215 (Abstract)
156. Thomas C H. Ulceration of the colon with a much enlarged fatty liver. Trans Path Soc Phil 1873; 4: 87–88
157. Lister J D. A specimen of diffuse ulcerative colitis with secondary diffuse hepatitis. Trans Path Soc Lond 1899; 50: 130–135
158. Chapin L E, Scudamore H H, Baggenstoss A H, Bargen J A. Regional enteritis: associated visceral changes. Gastroenterology 1956; 30: 404–415
159. Perrett A D, Higgins G, Johnston H H, Massarella G R, Truelove S C, Wright R. The liver in Crohn's disease. Q J Med 1971; 40: 187–209
160. Schrumpf E, Fausa O, Elgjo K, Kolmannskog F. Hepato-biliary complications of inflammatory bowel disease. Semin Liver Dis 1988; 8: 201–209
161. Vierling J M. Hepatobiliary complications of ulcerative colitis and Crohn's disease. In: Zakin D, Boyer T L, eds. Hepatology. A textbook of liver disease, 2nd edn. Philadelphia: W B Saunders, 1990: pp 1126–1158
162. Chapman R W, Angus P W. The effect of gastrointestinal diseases on the liver and biliary tract. In: McIntyre N, Benhamou J P, Bircher J, Rizzetto M, Rodes J, eds. Oxford textbook of clinical hepatology. Oxford: Oxford University Press, 1991: pp 1170–1174
163. Kastenberg D M, Friedman L S. Hepatobiliary complications of inflammatory bowel disease. In: Rustgi V K, van Thiel D H, eds. The liver in systemic disease. New York: Raven Press, 1993: pp 61–108
164. Mistilis S P. Pericholangitis and ulcerative colitis. I. Pathology, etiology and pathogenesis. Ann Int Med 1965; 63: 1–16
165. Mistilis S P, Skyring A P, Goulston S J M. Pericholangitis and ulcerative colitis. II. Clinical aspects. Ann Int Med 1965; 63: 17–26
166. Dordal E, Glasgov S, Kirsner J B. Hepatic lesions in chronic inflammatory bowel disease. I. Clinical correlations with liver biopsy diagnoses in 103 patients. Gastroenterology 1967; 52: 239–253
167. Eade M N. Liver disease in ulcerative colitis. I. Analysis of operative liver biopsy in 138 consecutive patients having colectomy. Ann Int Med 1970; 72: 475–487
168. Eade M N, Cooke W T, Brooke B N. Liver disease in ulcerative colitis. II. The long-term effect of colectomy. Ann Int Med 1970; 72: 489–497
169. Eade M N, Cooke W T, Brooke B N, Thompson H. Liver disease in Crohn's colitis. Ann Int Med 1971; 74: 518–528
170. Perrett A D, Higgins G, Johnston H H, Massarella G R, Truelove

S C, Wright R. The liver in ulcerative colitis. Q J Med 1971;
40: 211–238

171. Kern F. Hepatobiliary disorders in inflammatory bowel disease.
In: Schiff L, Schiff E R, eds. Diseases of the liver, 5th edn.
Philadelphia: Lippincott, 1976: pp 1603–1614

172. Chapman R W G, Arborgh B A M, Rodes J M et al. Primary
sclerosing cholangitis: a review of its clinical features,
cholangiographs and hepatic histology. Gut 1980;
21: 870–877

173. Ludwig J, Braham S S, LaRusso N F et al. Morphological
features of chronic hepatitis associated with primary sclerosing
cholangitis and chronic ulcerative colitis. Hepatology 1981;
1: 632–640

174. Wee A, Ludwig J. Pericholangitis in chronic ulcerative colitis:
Primary sclerosing cholangitis of the small bile ducts? Ann Int
Med 1985; 102: 581–587

175. MacSween R N M. Primary sclerosing cholangitis. In:
Anthony P P, MacSween R N M, eds. Recent advances in
histopathology, no. 12. Edinburgh: Churchill Livingstone, 1984:
pp 158–167

176. Desmet V J, Geboes K. Liver lesions in inflammatory bowel
disorders. J Pathol 1987; 151: 247–255

177. Dew M J, Thompson H, Allan R N. The spectrum of hepatic
dysfunction in inflammatory bowel disease. Q J Med 1979;
48: 113–135

178. Schrumpf E, Elgjo K, Fausa O, Gjone E, Kolmannskig F,
Ritland S. Sclerosing cholangitis in ulcerative colitis. Scand J
Gastroenterol 1980; 15: 689–697

179. Schrumpf E, Gjone E. Hepatobiliary disease in ulcerative colitis.
Scand J Gastroenterol 1982; 17: 961–964

180. Wewer V, Gluud C, Schlichting P, Burcharth F,
Binder V. Prevalence of hepatobiliary dysfunction in a regional
group of patients with chronic inflammatory bowel disease. Scand
J Gastroenterol 1991; 26: 97–102

181. Broome U, Glaumann H, Hultcrantz R. Liver histology and
follow-up of 68 patients with ulcerative colitis and normal liver
function tests. Gut 1990; 31: 468–472

182. Rabinovitz M, Demetris A J, Bou-Abboud C F, Van Thiel D H.
Simultaneous occurrence of primary sclerosing cholangitis and
autoimmune chronic active hepatitis in a patient with ulcerative
colitis. Dig Dis Sci 1992; 37: 1606–1611

183. Edwards P C, Truelove SC. The course and prognosis of
ulcerative colitis. Gut 1963; 4: 299–315

184. Palmer W L, Kirsner J B, Goldgraber M B, Fuentes S S. Disease
of the liver in chronic ulcerative colitis. Am J Med 1964;
36: 856–866

185. Kern F. Hepatobiliary disorders in inflammatory bowel disease.
In: Schiff L, Schiff E R, eds. Diseases of the liver, 4th edn.
Philadelphia: J B Lippincott, 1987: pp 1450–1460

186. Wiesner R H, LaRusso N F, Dozois R R, Beaver S J. Peristomal
varices after proctocolectomy in patients with primary sclerosing
cholangitis. Gastroenterology 1986; 90: 316–322

187. Ritchie J K, Allan R N, MacCartney J et al. Biliary tract
carcinoma associated with ulcerative colitis. Q J Med 1974; 43:
263–279

188. Mir-Jadjlessi S H, Farmer R G, Sivak M V. Bile duct carcinoma
in patients with ulcerative colitis. Dig Dis Sci 1987;
32: 145–154

189. Berman M D, Falchuk K R, Trey C. Carcinoma of the biliary tree
complicating Crohn's disease. Dig Dis Sci 1980; 25: 795–797

190. Ross A P, Braasch J W. Ulcerative colitis and carcinoma of the
proximal bile ducts. Gut 1973; 14: 94–97

191. Wheeler P G, Dawson J L, Nunnerley H et al. Newer techniques
in the diagnosis and treatment of proximal bile duct carcinoma —
an analysis of 41 consecutive cases. Q J Med 1981; 50: 247–258

192. Rosen C B, Nagomey D M. Cholangiocarcinoma complicating
primary sclerosing cholangitis. Semin Liver Dis 1991;
11: 26–30

193. Wee A, Ludwig J, Coffey R J, LaRusso N F, Wiesner R H.
Hepatobiliary carcinoma associated with primary sclerosing
cholangitis and chronic ulcerative colitis. Hum Pathol 1985;
16: 719–726

194. Christophi C, Hughes E R. Hepato-biliary disorders in

195. Starzl T E, Iwatsuki S, van Thiel D H et al. Evolution of liver
transplantation. Hepatology 1982; 2: 614–636

196. Stieber A C, Marino I R, Iwatsuki S, Starzl T E.
Cholangiocarcinoma in sclerosing cholangitis: the role of liver
transplantation. Int Surg 1989; 74: 1–3

197. Baker A, Kaplan M, Norton R A, Patterson J F. Gallstones in
inflammatory bowel disease. Am J Dig Dis Sci 1974;
19: 109–112

198. Lapidus A, Einasson K. Effects of ileal resection on biliary lipids
and bile acid composition in patients with Crohn's disease. Gut
1991; 32: 1488–1491

199. McClure J, Banerjee S S, Schofield P S. Crohn's disease of the
gallbladder. J Clin Pathol 1984; 37: 516–518

200. Fausa O, Nygaaard K, Elgjo K. Amyloidosis and Crohn's disease.
Scand J Gastroenterol 1977; 12: 657–662

201. Lowdell C P, Shousha S, Parkins R A. The incidence of
amyloidosis complicating inflammatory bowel disease. A
prospective survey of 177 patients. Dis Colon Rectum 1986;
29: 351–354

202. Gitkind M J, Wright S C. Amyloidosis complicating inflammatory
bowel disease: a case report and review of the literature. Dig Dis
Sci 1990; 35: 906–908

203. Mandelstam P, Simmons D E, Mitchell B. Regression of amyloid
in Crohn's disease after bowel resection: a 19 year follow-up.
J Clin Gastroenterol 1989; 11: 324–326

204. Fitchen J H. Amyloidosis and granulomatous ileocolitis:
Regression after surgical removal of the involved bowel. N Engl J
Med 1975; 292: 352–353

205. Maurer L H, Hughes R W, Folley J H, Mosenthal W T.
Granulomatous hepatitis associated with regional enteritis.
Gastroenterology 1967; 53: 301–305

206. Weinberg R J, Klish W J, Brown M R, Smalley J R, Emmens R W.
Hepatic abscess as a complication of Crohn's disease. J Ped
Gastroenterol Nut 1983; 2: 171–174

207. Mir-Madjlessi S H, McHenry M C, Farmer R G. Liver abscess in
Crohn's disease: report of four cases and review of the literature.
Gastroenterology 1986; 91: 987–993

208. Teague M, Baddour L M, Wruble L D. Liver abscess: a harbinger
of Crohn's disease. Am J Gastroenterol 1988; 83: 1412–1414

209. MacDonald P H, Mercer C D. Hepatic abscess associated with
subclinical ulcerative colitis. Can J Gastroenterol 1989;
3: 123–125

210. Chesner I M, Muller S, Newman J. Ulcerative colitis complicated
by Budd-Chiari syndrome. Gut 1986; 27: 1096–1100

211. Brinson R R, Curtis W D, Schuman B M, Mills L R. Recovery
from hepatic vein thrombosis (Budd–Chiari Syndrome)
complicating ulcerative colitis. Dig Dis Sci 1988;
33: 1615–1620

212. Maccini D M, Berg J C, Bell G A. Budd-Chiari Syndrome and
Crohn's disease. An unreported association. Dig Dis Sci 1989;
34: 1933–1936

213. Hagander B, Brandt L, Sjolund K et al. Hepatic injury in adult
coeliac disease. Lancet 1977; ii: 270–272

214. Jacobsen M B, Fausa O, Elgjo K, Schrumpf E. Hepatic lesions in
adult coeliac disease. Scand J Gastroenterol 1990; 25: 656–662

215. Mitchison H C, Record C O, Bateson M C, Cobden I. Hepatic
abnormalities in coeliac disease: three cases of delayed diagnosis.
Postgrad Med J 1989; 65: 920–922

216. Lindberg T, Berg N O, Borulf S, Jakobsson I. Liver damage in
coeliac disease and other food intolerances in childhood. Lancet
1978; i: 390–391

217. Pollock D J. The liver in coeliac disease. Histopathology 1977;
1: 421–430

218. Logan R F A, Ferguson A, Finlayson N D C, Weir D G. Primary
biliary cirrhosis and coeliac disease. Lancet 1978; i: 230–233

219. Hay J E, Wiesner R H, Shorter R G et al. Primary sclerosing
cholangitis and celiac disease: a novel association Gastroenterology
1988; 94: A545

220. Upton A C. Histochemical investigation of mesenchymal lesions in
Whipple's disease. Am J Clin Pathol 1952; 22: 755–764

221. Haubrich W S, Watson J H L, Sieracki J C. Unique morphologic

features of Whipple's disease. A study by light and electron microscopy. Gastroenterology 1960; 39: 454–468

222. Enzinger F M, Helwig E B. Whipple's disease. A review of the literature and report of fifteen cases. Virchows Archiv (A) 1963; 336: 238–269

223. Cornet A, Barbier J P, Henry-Biabaud E D et al. Maladie de Whipple. Localisations granulomateuses hépatiques décelées par ponction — biopsie du foie (a propos de deux observations). Ann Med Intern 1976; 127: 139–146

224. Misra P S, Lebwohl P, Laufer H. Hepatic and appendiceal Whipple's disease with negative jejunal biopsies. Am J Gastroenterol 1981; 75: 302–306

225. Sieracki C, Fine G. Whipple's disease — observations on systemic involvement. II. Gross and histologic observations. Arch Pathol 1959; 67: 81–93

226. Brisseau J M, Rodat O, Buizelin F, Le Bodic O, Lucas J, Harousseau J L, Alliot M. Localisations granulomateuses hepatiques au course de la maladie de Whipple. Sem Hop 1983; 59: 2889–2892

227. Cho C, Linscheer W G, Hirschkorn M A, Ashutosh K. Sarcoid-like granulomas as an early manifestation of Whipple's disease. Gastroenterology 1984; 87: 941–947

228. Saint-Marc Girardin M-F, Zafrani E S et al. Hepatic granulomas in Whipple's disease. Gastroenterology 1984; 86: 753–756

229. Robert F, Omura E, Durant J R. Mucosal eosinophilic gastroenteritis with systemic involvement. Am J Med 1977; 62: 139–143

230. Morrell M T, Keynes W M. Annular pancreas and jaundice. Br J Surg 1970; 57: 814–816

231. Braganza J M, Howat H T. Cancer of the pancreas. Clin Gastroenterol 1972; 1: 219–237

232. Weinstein B R, Korn R J, Zimmerman H J. Obstructive jaundice as a complication of pancreatitis. Ann Int Med 1963; 58: 245–258

233. Frieden J H. The significance of jaundice in acute pancreatitis. Arch Surg 1965; 90: 422–426

234. Masih B, Lowenfels A B, Pendse P D, Rohman M. Jaundice from pancreatic pseudocyst. NY State J Med 1971; 71: 2312–2313

235. Parbhoo S P, Welch J, Sherlock S. Acute pancreatitis in patients with fulminant hepatic failure. Gut 1973; 14: 428

236. Ham J M, Fitzpatrick P. Acute pancreatitis in patients with acute hepatic failure. Am J Dig Dis 1973; 18: 1079–1083

237. Riely C A. Acute fatty liver of pregnancy. Semin Liver Dis 1987; 7: 47–54

238. Kruszynska Y, McIntyre N. In: McIntyre N, Benhamou J-P, Bircher J, Rizzetto M, Rodes J, eds. Oxford textbook of clinical hepatology. Oxford: Oxford University Press, 1991: pp 129–143

239. Starzl T E, Watanabe K, Porter K A, Putnam C A. Effects of insulin, glucagon and insulin/glucagon infusion on liver morphology and cell division after complete portocaval shunt in dogs. Lancet 1976; i: 821–825

240. Starzl T E, Terblanche J. Hepatotrophic substances. In: Popper H, Schaffner F, eds. Progress in liver diseases, vol V. New York: Grune 8 Stratton, 1979: pp 135–151

241. Stone B G, van Thiel D H. Diabetes mellitus and the liver. Semin Liver Dis 1985; 5: 8–28

242. Cherrington A D, Stevenson R W, Steiner K E et al. Insulin, glucagon and glucose as regulators of hepatic glucose uptake and production in vivo. Diab Metab Rev 1987; 3: 307–332

243. Fagiuoli S, van Thiel D H. The liver in endocrine disorders. In: Rustgi V K, van Thiel D H, eds. The liver in systemic disease. New York: Raven Press, 1993: pp 285–301

244. Manougian E, Pollycove M, Linfoot J A, Lawrence J H. C14 glucose kinetic studies in normal diabetic and acromegalic subjects. J Nuc Med 1964; 5: 763–795

245. Wahren J, Felig P, Cerasi E, Luft R. Splanchnic and peripheral glucose and amino acid metabolism in diabetes mellitus. J Clin Invest 1972; 51: 1870–1878

246. Felig P. The liver in glucose homeostasis in normal man and in diabetes. In: Vallance-Owen J, ed. The biochemical and physiological basis of diabetes. Lancaster: MTP Press, 1977,

247. McGarry J D, Foster D W. Regulation of ketogenesis and clinical aspects of the ketotic state. Metabolism 1972; 21: 471–489

248. Newsholme E A. Role of the liver in integration of fat and carbohydrate metabolism and clinical implantations in patients with liver disease. In: Popper H, Schaffner F, eds. Progress in liver diseases, vol V. New York: Grune & Stratton, 1976: pp 125–135

249. Gerich J E, Lorenzi M, Bier D M et al. Prevention of human diabetic keto-acidosis by somatostatin. N Engl J Med 1975; 292: 985–989

250. Felig P, Sherwin R. Carbohydrate homeostasis, liver and diabetes. In: Popper H, Schaffner F, eds. Progress in liver diseases, vol V. New York: Grune & Stratton, 1976: pp 149–171

251. Kolterman O G, Insel J, Saekow M, Olefsky J M. Mechanisms of insulin resistance in human obesity. J Clin Invest 1980; 65: 1272–1284

252. Arner P A, Einarsson K, Backman L et al. Studies of liver insulin receptors in non-obese and obese human subjects. J Clin Invest 1983; 72: 1729–1736

253. Consoli A. Role of liver in pathophysiology of NIDDM. Diabetes Care 1992; 15: 430–441

254. Dunn F L. Hyperlipidemia and diabetes. Med Clin N Amer 1982; 66: 1347–1360

255. Creutzfeldt W, Frerichs H, Sickinger K. Liver diseases and diabetes mellitus. In: Popper H, Schaffner F, eds. Progress in liver diseases, vol III. New York: Grune & Stratton, 1970: pp 371–407

256. Feinegold K R, Siperstein M D. Abnormalities of glucose metabolism in liver disease. In: Zakim D, Boyer T D eds. Hepatology. Philadelphia: W B Saunders, 1979:

257. Blei A T, Robbins D C, Drobny E, Baumann G, Rubenstein A H. Insulin resistance and insulin receptors in hepatic cirrhosis. Gastroenterology 1982; 83: 1191–1199

258. Proietto J, Dudley F J, Aitken P, Alford F P. Hyper-insulinaemia and insulin resistance of cirrhosis: the importance of insulin hypersecretion. Clin Endocrinol 1984; 21: 657–665

259. Proietto J, Nankervis A, Aitken P, Dudley F J, Caruso G, Alford F P. Insulin resistance in cirrhosis: evidence for a post-receptor defect. Clin Endocrinol 1984; 21: 677–688

260. Taylor R, Heine R J, Collins J, James O F W, Alberti K G M. Insulin action in cirrhosis. Hepatology 1985; 5: 64–71

261. Kruszynska Y T, Home P D, MacIntyre N. Relationship between insulin sensitivity, insulin secretion and glucose tolerance in cirrhosis. Hepatology 1991; 14: 103–111

262. Muller M J, Willmann O, Rieger A et al. Mechanism of insulin resistance associated with liver cirrhosis. Gastroenterology 1992; 102: 2033–2041

263. Petrides A S, Schulze-Berge D, Vogt C, Matthews D E, Strohmeyer G. Glucose resistance contributes to diabetes mellitus in cirrhosis. Hepatology 1993; 18: 284–291

264. Olefsky J M. Insulin resistance in humans. Gastroenterology 1982; 83: 1313–1318

265. Cavallo Perin P, Cassader M, Bozzo C et al. Mechanism of insulin resistance in human liver cirrhosis: evidence of a combined receptor and post receptor defect. J Clin Invest 1985; 75: 1659–1665

266. Reaven G M. Role of insulin resistance in human disease. Diabetes 1988; 37: 1595–1607

267. Mauriac P. Hepatomegalie, nanisme, obesite dans le diabete infantile, pathogenie du syndrome. Presse Medicale 1946; 54: 826–827

268. Hildes J A, Sherlock S, Walshe V. Liver and muscle glycogen in normal subjects, in diabetes mellitus and in acute hepatitis. Clin Sci 1949; 7: 287–295

269. Goodman J I. Hepatomegaly and diabetes mellitus. Ann Intern Med 1953; 39: 1077–1087

270. Seef L B, Zimmerman H J. Relationship between hepatic and pancreatic disease. In: Popper H, Schaffner F, eds. Progress in liver diseases, vol V. New York: Grune & Stratton, 1976: pp 590–608

271. Caramia F, Ghergo F G, Branciari C, Menghini G. New aspects of hepatic nuclear glycogenosis in diabetes. J Clin Pathol 1968; 21: 19–23

272. Batman P A, Scheuer P J. Diabetic hepatitis preceding the onset of glucose intolerance. Histopathology 1985; 9: 237–243

273. Bernuau D, Guillot R, Durand A M et al. Ultrastructural aspects of the liver perisinusoidal space in diabetic patients with and without microangiopathy. Diabetes 1982; 31: 1061–1067

274. Latry P, Bioulac-Sage P, Echinard E, Gin H, Boussarie L, Grimaud J A, Balabaud C. Perisinusoidal fibrosis and basement membrane-like material in the livers of diabetic patients. Hum Pathol 1987; 18: 775–780

275. Jacques W E. The incidence of portal cirrhosis and fatty metamorphosis in patients dying with diabetes mellitus. N Engl J Med 1953; 249: 442

276. Seige K, Thierback V. Post hepatitische Schaden bei diabetes mellitus. Verhandlungen der Deutschen Gesellschaft für Innere Medizin 1959; 65: 705

277. Foster J H, Donohue T A, Berman M M. Familial liver cell adenomas and diabetes mellitus. N Engl J Med 1978; 299: 239–241

278. Thung S N, Gerber M A, Bodenheimer H C Jr. Nodular regenerative hyperplasia of the liver in a patient with diabetes mellitus. Cancer 1982; 49: 543–546

279. Ludwig J, Dyck J, LaRusso F N. Xanthomatous neuropathy of liver. Hum Pathol 1982; 13: 1049–1051

280. Alberti-Flor J J, Jeffers L, Schiff E R. Primary sclerosing cholangitis occurring in a patient with systemic lupus erythematosus and diabetes mellitus. Am J Gastroenterol 1984; 79: 889–891

281. Bruguera M, Bertran A, Bombi J A, Rodes J. Giant mitochondria in hepatocytes. A diagnostic hint for alcoholic liver disease. Gastroenterology 1977; 73: 1383–1387

282. Kreek M J. Female sex steroids and cholestasis. Semin Liver Dis 1987; 7: 8–23

283. Van Thiel D H, Gavaler J S. Pregnancy-associated sex steroids and their effects on the liver. Semin Liver Dis 1987; 7: 1–8

284. Porter L E, Van Thiel D H, Eagon P K. Estrogens and progestins as tumor inducers. Semin Liver Dis 1987; 7: 24–31

285. Ishak K G, Zimmerman H J. Hepatotoxic effects of the anabolic/androgenic steroids. Semin Liver Dis 1987; 7: 230–236

286. Salata R, Klein I, Levey G S. Thyroid hormone homeostasis and the liver. Semin Liver Dis 1985; 5: 29–34

287. Van Thiel D H. The liver and the endocrine system. In: Arias I M, Jakoby W B, Popper H, Schaffner D, Shafritz D A, eds. The liver: biology and pathobiology, 2nd edn. New York: Raven Press, 1988: pp 1007–1031

288. Babb R R. Association between diseases of the thyroid and liver. Am J Gastroenterol 1984; 79: 421–423

289. Johnson P J. The effects of liver disease on the endocrine system. In: McIntyre N, Benhamou J-P, Bircher J, Rizzetto M, Rodes J, eds. Oxford textbook of clinical hepatology. Oxford: Oxford University Press, 1991: pp 1214–1224

290. Van Thiel D H, Udani M, Schade R R, Sanghvi A, Starzl T E. Prognostic value of thyroid hormone levels in patients evaluated for liver transplantation. Hepatology 1985; 5: 862–866

291. Ashkar F S, Miller R, Smoak W M, Gilson A J. Liver disease in hyperthyroidism. S Med J 1971; 64: 462–465

292. Thompson P J K, Strum O, Boehm T, Wartofsky L. Abnormalities of liver function tests in thyrotoxicosis. Military Med 1978; 143: 548–551

293. Greenberger N J, Milligan F D, De Groot L J, Isselbacher K J. Jaundice and thyrotoxicosis in the absence of congestive cardiac failure. Am J Med 1964; 36: 840–846

294. Movitt E R, Gerstl B, Davis A E. Needle liver biopsy in thyrotoxicosis. Arch Int Med 1953; 91: 729–739

295. Piper J, Poulsen E. Liver biopsy in thyrotoxicosis. Acta Med Scand 1947; 127: 439–447

296. Dooner H P, Parada J, Aliaga C, Hoyl C. The liver in thyrotoxicosis. Arch Int Med 1967; 120: 25–32

297. Sola J, Pardo-Mindan F J, Zozaya J, Quiroga J, Sangro B, Prieto J. Liver changes in patients with hyperthyroidism. Liver 1991; 11: 193–197

298. Klion F M, Segal R, Schaffner F. The effect of altered thyroid function on the ultrastructure of the human liver. Am J Med 1971; 50: 317–324

299. Van Steenbergen W, Fevey J, De Vos R et al. Thyroid hormone and the hepatic handling of bilirubin. I. Effects of hypothyroidism and hyperparathyroidism on the hepatic transport of bilirubin mono- and diconjugates in the Wistar rat. Hepatology 1989; 9: 314–321

300. Ariza C R, Frate A C, Sierra I. Hypothyroidism-associated cholestasis. JAMA 1984; 252: 2392

301. Clancy R L, Mackay I R. Myxoedematous ascites. Med J Aus 1970; 2: 415–416

302. Baker A, Kaplan M, Wolfe H. Central congestive fibrosis of the liver in myxoedema ascites. Ann Int Med 1972; 77: 927–929

303. Ono M, Ishizaki T. A case of nodular regenerative hyperplasia of the liver in Hashimoto's struma. Acta Hepatol Jap 1984; 25: 682–687

304. Weldon A P, Danks D M. Congenital hypothyroidism and neonatal jaundice. Arch Dis Childh 1972; 47: 469–471

305. McCann V J, Fulton T T. Cortisol metabolism in chronic liver disease. J Clin Endocrinol Metab 1975; 40: 1038–1044

306. Soffer L J, Iannaccone A, Gabrilove J L. Cushing's syndrome: a study of 50 patients. Am J Med 1961; 30: 129–146

307. Hill R B Jr. Fatal fat embolism from steroid-induced fatty liver. N Engl J Med 1961; 265: 318–320

308. Jones J P, Engleman E P, Najarian J S. Systemic fat embolism after renal homotransplantation and treatment with corticosteroids. N Engl J Med 1965; 273: 1453–1458

309. Olsson R G, Lindgren A, Zettergren L. Liver involvement in Addison's disease. Am J Gastroenterol 1990; 85: 435–438

310. Iram S, Sidki K, Al-Marshedy A-R, Judzewitsch R. Addison's disease, hypertension, renal and hepatic microthrombosis in primary antiphospholipid syndrome. Postgrad Med J 1991; 67: 385–388

311. van Thiel D H, Gabeler J S, Schade R R. Liver disease and the hypothalamic pituitary axis. Semin Liver Dis 1985; 5: 35–45

312. Russel W E. Growth hormone, somatomedins and the liver. Semin Liver Dis 1985; 5: 46–58

313. Preisig R, Morris T Q, Shaver J C, Christy N P. Volumetric haemodynamic and excretory characteristics of the liver in acromegaly. J Clin Invest 1966; 45: 1379–1387

314. Orloff M J. Hyperparathyroidism, cirrhosis and portacaval shunt. A new clinical syndrome. Am J Surg 1988; 155: 76–81

315. Loeb J M, Hauger P H, Carney J D, Cooper A D. Refractory ascites due to POEMS syndrome. Gastroenterology 1989; 96: 247–249

316. Ulissi A, Ricci G L. Hepatic histology in a case of Turner's syndrome. Ital J Gastroenterol 1989; 21: 340–341

317. Burroughs A K. Liver disease and pregnancy. In: McIntyre N, Benhamou-J P, Bircher J, Rizzetto M, Rodes J, eds. Oxford textbook of clinical hepatology. Oxford: Oxford University Press, 1991: pp 1319–1332

318. MacSween R N M. Pathology of the liver and gallbladder in pregnancy. In: Fox H, ed. Haines' & Taylor's Obstetrical and gynaecological pathology, 4th edn. Edinburgh: Churchill Livingstone, 1995 (in press)

319. Rustgi V K, Fagiuoli S, Van Thiel D H. The liver in pregnancy. In: Rustgi V K, Van Thiel D H, eds. The liver in systemic disease. New York: Raven Press, 1993: pp 267–283

320. Varma R. Course and prognosis of pregnancy in women with liver disease. Semin Liver Dis 1987; 7: 59–66

321. Lee W M. Pregnancy in patients with chronic liver disease. Gastroenterol Clin N Amer 1992; 21: 889–903

322. McNair R D, Jaynes R V. Alterations in liver function during normal pregnancy. Am J Obstet Gyn 1960; 80: 500–503

323. Hytten F E, Leitch I. The physiology of human pregnancy, 2nd edn. Oxford: Blackwell Scientific Publications, 1971

324. Seymour C A, Chadwick V S. Liver and gastrointestinal function in pregnancy. Postgrad Med J 1979; 55: 343–352

325. Robson S C, Mutch E, Boys R J, Woodhouse K W. Apparent liver blood flow during pregnancy: a serial study using indocyanine green clearance. Br J Obstet Gyn 1990; 97: 720–724

326. Haemmerli U P. Jaundice during pregnancy with special emphasis on recurrent jaundice during pregnancy and its differential diagnosis. Acta Med Scand 1966; Suppl 444: 1–111

327. Krejs G J, Haemmerli U P. Jaundice during pregnancy. In: Schiff L, Schiff E R, eds Diseases of the liver, 5th edn. Philadelphia: Lippincott, 1982: pp 1561–1580

328. Krejs G J. Jaundice during pregnancy. Semin Liver Dis 1983; 3: 73–82

329. Gonzalez-Angulo A, Aznar-Ramos R, Marquez-Monter H, Bierzwinsky G S, Martinez-Manautou J. The ultrastructure of liver cells in women under steroid therapy. I. Normal pregnancy and trophoblastic growth. Acta Endocrinol 1970; 65: 193–206

330. Perez V, Gorodisch S, Casavilla F, Maruffo C. Ultrastructure of the human liver at the end of normal pregnancy. Amer J Obs Gyn 1971; 110: 428–431

331. Van Thiel D H, ed. Effects of pregnancy and sex hormones on the liver. Semin Liver Dis 1987; 7: 1–66

332. Sheehan H L. The pathology of hyperemesis and vomiting of late pregnancy. J Obs Gyn 1940; 46: 658–699

333. Ober W B, Le Compte P M. Acute fatty metamorphosis of the liver associated with pregnancy. A distinctive lesion. Am J Med 1955; 19: 743–758

334. Moore H C. Acute fatty liver of pregnancy. J Obs Gyn 1956; 63: 189–198

335. Davies M H, Wilkinson S P, Hanid M A et al. Acute liver disease with encephalopathy and renal failure in late pregnancy and the early puerperium. A study of fourteen patients. Br J Obstet Gyn 1980; 87: 1005–1014

336. Burroughs A K, Seong N H, Dojcinov D M et al. Idiopathic acute fatty liver of pregnancy in twelve patients. Q J Med 1982; 204: 481–497

337. Hague W M, Fenton D W, Duncan S L B, Slater D N. Acute fatty liver of pregnancy. A review of the literature and six further cases. J Roy Soc Med 1983; 76: 652–661

338. Pockros P J, Peters R L, Reynolds T B. Idiopathic fatty liver of pregnancy: findings in ten cases. Medicine 1984; 63: 1–11

339. Rolfes D B, Ishak K G. Acute fatty liver of pregnancy: a clinicopathologic study of 35 cases. Hepatology 1985; 5: 1149–1158

340. Schorr-Lesnick B, Lebovics E, Dworkin B, Rosenthal W S. Liver diseases unique to pregnancy. Am J Gastroenterol 1991; 86: 659–670

341. Mabie W C. Acute fatty liver of pregnancy. Gastroenterol Clin N Amer 1992; 21: 951–960

342. Rolfes D B, Ishak K G. Liver disease in pregnancy. Histopathology 1986; 10: 555–570

343. Campillo B, Bernuau J, Witz M O et al. Ultrasonography in acute fatty liver of pregnancy. Ann Int Med 1986; 105: 383–384

344. Mabie W C, Dacus J V, Sibai B M et al. Computed tomography in acute fatty liver of pregnancy. Amer J Obs Gyn 1988; 158: 142–145

345. Sheehan H L. Jaundice in pregnancy. Amer J Obs Gyn 1961; 81: 427–440

346. Bernau J, Degott C, Nouel O, Rueff B, Benhamou J P. Non-fatal acute fatty liver of pregnancy. Gut 1982; 24: 340–344

347. Ebert E C, Sun E A, Wright S H et al. Does early diagnosis and delivery in acute fatty liver of pregnancy lead to improvement in maternal and infant survival? Dig Dis Sci 1984; 29: 453–455

348. Riely C A. Acute fatty liver of pregnancy (editorial). Dig Dis Sci 1984; 29: 456–457

349. Ockner S A, Brunt E M, Cohn S M et al. Fulminant hepatic failure caused by acute fatty liver of pregnancy treated by orthotopic liver transplantation. Hepatology 1990; 11: 59–64

350. Amon E, Allen S R, Petrie R H et al. Acute fatty liver of pregnancy associated with pre-eclampsia; management of hepatic failure with postpartum liver transplantation. Am J Perinatol 1993; 8: 278–279

351. Woolf A J, Johnston A W, Stokes J F, Roberton N R C. Acute liver failure in pregnancy. Case report with survival of mother and child. J Obs Gyn 1964; 71: 914–918

352. Duma R J, Dowling E A, Alexander H C, Sibrons D, Dempsey H. Acute fatty liver of pregnancy: report of surviving patient studied with serial liver biopsies. Ann Int Med 1965; 63: 851–858

353. Breen K J, Perkins K W, Mistilis S P, Shearman R. Idiopathic acute fatty liver of pregnancy. Gut 1970; 11: 822–825

354. Jenkins W F, Darling M R. Idiopathic acute fatty liver of pregnancy: subsequent uncomplicated pregnancy. J Obs Gyn 1980; 1: 100–101

355. Barton J R, Sibai B M, Mabie W C et al. Recurrent acute fatty liver of pregnancy. Amer J Obs Gyn 1990; 163: 534–538

356. Schoeman M N, Batey R G, Wilcken B. Recurrent acute fatty liver of pregnancy associated with a fatty-acid oxidation defect in the offspring. Gastroenterology 1991; 100: 544–548

357. Vanjak D, Moreau R, Roche-Sicot J, Soulier A, Sicot C. Intrahepatic cholestasis of pregnancy and acute fatty liver of pregnancy: an unusual but favourable association. Gastroenterology 1991; 100: 1123–1125

358. Malatjalian D A, Badley B W D. Acute fatty liver of pregnancy. Light and electron microscopic studies. Gastroenterology 1983; 84: 1384 (Abstract)

359. Joske R A, McCully D J, Mastaglia F L. Acute fatty liver of pregnancy. Gut 1968; 9: 489–493

360. Weber F L, Snodgrass P J, Powell D E et al. Abnormalities of hepatic mitochondrial urea-cycle enzyme activities and hepatic ultrastructure in acute fatty liver of pregnancy. J Lab Clin Med 1979; 94: 27–41

361. Slater D N, Hague W M. Renal morphological changes in idiopathic acute fatty liver of pregnancy. Histopathology 1984; 8: 567–581

362. Liebman H A, McGhee W G, Patch M J, Feinstein D I. Severe depression of antithrombin III associated with disseminated intravascular coagulation in women with fatty liver of pregnancy. Ann Int Med 1983; 98: 330–333

363. Minakami H, Oka N, Sato T et al. Pre-eclampsia: a microvesicular fat disease of the liver? Am J Obs Gyn 1988; 159: 1043–1047

364. Killam A P, Dillard S H, Patton R C, Pedersen P R. Pregnancy-induced hypertension complicated by acute liver disease and disseminated intravascular coagulation. Am J Obs Gyn 1975; 123: 823–828

365. Long R G, Scheuer P J, Sherlock S. Pre-eclampsia presenting with deep jaundice. J Clin Pathol 1977; 30: 212–215

366. Barron W M. The syndrome of pre-eclampsia. Gastroenterol Clin N Amer 1992; 21: 851–872

367. Antia F P, Bharadwaj T P, Watsa M C, Master J. Liver in normal pregnancy, pre-eclampsia and eclampsia. Lancet 1958; ii: 776–778

368. Arias F, Manchilla-Jimenez R. Hepatic fibrinogen deposits in pre-eclampsia. Immunofluorescent evidence. N Engl J Med 1976; 295: 578–582

369. Weinstein L. Syndrome of hemolysis, elevated liver enzymes, and low platelet count: a severe consequence of hypertension in pregnancy. Am J Obs Gyn 1982; 142: 159–167

370. Barton J R, Sibai B M. Care of the pregnancy: complicated by HELLP syndrome. Gastroenterol Clin N Amer 1992; 21: 937–950

371. Sibai B M, Taslimi M M, El-Nazer A et al. Maternal-perinatal outcome associated with the syndrome of hemolysis, elevated liver enzymes, and low platelets in severe pre-eclampsia-eclampsia. Am J Obs Gyn 1986; 155: 501–509

372. Sibai B M. The HELLP syndrome (hemolysis, elevated liver enzymes and low platelets): Much ado about nothing? Am J Obs Gyn 1990; 162: 311–316

373. Abell T L, Riely C A. Hyperemesis gravidarum. Gastroenterol Clin North Amer 1992; 21: 835–849

374. Wallstedt A, Riely C A, Shaver D et al. Prevalence and characteristics of liver dysfunction in hyperemesis gravidarum. Clin Res 1990; 38: 970–976

375. Adams R H, Gordon J, Combes B. Hyperemesis gravidarum. I. Evidence of hepatic dysfunction. Obs Gyn 1968; 31: 659–664

376. Richards R L, Willocks J, Dow T G B. Jaundice in pregnancy. Scot Med J 1970; 15: 52–57

377. Neerhoff M G, Zelman W, Sullivan T. Hepatic rupture in pregnancy: a review. Obs Gyn Surg 1989; 44: 407–409

378. Smith L G, Moise K J, Dildy G A, Carpenter R J. Spontaneous rupture of liver during pregnancy: current therapy. Obs Gyn 1991; 77: 171–175

379. Golan A, White R G. Spontaneous rupture of the liver associated with pregnancy. A report of 5 cases. S Afr Med J 1979; 56: 133–136

380. Manas K J, Welsh J D, Rankin R A, Miller D D. Hepatic haemorrhage without rupture in pre-eclampsia. N Engl J Med 1985; 312: 424–426

381. Cornell E L, Lash A F. Abdominal pregnancy. Int Abs Surg 1933; 8: 98–104

382. Morley A H G. Liver pregnancies. Lancet 1956; i: 994–995

383. Meare Y, Ekna J B, Raolison S. Un cas de grossesse à implantation hépatique avec enfant virant. Sem des Hopitaux de Paris 1965; 41: 1430–1433

384. Kirby N G. Primary hepatic pregnancy. Br Med J 1969; 1: 296

385. Hietala S-O, Anderson M, Emdin S O. Ectopic pregnancy in the liver: report of a case and angiographic findings. Acta Chir Scand 1983; 149: 633–635

386. Mitchell R W, Teare A J. Primary hepatic pregnancy. A case report and review. S Afr Med J 1984; 65: 220–225

387. De Almeida Barbosa A Jr, Rodriguez de Freitas L A, Andrade Mota M. Primary pregnancy in the liver. A case report. Pathol Res Prac 1991; 187: 329–331

388. Green T W, Conley C L, Berthrong M. The liver in sickle cell anaemia. Bull Johns Hopkins Hosp 1953; 92: 99–127

389. Edington G M. The pathology of sickle-cell disease in West Africa. Trans Roy Soc Trop Med 1955; 49: 253–267

390. Song Y S. Hepatic lesions in sickle cell anemia. Am J Pathol 1957; 33: 331–351

391. Rosenblate H J, Eisenstein R, Holmes A W. The liver in sickle cell anemia. Arch Pathol 1970; 90: 235–245

392. Bauer T W, Moore G W, Hutchins G M. The liver in sickle cell disease: a clinicopathologic study of 70 patients. Am J Med 1980; 69: 833–837

393. Johnson C S, Omata M, Tong M J, Simmons J F, Weiner J, Tatter D. Liver involvement in sickle cell disease. Medicine 1985; 64: 349–356

394. Mills L R, Mwakyusa D, Milner P F. Histopathologic features of liver biopsy specimens in sickle cell disease. Arch Path Lab Med 1988; 112: 290–294

395. Sty J R. Hepatic vein thrombosis in sickle cell anaemia. Amer J Ped Haematol Oncol 1982; 4: 213–215

396. Heaton N D, Pain J, Cowan N C, Salisbury J, Howard E R. Focal nodular hyperplasia of the liver: a link with sickle cell disease. Arch Dis Childn 1991; 66: 1073–1074

397. Middleton J P, Wolper J C. Hepatic biloma complicating sickle cell disease. A case report and a review of the literature. Gastroenterology 1984; 86: 743–744

398. Avigan M I, Ishak K G, Gregg R E, Hoofnagle J H. Morphologic features of the liver in abetalipoproteinemia. Hepatology 1984; 4: 1223–1226

399. Grossman J A, McDermott W V. Paroxysmal nocturnal haemoglobinuria associated with hepatic and portal vein thrombosis. Am J Surg 1974; 127: 733–736

400. Liebowitz A I, Hartman R C. The Budd-Chiari syndrome and paroxysmal nocturnal haemoglobinuria. Br J Haematol 1981; 48: 1–6

401. Braude S, Portmann B, Gimson A E S, Williams R. Fulminant hepatic failure in non-Hodgkin's lymphoma. Postgrad Med J 1982; 58: 301–304

402. Colby T V, La Brecque D R. Lymphoreticular malignancy presenting as fulminant hepatic disease. Gastroenterology 1982; 82: 339–345

403. Zafrani E S, Leclerca B, Vernan J-P, Pinaudeau Y, Chomette G, Dhumeaux D. Massive blastic infiltrations of the liver: a cause of fulminant hepatic failure. Hepatology 1983; 3: 428–432

404. Nizalik E, Zayed E, Foyle A. Malignant lymphoma presenting as fulminant hepatic failure. Can J Gastroenterol 1989; 3: 111–114

405. Conway E E Jr, Santorineou M, Mitsudo S. Fulminant hepatic failure in a child with acute lymphoblastic leukemia. J Pediatr Gastroenterol Nutr 1992; 15: 194–197

406. Yam L T, Janckila A J, Chan C H, Chin-Yang L I. Hepatic involvement in hairy cell leukaemia. Cancer 1983; 51: 1497–1504

407. Zafrani E S, Degos F, Guigui B et al. The hepatic sinusoid in hairy cell leukemia: an ultrastructural study of 12 cases. Hum Pathol 1987; 18: 801–807

408. Bendix-Hansen K, Bayer Kristensen I. Granulomas of spleen and liver in hairy cell leukaemia. APMIS 1984; 92: 157–160

409. Nanba K, Soban E J, Bowling M C, Berard C W. Splenic pseudosinuses and hepatic angiomatous lesions. Distinctive features of hairy cell leukaemia. Am J Clin Pathol 1977; 67: 415–526

410. Roquet M-L, Zafrani E-S, Farcet J-P, Reyes F, Pinaudeau Y. Histopathological lesions of the liver in hairy cell leukemia: a report of 14 cases. Hepatology 1985; 5: 496–500

411. Grouls V, Stiers R. Hepatic involvement in hairy cell leukaemia: diagnosis by tartrate resistant acid phosphatase enzyme histochemistry on formalin-fixed and paraffin-embedded liver biopsy specimens. Path Res Pract 1984; 178: 332–334

412. Falini B, Schwarting R, Enber W et al. The differential diagnosis of hairy cell leukemia with a panel of monoclonal antibodies. Am J Clin Pathol 1985; 83: 289–300

413. Zafrani E S, Cazier A, Baudelot A M et al. Ultrastructural lesions of the liver in human peliosis. A report of 12 cases. Am J Pathol 1984; 114: 349

414. Rozman M. Chronic lymphatic leukaemia and portal hypertension. Med Clinics Barcelona 1989; 92: 26–28

415. Locasiulli A, Vergani G M, Uderzo C et al. Chronic liver disease in children with leukaemia in long-term remission. Cancer 1983; 52: 1080–1087

416. Barton J C, Conrad M E. Beneficial effects of hepatitis in patients with acute myelogenous leukemia. Ann Int Med 1979; 90: 188–190

417. Rosner F. Hepatitis and leukemia. Ann Int Med 1979; 90: 853

418. Brody S A, Russell W G, Krantz S B, Graber E. Beneficial effect of hepatitis in leukemic reticulo-endotheliosis. Arch Int Med 1981; 141: 1080–1081

419. Dubois A, Dauzat M, Pignodel C et al. Portal hypertension in lymphoproliferative and myeloproliferative disorders: hemodynamic and histological correlations. Hepatology 1993; 17: 246–250

420. Amos J A, Goodbody R A. Lymph node and liver biopsy in the myeloproliferative disorders. Br J Cancer 1959; 13: 173–180

421. Ligumski M, Polliak A, Benbassat J. Nature and incidence of liver involvement in agnogenic myeloid metaplasia. Scand J Haematol 1978; 21: 81–93

422. Pereira A, Bruguera M, Cervantes F, Rozman C. Liver involvement at diagnosis of primary myelofibrosis: a clinicopathological study of twenty-two cases. Eur J Haematol 1988; 40: 355–361

423. Scheuer P J. Liver biopsy interpretation, 4th edn. London: Bailliere Tindall, 1988: p. 243

424. Degott C, Capron J P, Bettan L et al. Myeloid metaplasia, perisinusoidal fibrosis, and nodular regenerative hyperplasia of the liver. Liver 1985; 5: 276–281

425. Bioulac-Sage P, Roux D, Quinton A, Lamouliatte H, Balabaud C. Ultrastructure of sinusoids in patients with agnogenic myeloid metaplasia. J Submicrosc Cytol 1986; 14: 815–821

426. Roux D, Merlio J P, Quinton A, Lamouliatte H, Balabaud C, Bioulac-Sage P. Agnogenic myeloid metaplasia, portal hypertension and sinusoidal abnormalities. Gastroenterology 1987; 92: 1067–1072

427. Hayes L W, Bennett W H, Hech F J. Extra-medullary lesions in multiple myeloma; review of literature and pathologic studies. Arch Pathol 1952; 53: 262–272

428. Thiruvengadam R, Penetranti R, Grolsky H J et al. Multiple myeloma presenting as space-occupying lesions of the liver. Cancer 1990; 65: 2784–2786

429. Thomas F B, Clausen K P, Greenberger N J. Liver disease in multiple myeloma. Arch Int Med 1973; 132: 195–202

430. Brooks A P. Portal hypertension in Waldenström's macroglobulinaemia. Br Med J 1976; 1: 689–690

431. Wanless I R. Micronodular transformation (nodular regenerative hyperplasia) of the liver: a report of 64 cases among 2,500 autopsies and a new classification of benign hepatocellular nodules. Hepatology 1990; 11: 787–797

432. Voinchet O, Degott C, Scoazec J-Y, Feldmann G, Benhamou J-P. Peliosis hepatis, nodular regenerative hyperplasia of the liver, and light chain deposition in a patient with Waldenström's macroglobulinemia. Gastroenterology 1988; 95: 482–486

433. Kim H, Dorfman R F. Morphological studies of 84 untreated patients subjected to laparotomy for the staging of non-Hodgkin's lymphomas. Cancer 1974; 33: 657–674

434. Kim H, Dorfman R F, Rosenberg S A. Pathology of malignant lymphomas in the liver: application in staging. In: Popper H, Schaffner F, eds. Progress in liver diseases, vol 5. New York: Grune & Stratton, 1976: pp 683–698

435. Lefkowitch J H, Falkow S, Whitlock R T. Hepatic Hodgkin's disease simulating cholestatic hepatitis with liver failure. Arch Path Lab Med 1985; 109: 424–426

436. Gunasekaran T S, Hassall E, Dimmick J E, Chan K W. Hodgkin's disease presenting with fulminant liver disease. J Pediatr Gastroenterol Nutr 1992; 15: 189–193

437. Abt A B, Kirschner R H, Belliveau R E, O'Connell M J, Schlansky B D, Greene W H, Wiernik P H. Hepatic pathology associated with Hodgkin's disease. Cancer 1974; 33: 1564–1571

438. Kaplan H S. Hodgkin's disease: unfolding concepts concerning its nature, management and prognosis. Cancer 1980; 45: 2439–2474

439. Jaffe E S. Malignant lymphomas: pathology of hepatic involvement. Semin Liver Dis 1987; 7: 257–268

440. Fialk M A, Janowski C I, Coleman M, Mouradian J. Hepatic Hodgkin's disease without involvement of the spleen. Cancer 1979; 43: 1146–1147

441. Gordon C D, Sidawy M K, Talarico L, Kondi E. Hodgkin's disease in the liver without splenic involvement. Arch Int Med 1984; 144: 2277–2278

442. Colby T V, Hopper R T, Warnke R A. Hodgkin's disease: a clinicopathological study of 659 cases. Cancer 1982; 49: 1848–1855

443. Rappaport H, Bernard C W, Butler J J, Dorfman R F, Lukes R J, Thomas L B. Report of the committees on histopathological criteria contributing to staging of Hodgkin's disease. Cancer Res 1971; 31: 1864–1865

444. Skovsgaard T, Brinckmeyer L M, Vesterager L et al. The liver in Hodgkin's disease. II. Histopathologic findings. Eur J Cancer Clin Oncol 1982; 18: 429–435

445. Cavalli G, Casali A M, Lambertini F, Busachi C. Changes in the small biliary passages in the hepatic localization of Hodgkin's disease. Virchows Arch (A) 1979; 384: 295–306

446. Leslie K O, Colby T V. Hepatic parenchymal lymphoid aggregates in Hodgkin's disease. Hum Pathol 1984; 15: 808–809

447. Kadin M E, Donaldson S S, Dorfman R F. Isolated granulomas in Hodgkin's disease. N Engl J Med 1970; 283: 859–861

448. Sacks E L, Donaldson S S, Gordon J, Dorfman R F. Epithelioid granulomas associated with Hodgkin's disease. Cancer 1978; 41: 562–567

449. Pak H Y, Friedman N B. Pseudosarcoid granulomas in Hodgkin's disease. Hum Pathol 1981; 12: 832–837

450. Johnson L N, Iseri O, Knodell R G. Caseating hepatic granulomas in Hodgkin's lymphoma. Gastroenterology 1990; 99: 1837–1840

451. Taxy J B. Peliosis: a morphologic curiosity becomes an iatrogenic problem. Hum Pathol 1978; 9: 331–340

452. Bruguera M, Aranguibel F, Ros E, Rodes J. Incidence and clinical significance of sinusoidal dilatation in liver biopsies. Gastroenterology 1978; 75: 474–478

453. Bain B J, Chong K C, Coghlan S J, Roberts S J. Hepatic sinusoidal ectasia in association with Hodgkin's disease. Postgrad Med J 1982; 58: 182–184

454. Bruguera M, Caballero T, Carreras E et al. Hepatic sinusoidal dilatation in Hodgkin's disease. Liver 1987; 7: 76–80

455. Birrer M J, Young R C. Differential diagnosis of jaundice in lymphoma patients. Semin Liver Dis 1987; 7: 269–277

456. Lieberman D A. Intrahepatic cholestasis due to Hodgkin's disease: an elusive diagnosis. J Clin Gastroenterol 1986; 8: 304–307

457. Hubscher S G, Lumley M A, Elias E. Vanishing bile duct syndrome: a possible mechanism for intrahepatic cholestasis in Hodgkin's lymphoma. Hepatology 1993; 17: 70–77

458. Man K M, Drejet A, Keefe E B. Primary sclerosing cholangitis and Hodgkin's disease. Hepatology 1993; 18: 1127–1131

459. Kahn L B, King H, Jacobs P. Florid epithelioid cell and sarcoid-type reaction associated with non-Hodgkin's lymphoma. S Afr Med J 1977; 51: 341–347

460. Saito K, Nakanuma Y, Ogawa S, Arai Y, Hayashi M. Extensive hepatic granulomas associated with peripheral T-cell lymphoma. Am J Gastroenterol 1991; 86: 1243–1246

461. Watterson J, Priest J R. Jaundice as a paraneoplastic phenomenon in a T-cell lymphoma. Gastroenterology 1989; 97: 1319–1322

462. Cozzolino G, Lonardo A, Fracica G, Cacciatore L. Three more cases of concurrent liver cirrhosis and non-Hodgkin's lymphoma. Ital J Gastroenterol 1984; 16: 235–237

463. Di Stasi M, Cavanna L, Fornari F et al. Association of non-Hodgkin's lymphoma and hepatocellular carcinoma. Oncology (Switzerland) 1990; 47: 80–83

464. Voigt J J, Vinel J P, Caveriviere P et al. Diagnostic immunohistochimique des localisations hepatiques des hemopathies lymphoides malignes; etude de 80 cas. Gastroent Clin Biol 1989; 13: 343–352

465. Wright D H. Burkitt's tumour. A post-mortem study of 50 cases. Br J Surg 1964; 51: 245–251

466. Banks P M, Arseneau J C, Gralnick H R et al. American Burkitt's lymphoma: a clinicopathologic study of 30 cases. Am J Med 1975; 58: 322–329

467. Gaulard P, Zafrani E S, Mavier P et al. Peripheral T-cell lymphoma presenting as predominant liver disease: a report of three cases. Hepatology 1986; 6: 864–868

468. Blayney D, Jaffe E, Blattner W et al. The human T-cell leukemia/lymphoma virus (HTLV) associated with American adult T-cell leukemia/lymphoma (ATL). Blood 1983; 62: 401–405

469. Fakunle Y M, Greenwood B M. The nature of hepatic lymphocytic infiltrates in the tropical splenomegal syndrome. Clin Exp Immunol 1982; 48: 546–550

470. Dacie J V, Brain M C, Harrison C V, Lewis S M, Worlledge S M. Non-tropical idiopathic splenomegaly (primary hypersplenism): a review of ten cases and their relationship to malignant lymphoma. Br J Haematol 1982; 17: 317–333

471. Sandilands G P, Cooney A, Grant R M et al. Lymphocytes with T- and B-cell properties in a lymphoproliferative disorder. Lancet 1974; i: 903–904

472. Kadin M E, Kamoun M, Lamberg J. Erythrophagocytic T gamma lymphoma. A clinicopathologic entity resembling malignant histiocytosis. N Engl J Med 1981; 304: 648–653

473. Kruskall M S, Weitzman S, Stossel T P, Harris N, Robinson S H. Lymphoma with autoimmune neutropenia and hepatic sinusoidal infiltration: a syndrome. Ann Int Med 1982; 97: 202–205

474. Paradinas F J, Harrison K M. Visceral lesions in an unusual case of Sezary's syndrome. Cancer 1974; 33: 1068–1074

475. Variakojis D, Rosas-Uribe A, Rappaport H. Mycosis fungoides. Pathologic findings in staging laparotomies. Cancer 1974; 33: 1589–1600

476. Rappaport H, Thomas L. Mycosis fungoides. The pathology of extracutaneous involvement. Cancer 1974; 34: 1198–1292

477. Cadranel J-F, Cadranel J, Buffet C et al. Nodular regenerative hyperplasia of the liver, peliosis hepatis, and perisinusoidal fibrosis. Association with angioimmunoblastic lymphadenopathy and severe hypoxemia. Gastroenterology 1990; 99: 268–273

478. Lafon M E, Bioulac-Sage P, Grimaud J A et al. Perisinusoidal fibrosis of the liver in patients with thrombocytopenic purpura. Virchows Arch (A) 1987; 411: 553–559

479. Neiman J C, Mant M J, Shnitka T K. Phagocytosis of platelets by Kupffer cells in immune thrombocytopenia. Arch Pathol Lab Med 1987; 111: 563–565

480. Croffy B, Kopelman R, Kaplan M. Hypereosinophilic syndrome. Association with chronic active hepatitis. Dig Dis Sci 1988; 33: 233–239

481. Foong A, Scholes J V, Gleich G J, Kephart G M, Holt P R. Eosinophil-induced chronic active hepatitis in the idiopathic hypereosinophilic syndrome. Hepatology 1991; 13: 1090–1094

482. Fauci A S, Harley J B, Roberts W C et al. The idiopathic hypereosinophilic syndrome. Clinical, pathophysiologic and therapeutic considerations. Ann Int Med 1982; 97: 78–92

483. Pfeifer U, Ormanns W, Klinge O. Hepatocellular fibrinogen storage in familial hypofibrinogenemia. Virchows Archiv (A) 1981; 36: 247–255

484. Wehinger H, Klinge O, Alexandrakis E, Schurmann J, Witts J, Seydewitz H H. Hereditary hypofibrinogenemia with fibrinogen storage in the liver. Eur J Ped 1983; 141: 109–112

485. Callea F, de Vos R, Togni R et al. Fibrinogen inclusions in liver cells: a new type of ground-glass hepatocyte: immune, light and electron microscopic characterisation. Histopathology 1986; 10: 65–74

486. Storch W, Riedel H, Trautmann B, Justus J, Hiemann D. Storage of the complement components C4, C3 and C3-activator in the human liver as PAS-negative globular hyaline bodies. Exp Pathol 1982; 21: 199–203

487. Storch W. Immunohistological investigation of PAS-negative intracisternal hyalin in human liver biopsy specimens. Virchows Arch (A) 1985; 48: 155–165

488. Mills P R, Sturrock R D. Clinical associations between arthritis and liver disease. Ann Rheum Dis 1982; 41: 295–307

489. Asherson R A, Hughes G R V. Musculoskeletal diseases and the liver. In: McIntyre N, Benhamou J-P, Bircher J, Rizzetto M, Rodes J, eds. Oxford textbook of clinical hepatology. Oxford: Oxford University Press, 1991: pp 1196–1201

490. Ayers A B, Fitchett D H. Hepatic haematoma in polyarteritis. Br J Radiol 1976; 49: 184–185

491. Haslock I. Spontaneous rupture of the liver in systemic lupus erythematosus. Ann Rheum Dis 1974; 33: 482–484

492. Hocking W G, Lasser K, Ungerer R, Bersohn M, Palos M, Spiegel T. Spontaneous hepatic rupture in rheumatoid arthritis. Arch Int Med 1981; 141: 792–794

493. Pettersson T, Lepantalo M, Frirnan C, Ahonen J. Spontaneous rupture of the liver in rheumatoid arthritis. Scand J Rheumatol 1986; 15: 348–349

494. Kendall M J, Cockel R, Becker J, Hawkins C F. Raised serum alkaline phosphatase in rheumatoid disease. Ann Rheum Dis 1970; 29: 537–540

495. Kendall M J, Cockel R, Becker J, Hawkins C F. Rheumatoid liver. Br Med J 1970; i: 221

496. Fernandes L, Sullivan, McFarlane I G et al. Studies on the frequency and pathogenesis of liver involvement in rheumatoid arthritis. Ann Rheum Dis 1975; 34: 198–199

497. Lowe J R, Pickup M E, Dixon J S et al. Gamma glutamyl transpeptidase levels in arthritis: a correlation with clinical and laboratory indices of disease activity. Ann Rheum Dis 1978; 37: 428–431

498. Spooner R J, Smith D H, Bedford D, Beck P R. Serum gamma-glutamyltransferase and alkaline phosphatase in rheumatoid arthritis. J Clin Pathol 1982; 35: 638–641

499. Siede W H, Seiffert U B, Merle S, Goll H G, Oremek G. Alkaline phosphatase isoenzymes in rheumatic diseases. Clin Biochem 1989; 22: 121–124

500. Webb J, Whaley K, MacSween R N M, Nuki G, Dick W C, Buchanan W W. Liver disease in rheumatoid arthritis and Sjögren's syndrome. Ann Rheum Dis 1975; 34: 70–81

501. Tiger L H, Gordon M H, Ehrlich G E, Shapiro B. Liver enlargement demonstrated by scintigraphy in rheumatoid arthritis. J Rheumatol 1976; 3: 15–20

502. Rau R, Pfenninger K, Boni A. Liver function tests and liver biopsies in patients with rheumatoid arthritis. Ann Rheum Dis 1975; 34: 198–199

503. Dietrichson O, From A, Christofferson P, Juhl E. Morphological changes in liver biopsies from patients with rheumatoid arthritis. Scand J Rheumatol 1976; 5: 65–69

504. Whaley K, Webb J. Liver and kidney disease in rheumatoid arthritis. Clin Rheum Dis 1977; 3: 527–547

505. Mills P R, MacSween R N M, Dick W C, More I A, Watkinson G. Liver disease in rheumatoid arthritis. Scot Med J 1980; 25: 18–22

506. Rau R, Karger T, Herborn G, Frenzel H. Liver biopsy findings in patients with rheumatoid arthritis undergoing longterm treatment with methotrexate. J Rheumatol 1989; 16: 489–493

507. Job-Deslandre C, Feldmann J L, Diyan Y, Meukes C J. Chronic hepatitis during rheumatoid arthritis. Clin Exp Rheumatol 1991; 9: 507–510

508. Laffon A, Moreno A, Gutierrez-Bucero A et al. Hepatic sinusoidal dilatation in rheumatoid arthritis. J Clin Gastroenterol 1989; 11: 653–657

509. Teh L G, Steven M M, Capell H A. Alpha-1-antitrypsin associated liver disease in rheumatoid arthritis. Postgrad Med J 1985; 61: 171–172

510. Sherlock S, Scheuer P J. The presentation and diagnosis of 100 patients with primary biliary cirrhosis. N Engl J Med 1973; 289: 674–678

511. Harris M, Rash R M, Dymock I W. Nodular non-cirrhotic liver associated with portal hypertension in a patient with rheumatoid arthritis. J Clin Pathol 1974; 27: 963–966

512. Stomeyer F W, Ishak K. Nodular transformation (nodular 'regenerative' hyperplasia) of the liver. Hum Pathol 1981; 12: 60–71

513. Reynolds W J, Wanless I R. Nodular regenerative hyperplasia of the liver in a patient with rheumatoid vasculitis: a morphometric study suggesting a role for hepatic arteritis in the pathogenesis. J Rheumatol 1984; 11: 838–842

514. Smits J G, Kooijman C D. Rheumatoid nodules in liver (letter). Histopathology 1986; 10: 1211–1212

515. Phillips C A, Cera P J, Mangan T F, Newman E D. Clinical liver disease in patients with rheumatoid arthritis taking methotrexate. J Rheumatol 1992; 19: 229–233

516. Hall P de la M, Ahern M J, Jarvis L R, Stott P, Jenner M A, Harley H. Two methods of assessment of methotrexate hepatotoxicity in patients with rheumatoid\arthritis. Ann Rheum Dis 1991; 50: 471–476

517. Landas S K, Mitros F A, Furst D E, La Brecque D R. Lipogranulomas and gold in the liver in rheumatoid arthritis. Am J Surg Pathol 1992; 16: 171–174

518. Bloch K J, Buchanan W W, Wohl M J, Bunin J J. Sjogren's syndrome. A clinical, pathological and serological study of 62 cases. Medicine 1965; 44: 187–231

519. Tsianos E V, Hoofnagle J H, Fox P C et al. Sjögrens syndrome in patients with primary biliary cirrhosis. Hepatology 1990; 11: 730–734

520. Montefusco P P, Geiss A C, Bronzo R L et al. Sclerosing cholangitis, chronic pancreatitis and Sjögren's syndrome: a syndrome complex. Am J Surg 1984; 147: 822–826

521. Blendis L M, Ansell I D, Lloyd-Jones K, Hamilton E, Williams R. Liver in Felty's syndrome. Br Med J 1970; 1: 131–135

522. Cohen M L, Marnier J W, Bredfeldt J E. Sinusoidal lymphocytosis of the liver in Felty's syndrome with a review of the liver involvement in Felty's syndrome. J Clin Gastroenterol 1989; 11: 92–94

523. Blendis L M, Parkinson M C, Shilkin K B, Williams R. Nodular regenerative hyperplasia of the liver in Felty's syndrome. Q J Med 1974; 43: 25–32

524. Blendis L M, Lovell D, Barris C G, Ritland S, Catton D, Vesia P. Esophageal variceal bleeding associated with nodular regenerative hyperplasia. Ann Rheum Dis 1978; 37: 183–186

525. Cohen M D, Ginsburg W W, Allen G L. Nodular regenerative hyperplasia of the liver and bleeding esophageal varices in Felty's syndrome: a case report and literature review. J Rheumatol 1982; 9: 716–728

526. Thorne C, Urowitz M B, Wanless I, Roberts E, Blendis L M. Liver disease in Felty's syndrome. Am J Med 1982; 73: 35–40

527. Young I D, Segura J, Ford P M, Ford S E. The pathogenesis of nodular regenerative hyperplasia of the liver associated with rheumatoid vasculitis. J Clin Gastroenterol 1992; 14: 127–131

528. Schaller J, Beckwith B, Wedgwood R J. Hepatic involvement in juvenile rheumatoid arthritis. J Pediatr 1970; 77: 203–210

529. Kornreich H, Malouf N N, Hanson V. Acute hepatic dysfunction in juvenile rheumatoid arthritis. J Pediatr 1971; 79: 27–35

530. Esdaile J M, Tannenbaum J, Hawkins D. Adult Still's disease. Am J Med 1980; 68: 825–830

531. Baker D G, Shumacher H R, Reginato A J. Fifteen patients with adult onset Still's disease: life-threatening liver failure in two. Arth Rheum 1979; 22: 590

532. Dubois E L, Wierzchowiecki M, Cox M B, Weirner J M. Duration and death in systemic lupus erythematosus. An analysis of 249 cases. JAMA 1974; 227: 1399–1402

533. Runyon B A, LeBrecqui D R, Anuras S. The spectrum of liver disease in systemic lupus erythematosus: report of 33 histologically-proved cases and review of the literature. Am J Med 1980; 69: 187–194

534. Gibson T, Myers A R. Subclinical liver disease in systemic lupus erythematosus. J Rheumatol 1981; 8: 752–759

535. Miller M H, Urowitz M B, Gladman D D, Blendis L M. The liver in systemic lupus erythematosus. Q J Med 1984; 211: 401–409

536. Matsumoto T, Yoshimine T, Shimouchi K, Shiotu H, Kuwabara N, Fukuda Y, Hoshi T. The liver in systemic lupus erythematosus: pathologic analysis of 52 cases and review of Japanese autopsy registry data. Hum Pathol 1992; 23: 1151–1158

537. Mackay I R. The hepatitis-lupus connection. Semin Liver Dis 1991; 11: 234–240

538. Colina F, Alberti N, Solis J A et al. Diffuse nodular regenerative hyperplasia of the liver (DNRH). A clinicopathologic study of 24 cases. Liver 1989; 9: 253–265

539. Hughes G R V. The antiphospholipid syndrome: ten years on. Lancet 1993; 342: 341–344

540. Perez-Ruiz F, Zea A C, Orte F J. Antiphospholipid antibodies may play a role in the pathogenesis of nodular regenerative hyperplasia of the liver. Br J Rheum 1990; 295: 107 (abstr)

541. Asherson R A, Thompson R P, MacLachlan N, Baguley E, Hicks P, Hughes G R. Visceral arterial occlusions, Budd-Chiari syndrome, recurrent fetal loss and the "lupus anticoagulant" in systemic lupus erythematosus. J Rheumatol 1989; 16: 219–224

542. Pelletier S, Landi B, Piette J C et al. The antiphospholipid syndrome as the second cause of non-malignant Budd-Chiari syndrome. Arthr Rheum 1992; 35 (suppl): S238 (abstr)

543. Khoury G, Tohi M, Oren M, Traub Y M. Massive hepatic infarction in systemic lupus erythematosus. Dig Dis Sci 1990; 35: 1557–1560

544. Haslock I. Spontaneous rupture of the liver in systemic lupus erythematosus. Ann Rheum Dis 1974; 33: 482–484

545. Robertson S J, Higgins R B, Powell C. Malakoplakia of liver: a case report. Hum Pathol 1992; 22: 1294–1295

546. Laxer R M, Roberts E A, Gross K R et al. Liver disease in neonatal lupus erythematosus. J Paed 1990; 116: 238–242

547. Bartholomew L G, Cain J C, Winkelmann R K, Baggenstoss A H. Chronic disease of the liver associated with systemic scleroderma. Am J Dig Dis 1964; 9: 43–55

548. D'Angelo W A, Fries J F, Masi A T, Shulman L E. Pathologic observations in systemic sclerosis (scleroderma). Am J Med 1969; 46: 428–440

549. Morris J S, Htut T, Read A E. Scleroderma and portal hypertension. Ann Rheum Dis 1972; 31: 316–318

550. Copeman P N M, Medd W D. Diffuse systemic sclerosis with abnormal liver and gallbladder. Br Med J 1967; ii: 353–354

551. Wildenthal K, Schenker S, Smiley J D, Ford K L. Obstructive jaundice and gastrointestinal haemorrhage in progressive systemic sclerosis. Arch Int Med 1968; 121: 365–368

552. Fraile G, Rodriguez-Garcia J L, Morena A. Primary sclerosing cholangitis associated with systemic sclerosis. Postgrad Med J 1991; 67: 189–192

553. Murray-Lyon I M, Thompson R P H, Ansell I D, Williams R. Scleroderma and primary biliary cirrhosis. Br Med J 1970; ii: 258–259

554. Barnett A J. The systemic involvement in scleroderma. Med J Aust 1977; 2: 659–662

555. Lurie B, Novis B, Banks J et al. CRST syndrome and nodular transformation of the liver. A case report. Gastroenterology 1973; 64: 457–461

556. McMahon H E. Systemic scleroderma and massive infarction of intestine and liver. Surg Gyn Obst 1972; 134: 10–14

557. Marshall J B, Ravendhran N, Sharp G C. Liver disease in mixed connective tissue disease. Arch Int Med 1983; 143: 1817–1818

558. Rolny P, Goobar J, Zettergren L. HBsAg-negative chronic active hepatitis and mixed connective tissue disease syndrome. An unusual association observed in two patients. Acta Med Scand 1984; 215: 391–395

559. Maeda M, Kanayama M, Hasumura Y, Takeuchi J, Uchida T. Case of mixed connective tissue disease associated with autoimmune hepatitis. Dig Dis Sci 1988; 33: 1487–1490

560. Singsen B H, Swanson V L, Bernstein B H et al. A histologic evaluation of mixed connective tissue disease in childhood. Am J Med 1980; 68: 710–717

561. Cosnes J, Robert A, Levy V G, Darnis F. Budd-Chiari syndrome in a patient with mixed connective tissue disease. Dig Dis Sci 1980; 25: 467–469

562. von Knorring J, Wasastjerna C. Liver involvement in polymyalgia rheumatica. Scand J Rheumatol 1976; 5: 179–204

563. Sattar M A, Cawley M I D, Hamblin T J, Robertson J C. Polymyalgia rheumatica and antimitochondrial antibodies. Ann Rheum Dis 1984; 43: 264–266

564. Thompson K, Roberts P F. Chronic hepatitis in polymyalgia rheumatica. Postgrad Med J 1976; 52: 236–238

565. Leong A S-Y, Alp M H. Hepatocellular disease in the giant cell arteritis/polymyalgia rheumatica. Scand J Rheumatol 1981; 5: 179–204

566. Long R, James O. Polymyalgia rheumatica and liver disease. Lancet 1972; i: 77–79

567. James O, Macklon A F, Watson A J. Primary biliary cirrhosis — a revised clinical spectrum. Lancet 1978; i: 1278–1281

568. Epstein O, Burroughs A K, Sherlock S. Polymyositis and acute onset systemic sclerosis in a patient with primary biliary cirrhosis: a clinical syndrome similar to the mixed connective tissue disease. J R Soc Med 1981; 74: 456–458

569. Milosevic M, Adams P C. Primary biliary cirrhosis and polymyositis. J Clin Gastroenterol 1990; 12: 332–335

570. Bitnum S, Daeschner C W, Travis L B, Dodge W F, Hopps H. Dermatomyositis. J Pediatr 1974; 64: 101–131

571. Sattar M A, Guindi R T, Khan R A, Tungekar M F. Polymyositis and hepatocellular carcinoma. Clin Rheumatol 1988; 7: 538–542

572. Oram S, Cochrane G M. Weber-Christian disease with visceral involvement. An example with hepatic enlargement. Br Med J 1958; 2: 281–284

573. Mowrey F H, Lundberg E A. The clinical manifestations of essential polyangiitis (periarteritis nodosa) with emphasis on the hepatic manifestations. Ann Intern Med 1954; 40: 1145–1164

574. Rousselet M-Ch, Kettani S, Rohmer V, Saint-Andre J-P. A case of temporal arteritis with intrahepatic arterial involvement. Path Res Prac 1989; 185: 329–331

575. Matsumoto T, Uekusa T, Fukuda Y. Vasculo-Behcet's disease: a pathologic study of eight cases. Hum Pathol 1991; 22: 45–51

576. Al-Dalaan A, Al-Balaa S, Ali M A et al. Budd-Chiari syndrome in association with Behcet's disease. J Rheumatol 1991; 18: 622–626

577. Ware A J, Luby J P, Hollinger B et al. Etiology of liver disease in renal transplant patients. Ann Int Med 1979; 91: 364–371

578. Ware A J, Gorder N L, Gurian L E et al. Value of screening for markers of hepatitis in dialysis units. Hepatology 1983; 3: 513–518

579. Chan M K, Moorhead J F. Hepatitis B and the dialysis and renal transplantation unit. Nephron 1981; 27: 229–232

580. Alter M J, Favero M S, Maynard J E. Impact of infection control strategies on the incidence of dialysis associated hepatitis in the US. J Inf Dis 1986; 153: 1149–1151

581. Briggs W A, Lazarus J M, Birch A G, Hampers C L, Hager E B, Merrill J P. Hepatitis affecting haemodialysis and transplant patients. Its considerations and consequences. Arch Int Med 1973; 132: 21–28

582. Anuras S, Piros J, Bonney W. Liver disease in renal transplant recipients. Arch Int Med 1977; 137: 42–48

583. Dusheiko G, Song E, Bowyer S et al. Natural history of hepatitis B virus infection in renal transplant recipients - a fifteen year follow-up. Hepatology 1983; 3: 330–336

584. Weir M R, Kirkman R L, Strom T B, Tilney N L. Liver disease in recipients of long-functioning renal allografts. Kidney Int 1985; 28: 839–844

585. Degos F, Lugassy C, Degott C et al. Hepatitis B virus and hepatitis B-related viral infection in renal transplant recipients. A prospective study of 90 patients. Gastroenterology 1988; 94: 151–156

586. Takahara S, Ihara H, Ichikawa Y et al. Prospective study and long-term follow-up of liver damage in renal transplant recipients. Transplant Proc 1987; 21: 2221–2224

587. Toussaint C, Kinnaert P, Vereerstraeten P. Late mortality and morbidity five to eighteen years after kidney transplantation. Transplantation 1988; 45: 554–558

588. Pol S, Debure A, Degott C et al. Chronic hepatitis in kidney allograft recipients. Lancet 1990; ii: 878–880

589. Rao K V, Kasiske B L, Anderson W R. Variability in the morphological spectrum and clinical outcome of chronic liver disease in hepatitis B-positive and B-negative renal transplant recipients. Transplantation 1991; 51: 391–396

590. Allison M C, Mowat A, McCruden E A B et al. The spectrum of chronic liver disease in renal transplant recipients. QJ Med 1992; 301: 355–367

591. Miller D J, Williams A E, Le Bouvier G L et al. Hepatitis B in hemodialysis patients: significance of HBeAg. Gastroenterology 1978; 74: 1208–1213

592. Degott C, Degos F, Jungers P et al. Relationship between liver histopathological changes and HBsAg in 111 patients treated by long-term hemodialysis. Liver 1983; 3: 377–384

593. Parfrey P S, Forbes R D C, Hutchinson T A et al. The clinical and pathological course of hepatitis B liver disease in renal transplant recipients. Transplantation 1984; 37: 461–466

594. Debure A, Degos F, Pol S et al. Liver diseases and hepatic complications in renal transplant patients. Adv Nephrol 1988; 17: 375–400

595. Crosnier J, Jungers P, Courouce A M et al. Randomised placebo-controlled trial of hepatitis B surface antigen vaccine in French haemodialysis units. I. Haemodialysis patients. Lancet 1981; i: 797–800

596. Carreno V, Mora I, Escuin F et al. Vaccination against hepatitis B in renal dialysis units: short or normal vaccination schedule? Clin Nephrol 1985; 24: 215–220

597. Quiroga J A, Castillo I, Porres J C et al. Recombinant gamma-interferon as adjuvant to hepatitis B vaccine in haemodialysis patients. Hepatology 1990; 12: 661–663

598. Esteban J I, Esteban R, Viladomiu L et al. Hepatitis C virus antibodies among risk groups in Spain. Lancet 1989; ii: 294–297

599. Schlipkoter U, Roggendorf M, Ernst G et al. Hepatitis C virus antibodies in haemodialysis patients. Lancet 1990; 335: 1409

600. Kallinowski B, Theilmann L, Gmelin K et al. Incidence and prevalence of antibodies to hepatitis C virus in kidney transplanted patients. J Hepatol 1991; 12: 404–405

601. Chan T M, Lok A S F, Cheng I K P, Chan R T. Prevalence of hepatitis C virus infection in hemodialysis patients: a longitudinal study comparing the results of RNA and antibody assays. Hepatology 1990; 11: 5–8

602. Glen J. Cytomegalovirus infection following renal transplantation. Rev Infect Dis 1981; 3: 1151–1178

603. Shiman-Chang R, Lewis J P, Reynolds R D, Sullivan M J, Neuman J. Oropharyngeal secretion of Epstein-Barr virus by patients with lymphoproliferative disorders and by recipients of renal homografts. Ann Int Med 1978; 88: 36–40

604. Anuras S, Summers R. Fulminant herpes simplex hepatitis in an adult. Report of a case in renal transplant recipient. Gastroenterology 1976; 70: 425–428

605. Taxy J B. Peliosis: a morphologic curiosity becomes an iatrogenic problem. Hum Pathol 1978; 9: 331–340

606. Hillion D, De Viel E, Bergue A et al. Peliosis hepatis in a chronic haemodialysis patient. Nephron 1983; 35: 205–206

607. Degott C, Rueff B, Kreis H et al. Peliosis hepatis in recipients of renal transplants. Gut 1978; 19: 748–753

608. Ihara H, Ichikawa Y, Nagano S, Fukunishi T, Shinji Y. Peliosis hepatis and nodular regenerative hyperplasia of the liver in renal transplant recipients. Med J Osaka Univ 1982; 33: 13–18

609. Bories P, Mourad G, Garnier T et al. Peliose et hyperplasie régénérative du foie: une seule maladie en rapport avec l'azathioprine ou le cytomégalovirus? Gastroenterol Clin Biol 1987; 11: 72–75

610. Mourad G, Bories P, Berthelemy C, Barneon G, Michel H, Mion C. Peliosis hepatis and nodular regenerative hyperplasia of the liver in renal transplants. Is cytomegalovirus the cause of this severe disease? Transplant Proc 1987; 19: 3697–3698

611. Buffet C, Cantarovitch M, Pelletier G et al. Three cases of nodular regenerative hyperplasia of the liver following renal transplantation. Nephrol Dial Transplant 1988; 3: 327–330

612. Morales J M, Prieto C, Mestre M J et al. Nodular regenerative hyperplasia of the liver in renal transplantation. Transplant Proc 1987; 19: 3694–3696

613. Naber A H J, Van Haelst U, Yap S H. Nodular regenerative hyperplasia of the liver: an important cause of portal hypertension in non-cirrhotic patients. J Hepatol 1991; 12: 94–99

614. Bredfeld J E, Harvey A L. Nodular regenerative hyperplasia of the liver following renal transplantation. Dig Dis Sci 1981; 26: 271–274

615. Capron J P, Degott C, Bernuau J et al. L'hyperplasie nodulaire regenerative du foie. Etude de 15 cas et revue de la literature. Gastroenterol Clin Biol 1983; 7: 761–769

616. Jones M C, Best P V, Catto G R D. Is nodular regenerative hyperplasia of the liver associated with azathioprine therapy after renal transplantation? Nephrol Dial Transplant 1988; 3: 331–333

617. Colina F, Alberti N, Solis J A, Martinez-Tello F J. Diffuse nodular regenerative hyperplasia of the liver (DNRH). A clinicopathologic study of 24 cases. Liver 1989; 9: 253–265

618. Marubbio A T, Danielson B. Hepatic veno-occlusive disease in a renal transplant patient receiving azathioprine. Gastroenterology 1975; 69: 739–743

619. Katzka D A, Saul S H, Jorkasky D et al. Azathioprine and hepatic venocclusive disease in renal transplant patients. Gastroenterology 1986; 90: 446–454

620. Read A E, Wiesner R H, LaBrecque D R et al. Hepatic veno-occlusive disease associated with renal transplantation and azathioprine therapy. Ann Int Med 1986; 104: 651–655

621. Gerlag P G G, Van Hoof J P. Hepatic sinusoidal dilatation with portal hypertension during azathioprine treatment: a cause of chronic liver disease after kidney transplantation. Trans Proc 1987; 19: 3699–3703

622. Nataf C, Feldman G, Lebrec D et al. Idiopathic portal hypertension (perisinusoidal fibrosis) after renal transplantation. Gut 1979; 20: 531–537

623. Sidi Y, Boner G, Bergamen D et al. Haemochromatosis in a renal transplant recipient. Clin Nephrol 1980; 13: 197–200

624. Rao K V, Anderson W R. Hemosiderosis and hemochromatosis in renal transplant recipients. Am J Nephrol 1985; 5: 419–430

625. Pahl M V, Vaziri N D, Dure-Smith B et al. Hepatobiliary pathology in hemodialysis patients: an autopsy study of 78 cases. Am J Gastroenterol 1986; 81: 783–787

626. Pritzker K. Neoplasia in renal transplant recipients. Can Med Ass J 1972; 107: 1059

627. Schroter G P J, Weil I R, Penn I, Speers W C, Waddell W R. Hepatocellular carcinoma associated with chronic hepatitis B virus infection after kidney transplantation. Lancet 1982; ii: 381–382

628. Gardner B P, Evans D B. Primary hepatocellular carcinoma arising in a renal transplant recipient with polycystic disease. Postgrad Med J 1983; 59: 120–121

629. Penn I. The occurrence of cancer in immune deficiencies. Current Problems in Cancer 1982; 6: 1–64

630. Boraa S, Kleinfeld M. Subcapsular liver hematomas in a patient on chronic haemodialysis. Ann Int Med 1980; 93: 574–575

631. Leong A S-Y, Disney A P S, Gove D W. Refractile particles in long-term haemodialysis patients. Lancet 1981; i: 889–890

632. Leong A S-Y, Gove D W. Foreign material in the tissues of patients on recurrent haemodialysis. Ultrastruct Pathol 1981; 2: 401–403

633. Parfrey P S, O'Driscoll J P, Paradinas F J. Refractile material in the liver of haemodialysis patients. Lancet 1981; i: 1101–1102

634. Hunt J, Farthing M J G, Baker L R I, Crocker P R, Levison D A. Silicone in the liver: possible late effects. Gut 1989; 30: 239–242

635. Kurumaya H, Kono N, Nakanuma Y, Tomoda F, Takazakura E. Hepatic granulomata in long-term hemodialysis patients with hyperaluminumemia. Arch Path Lab Med 1989; 113: 1132–1134

636. Sugiura H, Yoshida K, Nakanuma Y et al. Hepatic calcification in the course of hemodialysis. Am J Gastroenterol 1987; 82: 786–789

637. Sethi D, Cary N R B, Brown E A, Woodrow D F, Gower P E. Dialysis-associated amyloid: systemic or local? Nephrol Dial Transplant 1989; 4: 1054–1059
638. Campistol J M, Sole M, Munoz-Gomez J, Lopez-Pedret J, Revert L. Systemic involvement in dialysis-amyloidosis. Am J Nephrol 1990; 10: 389–396
639. Koch K M. Dialysis-related amyloidosis. Kidney Int 1992; 41: 1416–1429
640. Rokitansky C. Handbook der Pathologischen Anatomie, 1842; 3: 311
641. Glenner G G. Amyloid deposits and amyloidosis: the beta fibrilloses. N Engl J Med 1980; 302: 1283–1292 and 1333–1343
642. Kyle R A, Gertz M A. Systemic amyloidosis. Clin Rev Oncol Haematol 1990; 10: 49–87
643. McAdam K P W. Amyloidosis. In: McIntyre N, Benhamou J-P, Bircher J, Rizetto M, Rodes J, eds. Oxford textbook of clinical hepatology. Oxford: Oxford University Press, 1991: pp 779–787
644. Fievet P, Sevestre H, Boudjelal M et al. Systemic AA amyloidosis induced by liver cell adenoma. Gut 1990; 31: 361–363
645. Levine R A. Amyloid disease of the liver. Am J Med 1962; 3: 349–357
646. Kyle R A, Greipp P R. Amyloidosis (AL): clinical and laboratory features in 229 cases. Mayo Clin Proc 1983; 58: 665–683
647. Chopra S, Rubinow A, Koff R S, Cohen A S. Hepatic amyloidosis. A histopathologic analysis of primary (AL) and secondary (AA) forms. Am J Pathol 1984; 115: 186–193
648. Gertz M A, Kyle R A. Hepatic amyloidosis (primary AL): the natural history in 80 patients. Am J Med 1988; 85: 73–80
649. Looi L-M, Sumithran E. Morphologic differences in the pattern of liver infiltration between systemic AL and AA amyloidosis. Hum Pathol 1988; 19: 732–735
650. Kyle R A, Bayrd E D. Amyloidosis: a review of 236 cases. Medicine 1975; 54: 271–299
651. Melato M, Manconi R, Magris D et al. Different morphologic aspects and clinical features in massive hepatic amyloidosis. Digestion 1984; 29: 138–145
652. Levy-Lehad E, Steiner-Salz D, Berkman N et al. Reversible functional aplasia and sub-capsular liver haematoma: two distinctive manifestations of amyloidosis. Klin Wschr 1987; 65: 1104–1107
653. Kennan N M, Evans C. Case report: hepatic and splenic calcification due to amyloid. Clin Radiol 1991; 44: 60–61
654. Oliai A, Koff R S. Case report: primary amyloidosis presenting as 'sicca complex' and severe intrahepatic cholestasis. Am J Dig Dis 1972; 17: 1033–1036
655. Rubinow A, Koff R S, Cohen A S. Severe intrahepatic cholestasis in primary amyloidosis. A report of a few cases and a review of the literature. Am J Med 1978; 64: 937–946
656. Cox R. Amyloidosis of the liver causing jaundice. Postgrad Med J 1982; 58: 192–193
657. Pirovino M, Altorfer J, Maranta E, Haemmerli U P, Schmid M. Ikterus von Typ der intrahepatischen Cholestase bei Amyloidose der Leber. Zeitschrift fur Gastroenterologie 1982; 6: 321–331
658. Hoffman M S, Stein B E, Davidian M M, Rosenthal W S. Hepatic amyloidosis presenting as severe intrahepatic cholestasis: a case report and review of the literature. Am J Gastroenterol 1988; 83: 783–785
659. Itescu S. Hepatic amyloidosis: an unusual case of ascites and portal hypertension. Arch Int Med 1984; 144: 2257–2259
660. Kitazono M, Saito Y, Kinoshita M et al. Nodular regenerative hyperplasia of the liver in a patient with multiple myeloma and systemic amyloidosis. Arch Pathol Jpn 1985; 35: 961–967
661. Ades C J, Strutton G M, Walker N I, Furnival C M, Whiting G. Spontaneous rupture of the liver associated with amyloidosis. J Clin Gastroenterol 1989; 11: 85–87
662. Wright J R, Calkins E, Humphrey R L. Potassium permanganate reaction in amyloidosis: a histologic method to assist in differentiating forms of the disease. Lab Invest 1977; 36: 274–279
663. Shirahama T, Skinner M, Sipe J D, Cohen A S. Widespread occurrence of AP in amyloidotic tissues: an immunohistochemical observation. Virchows Arch (B) 1985; 48: 197–206
664. French S W, Schloss G T, Stillman A E. Unusual amyloid bodies in human liver. Am J Clin Pathol 1981; 75: 400–402

665. Kanel G C, Uchida T, Peters R L. Globular hepatic amyloid — an unusual morphologic presentation. Hepatology 1981; 1: 647–652
666. Sasaki M, Nakanuma Y, Terada T et al. Amyloid deposition in intrahepatic large bile ducts and peribiliary glands in systemic amyloidosis. Hepatology 1990; 12: 743–746
667. Randall R E, Williamson W C, Mullinax F, Tung M Y, Still W J S. Manifestations of systemic light chain deposition. Am J Med 1976; 60: 293–299
668. Silver M M, Hearn S A, Ritchie S et al. Renal and systemic kappa light chain deposits and their plasma cell origin identified by immunoelectron microscopy. Am J Pathol 1986; 122: 17–27
669. Confalonieri R, Barbiano di Belgioioso G, Banfi G et al. Light chain nephropathy: histological and clinical aspects in 15 cases. Nephrol Dial Transplant 1988; 3: 150–156
670. Maury C P J, Teppo A M. Massive cutaneous hyalinosis. Am J Clin Pathol 1984; 82: 543–551
671. Kijner C H, Yousem S Y. Systemic light chain deposition disease presenting as multiple pulmonary nodules. Am J Surg Pathol 1988; 12: 405–413
672. Stone G C, Wall B A, Oppliger I R et al. A vasculopathy with deposition of lambda light chain crystals. Ann Int Med 1989; 110: 275–278
673. Preud'homme J L, Morel-Maroger L, Brouet J C, Mihaesco E, Mery J P, Seligmann P M. Synthesis of abnormal heavy and light chains in multiple myeloma with visceral deposition of monoclonal immunoglobulin. Clin Exp Immunol 1980; 42: 545–553
674. Preud'homme J L, Morel-Maroger L, Brouet J C et al. Synthesis of abnormal immunoglobulins in lymphoplasmacytic disorders with visceral light chain deposition. Am J Med 1980; 69: 703–710
675. Case records of the Massachusetts General Hospital (Case 1-1981). N Engl J Med 1981; 304: 33–43
676. Droz D, Noel L H, Carnot F, Degos F, Ganeval D, Grunfeld J P. Liver involvement in non-amyloid light chain deposits disease. Lab Invest 1984; 50: 683–689
677. Bedossa P, Febre M, Paraf F, Martin E, Lemaigre G. Light chain deposition disease with liver dysfunction. Hum Pathol 1988; 19: 1008–1014
678. Pelletier G, Fabre M, Attali P, Ladouch-Badre A, Ink O, Martin E, Etienne J-P. Light chain deposition disease presenting with hepatomegaly: an association with amyloid-like fibrils. Postgrad Med J 1988; 64: 804–808
679. Faa G, Van Eyken P, De Vos R et al. Light chain deposition disease of the liver associated with AL-type amyloidosis and severe cholestasis. A case report and literature review. J Hepatol 1991; 12: 75–82
680. Feiner H D. Pathology of dysproteinemia: light chain amyloidosis, non-amyloid immunoglobulin deposition disease, cryoglobulinemia syndromes and macroglobulinemia of Waldenstrom. Hum Pathol 1988; 19: 1255–1272
681. Ganeval D, Noel L H, Droz D, Leibowitch J. Systemic lambda light chain deposition in a patient with myeloma. Br Med J 1981; 282: 681–683
682. Jacquot C, Saint-Andre J P, Toucard G et al. Association of systemic light chain deposition disease and amyloidosis: a report of three patients with renal involvement. Clin Nephrol 1985; 24: 93–98
683. Kirkpatrick C J, Curry A, Galle J, Melzner I. Systemic kappa light chain deposition and amyloidosis in multiple myeloma: novel morphological observations. Histopathology 1986; 10: 1065–1076
684. Smith N M, Malcolm A J. Simultaneous AL-type amyloid and light chain deposit disease in a liver biopsy: a case report. Histopathology 1986; 10: 1057–1064
685. Lefkowitch J H, Mendez L. Morphological features of hepatic injury in cardiac disease and shock. J Hepatol 1986; 2: 313–327
686. Klatt E C, Koss M N, Young T S, MacAuley L, Martin S E. Hepatic hyaline globules associated with passive congestion. Arch Pathol Lab Med 1988; 112: 510–513
687. Steiner P E. Nodular regenerative hyperplasia of the liver. Am J Pathol 1959; 35: 943–953
688. Ellenberg M, Osserman K E. Role of shock in production of central liver cell necrosis. Am J Med 1951; 11: 170–178

689. de la Monte S M, Arcide J M, Moore G W, Hutchins G M. Midzonal necrosis as a pattern of hepatocellular injury after shock. Gastroenterology 1984; 86: 627–631

690. Lancet 1985. Ischaemic hepatitis. Lancet 1985; i: 1019–1020

691. Gibson P R, Dudley F J. Ischaemic hepatitis: clinical features, diagnosis and prognosis. Aust NZeal J Med 1984; 14: 822–825

692. Gitlin N, Serio K M. Ischemic hepatitis: widening horizons. Am J Gastroenterol 1992; 87: 831–836

693. Garland J S, Werlin S L, Rice T B. Ischemic hepatitis in children: diagnosis and clinical course. Crit Care Med 1988; 16: 1209–1212

694. Sherlock S. The liver in heart failure. Relation of anatomical, functional and circulatory changes. Br Heart J 1951; 13: 273–293

695. Arcidi J R, Moore G W, Hutchins G M. Hepatic morphology in cardiac dysfunction. A clinicopathologic study of 1000 subjects at autopsy. Am J Pathol 1981; 104: 159–166

696. Nouel O, Herrion J, Degott C et al. Fulminant hepatic failure due to transient circulatory failure in patients with chronic heart disease. Dig Dis Sci 1980; 25: 49–52

697. Shibayama Y. The role of hepatic venous congestion and endotoxaemia in the production of fulminant hepatic failure secondary to congestive heart failure. J Pathol 1987; 151: 133–138

698. Shibuya A, Unuma T, Sugimoto T et al. Diffuse hepatic calcification as a sequela to shock liver. Gastroenterology 1985; 89: 196–201

699. Gore I, Isaacson N H. Pathology of hyperpyrexia; observations at autopsy in 17 cases of fever therapy. Am J Pathol 1949; 25: 1029–1046

700. Biabchi L, Ohnacker H, Beck K, Zimmerli-Ning M. Liver damage in heatstroke and its regression. Hum Pathol 1972; 3: 237–248

701. Hassanein T, Razack A, Gavaler J S, Van Thiel D H. Heat stroke; its clinical and pathological presentation, with particular attention to the liver. Am J Gastroenterol 1992; 87: 1382–1389

702. Murata K, Okudaira M, Akashio K. Mast cells in human liver tissue. Acta Derm Venereol (Stockh) 1973; 73: 157–178

703. Bardadin K A, Scheuer P J. Mast cells in acute hepatitis. J Pathol 1986; 149: 315–325

704. Celasun B, Crow B, Scheuer P J. Mast cells in granulomatous liver disease. Path Res Pract 1991; 188: 97–100

705. Lennert K, Parwaresch M R. Mast cells and mast cell neoplasia: a review. Histopathology 1979; 3: 349–365

706. Webb T A, Li C Y, Yam L T. Systemic mast cell disease: A clinical and hematopathologic study of 26 cases. Cancer 1982; 49: 927–938

707. Yam L T, Chan C H, Li C Y. Hepatic involvement in systemic mast cell disease. Am J Med 1986; 80: 819–826

708. Horny H-P, Kaiserling E, Campbell M, Parwaresch M R, Lennert K. Liver findings in generalized mastocytosis. A clinicopathologic study. Cancer 1989; 63: 532–538

709. Capron J-P, Lebrec D, Degott C, Chirrac D, Coevoet B, Delobel J. Portal hypertension in systemic mastocytosis. Gastroenterology 1978; 74: 595–597

710. Grundfest S, Cooperman A M, Ferguson R, Benjamin S. Portal hypertension associated with systemic mastocytosis and splenomegaly. Gastroenterology 1980; 78: 370–373

711. Sawers A H, Davson J, Braganza J, Geary C G. Systemic mastocytosis, myelofibrosis and portal hypertension. J Clin Pathol 1982; 35: 617–619

712. Ghandur-Mnaymneh L, Gould E. Systemic mastocytosis with portal hypertension. Autopsy findings and ultrastructural study of the liver. Arch Path Lab Med 1985; 109: 76–78

713. Bonnet P, Smadja C, Szekely A-M, Delage Y, Calmus Y, Poupon R, Franco D. Intractable ascites in systemic mastocytosis treated by portal diversion. Dig Dis Sci 1987; 32: 209–213

714. Narayanan M N, Liu Yin J A, Azzawi S, Warnes T W, Turck W P G. Portal hypertension and ascites in systemic mastocytosis. Postgrad Med J 1989; 65: 394–396

715. Korkij W, Chuang T-Y, Soltani K. Liver abnormalities in patients with lichen planus. A retrospective case-control study. J Am Acad Dermatol 1984; 11: 609–615

716. Cottoni F, Solinas A, Piga M R, Tocco A, Lissia M, Cerimele D. Lichen planus, chronic liver diseases, and immunologic involvement. Dermatol Res 1988; 280: S55–S60

717. del Olmo J A, Almenar E, Bagan J V et al. Liver abnormalities in patients with lichen planus of the oral cavity. Eur J Gastroenterol Hepatol 1990; 2: 479–481

718. Virgili A, Robert E, Rebora A. Hepatocellular carcinoma and lichen planus: report of two cases. Dermatology 1992; 184: 137–138

719. Meyer G W, Griffiths W J, Welsh J, Cohen L, Johnson L, Weaver M J. Brief reports: Hepatobiliary involvement in von Recklinghausen's disease. Ann Int Med 1982; 97: 722–723

720. Young S J. Primary malignant neurilemmoma (Schwannoma) of the liver in a case of neurofibromatosis. J Pathol 1975; 117: 151–153

721. Lederman S M, Martin E G, Laffey K T, Lefkowitch J H. Hepatic neurofibromatosis, malignant schwannoma and angiosarcoma in von Recklinghausen's disease. Gastroenterology 1987; 92: 234–239

722. Di Bisceglie A M, Hodkinson H J, Berkowitz I, Kew M C. Pityriasis rotunda. A cutaneous marker of hepatocellular carcinoma in South African Blacks. Arch Dermatol 1986; 122: 802–804

723. Berkowitz I, Hodgkinson H J, Kew M C, Di Bisceglie A M. Pityriasis rotunda as a cutaneous marker of hepatocellular carcinoma: a comparison with its prevalence in other diseases. Br J Dermatol 1989; 120: 545–549

724. Gilbert S C, Klintmalm G, Menter A, Silverman A. Methotrexate-induced cirrhosis requiring liver transplantation in three patients with psoriasis. Arch Int Med 1990; 150: 889–891

725. Pascual M, Widmann J-J, Schifferli J A. Recurrent febrile panniculitis and hepatitis in two patients with acquired complement deficiency and paraproteinemia. Am J Med 1987; 83: 959–962

726. Banerjee A K, Grainger S L, Davies D R, Thompson R P H. Active chronic hepatitis and febrile panniculitis. Gut 1989; 30: 1018–1019

727. Langley J M, Roberts E A, Ipp M, Laxer R M, Boxall L, Phillips M J. Pyoderma gangrenosum and autoimmune chronic active hepatitis in a 17 year old female. Can J Gastroenterol 1988; 2: 137–139

728. Caplan R M. Visceral involvement in lipoid proteinosis. Arch Dermatol 1967; 95: 149–155

729. Weedon D. Cutaneous deposits in the skin. In: Weedon D, ed. Systemic pathology, 3rd edn, vol 9. Symmers W St C. (Gen. Ed.) Edinburgh: Churchill Livingstone, 1993: pp 412–443

730. Welch W H. Cirrhosis hepatis anthracotica. Johns Hopkins Hospital Bulletin 1891; 2: 32

731. LeFevre M E, Green F H Y, Joel D D, Laquer W. Frequency of black pigment in livers and spleens of coal workers: correlation with pulmonary pathology and occupational information. Hum Pathol 1982; 13: 1121–1126

732. Eliakim R, Ligumsky M, Jurim O, Shouval D. Nodular regenerative hyperplasia with portal hypertension in a patient with myasthenia gravis. Am J Gastroenterol 1987; 82: 674–676

733. Theodore C, Cornud F, Mendez J et al. Cholestasis and myotonic dystrophy. N Engl J Med 1979; 301: 329–430

734. Poynard T, Bedossa P, Naveau S et al. Perisinusoidal cells (Ito cells) enlargement in a family with myotonic dystrophy. Liver 1989; 9: 276–278

735. Soderhall S, Gustafsson J, Bjorkhem I. Deoxycholic acid in myotonic dystrophy. Lancet 1982; i: 1046–1069

736. Shepherd N A, Lee G. Solitary necrotic nodules of the liver simulating hepatic metastases. J Clin Pathol 1983; 36: 1181–1183

737. Tsui W M S, Yuen R W S, Chow L T C, Tse C C H. Solitary necrotic nodule of the liver: parasitic origin? J Clin Pathol 1992; 45: 975–978

738. Berry C L. Solitary 'necrotic nodule' of the liver: a probable pathogenesis. J Clin Pathol 1985; 38: 1278–1280

18

Transplantation pathology
Including liver injury in graft versus host disease and in recipients of renal and other allografts

J. Ludwig   K. P. Batts

PATHOLOGY OF HEPATIC ALLOGRAFTS

GENERAL ASPECTS OF LIVER TRANSPLANTATION

Successful human liver transplantation was first performed by Dr T Starzl and Dr R Y Calne in the 1960s.[1] Extensive experimental work preceded and accompanied these achievements.[2,3] In the course of these studies, porcine liver grafts were found to survive with little or no immunosuppression; indeed, the grafts decreased the responsiveness of the pigs to other tissues from the same donor. Although other animals and man required immunosuppression to prevent cell-mediated rejection, humoral (hyperacute) rejection did not occur in the pre-sensitized recipients that were studied. In rat experiments, liver allografts were found to go through a rejection episode but, between certain strains,[4,5] the grafts eventually were tolerated although other grafted organs were acutely rejected. Here again, the grafts induced a state of donor-specific unresponsiveness. Interestingly, these effects were not observed if the recipient liver was left in place — that is, auxiliary grafts were rejected. These phenomena have not yet been explained in every detail. In any event, researchers established early on that the liver is to some extent immunologically 'privileged.'[5a,5b]

Morphological studies on experimental animals involved not only rats but untreated canine and porcine allografts[3] as well as dogs that had been immunosuppressed with azathioprine and heterologous antilymphocyte globulins. The portal cellular infiltrates and endotheliitis were clearly recognized as features of rejection. Even the experience with a chimpanzee-to-human heterograft was described; this is of particular interest because of the recent revival of this method, using baboon livers in an attempt to treat patients who had lost grafts after recurrent hepatitis B.[6] The first morphological descriptions of human allografts[3] revealed most of the complications that are described in this chapter; they included cellular and vascular rejection, hepatic artery and portal vein thrombosis, bile-duct damage, hepatic infarctions and tumour recurrence.

Terminology, surgical procedures, and results

Almost all liver transplantations today entail removal of the host liver and replacement by the donor liver. In this context, the host liver is termed the 'native liver' and the implanted donor liver the 'allograft'. Because the allograft is placed in the position formerly occupied by the native liver, the procedure is named orthotopic liver transplantation (OLT). Since its initiation in 1963 by Starzl,[1] this method has become the procedure of choice; in 1991, the United Network for Organ Sharing (UNOS) reported that 2647 cadaveric liver transplantations were performed in the USA alone.[7] In recent years, improved preservation fluids[8] have prolonged the viability of harvested livers to approximately 15–20 hours. At the same time, improved immunosuppression has decreased the loss of allografts from rejection.[9] Thus, in 1991, the 1-year survival at the Mayo Clinic was 90% and the 5-year survival was 83%.

Despite the undisputed successes of OLT, auxiliary heterotopic liver transplantation has also been done in selected cases.[10] With this procedure, a reduced-size donor liver is transplanted to the right sub-hepatic region; the host liver is left in place. Early results have been poor but, in principle, the method appears well suited for high-risk patients[10] or for patients with fulminant viral hepatitis or other types of massive hepatic necrosis where recovery of the failing liver might be expected.[10a]

With only a few exceptions, cadaveric donor organs are used for liver transplantation, intact or reduced[11] to suit the size of the right hypochondrial fossa in children. Recently, the shortage of donor organs, particularly for paediatric patients, has led to attempts to transplant liver segment(s) excised from living related donors; this has been successful in some instances.[12] UNOS reported that nine such procedures had been done in 1991.[7] In Japan, transplantation from living related donors is the only acceptable method; this may be changing.

Indications for liver transplantation

The indications for OLT[13] can be subdivided into three major groups — namely, non-neoplastic hepatobiliary diseases, primary or secondary hepatic tumours, and a small but enlarging cohort of genetic diseases. In the first group, the most common conditions are primary biliary cirrhosis, autoimmune or chronic viral hepatitis complicated by cirrhosis, primary sclerosing cholangitis, cryptogenic cirrhosis, alcoholic cirrhosis, and acute hepatic failure (massive hepatic necrosis) of any cause. Reported aetiologies of acute hepatic failure include fulminant viral hepatitis, toxic hepatitis, fulminant Wilson's disease, and acute fatty liver of pregnancy. Liver transplantation for hepatic vein thrombosis with Budd–Chiari syndrome can also be added here.[14]

Hepatic malignancies are another indication for OLT but the results so far have been marred by a high percentage of tumour recurrence, often within a few months of transplantation. Patients with metastatic carcinomas or primary cholangiocarcinomas fared worse than patients with hepatocellular carcinomas.[15] The prognosis was better if OLT was done for less aggressive malignant tumours such as epithelioid haemangioendotheliomas or primary or secondary carcinoid tumours.[16]

In genetic diseases, OLT may be indicated because of the liver damage or because the liver is the site of the genetically determined metabolic defect. For example, in α_1-antitrypsin deficiency, tyrosinaemia, and Wilson's disease, the overt liver damage is the indication for OLT, whereas in type I hyperoxaluria and ornithine carbamoyl transferase deficiency (urea cycle enzyme), the metabolic defect necessitates transplantation.[13,17] In the latter category, the livers may be morphologically normal or show only mild changes that would not interfere with liver function. In appropriate cases, the allograft promptly corrects the manifestations of the metabolic defect and thus may be life-saving. More than 16 genetic diseases have already been treated with OLT.[17,18,18a,18b]

Complications of OLT include surgical mishaps, preservation injury, unexplained acute graft failure, rejection, and hepatic artery thrombosis with related ischaemic lesions. Of particular importance in this context are complications affecting the bile ducts such as dehiscence and leaks, necrosis, strictures, accumulation of concrements, infection and rejection-associated damage. Other complications result from systemic infections, recurrence of conditions that led to OLT, adverse drug effects, and post-transplant lymphoproliferative disorders. The pathology of most of these complications is presented in the following pages.

REJECTION OF ALLOGRAFTS

Transplant immunology

Cellular immunity is thought to be accomplished through multiple effector pathways including delayed-type hypersensitivity responses, allogeneic cytotoxic T-lymphocytes, and antibody-dependent cell cytotoxicity which is mediated by killer cells.[2] In these processes, both CD8+ and CD4+ lymphocytes in the presence of interleukin-2 are involved, with B-lymphocytes and natural killer (NK) cells also playing a role. In liver transplantation, the principal antigen targets appear to be the major histocompatibility (MHC) antigens. It should be noted that in hepatic rejection, neutrophils and, in particular, eosinophils[19] also are an important part of the process; these granulocytes are found regularly among the mononuclear immunocytes.

Antibody-mediated immunity may also affect the liver, although it appears to play a lesser role than cellular immunity. The processes probably can occur together. Thus, in early cell-mediated rejection, anti-MHC antibodies may be involved. While MHC antibodies may be preformed or acquired, the antibodies against ABO blood group antigens are always preformed. In ABO incompatibility, these preformed antibodies may cause antibody-mediated graft failure,[20] usually 1–2 weeks after OLT. This process appears to be analogous to hyperacute rejection in kidneys and hearts. Lymphocytotoxic antibodies also have been implicated in a case of early graft failure.[21] Because 'hyperacute' hepatic rejection may occur as late as 4 weeks after OLT, as compared to minutes or hours in hyperacute renal rejection, the term 'primary humoral rejection' has been proposed for this type of liver injury.[20] It should be noted that anti-ABO antibodies also may be a cause of biliary and arterial complications that occur late in the post-operative course;[22,23] the ischaemic damage to ducts and arteries might be the result of antibody-mediated endothelial injury of small vessels in the vicinity of the anastomoses.

As stated in the first paragraphs of this chapter, the liver, in comparison with other vascularized allografts, is less susceptible to cellular rejection and responds more readily to anti-rejection treatment; the liver is also less often the target of primary humoral rejection. In contrast to the experience with hearts and kidneys, matching for human leucocyte antigen (HLA) prior to OLT seems to have little influence on graft or patient survival.[24] Furthermore, transplantation of livers across ABO barriers has yielded satisfactory results in many instances. However, because of decreased graft survival[20] and the aforementioned arterial and bile-duct complications,[22,23] ABO mismatches are regarded as a relative contraindication for liver transplantation.

The immunologically privileged properties of human hepatic allografts are poorly understood. One factor in primary humoral rejection may be the presence of a fenestrated sinusoidal microvasculature with Kupffer cells; the structure of hepatic sinusoids differs from the architecture of capillaries in hearts and kidneys, and this might help to impede antibody-mediated damage.[2] This hypothesis would explain why bile ducts, which are supplied by a hepatic-artery derived capillary system, can be injured after ABO mismatch, even if the remaining liver is not damaged.

The partial resistance of the liver to cell-mediated rejection might be related to the limited expression of the major histocompatibility antigens (MHC), the principal targets of the process. Normal hepatocytes express little or no class I MHC antigen but this antigen is expressed by biliary epithelium, endothelial cells, Kupffer cells, and dendritic cells.[2] The situation changes after infections and other complications, including rejection; these events induce expression of class I and class II antigens in hepatocytes and biliary epithelium and enhance the expression of class II antigens on endothelium.[2,24] Because the epithelium of bile ducts and the endothelium of arteries and veins are the principal sites of morphological injury, expression of class II antigens on these structures is assumed to participate in the initiation of rejection. The highly effective immunosuppressant cyclosporine. A appears to inhibit primarily interleukin-2, a mitogenic lymphokine. This immunosuppressant also may affect interleukin-1, interferons, and interleukin-2 receptor.[25] Steroids act mainly through their anti-inflammatory effects whereas azathioprine is immunosuppressive because of its cytotoxic effects. The monoclonal antibody OKT$_3$ inactivates T-cells by binding to the CD3 component of the CD3-T-cell receptor complex.[25]

Definitions and terminology

Rejection is best defined as the response of the recipient's immune system to the transplanted graft, leading to graft damage. In liver transplantation, rejection may be antibody-mediated or cell-mediated or both. Hyperacute rejection or its aptly termed synonym, primary humoral rejection,[20] can be defined as an antibody-mediated rejection in a pre-sensitized recipient. The definition requires that the process occurs within days or weeks of OLT and that the allograft contains donor-specific antibodies.

Cell-mediated rejection, the most common type of rejection after OLT, can be defined as any form of hepatic allograft rejection that is not caused by preformed cytotoxic antibodies.[26] This is meant to exclude 'hyperacute' rejection but acknowledges that antibodies may play a role in cell-mediated rejection. The main manifestations of cell-mediated rejection are cellular rejection, ductopenic rejection (rejection with duct loss), and vascular rejection (rejection-related foam-cell arteritis or arteriopathy). In resected grafts, vascular rejection is less common than ductopenic rejection[27] but if vascular rejection is found, ductopenic rejection is usually present as well.

Traditionally, a combined clinical/morphological terminology of rejection has been used — namely, hyperacute,[2] acute, and chronic.[28] Although definitions vary, all authors have considered acute rejection to be reversible or potentially reversible, and chronic rejection potentially irreversible. Indeed, irreversibility has been used as a criterion for chronic rejection.[28] Histologically, acute rejection generally corresponds to cellular rejection, and chronic rejection often corresponds to ductopenic rejection. However, cellular rejection is not always acute and ductopenic rejection is not always chronic or irreversible.[29,30] A schematic comparison of the three terminologies is presented in Figure 18.1. Because duct loss appears to be the most important sign of potentially irreversible rejection, a simplified terminology is being tested in five centres in the United States.[31] Essentially, only two categories are distinguished — namely, 'rejection without duct loss' and 'rejection with duct loss' (ductopenic rejection). In this terminology, vascular rejection is considered a coinci-

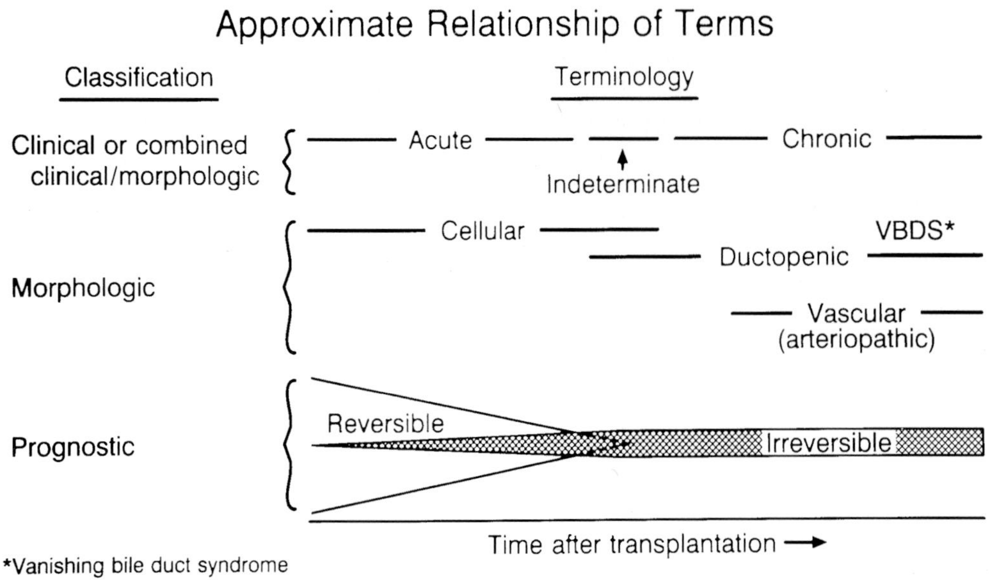

Approximate Relationship of Terms

Fig. 18.1 Schematic representation of three classes of rejection. The horizontal lines indicate the types of rejection as they relate to each other and to an approximate time line running from left to right. Note that 'indeterminate' in the clinical/morphological classification refers to the cases that cannot be assigned reliably to 'acute' or 'chronic'. The figure also shows that the morphological features of cellular and ductopenic rejection in the prognostic classification reach to the very beginning of the post-transplant period, suggesting that some cases of rejection never respond satisfactorily to treatment. Reproduced with permission from Wiesner et al.[9]

dental finding. Evidently, not all cases can be classified by such a simple scheme. On the other hand, detailed grading schemes have not stood the test of time because most histological features of rejection, such as the intensity of portal inflammation, have insufficient prognostic value. Furthermore, inter-observer and intra-observer variations in the diagnosis of various histological features of rejection may be considerable[32] and, thus, comparable results are difficult to obtain.

Histopathological features

Antibody-mediated (hyperacute) rejection

In antibody-mediated, hyperacute rejection, the liver shows widespread areas of coagulative and haemorrhagic necrosis, often with fibrin thrombi in intact or disrupted arteries and veins. Immunostaining reveals deposits of IgM and C1q. In the early stages of this condition, IgG and C3 also may be present.[33,34] Light microscopy reveals abundant erythrocytes and neutrophils in sinusoids as well as haemorrhages in the portal tracts. Neutrophilic or necrotizing arteritis is a rare finding but, as stated, thrombi are common both in arteries and in portal or hepatic vein branches. It should be noted that the described morphological features do not prove the presence of antibody-mediated rejection *unless* (i) they occur shortly after OLT, usually within 1 or 2 weeks, (ii) the pre-sensitized state of the recipient can be confirmed, and (iii) an eluate from the failed graft contains donor-specific antibodies.[33]

Cellular rejection

Biopsy specimens typically show the classic triad of portal or periportal hepatitis, endotheliis or phlebitis (venulitis), and non-suppurative cholangitiis.[35] The portal tract infiltrate consists of small and activated lymphocytes, immunoblasts, and plasma cells, neutrophils, and often many eosinophils (Fig. 18.2). Mitoses are common in these infiltrates. Immunostaining shows that most of the lymphocytes in affected portal tracts are T-cells (CD4+ and CD8+), but some B-cells are also present.[36] Periportal spillage and linkage of portal tracts by inflammatory cells is a rare feature, usually associated with cessation of immunosuppressive therapy, and indicates a severe rejection episode.

Endotheliitis or phlebitis (venulitis) is diagnostically the most reliable sign of rejection, provided it occurs in the appropriate clinical setting. However, endotheliitis often cannot be recognized in otherwise convincing cases of rejection; it appears to be a fleeting phenomenon, particularly after administration of steroid boluses. In endotheliitis, lymphocytes and other immunocytes are attached to the luminal surface of the endothelium, sometimes with a single cytoplasmic stalk, sometimes piling up in large cell clusters (Figs 18.3 and 18.4). The inflammation does not always involve the entire circumference of a vein but may affect only a small segment of a cross-section. Immunocytes also aggregate underneath the damaged endothelium which is then lifted from the basement membrane. In severe cases, the entire thickness of the venule may be infiltrated by mononuclear cells, imparting the features of phlebitis (venulitis). Immunostaining has shown that endotheliitis

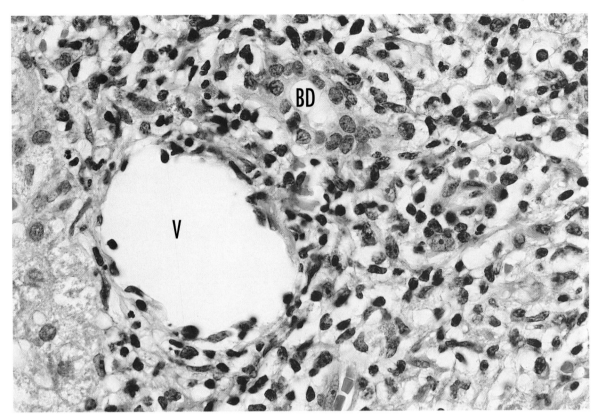

Fig. 18.2 Portal inflammatory infiltrates in cellular rejection. Note the mixture of small and activated lymphocytes, immunoblasts, and eosinophils. Mild endotheliitis is also present. V = portal vein; BD = bile duct. H & E.

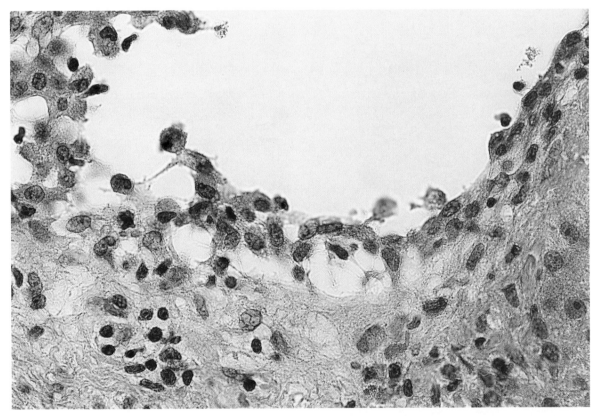

Fig. 18.3 Endotheliitis in cellular rejection. Numerous lymphocytes are present singly and in clusters both above and below the endothelium. The endothelial cells have become lifted so that the intima resembles a Roman aqueduct. H & E.

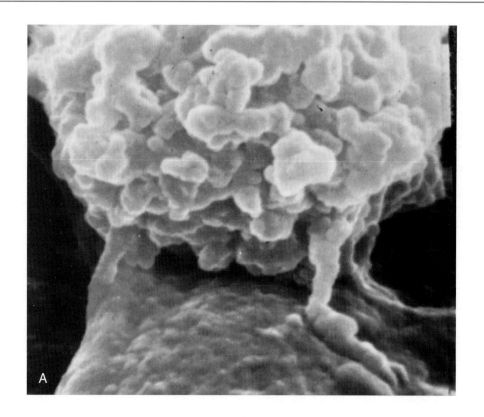

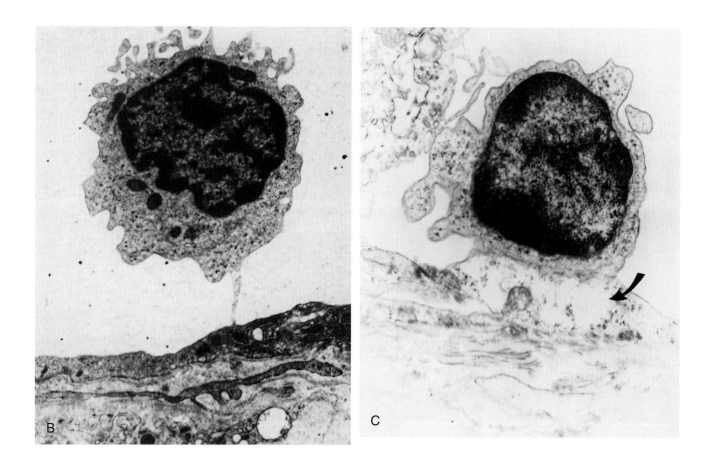

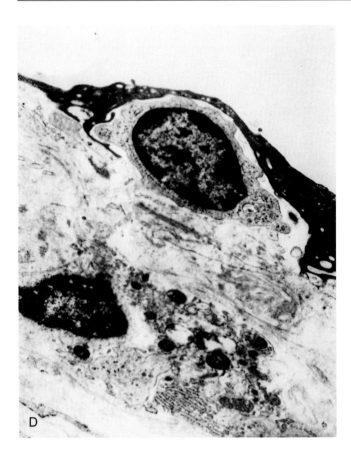

D

Fig. 18.4 Lymphocytes in endotheliitis — scanning (SEM) and transmission (TEM) electron micrographs. (a) Multiple cytoplasmic processes attach the lymphocyte to the underlying endothelial cell. (b) Circulating lymphocyte attached to endothelial cells by fine cytoplasmic processes. (c) Lymphocyte attached to an endothelial cell by a broad base, with associated (? cytokine-mediated) cytoplasmic swelling of the endothelial cell (arrow). (d) Lymphocyte beneath endothelial cell. (a) SEM, × 18 000; (b–d) TEM, × 8100. Reproduced with permission from Ludwig et al[37]

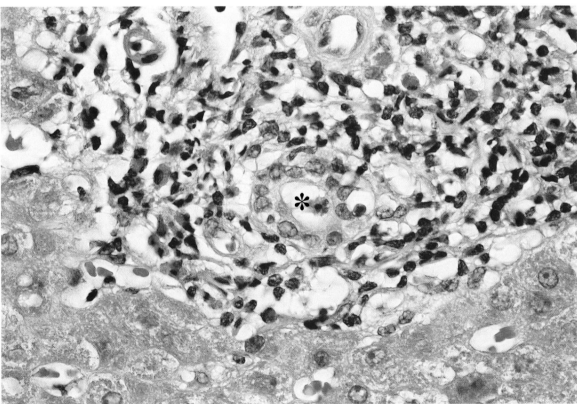

Fig. 18.5 Rejection cholangitis. A bile duct (asterisk) shows numerous intraepithelial lymphocytes as well as a dense mixed inflammatory infiltrate in the surrounding portal tract. Note biliary epithelial damage with cytoplasmic swelling and variation in size of nuclei. H & E.

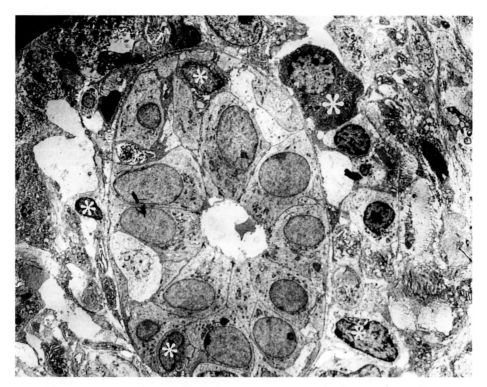

Fig. 18.6 Rejection cholangitis — TEM. Most lymphocytes line up along the inner and outer surfaces of the basement membrane (small asterisks). A plasma cell (large asterisk) can also be identified. Associated biliary epithelial damage is indicated by the irregular spacing of the cells and cytoplasmic vacuolization. TEM, × 7000

and phlebitis are caused mostly by T-cells (CD4+ and CD8+)[37] but, occasionally, even eosinophils can be found underneath the endothelium. Endotheliitis, like portal hepatitis and non-suppurative cholangitis, is not pathognomonic for cellular rejection; it may occur in conditions such as viral hepatitis, systemic Epstein–Barr virus (EBV) infections,[38] adverse drug reactions, and the syndrome of primary biliary cirrhosis; it also may be simulated by lymphoproliferative disorders ('pseudo-endotheliitis').

Non-suppurative cholangitis may be destructive or non-destructive and this distinction is the most important for the prognosis of rejection. Typically, ducts are surrounded by immunocytes which sometimes also are found between epithelial cells, inside the basement membrane or even in the lumen (Figs 18.5 and 18.6). Neutrophils also may surround and invade the ducts as part of the rejection process. This is important because that feature is easily confused with suppurative cholangitis in ascending infection. The clinical and radiological findings are often helpful. In cellular rejection, biliary epithelial cells often show evidence of damage such as cytoplasmic vacuolization or pyknosis of nuclei.[39] In severe rejection, ducts are sometimes overrun by inflammatory cells including neutrophils; cytokeratin stains may then be needed to locate the epithelium. In cases of this type, the distinction between 'rejection without duct loss' and 'rejection with duct loss' is often difficult, particularly if only one specimen is available for

study. In addition to ductopenia, portal arteritis (Fig. 18.7) may herald a poor prognosis of the graft.[40] However, this feature is uncommon and difficult to diagnose.

Cellular rejection also may be associated with inflammatory infiltrates (mostly T-cells) in sinusoids, hepatocanalicular cholestasis and clusters of acidophilic or apoptotic bodies. The presence of these necrotic cells or cell fragments should not be misinterpreted as a sign of viral hepatitis.

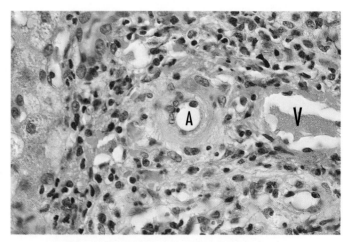

Fig. 18.7 Rejection arteritis. Lymphocytes are present on the endothelial surface. This feature is uncommonly seen in rejection and may herald a poor prognosis. A = artery; V = portal vein. H & E.

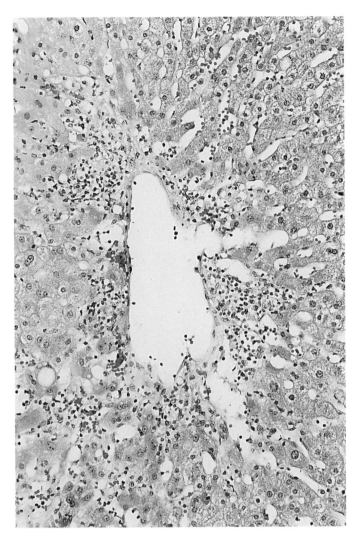

Fig. 18.8 Intra-acinar (lobular) cellular rejection. In this uncommon condition, sinusoidal lymphocytes abound, particularly in zone 3. Note drop-out of hepatocytes, a sign of incipient perivenular necrosis. This feature probably represents a severe rejection episode that may respond poorly to treatment. H & E.

Perivenular (zone 3) necrosis (Fig. 18.8) is found in many instances, particularly in progressive rejection with ductopenia and graft failure.[41,41a]

Ductopenic rejection (rejection with duct loss)

Generally, this condition evolves from cellular rejection, sometimes acutely as early as 2 weeks after OLT[42] but usually between 6 weeks and 6 months (delayed ductopenic rejection). The least common manifestation, late ductopenic rejection, appears after 6 months or more[33] following transplantation. Ductopenia is the defining histological feature. The diagnosis can be made with reasonable confidence if 20 or more portal tracts can be reviewed (often in consecutive specimens) and if 50% of these lack interlobular bile ducts.[26] It is important to note in this context that ductules (cholangioles) should not be counted

as ducts; this usually is not difficult because ductules generally run near the limiting plates, often lack a lumen, and display a 'Chinese-letter configuration' whereas interlobular bile ducts, the main targets of ductopenic rejection, run in the immediate vicinity of the hepatic artery branches,[43] always have a lumen, and lack the convoluted growth pattern of ductules. Ductopenia may be difficult to recognize in its early stage, when features of cellular rejection still prevail. However, as the condition progresses, inflammatory infiltrates tend to vanish and portal tracts emerge that contain only blood vessels (Fig. 18.9a). Even the hepatic artery branches may disappear in some instances[44] and then the distinction between portal tracts and terminal hepatic venules may become difficult (Fig. 18.9b). There is usually severe intra-acinar hepatocanalicular cholestasis, sometimes diffuse, sometimes primarily in zone 3. Perivenular necrosis prevails in many instances[41] (Fig. 18.9c). The sinusoids or perisinusoidal spaces often contain foam cells; they are lipid-laden macrophages that probably represent a response to the cholestasis (Fig. 18.9d). It is not clear whether these foam cells may also develop after immunological endothelial damage, akin to the putative pathogenesis of foam cell arteritis or arteriopathy described below.

Vascular rejection

This type of rejection is characterized solely by the presence of foam cell arteritis or arteriopathy; the diagnostic criterion is the presence of clusters of lipid-laden macrophages in the intima of affected arteries, often causing total occlusion of the lumen (Fig. 18.10a). The condition probably results from immunological damage of the arterial endothelium, leading to an influx of serum lipids that later are phagocytosed by host macrophages; these macrophages thus assume the features of foam cells. If vascular rejection is associated with intimal or transmural inflammation, the term 'foam cell arteritis' appears appropriate; the name 'foam cell arteriopathy' describes vessels with foam cells but without inflammatory changes. It should be noted that the arteritis that occurs in some cases of cellular rejection (Fig. 18.7) lacks foam cells and, by convention, is not considered under the name of vascular rejection. In some instances, vascular rejection may coexist with cellular rejection (Fig. 18.10b); this may represent both antibody-mediated and cell-mediated processes.

The diagnosis of vascular rejection can rarely be made from biopsy specimens because most affected arteries are outside the reach of the biopsy needle — namely, in large portal tracts and in the perihilar soft tissues. Even without biopsy confirmation, vascular rejection can be expected in many cases of ductopenic rejection although the relationship between these two conditions is not clear. Obliterative foam cell arteritis or arteriopathy appears to cause ischaemic duct injury in some cases and might even be a cause of ductopenia.[9,33] However, ductopenic rejection certainly can

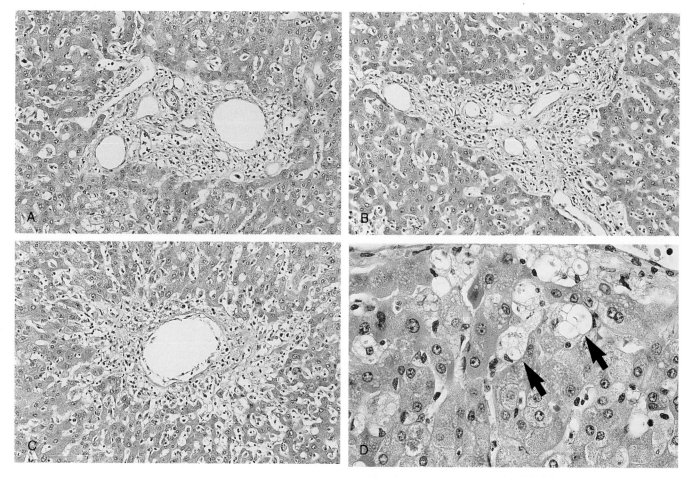

Fig. 18.9 Ductopenic rejection. (a) Portal tract without bile duct; numerous similar portal tracts were observed (ductopenia). Note the lack of inflammation which is typical of late-stage ductopenic rejection. H & E. (b) Portal tract without bile duct and without hepatic artery branches. Such a portal tract may be difficult to distinguish from perivenular necrosis as shown in (c). H & E. (c) Perivenular necrosis, a common finding in ductopenic rejection; the lesion may represent ischaemia complicating arteriopathy. H & E. (d) Widespread sinusoidal foam cells (arrows); they probably reflect cholestasis. H & E.

occur without evidence of vascular rejection and, therefore, duct loss in this setting does not require ischaemia; the immunological injury may suffice.

ALLOGRAFT PATHOLOGY OTHER THAN REJECTION

Acute graft failure

This condition is characterized by massive hepatic necrosis in the immediate post-transplant period, usually the first week; it is a rare but catastrophic event. Unless the criteria for 'hyperacute' rejection are met, the causes of acute graft failure are unknown. In some cases, preservation injury may have been responsible[44a]. In addition, donor livers with severe fatty changes[45] or hypertensive artery disease[46] appear to be prone to develop this condition. Histologically, the liver shows preserved architecture despite coagulative necrosis of most hepatocytes (Fig. 18.11a). The necrotic hepatocytes first have brick-red cytoplasm (Fig. 18.11b)

but, later, groups of regenerative hepatocytes with slightly basophilic cytoplasm can be identified in most instances. The mesenchymal portions of the liver remain intact; arteries and veins are patent. The damaged tissue is often infiltrated by neutrophils. In some cases, the necrosis is severely haemorrhagic.[47] At autopsy, pathologists should pay particular attention to the state of the hepatic artery anastomosis because this is an especially vulnerable site, and lesions are not always apparent clinically.[48]

Functional cholestasis

This condition is unique for hepatic allografts and typically occurs in the early post-transplant period. Specimens show hepatocanalicular cholestasis in zones 2 and 3, often associated with severe ballooning of hepatocytes in these areas. The cholestasis occurs independent of rejection, parenteral hyperalimentation, or the use of specific drugs. Subcellular organelle damage produced by cold ischaemia may play an aetiological role, leading to bile flow dysfunction,[49,50] hence

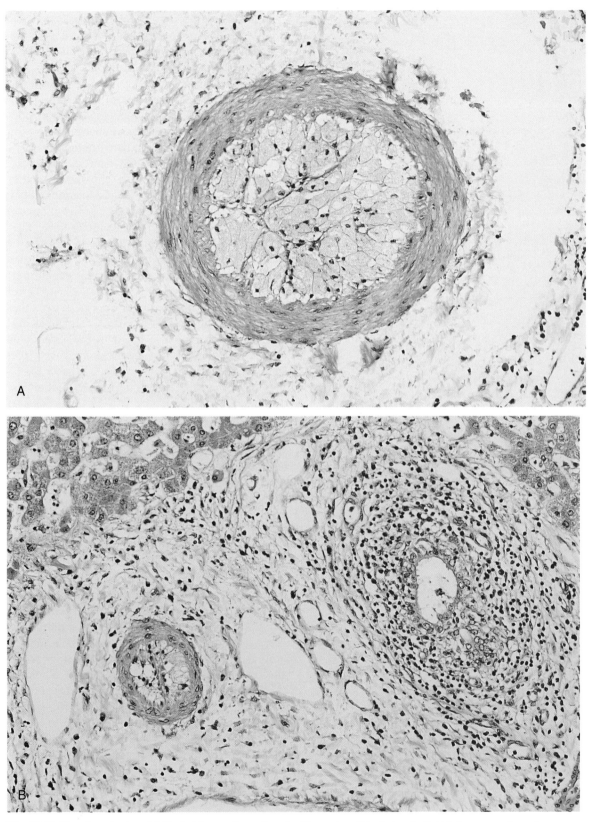

Fig. 18.10 Vascular rejection. (a) Typical foam cell arteriopathy. Expansion of the intima by lipid-laden macrophages has occluded the lumen. H&E. (b) Note presence of both foam cell arteritis (left) and mixed-cell cholangitis (right); this probably represents co-existent vascular and cellular rejection. H & E.

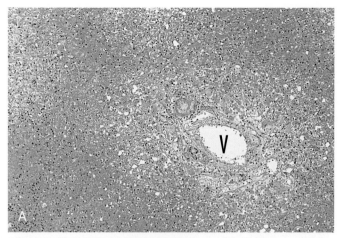

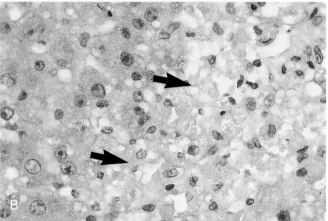

Fig. 18.11 Acute graft failure. (a) Note that the hepatic architecture is generally intact. V = portal vein. H & E. (b) The brick-red cytoplasm of the hepatocyte represents early coagulative necrosis (arrows). H & E.

the name functional cholestasis. In electron micrographs, prominent dilatation of the cisternae of the rough endoplasmic reticulum is found[51] and thus the changes differ from those in cholestasis of other causes. Whatever the cause, the condition is a benign, self-limited process. In rare instances, the features of functional cholestasis — hepatocanalicular cholestasis with ballooning — may appear weeks or months after OLT, usually in association with biliary disease.

Ischaemic lesions

Subcapsular infarcts develop in some allografts, probably because of transplant hypoperfusion. The condition may be associated with fatty change in the remaining liver but it often has no serious consequences.[52] However, catastrophic ischaemic injury with total or subtotal infarction of the liver may also occur, most commonly after hepatic artery thrombosis which may develop days, weeks, or months after OLT. Thus, liver biopsy specimens with evidence of infarction must be interpreted with caution because the

histological lesion may be inconsequential or it may herald widespread ischaemia and impending loss of the graft. Infarcts due to ischaemia should be distinguished from the changes seen in acute graft failure; in infarcts, the coagulation necrosis is complete, uniform, and often sharply demarcated. This differs from the typical changes in acute graft failure and in hyperacute rejection, as previously described.

An unusual ischaemic lesion, found almost exclusively in allografts, is ischaemic cholangitis which most commonly is another complication of hepatic artery thrombosis. Necrosis of ducts, cholangitis without necrosis, cholangiectases and strictures are the main pathological findings; neutrophilic cholangitis with cholangitic abscesses may also be present[53] (Fig. 18.12). Ischaemic cholangitis may be associated with widespread hepatic infarctions but it may also occur in an otherwise intact liver. The speed of the thrombus formation in the artery may be one of the factors that determines the ischaemic manifestations. Isolated ischaemic cholangitis probably occurs because bile ducts depend on a particularly rich, dedicated arterial blood supply which is provided by the peribiliary plexus. It should be noted, however, that bile-duct damage as described in this paragraph may also occur in the absence of demonstrable vascular lesions. In these instances, preservation injury seems to be the main cause;[54] in other cases, infection may have played a role but the cause is not always clear.

Infections

Bacterial, viral, fungal, and protozoal infections are common after OLT.[55] Enterobacteriaceae and other Gram-negative bacilli, cytomegalovirus, as well as Candida or Aspergillus species are commonly cultured. It should be noted that aspergillosis in this setting is almost always fatal. *Pneumocystis carinii* is the only common protozoon in this group although infections with *Toxoplasma gondii* have also been described. The manifestations of these infections do not differ from those in other immunosuppressed hosts; the typical changes in the liver are described in Chapter 7.

Bacterial and fungal infections may arise (i) from the allograft — for instance, from infected infarcts or infective ascending cholangitis, (ii) from exudates or infected haematomas in the vicinity of the graft, or (iii) *de novo* at any site, as exemplified by cases of cryptococcal meningitis after OLT. Fungal infections with zygomycetes and *Trichosporon beigellii* also have been encountered in liver transplant patients.[55]

Systemic viral infections that may affect allografts are caused by cytomegalovirus (CMV), EBV and, rarely, adenovirus or a herpesvirus. Hepatitis virus infections include hepatitis viruses B[55a], B with D, C, and possibly other rare non-B, non-C viruses. CMV hepatitis is the most common viral infection of allografts, and positive donor CMV serology appears to be the most important risk factor.[56] The diagnosis is reliably made by routine histology

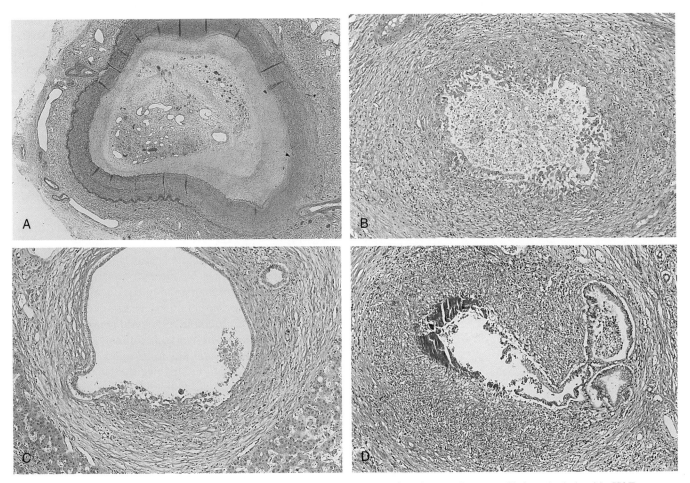

Fig. 18.12 Ischaemic cholangitis. (a) This hepatic artery thrombosis in the anastomotic region was the cause of ischaemic cholangitis. H&E. (b) Ischaemic cholangitis with bile-duct necrosis and both acute and chronic inflammatory changes. H&E. (c) Cholangiectasis with segmental ischaemic bile duct damage but only minimal inflammation. H&E. (d) Cholangitic abscess associated with ischaemic cholangitis. H&E. Fig. 18.12c reproduced with permission from Ludwig et al[53]

with immunostaining, using commercially available monoclonal mouse antibody directed against early and late CMV antigens (DAKO Corp, Carpenteria, California, USA).[57] DNA in situ hybridization and cell culture are less effective.[58] Microscopically, typical CMV inclusions may be found in hepatocytes, biliary epithelium, or endothelium. Infected hepatocytes are often surrounded by clusters of neutrophils, resembling a microabscess (Fig. 18.13). It should be noted that allograft biopsy specimens often contain clusters of neutrophils in the acini which are unexplained but clearly unrelated to CMV.[59] Although CMV hepatitis after OLT generally is not a threat to the graft, it indicates the presence of a potentially fatal systemic infection. Furthermore, persistent CMV infection of the graft has been considered to be a risk factor for irreversible rejection[60] although this association is still controversial.[61]

Adenoviral hepatitis is essentially confined to the paediatric age group.[62] The typical nuclear viral inclusions are indistinguishable from those seen in herpes simplex or varicella–zoster hepatitis which also may occur in paediatric OLT patients. Infections with EBV are discussed below

in relation to lymphoproliferative disorders. Infections with hepatitis viruses may develop de novo but more commonly represent a recurrence of the primary disease; they are discussed under that heading. Finally, transplanted infections[63] must be considered. Because of the immunosuppressed state of transplant recipients, infected grafts are a serious threat, even if the organisms would be harmless for most other patients.

Recurrence of primary disease

Hepatitis B often recurs after OLT if patients had been positive for HBsAg or HBcAg[64,65] and particularly if the virus replicated actively at the time of transplantation, as indicated by the presence of HBV DNA.[66,66a] Although long-term survival may occur,[67,68] collectively graft and patient survival decrease after two months.[64] Without immunoprophylaxis, recurrent hepatitis B often has an accelerated course; as early as 2–5 weeks after OLT, biopsy specimens may reveal cytoplasmic HBcAg or HBsAg,[64,65] and lobular hepatitis often develops 70–300

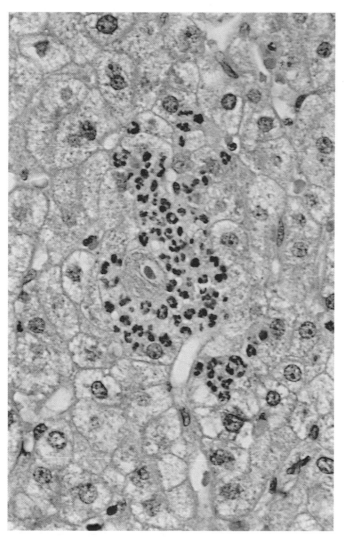

Fig. 18.13 Cytomegalovirus hepatitis. A hepatocyte with a typical intranuclear cytomegalovirus inclusion is surrounded by a cluster of neutrophils, resembling a microabscess. H & E.

days after OLT.[65] The condition may then evolve into a chronic carrier state but active chronic hepatitis B often develops, sometimes with swift progression to cirrhosis.[65,69] For a unique, rapidly progressing form of recurrent hepatitis B,[69,70] the names 'fibrosing cholestatic hepatitis'[70,70a] and 'fibrosing cytolytic hepatitis'[71] have been proposed. In this variant, inflammatory changes are often mild but ballooning degeneration and necrosis of hepatocytes, periportal fibrosis, postnecrotic multiacinar collapse, and cholestasis may be severe, and nuclear and cytoplasmic HBcAg and cytoplasmic HBsAg abound (Fig. 18.14). The virus may be cytopathic in these cases and not a trigger of immunologically mediated damage. Finally, hepatocellular carcinoma may develop de novo in patients with chronic hepatitis B and HBV-associated cirrhosis[72] (Fig. 18.15). If HBV does not replicate at the time of OLT and if patients had received an appropriate does of long-term HB immunoglobulin, the rate of recurrence is low.[73]

Hepatitis delta virus (HDV) infection recurs in up to 80% of patients with hepatitis B and HDV.[74] The HBV in this setting usually does not replicate, and after immunoprophylaxis the prognosis is good. Thus, HDV appears to impart some protection from B virus-related graft loss.[44] In auxiliary grafts, the HDV antigen has been detected as early as one week after OLT.[75] It is of interest that the presence of HDV does not seem to worsen graft and patient survival and that, in contrast to non-allograft livers, HDV does persist in the absence of detectable HBV and of tissue damage.[74,76,76a] However, after recurrence of HBV antigens, HDV antigens also re-accumulate massively, often accompanied by a lobular hepatitis.[76]

Hepatitis C infection appears to recur in nearly all patients after OLT[77–81] and it is also commonly acquired by patients who had not been infected prior to transplantation. Serological results may be difficult to interpret because immunosuppression may inhibit the formation of anti-HCV[78] and because seroconversion may occur as late as 6 months after OLT. Reliable results are obtainable with the polymerase chain reaction which can amplify HCV RNA both in serum and in liver biopsy samples.[79]

Hepatitis C tends to recur towards the end of the first year or in the second year after OLT. Acute progressive graft damage is rare.[82] Biopsy specimens often show mild periportal hepatitis with lymphoid aggregates in the portal tracts. Mild lymphoid cholangitis and endotheliitis may be found, and in these instances clinical information may be required to distinguish hepatitis C from cellular rejection. If fatty change is present, hepatitis C is the more likely diagnosis. Current experiences suggest that both recurrent and acquired post-transplant hepatitis C have a rather mild course[83,83a] although the long-term prognosis has not yet been sufficiently studied.

In patients with primary biliary cirrhosis (PBC), evidence is mounting that the condition indeed may reappear.[84–84c] It is conceivable that anti-rejection treatment delays, attenuates or even prevents the recurrence of PBC in many cases. Furthermore, many patients may not have lived long enough for the disease to recur. The histological diagnosis of PBC in allografts is bound to be difficult because PBC and rejection share many features. The diagnosis rests on the presence of classic destructive granulomatous cholangitis (florid duct lesion) as shown in Figure 18.16, but absence of this finding certainly does not preclude the diagnosis of recurrent PBC.

In primary sclerosing cholangitis (PSC), the diagnosis of recurrent disease is even more controversial than in PBC because ischaemic cholangitis[53] and possibly other conditions such as rejection or CMV cholangitis may cause comparable cholangiographic changes. The issue is further complicated by the fact that most patients who received an allograft for PSC have a Roux-en-Y anastomosis which has a higher rate or biliary complications than the more widely used duct-to-duct anastomosis.[84d] Fibro-

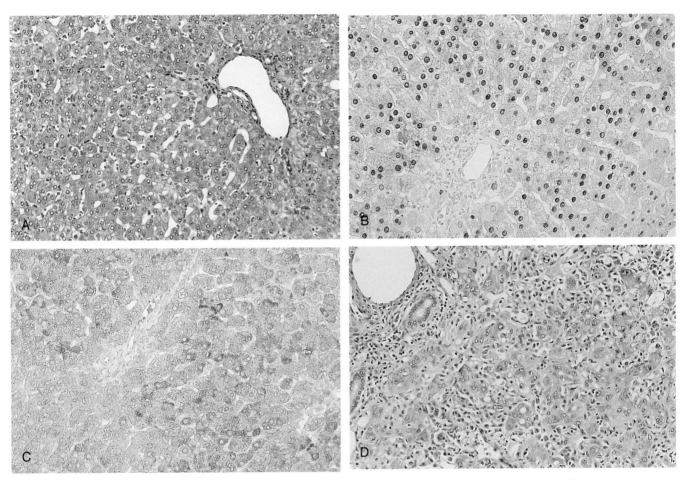

Fig. 18.14 Fibrosing cholestatic hepatitis B. (a) Seven weeks after OLT, the liver has a normal appearance in this haematoxylin–eosin stained specimen. Note the absence of portal inflammation. H&E. (b) Same specimen after immunostaining; note abundant nuclear HBcAg. Anti-HBcAg. (c) Same specimen after immunostaining; note abundant cytoplasmic HBsAg. Anti-HBsAg. (d) Same liver removed 10 days later because of fulminant hepatic failure. Massive necrosis of hepatocytes is now evident, with numerous neocholangioles which represent regenerating hepatocytes. This process might reflect cytolytic hepatocyte destruction. H&E.

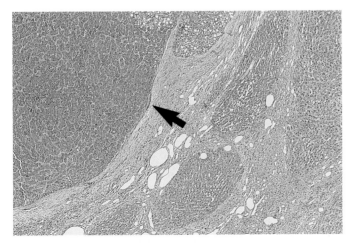

Fig. 18.15 Hepatitis B with cirrhosis and hepatocellular carcinoma, 5 years after OLT. A small, de novo hepatocellular carcinoma (arrow) was detected through serum α-fetoprotein screening. H&E.

obliterative cholangitis, the histological hallmark of PSC, has been documented in putative recurrent PSC,[84e] but might also be seen in cases of secondary sclerosing cholangitis.

Malignant hepatic tumours recur after OLT in most instances; thus results generally are poor.[15,85,86] However, long-term survival has been reported in some cases.[15,86] In patients with hepatocellular carcinoma (HCC), OLT occasionally is successful; tumour recurrence is particularly common if the neoplasm was large or multifocal[86a] or if macroscopic vascular invasion had been present.[86] Nevertheless, in some patients with cirrhosis and hepatocellular carcinoma, liver transplantation may offer a better chance for long-term survival than tumour resection.[87] Recurrence usually occurs within the first year after OLT, most often in the allograft or in the lungs.[64,86] Fibrolamellar hepatocellular carcinoma has a better prognosis after liver transplantation than other types of HCC, but approximately

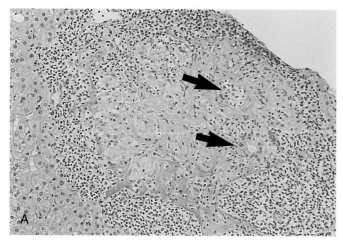

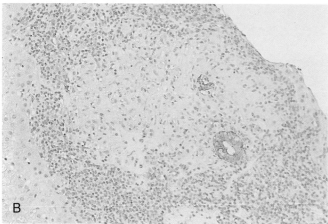

Fig. 18.16 Florid duct lesion in hepatic allograft, indicative of recurrent syndrome of primary biliary cirrhosis. (a) Non-caseating portal tract granuloma with evidence of duct destruction (arrows). PAS with diastase digestion. (b) Cytokeratin immunoperoxidase staining highlights the destructive cholangitis shown in (a). AE1/AE3. Reproduced with permission from Balan et al.[84a]

40–50% still recur.[15,86] Cholangiocarcinomas and bile-duct adenocarcinomas have recurred in most instances;[15,88,89] among the few exceptions were incidental carcinomas complicating primary sclerosing cholangitis.[86] In some patients with unresectable epithelioid haemangioendothelioma, OLT has resulted in long survival even if metastases had been present[90] but in other patients recurrence promptly ensued.[15,91]

Metastatic tumours in the liver also have been treated with OLT, either because they were presumed to be isolated[89,92] or because they represented slow-growing endocrine neoplasms. In patients with the carcinoid syndrome, symptomatic relief has been readily achieved but new metastases developed in many patients.[93]

Adverse drug effects

The evaluation of possible adverse drug effects in allografts after OLT is hampered by the many other abnormal findings that can be encountered in biopsy material. Thus, azathioprine,[94] cyclosporine,[95] and probably FK 506 can cause liver damage, but this can be evaluated reliably only in non-liver-transplant recipients. In one centre[96] some allografts showed convincing evidence of azathioprine-induced nodular regenerative hyperplasia with portal hypertension.

Lymphoproliferative disorders

The appearance of malignancies is a well-known complication of immunosuppression after organ transplantation.[97,97a] Most post-transplant lymphoproliferative disorders affect B-cells; they occur in approximtately 1–2% of liver transplant patients.[98] In the paediatric age group, up to 8% of patients are affected.[99] Most cases can be linked to infection with EBV. Presence of the EBV genome has been confirmed by in situ hybridization and by the demonstration of EBV DNA with the polymerase chain reaction.[100]

After OLT, primary EBV infection may occur or latent EBV may become reactivated. In this setting, EBV is integrated into B-cells and a mononucleosis-like disease can develop. Subsequently, B-cell clones may proliferate, probably because immunosuppressive therapy impairs T-cell regulation. During this phase, cellular infiltrates are still polyclonal and responsive to decreased immunosuppression or antiviral drugs.[99,101] The frank malignant phase of the lymphoproliferative disorder probably is the result of clonal mutations. At this stage, the condition is likely to be unresponsive to treatment.

Biopsy specimens from EBV-infected livers reveal mononuclear portal tract infiltrates composed of small lymphocytes, plasma cells, large cleaved and non-cleaved cells, and immunoblasts[102] (Fig. 18.17). The findings may resemble cellular rejection, but the composition of the infiltrate with the lack of eosinophils and the absence of prominent cholangitis favours the diagnosis of a systemic viral disease, particularly if lobular hepatitis is also present.[102] The transition from immunoresponsive to unresponsive disease is not accompanied by consistent histological changes and, thus, cannot be recognized reliably. Once overt EBV-associated lymphomas have developed, the large-cell type is most often found but Burkitt-like lymphomas have also been reported.[103]

ALLOGRAFT ABNORMALITIES IN RELATION TO TIME AFTER LIVER TRANSPLANTATION

Most complications tend to occur during a specific period after OLT and are rarely encountered or even non-existent at other times. This can be most helpful in the differential diagnosis of hepatic allograft abnormalities. Early complications, mostly in the first week after OLT, include hyperacute rejection (primary humoral rejection), acute cellular rejection, acute graft failure, and functional cholestasis.

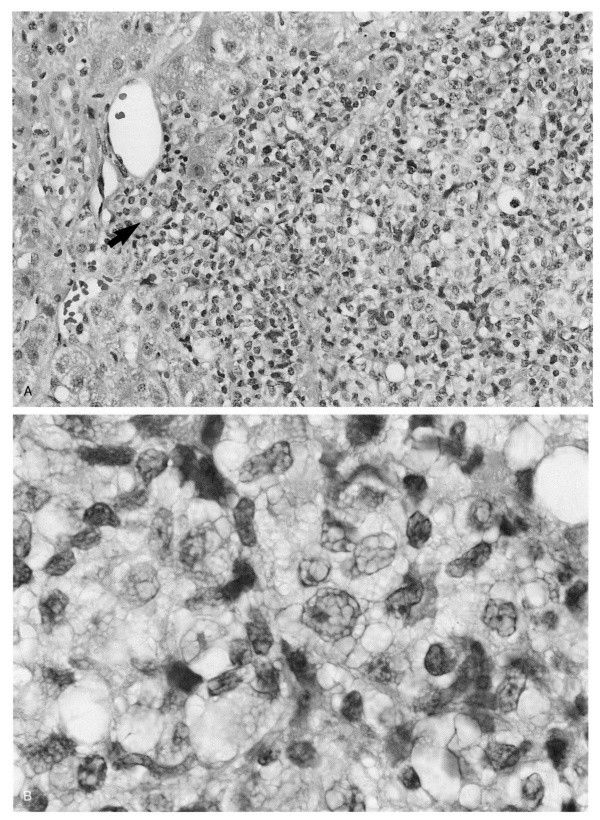

Fig. 18.17 Epstein–Barr virus infection with associated lymphoproliferative disorder, 21 months after OLT. (a) A dense mononuclear infiltrate expands this portal tract. The composition of the infiltrate and the preservation of the bile duct (arrow) make rejection unlikely. H&E. (b) The infiltrate is composed of a polymorphous infiltrate of mononuclear cells with many large lymphocytes and immunoblasts. H&E.

Delayed complications, anywhere between 3 weeks and 3 months after OLT, include cytomegalovirus and other systemic infections, cellular or ductopenic rejection or both, and ischaemic graft damage.[103a] Late complications, often 6 months or more after OLT, include unresolved or chronic viral hepatitis B and C, ductopenic or vascular rejection or both, tumour recurrence, and post-transplantation lymphoproliferative diseases. All these conditions have been discussed in this chapter.

LIVER PATHOLOGY AFTER BONE MARROW TRANSPLANTATION

Definitions and terminology

Graft versus host disease (GVHD) is characterized by the adverse effects on organs and tissues of transplanted immunologically competent cells. Thus, a patient with GVHD must have received a graft that contains such cells; the patient also must be genetically different and unable to reject the engrafted immunocytes. GVHD is most common in patients who received allogeneic bone marrow transplantation but other grafts, including transplanted livers,[104] also may induce the condition.

The main targets of immunocompetent cells causing GVHD are the gastrointestinal tract, the skin, and the liver. Usually, all these organs are involved but isolated hepatic GVHD also has been reported.[105] Customarily, acute GVHD, developing 20–100 days after engrafting, is distinguished from chronic GVHD, which is observed after 100 days. Acute GVHD is an important risk factor for the development of chronic GVHD.[106] Nevertheless, acute GVHD may be self-limited whereas chronic GVHD tends to be progressive. The two conditions appear to differ in the degree of organ involvement; chronic GVHD tends to spread beyond the gastrointestinal tract, the skin, and the liver, and the inflammatory response is often more severe. In addition to these morphological and corresponding clinical differences, acute and chronic GVHD might also differ pathogenetically.[106]

Histopathological features

The main histological features of hepatic GVHD are portal hepatitis, destructive non-suppurative cholangitis, cholestasis, and endotheliitis. Thus, the changes closely resemble those seen in cellular rejection. Lymphocytes are found to invade bile-duct epithelium (Fig. 18.18), probably because of aberrant expression of class II MHC antigens;[107] the affected cells show cytoplasmic vacuolation and, eventually, they drop out. This process continues until the attacked interlobular bile ducts are destroyed. Duct damage and the accompanying cholestasis are rather reliable diagnostic markers for GVHD; they usually allow a distinction between this condition and other types of

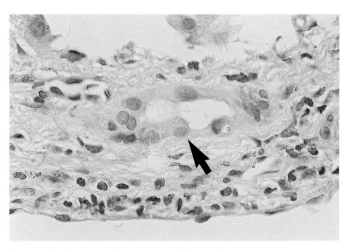

Fig. 18.18 Hepatic graft-versus-host disease. Non-suppurative cholangitis is evident with intraepithelial lymphocytes and damaged, atrophic biliary epithelium (arrow). In this case, endotheliitis is not present and portal inflammation is minimal. H&E.

hepatitis, e.g. drug-induced liver disease[108] and viral hepatitis. If intra-acinar inflammation predominates, viral hepatitis is the more likely diagnosis. The progressive duct destruction in GVHD may lead to biliary fibrosis and even cirrhosis.[109] The endotheliitis in GVHD can be found in both portal vein branches and in terminal hepatic venules; lymphocytes are found attached to the endothelium as well as underneath damaged endothelial cells that have been lifted from the basement membrane. Although endotheliitis is not specific, its presence is diagnostically helpful if found in patients with suspected GVHD.

Complications after bone marrow transplantation, unrelated to GVHD, include veno-occlusive disease, caused by chemoradiation therapy.[110] The prognosis is poor. Nodular regenerative hyperplasia is another common complication after bone marrow transplantation.[111] Although both nodular regenerative hyperplasia and veno-occlusive disease may cause ascites, the prognoses differ. In one series,[111] no patient with nodular regenerative hyperplasia died of liver disease. Veno-occlusive disease generally is fatal.

PATHOLOGY OF THE LIVER AFTER TRANSPLANTATION OF OTHER SOLID ORGANS

Pathogenetic mechanisms

Almost without exception, hepatic abnormalities after transplantation of non-liver solid organs, primarily kidneys and hearts, are direct adverse drug effects or are caused indirectly by drug-induced immunosuppression. This immunosuppression is the most common cause of complications; it may lead to infections, systemic viral infections in particular, and post-transplant lymphoproliferative disorders. Direct adverse drug effects are caused mainly by azathioprine, a hepatotoxic antineoplastic and immunosuppressant.

Infections and post-transplant lymphoproliferative disorders related to drug-induced immunosuppression

Post-transplant cytomegalovirus hepatitis and adenovirus hepatitis are observed in both liver and non-liver transplant recipients. Herpes simplex hepatitis, on the other hand, appears to be much more common in renal or heart transplant recipients. The condition may develop less than 3 weeks after transplantation, i.e. earlier than cytomegalovirus hepatitis would be expected. Diffuse hepatic involvement generally is fatal.[112] Adenovirus hepatitis is rare in adults[113] but should be expected in the paediatric age group. Cytomegalovirus hepatitis in transplant recipients rarely causes major morbidity; its histological manifestations are important mainly as a sign of systemic organ involvement. Finally, hepatic (visceral) bacillary epithelioid angiomatosis has been observed in a heart transplant recipient;[114] that condition had been found primarily in patients with the acquired immunodeficiency syndrome. The infective agent is the rickettsial organism *Rochalimaea henselae*.[115]

Pre-existing hepatitis B infection has played an important role in renal transplant patients; chronic hepatitis, cirrhosis, and hepatocellular carcinoma were the main complications.[116,117] With the possible exception of hepatocellular carcinoma, similar complications have been caused by hepatitis non-A, non-B infections after heart transplantation.[118] Experiences in non-transplant patients suggest that hepatocellular carcinoma may also develop.[119] It should be noted, however, that positive test results do not necessarily herald a poor prognosis because hepatitis B surface antigen positivity and hepatitis C antibody positivity alone did not affect mortality or graft survival in renal transplant patients.[120]

Post-transplant lymphoproliferative disease is most commonly observed in heart transplant patients, probably because they receive higher doses of immunosuppressive drugs. The liver may be one of the sites involved by lymphoma.[121]

Adverse drug effects unrelated to immunosuppression

In non-liver transplant recipients, adverse hepatic drug effects are caused primarily by azathioprine. Endothelial cell injury[94] by this this drug may lead to sinusoidal dilatation,[122] peliosis hepatis, veno-occlusive disease, perisinusoidal fibrosis, and nodular regenerative hyperplasia. Azathioprine-induced cholestasis[123] and hepatocellular carcinoma[124] have also been observed.

Other complications

Some liver diseases in renal transplant patients appear unrelated to adverse drug effects; they include haemosiderosis[125] and rare cases of focal hepatic calcification; the mineralization may be both dystrophic and metastatic.[126] It should be noted, however, that cyclosporine-induced hepatic calcification probably can occur also.[127]

REFERENCES

1. Starzl T E, Iwatsuki S, Van Thiel D H et al. Evolution of liver transplantation. Hepatology 1982; 2: 614–636
2. Demetris A J, Markus H. Immunopathology of liver transplantation. Crit Rev Immunol 1989; 9: 67–92
3. Porter K A. Pathology of the orthotopic homograft and heterograft. In: Starzl T E, Putnam C W, eds. Experience in hepatic transplantation. Philadelphia: W B Saunders, 1969; pp 422–471
4. Houssin D, Charpentier B, Gugenheim J et al. Spontaneous long-term acceptance of RT-1-incompatible liver allografts in rats. Transplantation 1983; 36: 615–620
5. Tamisier D, Houssin D, Gugenheim J et al. Spontaneous long-term survival of liver allografts in inbred rats: comparison between semi-allogeneic and fully allogeneic strain combinations. Eur Surg Res 1983; 15: 145–150
5a. Starzl T E, Demetris A J, Trucco M, et al. Cell migration and chimerism after whole-organ transplantation: The basis of graft acceptance. Hepatology 1993; 17: 1127–1152
5b. Calne R, Davies H. Organ graft tolerance: the liver effect. Lancet 1994; 343: 67–68
6. Starzl T E, Fung J, Tzakis A et al. Baboon-to-human liver transplantation. Lancet 1993; 341: 65–71
7. United Network of Organ Sharing (UNOS). 1992; 8
8. Todo S, Nery J, Katsuhiko Y, Podesta L, Gordon R D, Starzl T E. Extended preservation of human liver grafts with UW solution. JAMA 1989; 261: 711–714
9. Wiesner R H, Ludwig J, Van Hoek B, Krom R A F. Current concepts in cell-mediated hepatic allograft rejection leading to ductopenia and liver failure. Hepatology 1991; 14: 721–729
10. Terpstra O T, Schalm S W, Weimar W et al. Auxiliary partial liver transplantation for end-stage chronic liver disease. N Engl J Med 1988; 319: 1014–1022
10a. Boudjema K, Jaeck D, Siméoni U, Bientz J, Chenard M P, Brunot P. Temporary auxiliary liver transplantation for subacute liver failure in a child. (Short reports.) Lancet 1993; 342: 778–779
11. Emond J C, Whitington P F, Thistlewaite J R et al. Transplantation of two patients with one liver. Analysis of a preliminary experience with "split-liver" grafting. Ann Surg 1990; 212: 14–22
12. Broelsch C E, Whitington P F, Emond J C et al. Liver transplantation in children from living related donors. Surgical techniques and results. Ann Surg 1991; 214: 428–439
13. Dindzans V J, Schade R R, Gavaler J S et al. Liver transplantation. A primer for practicing gastroenterologists, part I. Dig Dis Sci 1989; 34: 2–8
14. Halff G, Todo S, Tzakis A G et al. Liver transplantation for the Budd–Chiari syndrome. Ann Surg 1990; 211: 43–49
15. O'Grady J G, Polson R J, Rolles K, Calne R Y, Williams R. Liver transplantation for malignant disease. Results in 93 consecutive patients. Ann Surg 1988; 207: 373–379
16. Arnold J C, O'Grady J G, Bird G L, Calne R Y, Williams R. Liver transplantation for primary and secondary hepatic apudomas. Br J Surg 1989; 76: 248–249
17. Starzl T E, Demetris A J, van Thiel D. Liver transplantation (first of two parts). N Engl J Med 1989; 321: 1249–1259
18. Smanik E, Tavill A, Jacobs G et al. Orthotopic liver transplantation in two adults with Niemann–Pick and Gaucher's diseases: Implications for the treatment of inherited metabolic disease. Hepatology 1993; 17: 42–49
18a. Holmgren G, Ericzon B G, Groth C G, et al. Clinical improvement and amyloid regression after liver transplantation in

hereditary transthyretin amyloidosis. Lancet 1993; 341: 1113–1116

18b. Skinner M, Lewis W D, Jones L A, et al. Liver transplantation as a treatment for familial amyloidotic polyneuropathy. Ann Intern Med 1994; 120: 133–134

19. Foster P F, Bhattacharyya A, Sankary H N, Coleman J, Ashmann M, Williams J W. Eosinophil cationic protein's role in human hepatic allograft rejection. Hepatology 1991; 13: 1117–1125

20. Demetris A J, Jaffe R, Tzakis A et al. Antibody-mediated rejection of human orthotopic liver allografts. A study of liver transplantation across ABO blood group barriers. Am J Pathol 1988; 132: 489–502

21. Hanto D W, Snover D C, Sibley R K, Noreen H J, Gajl-Pezalska K J, Najarian J S, Ascher N L. Hyperacute rejection of a human orthotopic liver allograft in presensitized recipient. Clin Transplantation 1987; 1: 304–310

22. Gugenheim J, Samuel D, Reynes M, Bismuth H. Liver transplantation across ABO blood group barriers. Lancet 1990; 336: 519–523

23. Sanchez-Urdazpal L, Sterioff S, Janes C, Schwerman L, Rosen C, Krom R A F. Increased bile duct complications in ABO incompatible liver transplant recipients. Transplant Proc 1991; 23: 1440

24. Steinhoff G. Major histocompatibility complex antigens in human liver transplants. J Hepatol 1990; 11: 9–15

25. Sher L S, Howard T K, Podesta L G et al. Liver transplantation. In: McIntyre N, Benhamou J-P, Bircher J, Rizetto M, Rodes J, eds. Oxford Textbook of Clinical Hepatology. Oxford: Oxford Medical Publications, 1991: vol 2, pp 1429–1449

26. Ludwig J. Terminology of hepatic allograft rejection (glossary). Semin Liver Dis 1992; 12: 89–92

27. Ludwig J, Weisner R H, Batts K P, Perkins J D, Krom R A F. The acute vanishing bile duct syndrome (acute irreversible rejection) after orthotopic liver transplantation. Hepatology 1987; 7: 476–483

28. Snover D C. Problems in the interpretation of liver biopsies after liver transplantation. Am J Surg Pathol 1989; 13: 31–38

29. Hubscher S G, Buckels J A C, Elias E, McMaster P, Neuberger J M. Reversible vanishing bile duct syndrome after liver transplantation: Report of 6 cases. Transplant Proc 1991; 23: 1415–1416

30. Wiesner R H, Ludwig J, Krom R A F, Hay J E, van Hoek B. Hepatic allograft rejection: New developments in terminology, diagnosis, prevention, and treatment. Mayo Clin Proc 1993; 68: 69–79

31. NIDDK Liver Transplant Database, presented by A J Demetris. Standardized nomenclature and grading system for acute cellular rejection of liver allografts. Gastroenterology 1992; (no. 4, part 2): A800

32. Demetris J A, Belle S H, Hart J et al. Intraobserver and interobserver variation in the histopathological assessment of liver allograft rejection. Hepatology 1991; 14: 751–755

33. Demetris A J, Qian S, Sun H, Fung J J. Liver allograft rejection: An overview of morphologic findings. Am J Surg Pathol 1990; 14: 49–63

34. Demetris A, Nakamura K, Yagihashi A et al. A clinicopathological study of human liver allograft recipients harboring performed IgG lymphocytoxic antibodies. Hepatology 1992; 16: 671–682

35. Snover D C, Sibley R K, Freese D K, Sharp H L, Bloomer J R, Najarian J S, Ascher N L. Orthotopic liver transplantation: A pathological study of 63 serial liver biopsies from 17 patients with special reference to the diagnostic features and natural history of rejection. Hepatology 1984; 4: 1212–1222

36. Perkins J D, Wiesner R H, Banks P M, LaRusso N F, Ludwig J, Krom R A F. Immunohistologic labeling as an indicator of liver allograft rejection. Transplantation 1987; 43: 105–108

37. Ludwig J, Batts K P, Ploch M, Rakela J, Perkins J D, Wiesner R H. Endotheliitis in hepatic allografts. Mayo Clin Proc 1989; 64: 545–554

38. Nonomura A, Mizukami Y, Matsubara F, Kobayashi K. Clinicopathologic study of lymphocyte attachment to endothelial cells (endothelialitis) in various liver diseases. Liver 1991; 11: 78–88

39. Vierling J M, Fennel R H Jr. Histopathology of early and late human hepatic allograft rejection: Evidence of progressive destruction of interlobular bile ducts. Hepatology 1985; 5: 1076–1082

40. Snover D C, Freese D K, Sharp H L, Bloomer J R, Najarian J S, Ascher N L. Liver allograft rejection. An analysis of the use of biopsy in determining outcome of rejection. Am J Surg Pathol 1987; 11: 1–10

41. Ludwig J, Gross J B Jr, Perkins J D, Moore S B. Persistent centrilobular necroses in hepatic allografts. Hum Pathol 1990; 21: 656–661

41a. Dhillon A P, Burroughs A K, Hudson M, Shah N, Rolles K, Scheuer P J. Hepatic venular stenosis after orthotopic liver transplantation. Hepatology 1994; 19: 106–111

42. Adams D H, Neuberger J M. Patterns of graft rejection following liver transplantation. J Hepatol 1990; 10: 113–119

43. Nakanuma Y, Ohta G. Histometric and serial section observations of the intrahepatic bile ducts in primary biliary cirrhosis. Gastroenterology 1979; 76: 1326–1332

44. Oguma S, Belle S, Starzl T E, Demetris A J. A histometric analysis of chronically rejected human liver allografts: insights into the mechanisms of bile duct loss: direct immunologic and ischemic factors. Hepatology 1989; 9: 204–209

44a. Chazouillères O, Calmus Y, Vaubourdolle M, Ballet F. Preservation-induced liver injury. Clinical aspects, mechanisms and therapeutic approaches. J Hepatol 1993; 18: 123–134

45. Todo S, Demetris A J, Makowka L et al. Primary nonfunction of hepatic allografts with preexisting fatty infiltration. Transplantation 1989; 47: 903–905

46. Wisecarver J, Radio S, Shaw B Jr, Langnas A, Fox I, Heffron T, Markin R. Intrahepatic arteriopathy associated with primary non-function of liver allografts. Mod Pathol 1993; 6 (no. 1): abstract 668

47. Hübscher S G, Adams D H, Buckels J A C, McMaster J A, Neuberger J, Elias E. Massive hemorrhagic necrosis of the liver after liver transplantation. J Clin Pathol 1989; 42: 360–370

48. Markin R S, Hollins S, Wood R P, Shaw B W Jr. Main autopsy findings in liver transplant patients. Mod Pathol 1989; 2: 339–348

49. Williams J W, Vera S, Peters T G et al. Cholestatic jaundice after hepatic transplantation. A nonimmunologically mediated event. Am J Surg 1986; 151: 65–70

50. Goldstein N S, Hart J, Lewin K J. Diffuse hepatocyte ballooning in liver biopsies from orthotopic liver transplant patients. Histopathology 1991; 18: 331–338

51. Ng I O I, Burroughs A K, Rolles K, Belli L, Scheuer P. Hepatocellular ballooning after liver transplantation: A light and electron microscopic study with clinicopathological correlation. Histopathology 1991; 18: 323–330

52. Russo P A, Yunis E J. Subcapsular hepatic necrosis in orthotopic liver allografts. Hepatology 1986; 6: 708–713

53. Ludwig J, Batts K P, MacCarty R L. Ischemic cholangitis in hepatic allografts. Mayo Clin Proc 1992; 67: 519–526

54. Li S, Stratta R J, Langnas A N et al. Diffuse biliary tract injury after orthotopic liver transplantation. Am J Surg 1992; 164: 536–540

55. Markin R S, Stratta R J, Woods G L. Infection after liver transplantation. Am J Surg Pathol 1990; 14: 64–78

55a. Chazouillères O, Mamish D, Kim M, et al. 'Occult' hepatitis B virus as source of infection in liver transplant recipients. Lancet 1994; 343: 142–146

56. Gorensek M J, Carey W D, Vogt D, Goormastic M. A multivariate analysis of risk factors for cytomegalovirus infection in liver-transplant recipients. Gastroenterology 1990; 98: 1326–1332

57. Theise N D, Birks E J, Grundy J E, Scheuer P. Detection of cytomegalovirus in liver allografts in the early posttransplant period: a study and review of the literature. Eur J Gastroenterol Hepatol 1992; 4: 727–732

58. Paya C V, Holley K E, Wiesner R H et al. Early diagnosis of cytomegalovirus hepatitis in liver transplant recipients: Role of

immunostaining, DNA hybridization and culture of hepatic tissue. Hepatology 1990; 12: 119–126

59. DelBuono E A, Frank T S, Wilson M et al. Posttransplant minimicroabscess disease (PTMMD). Mod Pathol 1992; (no. 5): abstract 565

60. Arnold J C, Portmann B C, O'Grady J G, Naoumov N V, Alexander G J M, Williams R. Cytomegalovirus infection persists in the liver graft in the vanishing bile duct syndrome. Hepatology 1992; 16: 285–292

61. Paya C, Wiesner R, Hermans P et al. Lack of association between cytomegalovirus infection, HLA matching and the vanishing bile duct syndrome. Hepatology 1992; 16: 66–70

62. Varki N M, Bhuta S, Drake T, Porter D D. Adenovirus hepatitis in two successive liver transplants in a child. Arch Pathol Lab Med 1990; 114: 106–109

63. Gottesdiener K M. Transplanted infections: Donor-to-host transmission with the allograft. Ann Intern Med 1989; 110: 1001–1016

64. Hart J, Busuttil R W, Lewin K J. Disease recurrence following liver transplantation. Ann J Surg Pathol 1990; 14: 79–91

65. Todo S, Demetris A J, Van Thiel D, Teperman L, Fung J J, Starzl T E. Orthotopic liver transplantation for patients with hepatitis B virus-related liver disease. Hepatology 1991; 13: 619–626

66. Martin P, Munoz S, Friedmann L. Liver transplantation for viral hepatitis: current status. Am J Gastroenterol 1992; 87: 409–418

66a. Samuel D, Muller R, Alexander G, et al. Liver transplantation in European patients with the hepatitis B surface antigen. N Engl J Med 1993; 329: 1842–1847

67. Feria G, Colledan M, Doglia M et al. B hepatitis and liver transplantation. Transplant Proc 1988; 20: 566–569

68. O'Grady J G, Smith H M, Davies S E et al. Hepatitis B virus reinfection after orthotopic liver transplantation. Serological and clinical implications. J Hepatol 1992; 14: 104–111

69. Demetris A J, Todo S, Van Thiel D H et al. Evolution of hepatitis B virus liver disease after hepatic replacement. Practical and theoretical consideration. Am J Pathol 1990; 137: 667–676

70. Davies S E, Portmann B C, O'Grady J G, Aldis P M, Chaggar K, Alexander G J M, Williams R. Hepatic histological findings after transplantation for chronic hepatitis B virus infection, including a unique pattern of fibrosing cholestatic hepatitis. Hepatology 1991; 13: 150–157

70a. Mason A L, Wick M, White H M, et al. Increased hepatocyte expression of hepatitis B virus transcription in patients with features of fibrosing cholestatic hepatitis. Gastroenterology 1993; 105: 237–244

71. Benner K G, Lee R G, Keeffe E B, Lopez R R, Sasaki A W, Pinson C W. Fibrosing cytolytic liver failure secondary to recurrent hepatitis B after liver transplantation. Gastroenterology 1992; 103: 1307–1312

72. Luketic V A, Shiffman M L, McCall J B, Posner M P, Mills A S, Carithers R L Jr. Primary hepatocellular carcinoma after orthotopic liver transplantation for chronic hepatitis B infection. Ann Intern Med 1991; 114: 212–213

73. Samuel D, Bismuth A, Mathieu D et al. Passive immunoprophylaxis after liver transplantation in HBsAg-positive patients. Lancet 1991; 813–815

74. Marzano A, Ottobrelli A, David E, Durazzo M, Rizzetto M. Hepatitis delta virus infection and disease; the lesson from the liver transplantation model. Prog Clin Biol Res 1991; 364: 439–446

75. ten Kate F J, Schalm S W. Course of hepatitis delta virus infection in auxiliary liver grafts in patients with delta virus cirrhosis. Prog Clin Biol Res 1991; 364: 429–437

76. Davies S E, Lau J Y N, O'Grady J G, Portmann B C, Alexander G J M, Williams R. Evidence that hepatitis D virus needs hepatitis B virus to cause hepatocellular damage. Am J Clin Pathol 1992; 98: 554–558

76a. David E, Rahier J, Pucci A, et al. Recurrence of hepatitis D (Delta) in liver transplants: Histopathological aspects. Gastroenterology 1993; 104: 1122–1128

77. Wright T, Donegan E, Hsu H et al. Recurrent and acquired hepatitis C viral infection in liver transplant recipients. Gastroenterology 1992; 103: 317–322

78. Poterucha J J, Rakela J, Lumeng L, Lee C-H, Taswell H F, Wiesner R H. Diagnosis of chronic hepatitis C after liver transplantation by the detection of viral sequences with polymerase chain reaction. Hepatology 1992; 15: 42–44

79. Nuovo G J, Lidonnici K, Lane B. Histological correlation of hepatitis cDNA in liver biopsies as detected by RT in situ PCR hybridization. Mod Pathol 1993; 6 (no. 1): abstract 612

80. Martin P, Munoz S J, Di Bisceglie A M et al. Recurrence of hepatitis C infection after orthotopic liver transplantation. Hepatology 1991; 13: 719–721

81. Read A E, Donegan E, Lake J et al. Hepatitis C in patients undergoing liver transplantation. Ann Intern Med 1991; 114: 282–284

82. König V, Bauditz J, Lobek H et al. Hepatitis C virus reinfection in allografts after orthotopic liver transplantation. Hepatology 1992; 16: 1137–1143

83. Shah G, Demetris A, Gavaler J et al. Incidence, prevalence, and clinical course of hepatitis C following liver transplantation. Gastroenterology 1992; 103: 323–329

83a. Shah G, Demetris A J, Irish W, Scheffels J, Mimms L, Van Thiel D H. Frequency and severity of HCV infection following orthotopic liver transplantation. Effect of donor and recipient serology for HCV using a second generation ELISA test. J Hepatol 1993; 18: 279–283

84. Polson R J, Portmann B, Neuberger J, Calne R Y, Williams R. Evidence of disease recurrence after liver transplantation for primary biliary cirrhosis. Clinical and histologic follow-up studies. Gastroenterology 1989; 97: 715–725

84a. Balan V, Batts K P, Porayko M K, Krom R A F, Ludwig J, Wiesner R H. Histological evidence for recurrence of primary biliary cirrhosis after liver transplantation. Hepatology 1993; 18: 1392–1398

84b. Wong P Y N, Portmann B, O'Grady J G, Devlin J J, Hegarty J E, Tan K-C, Williams R. Recurrence of primary biliary cirrhosis after liver transplantation following FK506-based immunosuppression. J Hepatol 1993; 17: 284–287

84c. Hubscher S G, Elias E, Buckels J A C, Mayer A D, McMaster P, Neuberger J M. Primary biliary cirrhosis: Histological evidence of disease recurrence after liver transplantation. J Hepatol 1993; 18: 173–184

84d. McEntee G, Wiesner R, Rosen C, et al. Comparative study of patients undergoing liver transplantation for primary sclerosing cholangitis and primary biliary cirrhosis. Transplantation Proceedings 1991; 23: 1563–1564

84e. Harrison R F, Davies M H, Neuberger J M, Hubscher S G, Sclerosing cholangitis in liver allografts: Histological evidence for disease recurrence. Abstract Book, 6th Congress ESOT, Greece, 1993.

85. Ringe B, Pichlmayr R, Wittekind C, Tusch G. Surgical treatment of hepatocellular carcinoma: Experience with liver resection and transplantation in 198 patients. World J Surg 1991; 15: 270–285

86. Yokoyama I, Todo S, Iwatsuki S, Starzl T E. Liver transplantation in the treatment of primary liver cancer. Hepatogastroenterology 1990; 37: 188–193

86a. McPeake J R, O'Grady J G, Zaman S, et al. Liver transplantation for primary heptocellular carcinoma: tumour size and number determine outcome. J Hepatol 1993; 18: 226–234

87. Belli L, Romani F, Belli L S et al. Reappraisal of surgical treatment of small hepatocellular carcinomas in cirrhosis: clinicopathological study of resection or transplantation. Dig Dis Sci 1989; 34: 1571–1575

88. Koneru B, Cassavilla A, Bowman J, Iwatsuki S, Starzl T E. Liver transplantation for malignant tumors. Gastroenterol Clin North Am 1988; 17: 177–193

89. Ringe B, Wittekind C, Bechstein W O, Bunzendahl H, Pichlmayr R. The role of liver transplantation in hepatobiliary malignancy. A retrospective analysis of 95 patients with particular regard to tumor stage and recurrence. Ann Surg 1989; 209: 88–98

90. Kelleher M B, Iwatsuki S, Sheahan D G. Epithelioid hemangioendothelioma of liver. Clinicopathological correlation

of 10 cases treated by orthotopic liver transplantation. Am J Surg Pathol 1989; 13: 999–1008

91. Jenkins R L, Pinson C W, Stone M D. Experience with transplantation in the treatment of liver cancer. Cancer Chemother Pharmacol 1989; 23(suppl): S104–S109

92. Olthoff K M, Millis J M, Rosove M H, Goldstein L I, Ramming K P, Busuttil R W. Is liver transplantation justified in the treatment of hepatic malignancies? Arch Surg 1990; 125: 1261–1268

93. Alsina A E, Bartus S, Hull D, Rosson R, Schweizer R T. Liver transplant for metastatic neuroendocrine tumor. J Clin Gastroenterol 1990; 12: 533–537

94. Haboubi N Y, Ali H H, Whitwell H L, Ackrill P. Role of endothelial cell injury in the spectrum of azathioprine-induced liver disease after renal transplant: Light microscopy and ultrastructural observations. Am J Gastroenterol 1988; 83: 256–261

95. Kassianides C, Nussenblatt R, Palestine A G, Mellow S D, Hoofnagle J H. Liver injury from cyclosporine A. Dig Dis Sci 1990; 35: 693–697

96. Gane E, Ramage J, Portmann B, Williams R. Nodular regenerative hyperplasia of the liver following liver transplantation. Gut 1993; 31: S44 (abstract)

97. Penn I. Cancers complicating organ transplantation (editorial). N Engl J Med 1990; 323: 1767–1769

97a. Craig F E, Gulley M L, Banks P M. Posttransplantation lymphoproliferative disorders. Am J Clin Pathol 1993; 99: 265–276

98. Nalesnik M A, Jaffe R, Starzl T E et al. The pathology of posttransplant lymphoproliferative disorders occurring in the setting of cyclosporin A-prednisone immunosuppression. Am J Pathol 1988; 133: 173–192

99. Malatack J J, Gartner J C, Urbach A H, Zitelli B J. Orthotopic liver transplantation, Epstein–Barr virus, cyclosporine, and lymphoproliferative disease: A growing concern. J Pediatr 1991; 118: 667–675

100. Telenti A, Smith T F, Ludwig J, Keating M R, Krom R A F, Wiesner R H. Epstein–Barr virus and persistent graft dysfunction after liver transplantation. Hepatology 1991; 14: 282–286

101. Stieber A C, Boillot O, Scotti-Foglieni C et al. The surgical implications of the posttransplant lymphoproliferative disorders. Transplant Proc 1991; 23: 1477–1479

102. Randhawa P S, Markin R S, Starzl T E, Demetris A J. Epstein–Barr virus-associated syndromes in immunosuppressed liver transplant recipients. Clinical profile and recognition on routine allograft biopsy. Am J Surg Pathol 1990; 14: 538–547

103. Wolford J F, Krause J R. Posttranplant mediastinal Burkitt-like lymphoma — diagnosis by cytologic and flow cytometric analysis of pleural fluid. Acta Cytol 1990; 34: 261–274

103a. Rubin R, Munoz S J. Clinicopathologic features of late hepatic dysfunction in orthotopic liver transplants. Hum Pathol 1993; 24: 643–651

104. Roberts J P, Ascher N L, Lake J et al. Graft vs. host disease after liver transplantation in humans: A report of four cases. Hepatology 1991; 14: 274–281

105. Gholson C F, Yau J C, LeMaistre C F, Cleary K R. Steroid-responsive chronic hepatic graft-versus-host disease without extrahepatic graft-versus-host disease. Am J Gastroenterol 1989; 84: 1306–1309

106. Snover D C. Acute and chronic graft versus host disease: Histopathologic evidence for two distinct pathogenetic mechanisms. Hum Pathol 1984; 15: 202–205

107. Miglio F, Pignatelli M, Mazzeo V et al. Expression of major histocompatibility complex class II antigens on bile duct epithelium in patients with hepatic graft-versus-host disease after bone marrow transplantation. J Hepatol 1987; 5: 183–190

108. Shulman H M, Sharma P, Amos D, Fenster L F, McDonald B. A coded histologic study of hepatic graft-versus-host disease after human bone marrow transplantation. Hepatology 1988; 8: 463–470

109. Stechschulte D J Jr, Fishback J L, Emami A, Bhatia P. Secondary biliary cirrhosis as a consequence of graft-versus-host disease. Gastroenterology 1990; 98: 223–225

110. McDonald G B, Sharma P, Matthews D E, Shulman H M, Thomas E D. Venocclusive disease of the liver after bone marrow transplantation: Diagnosis, incidence, and predisposing factors. Hepatology 1984; 4: 116–122

111. Snover D C, Weisdorf S, Bloomer J, McGlave P, Weisdorf D. Nodular regenerative hyperplasia of the liver following bone marrow transplantation. Hepatology 1989; 9: 443–448

112. Kusne S, Schwartz M, Breinig M K et al. Herpes simplex virus hepatitis after solid organ transplantation in adults. J Infect Dis 1991; 163: 1001–1007

113. Norris S H, Butler T C, Glass N, Tran R. Fatal hepatic necrosis caused by disseminated type 5 adenovirus infection in renal transplant recipient. Am J Nephrol 1989; 9: 101–105

114. Kemper C A, Lombard C M, Deresinski S C, Tompkins L S. Visceral bacillary epithelioid angiomatosis: Possible manifestations of disseminated cat scratch disease in the immunocom promised host: A report of two cases. Am J Med 1990; 89: 216–222

115. Reed J A, Brigati D J, Flynn S D et al. Immunocytochemical identification of *Rochalimaea henselae* in bacillary (epithelioid) angiomatosis, parenchymal bacillary peliosis, and persistent fever with bacteremia. Am J Surg Pathol 1992; 16: 650–657

116. Hiesse C, Cantarovich M, Charpentier B, Francais P, Benoit G, Fries D. Need for hepatocellular carcinoma screening before renal transplantation in HB$_s$+, HB$_e$+, western Africans. Clin Nephrol 1985; 24: 209–211

117. Rao K V, Kasiske B L, Anderson W R. Variability in the morphological spectrum and clinical outcome of chronic liver disease in hepatitis B-positive and B-negative renal transplant recipients. Transplantation 1991; 51: 391–396

118. Cadranel J F, Grippon P, Mattei M F et al. Prevalence and causes of long-lasting hepatic dysfunction after heart transplantation: A series of 80 patients. Artif Organs 1988; 12: 234–238

119. Hasan F, Jeffers L J, De Medina M et al. Hepatitis C-associated hepatocellular carcinoma. Hepatology 1990; 12: 589–591

120. Ranjan D, Burke G, Esquenazi Y et al. Factors affecting the ten-year outcome of human renal allografts. The effect of viral infections. Transplantation 1991; 51: 113–117

121. Kemnitz J, Cremer J, Gebel M, Uysal A, Haverich A, Georgii A. T-cell lymphoma after heart transplantation. Am J Clin Pathol 1990; 94: 95–101

122. Gerlag P G, Lobatto S, Driessen W M M et al. Hepatic sinusoidal dilatation with portal hypertension during azathioprine treatment after kidney transplantation. J Hepatol 1985; 1: 339–348

123. Sparberg M, Simon N, Del Greco F. Intrahepatic cholestasis due to azathioprine. Gastroenterology 1969; 57: 439–441

124. Gruber S, Dehner L P, Simmons R L. De novo hepatocellular carcinoma without chronic liver disease but with 17 years of azathioprine immunosuppression. Transplantation 1987; 43: 597–600

125. Rao K V, Anderson W R. Hemosiderosis and hemochromatosis in renal transplant recipients. Clinical and pathological features, diagnostic correlations, predisposing factors, and treatment. Am J Nephrol 1985; 5: 419–430

126. Ladefoged C, Frifelt J J. Hepatocellular calcification. Virchows Arch [A] 1987; 410: 461–463

127. Nanni G, De Gaetano A M, Boldrini G et al. Parenchymal calcifications in the liver of kidney allograft recipients: An unrecognized side effect of cyclosporine. Transplant Proc 1989; 21: 1558–1559

19

Liver biopsy

S. N. Thung   F. Schaffner

Significant progress has been made in the evaluation of liver dysfunction by non-invasive physical and biochemical test procedures. Liver biopsy, however, remains an important tool in the diagnosis, evaluation of prognosis, treatment and follow-up of patients with liver disease. Liver biopsy results are most useful when the biopsy is performed for well-defined indications following a complete work-up of the patient.

SURGICAL BIOPSY

Surgical biopsy specimens are obtained mainly in diseases for which a laparotomy is indicated. Surgical biopsies should not be used to diagnose or rule out extrahepatic biliary obstruction as this can be done effectively by imaging and cholangiographic procedures, but have been recommended routinely during cholecystectomy to ascertain if the patient has associated cholangitis[1] and to determine whether prolonged cholestasis has resulted in fibrosis. Surgical biopsies are also the best means of recognizing the nature of focal lesions seen during a laparotomy for some other purpose. The surgeon should be asked to include liver tissue adjacent to the lesion and to avoid taking superficial, small scoops of tissue.

Surgical biopsy specimens have several features not seen in needle biopsy specimens that may cause diagnostic difficulties. If the surgeon removes a small superficial wedge of liver tissue from the inferior margin, the triangular tissue fragment is covered on two sides by capsule. The fibrous connections between the superficial portal tracts and the capsule may mimic cirrhosis.[2,3] However, these changes usually do not extend more than 2 mm into the liver parenchyma. In biopsy specimens removed at the end of a surgical procedure, clusters of polymorphonuclear neutrophils are seen, probably as a result of minor trauma, in or under the capsule, in sinusoids, overlying individual necrotic liver cells, and around terminal hepatic venules.[4,5] This characteristic lesion must be recognized and distinguished from inflammatory liver diseases such as cholangitis, and in immunosuppressed patients with microabscesses associated with cytomegalovirus (CMV) infection. One advantage of surgical biopsy is the large amount of liver tissue, several grams in weight, which can be used for biochemical and tissue fractionation studies, in contrast to 10–30 mg of tissue obtained by needle biopsy.

NEEDLE BIOPSY

Percutaneous needle biopsy of the liver is the most widely and easily performed procedure. The goals of needle biopsy are to obtain a big enough piece of tissue, free of distortion artefacts, quickly and simply with minimum risk or discomfort for the patient. The Menghini procedure fulfils most of these aims, especially if a disposable modification such as the Jamshidi needle is used. The main shortcoming of the Menghini procedure is fragmentation of the specimen, particularly if it is from a cirrhotic liver. This problem has been best overcome with the Tru-cut needle, which is a variant of the punch biopsy technique. Its limitations are that the procedure is somewhat more complex and the specimen smaller for the same size of needle as used in the Menghini procedure. The pathologist must be given an adequate amount of tissue even if it requires several passes.[6] The problem of sampling variability can be partially overcome if consecutive biopsies are taken by redirecting the biopsy needle through a single entry site; morbidity is not increased, provided that standard precautions are taken, and the diagnostic yield of liver tissue is increased.[7,8]

TRANSJUGULAR LIVER BIOPSY

This is a safe alternative technique for obtaining adequate liver tissue for diagnosis in special clinical situations[9–13]. The usual indications for transjugular rather than percutaneous liver biopsy are: (i) a coagulation disorder, (ii) massive ascites, and (iii) work up of a patient with portal hypertension. Less common indications include failed percutaneous biopsy, massive obesity, a small cirrhotic liver (increased risk and lower success rate) and a suspected vascular tumour or peliosis hepatis. The biopsy is best performed by passing a Tru-cut needle inside a 45 cm cardiac catheter into the jugular vein, through the superior vena cava and directly into a hepatic vein. This must be done under fluoroscopic control and with electrocardiographic monitoring. After the catheter is wedged into a hepatic vein tributary, the needle is thrust into the parenchyma and is triggered via a coaxial cable. Samples obtained with this Tru-cut needle are almost the same size as percutaneous biopsy specimens. Adequate specimens are obtained in 77–97% of cases.[10,11] The femoral vein can also be used for transvenous biopsy with small biopsy forceps.[14]

LAPAROSCOPIC LIVER BIOPSY

Direct vision is sometimes necessary to sample focal lesions detected by ultrasonography and computed tomography, or suspected but not seen by these imaging techniques. It can be used to identify focal lesions such as primary liver tumour[15] and metastatic tumours[16] or a diffuse process such as cirrhosis.[17] The biopsy is best done percutaneously with a needle which can be guided by the laparoscopist into the site to be examined. A biopsy from the uninvolved liver can be taken at the same time. Morbidity following laparoscopy is minimal. Laparoscopic control compares favourably with ultrasonographic[18] and computed tomographic[19] control. Laparoscopic guided biopsies of the right and left lobes have been shown to reduce sampling error.[20]

FINE NEEDLE ASPIRATION

The field of fine needle aspiration cytology has grown remarkably in the past few years as a result of the combined impetus of increasing levels of diagnostic resolution and demand for outpatient diagnostic procedures. This technique is a refinement of the original liver sampling attempts. The needle most widely used is the Chiba needle, introduced for modern-day percutaneous transhepatic cholangiography. The needle is inserted through a small hole in the skin down to the lesion that has been visualized under sonographic or computed tomographic control. Because the procedure elicits little pain, multiple stabs can be done, each in a slightly different direction. Other advantages of fine needle aspiration are sampling of lesions otherwise unreachable by percutaneous liver biopsy and where a core biopsy has missed the tumour.[21] The material obtained consists of small fragments of tissue, isolated cells and clusters of cells. The material can be smeared on slides, ejected into fixatives for cell block preparation or placed in tissue culture media. The most common use has been for the differentiation of primary liver tumours, e.g. hepatocellular carcinoma (HCC)[22–24] and hepatoblastoma,[25] from tumour metastases to the liver.[26]

Since the amount of material obtained is small, recognition of the liver architecture may be difficult. A well-differentiated HCC may therefore be impossible to diagnose. Comparison of the sinusoidal stroma of material from the lesion and from the surrounding tissue is often useful.[22] Immunohistochemical staining has also been applied to these specimens to identify the site of origin of a carcinoma.[24] Haemangiomas can be recognized cytologically[27,28] and represent a condition that should not lead to a core biopsy. Computed tomographic guidance[29] has been compared with ultrasonic guidance; both seem to be equally effective, although the former was better when ascites was present.[30]

PRECAUTIONS, CONTRAINDICATIONS AND COMPLICATIONS

The complications of needle biopsy most often involve bleeding or bile leakage. Although a large series of biopsies has been reported from a single clinic without fatalities,[31] the overall mortality appears to be between 0.01 and 0.1% and the overall incidence of non-fatal bleeding or bile leakage is up to 10 times the mortality rate. Estimation of risk and benefits must be made prior to performing a liver biopsy. The risk part of the equation is examined first, since it applies to all biopsies, while benefits differ in the various conditions in which the procedure is used.

Needle biopsy of the liver should not be undertaken unless blood clotting is adequate because bleeding is the most frequent complication.[8,31,32] Unless the patient has a specific known defect in the clotting cascade, the demonstration of an acceptable prothrombin time and platelet count suffices. Platelet counts above 50 000 or 60 000 (if platelet function is normal), and prothrombin time not greater than 50% above control values (usually within 5 or 6 seconds from control values) are adequate. If the prothrombin time is unduly prolonged, correction can be attempted with vitamin K or fresh frozen plasma; severe thrombocytopenia can be corrected by platelet transfusions. Bleeding sometimes occurs after liver biopsy in myeloproliferative disorders, even when the platelet count and prothrombin time are normal. This risk is also higher when biopsies are performed in patients with malignancy and following bone marrow transplantation.[8,32] Bleeding may result in intrahepatic haematoma, haemoperitoneum or haemothorax,[31] or haemobilia[33] with its characteristic symptomatology.

Suspected haemangiomas are contraindications for biopsy;[34,35] ultrasonic examination and computed tomography should be helpful in the recognition of these lesions. Angiosarcomas, peliosis hepatis and focal nodular hyperplasia can bleed after biopsy, but the risk seems to be small. Many angiosarcomas have been recognized by needle biopsy without adverse effects. Bleeding can also originate from the puncture site when the liver is stiff as the result of tumour or amyloidosis, and the puncture hole fails to collapse. Amyloidosis of the liver is often a surprise and rare diagnosis, therefore this condition cannot be considered a contraindication.

Bile leakage occurs less often than bleeding and usually in adults in whom there is biliary obstruction; the risk of biliary peritonitis is greater when the biliary tree is obstructed, regardless of the type of needle used.[36,37] Penetration of the gallbladder, especially if it is distended, may lead to bile leakage. The problem of bile leakage should become rare as various imaging procedures are used to recognize biliary obstruction.

Air may also leak after biopsy, usually from the lung, causing pneumothorax, subcutaneous emphysema and, rarely, pneumoscrotum.[38] Bacteraemia and septicaemia[39-41] and even liver and subphrenic abscesses[42] have developed following liver biopsy. These complications are associated with fever and result from penetration of the colon, an infected biliary tree or an unsuspected abscess; they should be avoided by using imaging and other diagnostic procedures. Arteriovenous fistulas have occurred following liver biopsies, but they seem to have little clinical significance.[43] Fatal carcinoid crisis has been reported after fine needle biopsy of a metastatic carcinoid tumour.[44] Hydatid disease remains an absolute contraindication to liver biopsy.[45]

INDICATIONS FOR LIVER BIOPSY

Liver biopsy should only be performed where the patient can be expected to benefit from the information gained and where it cannot be obtained by less invasive means. Satisfying the intellectual curiosity of the physician is not an indication. Informed consent is necessary before doing a biopsy. It entails explanation of risks and, more importantly, the expected benefits to the patient. Indications for liver biopsy have changed since the procedure was introduced and will continue to do so. The major indications for liver biopsy are discussed below.

Acute viral hepatitis

Liver biopsy is rarely indicated in acute viral or drug-induced hepatitis. Acute hepatitis due to most of the hepatotropic viruses (hepatitis A, B, D and E) can be diagnosed serologically, except for hepatitis C virus, in which detectable antibodies (anti-HCV) are delayed.[46] Liver biopsy is often needed to confirm and to determine the extent of liver involvement in non-hepatotropic viruses, e.g. adenovirus, Epstein–Barr virus, and herpes viruses, particularly since extensive liver necrosis can occur rapidly and specific antiviral treatment is available for these viruses.[47,48] In drug-induced hepatitis, liver biopsy is performed when the clinical presentation is atypical or when hepatitis develops with new drugs.

Chronic hepatitis

In chronic hepatitis, liver biopsy is performed to determine: (i) the aetiology; (ii) the activity of the disease; (iii) the presence of fibrosis and/or cirrhosis; and (iv) the effect of treatment. Some histological features are characteristic for certain diseases, e.g. ground-glass hepatocytes for chronic hepatitis B, lymphoid follicles for chronic hepatitis C, severe piecemeal necrosis with abundant plasma cells for autoimmune chronic hepatitis.[49-53]

Immunohistochemical studies are useful in demonstrating viral antigens in the biopsy specimens[54-56]. The widely used classification of chronic hepatitis into chronic lobular hepatitis,[57] chronic persistent and chronic active hepatitis[58,59] was based on morphological criteria. The distinction between the two main forms, i.e. chronic persistent and chronic active hepatitis, has played an important role in the management of patients, since chronic active hepatitis was considered a precursor of cirrhosis and amenable to treatment. With the recognition of differences in natural history of chronic hepatitides of different aetiologies, however, this classification has lost some of its relevance[60,61] (see Ch. 9).

Alcoholic liver disease

Whether all patients with a clinical diagnosis of alcoholic liver disease should have a liver biopsy to help confirm the diagnosis remains controversial.[62] Clinicians have little difficulty in recognizing the end-stage cirrhotic, but the earlier stages cannot be clearly ascertained without a liver biopsy. The amount of fat, the degree of alcoholic hepatitis and the amount of fibrosis may be variably admixed in different patients; therefore, the biopsy is useful for prognostic reasons[63] (Ch. 8). The liver biopsy findings may also help to convince the patient of how far their drinking habit has affected their liver,[64,65] and to exclude coexistent non-alcoholic liver diseases that might otherwise be missed.[66–69]

Cholestatic liver diseases

The introduction of new tools for the differential diagnosis of jaundice such as ultrasonography, endoscopic retrograde cholangio-pancreatography (ERCP) and percutaneous transhepatic cholangiography has led to extensive changes in the approach to patients with cholestasis. As discussed earlier, liver biopsy is not to be used to diagnose or rule out extrahepatic biliary obstruction but should be reserved for jaundiced patients with (i) normal bile ducts as established by imaging procedures and cholangiography; (ii) a mass in the liver, to establish its nature (provided it is not cystic or a haemangioma); or (iii) to differentiate viral, drug, or alcoholic hepatitis. The pathologist cannot always distinguish 'surgical' from 'medical' jaundice and should not be expected to do so.

Liver biopsy is especially useful in neonatal and infantile jaundice. The differentiation of extrahepatic biliary atresia[70] from other causes such as neonatal hepatitis, paucity of intrahepatic bile ducts,[71] and heritable disorders like galactosaemia and tyrosinaemia, must be done as soon as possible so that appropriate treatment can be promptly instituted. The success of surgical intervention in extrahepatic biliary atresia depends on whether or not concomitant paucity of intrahepatic bile ducts is seen in the liver specimen.

In chronic cholestasis, liver biopsy is also recommended only after imaging procedures and cholangiography have been performed. Liver biopsy is useful in confirming the diagnosis of primary biliary cirrhosis. However, because of variation from one portal tract to the next, the results of biopsy are less reliable in establishing the histological stage of the disease.[72] Liver biopsy will continue to be needed for various therapeutic clinical trials in primary biliary cirrhosis. Biopsies are less helpful in chronic obstructive biliary tract disease, i.e. primary sclerosing cholangitis and postoperative sclerosing cholangitis or stricture. Whether biopsy findings are useful in predicting the need and the timing of liver transplantation in chronic cholestatic disease remains to be seen; these decisions are often made on clinical grounds.

Cirrhosis

Liver biopsy is still the only diagnostic means of establishing the presence of cirrhosis. The stage of development and activity of the necro-inflammatory process, as evidence of progression, can be assessed histologically. In patients in whom more than one condition may lead to cirrhosis, biopsy is helpful in determining the cause. The presence of dysplasia of hepatocytes and/or macroregenerative nodules may suggest malignant transformation.[73,74]

Immunodeficiency disorders

Although the liver is not the primary target of human immunodeficiency virus (HIV), several opportunistic infections and other histological abnormalities have been noted in the liver of patients with acquired immunodeficiency syndrome (AIDS — see Ch. 7)[75] and other forms of immunodeficiency. Infection with *Mycobacterium avium intracellulare* and cytomegalovirus can rapidly be diagnosed by liver biopsy (p. 794). All biopsy specimens from AIDS patients should be stained for acid-fast bacilli and fungi, even in the absence of granulomas. Patients with AIDS are also susceptible to viral hepatitis A, B, C and D, and this can be recognized in the liver biopsy specimens. Biopsies can help in establishing which condition is responsible for the changes noted in blood tests.

Fever of unknown origin

Occasionally, attention is directed to the liver as the organ to be investigated in order to establish the cause of a protracted fever. If caused by systemic granulomatous disease, hepatic granulomas are detected in a high percentage of cases. The application of liver biopsy for this purpose is diminishing with the continued development of microbiological and immunological methods, and of imaging procedures. The diagnosis of disseminated miliary tuberculosis, histoplasmosis, toxoplasmosis and sarcoidosis, however, can still be reliably made by liver biopsy. Geographically circumscribed diseases like Q fever[76,77] and coccidioidomycosis[78] can be recognized on liver biopsy. Results of needle biopsy are less rewarding in Hodgkin's disease and other lymphomas. In addition, small lesions of Hodgkin's disease are often difficult to separate from non-specific portal inflammation. While the diagnosis of amoebic and bacterial infections, especially with abscess formation, can be made by liver biopsy, this is an incorrect diagnostic approach.[45]

Metabolic disorders

The liver is often the site studied in many metabolic disorders like the genetic diseases of carbohydrate, fat, amino acid, copper and iron metabolism (Ch. 4). If a specific diagnosis is suspected, a portion of the biopsy or even the entire specimen must be used for the biochemical procedure to pinpoint the problem. Combined morphological, usually ultrastructural,[79] and biochemical studies continue to yield much information about these diseases. Sending the patient to a centre specializing in the management of some of these rare diseases is usually warranted. Since treatment is being developed for these conditions, liver biopsies will be useful in assessing its effect.

Focal lesions

Liver biopsy is a valuable tool for establishing the type of primary or metastatic neoplasms in the liver. The focal lesions should be first visualized either directly or by imaging techniques. Seeing the lesion first by these procedures often provides a clue as to its nature, so that puncture of haemangiomas, abscesses or cysts can be avoided. When a liver mass is felt or is large and readily accessible, blind percutaneous biopsy is the simplest procedure.[80] When a mass is small, biopsy directed by laparoscopy, ultrasonography or computed tomography reduces the number of false negative biopsies significantly. This procedure may also be indicated in patients with histological features in the liver suggestive of an adjacent space-occupying lesion.[21]

Concern has been expressed over the years about seeding of the needle tract with malignant cells. Indeed, such instances have been recorded with various carcinomas, but they are rare events and seldom of clinical importance. Similarly, concerns of post-biopsy bleeding should not deter proper diagnostic workup because the increased risk is very small. While the use of fine needles to minimize the risk is at the same time simple, safe and painless, it may lead to delays and inaccuracies.

Monitoring therapy

Patients undergoing potentially hepatotoxic treatment, e.g. methotrexate for psoriasis or jejuno-ileal bypass for morbid obesity, should be biopsied before and during therapy in order to determine liver damage and fibrosis. It is important to recognize the insidious development of fibrosis in these cases before it becomes irreversible cirrhosis.

Hepatic allografts (post liver transplantation)

Liver transplantation has made necessary the development of a new branch of hepatic pathology[41,81–86] (see Ch. 18). Some transplant centres perform protocol biopsies at one week after transplantation, before discharge from the hospital, and at periodic intervals such as one year. Liver biopsies are absolutely necessary in the assessment and differential diagnosis of graft dysfunction suggested by results of various tests. Graft dysfunction may result from acute or chronic rejection, drug reactions, opportunistic infections, recurrent or post-transfusion hepatitis, sepsis, ischaemic liver injury, or bile-duct problems. Biopsies are useful in determining the responsible factors and directing appropriate therapy.

Vascular disorders in liver

Veno-occlusive disease, when it involves small terminal hepatic venules, can be diagnosed by liver biopsy. Rarely, intrahepatic arteries may be involved in polyarteritis nodosa. In a few cases, pylephlebitis associated with intra-abdominal infection has been demonstrated in biopsy specimens.

Hepatomegaly and abnormal liver function tests

Hepatologists are frequently asked to evaluate patients with chronically elevated serum aminotransferase levels. In such cases, various non-invasive tests — including history, physical examination, blood tests and imaging procedures — are usually done to arrive at a clinical diagnosis. A liver biopsy is often recommended when, after an extensive diagnostic work-up, these abnormalities remain unexplained. The most frequent causes for isolated mild increases in transaminase levels include steatosis in alcohol abuse and obesity, and non-specific reactive hepatitis in non-B, non-C chronic hepatitis suspected because of a history of transfusion or drug abuse. Liver biopsy is helpful in identifying the cause of these abnormalities in many, but not all, cases.[87,88]

The higher the elevation of the transaminase values, the greater the possibility of making a more specific diagnosis. Aminotransferase activity in excess of three times the upper limit of normal is an indication for biopsy in the face of a negative examination and other laboratory work-up. Isolated increases in alkaline phosphatase or γ-glutamyltransferase activities are frustrating abnormalities. Alcohol, drugs and early cases of primary sclerosing cholangitis may cause elevation of these bile canalicular enzyme activities. Biopsy, however, is not always indicated in these conditions.

Increased hepatic content of fat, glycogen and blood can result in hepatomegaly in adults. Patients on drugs known to induce the metabolizing enzyme systems may have an enlarged liver due to hypertrophy of hepatocytes (induction cells). These causes are usually recognized clinically and therefore liver biopsy is not needed. In children, liver biopsy plays an important role in the diagnosis of storage diseases, if simple post-prandial glycogen deposition causing hepatomegaly is eliminated.

PROCESSING AND STAINING OF SPECIMEN

Immediately after the needle biopsy specimen has been obtained, it should be inspected at the bedside. If the amount of tissue is inadequate, i.e. less than 2 cm in total length, another pass should be done immediately. Adequate size of specimen minimizes sampling errors.[89] At this point, the clinician has to decide whether special studies which require separate handling of tissue are needed: e.g. fixation in 3% buffered glutaraldehyde for electron microscopy; fresh, unfixed tissue for viral and mycobacterial cultures; and rapid freezing in liquid nitrogen or a mixture of dry ice and isopentane for immunohistochemical and enzyme activity studies,[90] quantitative studies of hormone receptors, and isolation of genomic and viral DNA and RNA for molecular analyses.[91]

The specimen is carefully placed on filter paper in order to avoid fragmentation or distortion and fixed as quickly as possible in 10% phosphate-buffered formalin. The clinician should record gross characteristics of tissue such as colour, consistency, and its tendency to fragment or to float. Tumour or granulomas can be recognized as white areas in the otherwise reddish brown tissue. Failure to find comparable areas in stained sections calls for more sections to be cut. Greyish-black coloured specimens are seen in Dubin–Johnson syndrome, rusty brown in haemochromatosis, green in cholestasis, yellow in steatosis, and variegated or dark brown in melanoma. Fragmented specimens, especially with the Menghini needle, often indicate cirrhosis. Artefacts from squeezing or drying of the specimen should be avoided.

After fixation for at least 3 hours, the specimen is processed by standard histological methods and embedded in paraffin. The time taken for a small biopsy specimen is less than for a larger specimen. Liver biopsy tissue, therefore, should be processed separately with other small biopsy specimens in an automatic machine or by hand. Processing may be expedited by the use of microwaves. Sections should be cut at 3–5 μm thickness by an experienced technician with a sharp knife. Thin, well-stained sections without artefacts will make histological evaluation much easier. At least two stains are employed routinely: haematoxylin and eosin (H&E) and Masson's trichrome stain for connective tissue (Figs 19.1 and 19.2). Commonly used special stains include stains for iron and copper (Figs 19.3 and 19.4), Shikata's orcein stain or Victoria blue stain for hepatitis B surface antigen (HBsAg) (Fig. 19.5), copper-binding protein and elastic fibres,[92] silver impregnation for reticulin (Fig. 19.6), periodic acid–Schiff (PAS) reaction for glycogen followed by a diastase digestion for non-glycogenic carbohydrates such as α_1-antitrypsin, phagocytes laden with ceroid pigment and basement membrane (Fig. 19.7). Additional special stains may be employed as indicated (Fig. 19.8). Serial sections are necessary if focal lesions are suspected.

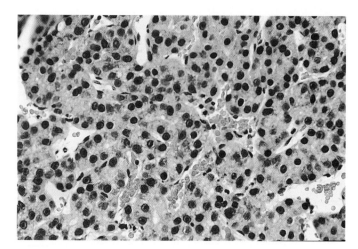

Fig. 19.1 A well-differentiated hepatocellular carcinoma. The tumour cells are arranged in several cell-thick plates and they have large, hyperchromatic nuclei. H & E.

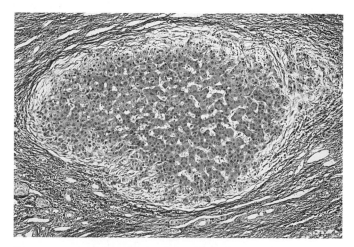

Fig. 19.2 A cirrhotic nodule in a liver with primary sclerosing cholangitis. The nodule is surrounded by fibrous tissue which is stained blue. A less dense fibrous tissue forming a 'halo' around the nodule is characteristic of a biliary type of cirrhosis. Trichrome.

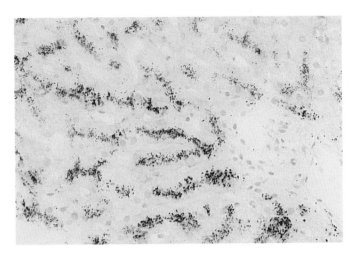

Fig. 19.3 Blue granules of iron in hepatocytes of a patient with haemochromatosis. The iron granules are deposited along the bile canaliculi. Prussian blue stain.

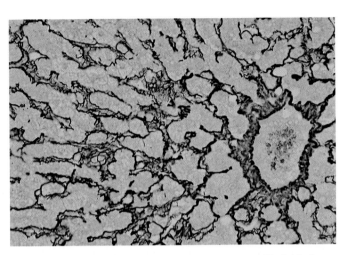

Fig. 19.6 Increased reticulin fibres stained brown around individual hepatocytes in a perivenular region of a liver with alcoholic liver disease. Silver impregnation.

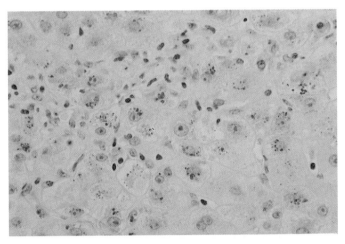

Fig. 19.4 Orange granules of copper in the cytoplasm of periportal hepatocytes in a liver with primary biliary cirrhosis. Rhodanine stain.

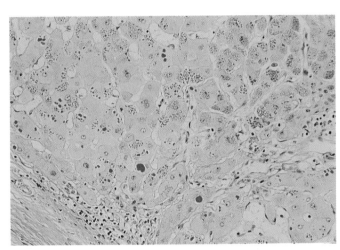

Fig. 19.7 Diastase-resistant periodic acid–Schiff stain (D–PAS) positive granules and globules (red) in cytoplasm of hepatocytes in a patient with α_1-antitrypsin deficiency. Diastase–PAS.

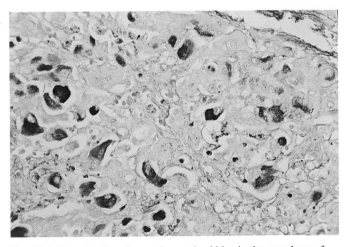

Fig. 19.5 Hepatitis B surface antigen stained blue in the cytoplasm of hepatocytes. Victoria blue stain.

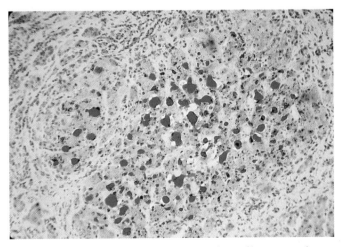

Fig. 19.8 Fat globules stained red in the cytoplasm of hepatocytes in a patient with alcoholic liver disease. Oil red O.

INTERPRETATION

Interpretation of liver biopsy specimens depends on the skill and experience of the observer.[93] Observer variation is considerably less among pathologists with experience in liver pathology than among general pathologists.[94] Sampling error is a major limitation of liver biopsies[95] since the needle biopsy specimen represents approximately 1/500 000 of the entire organ. A specimen should preferably be at least 2 cm in length and with more than four portal zones if a reliable opinion is to be given. Many liver diseases, such as acute hepatitis and drug-induced liver disease, however, are diffuse and involve every acinus. Sampling variability is more frequent in chronic hepatitis and cirrhosis,[96] and the chances of diagnosing focal lesions such as hepatic granulomas increase with the number of sections cut.

During the microscopic examination, the pathologist should follow a certain routine to avoid omissions. First, the acinar architecture and spatial arrangement between portal tracts and terminal hepatic venules are studied. Then the individual structures are evaluated: portal tract with bile duct, hepatic artery and portal vein, limiting plate, parenchyma with hepatocytes, sinusoids and sinusoidal lining cells, and terminal hepatic venules.[2] In order to avoid bias, the pathologist should examine the sections and interpret the histological changes without any knowledge of the clinical data. Subsequently, the case is discussed with the clinician in charge. Clinical information is essential before a final diagnosis can be reached.

SPECIAL STUDIES

Immunofluorescence studies for the detection of extracellular antigens and proteins sensitive to aldehyde-based fixatives are best performed on unfixed frozen sections. In liver allograft biopsy specimens, the presence of granular deposition of immunoglobulins and complement components within the sinusoids suggests humoral rejection.[97] Immunohistochemical studies are routinely used on liver biopsy and fine needle aspiration specimens. The sensitivity of the method has increased tremendously with the use of different enzymes and detergents to expose the antigens, the use of better polyclonal and monoclonal antibodies, and the use of amplified detection techniques. Different panels of antibodies to tumour markers are used to determine the origin of a tumour, depending on the differential diagnosis of a particular tumour.[98–100] Immunohistochemical studies are also used to detect viral antigens such as hepatitis B surface and core antigens, hepatitis D, Herpes simplex, varicella, adenovirus, cytomegalovirus and Epstein–Barr virus.[47,54,55,81] Other antibodies used are those directed against hormone receptors (androgen, progesterone and oestrogen), oncogene and tumour suppressor gene products, and HLA class I and II antigens.[101]

In situ hybridization techniques are used to detect different viruses in liver biopsy sections. This technique is sometimes, but not always, more sensitive than immunohistochemistry, the sensitivity depending on the available probe.

Morphometric studies can be performed on formalin-fixed paraffin-embedded sections although fresh tissue is preferred and gives better results. DNA content in hepatocellular nuclei in malignant tumours of liver and preneoplastic lesions has been studied using this method.[102,103] DNA ploidy can also be studied by flow cytometry.

DNA and RNA for molecular analyses can be isolated either from unfixed, frozen tissue or formalin-fixed, paraffin-embedded sections. The yield, however, is better from the unfixed specimens.[91] Identification of low levels of viral DNA and RNA can be achieved using the polymerase chain reaction. Polymerase chain reaction for hepatitis C virus has proved invaluable in liver allograft recipients.

FUTURE OF LIVER BIOPSY

Although liver biopsies are performed primarily for morphological diagnosis on patients with a wide variety of liver diseases, histological examination of liver specimens is frequently used in clinical research to assess responses to therapy. With improvement in specific therapies for different conditions, liver biopsy will be needed to evaluate and document the results. The role of liver biopsy is also changing as a variety of methods which increase sensitivity and specificity (described above) can be employed on a liver biopsy specimen, e.g. immunohistochemical studies to demonstrate the presence of viral antigens before liver injury occurs[81] and the persistence of viral infection by the polymerase chain reaction,[91,102] and morphometric studies to demonstrate aneuploidy of hepatocellular DNA to predict the risk of malignant transformation.[103,104]

REFERENCES

1. Scheegans H J. Die Intraoperative Leberbiopsie — ein Beitrag zur intraoperativen diagnosic. Dtsch Gesundheit Zeitschrift Klin Med 1983; 38: 857–860
2. Thung S N, Gerber M A. The liver. In: Sternberg S, ed. Histology for pathologists. New York: Raven Press, 1992: pp 625–637
3. Petrelli M, Scheuer P J. Variation in subcapsular liver structure and its significance in the interpretation of wedge biopsies. J Clin Pathol 1967; 20: 743–748
4. Keller T C, Smetana H F. Artefacts in liver biopsies. Am J Pathol 1950; 20: 738–741
5. Christoffersen P, Poulsen H, Skei E. Focal liver cell necrosis accompanied by infiltration of granulocytes arising during operation. Acta Hepato-Splenol 1970; 17: 240–245
6. Schaffner F, Thung S N. Liver biopsy. In: Haubrich W S, Schaffner F, eds. Bockus Gastroenterology, 5th ed. Philadelphia: WB Saunders, 1994 (in press)

7. Maharaj B, Leary W P, Naran A D et al. Sampling variability and its influence on the diagnostic yield of percutaneous needle biopsy of the liver. Lancet 1986; i: 523–525

8. Cohen M B, A-Kader H H, Lambers D, Heubi J E. Complications of percutaneous liver biopsy in children. Gastroenterology 1992; 102: 629–632

9. Lebrec D, Goldfarb G, Degott C, Rueff B, Benhamou J-P Transvenous liver biopsy. An experience based on 1000 hepatic tissue samplings with this procedure. Gastroenterology 1982; 83: 338–340

10. McAfee J M, Keeffe E B, Lee R G, Rosch J. Transjugular liver biopsy. Hepatology 1992; 14: 726–732

11. Corr P, Beningfield S J, Davey N. Transjugular liver biopsy: a review of 200 biopsies. Clin Radiol 1992; 45: 238–239

12. Lipchik E O, Cohen E B, Mewissen M W. Transvenous liver biopsy in critically ill patients: Adequacy of tissue samples. Radiology 1991; 181: 497–499

13. Bull H J M, Gilmore I T, Bradley R D, Marigold J H, Thompson R P H. Experience with transjugular liver biopsy. Gut 1983; 24: 1057–1060

14. Mewissen M W, Lipchik E O, Schreiber E R, Varma R R. Liver biopsy through the femoral vein. Radiology 1988; 169: 842–843

15. Jeffers L, Spieglman G, Reddy R et al. Laparoscopically directed fine needle aspiration for the diagnosis of hepatocellular carcinoma: a safe and accurate technique. Gastrointest Endosc 1988; 34: 235–237

16. Hansen S W, Jensen F, Pedersen N T et al. Detection of liver metastases in small cell lung cancer: a comparison of peritoneoscopy with liver biopsy and ultrasonography with fine needle aspiration. J Clin Oncol 1987; 5: 255–259

17. Dagnini G, Zotti S, Marin G et al. Laparoscopy and guided biopsy in the diagnosis of cirrhosis. Ital J Gastroenterol 1986; 18: 93–96

18. Fornari F, Rapaccini G L, Cavanna L et al. Diagnosis of hepatic lesions: ultrasonically guided fine needle biopsy or laparoscopy? Gastrointest Endosc 1988; 34: 231–234

19. Brady P G, Goldschmid S, Chappel G et al. A comparison of biopsy techniques in suspected focal liver disease. Gastrointest Endosc 1987; 33: 289–292

20. Jeffers L J, Findor A, Schiff E R et al. Minimizing sampling error with laparoscopic guided liver biopsy of right and left lobes. Gastroenterology 1991; 100: 555A

21. Gerber M A, Thung S N, Bodenheimer H C Jr, Kapelman B, Schaffner F. Characteristic histologic changes in liver adjacent to metastatic neoplasm. Liver 1986; 6: 85–88

22. Kung I T M, Chan S K, Fung K H. Fine needle aspiration in hepatocellular carcinoma: combined cytologic and histologic approach. Cancer 1991; 67: 673–680

23. Bru C, Maroto A, Bruix J et al. Diagnostic accuracy of fine needle aspiration biopsy in patients with hepatocellular carcinoma. Dig Dis Sci 1989; 34; 1763–1769

24. Bedrossian C W, Davile R M, Merenda G. Immunocytochemical evaluation of liver fine needle aspirations. Arch Pathol Lab Med 1989; 113: 1225–1230

25. Wakely P E, Silverman J F, Geisinger K R, Frable W J. Fine needle biopsy aspiration cytology of hepatoblastoma. Modern Pathol 1990; 3: 688–693

26. Servoll E, Viste A, Skaarland E et al. Fine needle aspiration cytology of focal liver lesions: advantages and limitations. Acta Chir Scand 1988; 154: 61–63

27. Caturelli E, Rapaccini G L, Sabelli C et al. Ultrasound-guided fine needle aspiration biopsy in the diagnosis of hepatic hemangioma. Liver 1986; 6: 326–330

28. Nakaizumi A, Iishi H, Yamamoto R et al. Diagnosis of cavernous hemangioma by fine needle aspiration biopsy under ultrasonic guidance. Gastrointest Radiol 1990; 15: 39–42

29. Luning M, Schroeder K, Wolff H et al. Percutaneous biopsy of the liver. Cardiovasc Intervent Radiol 1991; 14: 40–42

30. Murphy F B, Barefield K P, Steinberg H V, Bernardino M E. CT- or sonography-guided biopsy of the liver in the presence of ascites: frequency of complications. Am J Roent 1988; 151: 485–486

31. Wildhirt E, Moller E. Erfahrungen bei ngendhezu 20.000 Leberblindpunktionen. Med Klin 1981; 76: 254–255

32. McGill D B, Rakela J, Zinsmeister A R, Ott B J. A 21 year experience with major hemorrhage after percutaneous liver biopsy. Gastroenterology 1990; 99: 1396–1400

33. Levinson J D, Olsen G, Terman J W et al. Hemobilia secondary to percutaneous liver biopsy. Arch Intern Med 1972; 130: 396–400

34. Karpas C M, Parvon E E. Fatal haemorrhage following needle biopsy of hepatic hemangioendothelioma. NY State J Med 1971; 71: 770–772

35. Kato M, Sugawara F, Okada A et al. Hemangioma of the liver. Am J Surg 1975; 129: 698–704

36. Kelly M L, Mosenthal W T, Milne J. Bile leakage following Menghini needle liver biopsy. JAMA 1971; 216: 333

37. Conn H O. Liver biopsy in extrahepatic biliary obstruction and in other 'contraindicated' disorders. Gastroenterology 1975; 68: 817–821

38. Engelhard D, Ornoy A, Deckelbaum R J. Pneumoscrotum complicating percutaneous liver biopsy. Gastroenterology 1981; 80: 390–392

39. McCloskey R V, Gold M, Weser E. Bacteremia after liver biopsy. Arch Intern Med 1973; 132: 213–215

40. Moreira Vincente V F, Hernandez Ranz F M, Ruiz del Arbol L K, Bouza E P. Septicaemia as a complication of liver biopsy. Am J Gastroenterol 1981; 76: 145–147

41. Domingo M, Grau J, Vasquez A et al. Septic shock and bacteremia associated with laparoscopic guided liver biopsy: report on two cases. Endoscopy 1989; 21: 240–241

42. Ben-Itzhak J, Bassan H M. Subphrenic abscess following percutaneous liver needle biopsy. Israel J Med Sci 1983; 19: 356–358

43. Okud K, Kotoda K, Igarashi M, Karasawa E. Intrahepatic arteriovenous fistula resulting from needle biopsy: a case report. Acta Hepatogastroenterol 1974; 21: 422–425

44. Bissonnette R T, Gibney R G, Berry B R, Buckley A R. Fatal carcinoid crisis after percutaneous fine-needle biopsy of hepatic metastasis: case report and literature review. Radiology 1990; 174: 751–752

45. Sherlock S, Dick R, Van Leeuwen D J. Liver biopsy today. J Hepatology 1984; 1: 75–85

46. Hoofnagle J H. Acute viral hepatitis. Clinical features, laboratory findings, and treatment. In: Berk J E, Haubrich W S, Kalser M H, Roth J L A, Schaffner F, eds. Bockus Gastroenterology, 4th edn. Philadelphia: WB Saunders, 1985: pp 2856–2901

47. Thung S N, Gerber M A. Histopathology of liver transplantation. In: Fabry T L, Klion F M, eds. Guide to liver transplantation. New York: Igaku-Shoin, 1992: pp 265–298

48. Erice A, Jordan M C, Chace B A et al. Ganciclovir treatment of cytomegalovirus disease in transplant recipients and other immunocompromised hosts. JAMA 1987; 257: 3082–3087

49. Gerber M A, Thung S N. Viral hepatitis: pathology. In: Berk J E, Haubrick W S, Kalser M H, Roth J L A, Schaffner F, eds. Bockus Gastroenterology, 4th edn. Philadelphia: WB Saunders, 1985: pp 2825–2855

50. Bach N, Thung S N, Schaffner F. The histological features of chronic hepatitis C and autoimmune chronic hepatitis. A comparative analysis. Hepatology 1992; 15: 572–577

51. Scheuer P J, Ashrafzadeh P, Sherlock S, Brown D, Duksheiko G M. The pathology of hepatitis C. Hepatology 1992; 15: 567–571

52. Dienes H P, Popper H, Arnold W, Lobeck H. Histologic observations in human hepatitis non-A , non-B. Hepatology 1982; 2: 562–571

53. Hadziyannis S, Gerber M A, Vissoulis C, Popper H. Cytoplasmic hepatitis B antigen in 'ground glass' hepatocytes of carriers. Arch Pathol 1973; 96: 327–330

54. Gerber M A, Thung S N. The localisation of hepatitis virus in tissues. Int Rev Exp Pathol 1979; 29: 49–76

55. Gerber M A, Thung S N. Molecular and cellular pathology of hepatitis B. Lab Invest 1985; 52: 572–590

56. Thung S N, Gerber M A. Immunohistochemical study of delta antigen in an American metropolitan population. Liver 1983; 3: 392–397

57. Popper H, Schaffner F. The vocabulary of chronic hepatitis. N Engl J Med 1971; 284: 1154–1156

58. Review by an International Group. Morphological criteria in viral hepatitis. Lancet 1971; 1: 333–337

59. Review by an International Group. Acute and chronic hepatitis revisited. Lancet 1977; 2: 914–919

60. Scheuer P J. Classification of chronic hepatitis: A need for reassessment. J Hepatol 1991; 13: 372–374

61. Gerber M A. Chronic hepatitis C: the beginning of the end of a time-honored nomenclature? Hepatology 1992; 15: 733–734

62. Tally N J, Roth A, Woods J, Hench V. Diagnostic value of liver biopsy in alcoholic liver disease. J Clin Gastroenterol 1988; 10: 647–650

63. Pimstone N R, French S W. Alcoholic liver disease. Med Clin North Am 1984; 68: 39–56

64. Jeffers L J, Schiff E R. Evaluation of invasive diagnostic procedures in alcoholic liver disease. Alcoholism. Clin Exp Res 1981; 5: 131–136

65. Sanchez G C, Baunsgaard P, Lundborg C J. A comparison between clinical diagnosis and histopathological findings in liver biopsies. Scand J Gastroenterol 1980; 15: 985–991

66. Levin D M, Baker A L, Riddell R H, Rochman H, Boyer J L. Non-alcoholic liver disease. Overlooked causes of liver injury in patients with heavy alcohol consumption. Am J Med 1979; 66: 429–434

67. Goldberg S J, Mendenhall C L, Connell A M, Chedid A. Non-alcoholic chronic hepatitis in the alcoholic. Gastroenterology 1977; 72: 598–604

68. Crapper R M, Bhathal P S, Mackay I R. Chronic active hepatitis in alcoholic patients. Liver 1983; 3: 327–337

69. Marbet U A, Bianchi L, Meury U, Stalder G A. Long-term histological evaluation of the natural history and prognostic factors of alcoholic liver disease. J Hepatol 1987; 4: 364–372

70. Deutsch J. Die Stellung der perkutane Leberblindbiopsie in der praeoperativen differential Diagnose der extrahepatischen Gallengangsatresie. Mschr Kinderheilk 1987; 135: 763–769

71. Kahn E, Daum F, Markowitz J et al. Nonsyndromatic paucity of intralobular bile ducts: light and electron microscopic evaluation of sequential liver biopsies in early childhood. Hepatology 1986; 6: 890–901

72. Schaffner F, Popper H. Clinical–pathologic relations in primary biliary cirrhosis. In: Popper H, Schaffner F, eds. Progress in liver diseases, vol VIII. New York: Grune & Stratton, 1982: pp 529–554

73. Theise N D, Schwartz M, Miller C, Thung S N. Macroregenerative nodules and hepatocellular carcinoma in forty four sequential adult liver explants with cirrhosis. Hepatology 1992; 16: 949–955

74. Kondo F, Ebara M, Sugiura N et al. Histological features and clinical course of large regenerative nodules. Evaluation of their precancerous potentiality. Hepatology 1992; 12: 592–598

75. Lebovics E, Thung S, Schaffner F, Radensky P W. The liver in the acquired immunodeficiency syndrome. A clinical and histologic study. Hepatology 1985; 5: 293–298

76. Qizilbash A H. The pathology of Q fever as seen on liver biopsy. Arch Pathol Lab Med 1983; 107: 364–367

77. Thung S N, Gerber M A, Lebovics E, Reichman S. Granulomatous hepatitis in Q fever. Mt Sinai J Med 1986; 53: 293–295

78. Howard P F, Smith J W. Diagnosis of disseminated coccidioidomycosis by liver biopsy. Arch Intern Med 1983; 143: 1335–1338

79. Phillips M J, Poucell S, Patterson J, Valencia P. The liver. An atlas and text of ultrastructural pathology. New York: Raven Press, 1987

80. Nagato Y, Kondo F, Kondo Y et al. Histologic and morphometrical indicators for a biopsy diagnosis of well-differentiated hepatocellular carcinoma. Hepatology 1991; 14: 473–478

81. Theise N, Conn M, Thung S N. Localisation of CMV antigens in liver allografts. Hum Pathol 1994 (in press)

82. Thung S N, Gerber M A. Histologic features of liver allograft rejection. Do you see what I see? Hepatology 1991; 14: 949–951

83. Demetris A J. The pathology of liver transplantation. In: Popper H, Schaffner F, eds. Progress in liver diseases, vol IX. Philadelphia: Saunders, 1990: pp 687–717

84. Snover D C, Freese D K, Sharp H L et al. Liver allograft rejection. An analysis of the use of biopsy in determining outcome of rejection. Am J Surg Pathol 1987; 11: 1–10

85. Thung S N, Bach N, Miller C M, Schaffner F. Antibody-mediated liver allograft rejection is associated with poor prognosis. Hepatology 1989; 10: 673 (abstract)

86. Ludwig J. Classifications and terminology of hepatic allograft rejection. Whither bound? Mayo Clin Proc 1989; 64: 676–679

87. Van Ness M M, Diehl A M. Is liver biopsy useful in the evaluation of patients with chronically elevated liver enzymes? Ann Intern Med 1989; 111: 473–478

88. Riely C A. Liver biopsy shown useful in work-up of patients with chronically abnormal 'LFTs' — still. Gastroenterology 1990; 98: 797–798

89. Maharaj B, Maharaj R J, Leary W P et al. Sampling variability and its influence on the diagnostic yield of percutaneous needle biopsy of the liver. Lancet 1986; 1: 523–525

90. Thung S N, Gerber M A. Enzyme pattern and marker antigens in nodular regenerative hyperplasia of the liver. Cancer 1981; 47: 1796–1799

91. Shieh Y S C, Shim K S, Lampertico P et al. Detection of hepatitis C virus sequences in liver tissue by the polymerase chain reaction. Lab Invest 1991; 65: 408–411

92. Shikata T, Uzawa T, Yashiwara N, Akatsuka T, Yamazaki S, Staining methods of Australia antigen in paraffin sections. Detection of cytoplasmic inclusion bodies. J Exp Med 1974; 44: 25–36

93. Demetris A J, Belle S H, Hart J et al. Intraobserver and interobserver variation in the histopathological assessment of liver allograft rejection. Hepatology 1991; 14: 751–755

94. Theodossi A, Skeni A, Portmann B et al. Observer variation in assessment of liver biopsies including analysis of Kappa statistics. Gastroenterology 1980; 79: 232–241

95. Abdi W, Millan J C, Mezey E. Sampling variability on percutaneous liver biopsy. Arch Intern Med 1979; 139: 667–669

96. Kirschner E, Chalmers T C, Popper H et al. Observer error in biopsy interpretations and outcome in chronic hepatitis. Mt Sinai J Med 1982; 49: 472–474

97. Evrard H, Miller C, Schwartz M, Thung S N, Mayer L. Resistant hepatic allograft successfully treated with cyclophosphamide and plasmapheresis. Transplantation 1990; 50: 702–704

98. Thung S N, Gerber M A, Sarno E, Popper H. Distribution of five antigens in hepatocellular carcinoma. Lab Invest 1979; 41: 101–105

99. Lai Y-S, Thung S N, Gerber M A, Chen M-L, Schaffner F. Expression of cytokeratins in normal and diseased livers and in primary liver carcinomas. Arch Pathol Lab Med 1989; 113: 134–138

100. Thung S N. The development of ductular structures in diseased livers. An immunohistochemical study. Arch Pathol Lab Med 1990; 114: 407–411

101. Fukusato T, Gerber M A, Thung S N, Ferrone S, Schaffner F. Expression of HLA class I antigens on hepatocytes in liver disease. Am J Pathol 1986; 123; 264–270

102. Poterucha J J, Rakela J, Lumeng L, Lee C-H, Taswell H F, Wiesner F H. Diagnosis of chronic hepatitis C after liver transplantation by the detection of viral sequences with polymerase chain reaction. Hepatology 1992; 15: 42–45

103. Orsatti G, Theise N D, Thung S N, Paronetto F. DNA image cytometric analysis of macroregenerative nodules (adenomatous hyperplasia) of the liver: evidence in support of their preneoplastic nature. Hepatology 1993; 17: 621–627

104. Fyfe B, Toor A H, Thung S N, Dische M R, Kidron D, Gil J. Hepatoblastoma versus hepatocellular carcinoma. A morphometric analysis. Modern Pathol 1991; 4: 108A

Index